T0337393

SOCIAL WORK
ESSENTIALS

EDITORIAL BOARD

SOCIAL WORK
ESSENTIALS

Cynthia Franklin

Editor in Chief

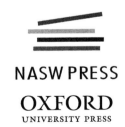

NASW PRESS

OXFORD
UNIVERSITY PRESS

2016

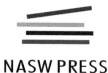

NASW PRESS

The NASW Press is a leading scholarly press in the social sciences. It serves faculty, practitioners, agencies, libraries, clinicians, and researchers throughout the United States and abroad. Known for attracting expert authors, the NASW Press delivers professional information through its scholarly journals, books, and reference works.

NASW Press is a registered trademark of the National Association of Social Workers, Inc.

OXFORD
UNIVERSITY PRESS

Oxford University Press is a department of the University of Oxford.
It furthers the University's objective of excellence in research, scholarship, and education by publishing worldwide. Oxford is a registered trade mark of Oxford University Press in the UK and certain other countries.

Published in the United States of America by

NASW Press
750 First Street, NE, Suite 800, Washington, DC 20002-4241
http://www.naswpress.org/

and

Oxford University Press
198 Madison Avenue, New York, NY 10016-4314
http://www.oup.com/us

Library of Congress Cataloging-in-Publication Data
Names: Franklin, Cynthia, editor.
Title: Social work essentials : selections from the Encyclopedia of social work / Cynthia Franklin, Editor in Chief.
Other titles: Encyclopedia of social work.
Description: Washington, DC : NASW Press, 2016. | Includes index.
Identifiers: LCCN 2016012887 | ISBN 9780190499624 ((hardback) : alk. paper)
Subjects: LCSH: Social service. | Social service—Practice.
Classification: LCC HV40 .S617826 2016 | DDC 361.3—dc23 LC record available at https://lccn.loc.gov/2016012887

1 3 5 7 9 8 6 4 2
Printed in the United States of America
on acid-free paper

Contents

List of Entries

Foreword

*Deciding to remember, and what to remember, is
how we decide who we are.*
　　　*—Robert Pinsky, former United States Poet
Laureate*

Sixty years is an achievement worth marking and celebrating for any movement or institution or individual
life. Sixty years provides a vantage point for reflection, to examine what has been and imagine a future
of making the world a better place. But beyond the
celebration of having made it this far, why should we
care about the history of our profession and NASW?
And what does that history have to do with motivating and influencing our profession's path forward?

In the first place, we have come a long way. We
can and should recognize the scope of our success
and the efforts that contributed to it. In 1955, when
seven social work organizations negotiated to form a
single, unified professional entity, NASW had 22,027
individual members. Today our organization's membership stands at 130,000. Thousands of social work
practitioners provide psychotherapeutic services independently and are reimbursed through insurance.
This is largely because of NASW's persistent advocacy and lobbying over more than twenty years to
eliminate requirements of referral and supervision
by a psychiatrist, and to have social workers named
providers in major insurance programs. Licensure
for social workers in some form now exists in all fifty
states. We have struggled long and hard to achieve
our place and with it society's understanding and acceptance of who we are. And the struggle continues.

Looking back, our nation's pressing problems of
poverty, inequality, and racism, so apparent today,
appear and recycle. As our profession engages again
in the struggle for an equitable society that is responsive to all, we can learn from our own past efforts. In
1968 NASW was a collaborating organization with
Reverend Dr. Martin Luther King, Jr.'s Poor People's
Campaign, an undertaking that ultimately brought

over 3,000 individuals to a Resurrection City of tents
on the National Mall. There they remained for six
weeks while campaign leaders petitioned Congress
and the federal government for jobs, housing, and
racial equity in aid programs—economic justice for
all. NASW's Metro DC chapter set up and staffed a
service tent throughout the campaign, offering help,
referrals, information, and tangible aid to the participants, many of whom lacked the resources to return
home. A stance for social justice and practical help to
achieve it have always been a key part of who we are.

The contributors to this volume crisscross a wide
landscape, creating an historical canvas of knowledge that forms a firm foundation for social work
in a global world—a world that has changed in profound ways during the past sixty years. Today we are
all interrelated and interconnected. The challenges
we recognize and confront as social workers require
an attitude of tolerance, compassion, devotion, persistence, and, above all, caring. They require dedication to effective practice and ongoing knowledge
creation for that practice. And they require a commitment to honor and uphold the entirety of our
historical development and unfolding.

Moving forward, constructing our future, always
mindful of the past, we can celebrate the wisdom of
coming together in 1955. We can embrace the accumulated knowledge, expertise, experiences, and efforts
that have enriched social work education, practice,
and research and have impacted the nation and the
world. We can remember the breadth and strength of
what our profession stands for and relish the fullness
of who we are in our many manifestations.

*Bernice Catherine Harper, LLD, ACSW, NASW
Social Work Pioneer®*

*Betsy Schaefer Vourlekis, Professor Emerita,
University of Maryland School of Social Work, and
NASW Social Work Pioneer®*

Preface

In 2015 the National Association of Social Workers (NASW) turned sixty years old, launching an eight-month celebration highlighting the many ways that social workers have *paved the way for change*. Fifty years ago, setting the stage for change through a unified profession, NASW launched the *Encyclopedia of Social Work*, a compendium of knowledge that is the premier reference guide for the social work profession. Since that time, the Encyclopedia has continuously repaved knowledge within social work, providing new generations with an important resource for both pedagogy and practice. In order to keep pace with the changing knowledge within the profession and in celebration of the anniversaries of NASW and the *Encyclopedia of Social Work*, it was decided that a one-volume print compilation of entries from the *Encyclopedia of Social Work* would be offered. This new volume, *Social Work Essentials*, handpicks for practitioners, academicians, and students important articles from the *Encyclopedia of Social Work*.

Development of *Social Work Essentials*

The articles within *Social Work Essentials* reflect the *Encyclopedia's* status as a provider of both fundamental knowledge for the social work profession and timely updates on the knowledge needed for social work practice, making this commemorative volume an excellent resource for all areas of social work history, values and ethics, and policy and practice. *Social Work Essentials* covers major areas of social work curricula and is a welcome resource for pedagogy and a useful source of information for licensing exam reviews. Approximately 70 percent of the articles in this volume represent new or updated content that cannot be found within the older, 2008 print version of the *Encyclopedia of Social Work*.

Social Work Essentials is the first print version of new material from the *Encyclopedia of Social Work* to appear since 2008. The previous print version of the 20th edition of the *Encyclopedia of Social Work* was published in partnership with Oxford University Press (OUP), a worldwide leader in reference publishing. With the advent of online platforms and digital publishing, NASW Press and OUP quickly agreed that the time had come to transition the *Encyclopedia of Social Work* to an online-first mentality. NASW Press appointed an Editor-in-Chief and a 13-member editorial board to guide the

Encyclopedia of Social Work online, with a goal of producing a digital product that could provide continuous updates of the social work knowledge base. Since that time nearly one hundred of the articles within the 2008 print version that are now online have received minor or substantive updates, and over one hundred and fifty new articles have been published. In addition, scholars within the field have worked to refresh the knowledge by proposing new and timely topics that are reviewed and approved by the editorial board. An international editorial board has also been appointed to increase global content. This results in articles that are refreshed and evolving as well as content that is more attuned to the immediate and global concerns of social workers.

For the *Social Work Essentials* volume, the editorial board from the *Encyclopedia of Social Work* concentrated on the selection of the new and revised articles along with a few core, unrevised articles from the 2008 print version with a goal of producing a brief reference guide for the social work profession. Inside *Social Work Essentials* readers will find topics that every social worker needs to know, including entries covering health care, clinical social work and mental health practice, substance use, child welfare, school social work, gerontology, policy interventions, community organization, international social work, and research, among others. Relevant and timely topics were also given priority, including articles on integrative health care, transdisciplinary teamwork, technology, immigration, restorative justice, human rights and social justice, human trafficking, military social work, changes in diagnosis within the DSM-5, suicide prevention, trauma-focused care, ethics, and evidence-based practice, just to name a few. A range of theoretical and practice orientations were also selected to be in *Social Work Essentials*, such as strength-based interventions, cognitive behavioral therapies, psychosocial perspectives, systems theories, motivational interviewing, couples and family interventions, group work, community development, and leadership. In keeping with the goals of the *Encyclopedia of Social Work* to provide comprehensive coverage of knowledge for the social work profession, attention was given to providing as much attention as possible to the many varied areas of social work while condensing that knowledge into one helpful volume, culminating in *Social Work Essentials* in its current form.

Organization and Finding Topics

The articles for *Social Work Essentials* are listed alphabetically with a quick and easy topical outline and index to help readers access the content that is of most interest. The topics are diverse, representing both the editorial board's efforts to include as many substantive topics as feasible and the broad transdisciplinary knowledge of the social work profession. Of course, every topic that may interest social workers could not be included in this one volume. For this reason, I encourage readers of *Social Work Essentials* to also explore the *Encyclopedia of Social Work* online, which provides greater breadth of content than could be included in this volume. Within the online *Encyclopedia of Social Work*, readers can access all of the articles that are in the 2008 *Encyclopedia* and their updated versions, in addition to new articles that are added monthly. The digital platform also makes research of the content within the *Encyclopedia of Social Work* more visual, accessible, and transmittable. Readers will appreciate the advanced search tools and hyperlinks that aid in the rapid exploration of related information and the additional resources that are excellent for pedagogy, such as videos about practice and other tools. If for some reason the *Encyclopedia* does not include a particular topic of interest, we strongly encourage our readers to propose a new article with the online proposal mechanism that is provided.

Acknowledgements

It is a privilege to work with such a distinguished group of my colleagues and the Oxford University Press in providing this important and commemorative volume to the social work profession. My special thanks go to the very extraordinary editorial board of the *Encyclopedia of Social Work*, consisting of Tricia Bent-Goodley, Elizabeth Clark, Larry Davis, Rowena Fong, Alberto Godenzi, Lynne Healy, James Kelly, Michael Kelly, Johnny Kim, Sadye Logan, Terry Mizrahi, Frederic Reamer, and Joan Zlotnik. All editorial board members are eminent scholars in our field and each member has given many hours in service to the social work profession through their work on the *Encyclopedia of Social Work* and the thoughtful selection of the articles for *Social Work Essentials*.

I would also like to thank the leadership and editors of NASW and OUP, especially Angelo McClain, Darrell Wheeler, Cheryl Bradley, Dana Bliss, Max Sinsheimer, Robyn Curtis, and Brianna Marron, who worked diligently at every stage of the development of the *Encyclopedia of Social Work* and helped us create the current print volume, *Social Work Essentials*.

There is no doubt that *Social Work Essentials* and the *Encyclopedia of Social Work* continue to set the pace for change by providing the premier reference guides for the social work profession. It is my best of hopes that social workers all over the world will make use of both of these resources.

Cynthia Franklin, PhD, LCSW
Editor in Chief, *Encyclopedia
of Social Work*
Assistant Dean for Doctoral Education
Stiernberg/Spencer Family Professor
in Mental Health
School of Social Work
The University of Texas at Austin

SOCIAL WORK
ESSENTIALS

ACTION RESEARCH

Abstract: Through cycles of systematic and purposeful iterative engagement with problems they face in specific practice settings, social workers engaging in action research build knowledge that is useful in advancing practice for the purposes of social betterment. This entry situates action research in the development of social-work knowledge and then examine variants of action research formed when degrees of participation and control vary among members of vulnerable populations, particularly within community situations involving coping with a degraded quality of life. The author identifies the importance of methodological pluralism and addresses how sound action research results in knowledge dissemination and utilization for the purposes of social betterment, often through alternative methods of inquiry. The entry concludes with caveats social workers engaged in action research should heed, and the author emphasizes the pivotal role social work can serve in local efforts to engage in knowledge development for social betterment.

Key Words: action learning; action research; community development; evaluation practice; knowledge development and management; practice advancement; social research and development

By its very purpose, social work is an action profession—it exists to undertake action for the avowed purposes of social betterment, and its knowledge has evolved to fulfill this end. Social work is a synthetic profession in that its knowledge base involves the absorption of ideas, models, and methods from other disciplines melded with content social workers generate. This melding of adopted and self-generated knowledge forms the profession's diverse instrumental knowledge base. It is diverse because social work's scope of action is broad and encompasses multiple social issues. It is also instrumental because of the profession's prioritization of ways to undertake meaningful and effective practice within particular fields of action.

Unlike other professions or disciplines, social work cuts across many fields of practice and engages multiple domains of knowledge. Consistent with a Deweyian perspective on action, social work's efforts are purposeful: it undertakes action for social betterment with the intent to improve people's well-being, foster functioning, or advance quality of life, particularly within groups and communities. The profession's distinctive focus involves those individuals, groups, and communities that experience considerable social distress because of discrimination and oppression and, because of those social forces, they come to experience a degraded quality of life. Social betterment, or efforts to improve quality of life, is a principal outcome the profession seeks to enact within the greater society.

What Lewin (1946, 1948) referred to as action research is a form of inquiry undertaken by practitioners for the purposes of understanding their practice and for advancing that practice through systematic methods addressing questions defined by practitioners. Action research offers social work a way of realizing its principal aim of progress toward social betterment consistent with the practice focus governing the profession. The principal mooring of action research is social learning: action research enables practitioners to address self-generated questions that they test out through their own practice by taking action to reveal the strengths and limitations of theory, context, models, methods, and discrete procedures. Learning involves knowledge acquisition, insight, and formulation and enactment of new ways of performing (Garvin, 2003), as well as anticipation of the emerging future (Scharmer, 2007).

This learning occurs directly from the enactment of action in organizational contexts in which practitioners see value in examining and advancing their effectiveness (Argyris, 1982, 1993) in anticipation of resolving the issues they face or those that are emerging. In advanced forms of action research, the contexts in which practitioners work are purposively designed to produce knowledge through reflection, experimentation, and innovation (Argyris, Putnam, & Smith, 1985). Action research recognizes the complexity of situations; hence, framing them is an important competence of inquiry (Fairhurst & Sarr, 1996) that invariably involves the resolution of conflicting frames among various stakeholders (Schon & Rein, 1994) when action research incorporates the involvement of diverse groups.

Action research has expanded its scope and diversity since Kurt Lewin's early conception of this model of inquiry. It is no longer confined to a narrow conception of a practitioner working alone, separated from other groups and disciplines. Increasingly, action research involves interdisciplinary or transdisciplinary teams working side by side with people who directly experience social issues in their immediate neighborhoods or communities.

As insights into the dynamics of oppression have increased within the helping professions, there has been a corresponding diversification of models of action research to incorporate interdisciplinary, collaborative, participatory empowerment, and community-based strategies. The basic purpose of action research, however, has not changed since Lewin's conception of this model and its methods. No matter in what form professions, groups, and practitioners undertake action research, it remains a way to enact social learning—as a means to learn from action and use that learning immediately within those contexts in which they practice.

This dynamic of taking action and learning from action is a fundamental property. In this sense, action research is both illuminatory and instrumental. Action research is illuminatory at one level, particularly early in a knowledge-building project, because it can reveal (or otherwise shed light on) the expression of a social issue within a given context. At the level of instrumental knowledge, practitioners (or others undertaking action research) can formulate and test promising practices for taking meaningful action for the purposes of social betterment. Action research is consistent with other models for improving social-work practice, including practice-based research, empirical practice, social research and development, and design and development. Learning from practice is a common thread connecting these multiple models. The focus on generating new forms of intervention, testing those forms in practice, and developing practice procedures imbues those models with common purpose.

Action research does not prescribe a particular set of research procedures. It promotes methodological pluralism and recognizes the importance of learning in group contexts using dialogic processes. These qualities make action research and social work compatible. Thus, action research is relevant to the profession's practice advancement aims. Practitioners of either action research or social work seek to learn through engagement, reflection, and the reformulation of action.

Ultimately, action research is an intervention helping people to better understand their situations and how to undertake action for the improvement of those situations. Both action research and social work value a continuous, engaged, synthetic, and developmental strategy of knowledge development undertaken for the purposes of achieving innovation. It is the purpose of this entry to communicate the distinctiveness of action research within social-work practice.

Situating Action Research in the Development of Social-Work Knowledge

Why does a professional social worker undertake research, particularly when there are likely no accountability requirements or external demands for engaging in such activity? This constitutes an important question given the necessity in the profession today and the issues facing social work and the human services for the development and utilization of knowledge (Fern, 2012). Where does the felt need for inquiry begin and what factors mobilize the effort of social workers to engage in this form of practice?

Social workers can engage in inquiry because they are motivated to do so, perhaps by a funder, an external source of accountability, or contractual requirements as inherent in some forms of evaluation. From my perspective and experience, such demands influence a different form of research engagement and process than that which is undertaken by social workers who find meaning in the advancement of their own work or in the advancement of the well-being of groups (Blair & Minkler, 2009; Gehlert & Coleman, 2010) or in improving institutional performance (Brown-Sica, 2012). When social workers bring research into their practice and involve others, and when those others experience difficult if not oppressive circumstances, then research itself can serve as a form of helping (Branom, 2012).

Here action research is invaluable because it plays off of the intrinsic motivation of the social worker. The questions steering action research often emerge from a social worker taking action in a particular context and domain. Context refers to those factors in which social-work practice is embedded, such as an organizational setting, service system, or particular community. Domain involves the coalescence of a practice arena in which the social worker takes action using policies, theories, structures, paradigms, and prevailing practices common to that domain. Mental health, child welfare, and aging are three such domains within the profession of social work.

Within a given domain or context, principal questions concerning the need for certain knowledge may prevail. The social worker may orient to such questions, particularly ones forming what we can identify as either products of commonly accepted perspectives or prevailing paradigms within a given domain. Imagination, particularly the social-work imagination, and its influence on what social workers select as issues to examine through action research is an important consideration. What I label as the social-work imagination is inspired by Mills's idea of the sociological imagination. Social workers are well socialized to raise critical questions about human need and its fulfillment. Social workers are astute observers of social conditions and how those conditions shape or otherwise produce human need. In addition, they often raise questions about practice improvement that suggest more creative avenues for addressing such needs than what may exist in current practice situations.

Cognitive–Emotional States Enabling Action Research

Both *wonder* and *criticism* are important cognitive–emotional states contributing to the surfacing of questions steering subsequent action research undertaken by social workers. Austen (2010) emphasizes the importance of such emotions to the process of innovation. Both cognition and emotion combine to produce more insight into situations than either cognition or emotion can produce alone. Wonder is a cognitive emotion in which human beings project images of what they seek to understand and it is highly influenced by feeling. The ancient Greek idea of theory is instructive because its origins as a way of seeing the world invoked "beholding" a phenomenon. By observing something closely, something many social workers accomplish naturally as part of their own process of problem solving or solution finding, many questions emerge that astute social-work professionals may simply wonder about in graphic detail.

Situations in which social workers enact practice suggest issues, barriers, problems, and opportunities influencing both the formulation of the purpose of inquiry and the subsequent design of investigation. One signature of action research, whether it is enacted in business, education, human services, or health care, is that it is undertaken by practitioners working alone or with others for the purpose of addressing questions that practitioners (and collaborators) hold about their practice in particular con-

texts (Bradbury, 2006; Butler, Feller, Pope, Emerson, & Murphy, 2008; Chung & Windsor, 2012; Draper et al., 2011; Etowa, Bernard, Oyinsan, & Clow, 2007; Schneider, 2012). One must appreciate the cognitive emotion of wonder because, without it, one may simply overlook opportunities to improve practice for the purposes of social betterment.

But criticism factors into the creative engagement in inquiry in an important way. It can go hand in hand with wonder. By criticism I am referring to the engagement in an analytic process of deciphering a given situation to begin the process of weighing factors that can inform subsequent action in meaningful ways. Having a critical perspective means that the practitioner is engaged in a situation he or she observes firsthand and comes to understand in rich detail, because in action research such a form of engagement fuels the realism and authenticity of inquiry (Schein, 2006). The action research process is bounded by investigators' wonder about the situations in which they practice or experience. By their criticism of those existing situations, they can generate practice knowledge from inquiry into questions, the intent of which is practice advancement.

A third kind of cognitive emotion may also prove important to launching and sustaining action research for the purposes of practice improvement. *Conjecture* implicates the need to appreciate evidence that is incomplete, necessitating more illumination of situations such that factors influencing the improvement of practice become explicit (Deutsch, 2011). Making an inference about such incompleteness is a critical influence on the origins of key questions. By adding conjecture to wonder and criticism, we appreciate the reasons for undertaking action research in given situations. We see the emergence of rationale for a given investigation animated by the motivation of the social worker to learn through action. For Senge and Scharmer (2006), action research is a way of learning, the potency of which is amplified when such inquiry is undertaken in community settings. A community can serve as a forum in which those social workers undertaking action research in context can experience a form of immersive learning in a given situation (Bassman & Harris, 2007; Congdon & Congdon, 2011). Action research can help participants to appreciate situations that are otherwise unknown to them (Hammond, 1998). Thus, action research and appreciative learning align here. But action research can also extend into the critical as a means for participants to critique existing structures and arrangements within a given context (Cahill,

Quijada Cerecer, & Bradley, 2010; Corbett, Francis, & Chapman, 2007).

This learning through action is the essence of the knowledge-building sequence of action research. The learning action research produces may be well focused and incremental or it may be transformational, resulting in the emergence of a whole new way of understanding practice in a given situation and within a given context and domain (Mezirow & Taylor, 2009). This new way, or what Bohm (2002) refers to as creativity, can bring about new structures of action; for social work such action may illuminate novel ways of helping.

Action Research as Dialogic Practice

Weaving dialogic practice throughout the action research sequence may prove strategic to knowledge development and subsequent use of that knowledge for practice improvement. Dialog requires interaction among equals who examine the nature of practice within organizational settings, service systems, or perhaps even whole domains. Questioning existing practices is inherent in structuring innovation (Bohm, 2003a) and in formulating organizational worldviews that direct subsequent action (Bohm, 2003b). The challenge here, according to Bohm (2000), is to engage an "implicate order" in which all factors are folded together, thereby producing considerable complexity such as found in social-work practice. Inquiry into such complexity can be addressed through interdisciplinary or transdisciplinary collaboration (Bore & Wright, 2009; Lang et al., 2012) and the development of communities of practice involving participants with diverse backgrounds (Wenger, 1998; Wenger, McDermott, & Snyder, 2002).

Collaboration among diverse stakeholders is a common approach to the practice of inquiry through action research (Sullivan & Willis, 2001). Such collaboration imbues community–university engagement with considerable relevance (Wergin, 2004). Collaboration among academic social work and community organizations underscores the synergy inherent in the integration of diverse capacities to support mutually beneficial knowledge development through engaged research (Dulmus & Cristalli, 2012; Percy, Zimpher, & Brukardt, 2004).

Dialog facilitates an engagement of this order through the exercise of multiple perspectives typically undertaken in teams so that the visibility of what constitutes practice comes into relief. This is likely why the participatory element has gained so much interest in action research. Multiplicity of perspective can induce a diversity of thought and thereby stimulate criticism of what exists (Bohm & Peat, 2000). The diversification of perspective that dialog can achieve once inclusion of diverse voices comes about resists the simplification of what are naturally complex situations (Bohm, 2003b).

Progress and Its Realization as an Organizing Value and Operational Aim

The ideas of improvement or social betterment are central to action research undertaken by social workers who invest the premium of knowledge with considerable importance. Improvement suggests that social-work practitioners can advance its knowledge base in definitive and even measurable ways through the systematic engagement of their own practice. Action research is likely a local form of knowledge development: it is undertaken by those practitioners who see learning about practice as a fundamental way of engaging in social betterment (Checkland & Poulter, 2006) within the immediate contexts in which they work.

The psychological state of engaging in such inquiry invokes the importance of practitioner self-efficacy: a belief that social workers can actually improve a given set of circumstances through the purposeful and intentional action they undertake. Combining such beliefs with wonder, criticism, and conjecture within team cultures that inspire both action and reflective dialog can embody improvement aims in explicit ways. This combination explains why some organizations may advance their knowledge base as a regular product of their work (Pfeffer & Sutton, 2000). Action research is a form of engaged inquiry undertaken by social workers who believe that knowledge formulation can make a positive difference in what they do and how they do it.

We cannot discount progress as an organizing value of action research undertaken for the purposes of practice improvement or social betterment. Many of us may simply assume that in social work progress is not a widely shared value. We may assume that things will stay the same until something more dramatic occurs in the domain or in the greater society, such as economic breakthroughs. But even the accumulation of small improvements can influence great breakthroughs.

Progress can be a central idea animating organizational culture in certain instances and, therefore, is fundamental to incremental practice improvement or even practice breakthroughs within a given domain. Practitioners who realize effective means for retaining youth in secondary schools, facilitating the transition of youth to higher education, and augmenting early child development programs in certain neighborhoods may set the foundation for subsequent progress emerging latently over time. Too often progress is a function of small incremental changes over what Horton (1997) calls the long haul of positive change induced by intentional social action.

New structures guiding both thought and action may emerge over the long haul, only to be taken for granted by practitioners as the right thing to do in a given situation. There is a close correspondence between action research and the development of intervention culture, which can take place when new practice knowledge displaces old. It is this process of displacement that may form what we consider practice advancement.

Yet social workers must also understand how wonder, criticism, and conjecture enter the picture: such cognitive emotions set the stage for how common knowledge can be destroyed organizationally, as when routines become displaced through new action. One can see the importance of cycles of action research (Stringer, 2007). The never-ending game of inquiry means that the new innovation may be over the proverbial hill waiting for discovery by those practitioners who practice an ethic of improvement or transformation. The idea of progress is linked to cognitive–emotional virtues like optimism and hope. Openness to change anticipates that something better is on the horizon or can be if action is taken to seek it out. Anticipation is an act of hope. Action is an expression of optimism.

Movement from Incipient to Mature Knowledge

Knowledge in its early stages and beginning to appear or coming into form is indicative of action research in its early stages (Scharmer, 2007). Incipient knowledge suggests that social work's understanding is not yet clear and the variables influencing a given situation and outcomes lack clarity. Practitioners can be ignorant of the determinants of a given situation, and they may be without either theory to explain the issue they face in practice or models that direct action. Practitioners may apply standard models to a new situation and come to learn of their strengths or limitations. Or, whole new situations may require novel models awaiting invention and trial use in actual practice situations. Such invention may be a product of the fusion of action research a social worker undertakes with developmental aims, implementing what Thomas (1984) conceived of as design and development in social work.

Action research serves as a way of uncovering or illuminating such knowledge early, particularly early in the innovation or organizational development process. Seeding action research in novel situations can stimulate further thought about subsequent action and feed new insights into practice. Those insights, informed by wonder, criticism, and conjecture, can amplify promising practices or stimulate hope that breakthroughs can occur. Practice questions can emanate from the greater context in which a social issue emerges, such as what practices (or models or discrete interventions) are needed to help seasoned corporate executives displaced from well-paying jobs and whole careers, assist families in moving across a country to take advantage of emerging job markets, and support immigrant families in sustaining indigenous communities while pursuing higher education in a host country.

Action researchers seeking mature intervention knowledge may introduce new questions, or even novel kinds of questions and designs, compared with what practitioners used previously in a knowledge-building process. Using mature knowledge, social workers invoke ideas that are commonly accepted within the practice community or domain in which practitioners address a given social issue with considerable certainty. Certainty may be a product of systematic trial use, such as that found in clinical trials, or in so-called rigorous research that establishes functional relationships linking context with intervention and subsequent outcome. An organization's knowledge base forms when organizational actors make that knowledge about which they are certain an elemental part of the culture, so newcomers come to learn about it as reality involving preferred ways of taking action (Schein, 2010).

In open and fluid cultures, such certainty is never settled. They are open to wonder, criticism, and conjecture. Progress is seen as progressive and continuous but never fully realized. The difference between what Carse (1987) refers to as finite and infinite culture is instructive. Finite cultures accept the rules as fixed and their members do not readily challenge them. Infinite cultures are open to critical questioning of what exists in anticipation of the next breakthrough in thought or practice. In their characterization of East Asian business organizations as infinite in their cultures, Hampden-Turner and Trompenaars (1997) indicate that such cultures are largely paradigmatic; that is, they largely describe a general approach to inquiry about the universe by trying to answer the question, *What should we assume when setting out to learn?* (p. 12).

Practice knowledge is contested in infinite cultures and dynamic flow ensues as a result. Ways of testing knowledge, translating it into action, treating it as provisional, and opening it to criticism do not make such organizations incoherent and tentative. It can make them dynamic and somewhat wild. Wild knowledge is difficult to tame because for those practitioners who engage in action research, the taming process is somewhat provisional, capable of only taking the organization so far in its quest for progress. The concept of innovation can substitute for that of wild. And in innovation we see the necessity of change instilled by a culture of learning through inquiry into action, and through considerable interaction among members of a given system to frame the action necessary to advance innovative ideas and the practices those ideas generate (Johnson, 2010).

Action research is differential—practitioners can apply it to any phase of knowledge development along the nascent-naive to mature continuum. Some practitioners may wrongly classify action research as exclusively qualitative. Actually, action research can handle considerable diversity in design, method, form of data, and analytic strategy. What makes action research distinctive is that knowledge emerges from action, and the action practitioners take to understand practice then changes both those practitioners and their contexts. So, for action researchers inquiry can effect considerable reflexive learning.

The change process that naturally flows from action is the basis of practitioner reflexivity (D'Cruz, Gillingham, & Melendez, 2007). Knowledge can mature organizationally as practitioners grow in their reflexivity and form common ways of understanding that stand independent of specific disciplinary perspectives (Loibl, 2006). To move from a naive understanding of a given practice situation to a mature one is the basis of organizational knowledge management. Purposefully managing organizational knowledge concerning intervention can produce system reflexivity: a shared way among practitioners of taking action in a given domain of practice, potentially culminating in a mature knowledge base that itself can become a focus of subsequent change through action research.

Moving from naive to mature knowledge in which certainty prevails merely sets the stage for a subsequent cycle of inquiry. Conditions and contexts change. Experience, particularly when mediated by thoughtful and critical dialog, can change how practitioners see their practice knowledge base. Bringing this kind of iterative knowing into practice is the aim of action research. Networks and groups may be important structures within which knowledge forms through action research (Johnson, 2010; Martin, 2006). Thus, increasingly, the maturation of action takes place within group structures.

Variants of Action Research

PARTICIPATORY ACTION RESEARCH Action research can incorporate diverse models or strategies that fit with different knowledge development aims sought by practitioners, teams, or organizations. One of the principal variants is participatory action research (PAR), in which people of varying organizational locations or positions can participate in the conception, design, enactment, and utilization of action. The positional or locational imperative is prominent in PAR, given how local concerns of practitioners influence the key questions, aims, and structures of inquiry (Jagosh et al., 2012). For social work the participation or involvement of the members of underrepresented groups is an important, if not defining, element of social work's code of ethics. Participatory action research advocates highlight inclusion as a valued end, offering people who are affected by research a say in the research. Other benefits of participation include cultural responsiveness of inquiry, productive intergroup relationships, and systemic change in problem conditions (Jagosh et al., 2012).

Although this ethic is important, if not central, to the spirit and integrity of PAR in that inclusion can correct for some aspects of oppression, such involvement does not necessarily mean control over the research project. Prominent within action research and its variants is the issue of who controls the research agenda, its enactment, and the subsequent products of inquiry. Action research emerges as a local, almost "bottom-up approach" to inquiry in which the people who have been too often omitted from the means and ends of inquiry are included, as a corrective measure to exclusion. The rationale is that those who are "closest" to the phenomenon that acts as the object of inquiry are in the best position to build knowledge through their proximity, which rises to almost a stipulation in PAR.

EMPOWERMENT-FOCUSED ACTION RESEARCH One can go farther, however, in articulating why and how inquiry is undertaken by those who have been traditionally "left out" of inquiry. We can frame yet another variant of action research when we elevate the "lived experience" as a qualification for empowering actual investigators who engage in inquiry. Social workers engaging in such empowerment strategies are mindful of the importance of allowing collaboration indicative of PAR to yield to yet another form: empowerment-focused action research. In this variant social workers can become advisors, consultants, or technical assistants using their expertise to support the empowerment of researchers who are not formally trained in inquiry (although they very well may be) and who may benefit from facilitation, expertise in a substantive area, or expertise in methods of inquiry.

For the so-called indigenous perspective, expertise may come from "knowing" how situations actually work, the sense of discrimination or oppression that emerges from how communities and professionals can devalue people with certain qualities or characteristics and how certain system archetypes can diminish the importance of alternative perspectives (Struthers, Lauderdale, Nichols, Tom-Orme, & Strickland, 2005). Empowerment-focused action research may not gain traction in more traditional types of human service entities or communities, particularly where professional ideologies and control are dominant. But it may find a welcoming environment in what social workers identify as alternative service organizations, that is, those entities founded by people whose expertise emanates out of the lived experience of oppression, who convert that experience into a form of knowing and then use this knowing as the basis of structuring and engaging in advocacy (Smith, 2005). Expertise is not confined to traditional sources within participatory forms of action research. Participants with direct experience can serve as technical assistants and consultants within action research projects (Fern & Kristinsdóttir, 2011) as well as the principal leaders of such inquiry (Ozer & Wright, 2012).

COMMUNITY-BASED PARTICIPATORY ACTION RESEARCH

Still another variant of action research is community-based participatory action research (CBPAR) attaching "community-based" to PAR. A whole community or a substantial part of it can become involved in developing the agenda of inquiry and then enacting it using traditional or alternative methods of inquiry (Minkler & Wallerstein, 2003). Typically in CBPAR the community serving as the locus of action is facing considerable distress and public neglect (Munford, Sanders, & Andrew, 2003). In some cases, given the severity of social indicators and scope and multiplicity of need, as well as infrastructure challenges, characterizing those communities as devastated may be accurate. The placement of action research into that community as a means of

correcting the ills it faces, amplifying participation or involvement of its citizens or residents in multiple venues, and increasing local control over the action–research nexus (in terms of specifying questions, developing methods, and fostering utilization) are essential if not defining properties of CBPAR.

Social workers steeped in community practice, development, or organization may find CBPAR a consequential and ethical approach to address community issues that are too often defined and controlled by external entities. The CBPAR project may embrace useful world views involving asset and appreciative approaches to inquiry that neutralize the characterization of the community in question as devastated or "a problem." Whole organizations may form to perpetuate and sustain the CBPAR initiative, and residents of the focal community may witness the emergence of innovative forms of provision, helping and assistance, and opportunities. Connecting community control to the CBPAR project may elevate the status of residents who find alternative careers, seek out additional education and training, find meaningful work through the CBPAR initiatives, and assume powerful roles as the actual governors of the project. Community-based participatory action research holds the promise of catalyzing multiple forms of change or social betterment that radiate out into the community.

Staying true to the intrinsic nature of inquiry, those who coordinate and/or govern the CBPAR project within the focal community underscore the local nature of questions, the benefits sought through the nexus formed between local action and research, and the nature of local action that emerges. Imposing academic requirements on the inquiry may undermine, if not falsify, local ends. The idea of rigor inappropriately asserted by those who see the CBPAR initiative in traditional research terms may dampen local enthusiasm and, as a consequence, such an assertion can strip a project of its authenticity.

Those social workers whose commitment to local empowerment can offset the propensity to make the inquiry something it is not—a way of addressing what Stake (1995) refers to as instrumental ends found in building knowledge potentially generalizable to the class or type of problem the community experiences. In research terms, CBPAR, along with other variants of action research, is likely idiographic in form, character, and principal aims. Inquiry that is idiographic requires appreciation of the rich, textured, and nuanced context in which inquiry unfolds, and so, as a result, the effort produces local knowledge for local use. In this sense, traditional researchers may dismiss action research as mere case study, although the case study character of such inquiry may be its very strength.

Knowledge development in CBPAR is likely local, producing lessons learned for an immediate community. This does not mean that other communities, investigators, and projects will fail to see the relevance of such local knowledge and experience. What it does mean is that CBPAR is first a form of knowledge development that combines community control, participation, local priorities, and local information for the purposes of advancing the quality of life (or some aspect of it) of the immediate locale. For the social-work profession, CBPAR can be a form of progressive and enlightened service in which inquiry is used as a vehicle for mobilization.

Social-work researchers steeped in traditional ideologies and tools may find CBPAR a difficult transition. The rules are somewhat different and its ethical framework suggests that involvement, participation, and control serve as primary and necessary avenues of local change. This local imperative makes action research and its variants distinctive in social-work inquiry. When one ponders the scope of action research expressed through its variants, one can see an expanding arena in which questions, strategies, information, and the ultimate aims of social betterment move beyond professional control, emanating into groups and communities in which empowerment is perhaps the ultimate end of inquiry.

Bohmian dialog (Bohm, 1996) expands in conjunction with this broadening scope. Social workers can have new kinds of conversations with the members of multiple stakeholder groups concerning the action that best brings about consensually shared conceptions of social betterment or, in situations of conflict, the specification of alternative world views of social betterment. Social workers likely will find such dialog empowering because it establishes within the field of local knowledge numerous possibilities for how to proceed in subsequent cycles when appreciating experience flowing from action becomes a defining element of inquiry.

The previous paragraph implies how action research and its variants can produce psychological benefits for those who are involved in the process. Such inquiry can clarify cognition that too often is confused by what appear to be chaotic factors operating in a given situation. This clarity can feed into emotional states, building motivation to engage in inquiry, facilitating new self-conceptions, and stimulating both optimism and hope. The utilization of the knowledge products of an action research cycle for advancing local quality of life can result in the empowerment of community or group members, a principle consistent with Patton's (2012) utilization-focused evaluation.

Socially, well-executed action research can bring people together in collaboration for social betterment or it can enable intergroup conflict to find a constructive outlet. Armed with local knowledge, participants can shape an agenda of change that catalyzes and unites groups or communities. Realizing potent action to advance social betterment in a given locale can make action research and its variants a potentially high-impact strategy of inquiry. This is not to say that such impact will result from this form of inquiry. It is important, however, to underscore the potential here given how action research and its variants focus on the local knowledge people need for social betterment.

The Design of Action Research

The variants of action research suggest three somewhat overlapping dimensions of a model of inquiry. The overlapping dimensions make the model somewhat fuzzy but the three dimensions are nonetheless building blocks of action research in organizations, communities, or complex systems. These are as follows:

1. *Collaboration*, in which an intergroup field likely forms, characterized by the members of differing groups cooperating with one another, sharing resources, and combining assets for use within a common project of inquiry. For this dimension collaboration may not exist or it may be quite high, imbuing the particular project with qualities of collaborative action research.

2. *Participation*, in which people or groups who have been omitted from inquiry are included as empowered actors who have a say in the research. Participation can come in many different forms and at many different levels of intensity. High levels of participation of groups or people typically omitted from inquiry will imbue the model with participatory features, thereby justifying the moniker of PAR.

3. *Control*, in which a group may engage in considerable decision making over the particular purpose, aims, strategies, methods, and uses of action research in a given setting or context. This dimension seeks to correct for a whole

host of social ills marginalizing the will, say, and qualities of the members of certain groups. Control is directly linked to empowerment. Without control, there is likely little, if any, empowerment.

The three dimensions not only serve as a road map to initiating inquiry in a given context but also actually operate as design factors. In helping groups shape their variant of action research in a given context, practitioners ask explicitly how much collaboration, participation, and control those groups seek in the design of their project. At first, the members of those groups may see such questions as lacking immediate relevance. They want to move fast in getting the information they want or need. But process is very important to action research and the process itself may require a quieting of emotions and a slowing of pace so that the right design emerges, thereby fulfilling the needs of the many actors an action research project typically involves. Within the design process, soft system methodologies, like those proposed by Checkland (1999) and the organizational learning school, may prove to be important. Conducting search conferences (Weisbord & Janoff, 2010), World Cafes (Brown & Isaacs, 2005), and other avenues of intergroup learning may prove pivotal in producing a relevant local design of CBPAR.

Design in this context does not implicate traditional forms of research design. Design in action research speaks to the human and intergroup arrangements supporting the knowledge development effort understanding that low levels of collaboration, participation, and control form a project that is very different from those in which there are high levels of such qualities. When the three dimensions intersect, the distinctive culture of a given action research project emerges and frames subsequent action on the part of those who are involved in such an enterprise.

Developmental Action Research as Variant

Yet another variant of action research is developmental action research (DAR). The aim of DAR, which involves the melding of action research with social research and development, is to develop local interventions to address social issues of immediate importance to devalued communities (Moxley & Washington, 2012). Developmental action research involves the application of action research to the development and testing of helping strategies. Moxley and Washington undertook PAR in collaboration with older homeless and formerly homeless African

American women. Collectively they engaged in sequences of intervention design and development, addressing issues the participants saw as possessing immediate value in their local community. The overall DAR project was multilevel and incorporated multiple methods, particularly alternative methods.

The DAR process Moxley and Washington (2012) developed is indicative of the melding process in which new variants of action research can emerge given the purposes participants formulate. At first, action research was dominant because the participants had few, if any, linkages with the recipient population early in the project. As they situated themselves in the problem space and domain, participants came to appreciate the situation of homelessness in late life among African American women through traditional methods involving survey research and interviews, followed by in-depth qualitative interviews with women who were able to overcome homelessness using their own resources and strategies. By the end of the initial stage, participants had gained insight into the developmental objectives they would pursue to bring about relevant helping strategies.

At this juncture, midway in the 10-year lifespan of the project, it shifted from action research to a participatory form in which a small group of self-selected participants became governors of the project and were highly engaged in controlling the agenda of inquiry and in assisting other participants in staging what came to be known as substudies of the parent project. In total, 530 women participated in some aspect of the project as the project moved from specific developmental objectives to concept formation and then into the design of prototypes and their subsequent testing in action.

Increased involvement among the governors of the project resulted in a strong community of support and they emerged as advocates for other minority women facing homelessness at mid- or late life, an indication of how empowerment can be a product of PAR (Washington, Moxley, Garriott, & Crystal, 2009). Inclusion of the arts facilitated the advocacy process and those methods became useful in helping women communicate to the broader community the issues, challenges, and barriers they faced while homeless (Washington & Moxley, 2008). The public awareness-building paralleled the cultural development of the project such that a strong local identity emerged among participants, bringing even more attention to the issue within the community. The participants collected a community exhibit incorporating art and narrative content as a vehicle for cultural development to tell the stories of the various pathways women took into, through, and out of homelessness (Moxley, Washington, & Feen, 2008). The art and narrative content were products of the action research and served as a principal strategy of action for illuminating issues and factors pushing older minority women into homelessness (Moxley, Feen-Calligan, & Washington, 2012; Washington & Moxley, 2009).

Developmental action research is useful in working directly with participants in testing, improving, and confirming promising practices. Particularly useful in local situations with little infrastructure to address an issue, the synthesis DAR reflects involves the systematic procedures of social research and development melding with action research geared to building discrete aspects of that infrastructure. Prototyping becomes an important part of the process of inquiry in which teams can build on existing best practices or use their own practice wisdom in fabricating promising practices, ones that they can submit to further development through testing the prototype in a process that research and development professionals refer to as proof of concept or principle. This testing can occur in convenient local organizations, in the protected or specialized settings of formal testing environments, or in the crucible of challenging situations, such as street outreach to those who are homeless.

The DAR project the author described previously shows how a long-haul local–intrinsic model can emerge from collaborative research and PAR, the intent of which is to develop knowledge for a particular purpose and in a particular context (Stake, 1995). Some may argue that knowledge takes the form of technology in DAR, and so intervention technology and its development can be a distinctive aim of this kind of variant. As the local–intrinsic model crystallizes within a given culture, in a particular place, and with a particular set of actors, transportation of that model may become difficult. Local model development is therefore intrinsic (Freeman, Brugge, Bennett-Bradley, Levy, & Carrasco, 2006). A different research model and process may be necessary to make the model more generalizable. By definition, seeking generalizable knowledge is not a principal aim of action research and its variants.

As social workers consider knowledge development, the sequencing of DAR is instructive. Knowledge management involves the intentional administration of this sequence and its products. Thus, connecting knowledge development and knowledge management

is an intentional strategy in the development of helping processes.

Knowledge development starts with a perception of a local issue, and as wonder, criticism, and conjecture take form, the research participants become more mindful of the dynamics of that issue. The criticism of immediate context (which we might call context evaluation) reveals the necessity of subsequent action to build a meaningful and potentially promising local response. Moving from concept formation to prototyping and then to testing and on to improvement and even confirmation is an intense and value-added sequence of action. Confidence about the promise of the design may gain traction in this process, or the actors may make critical decisions about merit and subsequently abandon the design but not the project. Those designs emerging over time as successful face the challenge of sustainability. By successfully addressing sustainability, the designs take root and their permanence blends into community life or into the life of an organization or system of helping. Sustainability can build intervention or helping culture and yield a permanent presence of a new technology for social betterment (Leonard, 2011a).

The culture that forms in relationship to this process may anticipate the creation of a future organization to achieve what Huston (2007) calls a "holding space." This holding space ensures a support system for the project and its designs. In addition, that holding space can emerge as a community of learning, fostering even more innovation in the near future (Wenger, 1998). The innovative holding space of the project may become known for its commitment to progress in the issue area or domain in which it is rooted. It translates knowledge that the organization values and finds effective into action by teaching members of the system how to enact that knowledge (Pfeffer & Sutton, 2000). The teaching–learning nexus is vital to action research because it fosters both dissemination and utilization internally within the host of the action and the research. If others emulate or otherwise model those innovative forms, then action research can stimulate a form of diffusion based on social learning (Leonard, 2011b, 2011c). Such is the potential relationship between action research and organizational or systems development (Pasmore, 2006).

Achieving a permanent response to the identified issue in a given community is the essence of sustainability. Managing the ensuing knowledge products and making them permanent (or abandoning them if they prove ineffective) within some kind of organizational structure is yet another expression of the crystallization of know-how in a given community. The tension forming between the retention of a given knowledge product and its abandonment is strategic. Participants may actively engage in such dialog as an important step in the cycle of knowledge-building through action research.

Methodological Pluralism

Methodological pluralism legitimizes the many diverse tools social-work researchers and evaluators have available for the purposes of knowledge development in organizational and community contexts. In addition to those methods one reads about in the principal social-work research textbooks, other approaches, particularly ones encouraging or otherwise facilitating participation, as well as the release of tacit or indigenous knowledge, have come to the fore in recent times (Leonard & Sensiper, 2011; Von Krogh, Ichijo, & Nonaka, 2000). Many of those methods are narrative in form, designed to release knowledge about social issues among those who are most intimate with challenging circumstances that can degrade daily life (Coles, 1990). Narrative methods are fundamental to releasing and organizing knowledge and may be fundamental to the achievement of innovation (Nonaka & Takeuchi, 1995). Action research can incorporate narrative as a means of interpreting data, disseminating findings, and transferring knowledge within community or organizational settings (Swap, Leonard, Shields, & Abrams, 2011).

Narrative methods amplify both the content of the issues and how people experience them, particularly their causes and consequences. They respect the emotional field that surrounds an issue—those emotions that leave an indelible mark on people, whose first-person accounts reveal them as survivors of a situation no one can fully understand outside of individuals who have lived through such challenging and life-altering situations. Often the narrative is a principal means for the documentation of trauma and the experience of deprivation.

Narrative methods can also induce reflection by practitioners and others experienced with helping processes and, as a result, make explicit practice wisdom that is often tacit among practitioners. Illuminating this tacit knowledge can serve as a principal aim of action research (Tsang, 2008) through the engagement of participants in narrative inquiry (Sheppard, 1995) to release their assumptive knowledge guiding social-work action in particular contexts (Dybicz, 2004). The explication of practice wisdom can produce practice ontologies: the organized portrayal of first principles and assumptions that influence a social worker's action. Illuminating those ontologies is essential to knowledge development, particularly in practice situations (Abbas, 2010).

Consistent with contemporary trends, action research methods often constitute alternative ones because they are not widely used, more traditional researchers may find them suspect, and they challenge prevailing norms of quality in terms of the kinds of data they produce. But such methods contribute to the formation of an interesting toolkit for helping people "tell their stories" of the situations that challenge, if not overwhelm, their coping and adaptive resources. Many of them are indicative of the growing use of narrative approaches for capturing the lived experience of people whose voices too often go unheard. Photography and photovoice are two methods that can help people amplify their experience, particularly when photographs and words are brought together, forming rich narrative portraits (Brinton Lykes, 2006).

A photograph is a potentially evocative image but it can produce static images. Alternatively, videography can capture stream of experience and amplify aspects of a given context in which a social issue is rooted. Videography combined with performance in which people enact their experience is yet another powerful means of portraying situations and how people experience them, for better or worse. Performative methods are powerful tools for the portrayal of situations. Often, those people who have first-person experience with an issue, and who have survived it, can make this personal knowledge explicit through evocative methods of storytelling, interpretative reading, poetry, and song.

Through such methods, experts in the lived experience of a social issue, the survivors who have transcended those circumstances, come to serve as primary witnesses (Mienczakowski & Morgan, 2006). Making this witnessing explicit in community forums is yet another expression of participation in inquiry. Arts and activism cohere for advancing public understanding of social issues (Campana, 2011). Emotional knowledge can become prominent in such public education forums in which participants express their experience through the arts before audiences (Kaplan, 2007). The use of the arts by social workers for the purposes of social activism extends back to the settlement-house movement (Stankiewicz, 1989).

Using methods from the arts and folk arts can result in forms of knowledge that take concrete or physical form, such as a quilt. Synthesizing the actual performances, photographs, narrative, song, and poems into an educational exhibit can challenge visitors with new ways of viewing and understanding a social issue in a specific community. The methods make explicit tacit knowledge and affirm people as local experts on the consequences of degrading experience.

Bringing the product of those methods into an exhibit offers a strategy of building a local knowledge base and communicating the contours of this knowledge to people who may have once found the experiences remote and unfamiliar. The methods and their products lend themselves to dissemination, and bringing them into an innovative form of dissemination within a given community context expands the scope and depth of sharing the products of inquiry with others. Building community awareness and expanding public empathy for the people who experience a particular social issue can be important outcomes of action research. Note, however, that through such methods action research participants are erecting an emotional field through purposeful action. Emotions are important properties of knowledge development, equal in standing to rationale engagement of an issue. To isolate knowledge from emotion risks the loss of authenticity and realism.

Assessing the Quality of Action Research in Social Work

By what parameters can we assess the quality of action research? The idea of metaevaluation is now a standard practice in much of evaluation and the standards from the American Evaluation Association offer considerable guidance in how to view and appraise the quality of a given evaluation (Yarbrough, Shulha, Hopson, & Caruthers, 2011). Those standards and the manner in which they are organized indicate that accuracy (or rigor) of the evaluation stands in a complementary relationship to several other dimensions in assessing the quality of evaluation. In addition to the accuracy dimension, those standards that focus on the quality of the research method and measurement, the American Evaluation Association system, includes utility, feasibility, and propriety. Without attending to those dimensions, any evaluation project and any evaluator can fall short. The principal implication here is that rigor alone does not determine the quality of evaluation.

In considering local and intrinsic requirements of action research, a practitioner can expand quality to embrace immediate usefulness emanating from realism and authenticity of the action research undertaken in some local context. Action research focuses

specifically on an immediate intrinsic system, and coming to understand it within a given context is of utmost importance if this form of inquiry is to gain local credibility and relevance. That it is likely for participants to relate first to their own human experience and to those experiences of others closely situated moves the project from the abstract and imbues it with concrete immediacy. The project's capacity to engage reality as people live it should in no way be confused with what researchers consider realistic (Bronfenbrenner, 1979). Indeed, the action research project may embrace idealism, motivating people to look to a desired horizon of possibility for inspiration and hope (Spretnak, 1999). As was suggested earlier, those cognitive emotions are fundamental to the realization of good action research.

Still, authenticity serves as yet another important quality. By authenticity I am referring to the absence of artificiality by connecting to the kind of knowledge participants seek. The emergence of the true spirit of the project founded in local social betterment and using immediate resources (or assets) of people and organizations that populate the community make the project authentic. Realism—addressing the real issues the community faces in all of their severity and complexity—and authenticity—thereby making the project reflective of the spirit of the community—are essential to both relevance and usefulness (Bammer, 2005; Carolo & Travers, 2005).

The achievement of usefulness likely emerges early on from design incorporating the dimensions of collaboration, participation, and control to whatever extent they are relevant in the given situation. Feasibility then takes on importance as the aims of the action research are clear and those individuals and groups who are involved in it take into consideration available time, required resources, and specific expertise. Like any research endeavor, and as the American Evaluation Association dimension of feasibility reminds practitioners, good inquiry is inherent in projects that groups can complete and use for the purposes of social betterment.

Propriety, or the ethical dimension, is also an important criterion in assessing quality. The design qualities of collaboration, participation, and control are, in part, ethical considerations. How people treat one another in the process of inquiry, the management of confidentiality or anonymity when needed, respect for boundaries, and dignity all are central ethical considerations that take on particular importance when people's identities (too often diminished by social forces) factor into the process of knowledge development. Action research is often linked to understanding the causes and consequences of diminished status; hence, ethical interactions and even ethical treatment of those the mainstream considers deviant become important qualities of good action research.

Ultimately, when we consider propriety an aspect of quality and when we take control seriously, issues of intellectual property and ownership of knowledge likely come to the fore. Traditional researchers may consider the data and products of research as their own possession because they are the ones who conceive of the inquiry and engage in its process, sometimes under contract with other entities or sometimes using their own resources. Nonetheless, intellectual property becomes part of a contractual relationship. As action researchers enter venues in which collaboration, participation, and control are important qualities of design, then retention of knowledge within and for the community becomes part of the research process itself. Indeed, well-executed action research will likely produce knowledge and products that enhance the quality of life of a given context, and the members of the context should exercise some kind of corporate claim to that knowledge and its subsequent control.

When considering accuracy, we see its juxtaposition to a whole spectrum of quality considerations. Accuracy, or the rigor of action research, is not a principal driving value because it corresponds to other essential aspects of quality. Indeed, one can argue that usefulness, relevance, realism, and authenticity trump accuracy. Accuracy or rigor may serve as a contingent factor when action research participants ask fundamental questions about how decisions of usefulness influence the kind and degree of rigor a project can achieve with a given set of resources and the ethical challenges participants face in the execution of an action research project.

Conclusion: Caveats for Social Workers Undertaking Action Research with Intrinsic Aims

As framed here, action research is an intrinsic endeavor in which practitioners and human service organizations undertake inquiry for the purposes of addressing their own needs or the issues they face in an immediate environment. This inquiry largely engages the immediate situation in which those practitioners or organizations find themselves so they can generate information or perhaps form knowledge to

achieve those aims they find important. Inquiry may expand when practitioners or organizations engage recipients of service or members of the immediate community in which the organization takes action.

THE SOCIAL WORKER AS PARTICIPANT The intrinsic aims of inquiry can be further developed when research is undertaken by members of the community itself or when the recipients of social-work services engage in research, an action inherent in empowerment-oriented approaches. Those research initiators may wish to engage professional social workers and their organizations in the process of inquiry. Perhaps too often social workers frame research as something they initiate and recruit partners to address those issues or fulfill those needs that their research aims require. Action research does not prescribe who is either the initiator or the catalyst of inquiry. Although this is a key step in any inquiry (that is, someone or some entity must awaken to their need for knowledge), many forms of action research, particularly those involving a broad band of participation, leave those decisions open in the early stages. In the case of empowerment forms of action research, initiators or catalysts may be those people or groups who experience directly the causes and consequences of oppression or marginalization. Social workers who operate within such fields may possess collegial or secondary status. They may neither initiate nor control the inquiry.

ROLE FLEXIBILITY OF SOCIAL WORKERS The intrinsic focus may demand considerable flexibility on the part of social workers who can enact diverse roles in situations in which there are multiple stakeholders. This situation raises important questions about power, ethics, and relationships among multiple actors in chartering, designing, enacting, and utilizing intrinsically focused action research. Certainly one of those issues involves the question of who owns the research undertaken within such a field of action. Social workers should remain mindful of this question when it comes to actions pertaining to the assignment of credit, the dissemination of findings, and the subsequent utilization of knowledge. The practice aim of social workers in such situations likely involves their commitment to helping participants gain the capacities to enact and use intrinsically oriented action research. Thus, for the social worker intrinsically oriented action research may involve community organizing and asset-based community development as principal practice strategies.

FORMATION OF THE LOCAL RESEARCH COMMONS In community-based action research, if a coalition of participants exists, it likely exercises control over how research products are put to use. Traditional approaches that imbue principal investigators with considerable authority and control are likely inappropriate in many forms of action research. Indeed, in more community-based models of action research the idea of principal investigator may not have relevance. Because multiple constituencies can be involved in founding and steering the research, shaping the research through the enactment of critical judgment calls, acquiring resources and building capacities, and facilitating various processes of inquiry, a more democratic setting may vitiate the traditional idea that there is a controlling, dominant, and singular principal investigator. This possibility invests community organizing or development with considerable relevance.

When community representatives are the initiators or catalysts of inquiry, their dissemination needs are likely first and foremost. Other forms of dissemination, ones more consistent with instrumental ends, such as conferences or publication, are likely secondary in action research. The investment in local dissemination and support for local utilization possess immediate importance because the aim of an action research project involves the satisfaction of the intrinsic needs and the potential resolution of issues operating within a specific community (Kramer, 2011). Developing capacities for local dissemination may prove critical when it is important for an action research project to get findings out to local groups. Helping them put those findings to work in the improvement of community or organizational life makes utilization an important aim of the action research design.

What appears obvious may not serve as a simple solution: that those individuals who conceive of and initiate the research own the product of inquiry. Yet, conception and initiation of such research may reside with a nonacademic or nonorganizational entity of people within a community who do not possess a formal identity. It may be diffuse and therefore become part of the commonweal of a given community. Here what practitioners can conceive as the research commons is important. Not only do the research findings fall within the commons but also the capacities a community has won through considerable struggle become part of that commons. A professional social worker becomes mindful of this collective ownership and understands that al-

though immediate knowledge objectives are important for producing local singular solutions, ultimately multiple action research projects can help construct such a local commons. Those multiple projects can facilitate community capacity building, another possibility of long-haul community change.

For social workers engaged in community-based action research the commons may serve as the principal asset of the effort they invest in local inquiry. A coalition may invite the social worker (who may or may not be a formally trained researcher) or the professional's sponsoring or host organization to participate. Social workers and their sponsoring organizations may see themselves as pivotal within community-based action research, but they really are not, given the multiple actors who work together early on to initiate the research.

This contingency simply underscores the following observation: that action research, when undertaken for intrinsic purposes, can raise ethical questions involving how multiple stakeholders, whose interests may differ and whose passions about the issue at hand may vary in intensity and form, must recognize that inherent here is the need to govern the project. When a coalition of multiple stakeholders comes to work together for the purposes of enacting intrinsic action research, governance is an essential competence.

THE VALUE OF COLLABORATIVE KNOWLEDGE BUILDING When collaboration is a principal design element of action research, social workers must consider how the involvement of multiple constituencies influences the purpose of inquiry, the aim of which is bringing about actionable knowledge for local use. By expanding the field of involvement and participation among multiple groups, various interests form to shape the agenda of inquiry. However, it may be difficult for research organizers to engage certain groups because their visibility may create considerable risk for them, such as in the case of undocumented workers (Lykes, Hershberg, & Brabeck, 2011). The propriety of the inquiry itself can drive many of the subsequent decisions participants make about the enactment of inquiry, the scope of inclusion, and the consequences of involvement for the members of various groups forming a local community. It is here that the very best of social work's principled forms of action meld well with what those groups seek because it is through knowledge and its use that the quality of life of a local community can improve in demonstrable ways.

REFERENCES

Abbas, J. (2010). *Structures for organizing knowledge: Exploring taxonomies, ontologies, and other schema.* Chicago, IL: Neal-Schuman.

Argyris, C. (1982). *Reasoning, learning and action: Individual and organizational.* San Francisco, CA: Jossey-Bass.

Argyris, C. (1993). *Knowledge for action.* San Francisco, CA: Jossey-Bass.

Argyris, C., Putnam, R., & Smith, D. (1985). *Action science.* San Francisco, CA: Jossey-Bass.

Austen, H. (2010). *Artistry unleashed.* Toronto, Ontario, Canada: University of Toronto Press.

Bammer, G. (2005). Integration and implementation sciences: Building a new specialization. *Ecology and Society, 10*(2), 6. Retrieved from http://www.ecologyandsociety.org/vol10/iss2/art6/

Bassman, M. F., & Harris, K. (2007). Narrating the journey: Immersion learning in the migrant Latino community. *Partnerships Perspectives, 4*, 62–69.

Blair, T., & Minkler, M. (2009). Participatory action research with older adults: Key principles in practice. *Gerontologist, 49*(5), 651–662.

Bohm, D. (1996). *On dialogue.* New York, NY: Routledge.

Bohm, D. (2000). *Wholeness and the implicate order.* New York, NY: Routledge.

Bohm, D. (2002). *On creativity.* New York, NY: Routledge.

Bohm, D. (2003a). *Thought as a system.* New York, NY: Routledge.

Bohm, D. (2003b). *The essential David Bohm.* New York, NY: Routledge.

Bohm, D., & Peat, F. D. (2000). *Science, order, and creativity* (2nd ed.). New York, NY: Routledge.

Bore, A., & Wright, N. (2009). The wicked and complex in education: Developing a transdisciplinary perspective for policy formulation, implementation, and professional practice. *Journal of Education for Teaching, 35*(3), 241–256.

Bradbury, H. (2006). Learning with the natural step: Action research to promote conversations for sustainable development. In P. Reason & H. Bradbury-Huang (Eds.), *Handbook of action research* (pp. 236–242). London, England: Sage.

Branom, C. (2012). Community-based participatory research as a social work research and intervention approach. *Journal of Community Practice, 20*(3), 260–273.

Brinton Lykes, M. (2006). Creative arts and photography in participatory action research in Guatemala. In P. Reason & H. Bradbury-Huang (Eds.), *Handbook of action research* (pp. 269–278). London, England: Sage.

Bronfenbrenner, U. (1979). *The ecology of human development: Experiments by nature and design.* Cambridge, MA: Harvard University Press.

Brown, J., & Isaacs, D. (2005). *The world café: Shaping our futures through conversations that matter.* San Francisco, CA: Berrett-Koehler.

Brown-Sica, M. (2012). Library spaces for urban, diverse commuter students: A participatory action research project. *College & Research Libraries, 73*(3), 217–231.

Butler, T. T., Feller, J. J., Pope, A. A., Emerson, B. B., & Murphy, C. C. (2008). Designing a core IT artifact for knowledge management systems using participatory action research in a government and a non-government organization. *The Journal of Strategic Information Systems, 17*(4), 249–267.

Cahill, C., Quijada Cerecer, D., & Bradley, M. (2010). "Dreaming of …": Reflections on participatory action research as a feminist praxis of critical hope. *Affilia: Journal of Women & Social Work, 25*(4), 406–416.

Campana, A. (2011). Agents of possibility: Examining the intersections of art, education, and activism in communities. *Studies in Art Education, 52*, 278–291.

Carolo, H., & Travers, R. (2005). Challenges, complexities and solutions: A unique HIV research partnership in Toronto. *Journal of Urban Health, 82*, ii42.

Carse, J. P. (1987). *Finite and infinite games: A vision of life as play and possibility.* New York, NY: Ballantine.

Checkland, P. (1999). *Systems thinking, systems practice.* Chichester, England: Wiley.

Checkland, P., & Poulter, J. (2006). *Learning for action: A short definitive account of soft systems methodology and its use for practitioners, teachers and students.* Chichester, England: Wiley.

Chung, J. Y., & Windsor, C. A. (2012). Empowerment through knowledge of accounting and related disciplines: Participatory action research in an African village. *Behavioral Research in Accounting, 24*(1), 161–180.

Coles, R. (1990). *The call of stories.* New York, NY: Mariner.

Congdon, G., & Congdon, S. (2011). Engaging students in a simulated collaborative action research project: An evaluation of a participatory approach to learning. *Journal of Further and Higher Education, 35*(2), 221–231.

Corbett, A. M., Francis, K., & Chapman, Y. (2007). Feminist-informed participatory action research: A methodology of choice for examining critical nursing issues. *International Journal of Nursing Practice, 13*(2), 81–88.

D'Cruz, H., Gillingham, P., & Melendez, S. (2007). Reflexivity, its meanings and relevance for social work: A critical review of the literature. *British Journal of Social Work, 37*, 73–90.

Deutsch, D. (2011). *The beginning of infinity: Explanations that transform the world.* New York, NY: Penguin.

Draper, R., Adair, M., Broomhead, P., Gray, S., Grierson, S., Hendrickson, S., et al. (2011). Seeking renewal, finding community: Participatory action research in teacher education. *Teacher Development, 15*(1), 1–18.

Dulmus, C. N., & Cristalli, M. E. (2012). A university–community partnership to advance research in practice settings: The HUB research model. *Research on Social Work Practice, 22*(2), 195–202.

Dybicz, P. (2004). An inquiry into practice wisdom. *Families in Society, 85*, 197–203.

Etowa, J., Bernard, W., Oyinsan, B., & Clow, B. (2007). Participatory action research (PAR): An approach for improving black women's health in rural and remote communities. *Journal of Transcultural Nursing, 18*(4), 349–357.

Fairhurst, G. T., & Sarr, R. A. (1996). *The art of framing: Managing the language of leadership*. San Francisco, CA: Jossey-Bass.

Fern, E. (2012). Developing social work practice through engaging practitioners in action research. *Qualitative Social Work, 11*(2), 156–173.

Fern, E., & Kristinsdóttir, G. (2011). Young people act as consultants in child-directed research: An action research study in Iceland. *Child & Family Social Work, 16*(3), 287–297.

Freeman, E., Brugge, D., Bennett-Bradley, W., Levy, J., & Carrasco, E. (2006). Challenges of conducting community based participatory research in Boston's neighborhoods to reduce disparities in asthma. *Journal of Urban Health, 83*, 1013–1021.

Garvin, D. A. (2003). *Learning in action*. Cambridge, MA: Harvard Business School Press.

Gehlert, S., & Coleman, R. (2010). Using community-based participatory research to ameliorate cancer disparities. *Health & Social Work, 35*(4), 302–309.

Hammond, S. A. (1998). *The thin book of appreciative inquiry*. Bend, OR: Thin Book Publishing.

Hampden-Turner, C., & Trompenaars, F. (1997). *Mastering the infinite game: How East Asian values are transforming business practices*. Oxford, England: Capstone.

Horton, M. (1997). *The long haul: An autobiography*. New York, NY: Columbia University Press.

Huston, T. (2007). *Inside out: Stories and methods for generating collective will to create the future we want*. Boston, MA: SoL.

Jagosh, J., Macaulay, A., Pluye, P., Salsberg, J., Bush, P., Henderson, J., et al. (2012). Uncovering the benefits of participatory research: implications of a realist review for health research and practice. *Milbank Quarterly, 90*(2), 311–346.

Johnson, S. (2010). *Where good ideas come from: The natural history of innovation*. New York, NY: Riverhead Books.

Kaplan, F. F. (2007). *Art therapy and social action*. Philadelphia, PA: Jessica King.

Kramer, J. (2011). Following through to the end: The use of inclusive strategies to analyze and interpret data in participatory action research with individuals with intellectual disabilities. *Journal of Applied Research in Intellectual Disabilities, 24*(3), 263–273.

Lang, D., Wiek, A., Bergmann, M. Stauffacher, M., Martens, P. Moll, P., et al. (2012). Transdisciplinary research in sustainability science: Practice, principles, and challenges. *Sustainability Science, 7*(Supplement), 25–43.

Leonard, D. A. (2011a). Implementation of mutual adaptation of technology and organization. In D. A. Leonard (Ed.), *Managing knowledge assets, creativity and innovation* (pp. 235–250). Singapore: World Scientific Publishing.

Leonard, D. A. (2011b). Diffusing innovations when the users are not the choosers: The case of dentists. In D. A. Leonard (Ed.), *Managing knowledge assets, creativity and innovation* (pp. 235–250). Singapore: World Scientific Publishing.

Leonard, D. A. (2011c). Innovation as a knowledge generation and transfer process. In D. A. Leonard (Ed.), *Managing knowledge assets, creativity and innovation* (pp. 541–560). Singapore: World Scientific Publishing.

Leonard, D. A., & Sensiper, S. (2011). The role of tacit knowledge in group innovation. In D. A. Leonard (Ed.), *Managing knowledge assets, creativity and innovation* (pp. 301–324). Singapore: World Scientific Publishing.

Lewin, K. (1946). Action research and minority problems. *Journal of Social Issues, 2*, 34–56.

Lewin, K. (1948). *Resolving social conflicts*. New York, NY: Harper & Row.

Lewis, H. M. (2006). Participatory research and education for social change: Highlander research and education center. In P. Reason & H. Bradbury-Huang (Eds.), *Handbook of action research* (pp. 262–268). London, England: Sage.

Loibl, M. (2006). Integrating perspectives in the practice of transdisciplinary research. In J. Voß, D. Bauknecht, & R. Kemp (Eds.), *Reflexive governance for sustainable development* (pp. 294–310). Northampton, MA: Edward Elgar.

Lykes, M., Hershberg, R. M., & Brabeck, K. M. (2011). Methodological challenges in participatory action research with undocumented Central American migrants. *Journal for Social Action in Counseling & Psychology, 3*(2), 22–35.

Martin, A. (2006). Large group processes as action research. In P. Reason & H. Bradbury-Huang (Eds.), *Handbook of action research* (pp. 166–175). London, England: Sage.

Mezirow, J., & Taylor, E. W. (2009). *Transformative learning in practice: Insights from community, workplace, and higher education*. San Francisco, CA: Jossey-Bass.

Mienczakowski, J., & Morgan, S. (2006). Ethnodrama: Constructing participatory, experiential and compelling action research through performance. In P. Reason & H. Bradbury-Huang (Eds.), *Handbook of action research* (pp. 176–184). London, England: Sage.

Minkler, M., & Wallerstein, N. (2003). *Community-based participatory research for health*. San Francisco, CA: Jossey-Bass.

Moxley, D., Feen-Calligan, H., & Washington, O. (2012). Lessons learned from three projects linking social work, the arts, and humanities. *Social Work Education, 31*, 703–723.

Moxley, D., & Washington, O. (2012). Using a developmental action research strategy to build theory for intervention into homelessness among minority women. *Social Work in Mental Health, 10*, 426–444.

Moxley, D., Washington, O., & Feen, H. (2008). The social action art installation as educational forum. *Journal of Cultural Research in Art Education, 26*, 95–106.

Munford, R., Sanders, J., & Andrew, A. (2003). Community development—Action research in community settings. *Social Work Education, 22*(1), 93–104.

Nonaka, I., & Takeuchi, H. (1995). *The knowledge-creating company: How Japanese companies create the dynamics of innovation*. New York, NY: Oxford University Press.

Ozer, E. J., & Wright, D. (2012). Beyond school spirit: The effects of youth-led participatory action research in two urban high schools. *Journal of Research on Adolescence*, 22(2), 267–283.

Pasmore, W. (2006). Action research in the workplace: The socio-technical perspective. In P. Reason & H. Bradbury (Eds.), *Handbook of action research* (pp. 38–50). Thousand Oaks, CA: Sage.

Patton, M. Q. (2012). *Essentials of utilization-focused evaluation*. Los Angeles, CA: Sage.

Percy, S. L., Zimpher, N. L., & Brukardt, M. J. (2004). Creating a new kind of university: Institutionalizing community-university engagement. In S. L. Percy, N. L. Zimpher, & M. J. Brukardt (Eds.), *Creating a new kind of university: Institutionalizing community–university engagement* (pp. 3–22). Bolton, MA: Anker.

Pfeffer, J., & Sutton, R. I. (2000). *The knowing–doing gap: How smart companies turn knowledge into action*. Cambridge, MA: Harvard Business School Press.

Scharmer, C. O. (2007). *Theory U: Leading from the future as it emerges*. Cambridge, MA: SoL.

Schein, E. H. (2006). Clinical inquiry/research. In P. Reason & H. Bradbury-Huang (Eds.), *Handbook of action research* (pp. 185–194). London, England: Sage.

Schein, E. H. (2010). *Organizational culture and leadership* (4th ed.). San Francisco, CA: Jossey–Bass.

Schneider, B. (2012). Participatory Action Research, Mental Health Service User Research, and the Hearing (our) Voices Projects. *International Journal of Qualitative Methods*, 11(2), 152–165.

Schon, D. A., & Rein, M. (1994). *Frame reflection: Toward the resolution of intractable policy controversies*. New York City, NY: Basic Books.

Senge, P., & Scharmer, O. (2006). Community action research: Learning as a community of practitioners, consultants, and researchers. In P. Reason & H. Bradbury-Huang (Eds.), *Handbook of action research* (pp. 195–206). London, England: Sage.

Sheppard, M. (1995). Social work, social science, and practice wisdom. *British Journal of Social Work*, 25, 265–293.

Smith, L. T. (2005). *Decolonizing methodologies: Research and indigenous peoples*. London, England: Zed.

Spretnak, C. (1999). *The resurgence of the real: Body, nature and place in a hypermodern world*. New York City, NY: Routledge.

Stake, R. E. (1995). *The art of case study research*. Thousand Oaks, CA: Sage.

Stankiewicz, M. A. (1989). Art at Hull House 1989–1901: Jane Addams and Ellen Gates Starr. *Woman's Art Journal*, 10, 35–39.

Stringer, E. T. (2007). *Action research* (3rd ed.). Thousand Oaks, CA: Sage.

Struthers, R., Lauderdale, J., Nichols, L. Tom-Orme, L., & Strickland, C. (2005). Respecting tribal traditions in research and publications: Voices of five Native American nurse scholars. *Journal of Transcultural Nursing*, 16, 193–201.

Sullivan, M., & Willis, M. (2001). Collaboration: A broad based methodology. In M. Sullivan & J. Kelly (Eds.), *Collaborative research: University and community partnerships* (pp. xix–xvi). Washington, DC: American Public Health Association.

Swap, W. C., Leonard, D. A., Shields, M., & Abrams, L. (2011). Using mentoring and storytelling to transfer knowledge in the workplace. In D. A. Leonard (Ed.), *Managing knowledge assets, creativity and innovation* (pp. 137–158). Singapore: World Scientific Publishing.

Thomas, E. (1984). *Designing interventions for the helping professions*. Thousand Oaks, CA: Sage.

Tsang, N. M. (2008). Kairos and practice wisdom in social work practice. *European Journal of Social Work*, 11, 131–143.

Von Krogh, G., Ichijo, K., & Nonaka, I. (2000). *Enabling knowledge creation*. New York, NY: Oxford University Press.

Washington, O., & Moxley, D. (2008). Telling my story: From narrative to exhibit in illuminating the lived experience of homelessness among older African American women. *Journal of Health Psychology*, 13, 154–165.

Washington, O., & Moxley, D. (2009). "I have three strikes against me": Narratives of plight and efficacy among older African American homeless women and their implications for engaged inquiry. In S. Evans et al. (Eds.), *African Americans and community engagement in higher education* (pp. 189–203). New York, NY: State University of New York Press.

Washington, O., Moxley, D., Gariott, L., & Crystal, J. (2009). Building a responsive network of support and advocacy for older African American homeless women through developmental action research. *Contemporary Nurse*, 33, 140–160.

Weisbord, M., & Janoff, S. (2010). *Future search. Getting the whole system in the room for vision, commitment and action*. San Francisco, CA: Berrett–Koehler.

Wenger, E. (1998). *Communities of practice: Learning, meaning, and identity*. Long, England: Cambridge University Press.

Wenger, E., McDermott, R., & Snyder, W. (2002). *Cultivating communities of practice*. Cambridge, MA: Harvard Business School Press.

Wergin, J. (2004). Elements of effective community engagement. In S. L. Percy, N. L. Zimpher, & M. J. Brukardt (Eds.), *Creating a new kind of university: Institutionalizing community–university engagement* (pp. 23–42). Bolton, MA: Anker.

Yarbrough, D. B., Shulha, L. M., Hopson, R. K., & Caruthers, F. A. (2011). *The program evaluation standards: A guide for evaluators and evaluation users*. Los Angeles, CA: Sage.

FURTHER READING

Chevalier, J. M., & Buckles, D. (2013). *Participatory action research*. London, England: Routledge.

Django Paris, J., & Winn, M. (2013). *Humanizing research: Decolonizing qualitative inquiry with youth and communities*. Los Angeles, CA: Sage.

McIntosh, P. (2010). *Action research and reflective practice*. London, England: Routledge.

McNiff, J. (2013). *Action research: Principles and practices* (3rd ed.). London, England: Routledge.

Reason, P., & Bradbury-Huan, H. (2007). *The SAGE handbook of action research: Participatory inquiry and practice*. Los Angeles, CA: Sage.

Santiago, J. (2013). *Action research: Getting the unheard voice heard*. Amazon Digital Services.

Stringer, E. (2007). *Action research*. Los Angeles, CA: Sage.

DAVID P. MOXLEY

ADOLESCENTS: A HISTORICAL OVERVIEW OF DEVELOPMENTAL THEORIES

ABSTRACT: This article begins with an overview of biological development based upon empirical research. The main focus of the article is the presentation of the major theoretical frameworks that have been employed to explain the processes involved in the psychological, cognitive, moral, social, and sexual development of the adolescent and empirical research findings where appropriate.

KEY WORDS: adolescent development; adolescence; psychological development in adolescence; cognitive development in adolescence; moral development in adolescence; social development in adolescence; sexual development in adolescence; biological development in adolescence

Introduction

The concept of adolescence—a period in the life cycle between childhood and adulthood—was introduced at the beginning of the 20th century by Hall (1904). Although Hall considered adolescence to extend from 12 years to between 22 and 25 years, most researchers and theorists consider the age span to be from 12 to 18 years. Adolescence has also been divided into phases or age groupings, most typically preadolescence, early adolescence, middle adolescence or adolescence proper, and late adolescence (Blos, 1941, 1979; Dunphy, 1963; Sullivan, 1953).

Although menarche (the onset of menstruation) serves as a fairly clear biological marker for the entry of girls into adolescence, no similar clear-cut criterion exists for boys. Adolescence appears to be a phenomenon primarily of postindustrial societies. However, puberty, "the biological and physiological changes associated with sexual maturation" (Muuss, 1962, p. 5), is formally or informally recognized across all cultures, and the developmental sequence is similar, although the time frame may vary (Brooks-Gunn & Reiter, 1990).

The criteria that can indicate the end of adolescence are even less clear. The lack of uniformity in the laws discriminating between the status of minors and the status of adults for activities that range from marriage to alcohol consumption is a pointed example.

Adolescent Development

BIOLOGICAL DEVELOPMENT The development of primary and secondary sexual characteristics during adolescence is the result of endocrine changes, which produce changes in hormone levels. Although the growth rate during infancy proceeds at a more accelerated rate, the magnitude and rate of change experienced during puberty is more significant because the adolescent is more cognizant of the changes he or she is experiencing (Tanner, 1972). The sequence of development is considered universal; however, individual timetables for the various stages differ, and the areas of development may not be synchronous (Paikoff & Brooks-Gunn, 1991; Peterson & Taylor, 1980).

Since the beginning of the 20th century (especially since the 1950s), physical maturation has continued to occur earlier with each successive generation. This "secular trend" is particularly evident in the earlier onset of menarche and in the increases in the rate of growth and full adult stature over the past century. In the United States, the average age of menarche at the beginning of the 20th century was slightly over 14 years; by mid-century, it was less than 13 years (Tanner, 1962). The average age after the turn of the 21st century was 12.4 years (Stang & Story, 2005). Factors hypothesized to explain these phenomena include improvements in health and nutrition as well as the "hybrid vigor" hypothesis, which attributes the changes to the intermarriage of various groups because of greater social mobility (Muuss, 1970). However the age at which menarche occurs is highly variable; occurring as early as 9 years of age or as late as 17 years of age with factors that delay the onset of menstruation being restricted caloric intake and body weight or competing athletically (Stang & Story, 2005). Reports have found that 6.7% of White girls and 27.2% of African American girls were showing some signs of puberty by age 7 (American Psychological Association, 2002).

Among the most dramatic of the physical changes during adolescence is the height spurt. Girls generally experience their increase in height between 9.5

and 14.5 years of age, with the major increase in height occurring approximately 6–12 months prior to menarche, or when they are around 12 years old, about two years before boys (Stang & Story, 2005). Boys experience their growth spurt between 12.5 and 15 years; on average the major increase occurs at 14.4 years of age. However, the length of the growth spurt has great variation so that for girls it usually lasts 24–26 months, ending by 16.5 years of age, while for boys it can continue at a slower rate ceasing between 18 and 21 years of age (Stang & Story, 2005).

Changes also occur in weight; girls develop increased subcutaneous fatty tissue and boys usually become heavier than girls. Although the hips and shoulders become wider in both boys and girls, the boys' shoulders become wider than their hips, and girls' hips wider than their shoulders. Changes in skin texture and oiliness take place, along with gradual changes in the timbre and pitch of the voices of both boys and girls (Faust, 1977; Peterson & Taylor, 1980; Tanner, 1972).

Early physical maturation generally has a positive effect on boys; boys who mature early are rated as more relaxed and poised, higher in self-esteem, less dependent, and more attractive to and popular with their peers than those who mature later (Clausen, 1975; Jones, 1965; Mussen & Jones, 1957; Peskin, 1967; Petersen, 1987; Simmons & Blyth, 1987). Girls seem to have the opposite experience; early maturation appears to result in negative evaluations, including feelings of isolation, submissive behavior, and less popularity with and leadership of their peers (Clausen, 1975; Jones & Mussen, 1958; Peskin, 1973; Simmons & Blyth, 1987; Weatherley, 1964). Perceived weight problems also lead to an increased risk in behaviors such as heavy dieting, caloric deprivation, use of diet pills or laxatives, severe body image distortions, and other eating disorders (Stang & Story, 2005). In any case, research indicates that the individual's idiosyncratic range of physical development and its mesh or lack of sync with cultural norms have an impact on his or her overall development.

Although research in the biological aspects of adolescent development is straightforward, the literature on other aspects of adolescent development is characterized by controversy and conflicting viewpoints. Theorists and researchers agree that adolescence is a period in the life cycle when notable development occurs in many areas. They differ, however, about the following aspects of adolescence:

1. Whether the development is continuous or discontinuous with the preceding and following stages in the life cycle,

2. Whether the period of adolescence is one of turmoil and stress or relatively uneventful,
3. Whether it is critical for adolescents to experience or resolve specific developmental tasks or issues during this time,
4. Whether internal or environmental factors have a more significant influence on the experiences and outcome of adolescent development, and
5. Whether there are specific adolescent responses (such as coping or defense mechanisms) to internal and external changes.

For example, Hall (1904), often referred to as the father of the psychology of adolescence, viewed adolescence as a discontinuous experience—a period that is qualitatively and quantitatively different from childhood and from adulthood. The discontinuity, along with the great physical changes that adolescents experience, caused Hall to label the period as one of *"sturm und drang"* (literally, "storm and stress"). Hall's biogenetic approach posited that adolescence was a "recapitulation" of one of mankind's stages of evolution—a turbulent time for the species and, therefore, for the individual.

PSYCHOLOGICAL DEVELOPMENT

Psychosexual Theories. Psychoanalytic theorists have posited a different recapitulation theory. Specifically, they see the developmental processes of adolescence as a recapitulation of earlier infantile stages of development through the reexperiencing of either oedipal or preoedipal conflicts (Blos, 1941, 1979; Freud, 1948; Freud, 1924/1973).

The physiological changes that bring about sexual-reproductive maturation are considered to usher in the genital stage, which disturbs the psychological equilibrium achieved during the latency period (Freud, 1924/1973). The sheer "quantity of the instinctual impulses" (Freud, 1948, p. 164) is thought of as rekindling a conflict over dominance between the ego and the id, the latter of which has predominated and matured during the latency period. The ego is conceptualized as torn between the impulses and demands of the id and the restrictions of the superego (Freud, 1948). Consequently, adolescence is viewed as a period of stress and turmoil and as discontinuous with other phases in the life cycle.

According to the psychosexual theorists, two tasks must be accomplished during this stage if psychological maturity is to be attained: (a) detachment from the opposite sex parent as an incestuous love object and (b) establishment of a nonantagonistic, nondominated relationship with the same sex parent. This process of detachment may result in negativism and hostility toward parents and other authority figures for a time. Freud (1924/1973) believed that this process is seldom completed ideally.

Blos (1941, 1979) modified traditional psychoanalytic theory, stressing the importance of the "cultural milieu and social stratum" (Blos, 1941, p. 7) in personality formation and positing a reciprocal influence between the individual and his or her environment. Although he insisted that adolescent development must be considered in the context of a particular culture and the family's "unique version of the culture" (Blos, 1941, p. 260), like his psychoanalytic predecessors, he saw adolescence as a transitional period that involves a recapitulation of earlier familial patterns of interaction. However, he considered this process to be qualitatively different from earlier developmental experiences because of the significant maturation of the ego (ego supremacy and ego differentiation) during the latency period (Blos, 1941). This ego development allows the adolescent in most cases to resolve the oedipal conflicts and the component infantile dependencies (Blos, 1979).

According to Blos (1979), the second individuation process that occurs during adolescence requires a "normative regression in the service of development" (p. 153); that is, only in adolescence is regression an essential and normal process. Though normal, this regression still produces turmoil, volatile behavior, and anxiety that, if it becomes unmanageable, may result in the use of a variety of defense mechanisms such as withdrawal and secrecy, fantasy, temporary compulsive habit formation, compensation, intellectualization, rationalization, projection, and changes in the ego ideal (Blos, 1941).

Chodorow (1974, 1978) has reinterpreted the individuation process, challenging the male sex bias of earlier formulations. According to Chodorow, because the male's first love object—the mother—is of the opposite sex, separation and individuation are critical to male gender identity and development but not to the progress of female identity development.

Psychosocial Theories. Psychosocial theories of adolescence, although based on Freud's psychosexual conceptualization of development, emphasize the impact of the sociocultural context on individual development. Erikson (1963, 1968) viewed development as proceeding through a sequence of stages, each of which is characterized by a specific crisis. Not only are the crises of each stage produced by internal mechanisms, they are the result of the interaction between the individual and his or her social environment, which makes cultural demands in the form of social expectations, norms, and values.

Erikson thought of identity formation as a process that continues throughout one's life; but he believed that identity "has its normative crisis in adolescence" (1968, p. 23). Like the psychosexual theorists, Erikson described adolescence as a time of turmoil and stress. However, he (1968) considered it to be the result of an "identity crisis" that typifies this stage, rather than of a conflict between the ego and the id. Furthermore, he viewed adolescence as a necessary and productive period during which the adolescent experiments with and works to consolidate his or her personal, occupational, and ideological identity. This identity is formed through the individual's psychological integration as well as through the social environment, which serves critical functions during this process. In the search for self-definition, conflict arises between the adolescent and his or her parents as a necessary movement toward establishing the adolescent's own view of self, of the world, and of his or her place in that world.

Erikson's conceptualization has been criticized for its sex bias in that he generalized changes in the life cycle from a male model of development (Chodorow, 1974, 1978; Gilligan, 1979). Gilligan (1979) noted that individuation and separation from the mother are accepted as critical for the development of gender identity among males, but she proposed the opposite dynamic for females: "Femininity is defined through attachment" (p. 434) to the mother. According to Gilligan (1979), "male gender identity will be threatened by intimacy while female gender identity will be threatened by individuation" (p. 434). Erikson viewed separation as a healthy sign of progressive development and attachment as a problem. However, Chodorow (1974, 1978) and Gilligan (1979) proposed that, in the course of female development, intimacy may more appropriately precede separation or at least be fused with identity formation.

Social Learning Theory. Social learning theorists describe adolescence as a period of development that, for the majority of individuals, proceeds from childhood with great continuity in behavior, interpersonal relationships, and self-evaluation (Bandura & Walters, 1963). The behavioral and social learning principles that apply in infancy and childhood remain the same, with the possible expansion of sources of reinforcement in the environment, a greater number and variety of models, and an expanded capacity for self-regulated behavior.

The process of socialization includes the development of behavioral repertoires through differential reinforcement, stimulus and response generalization, higher order conditioning, modeling, and rule learning (Bandura, 1969; Gagne, 1970). Differential reinforcement refers to the process whereby behavior that is reinforced increases in frequency and behavior that is punished or placed on extinction decreases. For example, adolescents shape each other's social behaviors by positively responding to specific mannerisms, dress, and the latest slang terms and by ostracizing or ridiculing behaviors that do not meet the norms of their peers. Response generalization involves the production of behaviors (responses) that have properties similar to the response that has been reinforced. Via stimulus generalization, the adolescent is likely to respond with the same repertoire of responses to other peers he or she perceives as being similar to those from whom he or she received reinforcement. In higher order conditioning, certain individuals, environments, objects, words, symbols, and the like become positive or negative stimuli for the individual and result in specific responses because they are associated with positive or negative events.

Modeling is a mode of imitative or vicarious learning that involves the observation, coding, and retention of a set of behaviors for their performance at a subsequent time. It is particularly efficient for learning complex behaviors, such as interpersonal skills. Furthermore, modeled behaviors are more readily learned in situations for which the individual has no prior repertoire of responses. Moreover, the adolescent also combines behaviors of various models into novel responses or abstracts a rule that allows him or her to act as the model would act in a novel situation for which specific responses have not been observed (Mehrabian, 1970). Hence, as one moves from childhood into adolescence and is exposed to a greater number and variety of models, one's potential behavioral repertoire increases substantially.

Finally, as an individual progresses through childhood into adolescence and adulthood, one notes an increase in self-regulatory behavior, most notably self-evaluation and self-reinforcement (Bandura, 1969, 1995). Self-reinforcement is generally established through modeling as the observer evaluates and reinforces his or her performance via the same criteria as the model. Over time, the responses become independent of the original learning experience and are generalized to other situations. Although self-evaluation and reinforcement can be independent of social norms, they often correspond (Bandura, 1977).

Bandura and Walters (1963) and Bandura (1964) noted that empirical research had not borne out the claim that adolescence constitutes a sudden and drastic change from childhood, particularly in parent–child relations. They indicated that the pattern instead appears to be one of gradual socialization toward independence by means of a gradual change in reinforcement conditions.

COGNITIVE DEVELOPMENT According to Piagetian theory, cognitive development consists of the progression through stages of quantitatively and qualitatively more complex thought processes and structures. Piaget and Inhelder (1958) emphasized the discontinuity between the concrete operational thinking of the child and the qualitatively different formal operations of the adolescent. Piaget (1972) viewed the progression from concrete to formal operations as the product of individual "spontaneous and endogenous factors" (p. 7) and experiences in the environment that stimulate intellectual growth.

Formal operational thought is characterized by hypothetico-deductive reasoning: As the adolescent's thinking is no longer tied to concrete objects, he or she is able to construct possibilities, to manipulate and reflect upon mental constructs, and to assess probabilities. According to Piaget and Inhelder (1958), this new capacity enables the adolescent to "analyze his [or her] own thinking and construct theories" (p. 340). The adolescent's thought is no longer tied to trial and error, but can generate hypotheses regarding all the possible relations among the various factors in solving a problem. Moreover, the adolescent systematically tests alternative hypotheses, varying one factor at a time while holding all other factors constant (Piaget & Inhelder, 1958).

Cognitive development also is conceptualized as a process of decentering. Decentering involves the reduction of egocentric thought that thereby allows for the generation and testing of hypotheses. Formal operations progress through transitional stages (generally from ages 11 to 14) in which the operations of formal thought are confounded by the adolescent's egocentrism. Elkind (1967, 1974, 1978) believes this results in the phenomenon he calls "the imaginary audience." That is, the adolescent feels as though his or her actions and appearance are constantly being scrutinized by others. Elkind (1978) believed that this egocentrism may explain the feelings of self-consciousness that are prevalent during adolescence and "a good deal of adolescent boorishness, loudness, and faddish dress" (p. 387).

Also demonstrative of cognitive egocentrism is the complementary development of the "personal fable" (Elkind, 1967, 1974, 1978; Inhelder & Piaget, 1978). The personal fable involves viewing one's thoughts and feelings as unique experiences, often ones that should be saved for posterity (via diaries or poetry). Feelings of invulnerability accompany this perception and have been linked to such adolescent problems as the failure to use contraceptives and risk-taking behavior (Elkind, 1967). This cognitive egocentrism also results in projecting one's preoccupation with and plans for the future onto the society as a whole and viewing oneself in a Messianic role (Inhelder & Piaget, 1978). Primarily because of reality testing and the sharing of perceptions and experiences with peers, the egocentrism of early adolescence gives away to full formal operations by age 15 or 16 (Elkind, 1978; Inhelder & Piaget, 1978).

MORAL DEVELOPMENT Moral development is incorporated in psychoanalytic theory via the development of a conscience in childhood and such conceptualizations as the "reexternalization" of the superego in adolescence (Settlage, 1972). The latter consists of a conscious appraisal, challenging, and discarding of values and an incorporation into the superego of reappraised ideals and values (which are no longer mirrors of parental values) (Hoffman, 1980). Erikson (1970) described the adolescent in the process of identity development as moving from the specific moral learnings of childhood to the pursuit of a moral ideology that facilitates identity formation.

Piaget (1965) formulated a simple two-stage dichotomous model, moving from moral realism to subjectivism. In the stage of moral realism, the child judges the moral value (rightness or wrongness) of an act by the magnitude of the damage or injury or simple conformity with stated rules, irrespective of intention. In the second or autonomous stage of subjectivism, intention becomes the foremost consideration in judging the moral value of an act. The subjective nature of rules and the concept of rules by mutual consent are recognized.

It is only with the attainment of formal operations in adolescence that the individual has the capacity for developing postconventional morality, recognizing individual and cultural differences as well as universal principles. Although Kohlberg and Gilligan (1975) propose that many adolescents regress to an instrumental level of moral development,

Turiel (1974) describes the extreme relativism of the adolescent as a transitional phase. With attainment of formal operations and the recognition of differences in perspectives, the adolescent questions the rigid law-and-order morality of the conventional stage and rejects the imposition of moral codes and values on the individual. The adolescent's extreme relativism results from the rejection of conventional criteria for moral judgment, which leaves the individual for a time with the sense that no basis exists for objectively verifying values.

Hoffman (1980) proposed that the development of empathy and its transformation during cognitive development is the fundamental basis of moral development. As a result of his or her cognitive development, the adolescent begins to conceptualize others not only as distinct, but to project the self into another's experiences beyond the immediate concrete situation and, therefore, to respond with empathic distress and "a more reciprocal feeling of concern for the victim" (Hoffman, 1980, p. 311). Moreover, this empathic distress can also be transformed into feelings of guilt if the victim's distress leads to self-blame with respect to one's action or inaction. Finally, one's empathic distress, sense of guilt, and impetus to relieve the distress perceived in another are viewed as the significant motivational components for moral action.

In social learning theory, moral values, judgments, and behaviors are viewed as being dependent on a variety of environmental factors, such as the long- and short-term consequences, the setting, the type of act, and the characteristics of the victim. Moral development involves a process of learning through direct instruction (rule learning), reinforcement contingencies, modeling, and evaluative feedback. By exposure to diverse situations and models, one learns which factors are important to consider in various situations when moral judgments are required (Bandura, 1977, 1995; Rosenthal & Zimmerman, 1978).

SOCIAL DEVELOPMENT The adolescent's social development is closely related to his or her psychological development, particularly identity formation and the need for intimacy. Sullivan (1953) viewed interpersonal relations as central to one's individual identity. He posited three stages of adolescent development, which are distinguished by different needs and expressions of interpersonal intimacy: preadolescence, early adolescence, and late adolescence. Preadolescence is characterized by the need for intimacy expressed through strong relationships, usually with persons of the same sex. These relationships differ from those of childhood in their exclusivity and extent of personal intimacy, evidenced by disclosure of one's secret thoughts, feelings, and aspirations.

The stage of early adolescence is ushered in by the physiological changes of puberty with the concomitant appearance of the lust dynamism (Sullivan, 1953). Lust – a psychological rather than a moralistic construct – refers to genital drives that impel the individual toward sexual satisfaction. This new integrating dynamism results in the shift to intimate relations with persons of the opposite sex for most adolescents, patterned, to some degree, after preadolescent same-sex relationships.

According to Sullivan (1953), a person enters late adolescence when he or she "discovers what he [she] likes in the way of genital behavior and how to fit it into the rest of life" (p. 297). By late adolescence, Sullivan claimed, the majority of adolescents have established their preferred mode of sexual relationships and continue to develop and expand their interpersonal skills. Intimacy is the core of what Sullivan (1953) described as the mature person; it involves "a very lively sensitivity to the needs of the other and to the interpersonal security or absence of anxiety in the other" (p. 310).

More recently, Attachment Theory (Bowlby, 1982) has been employed to elucidate the nature and development of interpersonal relationships in adolescence. Expanding her body of work on attachment in infancy, Ainsworth (1989) posits a significant, complex, and qualitative change in the behavioral systems related to attachment: "key changes in the nature of attachment may be occasioned by hormone, neurophysiological and cognitive changes, and not merely by socioemotional experience" (p. 710). Attachment to parent(s) is seen as the basis for peer attachments and supported by a body of empirical literature, although some adolescents are spurred to establish peer attachments to compensate for lack of attachment to parental figures (See Rice, 1990 and Schneider & Younger, 1996 for reviews of this literature; Freeman & Brown, 2001; Furman, Simon, Shaffer, & Bouchey, 2002). The relationship skills, competencies, and expectations learned in the relationship with parental attachment figures become the basis for relationship building with peers; however, parent and peer attachments may not be parallel and may vary along a number of dimensions and functions (Black & McCartney, 1997; Markiewicz,

Lawford, Doyle, & Haggart, 2006). Moreover, the increase in peer attachments does not totally replace primary attachment to parental figures or specific attachment functions (Black & McCartney, 1997; Freeman & Brown, 2001; Markiewicz et al., 2006).

Bandura (1964) and others (e.g., Harter, 1990; Steinberg, 1990) have indicated that increased peer interaction does not usually result in a simultaneous shifting away from parent relationships and values. Examining relationships across several decades, researchers found that adolescents and parents viewed each other positively and that only a limited percentage experienced disruption in their relationship (Bandura, 1964; Bandura & Walters, 1963; Harter, 1990; Hess & Goldblatt, 1957; Meissner, 1965; Offer, 1967; Offer & Sabshin, 1984; Offer, Sabshin, & Marcus, 1965; Steinberg, 1990).

As early as 1980, Coleman's review of the literature (1980) pointed out that the need for friendships changes and that the greatest need (especially for girls) occurs during middle adolescence. It is during middle adolescence that the dread of rejection and the lack of social confidence take their toll. Moreover, girls experience more feelings of anxiety about friendships than do boys, probably because the socialization of girls places greater emphasis on the fulfillment of emotional needs through relationships. In contrast, boys tend to be socialized to seek relationships that are focused on actions. Consistent gender differences have been noted in the literature, with females demonstrating greater intimacy, self-disclosure and communication in their relationships than males (Belle, 1989; Berndt & Perry, 1990; Brendgen, Markiewicz, Doyle, & Burkowski, 2001; Buhrmester, 1990; Fischer, 1981; Furman & Buhrmester, 1992; Macoby & Jacklin, 1974; Nickerson & Nagle, 2005).

SEXUAL DEVELOPMENT Sexual development is the result of the interaction of intrapsychic, sociocultural, and biological factors. The physiological changes initiated in puberty influence the individual in a social context (Miller & Simon, 1980) and via the personal evaluation of their meaning and significance.

Gender identity and gender role expectations form the foundation of the young adolescent's sexual identity "since the sexual and social scenarios of the society are organized around norms for gender-appropriate behavior" (Miller & Simon, 1980, p. 383). Particularly in early adolescence, motivations for sociosexual behavior may be nonerotic, impelled instead by what are considered gender-appropriate behaviors in the specific social context (Miller & Simon, 1980).

With the onset of puberty, the adolescent must add a sexual dimension to his or her gender identity. According to Miller and Simon (1980), the progress of psychosexual development and concomitant sexual behavior depend on two factors and their interaction: (1) "the intrapsychic history and life of the individual" and (2) "the interpersonal requirements of social life" (p. 388) – the social context. The intrapsychic life of the individual refers to idiosyncratic values that result in the eroticizing of events, attributes, relationships, and so forth. Interpersonal "scripts" are less idiosyncratic because they reflect the present social expectations and constraints, which vary with time and the individual's reference group (Gagnon, 1974; Gordon & Gilgun, 1987; Miller & Simon, 1980). Hence, majority and minority adolescent cohorts may have significantly different interpersonal scripts.

When there is congruence between intrapsychic and interpersonal factors, sexual identity formation proceeds smoothly. When these two factors are discordant, the adolescent must choose to risk either alienation from others or a sense of self-betrayal. Particularly vulnerable in this regard are individuals whose intrapsychic content is homoerotic, but who feel constrained by sociocultural norms and demands (Miller & Simon, 1980).

Conclusion

It is particularly important to be aware that developmental processes, though universal, have cultural variations in their manifestation, normative appraisal, and time frame. Adolescent development occurs within a cultural milieu, and, therefore, the cultural context must be taken into account if the developmental process and the group and individual issues that are generated during this process are to be understood. For ethnic minority youth, this is further complicated by the bicultural socialization process (de Anda, 1984), which results in development occurring in a dual cultural context, that of White mainstream American culture and their culture of origin. Further complicating this process are structural factors, such as individual and group social status and income, especially poverty, that create barriers to the "normal" course of adolescent development.

The application of theories or principles that address the impact of various sociocultural factors on an individual's behavior, values, and beliefs holds the most promise and is most consonant with the practice of social work, which ascribes to a person-in-the-environment perspective, viewing the individual within his or her psychosociocultural context.

REFERENCES

Ainsworth, M. D. S. (1989). Attachments beyond infancy. *American Psychologist, 44,* 709–716.

American Psychological Association. (2002). *Developing adolescents: A reference for professionals.* Washington, DC: Author.

Bandura, A. (1964). The stormy decade: Fact or fiction? Psychology in the Schools, 1, 224–231.

Bandura, A. (1969). *Principles of behavior modification.* New York: Holt, Rinehart & Winston.

Bandura, A. (1977). *Social learning theory.* Englewood Cliffs, NJ: Prentice-Hall.

Bandura, A. (Ed.). (1995). *Self-efficacy in changing societies.* Cambridge, New York: Cambridge University Press.

Bandura, A., & Walters, R. M. (1963). *Social learning and personality development.* New York: Holt, Rinehart & Winston.

Belle, D. (1989). Gender differences in children's social networks and social supports. In D. Belle (Ed.), *Children's social networks and social supports* (pp. 173–188). New York: Wiley.

Berndt, T. J., & Perry, T. B. (1990). Distinctive features and effects of early adolescent friendships. In R. Montemayor, G. R. Adams, & T. P. Gullota (Eds.), *From childhood to adolescence: A transitional period?* (pp. 269–187). Newbury Park, CA: Sage.

Black, K. A., & McCartney, K. (1997). Adolescent females' security with parents predicts the quality of peer interactions. *Social Development, 6*(1), 91–110.

Blos, P. (1941). *The adolescent personality.* New York: D. Appleton-Century Co.

Blos, P. (1979). *The adolescent passage: Developmental issues.* New York: International Universities Press.

Bowlby, J. (1982). *Attachment and loss* (Vol. 1). New York: Basic Books.

Brendgen, M., Markiewicz, D., Doyle, S. B., & Burkowski, W. M. (2001). The relations between friendship quality, ranked friendship preferences, and adolescents' behavior with their friends. *Merrill-Palmer Quarterly, 47,* 395–415.

Brooks-Gunn, J., & Reiter, E. O. (1990). The role of pubertal processes in early adolescent transition. In S. Feldman & G. Eliott (Eds.), *At the threshold: The developing adolescent.* Cambridge, MA: Harvard University Press.

Buhrmester, D. (1990). Intimacy of friendship, interpersonal competence, and adjustment during middle childhood and adolescence. *Child Development, 61,* 1101–1111.

Chodorow, N. (1974). Family structure and feminine personality. In M. Rosoldo & L. Lamphere (Eds.), *Women, culture and society.* Stanford, CA: Stanford University Press.

Chodorow, N. (1978). *The reproduction of mothering.* Berkeley: University of California Press.

Clausen, J. A. (1975). The social meaning of differential physical and sexual maturation. In S. E. Gragastin & G. E. Elder, Jr. (Eds.), *Adolescence in the life cycle: Psychological change and social context* (pp. 24–47). New York: Wiley.

Coleman, J. C. (1980). Friendship and the peer group in adolescence. In J. Adelson (Ed.), *Handbook of adolescent psychology*. New York: Wiley.

de Anda, D. (1984). Bicultural socialization: Factors affecting the minority experience. *Social Work, 29*(2), 101–107.

Dunphy, D. S. (1963). The social structure of urban adolescent peer groups. *Sociometry, 26*, 230–246.

Elkind, D. (1967). Egocentrism in adolescence. *Child Development, 38*, 1025–1034.

Elkind, D. (1974). *Children and adolescents: Interpretive essays on Jean Piaget* (2nd ed.). New York: Oxford University Press.

Elkind, D. (1978). Egocentrism in adolescence. In J. K. Gardner (Ed.), *Readings in developmental psychology* (2nd ed.). Boston, MA: Little, Brown & Co.

Erikson, E. H. (1963). *Childhood and society* (2nd ed.). New York: W. W. Norton & Co.

Erikson, E. H. (1968). *Identity, youth and crisis*. New York: W. W. Norton & Co.

Erikson, E. H. (1970). Reflections on the dissent of contemporary youth. *International Journal of Psychoanalysis, 51*, 11–22.

Faust, M. S. (1977). Somatic development of adolescent girls. In *Monographs of the Society for Research in Child Development, 42*(1), 1–90.

Fischer, J. L. (1981). Transitions in relationship style from adolescence to young adulthoood. *Journal of Youth and Adolescence, 10*, 11–23.

Freeman, H., & Brown, B. B. (2001). Primary attachment to parents and peers during adolescence: Differences by attachment style. *Journal of Youth and Adolescence, 30*, 653–674.

Freud, A. (1948). *The ego and the mechanisms of defense* (C. Baines, Trans.). New York: International Universities Press.

Freud, S. (1973). *A general introduction to psychoanalysis*. New York: Pocket Books. (Original work published 1924.)

Furman, W., & Buhrmester, D. (1992). Age and sex differences in perceptions of networks of personal relationships. *Child Development, 63*, 103–115.

Furman, W., Simon, V. A., Shaffer, L., & Bouchey, H. A. (2002). Adolescents' working models and styles for relationships with parents, friends, and romantic partners. *Child Development, 73*, 241–255.

Gagne, R. (1970). *The conditions of learning*. New York: Holt, Rinehart & Winston.

Gagnon, J. H. (1974). Scripts and the coordination of sexual conduct. In J. K. Cole & R. Deinstbrier (Eds.), *Nebraska Symposium on Motivation* (Vol. 21). Lincoln, NE: University of Nebraska Press.

Gilligan, C. (1979). Woman's place in man's life cycle. *Harvard Educational Review, 49*(4), 431–446.

Gordon, S., & Gilgun, J. F. (1987). Adolescent sexuality. In V. B. Van Husselt & M. Hersen (Eds.), *Handbook of adolescent psychology*. New York: Pergamon.

Hall, G. S. (1904). *Adolescence: Its psychology and its relations to physiology, anthropology, sociology, sex, crime, religion, and education* (Vols. 1 & 2). New York: D. Appleton-Century Co.

Harter, S. (1990). Adolescent self and identity development. In D. D. Feldman & G. R. Eliott (Eds.), *At the threshold: The developing adolescent*. Cambridge, MA: Harvard University Press.

Hess, R. D., & Goldblatt, I. (1957). The status of adolescents in American society: A problem in social identity. *Child Development, 28*, 459–468.

Hoffman, M. L. (1980). Moral development in adolescence. In J. Adelson (Ed.), *Handbook of adolescent psychology* (pp. 293–343). New York: Wiley.

Inhelder, B., & Piaget, J. (1978). Adolescent thinking. In J. K. Gardner (Ed.), *Readings in developmental psychology*. Boston, MA: Little, Brown & Co.

Jones, M. C. (1965). Psychological correlates of somatic development. *Child Development, 36*, 899–911.

Jones, M. C., & Mussen, D. H. (1958). Self-conceptions, motivations, and interpersonal attitudes of early- and late-maturing girls. *Child Development, 29*, 491–501.

Kohlberg, L., & Gilligan, E. C. (1975). The adolescent as a philosopher: The discovery of self in a post-conventional world. In J. Conger (Ed.), *Contemporary issues in adolescent development* (pp. 414–443). New York: Harper & Row.

Macoby, E. E., & Jacklin, C. N. (1974). *The psychology of sex differences*. Stanford, CA: Stanford University Press.

Markiewicz, D., Lawford, H., Doyle, A. B., & Haggart, N. (2006). Developmental differences in adolescents' and young adults' use of mothers, fathers, best friends, and romantic partners to fulfill attachment needs. *Journal of Youth and Adolescents, 35*(1), 127–140.

Mehrabian, A. (1970). *The tactics of social influence*. Englewood Cliffs, NJ: Prentice-Hall.

Meissner, W. W. (1965). Parental interaction of the adolescent boy. *Journal of Genetic Psychology, 107*, 225–233.

Miller, Y., & Simon, W. (1980). The development of sexuality in adolescence. In J. Adelson (Ed.), *Handbook of adolescent psychology* (pp. 383–407). New York: Wiley.

Mussen, P. H., & Jones, M. C. (1957). Self-conceptions, motivations, and interpersonal attitudes of late- and early-maturing boys. *Child Development, 28*, 243–256.

Muuss, E. (1962). *Theories of adolescent development*. New York: Random House.

Muuss, E. (1970). Adolescent development and the secular trend. *Adolescence, 5*, 267–286.

Nickerson, A. B., & Nagle, R. J. (2005). Parent and peer attachment in late childhood and early adolescence. *Journal of Early Adolescence, 25*(2), 223–249.

Offer, D. (1967). Normal adolescents: Interview strategy and selected results. *Archives of General Psychiatry, 17*, 285–290.

Offer, D., & Sabshin, M. (1984). *Normality and the life cycle: A critical integration.* New York: Basic Books.

Offer, D., Sabshin, M., & Marcus, I. (1965). Clinical evaluation of normal adolescents. *American Journal of Psychiatry, 21,* 864–872.

Paikoff, R. L., & Brooks-Gunn, J. (1991). Do parent-child relationships change during puberty? *Psychological Bulletin, 110,* 47–66.

Peskin, H. (1967). Pubertal onset and ego functioning. *Journal of Abnormal Psychology, 72,* 1–15.

Peskin, H. (1973). Influence of the developmental schedule of puberty on learning and ego development. *Journal of Youth and Adolescence, 2,* 273–290.

Petersen, L. L. (1987). Change in variables related to smoking from childhood to late adolescence: An eight-year longitudinal study of a cohort of elementary school students. *Canadian Journal of Public Health, 77* (Suppl. 1), 33–39.

Peterson, A. C., & Taylor, B. (1980). The biological approach to adolescence. In J. Adelson (Ed.), *Handbook of adolescent psychology* (pp. 117–155). New York: Wiley.

Piaget, J. (1965). *The moral judgment of the child.* New York: Free Press.

Piaget, J. (1972). Intellectual evolution from adolescence to adulthood. *Human Development, 15*(1), 1–12.

Piaget, J., & Inhelder, B. (1958). *The growth of logical thinking from childhood to adolescence* (A. Parsons & S. Seagrin, Trans.). New York: Basic Books.

Rice, K. G. (1990). Attachment in adolescence: A narrative and meta-analytic review. *Journal of Youth and Adolescence, 19,* 511–538.

Rosenthal, T. L., & Zimmerman, B. J. (1978). *Social learning and cognition.* New York: Academic Press.

Schneider, B. H., & Younger, A. J. (1996). Adolescent-parent attachment and adolescents' relations with their peers. *Youth and Society, 28*(1), 95–108.

Settlage, C. F. (1972). Cultural values and the superego in late adolescence. *Psychoanalytic Study of the Child, 27,* 57–73.

Simmons, R. G., & Blyth, D. A. (1987). *Moving into adolescence.* Hawthorne, NY: Aldine.

Stang J., & Story, M. (Eds.). (2005). *Guidelines for adolescent nutrition services.* Minneapolis, MN: Center for Leadership, Education and Training in Maternal and Child Nutrition, Division of Epidemiology and Community Health, School of Public Health, University of Minnesota.

Steinberg, L. D. (1990). Interdependence in the family: Autonomy, conflict and harmony in the parent-child relationship. In S. S. Feldman & G. R. Elliott (Eds.), *At the threshold: The developing adolescent* (pp. 255–276). Cambridge, MA: Harvard University Press.

Sullivan, H. S. (1953). *The interpersonal theory of psychiatry.* New York: W. W. Norton & Co.

Tanner, J. M. (1962). *Growth at adolescence.* Springfield, IL.: Charles C. Thomas.

Tanner, J. M. (1972). Sequence, tempo, and individual variation in growth and development of boys and girls aged twelve to sixteen. In J. Kagan & R. Coles (Eds.), *Twelve to sixteen: Early adolescence* (pp. 1–24). New York: W. W. Norton & Co.

Turiel, E. (1974). Conflict and transition in adolescent moral development. *Child Development, 45,* 14–29.

Weatherley, D. (1964). Self-perceived rate of physical maturation and personality in late adolescence. *Child Development, 35,* 1197–1210.

DIANE DE ANDA

ADVOCACY

ABSTRACT: Social work advocacy is "the exclusive and mutual representation of a client(s) or a cause in a forum, attempting to systematically influence decision-making in an unjust or unresponsive system(s)." Advocacy was identified as a professional role as far back as 1887, and social workers consider client advocacy an ethical responsibility. Social workers are increasing the use of electronic advocacy to influence client issues and policy development. As client and societal needs evolve, universities should emphasize advocacy in their curricula, and the National Association of Social Workers should promote electoral and legislative initiatives that reflect an emphasis on social and economic injustices.

KEY WORDS: advocacy; influence; policy practice; social action; representation; social justice; online advocacy

Social work is the one profession that has acknowledged, decade after decade, a healthy tension between individual needs and the policies of the larger society (Schneider & Netting, 1999). This recognition often results in "advocacy."

Definition of Advocacy

Litzelfelner and Petr (1997) stated unequivocally, "The social work profession considers client advocacy an ethical responsibility and a primary function of social work practice" (p. 393). However, some scholars (Blakely, 1991; Kutchins & Kutchins, 1978; Schneider & Lester, 2001) believe that advocacy, while long associated with exciting changes that benefit vulnerable groups, refers to all kinds of social action without any distinguishing or specific characteristics of its own. Sosin and Caulum (2003) noted that "the role of *advocate* seems to be practically synonymous with about all social work roles, and it is presented in such broad strokes that it cannot be systematically studied, described, *taught, or practiced* [authors'emphasis]" (p. 12). Haynes and Mickelson

(2006) stated, "Advocacy requires no additional skills other than the ability to aggregate data or mobilize clients" (p. 84). Bateman (personal communication, October 4, 2001) stated, "Advocacy was assumed to be something one just knew how to do."

Schneider and Lester (2001) contributed to the evolution of the term by analyzing over 90 definitions of *advocacy* in the social work literature. Differing emphases in individual definitions ranged from "pleading on behalf of someone" to "securing social justice" to "identifying with the client" to "promoting change" to "accessing rights and benefits" to "demonstrating influence and political skills." Since the term *advocacy* possesses multiple meanings, it has become a futile term because practitioners and researchers do not have a common understanding of the word. By failing to limit the term, the profession has neglected to sharpen practice efficacy, that is, how does one advocate well and what is effective. This failure may lead social workers to continue to believe that advocacy is defined primarily by working actively to meet client needs *by arranging services*, and not by partisan intervention when it is needed (Herbert & Mould, 1992)

Schneider and Lester (2001) developed a new definition of social work advocacy that appears to advance the ongoing struggle for specific conceptual clarity. Their definition of advocacy is clear, measurable, action oriented, and focuses on what one *does* as an advocate, and not just on outcomes. The definition is comprehensive because it can be applied to the myriad practice settings where social workers find themselves, such as working one-on-one with clients, working for community causes, in legislative arenas, and in agencies.

Definition: Social work advocacy is the exclusive and mutual representation of a client(s) or a cause in a forum, attempting to systematically influence decision-making in an unjust or unresponsive system(s) (Schneider & Lester, 2001, pp. 64–68). Let us examine the key words in the definition:

Exclusive: The relationship between the client and the advocate is singular, unique, prioritized solely on the client, primarily responsible to the client, and centered on client needs.

Mutual: The relationship between the client and the advocate is reciprocal, interdependent, joint, and equal; they exchange ideas and plans together, proceeding in an agreed-upon direction. Included in the term, *mutual*, is also the notion of *empowerment* that not only enables the clients to carry out an activity, but also motivates them and teaches them skills required to interact with the environment.

Representation: The advocate uses the activities of speaking, writing, or acting on behalf of another, communicating or expressing the concerns of a client, standing up for another person or group, and serving as an agent or proxy for another.

Client(s): The client(s) may be an individual person, small or large groups, a community association, an ethnic population, individuals with common concerns, or other loosely or tightly knit organizations. The "client(s)" is not restricted a priori to certain sizes or numbers.

Cause: A cause is usually a condition or problem affecting a group or class of people with similar concerns. Circumstances of an individual may be the basis for a larger group needing the same remedy. An example may be advocating for the rights for all domestic abuse victims, not just one client.

Forum: A forum is any assembly designated to discuss issues, regulations, rules, public matters, laws, or differing opinions, or to settle disputes. Examples are public hearings, legislative committees, agency board meetings, and supervisory sessions. Two features are usually present: (a) a set of specific procedures to guide the conduct of the participants, and (b) a decision-making mechanism (Kutchins & Kutchins, 1987).

Systematically: The advocate applies knowledge and skills in a planned, orderly manner, analyzing the circumstances and conditions before deciding how to proceed.

Influence: An advocate attempts to modify, change, affect, act on, or alter decisions by another person or group with the authority or power over resources or policies that impinge upon a client(s). Some "influential" activities consist of organizing client groups, forming coalitions, educating the public, contacting public officials and legislators, giving testimony, and appealing to review boards (Hepworth, Rooney, Dewberry-Rooney, Strom-Gottfried, & Larsen, 2006). The following are the principles of influence used to take action:

1. Identify the issues and set goals
2. Get the facts
3. Plan strategies and tactics
4. Supply leadership
5. Get to know decision makers and their staff
6. Broaden the base of support
7. Be persistent
8. Evaluate your advocacy effort (Schneider & Lester, 2001, pp. 116–147)

Decision-making: This refers to the conclusions, judgments, or actions of those who are authorized to allocate resources, define benefits, and determine eligibility and access to services, adjudicate grievances, establish appeals, or make policy for a government or an agency.

Unjust: Advocates believe that an action, stance, institution, regulation, procedure, or decision is not in accord with the law or the principles of justice. "Unjust" indicates that fairness, equity, lawfulness, justice, and righteousness are absent to some degree.

Unresponsive: Advocates identify persons or institutions that fail to reply, acknowledge, correspond, or answer inquiries, requests, petitions, demands, questions, letters, communiqués, or requests for appointments in a timely fashion if at all.

System(s): This refers to organized agencies designed and authorized to provide services to eligible persons, enforce laws and judgments, and be responsible for key areas of a society's allocation of resources. Examples are the criminal justice system, the mental health system, the legislative system, the welfare system, the health care system, and the transportation system.

This definition provides a coherent and distinguishing set of characteristics for the term *advocacy*, and offers a systematic foundation for implementing future advocacy practice, education, and research.

History of Social Work Advocacy

Organized social work emerged in the 1870s. The term *advocacy* was first evidenced in the *Proceedings of the National Conference of Charities and Corrections* (1917), where it was referred to as a social work role as far back as 1887. At that time, social workers targeted social legislation for children, prisons, immigration, the courts, and working conditions of the poor. During the Progressive years, the late 1800s until 1914, social work advocates fought for basic human rights and social justice for oppressed, vulnerable, and displaced populations, including immigrants, women, children, and minorities. Settlement houses such as the famous Hull House in Chicago promoted equality and social justice. Among the notable social workers of this era were Jane Addams, Edward T. Devine, Edith Abbott, Grace Abbott, Lillian Wald, Sophonisba Breckinridge, Julia Lathrop, Mary Richmond, Florence Kelley, Simon Patten, and Samuel M. Lindsay (Schneider & Lester, 2001; Trattner, 1999).

World War I and the postwar years presented numerous challenges, and many social workers focused their efforts on humanitarianism and international peace. Two social work advocates subsequently received the Nobel Peace Prize—Jane Addams in 1931

and Emily Greene Balch in 1946 (Bicha, 1986). However, the development and inclusion of psychology in social casework techniques had an adverse effect on advocacy. The individual and the person's inadequacies became the focus of attention, blame for poverty and hardship was attributed to the individual rather than the larger forces of society (Kurzman, 1974).

Following the stock market crash in October 1929, advocacy reemerged during the Great Depression. Social workers advocated for economic relief legislation and measures such as the Temporary Emergency Relief Administration and the Federal Emergency Relief Administration (FERA). Harry Hopkins led FERA and Frances Perkins was appointed Secretary of Labor in the Roosevelt administration, the first woman in a president's cabinet. Both were social workers.

After World War II, the word *advocacy* disappeared from the literature, replaced by the term *social action*. This term included other concepts such as "citizen participation," "social change," and "community organization." In the 1960s, civil rights, poverty, and inner city life took center stage. Important programs of President Lyndon Johnson's Great Society such as the Job Corps, the Youth Corps, Head Start, VISTA, family planning services, neighborhood legal services, and community health centers were developed (Ehrenreich, 1985), renewing interest in advocacy practice for vulnerable and oppressed populations.

Grosser (1965) provided the first contemporary outline of a social work advocate's role, as "co-opted from the field of law." He believed that an advocate *should not be* an "enabler, broker, expert, consultant, guide, or social therapist" but *should be* "a partisan in a social conflict" (p. 18). In 1969, the National Association of Social Workers (NASW) appointed an Ad Hoc Committee on Advocacy to *define* the term *advocacy*. One element of its definition reflected the lawyer-advocate role as "one who pleads the cause of another" and another element proposed advocacy practice in the political environment as "one who argues for, defends, maintains, or recommends a cause or proposal" (Ad Hoc Committee on Advocacy, 1969, p. 17).

During the 1970s, under President Richard Nixon, an era of benign neglect for social problems began and opposition to social reform gained strength. Social workers experienced obstacles in practicing advocacy because strict limitations were placed on programs funded through federal grants, diminishing social work's efficacy with their targeted populations. The 1980s were also a particular challenge to professional social work advocates, as President Ronald Reagan revealed his political agenda to include (a) reducing the federal deficit and balancing the nation's budget, (b) increasing emphasis on the military and national security, and (c) significantly reducing or eliminating "burdensome" social programs.

Under the Clinton administration in the 1990s, entitlement programs for the vulnerable and at-risk populations were devolved to the states, reducing the federal budget and transferring decision-making authority for social welfare programs to the states. "Welfare reform" was passed in 1996 under the Personal Responsibility and Work Opportunity Reconciliation Act, imposing tighter access to programs for the poor. During the George W. Bush administration, 2000–2008, the issues of the war in Iraq, terrorism, budget deficits, managed care, increased devolution of policy-making to the states, and faith-based initiatives posed a constant challenge to social work advocates in the public sector. At the turn of the 21st century, the Internet and advanced technology emerged as fundamental features in all sectors of society. Hick and McNutt (2002) stated, "just as the early social workers emerged and defined their practice within the Industrial Revolution, today's social workers must reinvent their practice to work within the Information Revolution" (p. 15) (see Electronic Advocacy).

Obligation to Be a Social Work Advocate

Are all social workers obliged to be advocates? Do licensed private practitioners have such an obligation? The ethical responsibility to be an advocate flows directly from the NASW Code of Ethics adopted in 1996 and revised in 1999. The word, *advocacy*, is found explicitly six times and implied in several other phrasings.

In the Preamble, the Code states, "[A]n historic and defining feature of social work is the profession's focus on individual well-being in a social context and the well-being of society. Social workers promote social justice and social change with and on behalf of clients...these activities may be in the form of direct practice, community organizing, consultation, administration, advocacy, social and political action, policy development and implementation, education, and research and evaluation."

Under Purpose of the Code, it is affirmed that "the Code is relevant to all social workers...regardless of their professional functions, the settings in which they work, or the populations they serve." It also states that "social workers should consider the NASW Code as their primary source" of information about ethical thinking.

Under Ethical Principles, the Code also states that "social workers challenge social injustice" and "pursue social change, particularly with and on behalf of vulnerable and oppressed individuals and groups of people." Further, "[s]ocial workers seek to enhance clients' capacity and opportunity to change and to address their own needs. Social workers are cognizant of their dual responsibility to clients and to the broader society."

Under the Code [Section 3.07(a)], Social Workers' Ethical Responsibility in Practice Settings, it is stated that "social work administrators should advocate within and outside their agencies for adequate resources to meet clients' needs," and in Section 3.07(b), "social workers should advocate for resource allocation procedures that are open and fair." Sections 3.09(c) and (d) state that social workers "ensure that employers are aware of social workers' ethical obligations as set forth in the NASW Code and the implications of these obligations for social work practice" and "[s]ocial workers should not allow...organization's policies, procedures, regulations...to interfere with their ethical practice of social work."

Code section 6.01 of the Social Worker's Ethical Responsibilities to the Broader Society/Social Welfare, states that "social workers should promote the general welfare of society, from local to global levels, and the development of people, their communities, and their environments. Social workers should advocate for living conditions conducive to the fulfillment of basic human needs and should promote social, economic, political, cultural values, and institutions that are compatible with the realization of social justice." Section [6.04(a)] states that "[s]ocial workers should be aware of the impact of the political arena on practice and should advocate for changes in policy and legislation to improve social conditions in order to meet basic human needs and promote social justice." Section [6.04(c)] states that "[s]ocial workers...should advocate for programs and institutions that demonstrate cultural competence, and promote policies that safeguard the rights of and confirm equity and social justice for all people."

Regardless of employment setting, social workers' commitment to practice advocacy flows directly from our Code of Ethics. It is not an option; it is an obligation.

Barriers to Practicing Social Work Advocacy

Despite a clearly defined professional obligation for *all* social workers to practice advocacy, numerous barriers and attitudes often inhibit them from pursuing it.

Advocacy takes too much time, energy, and personal finances (Ezell, 2001; Hoefer, 2006; Schneider & Lester, 2001). When social workers want to change local, state, or national policies and laws, they often do it "off the clock," using personal leave, and pay for travel and other out-of-pocket costs themselves.

Sheafor and Horejsi 2003, state that advocacy is misunderstood and often perceived by social workers as "confrontation" between professionals, agencies, and decision makers; it is also perceived as risking important and necessary collaborative relationships, or even losing one's job.

Clinical social workers do not prioritize the interrelationship of clients' needs and laws. Client efficacy often requires advocacy at the individual *and* the system levels.

Social work agencies and their staff often devote most of their energies to direct service programs (O'Connell, 1978). Although job descriptions may include an advocacy component, social workers may not be encouraged to take time away from service delivery.

Some social work practice is dictated de facto by managerial, not professional considerations. Efficiency is valued over effectiveness (Reisch, 1986).

Neither universities nor professional organizations provide sufficient education or training on how to actually do advocacy (Blakely, 1991). Agencies do not provide sufficient resources to promote or engage in advocacy practice (Ezell, 2001).

Some social workers stand in awe of politicians and are not comfortable with one-on-one lobbying (Ezell, 2001).

In one study, social work students substantively disagreed with the statement "advocacy is the main thrust of social work," suggesting an imprecise view of the profession (Csikai & Rozensky, 1997).

This list is not all-inclusive. In order to overcome such barriers and attitudes, professional and educational social work leaders must promote a renewed emphasis on the professional obligation to advocate, role model, and communicate core social work values, and provide efficacious education, training, and supervision on advocacy practice.

Electronic Advocacy

In the 21st century, social workers are engaging in electronic advocacy using new tools to address ongoing client issues and policy outcomes (McNutt, 2006). Electronic advocacy, often called *online advocacy* or *cyber activism*, refers to the use of e-mail lists, Web sites, message boards, petitions, blogs, social networking, cell phone text messaging, mapping, video and animation, really simple syndication, and other Internet communication tools to advocate, organize, and mobilize support for community causes, "get out the vote" campaigns, and coalition actions (AdvocacyDev.org, 2005). The Internet allows advocates to easily include participants on an equal basis, regardless of age, race, gender, or disability (Delany, 2006).

Queiro-Tajallil, Campbell, & McNutt (2003) identify four key processes characteristic of electronic advocacy:

Issue research: The Internet provides quick and efficient access to information, research findings, policy problems and issues, and knowledge about oppositional stances.

Information dissemination and awareness: Through e-mail and Web sites, advocates can contact supporters and the public to inform them about social problems or issues. Advocates can learn about issues, research, and strategies all on the same day.

Coordination and organizing: Although time-consuming, an electronic advocacy campaign to organize supporters is one of the most critical tasks. The lower costs of multiple transactions and communications are highly advantageous. Tracking events, raising funds, monitoring decision makers, conducting conference-call meetings, and coordinating personnel and volunteers are all features available through advanced technology.

Influence: Applying pressure on decision makers through electronic advocacy tools remains one of its outstanding features. Politics and policy issues at the federal, state, and local levels can be shared among advocates who can devise strategies and tactics for influencing elected and appointed officials (pp. 154–156) (see also Johnson, 2006).

As this technology-based advocacy expands among social work advocates, professional practice will still require the traditional commitment to addressing injustices and seeking equitable access to services for vulnerable populations.

Future Implications for Social Work Advocacy

Advocacy is an activity requiring patience, tenacity, compromise, long-term commitment, energy, broad bases of support, research, political skills, knowledge of government, and capacity to analyze (Schneider & Lester, 2001). Fortunately, the centrality of advocacy to the professional social work mission continues to evolve. The two major professional organizations, NASW and the Council on Social Work Education (CSWE) are vital partners in promoting increased integration of advocacy into social work practice and education.

Three areas are highlighted for continued support and future resources:

The CSWE, through its Educational Policy and Accreditation Standards (CSWE, 2001), requires that more emphasis be placed on policy advocacy practice in undergraduate and graduate curricula. Educational programs must build upon this standard and promote faculty and student involvement in advocacy practice and research. Innovative field internships in advocacy arenas such as local, state, and federal legislatures or agencies using electronic advocacy tools can be developed.

NASW has made significant investments in electoral and legislative domains at the national and state levels. This allows the profession to increase its influence and voice in the election of local, state, and federal officials. Chapters of NASW have also developed legislative campaigns to influence the evolving role of states in welfare policies that have an effect on traditional clientele populations. Continued expansion of such activities is necessary in order to permit members to use their expertise and creativity in informing lawmakers about laws that will actually meet client needs.

As of 2008, there were two U.S. Senators and eight U.S. Representatives in Congress who were social workers and over 60 social workers elected to state legislatures across the United States. Supporting and encouraging social workers to run for elective offices at local, state, and federal levels should be an urgent goal because these individuals will be the actual decision makers on policies affecting vulnerable populations served by social workers. This traditional, but often neglected, role can reinvigorate the profession in a most meaningful way.

REFERENCES

Ad Hoc Committee on Advocacy (NASW). (1969). The social worker as advocate: champion of social victims. *Social Work, 14*(2), 16–22.

AdvocacyDev.org. (2005). AdvocacyDev II convergence. San Francisco, CA, 11–13 July. Retrieved October 17, 2006, from http://www.advocacydev.org

Bicha, K. D. (1986). Emily Greene Balch. In W. I. Trattner (Ed.), *Biographical dictionary of social welfare in America* (pp. 46–48), New York: Greenwood Press.

Blakely, T. J. (1991). Advocacy in the social work curriculum. Unpublished paper.

Csikai, C., & Rozensky, C. (1997). Social work idealism and students' perceived reasons for entering social work. *Journal of Social Work Education, 33*(3), 529–538.

The Council on Social Work Education. (2001). *Educational policy and accreditation standards.* Alexandria, VA: Author.

Delany, C. (2006). The tools and tactics of online political advocacy: Online politics 101. Retrieved February 26, 2007, from http://www.epolitics.com

Ehrenreich, J. H. (1985). *The altruistic imagination: A history of social work and social policy in the United States.* Ithaca, NY: Cornell University Press.

Ezell, M. (2001). *Advocacy in the human services.* Belmont, CA: Wadsworth/Thomson Learning.

Grosser, C. F. (1965). Community development programs serving the urban poor. *Social Work, 7*, 15–21.

Haynes, K. S., & Mickelson, J. S. (2006). *Affecting change* (6th ed.). Boston: Allyn and Bacon.

Hepworth, D. H., Rooney, R. H., Dewberry-Rooney, G., Strom-Gottfried, K., & Larsen, J. A. (2006). *Direct social work practice: Theory and skills* (7th ed.). Pacific Grove, CA: Brooks/Cole.

Herbert, M. D., & Mould, J. W. (1992). The advocacy role in public child welfare. *Child Welfare, 71*, 114–130.

Hick, S. F., & McNutt, J. G. (2002). Communities and advocacy on the Internet: A conceptual framework. In S. F. Hick & J. G. McNutt (Eds.), *Advocacy, activism, and the internet: Community organization and social policy.* Chicago: Lyceum Books.

Hoefer, R. (2006). *Advocacy practice for social justice.* Chicago: Lyceum Books.

Johnson, D. W. (2006). Connecting citizens and legislators. Retrieved October 11, 2006, from http://www.connectingcitizens.org/

Kurzman, P. A. (1974). *Harry Hopkins and the New Deal.* Fair Lawn, NJ: R.E. Burdick.

Kutchins, H., & Kutchins, S. (1978). Advocacy and social work. In G. Weber & G. McCall (Eds.), *Social scientists as advocates: Views from the applied disciplines* (pp. 13–48). Beverly Hills, CA: Sage.

Kutchins, H., & Kutchins, S. (1987). Advocacy and the adversary system. *Journal of Sociology and Social Work, 14*, 119–133.

Litzelfelner, P., & Petr, C. G. (1997). Case advocacy in child welfare. *Social Work, 42*, 392–402.

McNutt, J. G. (2006). Building evidence-based advocacy in cyberspace: A social work imperative for the new millennium. *Journal of Evidence-based Social Work, 3*, 91–102.

National Association of Social Workers. (1999). *Code of Ethics.* Washington, DC: Author.

O'Connell, B. (1978). From service to advocacy to empowerment. *Social Casework, 59*(4), 195–202.

Queiro-Tajallil, I., Campbell, C., & McNutt, J. (2003). International social and economic justice and on-line advocacy. *International Social Work, 46*, 149–161.

Reisch, M. (1986). From cause to case and back again: The reemergence of advocacy in social work. *The Urban and Social Change Review, 19*, 20–24.

Schneider, R. L., & Netting, F. E. (1999). Influencing social policy in a time of devolution: Upholding social work's great tradition. *Social Work, 44*, 349–357.

Schneider, R. L., & Lester, L. (2001). *Social work advocacy: A new framework for action.* Belmont, CA: Wadsworth/Thomson Learning.

Sosin, M., & Caulum, S. (2003). Advocacy: A conceptualization for social work practice. *Social Work*, 28, 12–17.

Trattner, W. I. (1999). *From poor law to welfare state: A history of social welfare in America* (6th ed.). New York: Free Press

FURTHER READING

Bateman, N. (1995). *Advocacy skills: A handbook for human service professionals.* Brookfield, VT: Ashgate.

Briar, S. (1977). In summary. *Social Work*, 22, 415–416, 444.

Jansson, B. (2007). *Becoming an effective policy advocate: from policy practice to social justice* (5th ed.). Pacific Grove, CA: Brooks/Cole.

Schneider, R. L., & Lester, L. (2001). *Social work advocacy: a new framework for action.* Belmont, CA: Wadsworth/ Thomson Learning.

Shaefor, B. W., & Horejsi, C. R. (2003). *Techniques and guidelines for social work practice* (6th ed.). Boston: Allyn and Bacon.

Wolk, J. L. (1981). Are social workers politically active? *Social Work*, 26, 283–288.

SUGGESTED LINKS

http://www.socialworkers.org
http://www.statepolicy.org
http://internetadvocacycenter.com
http://advocacydev.org
http://www.connectingcitizens.org
http://thePetitionSite.com
http://www.mobileactive.org
http://backspace.com/action
http://citizenspeak.org
http://www.greatergood.com
http://www.globalexchange.org
http://www.politicsonline.com
http://www.stateline.org
http://www.techsoup.org
http://epolitics.com
http://www.advocacyguru.com
http://www.independentsector.org/programs/gr/lobbyguide.html

ROBERT L. SCHNEIDER, LORI LESTER, AND JULIA OCHIENG

AGING: OVERVIEW

ABSTRACT: The rapidly growing older population is more heterogeneous by health and economic status, gender, race, sexual orientation, and family and living arrangements than any other age group. Although many adults face vulnerabilities and inequities as they age, most elders are resilient. This entry reviews this diversity, discusses concepts of productive, successful, and active aging, and suggests leadership roles for social workers in enhancing the well-being of elders and their families.

KEY WORDS: life course; inequities; productive; successful and active aging; resilience

The dramatic growth of the population age 65 and older is referred to as a demographic imperative because it affects all social institutions—families, the workplace, educational settings, health and mental health care delivery systems, and the leisure industry. It also has far-reaching implications for social work. Social workers in all practice arenas and with all age groups increasingly work with older adults and their families: in child welfare, family services, schools, mental health centers, AIDS treatment clinics, and among the homeless. This entry reviews the demographics of aging; vulnerabilities and challenges faced by older adults; emerging opportunities for active, productive, and resilient aging; and concludes with a discussion of the implications for social work. Although the older population is growing worldwide, the focus here is on the United States.

Demography of Aging

Americans age 65 and older comprise 13.1% of the population, compared to 4% in 1900. The population age 65 and older increased by almost 13 times during this period compared with a threefold increase in the population under age 65. With the first Baby Boomers (that is, those born between 1946 and 1964) turning 65 in 2011, the population age 65 and older is increasing significantly. Demographers predict that older adults, who now number 40.4 million, may number 88.5 million by 2050, a 100% increase over 30 years compared with a 30% increase in the total population. Those age 85 and older—the oldest-old—are the most rapidly growing age group. Now forming 13% of the older population, they are projected to increase fourfold by 2050. The population of centenarians, people age 100 or older, will also grow substantially since baby boomers are expected to survive to age 100 at rates never before achieved. One in 26 Americans can expect to live to be 100 years by 2025, compared with only 1 in 500 in 2000 (Administration on Aging [AOA], 2012; Howden & Meyer, 2011; U.S. Census Bureau, 2011b).

These demographic shifts are occurring because of increases in life expectancy (average length of time that one can expect to live based on the year born). Life expectancy at birth is expected to grow from slightly more than 78 years in 2011 to the mid-80s by 2050. On average, females born today will live 80.8 years compared to 75.7, respectively. A fairly constant 5-year gender difference in life expectancy is projected well into the future (Federal Interagency Forum on Aging-Related Statistics, 2012; U.S. Census Bureau, 2011a). Most of the gains in life expectancy have occurred in the younger ages because of better medical care and eradication of childhood diseases.

Population aging is a global phenomenon, occurring in just about every country in every part of the world as older adults grow in both real numbers and in proportion to the larger population. In 2008, the number of people 65 years and older in the world was estimated to be 506 million, or about 7% of the world's population. By 2040, that number is projected to increase to 1.3 billion people, or 14% of the world's population. At that time, about 76% of people 65 and older are likely to be in developing countries (Kinsella & He, 2009). The two major reasons for global aging are increased life expectancy and declining birth rates. Japan has the highest proportion of elders in the world (22%), followed by Italy (20%). It is noteworthy that the projected increase in the numbers and proportion of persons age 60 and older is higher for developing nations than for the more developed ones—increasing from 475 million in 2009 to 1.6 billion in 2050, when about 80% of the world's older adults will be living in developing countries. Currently, 60% of older adults live in developing countries, which may increase to 75% by 2020 (United Nations, 2009).

Heterogeneity of the Older Population

Aging cannot be defined merely in chronological terms, which only partially reflects the biological, psychological, and social-cultural processes as people age. A more relevant distinction is functional age or the ability to perform activities of daily living (ADLs), such as eating, bathing, and dressing that require cognitive and physical well-being (World Health Organization [WHO], 2002). Because aging is a complex process that involves factors unique to each individual, older people are more diverse in their health and socioeconomic status, ethnicity and race, and family situations than other age groups. Some are employed; most are retired. Most are healthy; some are frail, homebound, or have dementia. Most still live in a house or apartment; a small percent are in nursing homes. Some receive large incomes from pensions and investments; most depend primarily on Social Security and have little discretionary income. Most men age 65 years and older are married, while women are more likely to be widowed and living alone. Intersections among these variables play out in the poorest group in our society: older women of color living alone in rural areas (AOA, 2012).

As adults live longer, they also tend to manage their chronic conditions without resulting in frailty or physical disability. Disability rates have declined since 2002 in all age groups 65 years and older, especially among the oldest-old (Crimmins & Beltrán-Sánchez, 2010; Fuller-Thomson, Yu, Nuru-Jeter, Guralnik, & Minler, 2009; Manton, Gu, & Lowrimore, 2008). Although more than 80% of older adults have at least one chronic condition and 37% report some type of disability, only about 2% are bedbound. The vast majority are functionally able to conduct activities of daily living (ADLs) (AOA, 2012). The need for assistance with ADLs, which generally increases with age, typically determines whether older adults can remain in their homes. Although the baby boomers are currently healthier than prior cohorts, their sheer numbers, combined with increasing obesity rates, mean that by 2030, about 30% of them will have activity limitations that require some assistance and 20% of this group will have severe limitations. In sum, while people are living longer, many are also living longer with chronic illness and disability (Manton, Gu, & Lamb, 2006; National Institutes of Health [NIH], 2011).

ETHNICITY, RACE, GENDER, AND SEXUAL ORIENTATION Ethnic minorities comprise slightly less than 20% of the total older population (8.4% African American, 6.9% Latino, 3.1% Asian or Pacific Islander, and less than 1% American Indian or Native Alaskan) (AOA, 2012). These low rates result from higher fertility and mortality rates among young adults and high rates of immigration of younger adults, creating a smaller proportion of elders compared with Caucasian population. In addition, elders of color have a lower life expectancy, as noted earlier, generally because of lifelong inequities in access to economic resources, health care, and preventive services. However, by 2050, the percent of people of color age 65 and older is projected to increase to almost 42%, faster than the rate of growth among the Caucasian population. This will occur because of the large percent of children in these groups, who, unlike their parents and especially their grandparents, are expected to reach old age (AOA, 2012).

Women form the fastest growing segment of the older population, especially among the oldest-old, making the aging society a largely female society: they represent 58% of the population age 65 and older and 70% of those ages 85 and older. Women at age 85 and older outnumber their male counterparts by five to two and among centenarians by three to one (U.S. Census Bureau, 2011b).

Estimates of the number of older gay, lesbian, bisexual, and transgender (GLBT) adults range from as low as 3% to as high as 18–20%. This translates into at least 2 million older lesbians and gay men, which will likely increase to over 6 million by the year 2030 (Fredriksen-Goldsen & Muraco, 2010). Prevalence rates are probably underestimates because of the taboo of identifying as GLBT in a survey. The general invisibility of being old in our society is heightened for those who are old and GLBT, the most "invisible of an already invisible minority" (Blando, 2001; Gates, 2011). Because of the double stigma of being "twice hidden," some studies find that the aging experience is more difficult for GLBT adults who may experience higher rates of social isolation and mental distress while others suggest that lifelong marginalization and skills in managing a stigmatized status may stimulate adaptive strategies to the challenges of aging (Fredriksen-Goldsen, Kim, Emlet, et al., 2011; Gabbay & Wahler, 2002; McFarland & Sanders, 2003; Thompson, 2006). Although gains have been made in many states in terms of domestic partnerships, GLBT elders still encounter legal and attitudinal obstacles in receiving and providing care in health and long-term care settings, largely because of lacking the legal protection of marriage, and service providers must have the knowledge and skills to work effectively with GLBT elders (Cahill, South, & Spade, 2001; SAGE, 2010; Zodikoff, 2006).

GEOGRAPHIC LOCATION AND TYPE OF LIVING SITUATION About 57% of all adults aged 65 and older live in 11 states, with the highest proportion in Florida (17.4%), followed by West Virginia (16.1%) and Maine (15.9%), and lowest in Alaska (7%) and Utah (8.8%). In some states, such as Florida, in-migration of older adults explains the increase, while in others, such as West Virginia and Maine, the increase is due to the migration of young people out of the state. These regional differences are expected to continue (AOA, 2012). Residential relocation is relatively rare; in a typical year, less than 6% of people age 65 and older move, usually within the same region, compared with nearly 17% of people under age 65. The vast majority of older persons (80%) live in metropolitan areas. The oldest-old are most likely to relocate, often into or near their children's homes, which is typically precipitated by widowhood, significant deterioration in health, or disability (AOA, 2012; Frey, 2010).

Most elders prefer to remain in their own home, regardless of its condition, which reflects the almost universal desire to "age in place." As a result, 93.5% of those ages 65 and older live in independent housing, which they typically own, followed by 41% in long-term care facilities, and 2.4% in senior housing with services, such as assisted living. The lifetime risk of admission to a nursing home increases with age and for women, who are the majority of residents. Of these residents, about 87% are White (AOA, 2012).

EDUCATIONAL, EMPLOYMENT, AND ECONOMIC STATUS Today's older population is better educated, with nearly 80% of those ages 65 and older having a high school degree, compared with less than 20% in 1960, and 22.5% holding a bachelor's degree or more. Racial and generational differences are striking, however. Among Whites, 84% of older adults have at least a high school diploma. Because of historical patterns of discrimination in educational opportunities, 65% of older African Americans and 47% of Latinos today have less than a high school education (AOA, 2012). Because educational level is so closely associated with economic well-being, these racial differences have a major impact on poverty levels of persons of color across the life course and particularly in old age. Not surprisingly, the baby boomers who began to turn 65 in 2010 and the adults currently aged 65–69 years are better educated than the oldest-old, which has implications for the economic well-being of future generations of elders. The proportion of older people in the labor force has increased to 17% in recent years, in part because of the recession and the financial necessity to keep working longer than many older adults had anticipated: approximately 22% of men and almost 14% of women age 65 and older now work full- or part-time outside the home. The majority of these are employed in a part-time or temporary capacity (Bureau of Labor Statistics, 2011; Hicks & Kingson, 2009).

Older adults' economic status has generally improved in the last 50 years, largely because of Social Security and its annual cost of living increases, although income has declined slightly due to the recession. Social Security is a source of income for 87% of elders. Today about 9% of older people subsist on incomes below the poverty level, compared with 35% in the late 1950s. Another 5.8% of older adults are classified as "near-poor." Poverty rates increase among women and elders of color (AOA, 2012; Johnson & Wilson, 2010).

FAMILIES AND FAMILY CAREGIVING The family is the primary source of social support for older adults: over 90% of elders have living family members and about 60% reside in a family setting, typically with a spouse/partner. Nearly 55% of those ages 65 and older are married and living with a spouse in an independent household, while about 4% have never married. Although 80% of adults ages 65 and older have children, only about 6% of older men and 17% of women live with children, siblings, or other relatives. Significant differences exist, however, in living arrangements by gender and age. Because of women's longer life expectancy, higher rates of widowhood, and fewer options for remarriage, only 41% of women over age 65 are married and living with a spouse as compared with nearly 70% of men. Accordingly, 37% of women live alone compared with 19% of men. The percentages living with a spouse also decline markedly with age and among African Americans and Latinos (AOA, 2012; Uhlenberg, 2004). Marital status affects living arrangements and the nature of caregiving readily available in case of illness. Marriage appears to be a protective factor, associated with physical and mental health, life satisfaction, and happiness, especially for men (Lyyra & Heikkinen, 2006). Although lacking the legal option of marriage, GLBT elders who have partners tend to be less lonely and enjoy better physical and mental health than those living alone (Metlife Mature Market Institute, 2006). The aging family of the future will be profoundly affected by the growing incidence of younger adults who are single and never-married, divorced, and single parents along with reduced fertility and smaller family size.

With increased life expectancy, multigenerational families—composed of four or even five generations—are more common now, a pattern that crosses racial and ethnic groups and social classes. The percent of Americans living in multigenerational households had declined from 1940 to 1980 to about 12% of the population. But from 1980 to 2000, such households increased by 39%. As a result, 16% of the total population—about 6.6 million U.S. households—now encompasses three or more generations. The percent of children under 18 who lived in a household that included a grandparent increased from 8% in 2001 to 10% in 2010. The growth of multigenerational families means that some parents and children now share five decades of life, siblings perhaps eight decades, and the grandparent–grandchild bond lasts three or more decades (Pew Research Center, 2010b).

Among parents ages 65 and older, 80% are grandparents, with some women experiencing grandmotherhood for more than 40 years. This is because the transition to grandparenthood typically occurs in middle age, not old age, with about 50% of all grandparents younger than 60 years. As a result, there is wide diversity among grandparents, who vary in age from their late 30s to over 100 years old, with grandchildren ranging from newborns to retirees. Most grandparents derive satisfaction from their role and interaction with grandchildren (Pew Research Center, 2010b; Reitzes & Mutran, 2004).

Grandparents have traditionally provided care for grandchildren, especially within families of color and immigrant families (Cox, 2002). What has shifted since the mid-1990s is the dramatic increase in grandparents who assume primary responsibility for their grandchildren. With almost 2.9 million custodial grandparents providing such primary care, skipped-generation households—the absence of the parent generation—are currently the fastest growing type. This means that about 7.8 million children live in households headed by grandparents or other relatives. Custodial grandparenting crosscuts social class, race, and ethnicity. The majority of sole grandparent caregivers are White (53%), but Latinos (18%) and African Americans (24%) are disproportionately represented, given their percentage of the total population. In most instances, the parents—an invisible middle generation—are absent because of substance use or incarceration. Most custodial grandparents are women, even among older couples, and are younger than 65; the 30% who are age 65 and older typically deal with age-related changes along with the emotional stress of feeling alone and isolated from age peers. Grandparent caregivers have been called the "silent saviors" of the family; in addition to a greater likelihood of living in poverty, they face numerous legal, health-care, and financial barriers. These challenges are even greater for grandparents who are raising a chronically ill or "special needs" child, which is common since the incidence of emotional or behavioral problems is high (Generations United, 2012; Hayslip & Kaminski, 2005; Kropf & Yoon, 2006; Musil, Warner, Zauszniewski, Jeanblanc, & Kercher, 2006; Pew Research Center, 2010a).

Generally, families experience a pattern of reciprocal support between older and younger members, with older adults providing support to children and grandchildren as long as they are able (Silverstein, Conroy, Wang, Giarrusso, & Bengston, 2002). As another example of this pattern, increasing numbers of elders are providing care for their adult children with developmental disabilities or mental illness who are now living longer (McCallion, 2006).

The reciprocal nature of caregiving shifts as more adults—especially the oldest-old—live longer with chronic illness and seek to remain in the community. Families, who provide 80% of such care, are a significant factor influencing whether an older adult will live in a long-term care facility home. Over 80% of older adults with limitations in three or more ADLs are able to live in the community primarily because of family assistance; moreover, 66% of older people who receive long-term services and supports at home get all their care exclusively from family members. Informal caregiving has been shown to help delay or prevent the use of skilled nursing home care. The economic value contributed by family caregivers to society is estimated to be $450 billion, far more than the total expenditures for formal services. Family caregivers, then, constitute a large and often overlooked component of the American economy and systems of health care and long-term services and supports (Feinberg, Reinhard, Houser, & Choula, 2011; Gonyea, 2008; Hargrave, 2008; Raphael & Cornwell, 2008; Van Houtven & Norton, 2008).

Among caregivers, about 36% of them care for a parent and about 23% for a partner. Women form about 66% of the caregivers who have primary responsibility, providing more hours of assistance than their male counterparts. Women are more likely to provide emotional support and personal care, while men assist with instrumental tasks such as transportation, home maintenance, and finances. The average caregiver is 47 years old, female, married, earning an income outside the home of $35,000, and has performed their role for 4.6 years, devoting 25 hours per week of care (Family Caregiver Alliance, 2009). Caregiving for elders occurs across the life course, however; a growing number of young caregivers, age 8–18, are helping a parent or grandparent and caregivers who are in their 60s or even 70s are caring for centenarians (NAC & AARP, 2009).

Although there are gains from caregiving, the physical and mental health, financial and emotional costs of care—conceptualized as objective and subjective burden—generally exceed benefits for the caregiver, with approximately 30% of caregivers experiencing stress or burden. Caregiving is associated with a range of illnesses, including higher rates of depression, anxiety, heart disease, and even mortality (Feinberg et al., 2011; Pinquart & Sorenson, 2006). Financial costs encompass the direct costs of medical care, adaptive equipment, or hired help and as indirect opportunity costs of lost income, missed promotions, or unemployment. Averaging 12 years out of the paid workforce to provide care to family members, women suffer long-term economic costs of caregiving, including higher rates of poverty in old age. The caregiver's appraisal of the situation or subjective burden, such as feeling alone and overwhelmed, is more salient than objective burden or the actual tasks performed. On the other hand, living with the care recipient, being a woman, coping with an elder's behavioral problems, especially those associated with dementia, and long hours of intensive levels of care are associated with increased caregiver stress (Family Caregiver Alliance, 2009; Family Caregiver Alliance & National Center on Caregiving, 2011).

Children and partners typically turn to skilled nursing care as a "last resort" when faced with their own illness or severe family strain. Although most caregivers do not use formal services, psycho-educational programs, support groups, and respite care are relatively effective interventions in reducing caregiver stress, all of which have implications for social work roles (Belle et al., 2006; Gonyea, Connor, & Boyle, 2006; Kuhn & Fulton, 2004; Mittelman, Roth, Coon, & Haley, 2004; Parker, Mills, & Abbey, 2008; Zarit & Femia, 2008).

Vulnerabilities and Challenges of Aging

INEQUITIES ACROSS THE LIFE COURSE The concept of *life course* is central to understanding the vulnerabilities faced by some groups of elders. A life course approach captures how earlier life experiences and decisions affect options in later life and for future generations within and across cultures and time. It recognizes that gender or racial inequities, which limit earlier opportunities, are intensified in old age, resulting in increased economic and health disparities and cumulative disadvantage for older women and persons of color. Gender, ethnic minority status, sexual orientation, low educational and socioeconomic levels, and increased age are all associated with reduced social capital and increased health disparities (Ferraro, Shippee, & Schafer, 2009; George, 2007; O'Rand, 2006; Williams, 2005). Nevertheless, many older adults who have experienced cumulative adversity lifetime inequities demonstrate remarkable resilience and optimism.

The overall economic status of older people masks growing rates of poverty among women, elders of color, the oldest-old, and those living alone. Older women (nearly 11%) are more likely to be poor than men (6.7%). Older African Americans (nearly 15%) and Latinos (18%) are far more likely to be poor than Whites (6.8%) (AOA, 2012). Women and persons of color are least likely to have held jobs with private pensions and most likely to depend on Social Security as the primary source of income. Because of economic, family caregiving, and health disparities experienced across the life course, older women, elders of color, and the oldest-old are most likely to experience disabling illness along with poverty and inadequate housing (Ferraro et al., 2009; Johnson & Wilson, 2010; Walker, 2009). Although the likelihood of chronic illness grows with age, the origins of risk for such conditions and early mortality begin in early childhood. Regardless of age, chronic disability then magnifies the risk of poverty throughout the life course. When the intersections among structural variables are examined, it is not surprising that poor women of color age 85 and older have the highest prevalence of multiple chronic illnesses and functional limitations (Centers for Disease Control and Health Promotion [CDC], 2010; Whitfield, Angel, Burton, & Hayward, 2006; Williams, 2005).

PHYSICAL AND MENTAL CHALLENGES More than 80% of persons age 65 and older have at least one chronic illness, and 66% have multiple illnesses. The most frequently reported chronic conditions, which limit ADLs among older adults and are rooted in health practices across the life course, are hypertension, arthritis, and heart disease. Heart disease, cancer, and strokes account for more than two-thirds of all deaths among people age 65 and older (CDC, 2010; Federal Interagency Forum on Aging-Related Statistics, 2012).

Heart disease is the number-one risk factor among adults age 65 and older, killing 40% more people than all forms of cancer combined, and accounting for 20% of adult disabilities, with the highest rates among the oldest-old and among African Americans (American Heart Association, 2012). Disabling chronic diseases tend to occur earlier among African Americans, Latinos, and American Indians than among Whites. Comorbidity—coping with two or more chronic conditions—is a concept central to understanding health status and its secondary consequences, such as depression and anxiety, and is more common in older women and elders of color than in Caucasian men.

Although normal aging does not result in significant declines in intelligence, learning, and memory, the prevalence of mental disorders ranges from 15 to 25% of the older population, depending on whether samples include older residents in institu-

tional settings. In some instances, these represent mental illnesses that have occurred across the life course, while others are often precipitated by losses of old age. Anxiety and depression are the most common mental disorders in late life, with minor depression estimated to be as high as 10 to 30% among community-dwelling elders (Gellis, 2006). This is of concern since depression often coexists with medical conditions such as heart disease, stroke, arthritis, cancer, diabetes, chronic lung disease, and Alzheimer's disease, compounding dysfunction and delaying a recovery process. Detecting depression is challenging, since older people often mask or hide symptoms; it is most frequently misdiagnosed among elders of color. Rates of depression are highest among women, those lacking social supports, and low-income elders (Blazer, 2003; Mitchell & Subramaniam, 2005).

Most older adults with chronic mental disorders live in the community, but fewer than 25% of those who need mental health services ever receive treatment, a pattern across all service areas (Gellis, 2006; Kaskie & Estes, 2001). The likelihood of irreversible dementia increases with advancing age, with some estimates as high as 50% for those age 85 and older and over 80% for those age 90 and older. Alzheimer's disease (AD), the most common dementia in late life, accounts for 60 to 80% of all dementias, and 13% of adults age 65 and older are diagnosed with AD. By 2050, 11 to 16 million people age 65 and older are projected to have AD, compared with 5.2 million currently, unless there are medical breakthroughs in its prevention and treatment (Alzheimer's Association of America, 2012; Alzheimer's Disease International, 2009).

LIVING ALONE Although the majority of elderly people live with others, about 19% of men and 37% of women age 65 and older live alone; after age 75, these rates increase. Those living alone are most likely to be women, elders of color, the oldest-old, low-income, and in rural areas (AOA, 2012). Among those living alone, the most vulnerable are the homeless. Homeless elders (defined as age 55 and older because they are often 10 to 20 years older physiologically than their chronological age) comprise 8 to 10% of the homeless population (Sermons & Henry, 2010). Those living alone and the oldest-old are most vulnerable to being placed in nursing homes, assisted living, adult family homes, and hospitals. Among older age 95 and older, 25 percent are skilled nursing facilities, for example, (U.S. Census Bureau, 2011c).

Opportunities, Resources, and Incentives for Productive Aging

With the aging of the baby boomers, who may live a third of their lives in a healthier and more financially secure retirement than previous cohorts, increasing attention is given to concepts of productive aging and civic engagement. These concepts recognize that elders are our society's most underutilized asset, with wisdom, skills, and life experience to contribute to addressing social problems. This has translated into growing numbers of civic engagement initiatives, such as voluntarism, intergenerational programs, and cross-generational political advocacy, which are typically associated with higher life satisfaction (Freedman, 2011; Metlife, 2008).

Another widely used concept is successful aging, defined as a combination of physical and functional health, high cognitive functioning, and active involvement with society. However, this concept is critiqued for conveying a middle-age, middle-class norm of remaining active as a way to show that one is an exception to their age peers, that is, "not really old, not aging." Strategies to avoid being seen as old are put forth by the mass marketing of exceptionally fit and physically attractive older adults and the growth of "lifestyle industries" to preserve "youthfulness." The concepts of productivity, civic engagement, and successful aging can implicitly assume that all elders have resources to age successfully and be productive, such as volunteering. They may overlook structural constraints, such as unhealthy communities, limited employment options, and daily preoccupation with economic survival, that prevent choosing healthy lifestyles. Both policies and social environments need to be modified so that all adults have opportunities to be productive in the broadest sense of the term (Hendricks & Hatch, 2006; Kahn, 2003; Martinson & Minkler, 2006; Wray, 2003).

An emphasis on activity characteristic of mainstream Western culture may also overlook elders—often from other cultures—who are spiritual and contemplative, and experience a high degree of subjective well-being. A narrow definition of successful aging can be stigmatizing to older adults with chronic illness who develop strategies to compensate for their functional disabilities and experience quality of life. Instead, models of successful aging need to recognize that older adults may experience subjective well-being, engage in personally meaningful activities, and "age well," even though they may not be classified as successful in terms of external factors (George, 2006).

Because of class, race, and gender biases implicit within successful aging, the concepts of active aging and resilience may be more useful for conceptualizing elders' strengths (for example, internal, family, social, community, and cultural capacities) when faced with adversity. In fact, many older adults find meaning in their lives because of adversity, not despite it. Even when impaired, they may contribute to society in diverse ways (Fredriksen-Goldsen, 2006; Zarit, 2009).

The concept of "active aging" is relevant to culturally and economically diverse populations since it focuses on improving quality of life for all people, including those who are frail, disabled, or require assistance. It is consistent with the growing emphasis on autonomy and choice with aging, regardless of physical and mental decline, that benefits both the individual and society. The determinants of active aging include individual behaviors, personal characteristics, the physical and social environment, structural variables such as gender and race, economic security, and access to and use of health and social services across the life course (WHO, 2002).

Role of Social Workers

Social workers are well positioned to promote active aging and well-being for all older adults. The opportunity and challenge for social work, with its social justice mission, is to address both increased longevity along with life course inequities for women, persons of color, and GLBT individuals. As a first step, social workers must be prepared to meet the geriatric workforce challenge, since the need for gerontologically competent social workers far exceeds the supply. With its person-in-environment perspective and strengths-based values, social work is pivotally placed to advocate for structural and policy changes to reduce lifetime inequities (for example, dependent care credits in Social Security) and to enhance the well-being of adults and their families as they age.

As the primary providers of mental health services, social workers are also central to addressing growing rates of depression, substance abuse, and mistreatment among elders. They are often the lead professionals supporting multigenerational families, particularly related to psychosocial interventions to reduce the stress of cross-generational caregiving across the life course. Social work assessments are strengths-based and take account of the needs of the total caregiving system, not just the elder person. Similarly, social workers can provide leadership in developing and testing innovative models of integrated care or service delivery and interventions with caregiving dyads. As more adults live longer with disability, social workers are central to community-based models for chronic disease management, rather than cure, and to fostering the social supports essential to health-promoting behaviors. Similarly, social workers, with their value of self-determination and dignity, play vital roles in changing the culture of care of institutional settings to be resident-centered and to empower the direct care staff. Social workers also can facilitate the use of assistive technology, including computer-based options, along with informal social networks to enable elders to remain in their homes. In times of shrinking public resources and increasing societal and moral issues affecting all ages, social workers can foster intergenerational alliances that crosscut traditional age-based approaches to services. And most important, social workers, by building on the strengths of all elders, even those with limited functional disability, will reaffirm older adults' dignity and worth.

REFERENCES

Administration on Aging (AOA). (2012). *Profile of older Americans: 2011*. Washington, DC.

Alzheimer's Association of America. (2012) *Alzheimer's disease: Facts and figures*. Retrieved October 30, 2012 from http://www.alz.org/downloads/facts_figures_2013.pdf

Alzheimer's Disease International. (2009). *The prevalence of dementia*. Retrieved from http://www.alz.co.uk/adi/pdf/prevalence.pdf

American Heart Association. (2012). *African Americans and cardiovascular disease* [Statistical Fact Sheet: 2012 Update]. Retrieved from http://www.heart.org/HEARTORG/Conditions/More/MyHeartandStrokeNews/African-Americans-and-Heart-Disease-Stroke_UCM_444863_Article.jsp

Belle, S. H., Burgio, L., Burns, R., Coon, D., Czaja, S. J., Gallagher-Thompson, D., et al. (2006). Enhancing the quality of life of dementia caregivers from different ethnic or racial groups: A randomized controlled trial. *Annals of Internal Medicine, 145*, 727–738.

Blando, J. A. (2001). Twice hidden: Older gay and lesbian couples, friends and intimacy. *Generations, 25*(2), 87–89.

Blazer, D. G. (2003). Depression in late life: Review and commentary. *Journals of Gerontology Series A: Biological and Medical Sciences, 58*, M249–M265.

Bureau of Labor Statistics. (2011). *Income security: Older adults and the 2007–09 Recession*. Washington, DC: U.S. General Accountabiltiy Office.

Cahill, S., South, K., & Spade, J. (2001). *Outing age: Public policy issues affecting gay, lesbian, bisexual and transgender elders*. New York, NY: The Policy Institute of the National Gay and Lesbian Task Force.

Centers for Disease Control and Health Promotion (CDC). (2010). *REACH U.S.: Finding solutions to health disparities: At a glance, 2010*. Retrieved from http://www.cdc.gov/chronicdisease/resources/publications/AAG/reach.htm

Cox, C. (2002). Empowering African American custodial grandparents. *Social Work, 47*(1), 262–267.

Crimmins, E. M., & Beltrán-Sánchez, H. (2010). Mortality and morbidity trends: Is there compression of morbidity? *Journal of Gerontology: Social Sciences, 66B*(1), 75–86.

Family Caregiver Alliance. (2009). *Fact sheet: Caregiving*. San Francisco, CA: Family Caregiver Alliance.

Family Caregiver Alliance & National Center on Caregiving. (2011). *Family caregiving 2010 year in review*. San Francisco, CA: Family Caregiver Alliance.

Federal Interagency Forum on Aging-Related Statistics. (2012). *Older Americans 2012: Key indicators of well-being*. Hyattsville, MD: Author.

Feinberg, L., Reinhard, S. C., Houser, A., & Choula, R. (2011). *Valuing the invaluable: 2011 update: The growing contributions and costs of family caregiving*. Washington, DC: AARP Public Policy Institute.

Ferraro, K. F., Shippee, T. P., & Schafer, M. H. (2009). Cumulative inequality theory for research on aging and the life course. In V. L. Bengtson, D. Gans, N. M. Putney, & M. Silverstein (Eds.), *Handbook of theories of aging* (2nd ed.). New York, NY: Springer.

Freedman, M. (2011). *The big shift: Navigating the new stage beyond midlife*. New York, NY: Public Affairs.

Fredriksen-Goldsen, K. (2006). Caregiving and resiliency: Predictors of well-being. *Journal of Family Relations, 55*, 625–635.

Fredriksen-Goldsen, K. I., Kim, H.-J., Emlet, C. A., Muraco, A., Erosheva, E. A., Hoy-Ellis, C. P., et al. (2011). *The aging and health report: Disparities and resilience among lesbian, gay, bisexual, and transgender older adults*. University of Washington, Seattle: Institute for Multigenerational Health.

Fredriksen-Goldsen, K. I., & Muraco, A. (2010). Aging and sexual orientation: A 25-year review of the literature. *Research on Aging, 32*(3), 372–413.

Frey, W. H. (2010). Baby boomers and the new demographics of America's seniors. *Generations: Journal of the American Society on Aging, 30*(3), 28–37.

Fuller-Thomson, E., Yu, B., Nuru-Jeter, A., Guralnik, J. M., & Minkler, M. (2009). Basic ADL disability and functional limitation rates among Older Americans from 2000–2005: The end of the decline? *The Journals of Gerontology Series A: Biological Sciences and Medical Sciences, 64*(12), 1333–1336.

Gabbay, S., & Wahler, J. (2002). Lesbian aging: Review of a growing literature. *Journal of Gay and Lesbian Social Services, 14*(3), 1–21.

Gates, G. J. (2011). *How many people are lesbian, gay, bisexual, and transgender?* Los Angeles, CA: The Williams Institute, University of California. Retrieved from http://williamsinstitute.law.ucla.edu/research/census-lgbt-demographics-studies/how-many-people-are-lesbian-gay-bisexual-and-transgender

Gellis, Z. D. (2006). Older adults with mental and emotional problems. In B. Berkman & S. D'Ambruoso (Eds.), *The handbook of social work in health and aging* (pp.129–140). New York, NY: Oxford University Press.

George, L. K. (2007). Age structures, aging, and the life course. In J. M. Wilmoth & K. F. Ferraro (Eds.), *Gerontology: Perspectives and issues* (3rd ed.). New York, NY: Springer.

Generations United. (2012). *Grandfamilies statistics*. Retrieved November 2, 2012, from www2.gu.org/OURWORK/Grandfamilies/GrandfamiliesStatistics.aspx

George, L. K. (2006). Perceived quality of life. In R. H. Binstock & L. K. George (Eds.), *Handbook of aging and the social sciences* (6th ed., pp. 320–336). New York, NY: Academic Press.

Gonyea, J. (2008). Foreword: America's aging workforce: A critical business issue. *Journal of Workplace Behavioral Health*, 23(1/2), 1–14.

Gonyea, J. G., O'Connor, M. K., & Boyle, P. A. (2006). Project CARE: A randomized controlled trial of a behavioral intervention group for Alzheimer's disease caregivers. *The Gerontologist*, 46, 827–832.

Hargrave, T. H. (2008). The worker's point of view VIII: Working conditions and morale. *Human Factors (London)*, 6(10), 382–384.

Hayslip, B., & Kaminski, P. L. (2005). Grandparents raising their grandchildren. In R. K. Caputo (Ed.), Challenges of aging in U.S. families: Policy and practice implications (pp. 147–169). New York, NY: The Haworth Press.

Hendricks, J., & Hatch, L. R. (2006). Lifestyle and aging. In R. Binstock & L. George (Eds.), Handbook of aging and the social sciences (pp. 301–319). New York, NY: Academic Press.

Hicks, J., & Kingson, E. (2009). The economic crisis: How fare older Americans. *Generations*, 33(3), 6–11.

Howden, L. M., & Meyer, J. A. (2011). *Age and sex composition: 2010. 2010 Census Briefs*. Washington, DC: U.S. Department of Commerce.

Johnson, K., & Wilson, K. (2010). *Current economic status of older adults in the United States: A demographic analysis*. Washington, DC: National Council on Aging (NCOA). Retrieved from http://www.ncoa.org/assets/files/pdf/Economic-Security-Trends-for-Older-Adults-65-and-Older_March-2010.pdf

Kahn, R. L. (2003). Successful aging: Intended and unintended consequences of a concept. In L. W. Poon, S. H. Gueldner, & B. M. Sprouse (Eds.), *Successful aging and adaptation with chronic diseases* (pp. 55–69). New York, NY: Springer.

Kaskie, B., & Estes, C. L. (2001). Mental health services policy and the aging. Journal of Gerontological Social Work, 36(3/4), 99–114.

Kinsella, K. & He, W. (2009). *An aging world: 2008* (P95/09-1). Washington, DC: U.S. Government Printing Office.

Kropf, N., & Yoon, E. (2006). Grandparents raising grandchildren. Who are they? In B. Berkman & S. D'Ambruoso (Ed.), *Handbook of social work in health and aging* (pp. 355–362). New York, NY: Oxford University Press.

Kuhn, D., & Fulton, B. (2004). Efficacy of an educational program for relatives of persons in the early stages of Alzheimer's disease. *Journal of Gerontological Social Work*, 42, 109–130.

Lyyra, T. M., & Heikkinen, R. L. (2006). Perceived social support and mortality in older people. *Journals of Gerontology B*, 61, S147–S153.

Manton, K. G., Gu, X., & Lamb, V. L. (2006). Long-term trends in life expectancy and active life expectancy in the United States. *Population and Development Review*, 32(1), 81–106.

Manton, K. G., Gu, X., & Lowrimore, G. R. (2008). Cohort changes in active life expectancy in the U.S. elderly populating: Experiences from the 1982–2004 national long-term care survey. *Journal of Gerontology: Social Sciences*, 63B, S269–S282.

Martinson, M., & Minkler, M. (2006). Civic engagement and older adults: A critical perspective. *The Gerontologist*, 46, 318–324.

McCallion, P. (2006). Older adults as caregivers to persons with developmental disabilities. In B. Berkman & S. Ambruoso (Ed.), *Handbook of social work in health and aging* (pp. 363–370). New York, NY: Oxford University Press.

McFarland, P. L., & Sanders, S. (2003). A pilot study about the needs of older gays and lesbians: What social workers need to know. *Journal of Gerontological Social Work*, 40, 67–80.

Metlife Foundation. (2008). *New face of work survey*. Westport, CT: Author.

Metlife Mature Market Institute. (2006). *Out and aging: The Metlife study of lesbian and gay baby boomers*. Westport, CT: Author.

Mitchell, A. J., & Subramaniam, H. (2005). Prognosis of depression in old age compared to middle age: A systematic review of comparative studies. *American Journal of Psychiatry*, 162, 1588–1601.

Mittelman, M., Roth, D., Coon, D., & Haley, W. (2004). Sustained benefit of supportive intervention for depressive symptoms in caregivers of patients with Alzheimer's disease. *American Journal of Psychiatry*, 161, 850–856.

Musil, C. M., Warner, C., Zauszniewski, J., Jeanblanc, A., & Kercher, K. (2006). Grandmothers, caregiving and family functioning. *Journals of Gerontology B*, 69, 89–98.

National Alliance for Caregiving and American Association of Retired Persons (NAC & AARP). (2009). *Caregiving in the U.S.: Executive summary*. Bethesda, MD: National Alliance for Caregiving.

National Institutes of Health (NIH). (2011). *Disability in older adults*. [Fact sheet]. Retrieved from http://report.nih.gov/nihfactsheets/ViewFactSheet.aspx?csid=37.

O'Rand, A. M. (2006). Stratification and the life course. Life course capital, life course risks and social inequality. In R. Binstock & L. K. George (Eds.), *Handbook of aging and the social sciences* (6th ed., pp. 146–165). San Diego, CA: Academic Press.

Parker, D., Mills, S., & Abbey, J. (2008). Effectiveness of interventions that assist caregivers to support people with dementia living in the community: A systematic review. *Journal of Evidence-based Health, 6,* 137–172.

Pew Research Center. (2010a). *Since the start of the great recession, more children raised by grandparents.* Retrieved November 2, 2012, from http://www.pewsocialtrends.org/2010/09/09

Pew Research Center. (2010b). *The return of the multigenerational family household.* Retrieved July 15, 2011, from http://pewresearch.org/pubs/1528/multigeneratioanl-family-household.pdf

Pinquart, M., & Sorensen, S. (2006). Gender differences in caregiver stressors, social resources and health: An updated meta-analysis. *Journal of Gerontology: Psychological Sciences, 61B,* P33–P45.

Raphael, C., & Cornwell, J. L. (2008). Influencing support for caregivers. *Journal of Social Work Education, 44,* 97–103.

Reitzes, D. C., & Mutran, E. J. (2004). Grandparent identity, intergenerational identity and well-being. *Journals of Gerontology B, 59,* S213–S220.

SAGE: Services and Advocacy for GLBT Elders. (2010). *Improving the lives of LGBT older adults.* New York, NY: Author.

Sermons, M. W., & Henry, M. (2010). *Demographics of homelessness series: The rising elderly population.* Washington, DC: National Alliance to End Homelessness.

Silverstein, M., Conroy, S., Wang, H., Giarrusso, R., & Bengston, V. (2002). Reciprocity in parent–child relationships over the adult life course. *Journals of Gerontology, 57*(2), S3–S13.

Thompson, E. (2006). Being women, then lesbians, then old: Feminities, sexualities and aging. *The Gerontologist, 46,* 300–305.

Uhlenberg, P. (2004). Historical forces shaping grandparent-grandchild relationships: Demography and beyond. *Health and Medical Complete, 24,* 77.

U.S. Census Bureau. (2011a). *Births, deaths, marriages and divorces. Statistical Abstract of the United States.* Retrieved from http://www.census.gov/prod/2011pubs/12statab/vitstat.pdf

U.S. Census Bureau. (2011b). *Resident population projections by sex and age: 2010 to 2050.* Retrieved July 6, 2011, from http://www.census.gov/population/projections/

U.S. Census Bureau (2011c). *The older population: 2010. U.S. Census Brief.* Retrieved July 6, 2011, from http://www.census.gov/prod/cen2010/briefs/c2010br-09.pdf

United Nations. (2009). *World population to exceed 9 billion by 2050.* Retrieved April, 2009, from http://www.un.org/esa/population/publications/wpp2008/pressrelease.pdf

Van Houtven, C. H., & Norton, E. C. (2008). Informal care and Medicare expenditures: Testing for heterogeneous treatment effects. *Journal of Health Economics, 27,* 134–156.

Walker, A. (2009). Aging and social policy: Theorizing the social. In V. L. Bengtson, D. Gans, N. M. Putney, & M. Silverstein (Eds.), *Handbook of theories of aging* (2nd ed.). New York, NY: Springer.

Whitfield, K., Angel, J., Burton, L., & Hayward, M. (2006). Diversity, disparities and inequalities in aging: Implications for policy. *Public Policy and Aging Report, 16,* 16–22.

Williams, D. (2005). The health of U.S. racial and ethnic populations. *Journals of Gerontology B, 60,* 53–62.

World Health Organization (WHO). (2002, April). Active aging: A policy framework. Paper presented at the second United Nations World Assembly on Aging, Madrid, Spain.

Wray, S. (2003). Women growing older: Agency, ethnicity and culture. *Sociology, 37,* 511–527.

Zarit, S. H. (2009). A good old age: Theories of mental health and aging. In V. L. Bengtson, M. Silverstein, N. M. Putney, & D. Gans (Eds.), *Handbook of theories of aging.* New York, NY: Springer.

Zarit, S., & Femia, E. (2008). Behavioral and psychosocial interventions for family caregivers. *American Journal of Nursing, 108,* 47–53.

Zodikoff, B. D. (2006). Services for lesbian, gay, bisexual and transgender older adults. In B. Berkman & S. D'Ambruoso (Ed.), *Handbook of social work in health and aging* (pp. 569–576). New York, NY: Oxford University Press.

FURTHER READING

Administration on Aging: http://www.aoa.gov

Alzheimer's Association: http://www.alz.org

American Society on Aging: http://www.asaging.org

Association for Gerontology Education in Social Work: http://www.agesocialwork.org

Berkman, B., & D'Ambruoso, S. (Eds.). (2006). *Handbook of social work in health and aging.* New York, NY: Oxford University Press.

Cox, C. (Ed.). (2007). *Dementia and social work practice: Research and interventions.* New York, NY: Springer.

Family Caregiver Alliance: http://www.caregiver.org

Gerontological Society of America: http://www.geron.org

Greene, R., Cohen, H., Galambos, C., & Kropf, N. (2007). *Foundations of social work practice in the field of aging: A competency-based approach.* Washington, DC: National Association of Social Workers.

Hooyman, N., & Kiyak, A. (2011). *Social gerontology: A multidisciplinary perspective* (9th ed.). Boston, MA: Pearson.

John A. Hartford Foundation: http://www.jhartfound.org

Geriatric Social Work Initiative: http://www.gswi.org

McInnis-Dittrich, K. (2002). *Social work with elders: A biopsychosocial approach to assessment and intervention.* Boston, MA: Allyn & Bacon.

National Alliance for Caregiving: http://www.caregiving.org/

Richardson, V., & Barusch, A. (2006). *Gerontological practice for the twenty-first century. A social work perspective.* New York, NY: Columbia University Press.

U.S. Census Bureau News. (2011). *Facts for features: Older Americans month: May 2011.* Retrieved July 31, 2011, from http://www.census.gov/newsroom/releases/pdf/cb11-ff08_olderamericans.pdf

NANCY R. HOOYMAN

ALCOHOL AND DRUG PROBLEMS: OVERVIEW

ABSTRACT: Social workers commonly encounter individuals and families that have problems resulting from alcohol and other drug (AOD) misuse, abuse, and dependence. This entry provides an overview of AOD problems in the general population and within such subpopulations as young people, the elderly, women, ethnic and racial minorities, and the gay and lesbian community. Clinical and policy responses to these problems in the United States, the roles of social workers in this field, and directions for the future are addressed.

KEY WORDS: substance abuse; alcohol and other drugs; AOD treatment; policy issues; impact on family; social work role

Problems resulting from AOD misuse, abuse, and dependence affect individuals, families, communities, and society as a whole. It is critical, therefore, that all social workers have some familiarity with the various substances of abuse and with relevant clinical and policy issues. Due to space limitations, treatment and policy issues related to tobacco use are not included.

Definition of Terms

Millions of Americans use alcohol, tobacco, or other drugs (ATOD), but most do not experience any negative consequences. It is therefore helpful to conceptualize ATOD use on a continuum from non-problematic experimental and social *use* to substance *misuse* (such as using pain medication in order to get high) to *abuse*, which indicates problematic use that affects individuals and their relationships, and finally, to *dependence or addiction*, which implies compulsive use that may require medically supervised detoxification and/or formal treatment to abstain or curtail use (Straussner, 2004).

Many substances tend to be abused. They include those that are legally obtained, such as alcohol, tobacco, and caffeine; prescription medications (for example, OxyContin, Vicodin, Ritalin, and Adderall); various forms of inhalants (for example, glue, paint, and aerosols); and illicit drugs, such as marijuana, heroin, cocaine or crack, methamphetamine (known as "ice" or "crystal meth"); and hallucinogens (for example, LSD, PCP, and psylocybin mushrooms). Anabolic steroids and "designer" (synthetically produced compounds that mimic other psychoactive substances) or "club" drugs, such as MDMA (that is, Ecstasy), GHB, or Rohypnol ("the date-rape" drug) are often misused or abused, particularly by adolescents (Substance Abuse and Mental Health Services Administration [SAMHSA], 2005).

The most recent American Psychiatric Association's (APA, 2000) *Diagnostic and Statistical Manual of Mental Disorders* (DSM IV-TR) uses the term *substance-related disorders* (SRD) to classify all disorders related to problematic consequences of substance use. The SRD category is further divided into *Substance-Induced Disorders* (SID) and *Substance Use Disorders* (SUD). SID includes 11 different disorders ranging from substance intoxication or withdrawal symptoms to substance induced mood, anxiety, psychotic, or sleeping disorders. It is assumed that once a person stops their abuse or dependence on a substance, SIDs will disappear within a relatively short time. Individuals whose psychiatric symptoms do not disappear over time are likely to have additional diagnoses, variously referred to as having coexisting, co-occurring, or comorbid substance and mental disorders.

SUD consists of two subcategories: *substance abuse* and *substance dependence*. *Substance abuse* is defined as "a maladaptive pattern of substance use leading to clinically significant impairment or distress" in *one or more* of the following within a 12-month time frame: the continued use of psychoactive substances despite experiencing social, occupational, psychological, or physical problems; inability to fulfill "major role obligations at work, school, or home"; recurrent use in situations in which use is physically hazardous, such as driving while intoxicated; and/or recurrent legal problems related to the use of a substance (APA, 2000, pp. 114–115). *Substance dependence* is defined as the existence of *at least three* of the following 7 symptoms within a 12-month period:

1. Tolerance, as defined by either a need for increased amounts of a substance to achieve a desired effect or diminished effect with use of the same quantity of substances
2. Withdrawal, as characterized by specific withdrawal syndromes, or using a substance in order to relieve or avoid withdrawal symptoms
3. Taking the substance in larger amounts or over a longer period than was intended
4. A persistent desire or unsuccessful efforts to reduce or control use
5. A great deal of time spent obtaining, using, and recovering from substance use
6. Important social, occupational, or recreational activities are given up or reduced because of the use of the substance

7. Continued substance use despite knowledge of resulting serious physical or psychological problems

Once diagnosed with substance dependence, an individual can never be diagnosed with the less severe diagnosis of substance abuse. A substance abuse or dependence diagnosis also calls for one of six "course specifiers" delineating the longer-term outcome of these disorders. These specifiers can only be given *after* the individual stops using a given substance for at least *1 month*. They include (1) *early full remission*, defined as being substance-free for more than 1 month, but less than 12 months; (2) *early partial remission*, where the individual resumes some use of a substance (sometimes referred to as having a "relapse"), and subsequently meets at least one criterion of abuse or dependence within the first year of recovery; (3) *sustained full remission*, defined as being substance-free for more than 1 year; and (4) *sustained partial remission*, in which the individual resumes substance use after 12 months of not having any symptoms, and then meets at least one criterion of substance abuse or dependence. The two final specifiers are (5) *on agonist therapy*, which is used when the individual is placed on an agonist medication (that mimics the action of a naturally occurring substance) or antagonist (that acts against and blocks an action) medication to treat the substance of choice, such as using methadone as a replacement for opiates; and (6) *in a controlled environment*, indicating that the individual is residing in a substance-free environment, such as a therapeutic community or prison.

The Scope and Impact of Substance Abuse Problems

Substance abuse causes more deaths, illnesses, accidents, and disabilities than any other preventable health problem (Robert Wood Johnson Foundation [RWJ], 2001). Worldwide, the use of substances is increasing most dramatically in low-income countries, which in the coming decades are expected to suffer from a disproportionate burden of substance-related disability and premature death (Anderson, 2006). According to research done for the World Health Organization, during the year 2000, tobacco was the number one addiction problem in the world, responsible for 4.9 million deaths, while an estimated 1.8 million people die annually due to alcohol-related problems; illegal drugs cause 223,000 deaths. However, over the past decade, "alcohol has become the number one risk factor in developing countries...above tobacco" (News in Science, 2003).

In the United States, according to 2005 data, an estimated 22.2 million persons (9.1% of the population aged 12 or older) were classified as abusing or dependent on a substance. Of these, 15.4 million were dependent on or abused alcohol, 3.6 million abused or were dependent on illicit drugs, and 3.3 million were classified with dependence on or abuse of both alcohol and illicit drugs (SAMHSA, 2005). An estimated 60.5 million persons or 24.9% of the population are current cigarette smokers (SAMHSA, 2006). It is expected that smoking will result in approximately 440,000 deaths each year, and an additional 8.6 million people will have at least one serious illness caused by smoking (Collins, 2005).

While the magnitude of alcohol problems has been overshadowed by the political and media preoccupation with illicit drugs, it is important to note that the consequences of alcohol-related problems are more devastating and widespread for both individuals and society.

ALCOHOL-RELATED PROBLEMS

1. Alcohol contributes to close to 100,000 U.S. deaths annually from drunk driving, stroke, cancer, cirrhosis of the liver, falls, and other adverse effects (Mokdad, Marks, Stroup, & Gerberding, 2004).
2. Nearly half of all violent deaths (accidents, suicides, and homicides), particularly of men below age 34, are alcohol related (RWJ, 2001).
3. Alcohol is a consistent factor in reports of child physical and sexual abuse, including incest, and in cases of rape and domestic violence (Isralowitz, 2004; RWJ, 2001).
4. Between 53% and 73% of homeless adults are affected by an alcohol disorder (Podymow, Turnbull, Coyle, Yetisir, & Wells, 2006).

DRUG-RELATED PROBLEMS

The 6.8 million persons aged 12 or older classified as abusing or dependent on *illicit* drugs use a wide variety of substances including heroin, methamphetamines, inhalants, sedative-hypnotics, and designer drugs such as Ecstasy. The largest number of individuals, however, use marijuana (4.1 million), followed by cocaine (1.5 million), and narcotic or opioid pain relievers, such as OxyContin (1.5 million) (SAMHSA, 2005).

Injecting drugs, such as heroin, with a contaminated needle leads to high risk of becoming infected with HIV and of developing AIDS. Having sex with an HIV-infected individual is also a high risk factor for HIV/AIDS. This mode of HIV transmission has become especially detrimental for women: Since the epidemic began, 58% of all AIDS cases in women have been attributed to injection drug use or sex with partners who inject drugs, compared with 34% in men. The transmission of HIV through drug injection or sex with an infected individual is disproportionally high among black and Hispanic men and women (Centers for Disease Control and Prevention [CDC], 2006).

Substance Abuse Problems Among Special Populations

Substance abuse and dependence vary according to age and gender, ethnic and racial factors, as well as sexual orientation.

SUBSTANCE ABUSE BY YOUTH Unlike the relatively constant rate of alcohol and drug abuse by adults over the years, young people's substance use has fluctuated over time, reflecting the availability of particular substances and their popularity among certain subgroups; some of the variation reported is also attributable to changes in government data collection methods (Straussner, 2004). After a relatively high use of illicit substances by young people in the 1960s and 1970s, the proportion of high-school and college students using any illicit drug has decreased significantly, with the exception of prescription opioids abuse (National Institute on Drug Abuse [NIDA], 2006). Currently, the most frequently abused substances by young people are alcohol, marijuana, the so-called club drugs, such as Ecstasy, and the nonmedical use of the pain reliever, Vicodin (NIDA, 2006).

The heavy use of alcohol by young people is often viewed as a "gateway" to other drugs; research studies have showed that among heavy drinking youths, 66% were also current illicit drug users, compared to only 4.2% nondrinkers who were current illicit drug users (RWJ, 2001). In addition, there is growing evidence of an association between young age of first use of alcohol or other drugs and problematic use of these substances during adulthood (SAMHSA, 2005). According to the RWJ (2001), "More than 40 percent of those who started drinking at age 14 or younger developed alcohol dependence, compared with 10 percent of those who began drinking at age 20 or older. High school students who use illicit drugs are also more likely to experience difficulties in school, in their personal relationships, and in their mental and physical health" (p. 30). Thus there is a growing focus on prevention programs aimed at postponing the age of initiation of drug use.

SUBSTANCE ABUSE BY OLDER ADULTS Compared to the general population, substance abuse problems are less common among older adults. However, the number of elderly persons who misuse or abuse illicit drugs and alcohol is increasing. This is due to the growing number of aging baby boomers who tend to have a history of higher rates of alcohol use, as well as abuse and misuse of prescription and over-the-counter medications (Bogunovic, Shelly, & Greenfield, 2004).

GENDER AND SUBSTANCE ABUSE Studies in the early twenty-first century show that adult males are about twice as likely to be classified with substance dependence or abuse as females (12.0% versus 6.4%) (SAMHSA, 2005). However, the rates of nonmedical use of psychotherapeutic drugs (pain relievers, tranquilizers, stimulants, and sedatives) were similar for both males and females (1.8% versus 1.7%, respectively) (RWJ, 2001). Gender differences in substance dependence are diminishing among young people, portending a growing substance abuse problem among younger women as they age (SAMHSA, 2006).

While there are numerous issues unique to substance abusing women (see Straussner & Brown, 2002), one important aspect is the impact of their substance use on their children. Although studies show that most women tend to reduce their substance use during pregnancy (SAMHSA, 2005), some women, especially those dependent on alcohol, crack cocaine, or methamphetamine, continue their substance use (Sampson et al., 1998). These substances are then transmitted to the fetus resulting in a child who may be born addicted and/or who may suffer permanent brain or other physiological damage (Azmitia, 2001).

It is important to keep in mind that the impact of fetal exposure to AOD is determined by many factors, including the type of substance, the gestation age of the fetus at exposure, the route and duration of exposure, the dosage and frequency of drug intake, other substances consumed simultaneously, as well as environmental factors including nutrition and prenatal care (Nadel & Straussner, 2006).

RACE AND ETHNICITY SUD rates vary by race and ethnicity. In 2005, the rate of substance dependence or abuse for those age 12 and over was highest among American Indians and Alaska Natives (21.0%), followed by Native Hawaiians or other Pacific Islanders (11.0%), persons reporting two or more races (10.9%), Whites (9.4%), Hispanics (9.3%), and Blacks (8.5%). The lowest rate was found among Asians (4.5%), although rates vary greatly among different Asian populations (SAMHSA, 2006; Straussner, 2001).

Studies also reveal that among young adults (aged 18–29), White males have the highest risk for alcohol problems, while among those who are middle aged and elderly rates are highest for Black men and women (Isralowitz, 2004). Socioeconomic factors also correlate with race and gender: Limited education and poverty are related to alcohol dependence in Black males but not in White males (RWJ, 2001).

SEXUAL IDENTITY There has been much controversy regarding the rates of AOD use among gay men and women. After a careful review of the literature on alcohol use, Bux (1996) lists the following four conclusions:

1. Gay men and lesbians are less likely to be abstainers from alcohol than heterosexuals.
2. Gay men appear to have little increased risk of alcoholism over heterosexual men.
3. Lesbians appear to be at higher risk than heterosexual women for alcohol abuse, and match both heterosexual and gay men in heavy and problematic drinking.
4. Gay men appear to have reduced their consumption of alcohol by the mid-1990s.

The pattern of drug use among this population is similar to that of alcohol use: Gay men have been found to be less likely to abstain from marijuana and cocaine, but have similar rates of heavy use of these substances as heterosexual men. Marijuana and cocaine use by lesbian women, however, exceeded that of heterosexual women, but was similar to that of heterosexual and gay men. Finally, the usage of drugs by older gay men and women did not decrease as much as usage among the older heterosexual population (McKirnan & Peterson, 1989).

Certain drugs have particularly high usage in the gay male community. Methamphetamine, for example, has increased dramatically among gay and bisexual men who report rates 10 times greater than the general population (Halkitis, Shrem, & Martin, 2005).

Etiology of Substance Use Disorders

There is no single etiological factor that accounts for why some people develop a SUD and others do not. Among the factors often cited in the literature are

1. *Biochemical and Genetic Factors.* Substance dependence is increasingly conceptualized as biologically and genetically based, and as a "brain disease" rather than a "moral weakness or lack of willpower" (Brain Chemicals Trump Willpower in Addicts, 2006).

2. *Familial Factors.* Early separation from one or both parents and inadequate care during childhood, as well as physical or sexual abuse during childhood are some of the familial factors contributing to substance abuse problems (Roberts, Nishimoto, & Kirk, 2003). Substance abuse has also been seen as serving as an important stabilizing force in dysfunctional families (Steinglass, Weiner, & Mendelson, 1971).

3. *Psychological Factors.* These factors encompass various perspectives, including classical and modern psychoanalytic theory, developmental and personality theories, and behavioral, conditioning, and cognitive theories (Beck, Wright, Newman, & Liese, 1993; Peele, 1998).

4. *Environmental and Sociocultural Factors.* This view links substance abuse to a variety of environmental, social, cultural, and economic factors (RWJ, 2001; Wagner & Anthony, 2002). Studies of female substance abusers, in particular those in lower socioeconomic classes, show a high correlation between their substance abuse and that of their spouses or boyfriends (Straussner & Attia, 2002).

5. *Multifactorial Perspective.* This perspective views substance abuse and dependence as resulting from a combination of factors, including biochemical, genetic, familial, environmental, and cultural ones, as well as personality dynamics. SUDs are thus seen as a multivariate syndrome in which multiple patterns of dysfunctional substance abuse occur in various types of people with varying prognoses requiring a variety of interventions (Pattison & Kaufman, 1982; Straussner, 2004).

Clinical Issues

Less than one-fourth of all individuals who need help for their abuse or dependence on alcohol or other drugs receive treatment (SAMHSA, 2005). Nonetheless, studies indicate that for those who do obtain treatment, treatment does work (RWJ, 2001). Horgan (1995) notes: "The improvement rate for people completing substance abuse treatment is comparable to that of people treated for asthma and other chronic, relapsing health conditions." During 2005, almost 4 million persons aged 12 or older (1.6% of the population) received treatment for SUD.

Clinical interventions with substance abusers, as with all clients, need to begin with a comprehensive screening and assessment followed by appropriate intervention. A growing number of social workers are using standardized screening and assessment instruments (King & Bordnick, 2002). Among the most frequently used are various versions of the CAGE for assessing alcohol problems and the CAGE-AID that assesses for other drugs (Brown & Rounds, 1995; Mayfield, McLeod, & Hall, 1974); the Substance Abuse Subtle Screening Inventory (SASSI) (Feldstein & Miller, 2007); the Michigan Alcohol Screening Test (MAST) (Selzer, 1971); the Alcohol Use Disorders Identification Test (AUDIT) (Babor et al., 1992); the Drug Abuse Screening Test (DAST); the Addiction Severity Index (ASI) (McLellan et al., 1992), and CRAFFT for assessing adolescents (Knight et al., 1999).

An important area of assessment is differentiating between substance abuse and other psychopathology. Individuals with a diagnosis of SUD may also suffer from another major psychiatric (Axis I on DSM VI-R) disorder and/or have an underlying personality disorder (Axis II) necessitating a comprehensive psychiatric assessment in addition to assessment of their substance abuse (Straussner & Nemenzik, 2007).

A comprehensive assessment must also consider the client's motivation for treatment. As a rule, substance abusers do not enter treatment voluntarily. While a highly motivated client is likely to make better use of treatment, recovery from substance abuse is not always dependent upon whether or not the initial contact with treatment was voluntary. In fact, studies show that some individuals who are coerced into treatment have as good a recovery rate as those entering treatment voluntarily (Kelly, Finney, & Moos, 2005).

Practice Interventions

An important task for social workers is to determine appropriate forms of treatment for clients with SUDs. Medically supervised *detoxification* is often the first step in the treatment of those physically addicted to opioids, alcohol, barbiturates and other sedative hypnotics, and amphetamines. It is not required for those dependent on cocaine, crack, or marijuana.

Traditionally, all detoxification had been carried out on a medical or psychiatric inpatient unit, however with the advent of managed care, it is now often provided in outpatient clinics or by physicians in private practice. Heroin addicts can be detoxified on an outpatient basis with the help of such chemicals as clonodine or decreasing doses of methadone.

Detoxification is usually only the beginning of a long process of recovery. Short- and long-term inpatient and outpatient rehabilitation programs, drug-free residential therapeutic communities, and ongoing supportive counseling can help substance abusers examine the impact of alcohol and/or other drugs upon their lives and the necessary changes in their lifestyle that they must undertake if they want to recover from substance abuse (Straussner, 2004).

The use of methadone as a substitute for opiates or narcotics can lead to better prognosis for rehabilitation and allow narcotic addicts to avail themselves of counseling and educational or vocational training; it can also help them improve the overall quality of their lives once the daily concern about obtaining drugs is alleviated (Friedman & Wilson, 2004). Moreover, the potential for becoming infected with HIV is an important factor in referring intravenous narcotic users to methadone maintenance programs. While used less extensively, opioid antagonists such as naltrexone can prevent addicts from experiencing the effects of narcotics. Unlike methadone, naltrexone has no narcotic effect of its own and is not physiologically addictive. Under the trade name of ReVia, it also is being used for people with alcohol dependence. The use of other medications, such as Acamprosate (for alcohol dependence) and buprenorphine (for opioid dependence), has been increasing (Erickson & Wilcox, 2001). A chemical that is sometimes used to help alcoholics is disulfiram, commonly known as Antabuse. This medication blocks the normal oxidation of alcohol so that acetaldehyde, a by-product of alcohol, accumulates in the bloodstream and causes unpleasant, and at times even life-threatening, symptoms, such as rapid pulse and vomiting. The use of Antabuse thus serves as a conscious deterrent to drinking. A number of substance abuse treatment settings have also incorporated nontraditional treatment approaches such as acupuncture, yoga, and meditation.

Twelve-Step Programs, such as Alcoholics Anonymous (AA), Narcotics Anonymous (NA), Pills Anonymous, and Cocaine Anonymous, have proven to be particularly helpful and are free and available in every community. These groups allow members not only to receive help but also to give help to others, thereby enhancing self-esteem (Spiegel & Fewell, 2004). Other self- or mutual-help groups for substance abusers, such as Women for Sobriety, Rational Recovery, SMART groups, Social Workers Helping Social Workers, and Double Trouble/Recovery groups for those with co-occurring mental disorders, are available in many communities.

Patients with SUDs also experience various social problems. Thus, an essential aspect of helping this population is the provision of financial and social supports, including adequate housing, vocational rehabilitation, and legal assistance.

Harm-reduction approaches, which can range from needle exchange programs to the provision of housing, social and psychological services without focusing directly on the elimination of substance use, have been increasing throughout the United States (Sieger, 2004). These approaches remain controversial since abstinence is not their primary goal.

Treatment of substance abusers must take into account the clients' ethnocultural norms and values (see Straussner, 2001), history of trauma, as well as issues of sexual behavior including safe sex practices. Treatment of minorities, particularly African Americans, needs to take into account that they are more likely to enter treatment through the courts than through formal intervention processes or 12-step programs. Also, they are more likely to access treatment much later and thus have a more difficult recovery process (O'Connell, 1991). Lastly, it is important to remember that substance abuse, "like many other medical problems, is a chronic disorder in which recurrences are common and repeated periods of treatment are frequently required" (U.S. Department of Health and Human Services [USDHHS], 1991, p. 4).

Impact of Substance Abuse on the Family

Between 9% and 29% of all children in the United States are exposed to familial drug or alcohol abuse (SAMHSA, 2003). While many children from substance abusing families are highly resilient and do not exhibit blatant problems (Peleg-Oren & Teichman, 2006; Werner & Johnson, 2000), research indicates that a large number are at risk of developing a variety of physical, psychological, and social problems (Anda et al., 2002; Gruber & Taylor, 2006; Johnson & Leff, 1999).

Child neglect and, in more disturbed families, violence between parents, child abuse, and incest are some of the consequences and correlates of substance abuse. Substance abuse is present in at least two-thirds of the families known to public child welfare agencies (Hampton, Senatore, & Gullotta, 1998). Studies highlight the need to address the intergenerational cycle of substance abuse and child abuse if effective progress is to be made on either problem. During 2006, expert panels of social work educators, practitioners, and researchers, working under the auspices of the National Association for Children of Alcoholics (NACoA) and chaired by one of the authors (Straussner), developed a set of core competencies needed by social workers in order

to work effectively with this population (NACoA, 2006).

Couples and family therapy, including multifamily groups, are effective modalities for families with substance abusers who are already chemically free or working on their recovery. One evidence-based family-oriented treatment approach is Community Reinforcement and Family Training (CRAFT) (Miller, Meyers, & Tonigan, 1999). It is also beneficial to refer family members to such mutual-help groups as Al-Anon, Pill-Anon, Co-Anon, or Nar-Anon. These groups help adult family members examine their own role in the "enabling" behavior. There are also support groups for adolescent children of alcohol- and narcotic-abusing parents, such as Alateen and Narateen. Adult Children of Alcoholics (ACOA) groups may be helpful for mature adolescents and adult children of alcoholics.

Policy History

Treatment programs and practices are driven not only by clinical needs, but also by social policies. Substance abuse policies in the United States are generally consistent with prevailing ideology and tend to parallel public attitudes, and not necessarily the prevalence of a particular substance (Isralowitz, 2004). For example, in Colonial America and the early 1800s, drinking and even drunkenness were seen as acceptable behaviors. It was only during the latter part of the nineteenth century that any use of alcohol was perceived as problematic, resulting in the growth of the temperance movement. At the same time, during the 1800s, opiates and cocaine were legal and used widely, particularly as patent medicine by middle-class women (Straussner & Attia, 2002).

Beginning in 1906 the Pure Food and Drug Act, the Harrison Narcotic Act of 1914, the Volstead Act that ushered in Prohibition in 1919, and the 1937 Marijuana Tax Act led to public policies that criminalized the users of various substances while at the same time limiting their access to medical treatment (Isralowitz, 2004). Following the repeal of Prohibition in 1933, the social use of alcohol once again became widely acceptable, while problematic alcohol use was seen as a sign of an individual's shortcoming (Nadel & Straussner, 2006).

The passage of the Hughes Act in 1970, authorizing the establishment of the National Institute on Alcohol Abuse and Alcoholism (NIAAA) and the National Institute on Drug Abuse (NIDA), had a profound impact on the treatment of both drug and alcohol abusers. It provided the impetus for the decriminalization of public drunkenness; increased federal funding for substance abuse research and model treatment programs; and prompted coverage by health insurance companies for AOD treatment.

Faced with growing drug use among young people and concern about heroin-addicted servicemen returning from Vietnam, on June 17, 1971, President Nixon declared that drugs were America's number one enemy, marking the start of the United States' "War on Drugs." Nixon appointed Dr. Jerome Jaffe to head the new Special Office for Drug Abuse Prevention. Between 1971 and 1973, Jaffe developed a network of methadone treatment facilities all over the United States, and in 1973, the Drug Enforcement Administration (DEA), whose mission was to fight the drug war, was established (Frontline: Interview with Dr. Jerome Jaffe, n.d.)

In 1988, under the Reagan administration, the Office of National Drug Control Policy (ONDCP) was created to coordinate drug-related legislation, security, research, and health policy throughout the government. The director of ONDCP, commonly known as the Drug Czar, was raised to cabinet-level status by Bill Clinton in 1993 (A History of the War on Drugs, n.d.).

Other important legislation has been the passage of the 1997 Adoption and Safe Families Act (ASFA) [P.L. 105–8.9] that addressed the need for children in out-of-home placements to have a permanent home. Child protection workers are mandated to terminate clients' parental rights and free their children for adoption if substance abusing parents/caregivers do not improve within 15 months. Although ASFA identified the need for addiction treatment, few new resources have been provided to meet this need (Gustavsson & MacEachron, 1997).

Current federal policy efforts, under the auspices of The White House ONDCP and the Substance Abuse Mental Health Service Administration (SAMHSA), may be conceptualized as consisting of a three-pronged approach: domestic and international law enforcement, or interdiction, focusing on the "supply" of drugs to the United States public; and two approaches addressing the "demand" side: (1) drug prevention and prevention research and (2) drug treatment and treatment research (Nadel & Straussner, 2006).

The "Supply-Side" approach tries to prevent drugs from reaching U.S. consumers and focuses on foreign crop eradication, border and marine interdiction, and arrests of distributors and drug dealers. These programs claim the largest percentage of the federal substance-abuse budget—more than the other two areas combined (Veillette, 2006). Substance abuse

prevention and treatment, the "demand-side," seeks to prevent or decrease the use of drugs through various education/prevention activities, treatment programs, and research on treatment effectiveness and program evaluation (Nadel & Straussner, 2006).

Roles of Social Workers

Despite the historically limited focus on substance abuse education in schools of social work (Amodeo & Litchfield, 1999; Straussner & Senreich, 2002), social workers in the United States have always been involved with addicted individuals and their families. As early as 1917, Mary Richmond, one of the founders of social work, rejected the moral definition of alcoholism of her day with its characteristic view of alcoholics as "sinners." In her groundbreaking book, Social Diagnosis, Richmond (1917) stated that "inebriety is a disease" and provided a description that is entirely consistent with the disease model of alcoholism as described almost half a century later by Jellinek (1952) and reflected in the latest version of the APA's (2000) DSM IV-TR. Richmond viewed social workers as having an "important role to play in gathering the pertinent social data," offering the assistance necessary to supplement the medical treatment, and "providing the long period of after-care which is usually necessary" (Richmond, 1917/1944, p. 430).

Currently, social workers contribute greatly to the field of addictions. The profession's unique biopsychosocial perspective, its flexibility in adapting to new streams of thought and incorporating them into practice, and its ability to integrate disparate programming into a systemic whole make it a profession extremely well suited to the ever changing field of addictions. Thus, social workers are important players in program development, organizing community collaborations, administration, and treatment of substance abusers and their families, and are increasingly involved in addictions research, education, and policy development. Concern regarding the spread of HIV and AIDS among their clients has led many social workers to become active in the growing harm-reduction movement and in various prevention programs.

As the largest group of mental health professionals in the United States, all social workers must become knowledgeable about screening, assessment, motivational interviewing, treatment, and referrals of those with substance abuse problems. They also need to have a much greater role in primary and secondary prevention. The currently diminished role of social workers with families of substance abusers resulting from the lack of managed care payments for such services calls for greater advocacy in this area and for greater innovative practices to help families. Finally, social workers need to demand federal and state drug policies that are more equitable and effective in addressing this tremendous individual, familial, and social problem.

Current health insurance benefits for substance abuse treatment are unequal to mandated medical insurance for other medical and mental health conditions. This lack of parity continues to be a serious concern as it excludes many from needed substance abuse treatment. The lack of insurance coverage is partly responsible for the ethnic treatment disparities with African Americans less likely than Whites to have access to substance abuse or mental health care (25.4% versus 12.5%), and with Hispanics receiving delayed or less care than Whites (22.7% versus 10.7%) (Wells, Klap, Koike, & Sherbourne, 2001).

Another challenge for social workers is addressing the impact of drug-related arrests. The United States has the highest incarceration rate in the world. As of 2006, a record 7 million people were behind bars, on probation, or on parole (compared with second-ranked China, with 1.5 million people). At the end of 2003, federal prisons held a total of 158,426 inmates, the majority (55%) of whom were drug offenders. It is important to note that more than two-thirds (70%) of the 260,000 people in state prisons serving time for nonviolent drug-related charges are Black or Latino (Huffington, 2007), vastly over-representing their numbers in the general populations.

Trends and Future Directions

The field of substance abuse or addictions is constantly evolving with new substances of abuse, new populations to treat, new treatment approaches, and changing policies. An important current issue is the incorporation of *evidence-based practice* (EBP). The harm reduction movement, well established in most of western Europe, Canada, and Australia, appears to be growing rapidly in the United States, although how it will be incorporated within traditional AOD treatment facilities in this country remains to be seen.

From an international perspective, illicit substance use and its consequences (for example, crime and violence, military and police intervention, lost work, family destruction, property confiscation, and massive allocations of funding resources for treatment and health maintenance) constitute a major public concern. For the drug trade, nationalities and borders do not exist, and its negative impact on individuals and communities in the United States, as well as on our public policies will continue to be an issue for social workers in the future (Isralowitz, 2004).

REFERENCES

A History of the War on Drugs (n.d). Retrieved November 5, 2007, from http://faculty.ncwc.edu/toconnor/pol/495lect03.htm

Amodeo, M., & Litchfield, L. (1999). Integrating substance abuse content into social work courses: Effects of intensive faculty training. *Substance Abuse, 20*(1), 5–16.

American Psychiatric Association. (2000). *Diagnostic and statistical manual of mental disorders* (Rev. 4th ed.). Washington, DC: Author.

Anda, R. F., Whitfield, C. L., Felitti, V. J., Chapman, D., Edwards, V. J., Dube, S. R., et al. (2002). Adverse childhood experiences, alcoholic parents, and later risk of alcoholism and depression. *Psychiatric Services, 53*(8), 1001–1009.

Anderson, P. (2006). Global use of alcohol, drugs and tobacco. *Drug and Alcohol Review, 25*, 489–502.

Azmitia, E. C. (2001). Impact of drugs and alcohol on the brain through the life cycle: Knowledge for social workers. *Journal of Social Work Practice in the Addictions, 1*(3), 41–63.

Babor, T. F., de la Fuente, J. R., Saunders, J., & Grant, M. (1992). AUDIT: *The alcohol use disorders identification tests: Guidelines for use in primary health care.* Geneva, Switzerland: World Health Organization.

Beck, A. T., Wright, F. D., Newman, D. F., & Liese, B. S. (1993). *Cognitive therapy of substance abuse.* New York: Guilford.

Bogunovic, O. J., Shelly, F., & Greenfield, S. F. (2004). Practical geriatrics: Use of benzodiazepines among elderly patients. *Psychiatric Services, 55*, 233–235.

Brain Chemicals Trump Willpower in Addicts, NIDA Director Says (2006, April 4) Retrieved January 5, 2007, from http://www.drugfree.org/join-together/addiction/brain-chemicals-trump.

Brown, R. L., & Rounds, L. A. (1995). Conjoint screening questionnaires for alcohol and drug abuse. *Wisconsin Medical Journal, 94*, 135–140.

Bux, D. A. (1996). The epidemiology of problem drinking in gay men and lesbians: A critical review. *Clinical Psychology Review, 16*, 277–298.

Centers for Disease Control and Prevention (2006, February 1). Trends among IDUs. Retrieved January 30, 2007, from http://www.cdc.gov/hiv/resources/reports/hiv3rddecade/chapter4.htm

Collins, J. L. (2005). The director's perspective: The challenge and promise of tobacco control. Retrieved November 5, 2007, from http://www.cdc.gov/nccdphp/publications/cdnr/pdf/CDNRDec05.pdf

Erickson, C. K., & Wilcox, R. E. (2001). Neurobiological causes of addictions. *Journal of Social Work Practice in the Addictions, 1*(3), 7–22.

Feldstein, S. W., & Miller, W. R. (2007). Does subtle screening for substance abuse work? A review of the substance abuse subtle screening inventory (SASSI). *Addiction, 102*(1), 41.

Friedman, E. G., & Wilson, R. (2004). Treatment of opiate addictions. In S. L. A. Straussner (Ed.), *Clinical work with substance abusing clients* (2nd ed., pp. 187–208). New York: Guilford Press.

Frontline: Interview with Dr. Jerome Jaffe (n.d.). Retrieved October 30, 2007, from http://www.pbs.org/wgbh/pages/frontline/shows/drugs/interviews/jaffe.html

Gruber, K. J., & Taylor, M. F. (2006). A family perspective for substance abuse: Implications from the literature. *Journal of Social Work Practice in the Addictions, 6* (1/2), 1–30.

Gustavsson, N. S., & MacEachron, A. E. (1997). Criminalizing women's behavior. *Journal of Drug Issues, 27,* 673–687.

Halkitis, P. N., Shrem, M. T., & Martin, F. W. (2005). Sexual behavior patterns of methamphetamine-using gay and bisexual men. *Substance Use & Misuse, 40,* 703–719.

Hampton, R. L., Senatore, V., & Gullotta, T. (Eds.). (1998). *Substance abuse, family violence and child welfare: Bridging perspectives.* Thousand Oaks, CA: Sage.

Horgan, C. M. (1995, Spring). Cost of untreated substance abuse to society. *The Communique.* Rockville, MD: Center for Substance Abuse Treatment.

Huffington, A. (2007). The war on drugs' war on minorities. Retrieved November 5, 2007, from http://www.latimes.com/news/opinion/commentary/la-oe-huffington24mar24,0,175250,print.story?coll=la-home-commentary

Isralowitz, R. (2004). *Drug use.* Santa Barbara, CA: ABC-CLIO.

Jellinek, E. M. (1952). Phases of alcohol addiction. *Quarterly Journal of Studies on Alcohol, 13,* 673–684.

Johnson, J. L., & Leff, M. (1999). Children of substance abusers: Overview of research findings. *Pediatrics, 103* (Suppl. 5), 1085–1099.

Kelly, J. F., Finney, J. W., & Moos, R. (2005). Substance use disorder patients who are mandated to treatment: Characteristics, treatment process, and 1- and 5-year outcomes. *Journal of Substance Abuse Treatment, 28*(3), 213–223.

King, M. E., & Bordnick, P. S. (2002). Alcohol use disorders: A social worker's guide to clinical assessment. *Journal of Social Work Practice in the Addictions, 2*(1), 3–32.

Knight, J. R., Shrier, L. A., Bravender, T. D., Farrel, M., Vander Bilt, J., & Shaffer, H. J. (1999). A new brief screen for adolescent substance abuse. *Archives of Pediatric Adolescent Medicine, 153,* 591–596.

Mayfield, D., McLeod, G. N., & Hall, P. (1974). The CAGE questionnaire: Validation of a new alcoholism screening instrument. *American Journal of Psychiatry, 131*(10), 1121–1123.

McLellan, A. T., Kushner, H., Peters, F., Smith, I., Corse, S. J., & Alterman, A. I. (1992). The addiction severity index ten years later. *Journal of Substance Abuse Treatment, 9,* 199–213.

Miller, W. R., Meyers, R. J., & Tonigan, J. S. (1999). Engaging the unmotivated in treatment for alcohol problems: A comparison of three strategies for intervention through family members. *Journal of Consulting and Clinical Psychology, 67,* 688–697.

Mokdad, A. H., Marks, J. S., Stroup, D. F., & Gerberding, J. L. (2004). Actual causes of death in the United States, 2000. *Journal of American Medical Association, 291*(10), 1238–1245.

Nadel, M., & Straussner, S. L. A. (2006). Children in substance-abusing families. In N. K. Phillips & S. L. A. Straussner (Eds.), *Children in the urban environment: Linking social policy and clinical practice* (2nd ed., pp 169–190). Springfield, IL: Charles C. Thomas.

National Association of Children of Alcoholics. (2006). Core competencies for social workers in addressing the needs of children of alcohol and drug dependent parents. Retrieved from http://www.nacoa.org/pdfs/SW_report_web.pdf.

National Institute on Drug Abuse. (2006). *NIDA Infofacts: High school and youth trends.* Retrieved, July 5, 2007, from http://www.drugabuse.gov/infofacts/HSYouthtrends.html

News in Science. (2003). Tobacco, alcohol, drugs killing 7 million a year. Retrieved February 10, 2006, from http://www.abc.net.au/science/news/stories/2003/792982.htm

O'Connell, T. (1991). Treatment of minorities. *Drug and Alcohol Dependence, 15*(10), 13.

Pattison, E. M., & Kaufman, E. (1982). Alcoholism syndrome, definition and models. In E. M. Pattison & E. Kaufman (Eds.), *Encyclopedic handbook of alcoholism.* New York: Gardner.

Peele, S. (1998). *The meaning of addiction* (2nd ed.). San Francisco: Jossey-Bass.

Peleg-Oren, N., & Teichman, M. (2006). Young children of parents with substance use disorders (SUD): A review of the literature and implications for social work practice. *Journal of Social Work Practice in the Addictions, 6*(1/2), 49–62.

Podymow, T., Turnbull, J., Coyle, D., Yetisir, E., & Wells, G. (2006). Shelter-based managed alcohol administration to chronically homeless people addicted to alcohol. *Canadian Medical Association Journal, 174*(1), 45–49.

Richmond, M. E. (1917/1944). *Social diagnosis.* New York: The Free Press.

Robert Wood Johnson Foundation (RWJ) (2001, March 9). *Substance abuse: The nation's number one health problem.* Princeton, NJ: The Robert Wood Johnson Foundation, Substance Abuse Resource Center.

Roberts, A. C., Nishimoto, R., & Kirk, R. S. (2003). Cocaine abusing women who report sexual abuse: Implications for treatment. *Journal of Social Work Practice in the Addictions, 3*(1), 5–24.

Sampson, P. D., Ann, P., Streissguth, A. P., Bookstein, F. L., Little, R. E., Clarren, S. K., et al. (1998). Incidence of fetal alcohol syndrome and prevalence of alcohol-related neurodevelopmental disorder. *Teratology, 56*(5) 317–326.

Selzer, M. L. (1971). Michigan alcohol screening test: The quest for a new diagnostic. *American Journal of Psychiatry*, 127, 1653–1658.

Sieger, B. H. (2004). The clinical practice of harm reduction. In S. L. A. Straussner (Ed.), *Clinical work with substance abusing clients* (2nd ed., pp. 65–81). New York: Guilford.

Spiegel, B. R., & Fewell, C. H. (2004). 12-Step programs as a treatment modality. In S. L. A. Straussner (Ed.), *Clinical work with substance abusing clients* (2nd ed., pp. 125–145). New York: Guilford.

Steinglass, P., Weiner, S., & Mendelson, H. (1971). A systems approach to alcoholism: A model and its clinical application. *Archives of General Psychiatry*, 24, 401–408.

Straussner, S. L. A. (Ed.). (2001). *Ethnocultural factors in the treatment of addictions*. New York: Guilford.

Straussner, S. L. A. (2004). Assessment and treatment of clients with alcohol and other drug abuse problems: An overview. In S. L. A. Straussner (Ed.), *Clinical work with substance abusing clients* (2nd ed., pp. 3–35). New York: Guilford.

Straussner, S. L. A., & Attia, P. R. (2002). Women's addiction and treatment through a historical lens. In S. L. A. Straussner & S. Brown (Ed.), *The handbook of addictions treatment for women* (pp. 3–25). San Francisco: Jossey-Bass.

Straussner, S. L. A., & Brown, S. (Ed.). (2002). *The handbook of addiction treatment for women*. San Francisco: Jossey Bass.

Straussner, S. L. A., & Nemenzik, J. M. (2007). Co-occurring substance use and personality disorders: Current thinking on etiology, diagnosis and treatment. *Journal of Social Work Practice in Addictions*, 7(1–2), 5–23.

Straussner, S. L. A., & Senreich, E. (2002). Educating social workers to work with individuals affected by substance use disorders. *Substance Abuse*, 23(Suppl. 3), 319–340.

Substance Abuse and Mental Health Services Administration. (2003). *National household survey on drug abuse report: Children living with substance-abusing or substance dependent parents* [Electronic version]. Rockville, MD: Author. Retrieved December 26, 2006, from http://www.drugabusestatistics.samhsa.gov/2k3/children/children.cfm

Substance Abuse and Mental Health Services Administration. (2005). *National survey of substance abuse treatment services, 2002–2005* (Office of Applied Statistics, Substance Abuse and Mental Health Services Administration). Rockville, MD: Author.

Substance Abuse and Mental Health Services Administration [SAMHSA]. (2006). *Results from the 2005 national survey on drug use and health: national findings* (Office of Applied Studies, NSDUH Series H-30, DHHS Publication No. SMA 06-4194). Rockville, MD: Author.

U.S. Department of Health and Human Services. (1991). *Drug abuse and drug abuse research: The third triennial report to congress from the secretary, DHHS*. Washington, DC: U.S. Government Printing Office.

Veillette, C. (2006). Andean Counter Drug Initiative (ACI) and related funding programs: FY 2006 Assistance. Congressional Research Service, the Library of Congress. Retrieved February 10, 2006, from http://fpc.state.gov/documents/organization/60720.pdf

Wagner, F. A., & Anthony, J. C. (2002). Into the world of illegal drug use: Exposure opportunity and other mechanisms linking the use of alcohol, tobacco, marijuana, and cocaine. *American Journal of Epidemiology*, 155, 918–925.

Wells, K., Klap, R., Koike, A., & Sherbourne, C. (2001). Ethnic disparities in unmet need for alcoholism, drug abuse, and mental health care. *American Journal of Psychiatry*, 158, 2027–2032.

Werner, E. E., & Johnson, J. L. (2000). The role of caring adults in the lives of children of alcoholics. In S. Abbott (Ed.), *Children of alcoholics: Selected readings* (Vol. 2, pp. 119–141). Rockville, MD: National Association of Children of Alcoholics.

FURTHER READING

Bowman, L., Hoffman, L., & Bowman, T. (2007, January 24). Boomer doom: Falling victim to the culture of youth. Scripps News. Retrieved February 10, 2007, from http://www.scrippsnews.com/node/18878

Centers for Disease Control and Prevention. (1996). *HIV/AIDS Surveillance Report*, 8(2). Atlanta, GA: Author.

Ellis, A., McInterney, J. F., DiGiuseppe, R., & Yeager, R. J. (1988). *Rational emotive therapy with alcoholics and substance abusers*. New York: Pergamon Press.

Freud, S. (1954). Letter 79, December 22, 1897. In M. Bonaparte, A. Freud, & E. Kris (Eds.), E. Mosbacher & J. Strachey, (Trans.), *The origins of psycho-analysis: Letters to Wilhelm Fliess, drafts and notes: 1887–1902*. London: Imago. (Original work published 1897.)

Grant, B. F. (2000). Estimates of US children exposed to alcohol abuse and dependence in the family. *American Journal of Public Health*, 90(1), 112–115.

Khantzian, E. J. (1981). Some treatment implications of ego and self-disturbances in alcoholism. In M. H. Bean & N. E. Zimberg (Eds.), *Dynamic approaches to the understanding and treatment of alcoholism*. New York: Free Press.

Kohut, H. (1971). *The analysis of the self: A systematic approach to the psychoanalytic treatment of narcissistic personality disorders*. New York: International Universities Press.

Kohut, H. (1977). Preface. In *Psychodynamics of drug dependence* (NIDA Research Monograph No. 12). Washington, DC: U.S. Government Printing Office.

Lawental, E., McLellan, A. T., Grissom, G. R., Brill, P., & O'Brien, C. (1996). Coerced treatment for substance abuse problems detected through workplace urine surveillance: Is it effective? *Journal of Substance Abuse*, 8(1), 115–128.

Marlatt, G. A., Baer, J. S., Donovan, D. M., & Kivlahan, D. R. (1988). Addictive behaviors: Etiology and treatment. *Annual Review of Psychology, 39,* 223–252.

Maisto, S. A., Carey, M. P., Carey, K. B., Gordon, C. M., & Gleason, J. R. (2000). Use of the AUDIT and the DAST-10 to identify alcohol and drug use disorders among adults with a severe and persistent mental illness. *Psychological Assessment, 12*(2), 186–192.

McClelland, D. C., Davis, W., Kalin, R., & Wanner, E. (1972). *The drinking man: Alcohol and human motivation.* New York: Free Press.

McKirnan, D. J., & Peterson, P. L. (1989). Alcohol and drug use among homosexual men and women: epidemiology and population characteristics. *Addictive Behaviors, 14,* 545.

SHULAMITH LALA ASHENBERG STRAUSSNER
AND RICHARD ISRALOWITZ

C

CHILD ABUSE AND NEGLECT

ABSTRACT: The true extent of child abuse and neglect is unknown but reports to state agencies indicate over 3 million cited cases concerning maltreatment of 6 million children made each year. Confirmed reports involved almost 900,000 children in 2005. Yet, less than 30% of the children known to professionals in the community (for example, teachers, physicians in emergency rooms, day care providers) as maltreated are investigated by child protective services. The perplexing dilemma in surveillance and service delivery is how to identify those that need help without spuriously including those who do not. This entry focuses on the definition of maltreatment and provides an overview of the history, etiology, and consequences of child abuse and neglect as well as the current trends and dilemmas in the field.

KEY WORDS: child abuse and neglect; child maltreatment; definitions of maltreatment; etiology of child maltreatment; consequences of child maltreatment; evidence-based practice; disproportionality; cultural competence

The World Health Organization estimates 40 million children are abused each year around the world. Estimated annual rates of child homicide vary from 6 per 100,000 in Japan to 7 per 100,000 in the United States and 25 per 100,000 in Estonia (WHO, 2001). While much can be said about differences in definitions and data collection methods among various political and geographic entities, concern regarding children's health and safety is universal. Yet any type of maltreatment short of the most severe physical battering or deprivation is often subject to wide-ranging definitions. In one comparative analysis, Freysteinsdóttir (2004) reported that parents in Iceland generally do not use physical force (a commonly cited risk factor for abuse) to discipline children. On the other hand, due to the safety of the communities there, leaving children alone at a relatively young age is commonly practiced and not regarded as maltreatment to the extent that it is in the United States. This international context sets the stage for understanding the wide-ranging differences in standards and laws within the United States as well as internationally.

History

In the Western European tradition, child protection concerns centered more on children who were orphans and paupers than on their maltreatment. Gradually attention shifted to maltreatment. By the mid- to late 1800s, agencies had been established to protect children from excessive harm in their own homes. In Philadelphia, for example, children needing out-of-home placement were described as being from families who were either "too poor or too vicious" to care for them (Clement 1978, as per Lindsey, 2004). From that time through the 1950s, a complex network of private and public agencies developed to protect children from harm at the hands of their caretakers. These agencies were supported by a mix of public and private funds within the framework of state laws and local ordinances prohibiting the maltreatment of children. Until 1974, no federal laws existed to enforce national standards throughout the United States. Many state laws of the 1960s and, later, the Child Abuse Prevention and Treatment Act of 1974 (CAPTA) were prompted by a public outcry following the documentation of child abuse through the study of x-rays of children's multiple fractures (Kempe, Silverman, Steele, Droegmueller, & Silver, 1962). CAPTA signaled federal interest in mandated reporting of maltreatment by professionals and mandatory investigation of reports. As a result, recorded reports of child maltreatment serious enough to trigger an investigation rose from 60,000 in 1974 to 3.3 million in 2005.

Definitions

Definitions of child maltreatment in the United States focus on three major forms of abuse or neglect: physical abuse, sexual abuse, and neglect. Further, child abuse and neglect are defined by the fact that the maltreatment is perpetrated by a parent or caretaker (see the Child Welfare Information Gateway sponsored by the United States Children's Bureau for further information on definitions [http://www.childwelfare.gov]). For example, a beating by a stranger would be considered a matter for law enforcement. CAPTA, "as amended by the Keeping Children and Families Safe Act of 2003, defines child abuse and neglect as: (1) any act or failure to act on the part of a parent or caretaker which results in death, serious

TABLE 1

*Actions or Inactions of Caretakers Defined as Abusive or Neglectful by the National Incidence Studies
on Child Abuse and Neglect*

- Physical assault
- Sexual abuse or exploitation such as forcible or consensual rape, incest, intercourse, molestation
- Close confinement such as tying or binding of arms or legs, locking in a closet
- Any other pattern of assaultive, exploitative, or abusive treatment, such as threatened or attempted assault, habitual or extreme verbal abuse
- Abandonment or other refusal to maintain custody
- Permitting or encouraging chronic maladaptive behavior, such as delinquency
- Refusal to allow needed treatment for a professionally diagnosed physical, educational, emotional, or behavioral problem
- Failure to seek or unwarranted delay in seeking competent medical care
- Consistent or extreme inattention to the child's physical or emotional needs
- Failure to register or enroll the child in school, as required by state law

The definition of maltreatment is further defined by the type of injury sustained.
Harm is defined as: *fatal, serious, moderate,* or *probable*
    Fatal—the abuse or neglect is suspected to have been the cause of the child's death
    Serious injury/condition—injury or impairment serious enough to significantly impair the child
    Moderate injury/condition—behavior problem or physical/ mental/emotional condition with observable symptoms lasting at least 48 hours
    Probable impairment—maltreatment that is so extreme or inherently traumatic in nature that significant emotional injury or impairment may reasonably be assumed to have occurred
Additional cases may be identified by determining whether the child was *endangered*:
    Endangered—child's health or safety was or is seriously endangered, but child does not appear to have been harmed.

From Westat, Inc. (2007). NIS-4. A Web site sponsored by the Administration for Children and Families. Washington, DC: U.S. Department of Health and Human Services. Retrieved July 9, 2007, from https://www.nis4.org/DefAbuse.asp. Adapted with permission.

physical or emotional harm, sexual abuse or exploitation; or (2) an act or failure to act which presents an imminent risk of serious harm" (Child Welfare Information Gateway, 2006). More specifically, in defining maltreatment for the purpose of measuring the prevalence of child abuse and neglect in the United States, Westat Inc. developed the definitions in Table 1. These definitions have changed very little since the first National Incidence Study on Child Abuse and Neglect (NIS-1) in 1980 and are also reflected in the 19th edition of the *Encyclopedia of Social Work*.

State laws may or may not include all of the situations described in Table 1. The parameters of the federal definition of maltreatment are addressed in the CAPTA, referenced earlier. The states may vary on a number of dimensions including the definition of the term "caretaker," what is included in medical neglect, and whether certain specific acts constitute maltreatment. For example, the definition of caretaker may or may not include a school bus driver. Other sources of variation concern the types of incidents that are disallowed, often combined with the age of the child. In one state, for example, educational neglect or truancy is not reportable to child protective services (CPS). School attendance is handled by another governmental agency. Conversely, in another, if a child is under 12 and has 7 days of unexcused absences that child will, by law, be reported to CPS as neglected (Child Welfare Information Gateway, 2005; Zuel & Larson, 2005). In addition, localities may vary in how state laws are applied.

Prevalence

The National Child Abuse and Neglect Data System (NCANDS) reports 3.3 million referrals to CPS in 2005 involving 6 million children in the United States and Puerto Rico. Sixty-two percent were screened in for investigation or assessment by CPS (see also Child Care Services). Almost 30% of the investigated reports were substantiated or indicated cases of maltreatment. These reports involved 889,000 children or 12.1 per 1,000 children. Table 2 details the types of abuse experienced by these children. Children known to CPS, however, do not tell the whole story of children who are victimized by child maltreatment. In a 1993 survey of child serving professionals such as teachers, day care providers, and emergency room physicians, the Third National Incidence Study on Child Abuse and Neglect (NIS-3) found over 1.5 million children were harmed by maltreatment (fatal, serious, moderate, or probable injury, as described in Table 1) and less than 30% of these children were investigated by CPS. The children whose maltreatment was not investigated may have never been referred to CPS or

TABLE 2

Types of Maltreatment Experienced by Children Found to Have Been Maltreated in 2005 by a CPS agency

TYPE OF MALTREATMENT	PERCENT[a]
Neglect	62.8
Physical abuse	16.6
Sexual abuse	9.3
Psychological maltreatment	7.1
Medical neglect	2.0
Other (for example, abandonment, threats of harm, drug-exposed infants)	14.3

[a]Adds up to over 100% because a child may have more than one type of maltreatment.

they may have been referred and screened out before investigation. The Fourth National Incidence Study on Child Abuse and Neglect (NIS-4) was reported to Congress and on the World Wide Web in 2010. It should be noted that there is some discussion regarding the "true" prevalence of maltreatment due to the methodological variations in counting in various studies. For example, the NIS studies miss counting those cases known only to family or neighbors if they are not also reported to CPS.

NCCANDS recorded 1,460 child fatalities from maltreatment in 2005. These include only those known to CPS. With data from other sources the number is estimated to be fairly consistent at about 2,000 annually (McClain, Sacks, Froehlke, & Ewigman, 1993). The same researchers report children under 5 years old account for 90% of fatal maltreatment; 41% of the maltreatment deaths are those of infants. They also report about 85% of child maltreatment deaths are reported to be from other causes and recommend changes to reporting of child deaths to capture more accurate information.

Characteristics of Children and Families

Younger children are more likely to be maltreated than older children and more likely to experience neglect. Although African American children are no more likely to be maltreated than white children they are most likely to be reported and found as maltreated (19.5 per 1,000) compared to white children (10.8 per 1,000) (Sedlak & Broadhurst, 1996). This disproportionate reporting and CPS system involvement for children of color is being addressed through a number of initiatives described elsewhere in this encyclopedia.

American Indians, Alaskan Natives, and Pacific Islanders are also dramatically overrepresented in the child welfare system compared with their proportionate representation in the population. The NIS-3 (Sedlak & Broadhurst, 1996) found slightly more females than males are maltreated, more males than females are killed or seriously injured, and children of single parents are at higher risk of maltreatment and injury. Compared to families with incomes over $30,000 per year in 1993, those with incomes under $15,000 per year were 22 times more likely to be harmed by maltreatment and 44 times more likely to be neglected. The issue of poverty and neglect is of particular concern due to the potential confounding of the two. Sometimes families will be referred to CPS due to lack of food, shelter, or clothing that is solely due to lack of money and not a result of maltreatment. In Illinois, the *Norman v. McDonald* lawsuit, settled in 1991, led to a special fund to aid families who were in danger of child placement due to economic distress (for example, lacking food or housing) but who were not maltreating their children, thus keeping children and families out of CPS when there is no suspicion of maltreatment.

Causes and Consequences of Child Abuse and Neglect

One of the most thorough treatments of etiology of maltreatment is the National Research Council's 1993 book on *Understanding Child Abuse and Neglect*. In addition to poverty, risk factors for maltreatment include parental drug abuse, parental history of having been maltreated, unresolved or untreated parental mental health problems, age of the mother at the birth of her first child, child behavior problems, child disability, lack of familial social supports, situations perceived by family members as causing high stress, and family violence among adults in the household. Different types of maltreatment will have differing dynamics. For example, physical abuse in some families may be characterized by unrealistic expectations of the children, feelings of helplessness in responding to the child's needs, and situations of high perceived stress. Examples of social structural and institutional factors creating environments within which maltreatment may be more likely to occur or to be reported include poverty and low wages requiring longer hours of work, a culture that promotes violence through the media, a culture of substance abuse, negative peer influences, and racism.

The sequel of child maltreatment are well documented and include but are not limited to higher risk of drug abuse, behavior problems, delinquency, arrest and incarceration, failed relationships, and maltreatment of offspring. Protective factors are now known to be critically important in determining vulnerability to, and outcomes of, child maltreatment. Fraser and Terzian (2005) report that communication and problem solving and parental competence in child discipline and supervision are important factors mediating the effects of poverty. Sources of resilience come not only from one's own biological, cognitive, and personal experiences but also from the school, the neighborhood, and the community at large. The child who is most likely to fend off or minimize deleterious consequences is able to use resources available, engage in opportunities for support from others, and has a source of support in the larger environment (Fraser & Terzian, 2005).

Best Practices

Effective interventions may focus on prevention or remediation; and may involve broad-based social change, community organization or development, social policy change, or direct intervention with children and families. They may, for example, address the reduction of poverty, building social and support networks, changing child welfare laws and policies to enable family maintenance, or interventions in parenting styles, respectively. Most importantly, they should combine attention to both the evidence base of the practice to be used in concert with the degree to which the intervention is culturally competent (Wells, 2007). The evidence may be developed based on large-scale policy interventions such as subsidized guardianship for kinship caretakers or may be more specific to direct interventions with children and families (see Chaffin & Friedrich, 2004; DePanfilis, 2005; Kauffman Best Practices Project, 2004; Testa, n.d.).

Challenges and Debates

The challenges in preventing and responding to child maltreatment are many. The first is the definition of maltreatment itself. Definition affects every part of society's response with respect to funding, court intervention, and even out-of-home placement. There is a constant push/pull relationship between families who are at lower levels of risk within the CPS system to ensure they receive services or helping them through voluntary services which, in many cases, are less well funded. This leads to the second concern, the degree to which governmental agencies should be intervening in family life. The disproportionate representation of children of color in the system, particularly African American and aboriginal peoples, argues for a more circumspect look at reporting, intake, and placement of children and families in difficulty. Studies of alternative response to reports of maltreatment determined to be at lower risk have been important in guiding state laws and policies (Loman & Siegel,

2004). Alternative response systems allow the government agency to respond to a low-risk report by doing a voluntary assessment of the family's needs. In this case, the family is not compelled to cooperate unless, upon further inquiry, the worker refers the situation back to child protection services for a nonvoluntary or mandatory investigation. A third concern is the relative cost-effectiveness of focusing on prevention versus remediation and treatment. With limited resources available because of the less-than-favorable public sentiments toward public social services, the argument is not frivolous.

Trends include ongoing social concerns, the proliferation of violent media that reinforce all forms of violence, and the concurrent dwindling support for families in their communities. At the level of individual and family intervention, the question is whether basic services such as housing and substance abuse treatment are available. In addition, practitioners and policy makers are questioning whether evidence-based practices are known and readily available to all families in need. The need for evidence-based practices is great and the research capacity to meet the need is severely limited by the available funding.

Role of and Implications for Social Work Profession and Interdisciplinary Connections

The social work profession has historically been involved in the design and delivery of CPS as well as in addressing the social conditions that perpetuate the problem. A current challenge is to improve practice by understanding and applying research and by opening the door for ongoing practice evaluation. In addition to ongoing quality improvement, addressing public perceptions regarding funding of social services and preventive efforts could be tackled through the conducting and use of cost-effectiveness studies to show how much financial and societal cost can be saved by early intervention. At the same time, efforts to address the social issues that perpetuate risk cannot be neglected. All of this work will continue to be done in the context of interdisciplinary relationships. Child maltreatment touches all professions—medicine, law, education, child care, and many others. It is only through an interdisciplinary focus that progress can be made.

REFERENCES

Chaffin, M., & Friedrich, B. (2004). Evidence-based treatments in child abuse and neglect. *Children and Youth Services Review, 26,* 1097–1113.

Child Welfare Information Gateway. (January 2005). Definitions of child abuse and neglect: Summary of state laws.

Washington, DC: Author, Children's Bureau, Administration for Children Youth and Families, U.S. Department of Health and Human Services. Retrieved July 9, 2007, from: http://www.childwelfare.gov/systemwide/laws_policies/statutes/defineall.pdf

Child Welfare Information Gateway. (April 2006). What is child abuse and neglect? Washington, DC: Author, Children's Bureau, Administration for Children Youth and Families, U.S. Department of Health and Human Services. Retrieved July 9, 2007, from: http://www.childwelfare.gov/pubs/factsheets/whatiscan.cfm

Clement, P. F. (1978). Families in foster care: Philadelphia in the late nineteenth century. *Social Service Review, 53,* 406–420 as cited by Lindsey, D. (2004). *The welfare of children* (p. 17). New York: Oxford University Press.

DePanfilis, D. (2005). Family connections: A program for preventing child neglect. *Child Maltreatment, 10*(2), 108–123.

Freysteinsdóttir, F. J. (2004). Risk factors for repeated maltreatment. PhD Thesis, University of Iowa, Iowa City, IA, 2004. Retrieved July 9, 2007, from http://etd.lib.uiowa.edu/2004/ffreysteinsdottir.pdf

Fraser, M. W., & Terzian, M. A. (2005). Risk and resilience in child development. In G. P. Mallon & P. M. Hess (Eds.), *Child welfare for the 21st century.* New York: Columbia University Press.

Kauffman Best Practices Project. (2004). Closing the quality chasm in child abuse treatment: Identifying and disseminating best practices. Charleston, SC: National Crime Victims Research and Treatment Center.

Kempe, C. H., Silverman, F., Steele, B., Droegmueller, W., & Silver, H. (1962). The battered-child syndrome. *Journal of the American Medical Association, 181,* 17–24.

Loman, L. A., & Siegel, G. L. (2004). Minnesota alternative response evaluation: Final report. St. Louis, MO: Institute of Applied Research.

McClain, P. W., Sacks, J. J., Froehlke, R. G., & Ewigman, B. G. (1993). Estimates of fatal child-abuse and neglect, United-States, 1979–1988. *Pediatrics, 91*(2), 338–343.

National Academy Press. (1993). *Understanding child abuse and neglect.* Washington, DC: National Academy Press.

Norman v. McDonald, 930 F. Supp. 1219, 1227 (N.D. Ill 1996).

Sedlak, A., & Broadhurst, D. (1996). *The third national incidence study on child abuse and neglect.* Washington, DC: Children's Bureau, Administration for Children, Youth and Families, U.S. Department of Health and Human Services.

Testa, M. (n.d.). *Encouraging child welfare intervention through IV-E waivers.* Urbana: Children and Family Research Center, University of Illinois at Urbana-Champaign.

Wells, S. J. (2007). Evidence-based practice in child welfare in the context of cultural competency. Presentation at an invitational forum of the same name hosted by the School of Social Work in the College of Education and Human Development at the University of Minnesota in Minneapolis, Minnesota, June 11, 2007.

Westat Inc. (2007). NIS-4. A Web site sponsored by the Administration for Children and Families, U.S. Department of Health and Human Services, Washington, DC. Retrieved July 9, 2007, from: https://www.nis4.org/DefAbuse.asp.

World Health Organization (WHO). (2001). Prevention of child abuse and neglect; Making the links between human rights and public health. Paper submitted to the Committee on the Rights of the Child for its Day of General Discussion, September 28, 2001. Geneva, Switzerland: Author, Department of Injuries and Violence Prevention.

Zuel, T., & Larson, A. (December 15, 2005). Child protection and educational neglect: A preliminary study. An unpublished manuscript posted on the WWW. St. Paul, MN: Center for the Advanced Study of Child Welfare, School of Social Work, University of Minnesota. Retrieved July 9, 2007, from: http://ssw.che.umn.edu/img/assets/4467/Final%2012-15-05.pdf

SUSAN J. WELLS

CHILD AND ADOLESCENT MENTAL-HEALTH DISORDERS

ABSTRACT: Mental-health disorders are widely prevalent in children and adolescents, and social workers are the primary service providers for children and families experiencing these disorders. This overview examines some of the most commonly seen disorders in children and adolescents: attention deficit hyperactivity disorder, oppositional defiant disorder, conduct disorder, separation anxiety disorder, and specific learning disorders. The prevalence, course, diagnostic criteria, assessment guidelines, and treatment interventions are reviewed for each disorder. In addition, the key role of social workers in the identification and intervention of these disorders, as well as ways social workers can support the children and families experiencing these disorders, is discussed.

KEY WORDS: children; adolescents; mental-health disorders; diagnosis; treatment

Mental-health disorders are widely prevalent in children and adolescents, with estimates indicating that as many as 2.7 million children in the United States have a mental-health disorder (Federal Interagency Forum on Child and Family Statistics, 2007), and approximately 13% (13.1%) of all children will experience a diagnosable mental-health disorder in a given year (Merikangas et al., 2010). There is not a clear distinction between childhood and adult disorders because disorders commonly diagnosed in childhood often continue into adulthood, and adult disorders are typically rooted in early childhood conditions and experiences. For convenience, the *Diagnostic and Statistical Manual of Mental Disorders–IV* (DSM-IV; American Psychiatric Association [APA], 2000) included a separate diagnostic category for disorders that were usually first diagnosed in infancy, childhood, or adolescence. However, *DSM-5* (APA, 2013) no longer includes this category, and so disorders formerly included in the category have been moved to categories more reflective of related symptomology, presentation, and etiology. These new categories include neurodevelopmental disorders and disruptive, impulse control, and conduct disorders.

The focus here is on some of the most commonly diagnosed and recognized mental-health disorders in children and adolescents, including attention deficit hyperactivity disorder (ADHD), oppositional defiant disorder (ODD), conduct disorder (CD), separation anxiety disorder (SAD), and specific learning disorders. This is a broad overview of these diagnoses and is not meant to be used for diagnostic purposes. When making a diagnosis, the *DSM-5* (APA, 2013) should be consulted for a listing of full diagnostic criteria related to each disorder.

Attention Deficit Hyperactivity Disorder

Attention deficit hyperactivity disorder is a neurodevelopmental disorder characterized by behaviors relating to hyperactivity, impulsivity, and inattention that interfere with a child's ability to function in daily life (APA, 2013). The behaviors are severe enough to cause problems at home, in school, and with peers. In the past, ADHD was referred to as attention deficit disorder (ADD) with or without hyperactivity. However, in the *DSM-IV*, the name of the disorder was changed to ADHD, which was used even if there is no hyperactivity, and that name remains.

PREVALENCE Prevalence estimates of ADHD range from approximately 5% to 8% of children and adolescents, making it the most common neurobehavioral disorder in children (American Academy of Child and Adolescent Psychiatry [AACAP], 2011; APA, 2013). Attention deficit hyperactivity disorder is observed more predominately in males, with approximately 3% of males receiving an ADHD diagnosis for every female in the general population (Hinshaw & Blachman, 2005). One major limitation is that few studies of high quality have been conducted to explore the prevalence of ADHD across racial and ethnic groups.

DIAGNOSIS In the *DSM-5* (APA, 2013), ADHD is included in the new diagnostic category called neurodevelopmental disorders. In the prior edition, ADHD was included in the diagnostic category disorders usually first diagnosed in infancy, childhood, or adolescence, which has been removed as a category. The *DSM-5* (APA, 2013) diagnostic criteria for ADHD specify that there must be six or more symptoms of inattention or hyperactivity and impulsivity that interfere with functioning and are inconsistent with developmental level for at least six months. Common symptoms of inattentiveness include difficulty sustaining attention in tasks or play activities, difficulty following instructions and failing to finish schoolwork, and difficulty organizing tasks and activities. Symptoms of hyperactivity and impulsivity include frequent fidgeting or squirming in seat, excessive talking and interrupting others to blurt out an answer, and appearing "driven by a motor."

The *DSM-5* (APA, 2013) also specifies that symptoms must be present prior to age 12 and must occur in two or more settings (home, school, work) with evidence of clinically significant impairment in social, academic, or occupational functioning. Additionally, symptoms should not be better accounted for by another mental disorder and should not occur exclusively within the course of pervasive developmental disorder, schizophrenia, or another psychotic disorder.

Based on the varying combinations of presenting symptoms, there are three types of ADHD specified in the *DSM-5* (APA, 2013). Attention deficit hyperactivity disorder, combined type, is diagnosed if there are six or more inattentive symptoms and six or more hyperactive or impulsive symptoms. Attention deficit hyperactivity disorder, predominantly inattentive type, is diagnosed if there are six or more inattentive symptoms but hyperactive–impulsive symptom requirements are not met. Attention deficit hyperactivity disorder, predominantly hyperactive–impulsive type, is diagnosed if there are six or more hyperactive and impulsive symptoms but inattentive symptom requirements are not met. Clinicians should also specify that ADHD is "in partial remission" when complete criteria were previously met but have not been met for the past six months, but the symptoms still impair academic or occupational functioning. Specification is also required to describe symptoms as mild, moderate, or severe.

Attention deficit hyperactivity disorder is co-morbid with a number of other internalizing and disruptive behavior disorders in numbers that are above chance (Angold, Costello, & Erkanli, 1999). In particular, ODD and CD co-occur with one quarter to one half of children who have the combined presentation of ADHD (APA, 2013).

RISK FACTORS There does appear to be a genetic component to ADHD because the biological relatives of individuals with ADHD are substantially more likely to develop ADHD themselves. However, although ADHD does appear to be correlated with specific genes, those genes alone are not enough to cause ADHD (APA, 2013). A variety of environmental factors may increase the chances of a child developing ADHD (Rowland, Lesesne, & Abramowitz, 2002), including very low birth weight, smoking during pregnancy, a history of child abuse or neglect, drug and alcohol exposure in utero, and exposure to lead.

COURSE Although symptoms of ADHD, such as excessive physical activity, are often reported by parents in children as young as toddlers, ADHD is typically not diagnosed until children begin elementary school. At that point, a child's inattention becomes more apparent and likely to interfere with achievement and functioning (APA, 2013). The symptoms of ADHD tend to be consistent through early adolescence. For many children with ADHD, the motor hyperactivity subsides somewhat during adolescence but impulsivity, inattention, restlessness, and difficulty planning remain persistent (APA, 2013). As teenagers, a limited number of children will no longer meet diagnostic criteria, but somewhere between 43% and 80% will continue to have ADHD (Mannuzza, Klein, Bonagura, Malloy, Giampino, & Addalli, 1991). With treatment, symptoms of ADHD can be managed successfully, but the disorder often persists into adulthood.

ASSESSMENT Evaluation for ADHD should include information from multiple sources across settings including parents, schools, and the child, if possible. Several commonly used behavior rating scales are used in the assessment of ADHD. Parent rating scales include Conners Parent Rating Scale–Revised (Conners, 1997), Eyberg Child Behavior Inventory (Eyberg, 1999), and the Home Situations Questionnaire–Revised (Barkley, 1990). Rating scales for the school setting include the Academic Performance Rating Scale (Barkley, 1990), Conners Teacher Rating Scale–Revised (Conners), School Situations Questionnaire–Revised (Barkley, 1990), and Vanderbilt ADHD Diagnostic Parent and Teacher Scales (Wolraich et al., 2003).

In addition, clinicians should consider cultural factors when conducting an assessment because various cultural groups have differing norms regarding child behavior (APA, 2013). Concern has also been raised that even when displaying similar symptoms, African American children are more likely to enter the juvenile justice system instead of receiving mental-health services (Mattox & Harder, 2007).

TREATMENT Pharmacological treatment has demonstrated effectiveness in treating ADHD. The AACAP's (American Academy of Pediatrics, 2007) Practice Parameters for ADHD recommend that initial psycho-pharmacological treatment of ADHD should be a trial of one of the medications approved by the Food and Drug Administration for ADHD treatment. These include Adderall, Ritalin, Concerta, and Strattera. If none of the approved medications results in satisfactory improvement, the Practice Parameters recommend a review of the diagnosis and then consideration of behavior therapy or use of medications not approved by the Food and Drug Administration for ADHD treatment. These may include antidepressants such as bupropion, imipramine, nortriptyline, or 2-adrenergic agonists such as clonidine or guanfacine. Dosages should be adjusted to ensure the child is obtaining the greatest benefit from the medication with minimal adverse side effects (American Academy of Pediatrics, 2007).

For many children, pharmacological treatment combined with behavioral therapy is more effective than either one alone (Power et al., 2012). Behavioral interventions typically include components such as token economies, time-outs, and other incentives and interventions to which the child is individually responsive. Classroom behavioral interventions are also often required to assist children with ADHD in managing their behaviors at school and improving academic performance. Barkley (2005) has observed that ADHD treatment tends to be most helpful when it is directed at behaviors at the point of performance in the natural environment.

Although behavioral therapies have garnered support and are most commonly used to treat ADHD, parent training is often recommended (Mattox & Harder, 2007). Parent training is a form of therapy that not only works with the parent to manage a child's behavior, but also provides an educational component, includes the child, and assists in the reduction of parent–child conflict and family relationship building. Parent training is most likely to be helpful when combined with psychopharmacological and behavioral therapies in a holistic fashion.

Oppositional Defiant Disorder

Children with ODD typically display an irritable or angry mood, are frequently defiant or argumentative, and are vindictive toward others (APA, 2013). The symptoms of ODD can occur in one or more settings, typically including the home and school, and interfere with a child's ability to develop positive social relationships. The behavioral manifestation of ODD often makes it difficult for a child to perform at his or her full potential.

PREVALENCE Community prevalence of ODD has been reported between 1% and 16% depending on criteria used and methods of assessment (Loeber, Burke, Lahey, Winters, & Zera, 2000). The average prevalence rate appears to be approximately 3.3% (APA, 2013). Oppositional defiant disorder seems to be more common in males than in females during early childhood, but in adolescence it appears equally prevalent in males and females (APA, 2013).

DIAGNOSIS In the *DSM-5* (APA, 2013), ODD is included in the new diagnostic category of disruptive, impulse control, and conduct disorders. In the prior edition, ODD was included in the diagnostic category of disorders usually first diagnosed in infancy, childhood, or adolescence, which has been removed as a category. The *DSM-5* (APA, 2013) criteria for ODD specify that there must be a pattern of negativistic, hostile, and defiant behavior operationalized by the presence of four or more symptoms that occur for at least six months. These symptoms include often losing temper, frequently defying or refusing to comply with adult requests, and deliberately annoying others. For children under the age of five, the behaviors should occur on most days, and for individuals older than five, the behaviors should occur at least once per week. These behaviors should occur more frequently than is typical for the age and developmental level of the individual. The *DSM-5* (APA, 2013) also specifies that these behaviors must be causing clinically significant impairment in social, academic, or occupational functioning and must not occur exclusively during a psychotic or mood disorder. If criteria for both ODD and CD are met, then only a diagnosis of CD should be given. Oppositional defiant disorder is

often comorbid with ADHD, but can be distinguished by a child's display of anger or oppositional behavior in situations not solely requiring sustained attention or effort.

RISK FACTORS Oppositional defiant disorder is believed to stem from a mix of biological, psychological, and social factors. Understanding of the protective and risk factors for ODD relies heavily on the research on CD, and there is little separate research focusing specifically on ODD (American Academy of Pediatrics, 2007). It does appear that various temperamental factors, such as limited frustration tolerance and emotional reactivity, are related to ODD. In addition, inconsistent or harsh child-rearing practices may contribute to the development of ODD. Certain neurobiological markers have been associated with ODD as well, but again, those markers have not been distinguished from those of CD (APA, 2013).

COURSE Oppositional defiant disorder is usually manifest by age eight (Connor, 2002) and is relatively stable over time. However, most children no longer meet criteria of the diagnosis after a three-year follow up (Connor; Hinshaw & Anderson, 1996; Loeber et al., 2000). Oppositional defiant disorder is often a developmental antecedent of CD but many children with ODD do not ever develop CD (APA, 2000). It seems that earlier age of onset of ODD symptoms leads to a poorer prognosis with progression into CD (Connor; Loeber et al.). With increasing age, comorbidities with diagnoses such as ADHD, learning disorders, communication disorders, anxiety disorders, and mood disorders begin to appear (APA, 2013; Lavigne et al., 2001). Children with ODD often experience challenges academically and have difficulty forming social relationships with peers (Frankel & Feinberg, 2002).

ASSESSMENT A wide range of interviews and instruments are available for assessing oppositional behavior and aggression in children and adolescents in different settings. A number of assessment batteries have also been developed to aid in assessment. Parent or teacher report measures include the Conners Rating Scale (parent and teacher versions) (Conners, Sitatenios, Parker, & Epstein, 1998), Children's Aggression Scale (Halperin, McKay, & Newcorn, 2002), Parent Daily Report (Kazdin & Esveldt-Dawson, 1986), and Interview for Antisocial Behavior (Chamberlain & Reid, 1987).

Youth self-report measures include Youth Self-Report (Achenbach, 1991), Buss–Durkee Hostility Inventory (Buss & Durkee, 1957), Buss–Perry Aggression Questionnaire (Buss & Perry, 1992), and Conners/Wells Adolescent Self-Report of Symptoms (Conners et al., 1997). One of the challenges of assessment is that children often do not display the same behaviors during a clinical interview as they do in their natural environments. Therefore, the reports of parents, teachers, and other appropriate observers are particularly critical to obtaining a complete clinical picture (APA, 2013).

TREATMENT Interventions can be delivered in schools, clinics, and other community locations with differing approaches depending on the child's age. In preschool children, programs such as Head Start (Connor, 2002) and home visitation to high-risk families have produced positive outcomes (Eckenrode et al., 2000). In school-age children, parent management strategies have strong empirical support for disruptive behavior. In general, these approaches focus on the following four principles: (a) reduce positive reinforcement of disruptive behavior; (b) increase reinforcement of prosocial and compliant behavior; (c) apply consequences or punishment for disruptive behavior; and (d) make parental response predictable, contingent, and immediate (American Academy of Pediatrics, 2007). These approaches have been found to be effective in community and clinical samples, and examples of parent management training packages include Incredible Years (Webster-Stratton, Reid, & Hammond, 2004), Triple P-Positive Parenting Program (Sanders, Markie-Dadds, Tully, & Bor, 2000), and Parent–Child Interactional therapy (Brinkmeyer & Eyberg, 2003).

Conduct Disorder

Conduct disorder is characterized by a persistent pattern of behavior that violates age-appropriate social norms and interferes with the basic rights of others. Behaviors typically observed in CD include aggression and violence to others, property damage, deceitfulness, and serious rule violations (APA, 2013). These behaviors exceed what is developmentally appropriate and interfere with social, school, and occupational functioning.

PREVALENCE Estimates of the prevalence of CD range from 2% to 10% (APA, 2013), with an average of 6% (AACAP, 2004). Conduct disorder is typically seen more frequently as children enter adolescence and boys have higher prevalence rates of CD than girls.

Rates of CD appear relatively stable across countries that differ with respect to race and ethnicity (APA, 2013).

DIAGNOSIS In the DSM-5 (APA, 2013), CD is included in the new diagnostic category of disruptive, impulse control, and conduct disorders. In the prior edition, CD was included in the diagnostic category of disorders usually first diagnosed in infancy, childhood, or adolescence, which has been removed as a category. The DSM-5 (APA, 2013) criteria for CD specify that there must be a repetitive pattern of behavior that violates the basic rights of others or major age-appropriate societal norms as evidenced by the presence of three or more of the identified symptoms in a period of 12 months, with at least one of the criterion present in the past 6 months. Those symptoms include aggression to people or animals, destruction of property, and serious rule violations such as running away repeatedly and school truancy. The behavior must be causing clinically significant impairment in social, academic, or occupational functioning. If criteria for both ODD and CD are met, then only a diagnosis of CD should be given. The disorder is considered to have childhood onset if behavior occurred prior to age 10 and adolescent onset if behavior did not occur until after age 10. There is a diagnostic specifier included in the DSM-5 (APA, 2013) for callous–unemotional presentation, which is given if the person displays at least two of the following traits in the past 12 months: lack of remorse or guilt, callous–lack of empathy, unconcerned about performance, or shallow or deficient affect. Severity is specified as mild, moderate, or severe. Conduct disorder shares similar symptoms with ODD, but can be distinguished by the severity of the symptoms presented in CD.

RISK FACTORS A variety of factors have been associated with an increased risk of developing CD. There does appear to be a genetic component to CD. Children with a parent or sibling previously diagnosed with CD are more likely to develop it themselves (APA, 2013). Difficulties with impulse control, such as that seen in children with the hyperactive type of ADHD, can contribute to antisocial behaviors (Holmes, Slaughter, & Kashani, 2001). Child temperament also appears to play a role in the formation of CD, with children who display aggression at very young ages being more likely to manifest CD in adolescence (Mandel, 1997). Research has also demonstrated that a number of factors in a child's familial environment can contribute to later development of CD. These factors include inconsistent supervision, family alcoholism, parental conflict and violence, socioeconomic status, and physical or sexual abuse (APA, 2013; Campbell, 1990; Williams, Anderson, McGee, & Silva, 1990). Difficulties forming friendships and peer rejection have also been linked to CD (Holmes et al.). At the community level, high rates of violence are a risk factor as well (APA, 2013).

COURSE Conduct disorder can develop as early as the preschool years, but symptoms most typically begin to present during the middle childhood years through adolescence (APA, 2013). The course of CD varies significantly. It is common for many individuals diagnosed with CD, particularly those with an adolescent onset and mild symptoms, to become adjusted adults with stable social and occupational functioning. However, individuals with an early onset and more severe behaviors have a worse prognosis and are at risk of criminal behavior, substance-related disorders, and a variety of additional psychiatric disorders as adults (APA, 2013). For those individuals whose CD extends into adulthood and involves continued aggression, violence, deceitfulness, and rule violation at home and work, a diagnosis of antisocial personality disorder may be appropriate (APA, 2013).

ASSESSMENT The assessment of CD requires a comprehensive evaluation. Interviews with parents, teachers, and other sources familiar with a child's behavior across settings are useful in obtaining a full picture of a child's behaviors. In addition, various assessment scales, such as the Conners Rating Scale (parent and teacher versions) (Conners et al., 1998), Children's Aggression Scale (Halperin et al., 2002), Parent Daily Report (Kazdin & Esveldt-Dawson, 1986), and Interview for Antisocial Behavior (Chamberlain & Reid, 1987), can be helpful. Children can complete self-report assessments including the Youth Self-Report (Achenbach, 1991), Buss–Durkee Hostility Inventory (Buss & Durkee, 1957), Buss–Perry Aggression Questionnaire (Buss & Perry, 1992), and Conners/Wells Adolescent Self-Report of Symptoms (Conners et al., 1997). All sources of information should be considered when completing the assessment.

TREATMENT Intervention with children and adolescents diagnosed with CD is generally most effective when it takes a biopsychosocial approach, is multimodal, and is multisystemic (Gerten, 2000). Primary components of treatment for CD include the development of prosocial skills and prosocial peer relationships. A combination of behavioral therapy and psychotherapy is often needed to assist children and adolescents with CD in learning to express emotions and manage their behaviors. Social skills training can also be used to develop problem-solving abilities and form supportive relationships (AACAP, 2004). In addition, family therapy, parent training, and support are needed to implement behavioral interventions, build positive relationships, and cope with the child's challenging behaviors. Treatment interventions demonstrating effectiveness include Multisystemic Therapy, the Oregon Model Parent Management Training, and Functional Family Therapy (California Evidence-Based Clearinghouse for Child Welfare, 2013). For some children, medication may also be used to address impulse-control problems and stabilize aggressive outbursts (AACAP, 2004).

Separation Anxiety Disorder

PREVALENCE Separation anxiety disorder is one of the earliest and most common mental-health disorders of childhood (Kessler et al., 2005). Separation anxiety disorder is typically seen more frequently in early childhood and prevalence rates tend to decline as children move into adolescence (Eisen & Schaefer, 2005). The overall prevalence rate of SAD is estimated to be approximately 4% of children and 1.6% of adolescents in the United States (APA, 2013). Research regarding the prevalence of SAD among girls and boys has yielded mixed results. Generally, SAD appears to be equally common among girls and boys in clinical samples, whereas it is more frequently seen in females in community samples (APA, 2013). However, some studies have indicated a greater prevalence of SAD among girls in both community and clinical samples (Hale, Raaijmakers, Muris, & Meeus, 2005; Last, Hersen, Kazdin, Finkelstein, & Strauss, 1987; Ogliari et al., 2006), whereas other studies have discovered equal gender prevalence of SAD in clinical (Last, Perrin, Hersen, & Kazdin, 1992) and community samples (Cohen et al., 1993). Explanations for the varying prevalence rates of SAD among girls and boys include differences according to whether the parent or child is acting as the primary informant and greater social acceptance of anxiety disorders in females (Compton, Nelson, & March, 2000; Foley et al., 2004).

DIAGNOSIS The DSM-5 (APA, 2013) diagnostic criterion for SAD requires the existence of developmentally inappropriate and excessive anxiety concerning separation from those to whom the individual is attached. This anxiety is evidenced by at least three symptoms such as the following: recurrent excessive distress when anticipating or experiencing separation from home or from major attachment figures; persistent and excessive worry about losing major attachment figures or about possible harm to them, such as illness, injury, disaster, or death; persistent and excessive worry about experiencing an untoward event that causes separation from a major attachment figure; and persistent reluctance or refusal to go out, away from home, to school, to work, or elsewhere because of fear of separation. In addition, the fear, anxiety, or avoidance must be persistent for at least four weeks in children and adolescents. The anxiety must also cause clinically significant distress or impairment in social, academic, occupational, or other important areas of functioning. Finally, the anxiety and distress must not be better explained by another mental-health disorder (APA, 2013).

One of the particular difficulties in accurately diagnosing SAD is the challenge of distinguishing it from other mental-health disorders, particularly generalized anxiety disorder (GAD). One key to making the distinction between SAD and GAD is that in SAD the source of distress will be focused predominantly on situations where the child specifically fears separation from the caregiver, whereas in GAD the child's worries and fears are spread across a variety of situations and are more focused on harm that the child may experience, rather than being away from the caregiver or child's home (APA, 2013; Eisen & Schaefer, 2005). Separation anxiety disorder is also commonly seen with specific phobia (APA, 2013).

RISK FACTORS Separation anxiety disorder seems to have a heritable component, with a heritability rate of 73% in a community sample of six-year-old twins (APA, 2013). Compared with the general population, SAD is more common among first-degree relatives, and children whose mothers have anxiety disorders are more frequently diagnosed with SAD (Cooper, Fearn, Willetts, Seabrook, & Parkinson, 2006). Children who have experienced some form of early separation trauma, such as the death or military deployment of a caregiver, or have not developed a secure attachment to their caregiver, may be at increased risk of developing SAD. In addition, parenting styles that reward and reinforce excessive attachment rather than child independence might also act as contributing factors in the development of SAD (Eisen & Schaefer, 2005). Children of lower socioeconomic status appear to be at increased risk of developing SAD, with 50% to 75% of children diagnosed with SAD coming from lower-income homes (Last et al., 1992).

COURSE Although research indicates that some children with SAD may be at increased risk of developing another anxiety disorder as adults, the majority of children who experience SAD do not have a diagnosable anxiety disorder after extensive follow-up (APA, 2013). Separation anxiety disorder may develop in children as young as preschool age and onset can occur any time during childhood and adolescence before the age of 18. However, the first occurrence of SAD during adolescence is relatively uncommon. Separation anxiety disorder is often first recognized when a child exhibits school refusal, and studies suggest that even when school refusal symptoms subside, additional social and affective SAD symptoms can remain (Masi, Mucci, & Millepiedi, 2001). Separation anxiety disorder may also develop after a significant life stressor (for example, parental divorce, death of a pet, change of schools). The typical course of SAD involves fluctuating periods of remission and exacerbation (APA, 2013).

ASSESSMENT The assessment of SAD can be complicated and is best accomplished using a multimethod approach and a variety of informants. Particular challenges in assessment include distinguishing SAD from the typical anxiety sometimes experienced by children and youth as part of the developmental process. Recent research indicates that parents may be most able to determine a child's level of impairment and make behavioral observations, whereas children are best at reporting internal distress (Allen, Lavallee, Herren, Ruhe, & Schneider, 2010). Semistructured interviews prepared for clinical work with children can be useful in making an accurate diagnosis and include the Diagnostic Interview for Children and Adolescents–Revised (Reich, 1997) and the Anxiety Disorders Interview Schedule for Children (Silverman & Nelles, 1988), which is designed specifically for the diagnosis of anxiety disorders and can assist clinicians in distinguishing SAD from other potential anxiety disorders the child may be experiencing. Questionnaires such as the Multidimensional Anxiety Scale for Children (March, Parker, Sullivan, Stallings, & Conners, 1997) are also helpful in gathering information about the child's emotions and behaviors across settings. Finally, behavioral observations from a variety of informants, including parents, school staff, child-care providers, and others as appropriate, are extremely valuable in getting a full picture of the child's manifestation, pattern, and level of anxiety. Such information can also prove useful in developing an initial, child-focused treatment plan. In addition, a consideration of cultural factors is critical in conducting an accurate assessment because there is substantial variation across countries and cultural groups regarding the degree of interdependence among family members that is considered culturally acceptable (APA, 2013).

TREATMENT A variety of therapeutic interventions have demonstrated effectiveness in treating SAD. Psychoeducation for the whole family can be a useful first step to increase child and caregiver understanding of SAD and related treatments. Targeted parent training on the management of SAD and related behaviors appears to reduce parental stress and enhance parents' sense of self-efficacy (Eisen, Raleigh, & Neuhoff, 2008). Cognitive–behavioral interventions have shown promise by improving children's coping skills, challenging thought distortions, and alleviating the symptoms of SAD (Schneider et al., 2011). In particular, the Coping Cat Program is an evidence-based treatment for anxiety in children that has demonstrated significant success. Research also suggests that Parent–Child Interaction Therapy may be efficacious, especially for treating young children with SAD (Choate, Pincus, Eyberg, & Barlow, 2005; Pincus, Santucci, Ehrenreich, & Eyberg, 2008). Pharmacological treatment, although not recommended as the first choice in treating SAD, has demonstrated usefulness as an adjunctive treatment, particularly in children who have not responded well to other interventions or who demonstrate severe distress (Masi et al., 2001). Fluoxetine, fluvoxamine, and sertraline have all demonstrated clinical effectiveness (Birmaher, Axelson, & Monk, 2003; RUPP Anxiety Study Group, 2001; Walkup et al., 2008). Consultation with and the inclusion of school staff in treatment planning is also essential if school avoidance is a part of a child's clinical presentation of SAD (Eisen & Schaefer, 2005).

Specific Learning Disorders

Specific learning disorders are neurodevelopmental disorders that impact the brain's ability to attend to and process verbal or nonverbal information with accuracy and efficiency (APA, 2013). Children with learning disorders typically experience difficulties with learning and achievement in academic settings and often try very hard to concentrate and succeed in school, yet still struggle to master and maintain academic performance and fall behind grade-level

expectations (AACAP, 2011). Specific learning disorders can appear in the areas of reading, written expression, mathematics, or some combination thereof (APA, 2013).

PREVALENCE Current estimates regarding the prevalence of learning disorders vary from 5% to 15% among school-age children, depending upon the specific population and how a learning disorder is defined in the epidemiological study (APA, 2013). The AACAP estimates learning disabilities affect approximately 10% of all children (AACAP, 2011). No significant differences in prevalence of learning disorders have been identified between boys and girls. However, there are more than two times as many boys in special education programs than girls because boys are more likely to be evaluated, identified, and placed in special education (AACAP, 2011).

DIAGNOSIS To be diagnosed with a specific learning disorder according to DSM-5 criteria (APA, 2013), a child must demonstrate difficulty learning and applying academic skills for at least six months, despite attempts to target those difficulties. At least one of the following symptoms must be present: inaccurate or slow and effortful word reading; difficulty understanding the meaning of what is read; difficulties with spelling; difficulties with written expression; difficulties mastering number sense, number facts, or calculation; or difficulties with mathematical reasoning. The academic skills impacted must be substantially and quantifiably below those expected for the child's chronological age and significantly interfere with academic or occupational performance or activities of daily living. Underperformance in the specific learning area must be documented through standardized achievement measures and a thorough clinical assessment. The learning challenges must begin during a child's school-age years but may not become apparent until academic demands exceed the child's individual capacities (APA, 2013). The diagnosis of a specific learning disorder should also include specification of the academic domain(s) and subskills that are impacted. A full diagnosis will also include specification of the current severity of the specific learning disorder as mild, moderate, or severe (APA, 2013).

Because academic skills exist along a continuum and can vary significantly, psychometric evaluation is required to confirm a learning disorder diagnosis. Although score cutoffs will vary based on the standardized test used and additional information regarding the child's learning skills and performance, a score at least 1.5 standard deviations from the mean (or roughly the 7th percentile) is recommended by the APA (2013). Learning disorders often co-occur or may be preceded by developmental delays in language, attention, or motor skills, but the relationship between these delays and learning disorders is not clear (APA, 2013).

ASSESSMENT Professionals disagree about how to consistently and accurately assess learning disorders in children (Fletcher, Francis, Morris, & Lyon, 2005). To make the most accurate diagnosis possible, an assessment should include a comprehensive evaluation incorporating multiple informants who can gauge the full spectrum of issues that may be impacting a child's learning and academic performance (AACAP, 2011). A child psychiatrist or school psychologist can conduct the intellectual and education testing required to determine whether a learning disorder is present (AACAP, 2011). In addition, family members, teachers, and other school staff, such as speech and language pathologists or audiologists, should also be included to develop a full understanding of the child's environment and other potential contributing factors to a child's learning difficulties. In addition, when conducting assessment of learning disorders, it is extremely important to consider how ethnic and racial background and other cultural factors may impact results and seek to avoid bias (APA, 2013).

RISK FACTORS Genetic disposition and general medical conditions, such as perinatal injury, can be associated with the development of learning disorders, but many individuals with those conditions do not develop learning disorders and, conversely, individuals with learning disorders often have no such risk factors in their history. A history of lead poisoning, fetal alcohol syndrome, and fragile X syndrome do appear to substantially increase the chances of developing a learning disorder (APA, 2013). Litt, Taylor, Klein, and Hack (2005) discovered an increased risk of developing learning disorders among children with a very low birth weight. Although males are sometimes diagnosed with learning disorders more frequently in school settings, stringent criteria have found no sex-related differences (APA, 2013).

COURSE Specific learning disorder symptoms can occur as early as preschool or kindergarten, but learning disorders are not often diagnosed before the first grade because formal reading, writing, or mathe-matical instruction does not occur until that point in many educational settings. Early identification and intervention are crucial in achieving optimal outcomes and many children with learning disabilities, with proper assistance, are able to perform at grade level. However, children with learning disabilities are at an increased risk of not completing high school (APA, 2013). In addition, without intervention, children with learning disorders are also at increased risk of conduct and behavioral problems and the development of other mental-health disorders throughout the life course (Bennett, Brown, Boyle, Racine, & Offord, 2003).

TREATMENT Although social workers are not qualified to conduct the psychometric testing required to formally diagnose learning disorders, they play an active role in providing support and intervention services for children with learning disabilities and their families. A few of the tasks social workers frequently perform include providing needed information to families; McGill, Tennyson, and Cooper (2006) have noted that many families of children with learning disabilities experience frustration and a lack of adequate education regarding their child's educational needs and related options. Coordinated identification and planning of services, child and family advocacy, social and emotional support, and longer range educational planning are also key intervention components (Rosenkoetter, Hains, & Dogaru, 2007). Sometimes individual, family, or group psychotherapy is recommended to assist a child and his or her family in coping with a learning disorder and assuring a child's sense of self-esteem, self-efficacy, and social supports are not adversely impacted (AACAP, 2011). Group interventions have also shown promise in increasing students' knowledge of their disability, fostering self-advocacy skills, and increasing self-esteem and self-confidence (Mishna, Muskat, & Wiener, 2010). Although relatively rare and not consistent with current efforts to keep children in their families and local communities, some children, particularly those with more severe learning disabilities or additional behavioral needs, attend residential schools (McGill et al., 2006).

Social-Work Role in Child and Adolescent Mental-Health Disorders

Social workers who work with children and families in clinical and educational settings will likely encounter children with the various mental-health disorders discussed in this entry on a regular basis. Social workers in those areas of practice should be prepared to recognize the emotional, social, and behavioral symptoms of ADHD, ODD, SAD, and CD, as well as the cognitive and academic symptoms associated with the specific learning disorders. Social workers can play a key role in assessment using a biopsychosocial perspective and, using a family-centered approach, can act collaboratively with children, parents, teachers, and others to identify all factors impacting a child's behavior (Markward & Bride, 2001). In addition, social workers with proper training, experience, and credentials are qualified to diagnose all of the children's mental-health disorders discussed in this entry except specific learning disorders. The particular functions served by a social worker will depend on the work setting and the position of the social worker within that setting. Social workers with advanced clinical training can provide specialized individual and family therapy to address the child's diagnosis and its impact on the family. Social workers who provide case management play a vital role in service coordination, resource and referral, support, and advocacy. Social workers in school, hospital, and other interdisciplinary settings can also act as consultants to colleagues from other professions and assist them in understanding and properly managing the child's diagnosis and related social and emotional behaviors. Social workers should also be knowledgeable regarding the laws and policies impacting mental-health care in their treatment setting. In particular, social workers in school settings should be aware of the Individuals with Disabilities Education Improvement Act (P.L. 108–446; 2004). All child and family social workers will benefit from continuing education regarding the presentation, diagnosis, and treatment of these common childhood mental-health disorders.

Contribution

This review presented several childhood disorders that child and family social workers will encounter in their practice, including ADHD, ODD, SAD, and specific learning disorders. Although these disorders appear with varying frequency among children, social workers who work with children and families should be familiar with the general presentation of these disorders and prepared to identify, intervene, and provide appropriate referrals and support to children and families experiencing these disorders as needed. Ongoing research continues to inform our knowledge regarding how these disorders develop, present, and are effectively treated. Social workers will benefit from continued education to support their work with children and families impacted by these disorders, particularly those disorders most commonly seen in the social worker's particular practice setting.

REFERENCES

Achenbach, T. M. (1991). Manual for child behavior checklist 4–18, 1991 profile. Burlington, VT: Department of Psychiatry, University of Vermont.

Allen, J. L., Lavallee, K. L., Herren, C., Ruhe, K., & Schneider, S. (2010). DSM-IV criteria for childhood separation anxiety disorder: Informant, age, and sex differences. Journal of Anxiety Disorders, 24, 946–952.

American Academy of Child and Adolescent Psychiatry. (2004). Facts for families: Conduct disorder. Retrieved May 12, 2013, from http://www.aacap.org

American Academy of Child and Adolescent Psychiatry. (2011). Children with learning disabilities. Facts for Families, 16. Retrieved April 14, 2013, from http://www.aacap.org

American Academy of Pediatrics. (2007). Practice parameter for the assessment and treatment of children and adolescents with attention-deficit-hyperactivity disorder. Journal of the American Academy of Child and Adolescent Psychiatry, 46(7), 895–921.

American Psychiatric Association. (2000). Diagnostic and statistical manual of mental disorders (4th ed. revised). Washington, DC: Author.

American Psychiatric Association. (2013). Diagnostic and statistical manual of mental disorders (5th ed.). Washington, DC: Author.

Angold, A., Costello, E., & Erkanli, A. (1999). Comorbidity. Journal of Child Psychology and Psychiatry, 40, 57–87.

Barkley, R. A. (1990). Attention deficit hyperactivity disorder: A handbook for diagnosis and treatment. New York, NY: Guilford Press.

Barkley, R. A. (2005). Attention deficit hyperactivity disorder: A handbook for diagnosis and treatment (3rd ed.). New York, NY: Guilford Press.

Bennett, K. J., Brown, K. S., Boyle, M., Racine, Y., & Offord, D. (2003). Does low reading achievement at school entry cause conduct problems? Social Science and Medicine, 56, 2443–2448.

Birmaher, B., Axelson, D. A., & Monk, K. (2003). Fluoxetine for the treatment of childhood anxiety disorders. Journal of the American Academy for Child and Adolescent Psychiatry, 42, 415–423.

Brinkmeyer, M., & Eyberg, S. M. (2003). Parent–child interaction therapy for oppositional children. In A. E. Kazdin & J. R. Weisz (Eds.), Evidence-based psychotherapies for children and adolescents (pp. 204–223). New York, NY: Guilford Press.

Buss, A. H., & Durkee, A. (1957). An inventory for assessing different kinds of hostility. Journal of Consulting Psychology, 21, 343–348.

Buss, A. H., & Perry, M. (1992). The aggression questionnaire. Journal of Personality and Social Psychology, 63, 452–459.

California Evidence-Based Clearinghouse for Child Welfare. (2013). Disruptive behavior treatment (child and adolescent).

Retrieved from http://www.cebc4cw.org/topic/disruptive-behavior-treatment-child-adolescent/

Campbell, S. B. (1990). *Behavior problems in preschool children: Clinical and developmental issues.* New York, NY: Guilford Press.

Chamberlain, P., & Reid, J. B. (1987). Parent observation and report of child symptoms. *Behavioral Assessment, 9*(2), 97–109.

Choate, M. L., Pincus, D. B., Eyberg, S. M., & Barlow, D. H. (2005). Parent–child interaction therapy for treatment of separation anxiety disorder in young children: A pilot study. *Cognitive and Behavioral Practice, 12,* 126–135.

Cohen, P., Cohen, J., Kasen, S., Velez, C. N., Hartmark, C., Johnson, J., et al. (1993). An epidemiological study of disorders in late childhood and adolescence: Age and gender specific prevalence. *Journal of Child Psychology and Psychiatry, 34,* 851–867.

Compton, S. N., Nelson, A. H., & March, J. S. (2000). Social phobia and separation anxiety symptoms in community and clinical samples of children and adolescents. *Journal of the American Academy of Child and Adolescent Psychiatry, 39*(8), 1040–1046.

Conners, C. K., Sitatenios, G., Parker, J. D., & Epstein, J. N. (1998). The revised Conners Parent Rating Scale (CPRS-R): Factor structure, reliability, and criterion validity. *Journal of Abnormal Child Psychology, 26,* 257–268.

Conners, C. K., Wells, K. C., Parker, J., Sitarenios, J. M., Diamond, J. M., & Powell, J. W. (1997). A new self-report scale for assessment of adolescent psychopathology: Factor structure, reliability, validity, and diagnostic sensitivity. *Journal of Abnormal Child Psychology, 25,* 487–497.

Connor, D. F. (2002). *Aggression and antisocial behavior in children and adolescents: Research and treatment.* New York, NY: Guilford Press.

Cooper, P. J., Fearn, V., Willetts, L., Seabrook, H., & Parkinson, M. (2006). Affective disorder in the parents of a clinic sample of children with anxiety disorders. *Journal of Affective Disorders, 93,* 205–212.

Eckenrode, J., Ganzel, B., Henderson, C. R., Smith, E., Olds, D. L., Powers, J., et al. (2000). Preventing child abuse and neglect with a program of nurse home visitation: The limiting effects of domestic violence. *Journal of the American Medical Association, 284,* 1385–1391.

Eisen, A. R., Raleigh, H., & Neuhoff, C. C. (2008). The unique impact of parent training for separation anxiety disorder in children. *Behavior Therapy, 39,* 195–206.

Eisen, A. R., & Schaefer, C. E. (2005). *Separation anxiety disorder in children and adolescents: An individualized approach to assessment and treatment.* New York, NY: Guilford Press.

Eyberg, S. M. (1999). *Eyberg child behavior inventory.* Odessa, FL: Psychological Assessment Resources.

Federal Interagency Forum on Child and Family Statistics. (2007). *America's children: Key national indicators of well-being, 2007.* Washington, DC: U.S. Government Printing Office.

Fletcher, J. M., Francis, D. J., Morris, R. D., & Lyon, R. (2005). Evidence-based assessment of learning disabilities in children and adolescents. *Journal of Clinical Child and Adolescent Psychology, 34*(3), 506–522.

Foley, D., Rutter, M., Pickles, A., Angold, A., Maes, H., Silberg, J., et al. (2004). Informant disagreement for separation anxiety disorder. *Journal of the American Academy of Child and Adolescent Psychiatry, 42*(4), 452–460.

Frankel, F., & Feinberg, D. (2002). Social problems associated with ADHD vs. ODD in children referred for friendship problems. *Child Psychiatry and Human Development, 33*(2), 125–146.

Gerten, A. (2000). Guidelines for intervention with children and adolescents diagnosed with conduct disorder. *Social Work in Education, 22*(3), 132–144.

Hale, W. W., Raaijmakers, Q., Muris, P., & Meeus, W. (2005). Psychometric properties of the screen for child anxiety related emotional disorders (SCARED) in the general adolescent population. *Journal of the American Academy of Child and Adolescent Psychiatry, 42,* 30–40.

Halperin, J. M., McKay, K. E., & Newcorn, J. H. (2002). Development, reliability, and validity of the Children's Aggression Scale-Parent Version. *Journal of the American Academy of Child and Adolescent Psychiatry, 41,* 245–252.

Hinshaw, S. P., & Anderson, C. A. (1996). Conduct and oppositional defiant disorders. In E. J. Mash & R. A. Barkley (Eds.), *Child psychopathology* (pp 113–149). New York, NY: Guilford Press.

Hinshaw, S. P., & Blachman, D. R. (2005). Attention-deficit-hyperactivity disorder. In D. Bell-Dolan, S. Foster, & E. J. Mash (Eds.), *Handbook of behavioral and emotional problems in girls* (pp. 117–147). New York, NY: Kluwer Academic/Plenum Press.

Holmes, S. E., Slaughter, J. R., & Kashani, J. (2001). Risk factors in childhood that lead to the development of conduct disorder and antisocial personality disorder. *Child Psychiatry and Human Development, 31*(3), 183–193.

Individuals with Disabilities Education Act, 20 U.S.C. § 1400 (2004).

Kazdin, A. E., & Esveldt-Dawson, K. (1986). The interview for antisocial behavior: Psychometric characteristics and concurrent validity with child psychiatric inpatients. *Journal of Psychopathology and Behavioral Assessment, 8,* 289–303.

Kessler, R. C., Berglund, P., Demler, O., Jin, R., Merikangas, K. R., & Walters, E. E. (2005). Lifetime prevalence and age-of-onset distributions of DSM-IV disorders in the national comorbidity survey replication. *Archives of General Psychiatry, 62,* 593–602.

Last, C. G., Hersen, M., Kazdin, A. E., Finkelstein, R., & Strauss, C. C. (1987). Comparison of DSM-III separation anxiety and overanxious disorders: Demographic characteristics and patterns of comorbidity. *Journal of the American Academy of Child and Adolescent Psychiatry, 26,* 527–531.

Last, C. G., Perrin, S., Hersen, M., & Kazdin, A. E. (1992). DSM-III-R anxiety disorders in children: Sociodemographic and clinical characteristics. *Journal of the American Academy of Child and Adolescent Psychiatry, 31,* 1070–1076.

Lavigne, J. V., Cicchetti, C., Gibbons, R. D., Binns, H. J., Larsen, L., & DeVito, C. (2001). Oppositional defiant disorder with onset in preschool years: Longitudinal stability and pathways to other disorders. *Journal of the American Academy of Child and Adolescent Psychiatry*, 40, 1393–1400.

Litt, J., Taylor, H. G., Klein, N., & Hack, M. (2005). Learning disabilities in children with very low birth weight: Prevalence, neuropsychological correlates, and educational interventions. *Journal of Learning Disabilities*, 38(2), 130–141.

Loeber, R., Burke, J. D., Lahey, B. B., Winters, A., & Zera, M. (2000). Oppositional defiant and conduct disorder: A review of the past ten years, part I. *Journal of the American Academy of Child and Adolescent Psychiatry*, 39, 1468–1484.

Mandel, H. P. (1997). *Conduct disorder and under-achievement: Risk factors, assessment, treatment, and prevention*. New York, NY: Wiley.

Mannuzza, S., Klein, R. G., Bonagura, N., Malloy, P., Giampino, H., & Addalli, K. A. (1991). Hyperactive boys almost grown up: replication of psychiatric status. *Archives of General Psychiatry*, 48, 77–83.

March, J. S., Parker, J. D. A., Sullivan, K., Stallings, P., & Conners, K. C. (1997). The Multidimensional Anxiety Scale for Children (MASC): Factor structure, reliability, and validity. *Journal of the American Academy of Child and Adolescent Psychiatry*, 36(4), 554–565.

Markward, M. J., & Bride, B. (2001). Oppositional defiant disorder and the need for family-centered practice in schools. *Children and Schools*, 23(2), 73–83.

Masi, G., Mucci, M., & Millepiedi, S. (2001). Separation anxiety disorder in children and adolescents: Epidemiology, diagnosis and management. *CNS Drugs*, 15(2), 93–104.

Mattox, R., & Harder, J. (2007). Attention deficit hyperactivity disorder (ADHD) and diverse populations. *Child and Adolescent Social Work Journal*, 24(2), 195–207.

McGill, P., Tennyson, A., & Cooper, V. (2006). Parents whose children with learning disabilities and challenging behavior attend 52-week residential schools: Their perceptions of services received and expectations of the future. *British Journal of Social Work*, 36, 597–616.

Merikangas, K. R., He, J. P., Brody, D., Fisher, P. W., Bourdon, K., & Koretz, D. S. (2010). Prevalence and treatment of mental disorders among US children in the 2001–2004 NHANES. *Pediatrics*, 125(1), 75–81.

Mishna, F., Muskat, B., & Wiener, J. (2010). "I'm not lazy, it's just that I learn differently": Development and implementation of a manualized school-based group for students with LD. *Social Work with Groups*, 33, 1–21.

Ogliari, A., Citterio, A., Zanoni, A., Fagnani, C., Patriarca, V., Cirrincione, R., et al. (2006). Genetic and environmental influences on anxiety dimensions in Italian twins evaluated with the SCARED questionnaire. *Journal of Anxiety Disorders*, 20, 760–777.

Pincus, D. B., Santucci, L. C., Ehrenreich, J. T., & Eyberg, S. M. (2008). The implementation of modified parent–child interaction therapy for youth with separation anxiety disorder. *Cognitive and Behavioral Practice*, 15, 118–125.

Power, T. J., Mautone, J. A., Soffer, S. L., Clarke, A. T., Marshall, S. A., Sharman, J., et al. (2012). A family–school intervention for children with ADHD: Results of a randomized clinical trial. *Journal of Consulting and Clinical Psychology*, 80(4), 611–623. doi:10.1037/a0028188.

Reich, W. (1997). *Diagnostic Interview for Children and Adolescents—Revised DSM-IV version*. Toronto, ON, Canada: Multi-Health Systems.

Rosenkoetter, S., Hains, A., & Dogaru, C. (2007). Successful transitions for young children with disabilities and their families: Roles of school social workers. *Children and Schools*, 29, 25–34.

Rowland, A. S., Lesesne, C. A., & Abramowitz, A. J. (2002). The epidemiology of attention-deficit-hyperactivity disorder (ADHD): A public health view. *Mental Retardation and Developmental Disabilities Research Reviews*, 8, 162–170.

RUPP Anxiety Study Group. (2001). Fluvoxamine for the treatment of anxiety disorders in children and adolescents. *New England Journal of Medicine*, 344, 1279–1285.

Sanders, M. R., Markie-Dadds, C., Tully, L., & Bor, B. (2000). The Triple-P-Positive Parenting Program: A comparison of enhanced, standard, and self-directed behavioral family interventions for parents of children with early onset conduct problems. *Journal of Consulting and Clinical Psychology*, 68, 624–640.

Schneider, S., Blatter-Meunier, J., Herren, C., Adornetto, C., In-Albon, T., & Lavallee, K. (2011). Disorder-specific cognitive–behavioral therapy for separation anxiety disorder in young children: A randomized waiting-list-controlled trial. *Psychotherapy and Psychosomatics*, 80, 206–215.

Silverman, W. K., & Nelles, W. B. (1988). The anxiety disorders interview schedule for children. *Journal of the American Academy of Child and Adolescent Psychiatry*, 27(6), 772–778.

Walkup, J. T., Albano, A. M., Piacentini, J., Birmaher, B., Compton, S., Sherrill, J. T., et al. (2008). Cognitive-behavioral therapy, sertraline, or a combination in childhood anxiety. *The New England Journal of Medicine*, 359(26), 2753–2766.

Webster-Stratton, C., Reid, M. J., & Hammond, M. (2004). Treating children with early-onset conduct problems: Intervention outcomes for parent, child, and teacher training. *Journal of Clinical Child and Adolescent Psychology*, 33, 105–124.

Williams, S., Anderson, J., McGee, R., & Silva, P. A. (1990). Risk factors for behavioral and emotional disorder in preadolescent children. *Journal of the American Academy of Child and Adolescent Psychiatry*, 29, 413–419.

Wolraich, M. I., Lambert, W., Doffing, M. A., Bickman, L., Simmons, T., & Worley, K. (2003). Teachers' screening for attention deficit-hyperactivity disorder: Comparing multinational samples on teacher ratings of ADHD. *Journal of Abnormal Child Psychology*, 31, 445–455.

FURTHER READING

American Academy of Child and Adolescent Psychiatry, Children with Oppositional Defiant Disorder: http://www.aacap.org/AACAP/Families_and_Youth/Facts_for_Families/Facts_for_Families_Pages/Children_With_Oppositional_Defiant_Disorder_72.aspx

American Academy of Child and Adolescent Psychiatry, Conduct Disorder: http://www.aacap.org/cs/root/facts_for_families/conduct_disorder

American Academy of Child and Adolescent Psychiatry, Specific Learning Disorders: http://www.aacap.org/

Anxiety Disorders Association of America: http://www.adaa.org/

Children and Adults with Attention-Deficit-Hyperactivity Disorder: http://www.chadd.org/

Individuals with Disabilities Education Act (IDEA): http://idea.ed.gov/

National Institute of Mental Health, Anxiety Disorders: http://www.nimh.nih.gov/health/topics/anxiety-disorders/index.shtml

National Institute of Mental Health, Attention-Deficit-Hyperactivity Disorder: http://www.nimh.nih.gov/health/publications/attention-deficit-hyperactivity-disorder/complete-index.shtml

U.S. National Library of Medicine, Conduct Disorder: http://www.ncbi.nlm.nih.gov/pubmedhealth/PMH0001917/

U.S. National Library of Medicine, Oppositional Defiant Disorder: http://www.ncbi.nlm.nih.gov/pubmedhealth/PMH0002504/

SUSAN FRAUENHOLTZ AND AMY MENDENHALL

CHILDREN: OVERVIEW

ABSTRACT: Children are interesting, resilient people, whose lives are often perilous. Social workers deal extensively with children and families, and with policies that affect children, to help children and families overcome family disruption, poverty, and homelessness. Social workers also provide mental health care while working to ensure that children get medical care. Schools are areas of practice for social workers dealing with children. The issues of ethical practice and social justice for children are complex.

KEY WORDS: children's behavior; theories of behavior; child development; child poverty; substandard housing; homelessness; medical care for children; health impacts of diet and exercise on children; family break-up and reconfiguration; children functioning as parents; living with grandparents; children's mental well-being; common childhood mental disorders; children's responses to trauma; drug use among children; education; testing; bullying; ethics

Children in Society

Children, ideally, should enjoy life, with time to imagine, play, learn, and develop in safety and love, but many children's lives fall short of that ideal. Social workers work to enrich children's relationships and experiences, and to help adults understand that a child's behavior is a complex, interactive system affected by physical and mental health, family and home factors, spiritual influences, community and societal concerns, and economic issues. Adults who want to help children must take a broad perspective, creating strategies that integrate these various factors. However, children are amazingly resilient, and often develop their own successful strategies to deal with difficulties.

Approximately 73.5 million children under 18 live in the United States, and that number is expected to grow to 85.7 million by 2030 (Child Trends Data Bank, 2007). Worldwide, children number a staggering 2.2 billion (Shah, 2006).

Child Development

Children, because they are unique human beings living in and reacting to unique circumstances, defy easy classification of their development. Professionals classify child development, drawing on several theoretical frameworks, including Multicultural Theory, which maintains that the child should be viewed as developing within the context of family, community, and culture (Ashford, LeCroy, & Lortie, 2001). It is critical to be sensitive to the child's cultural identity, verbal and nonverbal communication, language, and spiritual beliefs.

Several major theories guide professional thinking about how children develop.

Psychodynamic Theory presumes that behavior is conscious (the person is aware of the behavior and its meaning); unconscious (the person is not aware of what is driving behavior, but senses feelings that influence behavior); or preconscious (thoughts and feelings can be brought into the conscious realm). The individual relives the past in present relationships, and is driven by the id (in which human drive is born), the ego (in which the individual makes executive decisions about how to behave), and the superego (the individual's conscience).

Ego Psychology Theory focuses on the ego, the personality's executive, highlighting ego functions (ranging from weak to strong) such as testing reality, making judgments, developing thought processes, and mastering behavior. This theory divides development into eight stages in which the child: (1) learns to trust or mistrust; (2) learns to feel autonomous or to feel shame and doubt; (3) initiates activities or feels guilty; (4) becomes industrious or feels inferior; (5) the adolescent develops personal identity or becomes confused in role identity; (6) the young adult learns to be intimate or feels isolated; (7) the adult generates productivity or stagnates; and (8) develops integrity or descends into despair.

Object Relations Theory posits that children seek stimulation, establish connections, and promote attachments by relating to people or objects as a function of their inborn drive to survive. Developing children learn to identify with objects or people, and learn to separate from them. Their feelings are split (like both loving and hating a parent) until they develop object constancy, allowing them to internalize the parent and hold that idea in their minds.

Cognitive Theory maintains that individuals' behaviors are determined by the way they structure their world. People's emotions flow out of what they believe or assume, and those assumptions may be outside their conscious thinking. Dysfunctional thoughts may result from organic, psychological, or chemical problems.

Behavioral Theory centers on how people learn to behave and change behavior. Behavior is conditioned by particular responses (classical conditioning) while operant conditioning refers to a person's ability to change a behavior when the behavior's antecedent or consequence is changed. Social learning theory indicates that behaviors are learned through imitating, modeling, and observing. Cognitive behavioral constructivist theory focuses on how and why people develop and are affected by stories about important life events.

Feminist Theory maintains that females develop largely in response to relationships. Healthy children develop by enhancing connection with others through engagement, empathy, and empowerment.

The Economic Circumstances of Children

In the United States, 13 million children live in poverty, according to the U.S. Census Bureau in 2004. Throughout the world, almost every other child, or about 1 billion children, exists in poverty (Shah, 2006; http://www.globalissues.org/TradeRelated/Facts.asp). Social workers are committed to helping people escape the negative consequences of poverty through working directly with the poor, and working with policy makers to develop societal strategies that attack poverty. Poverty's effects on children range from the obvious to the subtle, but are universally negative and become increasingly negative the longer a child lives in poverty (Downs, Moore, McFadden, & Costin, 2000). Poverty breeds housing and food insecurity, poses real barriers to getting a strong education, and factors into the development of serious health issues. And poverty has racial implications: the National Center for Children and Poverty stated in 2006 that, of U.S. children living in poverty, 10% are White; 35% are Black; 28% are Latino; 11% are Asian; and 29% are American Indian (http://www.nccp.org/state_detail_demographic_poor_US.html).

SUBSTANDARD HOUSING AND HOMELESSNESS

Poverty usually leads to substandard housing. An estimated 1.35 million American children, according to Horizons for Homeless, will experience homelessness over the course of a year (http://www.horizonsforhomelesschildren.org/Statistics_National_Statistics.asp), while, according to Shah (2006), 1 in 3 children (640 million) worldwide go without adequate shelter in a year (http://www.globalissues.org/TradeRelated/Facts.asp). Children who are homeless—or afraid of being homeless—are often depressed and frightened. Homelessness interrupts schooling and makes life more dangerous. Children living on the streets or in poor neighborhoods are more at risk of gunshot wounds, the second most frequent cause of death in children aged 10–19 after vehicular accidents, according to the Children's Defense Fund (January 31, 2005).

Poor children often live in and attend school in crowded, moldy, vermin-infested conditions where they are more susceptible to contagious diseases, respiratory illness, and injuries (Gracey, 2002). Children exposed (even before birth) to toxins such as lead, mercury, or pesticides are at risk of serious developmental damage. The majority of children live in cities where such substances are found (Gracey, 2002). Megacities with the most uncontrolled growth (such as São Paulo, Brazil; Mexico City; and Shanghai) have populations larger than nations such as Australia and, because they are overwhelmed with new residents, cannot keep up with the infrastructure necessary to protect children from disease and injury. As urban areas spread, creating more impervious surfaces such as roads and parking lots, water supplies increasingly collect pathogens, metals, and chemical pollutants, contributing to the growth of waterborne diseases to which children are particularly susceptible. According to Shah (2006), 1 in 5 children worldwide have no access to safe drinking water.

Children who have been living in foster care or other substitutes for parental care face acute housing problems when they "age" out of foster care, typically at age 18. They need transitional services, such as those authorized by the John Chafee Foster Care Independence Program of 1999, which funds states to assist foster care youths up to age 21 with educational and vocational services. Numerous child-caring agencies have "transitional living" programs for aging-out children.

SINGLE PARENTS AND POVERTY Currently 26% of American children under 18 live or have lived in a single-parent home, typically headed by a woman (Factbook, http://www.pobronson.com/factbook/pages/43.html). Sixty percent of births to black women in their 20s are to single women; 13% of births to 20-something white women are to single women (U.S. Census Bureau, 2004). Fewer than half the young men who father children with teen moms finish high school, so their earning potential is low (Kids Count Data Book, 2004).

Statistically, three elements increase a newborn's risk of child poverty: being born to a teenager, being born to a mother who has not completed high school, and being born to a mother who never married. Women who give birth as teens attain, on average, three years less education than women who delay childbearing till after their teen years, and only an estimated one-third of teen mothers go on to graduate high school (Kids Count Data Book, 2004). Raising children is expensive, and teen moms are ill prepared to pay the bills. Because they have had less time to mature through adolescence, they often lack adult skills in their decision making and behaviors.

ACCESS TO MEDICAL CARE Worldwide, 270 million (1 in 7 children) have no access to health services (Shah, 2006). In the U.S., poor children often do not receive the immunizations or medical care they need because of lack of funds or insurance, lack of transportation, confusing communication or language distinctions, and differences in cultural values.

Children of color, particularly, often have lower access to medical care because of poverty. They are more likely to visit emergency rooms rather than medical offices or clinics, and are less likely than White children to have completed their immunizations (Moniz & Gorin, 2003). Children of immigrants may lack immunizations and health care if their parents are afraid of seeking care and thereby exposing themselves to questions about their immigration status.

DIET AND EXERCISE Poverty also affects children's diets and their ability to exercise sufficiently. In 2002, the U.S. Department of Agriculture reported that nearly 35 million Americans—including over 13 million children—worried about how to secure their next meal (Children's Defense Fund, 2004). Fast food chains, with their inexpensive "extra value meals" and high saturated fats, are quite popular in low-income neighborhoods, while nutritious fresh vegetables and fish are too costly for many poor people to buy—and they may not have the kitchen appliances, electricity, and equipment to prepare foods in healthy ways. Nutrition-related problems, such as obesity and diabetes, are increasing in the United States. Lack of exercise contributes to the "super-sizing" of American children. Parents in poor neighborhoods may not allow children to play outside because play areas are limited or unsafe. Increasingly, children entertain themselves with sedentary pleasures, such as television. Lack of imaginative play with other children may increase a child's sense of isolation, decrease creativity, and limit opportunities to "practice" relating to others (Noble & Jones, 2006).

EDUCATION AND POVERTY Children of poverty often are not well prepared for school because their opportunities "to learn how to learn" are limited, they may be hungry and tired because of crowded and inadequate home conditions, and their families may not understand how to help them learn. Such children may be more likely to end up in special education programs, a stigmatizing experience (Oswald, Coutinho, Best, & Singh, 1999). Cultural issues, such as the child's most familiar language and patterns of eye contact, can unnerve teachers. Poor African American children are 2.3 times more likely to be identified by their teacher as having mental retardation than poor White children, and in some regions, Latino/a and Native American children are also overrepresented in special education (Oswald, Coutinho, Best, & Singh, 1999).

How Family Configuration Affects Children

Children are usually reared in families, but family configurations vary and affect the type of care children receive. Families, for instance, may be headed by divorced parents or by grandparents, while children in the family may be half-siblings or step-siblings; sometimes people who are not related by genetics or by law function as families. Social workers help parents and caregivers develop the best plans possible for children while securing the resources they need for the children. Social workers conduct home studies, mediate between parties seeking custody and child support, and testify in court (Noble & Ausbrooks, 2007).

FAMILY BREAK-UP AND FAMILY BLENDING Every year, more than 1 million children have parents who separate or divorce (Women's Educational Media in 2007; http://www.womedia.org/taf_statistics.htm). When families break up, children usually experience lowered family financial resources, and child support issues are troublesome (Downs, Moore, McFadden, & Costin, 2000). Children caught in highly emotional arguments between parents may experience fear, anger, and even physical danger (Noble & Ausbrooks, 2007). Children often see parents leaving one relationship for another relationship. Two-thirds of divorced parents marry again (Hetherington & Kelly, 2003), and children in blended families must adapt to step-parents and step-siblings.

PARENTS' EMPLOYMENT Work provides not only money to care for the family; it also gives people a sense of meaning and identity. When parents are unemployed, the strain on the family is both financial and emotional, and children may be confused, angry, or fearful. Often, employed parents have to place children in child care, which can be very costly. Some employed parents are forced to rely on child care arrangements that do not offer optimal safety and mental stimulation for developing children (Downs, Moore, McFadden, & Costin, 2000).

CHILDREN WHO FUNCTION AS PARENTS When parents have drug or alcohol habits, or mental or physical disabilities, children may be "parentified" by helping their parents take care of themselves, tending to younger siblings, and seeking ways to bring money into the family (Winton, 2003). Particularly in poor families, when adults are working and cannot purchase or otherwise provide child care, children may be left to fend for themselves while tending to siblings (Winton, 2003).

INCARCERATED PARENTS Children may also have to function as parents when their parents are incarcerated. At the beginning of the 21st century, 1,498,800 children had at least one parent in prison (Temin, 2001). Mothers, when arrested, sometimes do not reveal that they have children, fearing that the state will remove the children from their custody. During a father's incarceration, 89% of children will live with their mothers. During the incarceration of a mother, about 25% of children live with their fathers; 51% live with their grandparents; 20% live with other relatives, 9% live in foster homes, 4% live with friends, 2% live in an institution, and 2% live alone (Young & Smith, 2000).

LIVING WITH GRANDPARENTS In the United States, about 6 million children live in households headed by grandparents or other relatives. About 2.5 million of these children live in homes in which neither parent is present, so the relative is in charge of rearing the child, a steep assignment for grandparents who are on a fixed income and have limited energy or resources (Financial assistance for grandparents, 2004). Depending on state regulations, caregiving relatives may be eligible for financial assistance through Temporary Assistance for Needy Families (TANF), foster care payments, subsidized guardianship or kinship care payments, subsidized adoption arrangements, or Earned Income Tax Credit. The child who is disabled, poor, and under 18 may be eligible for Supplemental Security Income (SSI) payments (Financial assistance for grandparents, 2004).

GAY AND LESBIAN FAMILIES Children sometimes live with gay or lesbian parents, having been born during a parent's previous heterosexual relationship, conceived through reproductive technology, or adopted. They often face questions and misunderstanding from community members, as well as teasing or oppression from their contemporaries. Since, in most jurisdictions, gay and lesbian families lack typical family legal protections, children of gays or lesbians face unique family issues when parents break up and argue about custody, or parents become ill or die.

Children's Physical Well-Being
How well children reach developmental milestones is directly related to their physical well-being. Social workers have been active in developing and delivering health-related programs, such as Medicaid (health coverage for qualifying poor families) and the Women, Infants, and Children's Program (WIC) (health in infants).

INJURIES Historically, the biggest killer of children has been infectious disease, for example, diphtheria. Now the most common cause of child death in industrialized countries is injury (Gracey, 2002), particularly in areas where children must cope with poisonous substances, heavy traffic, the risks of falling from tall structures, limited play space, exposure to drugs and alcohol or users, and violent actions from others (Noble & Jones, 2006.)

PUBLIC PROGRAMS FOR POOR CHILDREN'S HEALTH CARE Of all the industrialized countries, the United

States is the only one that has no universal health care. Twelve percent of American children are not covered by any health insurance (Kids Count Data Book, 2004). Medicaid, established by Congress in 1967 and financed through federal and state taxes, provides medical assistance (as well as screening for certain health conditions) to qualifying low-income families. In 1997 Congress created the State Children's Health Insurance Program (SCHIP) to help states insure children whose parents are too poor to buy insurance but who are not poor enough to qualify for Medicaid. This program varies widely between states in structure and eligibility criteria. Some states have been slow to implement the program, and many families which might be eligible for coverage do not know about or understand how to apply for the program. Nonetheless, SCHIP has made a difference in children's access to health care; 6 million children nationwide are covered (The State Children's Health Insurance Program).

Most states have adopted some form of "Baby Moses" laws, which allow parents to legally abandon an infant 60 days old or younger at a "safe baby site," such as a fire station or hospital. Such legislation provides parents a way to legally give a child to an emergency care provider, rather than illegally abandon the child in a dangerous or unprotected location.

Children's Mental Well-Being

Not only do children need to be physically safe, cared for, and healthy, but they also need environments that support their mental and emotional needs. From 12% to 22% of all children under age 18 in the United States need services for mental, emotional, or behavioral problems, and approximately 1 out of every 50 children (1.3 million) receive mental health services (Latest Findings in Children's Mental Health, 2004; UCLA Center Report, 2003). Many of those services are designed and delivered by social workers.

Insurance or Medicare coverage is typically limited for mental health services. Social workers, however, have been instrumental in crafting legislation such as the Juvenile Justice and Delinquency Prevention Act, which established juvenile drug courts to help youngsters conquer alcohol and drug use, as well as advocating for more community-based programs to help children avoid and deal with mental and emotional difficulties.

A child's mental and emotional health is affected by complex interactions between physical environmental factors (such as overcrowding), family issues (such as the parent's mental health status), emotional environmental elements (such as parents' knowledge of appropriate discipline), and the child's inborn char-

acteristics (such as genetic make-up). Social workers develop and deliver mental health programs, work with children and parents to overcome problems, participate in emergency response teams during traumas, and advocate for public policies that help enhance children's mental health. Children need positive, stable support from family members, social workers, school officials, clergy and religious groups, and community programs and priorities that help them build buffers against mental problems.

COMMON CHILDHOOD MENTAL DISORDERS Anxiety disorders, attention deficit hyperactivity disorder, posttraumatic stress disorder, depression, and conduct disorder are common among children who have been maltreated; have lost a family member to death, military deployment, or incarceration; or have witnessed violence (Noble & Jones, 2006). Learning disorders and pervasive developmental disorders (such as autism and Asperger's Disorder) are linked to toxins such as environmental pollutants and fetal alcohol syndrome (APA, 2000). Environmental toxins, drug exposure in utero, and a history of child abuse and multiple foster care placements are related to Attention Deficit Hyperactivity Disorder (ADHD) (Harvard Mental Health Letter, 2004). Conduct disorder is associated with such inconsistent child-rearing practices as harsh discipline, lack of supervision, maternal smoking during pregnancy, and exposure to violence (APA, 2000). Oppositional defiant disorder is more prevalent in children who have had a succession of different caregivers or who live in families with harsh, inconsistent, neglectful child-rearing practices (American Psychiatric Association [APA], 2000). Almost a third of all children receiving mental health services suffer from two or more psychiatric disorders, making treatment more difficult. The most common diagnostic combination is ADHD and mood disorders (Latest Findings, 2004).

RESPONSES TO TRAUMA Children can view natural disasters, terrorist acts, school shootings, and other distressing events on television and the Internet at any time. Some trauma is time-limited (such as a sudden change in living situation) and may result in posttraumatic stress disorder. When the trauma is chronic (such as long-term incest), its cumulative effects open the child to additional psychopathology. A child may react to trauma by internalizing the pain and experiencing depression, withdrawal, and self-injury, or the child may externalize the pain and act it out in aggression—all reactions that interfere with normal social, educational, and physical development (Noble & Jones, 2006).

Children who suffer maltreatment, witness frequent family violence, or exist in dangerous living conditions are also more likely to suffer intellectual deficits (Noble & Jones, 2006). The child who is desensitized to violence may expect violence and become aggressive. Traumatized children can experience impaired memory or speech development, fear and guilt, unpleasant memories, repetitive behavior, emotional numbing, and a sense of hopelessness. Traumatized children are also more vulnerable to suicide attempts (Noble & Jones, 2006). On an average day, four American teens commit suicide (Kids Count Data Book, 2004), though the actual number may be higher because some suicides are listed as accidental deaths.

INTELLECTUAL DISABILITY Intellectual disability is a physical and mental condition rather than a psychiatric illness, but children with intellectual disabilities (once called "mental retardation") may also have psychiatric and physical difficulties. Intellectual disabilities can originate in biological factors, prenatal damage due to toxins, deprivation of nurturance or stimulation, fetal malnutrition, premature birth, viral infections during pregnancy, and childhood infections, injuries, or poisonings (APA, 2000). These children may also exhibit anxiety, conduct disorders, or impaired development.

USE OF ILLEGAL DRUGS AND PSYCHOTROPIC MEDICATIONS Children easily learn how to acquire illegal drugs and alcohol, and some indulge in these substances. Such behavior can trigger a downward spiral, bringing children into contact with criminals, stunting their development and education, impairing their judgment, making them more vulnerable to sexual activities and sexually transmitted diseases, and increasing their chances of dangerous behavior, injury, or death (Gracey, 2002; Noble & Jones, 2006). Educating children about the dangers of drugs and alcohol, limiting their chances of acquiring these substances, and supporting children in healthy drug and alcohol-free activities are strategies that go hand-in-hand with enforcing laws designed to stop drug commerce and keep alcohol off-limits for children.

Using psychotropic medications to treat children is controversial (FDA requires warnings for use of antidepressants on children, December 10, 2004).

Most antidepressants, for instance, have not been widely tested on children, though physicians may still prescribe such medications "off-label" (for a use other than that approved by government regulations). Prescribing medications "off-label" for children requires

caregivers to guess about dosage and duration of treatment. Some authorities blame some antidepressants for sparking suicidal or violent actions in children (Antidepressant medications for children and adolescents, February 2, 2005). Medical authorities across the world are examining whether to ban prescribing antidepressants for children (as Britain recently did), while the U.S. Food and Drug Administration now requires that antidepressants commonly prescribed for children carry strong warning labels that the drugs can spur suicidal behavior. Nonetheless, one-third of all children in mental heath services are treated with psychotropic drugs, particularly if they suffer from more than one diagnosis (Latest Findings, 2004). Using seclusion, physical restraints, or chemical restraints on children is controversial and open to legal challenge (Latest Findings, 2004). The cost of treating children and adolescents for mental health concerns is estimated at nearly $12 billion (UCLA Report, 2003).

How Educational Realities Affect Children
All the challenges that children face merge in their educational settings. In order to learn, children need to feel safe in their schools and their neighborhoods, and they need to be healthy and cognitively able to focus on schoolwork. While some social workers operate directly in school settings, many other social workers are also involved in school issues that affect children. Social workers help teachers understand the impact of culture and family resources on children's and parents' behavior, while emphasizing positive development in children. They work with children who are suddenly removed from their homes because of danger and are now in an unfamiliar foster home and a strange school with different classmates. In cases of sudden traumatic events, such as school violence, social workers are invaluable in helping children stay safe and cope with their fear and anger.

Social workers also advocate for programs such as Head Start, a comprehensive child development program authorized through the Economic Opportunity Act of 1965, which has helped millions of disadvantaged children get a head start in school, and the National School Lunch and Breakfast programs, which feed hungry children in school. Social workers also assist schools, as well as children and their families, to protect children's confidentiality under the Family Educational Rights and Privacy Act (FERPA) and the Health Insurance Portability and Accountability Act (HIPAA).

CHILDREN WITH SPECIAL NEEDS Children who primarily speak a language other than English need particular attention in the U.S. educational arena. How best to teach limited English-speaking (LEP) children is controversial, particularly in light of emotional responses to immigration (Meyer & Patton, 2001).

Various federal education laws, such as the Improving America's Schools Act of 1994 and the No Child Left Behind Act of 2002, address strategies to teach LEP children. Social workers can build bridges between LEP families and the school.

Social workers are often involved with processes generated by the Individuals with Disabilities Education Act (IDEA) of 1990 (P.L. 94–142), which provides federal money to states to augment special education for children with mental, physical, or emotional disabilities. This legislation states that every child is entitled to a free, appropriate public education, and that parents should be included in making their children's educational plans. Children, who are guaranteed procedural due process under the law, are to be placed in the "least restrictive environment" that can meet their educational needs. IDEA also includes a provision for the Handicapped Infant and Toddlers Program, an interdisciplinary system of early intervention for disabled babies and their families.

Because children with special education needs are often economically and socially disadvantaged, social workers deal with them to solve a broad array of social service needs. For instance, because poor children sometimes come to school wearing hand-me-down, ill-fitting shoes and thus cannot participate effectively in physical activities, social workers have helped develop resources to meet clothing needs.

TESTING Children are often grouped and labeled by standardized tests—the results of which tend to shape students' careers. The U.S. Department of Education presses school districts to meet testing standards in order to access federal funds, and the No Child Left Behind initiative relies heavily on testing for accountability and for determining whether children progress in school. The stress of this high-stakes testing takes a toll on school districts, families, and children (Children's Defense Fund, September 2004).

Children who have some hope of doing well in tests tend to study hard. But children who are not academically oriented and are depressed about testing may remove themselves, either by literally dropping out or by disengaging from studying and perhaps indulging in escape behaviors such as drugs. If students look like poor risks for success on these high-stakes exams, schools may encourage them to move into a General Education Diploma (GED) program to avoid the testing, or may retain them in the grade preceding the testing grade to avoid having the students pull down the test score (Children's Defense Fund, September 2004). Reports are widespread of schools "teaching to the test" and shifting time away from untested subjects, such as health. Testing may more accurately test the adults who operate schools than the children in the school. Social workers help students and teachers to cope with the pressures of this test-intensive environment.

Success in school is critical. As the United States becomes more mechanized, the job market and potential earnings for people without high school diplomas are grim (Children's Defense Fund, August 6, 2004).

Social workers help school children stay in school, find jobs, and plan for their future. They may train children how to interview for jobs, for instance, and how to develop habits like timeliness, required in the workplace.

BULLYING One reason children may stop engaging in their studies or even going to school is fear of violence, including the everyday possibility of being bullied by classmates (Duncan, 2004). Bullying attacks a child's self-esteem and interferes with schooling. Social workers have been instrumental in developing and delivering "stop bully abuse" programs for students, and in developing strategies to help children treat others with respect. Social workers involve parents of the "bully" to stop the discourteous and dangerous behavior; they also deal with people who witness or are victims of bullying.

Issues of Ethics and Social Justice in Children's Work

Children's legal rights have grown over the last century, and those rights often create tension between children, adults, and social institutions. Society continues to debate whether children are mentally and emotionally prepared to make decisions, and which person or entity is best prepared to make appropriate decisions concerning children (Noble & Ausbrooks, 2007). The court system has become increasingly important as the arbiter of decisions in child custody, the extent to which children should be held culpable for criminal behavior, child medical issues, child discipline, abortion, religious practices that affect children, educational priorities, sex education and sexual activity, children's rights to free speech, censorship of materials available to children, financial liabilities for children's behavior, inheritance, and other complex situations (Badeau, 2003). Social workers in various service systems are involved in all these issues.

The limits and boundaries of ethical behavior in working with children are often hard to determine. A social worker must always think through how children and parents may interpret activities such as hugging the child, discussing spiritual or religious issues with children, or transporting a child in a vehicle. Social workers are also obliged to understand state and federal regulations regarding confidentiality of children's medical or educational records and the circumstances under which release of children's records is allowed. They should be aware of laws related to children, such as children's rights to seek different medical treatments without parental consent.

Social workers should also keep focused on the rewards of working with children. Children are fascinating, and working with them is always interesting and challenging—and it is an investment in the future of the world.

REFERENCES

American Psychiatric Association Diagnostic Classification *DSM-IV-TR*. (2000). Retrieved May 1, 2007, from http://www.behavenet.com/capsules/disorders/dsm4TR classification.htm

Antidepressant medications for children and adolescents. (February 2, 2005). Retrieved from http://www.nimh.nih.gov/about/updates/2005/antidepressant-medications-for-children-and-adolescents-information-for-parents-and-caregivers.shtml.

Badeau, S. (2003). Child welfare and the courts. Retrieved August 8, 2005, from http://pewfostercare.org/docs/index.

Children's Defense Fund. (2004, June 2). 13 million children face food insecurity. Retrieved January 30, 2005, from http://www.childrensdefense.org

Children's Defense Fund. (2004, August 6). Joblessness for minority youth reaches historic. high. Retrieved May 15, 2005, from http://www.childrensdefense.org.

Children's Defense Fund. (September 2004). High School Exit Exams. Retrieved May 21, 2005, from http://www.childrensdefense.org.

Children's Defense Fund. (2005, January 31). A moral outrage: One American child or teen killed by gunfire nearly every 3 hours. Retrieved January 1, 2006, from http://www.childrensdefense.org

Child Trends Data Bank. (n.d). Retrieved May 10, 2007, from http://www.childtrendsdatabank.org

Downs, S. W., Moore, E., McFadden, E. J., & Costin, L. B. (2000). *Child welfare and family services: Policies and practices* (6th ed.). Boston: Allyn & Bacon.

Duncan, K. A. (2004). Bullying as child abuse: Intervention strategies schools can employ. American Counseling Association: Retrieved July 30, 2005, from http://www.counseling.org.

Factbook: Eye-opening memos on everything family. (n.d.). Retrieved May 10, 2007, from http://www.pobronson.com/factbook/pages/43.html

FDA requires warnings for use of antidepressants on children. (December 10, 2004). *New York Times*, p. A 36.

Financial assistance for grandparents and other relatives raising children. (July 2004). Children's Defense Fund. Retrieved January 1, 2006, from http://www.childrensdefense.org

Gracey, M. (2002). Child health in an urbanizing world. *Acta Paediatrica*, 91, 1–8.

Harvard Medical School (2004). An update on attention deficit disorder. *Harvard Mental Health Letter*, 20(11), 4–7.

Hetherington, E. M., & Kelly, J. (2003). *For better or worse: Divorce reconsidered*. New York: Norton.

Horizons for Homeless Children. (n.d.). Retrieved May 10, 2007, from http://www.horizonsforhomelesschildren.org/Statistics_National_Statistics.asp

Kids Count Data Book. (2004). Baltimore, MD: Annie E. Casey Foundation.

Latest Findings in Children's Mental Health. (Winter 2004). Institute for Health, Health Care Policy, and Aging Research: Rutgers University. Retrieved January 1, 2006, from http://www.ihhcpar.rutgers.edu

Meyer, G., & Patton, J. (2001). On the nexus of race, disability, and overrepresentation: What do we know? Where do we go? National Institute for Urban School Improvement. Retrieved May 15, 2005, from http://www.inclusiveschools.org.

Moniz, C., & Gorin, S. (2003). *Health and health care policy: A social work perspective*. Boston: Allyn & Bacon.

National Center for Children and Poverty. (2006). Columbia University, Mailman School of Public Health. Retrieved May 10, 2007, from http://www.nccp.org/state_detail_demographic_poor_US.html

Noble, D. N., and Ausbrooks, A. (2008). Serving Children. In D. M. DiNitto & C. A. McNeece, *Social Work: Issues and Opportunities in a Challenging Profession* (3rd ed.). Chicago: Lyceum.

Noble, D. N., & Jones, S. H. (2006). Mental health issues affecting urban children. In N. K. Phillips & S. L. A. Straussner (Eds.), *Children in the urban environment: Linking social policy and clinical practice* (2nd ed., pp. 97–121). Springfield, IL: Thomas.

Oswald, D. P., Coutinho, M. J., Best, A. M., & Singh, N. N. (1999). Ethnic representation in special education: The influence of school-related economic and demographic variables. *Journal of Special Education*, 32(4), 194–206.

Shah, A. (2006). Poverty: Facts and stats. Retrieved May 10, 2007, from http://www.globalissues.org/TradeRelated/Facts.asp

Temin, C. (2001). Let us consider the children. *Corrections Today*, 63, 66–68.

The State Children's Health Insurance Program (SCHIP). (n.d.). Retrieved from May 10, 2007, from http://www.results.org/website/article.asp?id=1561

UCLA Mental Health in Schools Center Report. (December 2003). Youngsters' mental health and psychosocial problems: What are the data? Retrieved January 1, 2006, from http://smhp.psych.ucla.edu

U.S. Census Bureau. (2004). Poverty: 2004 Highlights. Retrieved January 1, 2006, from http://www.census.gov/hhes/www/poverty/poverty04/pov04hi.html

Winton, C. A. (2003). *Children as caregivers: Parental and parentified children*. Boston: Allyn & Bacon.

Women's Educational Media: That's a Family! (2007). Retrieved May 10, 2007, from http://www.womedia.org/taf_statistics.htm

Young, D., & Smith, C. (2000). When Moms are incarcerated: The needs of children, mothers, and caregivers. *Families in Society, 81*, 130–141.

FURTHER READING U.S. Department of Justice. (1998). Bureau of Justice statistics sourcebook of criminal justice statistics. Washington, DC: US Government Printing Office.

DORINDA N. NOBLE

COGNITIVE BEHAVIORAL THERAPY

ABSTRACT: This is an overview of cognitive behavioral therapy (CBT). Cognitive behavioral therapy is introduced and its development as a psychosocial therapeutic approach is described. This overview outlines the central techniques and intervention strategies utilized in CBT and presents common disorder-specific applications of the treatment. The empirical evidence supporting CBT is summarized and reviewed. Finally, the impact of CBT on clinical social work practice and education is discussed, with attention to the treatment's alignment with the profession's values and mission.

KEY WORDS: cognitive behavioral therapy; evidence-based practice; clinical social work; mental health; psychosocial treatment; CBT

Definition/Description

Cognitive behavioral therapy (CBT) is a structured, time-limited approach to psychotherapy that aims to address clients' current problems (Dobson & Dobson, 2009). CBT uses problem-focused cognitive and behavioral strategies guided by empirical science and derived from theories of learning and cognition (Craske, 2010). These interventions are delivered within a collaborative context where therapists and clients work together to identify problems, set goals, develop intervention strategies, and evaluate the effectiveness of those strategies.

CBT represents a broad approach to treatment that encompasses various theoretical models, including cognitive therapy (CT; Beck, 1976; Beck, Rush, Shaw, & Emery, 1979; Beck, 1995), rational-emotive behavioral therapy (REBT; Ellis, 1962, 1979; 1994; Ellis & Dryden, 1997), problem-solving therapy (D'Zurilla & Nezu, 2007; Haley, 1987), stress inoculation training (SIT; Meichenbaum, 1993; Meichenbaum & Deffenbacher, 1988), schema-focused therapy (Young, 1994;

Young, Klosko, & Weishaar, 2003), and dialectical behavioral therapy (DBT; Linehan, 1987, 1993). Though individual cognitive behavioral treatment models may vary in their emphasis on behavioral and cognitive principles and methodologies, interventions under the CBT umbrella are unified by an empirical foundation, reliance on the theory and science of behavior and cognition, and a problem-focused orientation (Dobson & Dobson, 2009).

CBT can be defined by common features that cut across individual treatment models or variations.

Most notably, the cognitive behavioral approach emphasizes a person's thinking as the prime determinant of emotional and behavioral responses to life events (Beck, 1976; Ellis, 1994; Meichenbaum, 1993). Dobson and Dozois (2001) offer three basic principles that are common to most CBT models:

1. The access hypothesis, which asserts that the content and process of our thinking is knowable and, with appropriate training and attention, persons can become aware of their own thinking

2. The mediation hypothesis, positing that there is cognitive mediation between events and persons' typical responses to them. CBT maintains that the way people think about or interpret their experiences has a profound impact on how they feel about those experiences. Therefore, thoughts and beliefs strongly influence behavioral patterns. CBT suggests that thoughts and corresponding emotional and behavioral responses may become routine and automatic over time.

3. The change hypothesis asserts that, because cognitions are knowable and mediate the response to different situations, it is possible to intentionally modify how people respond to events. CBT maintains that an increased recognition and understanding of emotional and behavioral reactions, through the systematic use of cognitive strategies, leads to more functional and adaptive responses.

Additionally, CBT generally asserts that a more realistic, or accurate, appraisal of the world, and the ability to adapt to the real world, is one indication of good mental health. Conversely, maladaptive or dysfunctional assessments of reality lead to a distorted view of the world and more emotional and behavioral problems. As the mediation hypothesis suggests, CBT asserts that patterns of thinking, including general ideas, assumptions, and schemas (firmly held basic beliefs about the self, others, and the world), are derived over time based upon persons' experiences interacting with their social environment (Dobson & Dobson, 2009). These assumptions and schemas affect how people view the world around them, potentially predisposing them to certain ways of thinking that become self-fulfilling prophesies (Beck, 1976). Once schemas became established, they not only affect memories of past experiences, but also influence future development by restricting the situations and activities people choose to engage in (Beck, 1976; Dobson & Dobson, 2009).

However, CBT contends that people do not just passively react to events and triggers in the world around them; rather, they have the potential to actively shape the course of their lives (i.e., change hypothesis). Therefore, CBT utilizes cognitive and behavioral strategies to help clients identify and replace maladaptive behaviors, emotions, and cognitions with more adaptive ones. Behavioral interventions, including behavioral activation, exposure, problem solving, social skills training, and relaxation training, focus on decreasing maladaptive behaviors and increasing adaptive ones by modifying their antecedents and consequences in ways that lead to new learning. Cognitive interventions, such as thought recording, reality testing, and reattribution or reappraisal, aim to restructure maladaptive or distorted thoughts and generate alternative, more evidence-based appraisals and beliefs.

Origins, Major Developers, and Contributors
CBT emerged as an approach to psychotherapy during the mid-20th century. The philosophical foundations of CBT were informed by Greek and Roman Stoicism, Buddhism, and Taoism, all of which emphasize reason, logic, and acceptance (Beck et al., 1979; Dryden, David, & Ellis, 2010). Influenced by the shift from psychodynamic theory to more scientific approaches to treatment (Beck, 1967; Ellis, 1979), CBT derived from advances in behavioral and cognitive theory and science (e.g., Eysenck, 1960; Lazarus, 1966). Behavioral approaches drew from the classical conditioning theory of Watson (Watson & Raynor, 1920; Watson, 1925) and Mowrer (1960) and the operant conditioning theory of Pavlov (1927) and B. F. Skinner (1938, 1963), both of which focus on antecedents and reinforcers of behavior and advocate an empirical approach to evaluating behavior. In the 1950s and 1960s, pioneers in behavior therapy developed these theories further into models for intervening in various mental health problems, such as mood (depression, anxiety) and behavioral problems in children and adults (for review, see Clark & Fairburn, 1997). A few of these models and methods are noted below.

Early exposure methods for treating anxiety were derived from the animal models of reciprocal inhibition of Wolpe (1958), which he adapted for use in humans, developing and testing systematic desensitization, or brief exposures to feared cues offset by carefully trained relaxation responses (or other fear inhibitors). His methods were supported by Lang's (1968) studies documenting the fear reducing effects of desensitization and further outlining the nature of fear. The two-stage model of fear and avoidance of Mowrer (1960) proposed that human fear was conditioned through the pairing of ordinary cues with actual fear and that avoidance persisted because it was negatively reinforced. This model was used extensively to develop interventions for anxiety and obsessive-compulsive disorders. Skinner's operant conditioning models were further developed for application of reinforcement and contingencies applied to a variety of child and adult behaviors. Examples include Azrin's token economy, time out, and habit reversal procedures for motor disorders (see Hersen, 2005), as well as Kazdin's (1978) work on skills training and parent management for child behavior problems.

The social learning theory of Albert Bandura (1977) and social cognitive theory (1986), which focused on observational or vicarious learning, promoted both behavioral and cognitive models for understanding mental health. Albert Ellis (1962) and Aaron Beck (1976) developed early models of cognitive behavioral therapy that established the philosophical, theoretical, and practice foundations of this approach. While Ellis (1962) and Beck (1976; Beck et al., 1979) developed their models independently, both focused on the relationship between cognition and emotional disturbance, concluding that distorted and dysfunctional thinking is the primary determinant of mood and behavior (Craske, 2010). These early cognitive behavioral approaches also shared an emphasis on the importance of eliciting clients' reports of situations and events occurring in daily life and assigning common sense meanings to clients' problems (Dobson & Dobson, 2009).

Ellis's rational emotive behavior therapy (REBT; Ellis, 1962, 1979, 1994; Ellis & Dryden, 1997) was built upon the ancient Greek and Roman Stoic philosophers, such as Epictetus, Epicurus, and Marcus Aurelius, and Asian philosophers, such as Confucius, Lao-Tsu, and Gautama Buddha, all of whom maintained that people are not disturbed by things but by their view of things (Ellis & Dryden, 1997). Ellis asserted that people's beliefs, or how they think, strongly affect their emotional functioning. The REBT model maintained that emotional reactions were mediated by "internal sentences" or thoughts, and that holding certain irrational beliefs (e.g., absolutism, demand for love and approval, and demand for comfort) resulted in internal self-statements that were maladaptive responses to situations (Ellis, 1962). Ellis suggested that irrational beliefs lead to mislabeling of situations that ultimately create psychological problems and emotional distress. Ellis (1962) developed the ABC model to guide this process, wherein an activating event (A) happens in the environment around you; you hold a belief (B) about that event; and your belief elicits an emotional response or consequence (C). As a result, Ellis maintained that rational beliefs elicit appropriate emotional and behavioral response while irrational beliefs lead to inappropriate and dysfunctional response (Ellis & Dryden, 1997). Therefore, a goal of REBT is to help clients identify, challenge, and alter their irrational beliefs and negative thinking patterns to be more rational and realistic. REBT also focuses on targeting emotional responses that accompany irrational thoughts and encourages clients to change unwanted behaviors through meditation, journaling, and guided imagery.

Similarly, Beck based his cognitive therapy (CT) model (1976; Beck et al., 1979) on the idea that critical or negative automatic thoughts and unpleasant physical or emotional symptoms combine to form maladaptive cycles that maintain symptoms and result in emotional distress. Beck (1976) asserted that a person's fundamental beliefs about themselves and the world predispose them to either psychological health or distress. CT suggests that a person's way of organizing themselves and the world, or cognitive schema, results in automatic thoughts about situations and events (Dobson & Dobson, 2009). Beck identified common cognitive distortions (e.g., all-or-nothing thinking, overgeneralization, jumping to conclusions, should statements, labeling and mislabeling) that often operate as automatic thoughts (Beck, 1963, 1976; Beck et al., 1979). He argued that cognitive distortions lead to faulty assumptions and misconceptions that inform both emotional and behavioral responses to an event or situation (Beck, 1963). CT aims to help clients identify automatic thoughts, understand how cognitive distortion or negative thinking influence feelings and behavior, develop a more realistic appraisal of situations and events, and modify dysfunctional beliefs and assumptions that predispose cognitive distortions (Beck, 1976; Beck et al., 1979).

Other popular therapeutic approaches under the CBT umbrella include Meichenbaum's (1993; Meichenbaum & Deffenbacher, 1988) stress inoculation training (SIT), and problem-solving therapy (PST; D'Zurilla & Nezu, 2007; Haley, 1987). SIT helps persons develop skills, such as self-instruction, relaxation, behavioral rehearsal, and in vivo exposure, to protect themselves against the effects of anxiety and trauma and against future stressors. PST focuses on training individuals to effectively use problem-solving skills, which encourages and increases healthy coping and the ability to adapt.

It is also important to note the more recent development of third wave behavioral therapies. Since the 1990s a number of new interventions, referred to as the third wave of behavioral therapy, have emerged. Though rooted in CBT, third wave behavioral therapies emphasize the role of mindfulness and acceptance in the healing process. Dialectical behavior therapy (DBT; Linehan, 1987, 1993), acceptance and commitment therapy (ACT; Hayes, 2004; Hayes et al., 2006), mindfulness-based cognitive therapy (MBCT; Segal, Williams, & Teasdale, 2002), and mindfulness-based stress reduction (MBSR; Kabat-Zinn, 1990) are commonly considered part of the third wave. While still acknowledging the mediation between thoughts, behavior, and emotions, third wave interventions focus less on challenging clients' irrational or negative thoughts and more on changing clients' relationship to thoughts and feelings (Hayes, 2004; Singh, Lancioni, Wahler, Winton, & Singh, 2008). To this end, third wave behavioral therapies incorporate contextual and experiential change strategies such as mindfulness, acceptance, and cognitive defusion, and encourages a focus on relationships, values, emotional deepening, and contact with the present moment (Hayes, 2004), While proponents of third wave behavioral therapies assert that they maintain CBT's commitment to an empirical, scientific approach to treatment (Hayes, 2004; Hayes, Masuda, Bissett, Luoma & Guerrero, 2004), some scholars have argued that third wave behavioral therapies may be getting ahead of the data (Corrigan, 2001) and do not yet meet established criteria to be considered empirically supported treatments (EST; Ost, 2008).

CBT Techniques

Cognitive behavioral therapists utilize a combination of cognitive and behavioral intervention strategies to address clients' presenting problems. Clinicians select appropriate intervention strategies after conducting a thorough initial assessment to clarify how thoughts, emotions, and behaviors are interrelated. The intervention strategies employed may vary based upon clients' presenting problem and skill level, as well as the treatment model. Behavioral interventions are often employed earlier in treatment as they are likely to address symptoms quickly, leaving clients better equipped to start focusing on cognitive aspects of problems (Dobson & Dobson, 2009); however, some approaches reverse this order. All CBT techniques are implemented within the context of therapist and client collaboration. Cognitive behavioral therapists emphasize and reward the clients' effort when implementing intervention strategies, regardless of their outcome.

The central techniques and intervention strategies used in CBT are described below in the order they are generally implemented in treatment, beginning with psychoeducation, followed by behavioral interventions, and then cognitive restructuring. Finally, homework, a key aspect of CBT that is implemented across intervention strategies, is discussed.

Psychoeducation. Psychoeducation is defined as teaching relevant psychological principles and knowledge to clients (Anderson, Hogarty, & Reiss, 1980). Helpful materials include information about the diagnosis, the treatment rationale, and research findings (Anderson et al., 1980), which can be presented in a variety of ways, depending on clients' learning needs. Cognitive behavioral therapists often recommend a combination of didactic materials, including pamphlets, books, videos, and websites, that are tailored to a client's education, language, literacy, skills, interests, resources, privacy needs, distress level, concentration ability, and quality of materials (Dobson & Dobson, 2009). Psychoeducation lets clients know that they are not alone and that their problems have been widely identified, researched, and discussed (Anderson et al., 1980). This can lead to feelings of support, hope, and validation, as well as a sense of control over problems that may begin to shift beliefs.

Behavioral Interventions: Reinforcement and response contingencies. A variety of behavioral techniques are subsumed within this broad category of interventions that derive from operant (Skinnerian) models of human behavior. Following a careful behavioral analysis of the stimulus and responses in the problem context, therapists may apply direct reinforcements (rewards) for positive behaviors and costs (e.g., time out, loss of a privilege) for performance of problematic behaviors. In the case of child behaviors within a family context, parents are typically trained to observe the child's behavior and apply appropriate positive and negative reinforcements.

Behavioral activation. Behavioral activation encourages clients to engage in pleasurable or mastery (e.g., self-care, chores, paying bills) activities in a scheduled, monitored way. Originally developed by Ferster (1973) and Lewinsohn, Sullivan, & Grosscup (1980) as a depression treatment, behavioral activation has been implemented widely with clients experiencing decreased activity and reduced reinforcement across a range of diagnostic categories. Behavioral activation is used to help clients increase the quantity and quality of positively reinforced behavior and improve coping behaviors to deal more adaptively with negative life situations (Dobson & Dobson, 2009). Implementing behavioral activation early in therapy is likely to result in improved mood and higher levels of energy.

The first step in behavioral activation involves having clients create a simple, concrete list of their current activities, or, if they don't engage in any current activities, a list of activities they enjoyed in the past or imagine would be helpful (Dobson & Dobson, 2009). Clients then identify an activity that they would like to increase (e.g., spending time with friends, cleaning the house) and choose small, incremental steps in support of their goal (e.g., call a friend; invite a friend to lunch). Throughout the intervention, clients are asked to complete an Activity Schedule, where activities are systematically recorded until they become more habitual. Clients' efforts, rather than outcomes, are verbally reinforced, and clients are asked to make positive statements about their efforts as well (Dobson & Dobson, 2009).

Social skills training. Social skills training, also referred to as communication skills training and assertiveness training, is a core component of behavior therapy and is used in CBT as needed (Dobson & Dobson, 2009). Social skills training includes the teaching and practice of basic communication and verbal skills (e.g., how to start conversations; how to make and respond to requests; pacing, rate of speech; loudness of voice; extraneous or habitual voice patterns, tone of voice), and nonverbal communication skills such as appropriate body language (e.g., physical proximity, facial expressiveness, hand gestures). More advanced skills such as assertive communication, dealing with conflict, and communicating in intimate relationships may also be addressed through social skills training (Dobson & Dobson, 2009). When providing this training, therapists must consider the variability in social expression (e.g., across culture and age groups) to ensure clients are able to communicate their needs and desires in an appropriate, acceptable manner (Dobson & Dobson, 2009).

Problem solving training. CBT uses a general problem-solving format that is distinct from problem solving as a stand-alone treatment. In the problem-solving behavioral intervention strategy, clients identify a specific problem, generate strategies for addressing the problem, implement the strategy, and evaluate its effectiveness for addressing the identified problem (D'Zurilla & Goldfried, 1971).

The problem solving process begins with identifying and naming a specific problem (e.g., symptom of psychological disorder, psychosocial stressor) (D'Zurilla & Goldfried, 1971). The therapist and client determine the parameters of the problem, such as frequency, duration, triggers, and resolution, and develop an assessment strategy (Dobson & Dobson, 2009). During this process clients are encouraged to consider the idea of change and how to promote change. The therapist and client collectively generate a variety of possible strategies without initial evaluation of the approaches in order to think broadly and creatively about potential solutions. Then, they conduct cost-benefit analyses to evaluate each alternative and its likelihood of solving the original problem (D'Zurilla & Goldfried, 1971). The optimal strategy is selected and its implementation is discussed in detail (e.g., when it will begin, how it will be conducted, for how long) (Dobson & Dobson, 2009). The client then implements the selected strategy as homework. Finally, the client and therapist evaluate the outcome of the problem-solving strategy. If the problem was solved, they move to the next issue. If the problem was not solved, only partially solved, or changed, then the therapist and client circle back to reevaluate the problem and consider other alternative strategies (Dobson & Dobson, 2009).

Relaxation training. CBT utilizes relaxation training to provide a personal self-care activity for clients, either as a strategy to decrease physical tension, calm down when agitated, or regulate internal sensations (Dobson & Dobson, 2009). Therapists can teach clients to use several different types of relaxation training, including progressive muscle relaxation, breathing retraining, autogenic relaxation, and visualization exercises (Jacobson, 1938, 1970; Wolpe, 1969). It is often helpful to create personalized audio files for clients that include collaboratively planned relaxation strategies (Dobson & Dobson, 2009). CBT encourages frequent practice of relaxation strategies, and strategies are often tied to visual reminders or paired with regular daily activities to facilitate clients' ability to call on these skills when needed.

Exposure. Exposure-based interventions are among the most empirically tested and effective components of CBT (Barlow, 2002; Farmer & Chapman, 2008; Richard & Lauterbach, 2007). Exposure encourages clients to confront a feared stimulus (e.g., thoughts, emotional responses, activities, situations) in order to manage physiological anxiety and decrease fears. As exposure requires clients to take risks, cognitive behavioral therapists must ensure a good therapeutic alliance and communicate a solid rationale for the intervention strategy prior to its implementation (Dobson & Dobson, 2009).

The ultimate goal of exposure is to help clients recognize that a feared stimulus is not as scary, unpredictable, or out of control as they imagined and let them know that they can cope with previously avoided situations (Dobson & Dobson, 2009). Exposure-based interventions increase clients' self-efficacy. Gradual and systematic exposure over time has been shown to diminish avoidance patterns, which indicates new learning (D'Zurrilla, Wilson, & Nelson, 1973; Watson, Gaind, & Marks, 1971). More recently, Craske, Kircanski, Zelikowsky, Mystkowski, Chowdhury, & Baker (2008), noting that fear levels at the time of exposure have not been shown to be reliable indicators of learning, have posited the evocation of inhibitory learning and fear toleration as shown at episodes of reexposure.

Exposure targets should be hierarchical, starting with a stimulus expected to trigger low levels of anxiety and gradually moving to stimuli likely to result in higher levels of anxiety (Dobson & Dobson, 2009). Effective exposure typically produces feelings of moderate anxiety intensity and should not produce extreme or overwhelming anxiety. Exposure is most effective when used frequently and continuously until anxiety is reduced; accordingly, exposure-based interventions may require longer and/or more frequent sessions (Foa, Jameson, Turner, & Payne, 1980). Though exposure interventions can occur in vivo or in imagery, in vivo exposure leads to greater benefits (Emmelkamp & Wessels, 1975). Clients are encouraged to practice exposure in a variety of situations and settings to promote generalization, with clients keeping a record of exposures and outcomes (Dobson & Dobson, 2009). Practice should occur both in-session and outside of sessions as part of homework.

COGNITIVE RESTRUCTURING CBT clinicians use cognitive restructuring to help clients become aware of the connection between their thoughts, emotions, and behaviors. Cognitive restructuring consists of intervention strategies to help clients recognize, evaluate, and effectively respond to dysfunctional, negative, or distorted thoughts. The intervention strategies commonly employed during cognitive restructuring are described below.

Identification of problematic thoughts: *Thought recording.* Cognitive behavioral therapists must help clients develop an awareness of their dysfunctional or negative thoughts before they can employ interventions to change these thoughts. Thought recording helps increase clients' awareness of dysfunctional or negative thoughts, while also providing a way for them to share and communicate experiences with their therapist (Dobson & Dobson, 2009). A daily dysfunctional thought record (DTR; Beck et al., 1979; Beck, 1995) is often used for this purpose. The DTR includes columns in which clients can record situations (e.g., date, time, event), as well as the automatic thoughts, emotions (e.g., type and intensity), and behaviors (e.g., actions and tendencies) the situations elicit. Later in treatment, clients are often given another version of the DTR that includes columns in which alternative (more adaptive) thoughts and behavioral outcomes are recorded as well.

Because identifying and recording dysfunctional and negative thoughts can be challenging for clients, their abilities and skill levels must be considered. Further, some clients may respond negatively to the term "dysfunctional" thought, so clinicians may need to modify their language to ensure that it is acceptable to clients (Dobson & Dobson, 2009). Therapists must be sure that clients clearly understand the linkage between their thoughts and responses before encouraging them to engage in thought recording.

Labeling cognitive distortions. Once clients have identified and recorded their negative thoughts, clinicians can help clients identify cognitive distortions and discuss them. Driven by core beliefs, assumptions, or schemas, cognitive distortions interact with situational facts or circumstances, leading to automatic thoughts and situation-specific thinking (Beck, 1963). Cognitive behavioral therapists must recognize clients' distorted thinking in order to plan effective intervention strategies (Dobson & Dobson, 2009). It is common for therapists and clients to review a list of cognitive distortions together. The dysfunctional thought record (DTR), described above, can be modified to include an additional column where clients name the cognitive distortions underlying their negative and dysfunctional thoughts.

Evaluating problematic thoughts: *Reality testing and Socratic questioning.* To counter cognitive distortions and negative or dysfunctional thoughts, CBT encourages clients to evaluate their thoughts through empirical hypothesis testing. Thoughts are viewed as hypotheses, rather than facts, and therefore can be questioned and challenged. Reality testing refers to intervention strategies that offer opportunities for clients to compare their thoughts to the actual evidence.

One of the most straightforward strategies for countering negative thoughts and distortions is simply asking clients to examine the evidence (e.g., type, quality, amount) that supports and refutes their original thought (Dobson & Dobson, 2009). Therapists use Socratic questioning (Beck et al., 1979) to help clients make guided discoveries and question their thoughts (Craske, 2010). Socratic questioning simply follows the client's own logic, as if their assumption were true and corollaries to their reasoning would follow: "If what you say is true, then it seems like X would also be true. Do you think that's correct?" This process often leads clients to realize that they do not have all of the information necessary to draw conclusions. It introduces data that does not fully support or is inconsistent with the original thought, and it may inform an alternative explanation for events (Beck et al., 1979). In addition to helping clients change their beliefs and assumptions, reality testing and Socratic questioning support clients' ability to confront, rather than avoid, problem situations (Dobson & Dobson, 2009).

Reattribution. Clients who have cognitive distortions or negative, dysfunctional thoughts often falsely attribute the cause of certain events or situations. It is common for clients to relate events and situations to themselves and to blame themselves for perceived negative outcomes associated with events or situations. Three well-recognized dimensions of attributions are locus (internal v. external), stability (single occurrence/unstable v. permanent/stable), and specificity (specific to one situation v. global) (Dobson & Dobson, 2009). For example, someone with depression may have the tendency to make internal, stable, and global attributions for failure (e.g., I am a failure), but external, unstable, and specific attributions for success (e.g., I was lucky that time) (Alloy, Abramson, Whitehouse, Hogan, Panzarella, & Rose, 2006).

CBT seeks to assist clients in recognizing and addressing attributional biases. Once clients are able to recognize attributional biases, they can compare their thoughts to factual evidence. Reattributional pie charts may be used to address attribution biases. First, the clinician and client construct a pie chart reflecting the factors that the client believes contributed to an event or situation (usually a negative one). Next, other potential causes of the event or situation are identified. The clinician asks the client whether any other factors may help to explain the situation or if any additional information may be important to consider. Finally, the pie chart is modified to reflect this reattribution. The exercise can be completed without pie charts using a percentage metaphor to attribute causes or by simply naming various causes of an outcome without determining the proportions for each causal factor (Dobson & Dobson, 2009).

De-catastrophizing/Identifying unrealistic expectations. Clients with cognitive distortions and negative or dysfunctional thoughts may predict negative futures and create self-fulfilling prophecies. This is particularly common among clients with anxiety. CBT utilizes an evaluation process to facilitate clients' ability to identify self-fulfilling prophecies and examine evidence related to their predictions (Dobson & Dobson, 2009). Results of the evaluation are used to challenge negative or unrealistic expectations.

The evaluation process involves hypothesis testing implemented through homework. Clients are first asked to clearly identify their predictions. Then clients establish what evidence will be necessary to either confirm or reject their prediction and develop a procedure for collecting relevant evidence (Dobson & Dobson, 2009). Next, clients collect evidence as part of homework. At the next session, clients' predictions are compared to the evidence and evidence-based outcomes. This evaluation-based cognitive intervention strategy may help clients realize that engaging in situations, rather than avoiding them, results in more accurate information and, therefore, may encourage them to collect and evaluate evidence when making predictions in the future (Dobson & Dobson, 2009).

Downward arrow. The downward arrow is a common CBT strategy used to address implications of specific negative thoughts to help identify strongly held beliefs or catastrophic fears (Beck et al., 1979; Beck, 1995; Burns, 1989). The downward arrow technique helps clients think of their thoughts as hypotheses that can be evaluated rather than facts (Dobson & Dobson, 2009). Clinicians ask a series of questions about the meaning that clients attach to their thought until the client has no additional responses: "So if that happened, what would it mean?"; "What's the worst part about that?"; "What would that mean about you?" The downward arrow method can serve as an initial assessment tool to identify problematic beliefs, and later in treatment as a way to examine and change intermediate and/or core beliefs when they occur during sessions.

Generating alternative thoughts. Once clients have identified and evaluated dysfunctional, negative, or distorted thoughts, CBT employs cognitive strategies to generate, evaluate, and ultimately routinize more

adaptive, alternative thoughts (Dobson & Dobson, 2009). Alternative thoughts can be introduced by the client, the therapist, or collaboratively. Clients may be asked to generate alternative thoughts after evaluating and reviewing evidence related to their original problematic thoughts. If clients have difficulty coming up with alternatives, therapists can offer suggestions for the client to consider. During this process, therapists must respect clients' original problematic thoughts and acknowledge that generating alternative thoughts can be difficult.

After an alternative thought has been identified, the advantages of both the original and the alternative thought are evaluated. The evaluation process often includes an assessment of the negative thought and the alternative response (e.g., how useful, how helpful they are to clients), as well as cost-benefit analyses of the original thought and the alternative. Clinicians may also ask clients to consider how they would advise a friend with this type of thinking. Once acceptable alternative thoughts have been identified and evaluated, several strategies can be utilized to help clients respond to their original problematic thoughts with the more adaptive, alternative thoughts.

Point-counterpoint. A point-counterpoint approach is used to help clients respond to negative thoughts. This technique utilizes cue cards with the original thought on one side and the alternative thought on the other side. Therapists then state or read the original thought while clients practice saying the alternative.

Rational role play. Rational role play can be used to reinforce clients' use of alternative thoughts and to increase clients' confidence and ease in responding to negative, dysfunctional, or distorted thinking. This strategy calls for therapists and clients to engage in a role play between negative and more adaptive thinking, with the therapist articulating the problematic thoughts and the client verbalizing the alternative responses.

Task-interfering cognitions—task-orienting cognitions (TIC-TOC). Another strategy used in CBT to encourage clients' use of alternative thoughts is the task-interfering cognitions—task-orienting cognitions, or TIC-TOC intervention. The TIC-TOC approach, which refers to the sound of a clock's pendulum, focuses on going back and forth between task-interfering cognitions (e.g., "I will never get this done") and task-orienting cognitions (e.g., "If I just get started, it will likely get easier"). TIC-TOC helps clients develop an automatic, alternative response to negative thoughts. The TIC-TOC strategy is most appropriate for clients who experience repetitive thoughts that interfere with specific tasks (Dobson & Dobson, 2009).

HOMEWORK ASSIGNMENTS Homework is an essential part of CBT. Goals for homework include learning and generalizing change beyond therapy sessions (Beck & Tompkins, 2007; Lambert, Harmon, & Slade, 2007). Homework assignments may consist of reading educational materials, completing activity schedules and dysfunctional thought records, conducting behavioral experiments, practicing communication skills, or evaluating problematic thoughts (Dobson & Dobson, 2009). Homework assignments are collaboratively developed by therapists and clients, increasing the likelihood of compliance and success. The meta-analytic review of Kazantzis, Whittington, and Dattilio (2010) suggests that extra-therapy assignments enhance treatment outcomes, although homework compliance has not been positively associated with outcome in all studies (Kazantzis & Dattilio, 2007).

Current Applications
Various models of CBT have been applied to a wide range of mental health problems, substance abuse disorders, and other problems. The most common, empirically supported applications of CBT are identified and described below.

ADULT DISORDERS: DEPRESSION
Unipolar depression. CBT treatments for depression have typically employed behavioral activation to increase natural reinforcers in the environment and cognitive restructuring to reduce negative automatic thoughts and increase positive ones, which in turn improve mood and behavior. Meta-analytic studies on treatment outcomes of such CBT methods for depression concluded that most studies show CBT to be superior to waitlist control and placebo treatments (e.g., Beltman, Oude Voshaar, & Speckens, 2010; Butler, Chapman, Forman, and Beck, 2006). When compared to pharmacological approaches, CBT and pharmacotherapy independently produced similar benefits for depression symptoms within the moderate to large range (Vos et al., 2004). Research also demonstrates that medications combined with CBT are associated with better outcomes than CBT as a standalone treatment (Chan, 2006), however, Butler, Chapman, Forman, and Beck (2006) concluded that CBT was moderately superior to medication treatment. Additionally, Hofmann, Asnaani, Vonk, Sawyer, and

Fang (2012) suggest that CBT is as effective as other psychological treatments, such as psychodynamic psychotherapy, problem-solving therapy, and interpersonal psychotherapy, although CBT did not appear to improve upon behavioral treatments that lacked cognitive components. Similarly, findings for adolescents showed much larger effects for CBT than waitlist and other forms of treatment, including relaxation and supportive therapy. Hundt, Mignogna, Underhill, and Cully (2013) examined skill use as a component of CBT and found evidence that CBT skill practice has a mediating effect on depression.

Bipolar disorder. CBT for bipolar disorder commonly includes psychoeducation of patients and families, monitoring manic and depressive symptoms, encouraging medication adherence, stress management strategies (e.g., control of the circadian rhythm, daily thought records, social skills training, problem solving), and reduction of stigma. CBT methods produced only moderate benefits for manic and depressive symptoms in meta-analyses of pre-post outcomes, and these effects tended to diminish during the follow-up period (Hofmann et al., 2012). While evidence that CBT works well as a stand-alone treatment unaccompanied by medications is limited (as psychopharmacotherapy is the most common form of treatment), CBT did appear to help delay or prevent relapse when compared to medications (Beynon, Soares-Weiser, Woolacott, Duffy, & Geddes, 2008). The analysis of da Costa et al. (2010) found that the majority of studies indicated better outcomes when CBT was combined with medication compared with medication alone. However, they caution that more studies are needed.

ADULT DISORDERS: ANXIETY DISORDERS CBT methods have been especially well studied for anxiety disorders. Reviews on meta-analytic studies of psychotherapies for a range of anxiety disorders conclude that behavioral and cognitive treatments are efficacious whether delivered separately or combined (Deacon & Abramowitz, 2004; Hofmann et al., 2012). Hofmann and Smits (2008) conducted a meta-analysis of CBT versus placebo-controlled studies and found that CBT was effective for adult anxiety disorders, with the strongest effect among those with OCD and acute stress disorder. Norton and Price (2007) found similar results in another meta-analysis of CBT across the anxiety disorders.

Panic and agoraphobia. Effective treatments for panic, with or without agoraphobia, have included the following elements: education about the nature and physiology of anxiety and panic, correction of misinterpretations of body sensations (for example, bodily signals of catastrophic outcomes like heart attack or suffocation), exposure to feared body sensations that trigger these misinterpretations, as well as coping skills to manage discomfort. These CBT methods show substantial advantages over waitlist and pill-form or psychological placebo conditions (Deacon & Abramowitz; 2004; Hofmann et al., 2012). In some studies, combined CBT showed advantages over behavioral methods alone (Gould, Otto, & Pollack, 1995), although Deacon and Abramowitz (2004) noted that cognitive and behavioral methods could not always be differentiated from each other.

Social phobia. CBT for social anxiety typically includes exposure, cognitive restructuring, and social skills training that are delivered in either group or individual formats, or both. Meta-analytic findings indicated that CBT produced better outcomes than waitlist or placebo/attention control comparisons with evidence from follow-up measures demonstrating that medium-to-large effects were maintained or increased (Gould, Buckminster, Pollack, Otto, & Yap, 1997; Hofmann et al., 2012). Behavioral treatments using exposure were quite effective, and the addition of cognitive restructuring produced slightly higher effect sizes, but not significantly so; CT alone was less beneficial (Taylor, 1996). In reviewing the meta-analyses for CBT for social phobia, Deacon and Abramowitz (2004) concluded that behavioral elements were essential to effective treatment. In general, CBT methods showed more benefits over time than medication treatments (Hofmann et al., 2012).

Obsessive-compulsive disorder. Similarly, early studies on OCD showed clear efficacy of behavioral treatments that included exposure to feared cues plus response prevention of rituals and avoidance behaviors, commonly abbreviated as ERP (e.g., Abramowitz, 1997; van Balkom et al., 1994). More recently, cognitive therapy models have applied cognitive restructuring to misinterpretations of intrusive thoughts, images, or impulses. A meta-analysis by Abramowitz, Foa, and Franklin (2002) indicated a stronger overall effect size from ERP versus CT, though the difference between these two methods was not significant. Practitioners often combine both methods for clients with OCD, especially in the form of behavior experiments that contain elements of both cognitive therapy and behavior therapy. Deacon and Abramowitz (2004) concluded that for both OCD and social phobia, behavioral methods without cognitive elements appeared to be the critical factor in therapy outcomes.

Generalized anxiety disorder. Specific external triggers for GAD are more difficult to identify, and so it is challenging to apply standard exposure therapy used for other anxiety disorders. Thus, a wider variety of CBT methods have been studied. These include progressive muscle relaxation, self-monitoring and early cue detection, applied relaxation, self-control desensitization, and cognitive restructuring (Borkovec & Costello, 1993). Overall, meta-analyses strongly support the effectiveness of combined cognitive-behavioral interventions for GAD (Deacon & Abramowitz, 2004; Gould, Otto, Pollack, & Yap, 1997). A meta-analysis by Covin, Ouimet, Seeds, and Dozois (2008) found that combined cognitive and behavioral interventions were effective in treating pathological worry, a core component of GAD. Too few studies provide an adequate test of the benefits of strictly cognitive or strictly behavioral methods to indicate clearly that these are as effective as combined treatments.

Post-traumatic stress disorder. Post-traumatic stress disorder (PTSD) is usually treated with a combination of behavioral and cognitive methods, including exposure to fear evoking memories and situational cues, cognitive restructuring, and anxiety-management skills. Other interventions include education, relaxation, and cognitive interventions to help manage anxiety symptoms and modify maladaptive beliefs. Eye-movement desensitization and reprocessing (EMDR; Shapiro, 1991) includes imagined exposure to traumatic memories plus coping statements during trauma recall, accompanied by therapist-guided saccadic eye movements. The review of Butler et al. (2006) indicated strong benefits of CBT over waitlist, EMDR, as well as stress management and other therapies. Other studies suggest that CBT methods produce similar effects to EMDR (Bisson et al., 2007), but agree that the actual benefit of the eye movement element is highly questionable. Deacon and Abramowitz (2004) concluded that the effectiveness of behavioral versus cognitive strategies could not be determined from meta-analyses, as most interventions for PTSD involved combinations of these two methods.

PSYCHOSIS A number of meta-analyses have examined the efficacy of CBT for psychosis, also known as CBTp. CBTp includes cognitive and behavioral methods such as skills training, problem solving, Socratic questioning, exposure, and coping strategy enhancements (Lincoln et al., 2012). The largest of these meta-analyses reviewed 34 studies (Wykes, Steel, Everitt, & Tarrier, 2008). CBT showed a larger effect size for pre-post-treatment than treatment as usual (i.e., pharmacotherapy using anti-psychotic drugs) (Butler et al., 2006; Hofmann, Asmundson, & Beck, 2013; Hofmann et al., 2012). Beneficial effects were found for both positive and negative symptoms of schizophrenia, although the effects were larger overall for positive symptoms (Kingdon & Dimech, 2008). The Wykes et al. (2008) meta-analytic review also showed improvement in functioning, mood, and social anxiety for CBTp interventions compared to medications. A recent community-based clinical study by Lincoln et al. (2012) found that CBTp for positive symptoms was effective for a variety of clients, treatment settings, and providers. Gould, Mueser, Bolton, Mays, & Goff (2001) reviewed studies in which cognitive therapy for psychotic symptoms in schizophrenia targeted recognition of, and distorted thinking about, positive symptoms of hallucinations and delusions. Five of seven studies showed a significant decrease in these symptoms and two showed non-significant decreases. Butler et al. (2006) noted that other methods of treatment, such as befriending clients and supportive therapy, had an intermediate degree of effect, falling between CBT and routine care. Interestingly, Hofmann et al. (2012) reported that early intervention services and family treatment had a greater impact in reducing hospital admission and relapse than did CBT.

SUBSTANCE ABUSE CBT for substance abuse integrates principles of harm reduction, motivation, and relapse prevention by applying a combination of skills training and operant conditioning, to manage cues and control urges, with cognitive therapy and motivational interviewing. CBT has been shown to be an effective intervention for alcohol and other drug use disorders (Dutra et al., 2008; Magill & Ray, 2009). A CBT study of substance abuse found that the quality of skills was more important than quantity, and that having even a few coping skills can often produce positive outcomes (Kiluk, Nich, Babuscio, & Carroll, 2010). Hofmann et al. (2012) summarized evidence that multiple sessions of CBT worked only moderately well for cannabis dependence and noted that other psychosocial interventions that are also associated with behavioral (i.e., contingency management) and cognitive strategies (i.e., relapse prevention, motivational interviewing) as well as medication treatments showed more benefit for dependence on

opioids and alcohol (see Powers, Vedel, & Emmelkamp, 2008).

EATING DISORDERS CBT methods for treating eating disorders typically include developing a shared formulation of the problem, self-monitoring, weekly weighing, establishing regular eating patterns, involving others, and cognitive therapy to resolve the overvaluing of shape and weight and to reduce perfectionism and rigid dietary rules. Summaries of meta-analytic studies indicated that CBT showed strong effects for bulimia nervosa in pre-post trials (Butler et al., 2006) and medium effects compared to control therapies, such as interpersonal psychotherapy, dialectical behavioral therapy, hypno-behavioral therapy, supportive psychotherapy, weight loss strategies, and self-monitoring (Hay, Bacaltchuk, Stefano, & Kashyap, 2009; Hofmann et al., 2012). Behavioral treatments appeared to show more benefit than combined cognitive and behavioral methods (Thompson-Brenner, 2003). Binge eating disorder responded well to psychotherapy that typically included CBT methods as well as structured self-help with larger effect sizes than medications (Vocks et al., 2010). Combining these treatments did not improve binge eating specifically but appeared to increase weight loss somewhat (Reas & Grilo, 2008).

CHRONIC PAIN Cognitive behavioral interventions for chronic pain and/or fibromyalgia typically involve a number of CBT-based interventions including but not limited to: progressive muscle or imagery-based relaxation, sleep hygiene techniques (e.g., consistent times in/out of bed; evening wind-down activities); cognitive interventions aimed at negative automatic thoughts related to sleep (e.g., "I will be a mess tomorrow if I don't get to sleep"); pleasant activity scheduling; and activity pacing (e.g., limiting activities on days when feeling well and continuing some level of activity on higher pain days) (Williams, 2003). A recent meta-analysis of psychological treatment studies for fibromyalgia found modest effect sizes on short-term pain for a range of psychological interventions but found that CBT-based interventions were associated with the largest treatment effect sizes compared to other psychological approaches (Glombiewski et al., 2010).

INTIMATE PARTNER VIOLENCE (IPV) PERPETRATORS AND SURVIVORS Cognitive behavioral interventions for IPV perpetrators typically include cognitive approaches aimed at modifying attitudes and beliefs related to women, problem solving strategies, social skills training (e.g., assertiveness training) and anger management (e.g., timeout from anger-inducing situations, relaxation) approaches (Eckhardt et al., 2013). A single meta-analytic review involving psychosocial treatment for batterers found relatively small effects on a range of outcomes, including continued perpetration (Babcock, Green, & Robie, 2004). CBT-based approaches for batterers are typically delivered in small groups.

Studies of CBT-based approaches for IPV survivors are more limited in number but generally find positive impact on a range of targets including PTSD-related and depressive symptoms. In the largest of these studies, Kubany and colleagues (Kubany et al., 2004) compared immediate versus delayed cognitive trauma therapy for battered women (an approach that includes but is not limited to PTSD-related psychoeducation, prolonged exposure to abuse-related stimuli, cognitive approaches, assertiveness training and perpetrator identification training, and trauma history exploration) and found robust positive effects on PTSD symptoms, depression, guilt, and self-esteem in the immediate versus the delayed treatment group.

SMOKING CESSATION AND WEIGHT LOSS CBT for smoking cessation often combines principles of motivational interviewing to address early stage ambivalence/barriers related to quitting with a range of CBT-informed interventions (Perkins, Conklin, & Levine, 2008). Core CBT strategies typically include analysis of smoking triggers, stimulus control-related strategies for avoiding smoking triggers, responding to smoking-related cognitions, and learning coping strategies for craving (e.g., observe craving changes, relaxation). A meta-analysis of the best-designed randomized controlled intervention trials for smoking cessation indicated that intensive behavioral interventions are associated with substantial increases in smoking abstinence compared to control (Mottillo et al., 2009). Finally, augmenting behavioral interventions with pharmacological interventions is likely more effective than behavioral interventions alone and sustained abstinence from smoking remains challenging even with best-practice treatment (Hall et al., 2002).

CBT-based strategies also dominate the literature on the psychosocial treatment of obesity. CBT techniques for weight control are in many ways similar to those used for smoking cessation and other addictive behaviors and include increasing motivation to control eating, increasing awareness of over-eating triggers, increasing active behaviors and exercise, identifying and challenging maladaptive cognitions related to

eating, and self-monitoring (Cooper, Fairburn, & Hawker, 2003). A recent meta-analysis of randomized, controlled trials of psychosocial interventions (all but one involving either BT or CBT) found large and significant effect sizes for eating behavior and modest weight reductions post-treatment (Moldovan & David, 2011). Follow-up effect sizes are reduced for both eating and weight loss but remain significant.

COUPLES THERAPY Cognitive behavioral couples therapy (CBCT) employs guided behavior change, social skills training emphasizing constructive communication, and cognitive restructuring interventions (e.g., guided discovery; reattribution, downward arrow) to address dysfunctional or distorted thoughts (Baucom, Epstein, Kirby, & LaTaillade, 2010). Socratic questioning should be used cautiously in CBCT, as the therapists' questioning of one partner's thoughts in the presence of the other partner may further contribute to negative outcomes (Baucom et al., 2010). Recent enhancements to CBCT, influenced by systems and ecological models of relationship functioning (e.g., Brofenbrenner, 1989) and a strengths-based perspective, place increased attention to macro-level interaction patterns as well as to personality, motives, and more stable individual characteristics (Epstein & Baucom, 2002). The meta-analytic review of Butler et al. (2006) found that cognitive behavioral marital therapy had a moderate effect on marital distress; however, their review included only one meta-analysis (Dunn & Schwebel, 1995) on cognitive behavioral therapy for couples.

CHILD BEHAVIORAL MANAGEMENT The meta-analytic review of Hofmann et al. (2012) concluded that CBT was associated with large effects in treating internalizing symptoms in children and adolescents with anxiety disorders. This was especially true for children with OCD, as CBT improved these symptoms more than other forms of psychotherapy and serotonergic medications. Improvements in depressive symptoms were evident but not as strong, with medium effects. In the case of depression, CBT was as effective as interpersonal and family systems therapies but more effective than selective serotonin and other reuptake medications.

With regard to externalizing behaviors (e.g., disruptive classroom behaviors, aggressive/antisocial behaviors), CBT was as effective as other forms of psychosocial treatments and showed more benefit compared to treatment as usual, but not compared to pharmacotherapy. Very similar findings were also evident in meta-analyses of CBT for attention deficit hyperactivity disorder. Behavioral techniques such as motivational enhancement and application of contingencies showed modest benefits for adolescent smoking and substance use behaviors compared to no treatment, but not compared to other forms of psychotherapy.

Evidence-Based Practice

Given its scientific approach to treatment, it is not surprising that CBT is one of the most thoroughly researched forms of psychotherapy. The results of 120 clinical trials examining the effect of CBT were published between 1986 and 1993 (Hollon & Beck, 1994), by 2004 Butler et al. (2006) identified more than 325 published outcome studies on CBT's efficacy (Butler et al., 2006), and Hofmann et al. (2012) found 269 meta-analytic studies of CBT published since 2000.

The extensive research suggests a strong empirical basis for CBT across a wide range of disorders (Butler et al., 2006; Hofmann et al., 2012). A review of 16 meta-analyses by Butler et al. (2006) found CBT effective for treating adult unipolar depression, generalized anxiety disorder, panic disorder with and without agoraphobia, social phobia, obsessive-compulsive disorder, PTSD, schizophrenia, marital distress, anger, bulimia nervosa, sexual offending, and chronic pain as well as adolescent unipolar depression, childhood depressive and anxiety disorders, and childhood somatic disorders. The meta-analytic review of Hofmann et al. (2012) suggests CBT has the strongest support for treating anxiety disorders, somatoform disorders, bulimia, anger control problems, and general stress. Results suggest that treatment gains are generally maintained over follow-up intervals ranging from 6 to 24 months (Butler et al., 2006; Norton & Price, 2007). It should be noted that comparisons were usually with control conditions receiving no treatment or nondirective supportive counseling as a placebo. Limited research has compared CBT to other active psychotherapies (Butler et al., 2006; Hofmann et al., 2012).

Evidence also suggests the versatility of CBT. CBT is effective when delivered in both individual and group formats (e.g., Butler et al., 2006; Hofmann et al., 2012) and findings indicate that frequency and duration of sessions are not related to outcomes (Norton & Price, 2007). Research demonstrates that CBT is effective among diverse populations, including participants of different racial and ethnic backgrounds, ages, and socioeconomic status (e.g., Ayers, Sorrell, Thorp, & Wetherell, 2007; Cartwright-Hatton, Roberts, Chitsabesan, Fothergill, & Harrinton, 2004; Compton et al., 2004; Hays, 2009; Horrell, 2008; Schraufnagel, Wagner, Miranda, & Roy-Bryne, 2006; Scogin, Welsh, Hanson, Stump, & Coates, 2005; Wilson & Cottone, 2013).

Additionally, literature suggests that CBT is effective when implemented in non-mental health settings, such as primary care offices, schools, and vocational rehabilitation centers (e.g., Brown & Schulberg, 1995; Hoagwood & Erwin, 1997; Rose & Perz, 2005; Roy-Byrne et al., 2005). Further, evidence is growing indicating that CBT can be effectively delivered with technology, with computerized CBT (cCBT) and CBT delivered via videoconferencing garnering empirical support (e.g., Andrews et al., 2010; Antonacci, Bloch, Saeed, Yildirim, & Talley, 2008; Kaltenthaler et al., 2006; Simpson, 2009).

CBT AND SOCIAL WORK Enhancing human well-being and helping to meet basic human needs of all people, with particular attention to vulnerable populations, is the primary mission of the social work profession (NASW, 1996). Additionally, the *NASW Code of Ethics* (1996) states that social workers should advance the professional mission by working toward the maintenance and promotion of high standards of practice. Therefore, it is not surprising that social work has long emphasized the need for a scientific foundation to inform and guide practice (Cheney, 1926; Reynolds, 1942). The movement toward evidence-based practice (EBP), or "the integration of best research evidence with clinical expertise and client values" has further influenced the social work profession (Sackett, Straus, Richardson, Rosenberg, & Haynes, 2000, p.1).

Eileen Gambrill, one of the earliest, most influential scholars to introduce and advocate the use of EBP within the social work profession (Thyer, 2002), was also instrumental in studying and encouraging the implementation of behavioral approaches in social work (e.g., Gambrill, 1977; Gambrill, Thomas, & Carter, 1971). In the late 1960s and early 1970s, scholars at the University of Michigan School of Social Work, including Edwin Thomas, Richard Stuart, and Gambrill, began applying behavioral approaches to social work practice (Gambrill, 1995). Gambrill (1995) notes the expansion of behavioral methods, including CBT, within social work, and she attributes this to their compatibility with professional interests as well as their commitment to a scientific approach, including the use of empirical research, to guide practice.

CBT has arguably the best evidence for effectiveness of mental and behavioral health problems among all psychotherapies (Hollon & Beck, 1994; Dobson, 2010; Butler et al., 2006; Hofmann et al., 2012), and has become one of the most frequently used psychosocial interventions. Given the increasing emphasis on EBP, CBT has had a distinct impact on social work practice. Social workers make up the largest group of behavioral health providers in the United States (NASW, 2005) and deliver more than 60% of mental health treatment (NASW, 2006). An increasing number of social workers report using CBT as their preferred model of practice (Granvold, 2011; Thyer & Myers, 2011). Between 1987 and 2007, the percentage of social workers practicing from a CBT-perspective more than tripled (Bike, Norcross, & Schatz, 2009; Norcross, Garofalo, & Koocher, 2006). Evidence suggests that between 30% and 43% of social workers practicing in the United States report using CBT (Pignotti & Thyer, 2009; Prochaska & Norcross, 2010). The need for clinical social workers in the fields of mental health and substance abuse is expected to rise by 20% between 2008 and 2018 (Bureau of Labor Statistics, 2010), and expert forecasts indicate that CBT will be increasingly in demand and used among social workers (Prochaska & Norcross, 2010). However, an acute shortage of qualified CBT therapists exists in many countries relative to demand and the treatment's potential value to society (Chambless & Ollendick, 2001).

Though social workers indicate CBT is a preferred method of practice, a large gap remains between the availability of EBPs and their use in clinical practice (Weissman & Sanderson, 2002; New Freedom Commission, 2003). One proposed reason for this persistent gap is mental health professionals' lack of training in EBPs, such as CBT. While the combination of didactic content and supervised clinical work is considered the gold standard for learning a new treatment, a survey of randomly selected CSWE-accredited MSW programs suggests that 62% did not require both didactic training and clinical supervision for any EBP (Weissman et al., 2006). Didactic content related to CBT was offered and required at substantially higher rates than other evidence-based psychotherapies (e.g., interpersonal psychotherapy, multisystemic therapy), with 93% of MSW programs offering didactic training in CBT and 80% requiring didactic training in CBT. Though 66% of MSW programs reported offering clinical supervision for CBT, only 21% of programs required it (Weissman et al., 2006). Restructuring the organizational framework of social work curriculum to provide students with intensive training seminars and practicum devoted to EBPs and the systematic monitoring of clinical outcomes may help to address this gap within social work education (Thyer & Myers, 2011).

The widespread use of CBT among social workers and its inclusion in social work curriculum has led to attention to the fit between CBT as a thera-peutic approach and social work's professional mission and values. The critical analysis of CBT and social work values undertaken by Gonzalez-Prendes and Brisebois (2012) suggests that CBT promotes equality within the therapeutic relationship, aims to understand the context that has shaped a person's reality, and promotes a healthy level of social interest (e.g., protecting the rights of others and addressing unfair or unjust treatment that diminishes the quality of a person's social environment). Therefore, the analysis concludes that CBT, grounded in a non-judgmental, strength-based, empowering philosophy and focused on promoting unconditional acceptance and respect of self and others, aligns with the social work profession's mission of social justice (Gonzalez-Prendes & Brisebois, 2012).

Assessment

CBT refers to a family of short-term, problem-focused interventions rooted in behavioral and cognitive traditions that acknowledge the primary role thoughts have in shaping behaviors and emotions. CBT employs behavioral and cognitive intervention strategies aimed at identifying and challenging maladaptive or dysfunctional thoughts, behaviors, and emotions with more adaptive alternatives. Evidence supporting the effectiveness of CBT has grown substantially since the 1980s and, as such, the treatment has been increasingly used by mental health professionals, including social workers. Social workers provide a large proportion of mental health services and most commonly endorse CBT as their preferred model of practice. However, a documented shortage of providers qualified to deliver CBT has been registered, and social workers could be better prepared to provide CBT if more schools of social work offered both didactic and supervised clinical training. CBT aligns with social work's guiding values and mission, and it has been found to effectively treat mental disorders across diverse populations and settings, further supporting its relevance to the social work profession.

REFERENCES

Abramowitz, J. S. (1997). Effectiveness of psychological and pharmacological treatments for obsessive-compulsive disorder: A quantitative review. *Journal of Consulting and Clinical Psychology, 65*, 44–52.

Abramowitz, J. S., Foa, E. B., & Franklin, M. E. (2002). Empirical status of cognitive-behavior therapy for obsessive-compulsive disorder: A meta-analysis. *Romanian Journal of Cognitive and Behavioral Therapy, 2*, 89–104.

Alloy, L. B., Abramson, L. Y., Whitehouse, W. G., Hogan, M. E., Panzarella, C., & Rose, D. T. (2006). Prospective incidence of first onsets and recurrences of depression in indivduals at high and low cognitive risk for depression. *Journal of Abnormal Psychology, 115*, 145–156.

Anderson, C. M., Hogarty, G. E., & Reiss, D. J. (1980). Family treatment of adult schizophrenic patients: A psychoeducational approach. *Schizophrenia Bulletin, 6*, 490–505.

Andrews, G., Cuijpers, P., Craske, M. G., McEvoy, P., & Titov, N. (2010). Computer therapy for the anxiety and depressive disorders is effective, acceptable and practical health care: A meta-analysis. *PloS One, 5*, e13196.

Antonacci, D. J., Bloch, R. M., Saeed, S. A., Yildirim, Y., & Talley, J. (2008). Empirical evidence on the use and effectiveness of telepsychiatry via videoconferencing: Implications for forensic and correctional psychiatry. *Behavioral Sciences & the Law, 26*, 253–269.

Ayers, C. R., Sorrell, J. T., Thorp, S. R., & Wetherell, J. L. (2007). Evidence-based psychological treatments for late-life anxiety. *Psychology and Aging, 22*, 8.

Babcock, J. C., Green, C. E., & Robie, C. (2004). Does batterers' treatment work? A meta-analytic review of domestic violence treatment. *Clinical Psychology Review, 23*, 1023–1053.

Bandura, A. (1977). *Social learning theory.* Englewood Cliffs, NJ: Prentice Hall.

Bandura, A. (1986). *Social foundations of thought and action: A cognitive social theory.* Englewood Cliffs, NJ: Prentice Hall.

Barlow, D. (2002). *Anxiety and its disorders: The nature and treatment of anxiety and panic.* New York, NY: Guilford Press.

Baucom, D. H., Epstein, N. B., Kirby, J. S., & LaTaillade, J. J. (2010). In K. S. Dobson (Ed.), *Handbook of cognitive behavioral therapies* (pp. 411–444). New York, NY: Guilford Press.

Beck, A. T. (1963). Thinking and depression: I. Idiosyncratic content and cognitive distortions. *Archives of General Psychiatry, 9*, 324.

Beck, A. T. (1967). *Depression: Causes and treatment.* Philadelphia: University of Pennsylvania Press.

Beck, A. T. (1976). *Cognitive therapy of the emotional disorders.* New York, NY: Penguin Books.

Beck, A. T., Rush, A. J., Shaw, B. F., & Emery, G. (1979). *Cognitive therapy of depression.* New York, NY: Guilford Press.

Beck, J. S. (1995). *Cognitive therapy: Basics and beyond.* New York, NY: Guilford Press.

Beck, J. S., & Tompkins, M. A. (2007). Cognitive therapy. In N. Kazantzis & L. L'Abate (Eds.), *Handbook of homework assignments in psychotherapy: Research, practice, and prevention* (pp. 51–63). New York, NY: Springer.

Beltman, M. W., Oude Voshaar, R. C., & Speckens, A. E. (2010). Cognitive-behavioural therapy for depression in people with a somatic disease: Meta-analysis of randomised controlled trials. *British Journal of Psychiatry, 197*, 11–19.

Beynon, S., Soares-Weiser, K., Woolacott, N., Duffy, S., & Geddes J. R. (2008). Psychosocial interventions for the prevention of relapse in bipolar disorder: Systematic review of controlled trials. *British Journal of Psychiatry, 192*, 5–11.

Bike, D. H., Norcross, J. C., & Schatz, D. M. (2009). Processes and outcomes of psychotherapists' personal therapy: Replication and extension 20 years later. *American Psychological Association, 46*, 19–31. doi:10.1037/a0015139

Bisson, J. I., Ehlers, A., Matthews, R., Pilling, S., Richards, D., & Turner, S. (2007). Psychological treatments for chronic post-traumatic stress disorder: Systematic review and meta-analysis. *British Journal of Psychiatry, 190*, 97–104.

Borkovec, T. D., & Costello, E. (1993). Efficacy of applied relaxation and cognitive behavioral therapy in the treatment of generalized anxiety disorder. *Journal of Consulting and Clinical Psychology, 61*, 611–619.

Bronfenbrenner, U. (1989). *Ecological systems theory.* Greenwich, CT: JAI Press.

Brown, C., & Schulberg, H. C. (1995). The efficacy of psychosocial treatments in primary care: A review of randomized clinical trials. *General Hospital Psychiatry, 17*, 414–424.

Bureau of Labor Statistics. (2010). *U.S. Department of Labor, Occupational Outlook Handbook, 2010–11 Edition, Social Workers.* Washington, DC: Bureau of Labor Statistics. Retrieved June 3, 2014, from http://www.bls.gov/ooh/community-and-social-service/social-workers.htm#tab-6

Burns, D. D. (1989). *The feeling good handbook: Using the new mood therapy in everyday life.* New York, NY: Morrow.

Butler, A. C., Chapman, J. E., Forman, E. M., & Beck, A. T. (2006). The empirical status of cognitive-behavioral therapy: A review of meta-analyses. *Clinical Psychology Review, 26*(1), 17–31. doi:10.1016/j.cpr.2005.07.003

Cartwright-Hatton, S., Roberts, C., Chitsabesan, P., Fothergill, C., & Harrington, R. (2004). Systematic review of the efficacy of cognitive behaviour therapies for childhood and adolescent anxiety disorders. *British Journal of Clinical Psychology, 43*, 421–436.

Chambless, D. L., & Ollendick, T. H. (2001). Empirically supported psychological interventions: Controversies and evidence. *Annual Review of Psychology, 52*(1), 685–716.

Chan, E. K.-H. (2006). *Efficacy of cognitive-behavioral, pharmacological, and combined treatments of depression: A meta-analysis.* Calgary: University of Calgary Press.

Cheney, A. (1926). *The nature and scope of social work.* New York, NY: American Association of Social Workers.

Clark, D. M., & Fairburn, C. G. (1997). *Science and practice of cognitive behavior therapy.* Oxford: Oxford University Press.

Compton, S. N., March, J. S., Brent, D., Albano, A., Weersing, V. R., & Curry, J. (2004). Cognitive-behavioral psychotherapy for anxiety and depressive disorders in children and adolescents: An evidence-based medicine review. *Journal of the American Academy of Child & Adolescent Psychiatry, 43*, 930–959.

Cooper, Z., Fairburn, C. G., & Hawker, D. M. (2003). *Cognitive-behavioral treatment of obesity: A clinician's guide.* New York, NY: Guilford Press.

Corrigan, P. W. (2001). Getting ahead of the data: A threat to some behavior therapies. *The Behavior Therapist, 24*, 189–193.

Covin, R., Ouimet, A. J., Seeds, P. M., & Dozois, D. J. (2008). A meta-analysis of CBT for pathological worry among clients with GAD. *Journal of Anxiety Disorders, 22*(1), 108–116. doi:10.1016/j.janxdis.2007.01.002

Craske, M. G. (2010). *Cognitive-behavioral therapy.* Washington, DC: American Psychological Association.

Craske, M. G., Kircanski, K., Zelikowsky, M., Mystkowski, J., Chowdhury, N., & Baker, A. (2008). Optimizing inhibitory learning during exposure therapy. *Behaviour research and therapy, 46,* 5–27.

da Costa, R. T., Rangé, B. P., Malagris, L. E., Sardinha, A., de Carvalho, M. R., & Nardi, A. E. (2010). Cognitive-behavioral therapy for bipolar disorder. *Expert Review of Neurotherapeutics, 10*(7), 1089–1099. doi:10.1586/ern.10.75

Deacon B. J., & Abramowitz, J. S. (2004). Cognitive and behavioral treatments for anxiety disorders: A review of meta-analytic findings. *Journal of Clinical Psychology, 60*(4), 429–441. doi:10.1002/jclp.10255

Department of Health and Human Services (2003). New Freedom Commission on Mental Health: Achieving the Promise: Transforming Mental Health Care in America. Final Report. SMA-03-3832. Rockville MD: DHHS. Retrieved October 27, 2013, from http://govinfo.library.unt.edu/mentalhealthcommission/reports/FinalReport/downloads/downloads.html

Dobson, D., & Dobson, K. S. (2009). *Evidence-based practice of cognitive-behavioral therapy.* New York, NY: Guilford Press.

Dobson, K. S. (Ed.). (2010). *Handbook of cognitive-behavioral therapies* (3d ed.). New York, NY: Guilford Press.

Dobson, K. S., & Dozois, D. J. (2001). Historical and philosophical bases of cognitive-behavioral therapies. In K. S. Dobson (Ed.), *Handbook of cognitive-behavioral therapies* (2d ed., pp. 3–38). New York, NY: Guildford Press.

Dryden, W., David, D., & Ellis, A. (2010). Rational emotive behavior therapy. In K. S. Dobson (Ed.), *Handbook of cognitive-behavioral therapy* (pp. 226–276). New York, NY: Guilford Press.

Dunn, R. L., & Schwebel, A. I. (1995). Meta-analytic review of marital therapy outcome research. *Journal of Family Psychology, 9,* 58–68.

Dutra, L., Stathopoulou, G., Basden, S. L., Leyro, T. M., Powers, M. B., & Otto, M. W. (2008). A meta-analytic review of psychosocial interventions for substance use disorders. *American Journal of Psychiatry, 165,* 179–187.

D'Zurilla, T. J., & Goldfried, M. R. (1971). Problem solving and behavior modification. *Journal of Abnormal Psychology, 78,* 107.

D'Zurilla, T. J., & Nezu, A. M. (2007). *Problem-solving therapy: A positive approach to clinical intervention.* New York, NY: Springer.

D'Zurilla, T. J., Wilson, T., & Nelson, R. (1973). A preliminary study of the effectiveness of graduate prolonged exposure in the treatment of irrational fear. *Behavior Therapy, 4,* 672–685.

Eckhardt, C. I., Murphy, C. M., Whitaker, D. J., Sprunger, J., Dykstra, R., & Woodard, K. (2013). The effectiveness of intervention programs for perpetrators and victims of intimate partner violence. *Partner Abuse, 4,* 196–23

Ellis, A. (1962). *Reason and emotion in psychotherapy.* New York, NY: Citadel Press.

Ellis, A. (1979). Rational-emotive therapy. In A. Ellis & J. M. Whitley (Eds.), *Theoretical and empirical foundations of rational-emotive therapy* (pp. 1–60). Monterey, CA: Brooks/Cole.

Ellis, A. (1994). *Reason and emotion in psychotherapy: A comprehensive method of treating human disturbances: Revised and updated.* New York, NY: Citadel Press.

Ellis, A., & Dryden, W. (1997). *The practice of rational emotive therapy* (2d ed.). New York, NY: Springer.

Emmelkamp, P. M. G., & Wessels, H. (1975). Flooding in imagination versus flooding in vivo: A comparison with agoraphobics. *Behavioral Research and Therapy, 13,* 7–15.

Epstein, N. B., & Baucom, D. H. (2002). *Enhanced cognitive-behavioral therapy for couples: A contextual approach.* Washington, DC: American Psychological Association.

Eysenck, H. J. (1960). *Behavior therapy and the neuroses.* Oxford: Pergamon.

Farmer, R. F., & Chapman, A. L. (2008). *Behavioral interventions in cognitive behavior therapy: Practical guidance for putting theory into action.* Washington, DC: American Psychological Association.

Ferster, C. B. (1973). A functional analysis of depression. *American Psychologist, 28,* 857–870.

Foa, E. B., Jameson, J. S., Turner, R. M., & Payne, L. L. (1980). Massed vs. spaced exposure sessions in the treatment of agoraphobia. *Behaviour Research and Therapy, 18*(4), 333–338.

Gambrill, E. (1977). *Behavior modification: Handbook of assessment, intervention, and evaluation.* San Francisco: Jossey-Bass.

Gambrill, E. (1995). Behavioral social work: Past, present, and future. *Research on Social Work Practice, 4,* 460–484.

Gambrill, E., Thomas, E. J., & Carter, R. D. (1971). Procedure for socio-behavioral practice in open settings. *Social Work, 16,* 51–62.

Glombiewski, J. A., Sawyer, A. T., Gutermann, J., Koenig, K., Rief, W., & Hofmann, S. G. (2010). Psychological treatments for fibromyalgia: A meta-analysis. *Pain, 151,* 280–295.

Gonzalez-Prendes, A. A., & Brisebois, K. (2012). Cognitive-behavioral therapy and social work values: A critical analysis. *Journal of Social Work Values & Ethics, 9,* 21–33.

Gould, R. A., Buckminster, S., Pollack, M. H., Otto, M. W., & Yap, L. (1997). Cognitive-behavioral and pharmacological treatment for social phobia: A meta-analysis. *Clinical Psychology: Science and Practice, 4,* 291–306.

Gould, R. A., Mueser, K. T., Bolton, E., Mays, V., & Goff, D. (2001). Cognitive therapy for psychosis in schizophrenia: An effect size analysis. *Schizophrenia Research, 48,* 335–342.

Gould, R. A., Otto, M. W., & Pollack, M. H. (1995). A meta-analysis of treatment outcome for panic disorder. *Clinical Psychology Review, 8,* 819–844.

Gould, R. A., Otto, M. W., Pollack, M. H., & Yap, L. (1997). Cognitive behavioral and pharmacological treatment of generalized anxiety disorder: A preliminary meta-analysis. *Behavior Therapy, 28,* 285–305.

Granvold, D. K. (2011). Cognitive-behavioral therapy with adults. In J. R. Brandell (Ed.), *Theory and practice in clinical social work* (2d ed., pp. 179–212). Thousand Oaks, CA: SAGE.

Haley, J. (1987). *Problem-solving therapy.* San Francisco: Jossey-Bass.

Hall, S. M., Humfleet, G. L., Reus, V. I., Munoz, R. F., Hartz, D. T., & Maude-Griffin, R. (2002). Psychological intervention and antidepressant treatment in smoking cessation. *Archives of General Psychiatry, 59,* 930–936.

Hay, P. P., Bacaltchuk, J., Stefano, S., & Kashyap, P. (2009). Psychological treatments for bulimia nervosa and binging. *Cochrane Database of Systematic Reviews, 4,* CD000562.

Hayes, S. C. (2004). Acceptance and commitment therapy, relational frame theory, and the third wave of behavioral and cognitive therapies. *Behavior Therapy, 35,* 639–665.

Hayes, S. C., Luoma, J. B., Bond, F. W., Masuda, A., & Lillis, J. (2006). Acceptance and commitment therapy: Model, processes and outcomes. *Behaviour Research and Therapy, 44,* 1–25.

Hayes, S. C., Masuda, A., Bissett, R., Luoma, J., & Guerrero, L. F. (2004). DBT, FAP, and ACT: How empirically oriented are the new behavior therapy technologies? *Behavior Therapy, 35,* 35–54.

Hays, P. A. (2009). Integrating evidence-based practice, cognitive–behavior therapy, and multicultural therapy: Ten steps for culturally competent practice. *Professional Psychology: Research and Practice, 40,* 354–360.

Hersen, M. (Ed.). (2005). *Encyclopedia of behavior modification and cognitive behavior therapy.* Thousand Oaks, CA: SAGE.

Hoagwood, K., & Erwin, H. D. (1997). Effectiveness of school-based mental health services for children: A 10-year research review. *Journal of Child and Family Studies, 6,* 435–451.

Hofmann, S. G., Asmundson, G. J. G., & Beck, A. (2013). The science of cognitive therapy. *Behavior Therapy, 44(2),* 199–212. doi:10.1016/j.beth.2009.01.007

Hofmann, S. G., Asnaani, A., Vonk, I. J., Sawyer, A. T., & Fang, A. (2012). The efficacy of cognitive behavioral therapy: A review of meta-analyses. *Cognitive Therapy and Research, 36(5),* 427–440. doi:10.1007/s10608-012-9476-1

Hofmann, S. G., & Smits, J. A. (2008). Cognitive-behavioral therapy for adult anxiety disorders: A meta-analysis of randomized placebo-controlled trials. *Journal of Clinical Psychiatry, 69(4),* 621–632.

Hollon, S. D., & Beck, A. T. (1994). Cognitive and cognitive-behavioral therapies. In A. E. Bergin & S. L. Garfield (Eds.), *Handbook of psychotherapy and behavior change* (4th ed., pp. 428–466). New York, NY: J. Wiley.

Horrell, S. C. V. (2008). Effectiveness of cognitive-behavioral therapy with adult ethnic minority clients: A review. *Professional Psychology: Research and Practice, 39,* 160.

Hundt, N. E., Mignogna, J., Underhill, C., & Cully, J. A. (2013). The relationship between use of CBT skills and depression treatment outcome: A theoretical and methodological review of the literature. *Behavior Therapy, 44(1),* 12–26. doi:10.1016/j.beth.2012.10.001

Jacobson, E. (1938). *Progressive relaxation.* Chicago: University of Chicago Press.

Jacobson, E. (1970). *Modern treatment of tense patients.* Springfield, IL: Charles C Thomas.

Kabat-Zinn, J. (1990). *Full catastrophe living: Using the wisdom of your body and mind to face stress, pain, and illness.* New York, NY: Delacorte.

Kaltenthaler, E., Brazier, J., De Nigris, E., Tumur, I., Ferriter, M., Beverley, C., et al. (2006). Computerised cognitive behaviour therapy for depression and anxiety update: A systematic review and economic evaluation. *Health Technology Assessment, 10,* 1–186.

Kazantzis, N., & Dattilio, F. M. (2007). Beyond basics: Using homework in cognitive behavior therapy with challenging patients. *Cognitive and Behavioral Practice, 14,* 249–251.

Kazantzis, N., Whittington, C., & Dattilio, F. (2010). Meta-analysis of homework effects in cognitive and behavioral therapy: A replication and extension. *Clinical Psychology: Science and Practice, 17,* 144–156.

Kazdin, A. E. (1978). *History of behavior modification: Experimental foundations of contemporary research.* Baltimore: University Park Press.

Kiluk, B. D., Nich, C., Babuscio, T., & Carroll, K. M. (2010). Quality versus quantity: Acquisition of coping skills following computerized cognitive-behavioral therapy for substance use disorders. *Addiction, 105(12),* 2120–2127. doi:10.1111/j.1360-0443.2010.03076.x

Kingdon, D., & Dimech, A. (2008). Cognitive and behavioural therapies: The state of the art. *Psychiatry, 7(5),* 217–220. doi:10.1016/j.mppsy.2008.03.002

Kubany, E. S., Hill, E. E., Owens, J. A., Iannce-Spencer, C., McCaig, M. A., Tremayne, K. J., & Williams, P. L. (2004). Cognitive trauma therapy for battered women with PTSD (CTT-BW). *Journal of Consulting and Clinical Psychology, 72,* 3–18.

Lambert, M. J., Harmon, S. C., & Slade, K. (2007). Directions for research on homework. In N. Kazantzis & L. L'Abate (Eds.), *Handbook of homework assignments in psychotherapy: Research, practice, and prevention* (pp. 407–423). New York, NY: Springer.

Lang, P. (1968). Appraisal of systematic desensitization techniques with children and adults. In C. M. Franks (Ed.), *Assessment and status of behavior therapies and associated developments.* New York, NY: McGraw Hill.

Lazarus, R. S. (1966). *Psychological stress and the coping process.* New York, NY: McGraw-Hill.

Lewinsohn, P. M., Sullivan, J. M., & Grosscup, S. J. (1980). Changing reinforcing events: An approach to the treatment of depression. *Psychotherapy: Theory, Research and Practice, 47,* 322–334.

Lincoln, T. M., Ziegler, M., Mehl, S., Kesting, M. L., Lüllmann, E., Westermann, S., & Rief, W. (2012). Moving from efficacy to effectiveness in cognitive behavioral therapy for psychosis: A randomized clinical practice trial. *Journal of Consulting and Clinical Psychology, 80(4),* 674–686. doi:10.1037/a0028665

Linehan, M. M. (1987). Dialectical behavior therapy for borderline personality disorder: Theory and method. *Bulletin of the Menninger Clinic, 51,* 261–276.

Linehan, M. M. (1993). *Skills training manual for treating borderline personality disorder.* New York, NY: Guilford Press.

Magill, M., & Ray, L. A. (2009). Cognitive-behavioral treatment with adult alcohol and illicit drug users: A meta-analysis of randomized controlled trials. *Journal of Studies on Alcohol and Drugs, 70(4),* 516–527.

Meichenbaum, D. H. (1993). Stress inoculation training: A 20-year update. In P. M. Lehrer & R. L. Woolfolk (Eds.), *Principles and practice of stress management* (2d ed., pp. 373–406). New York, NY: Guilford Press.

Meichenbaum, D. H., & Deffenbacher, J. L. (1988). Stress inoculation training. *The Counseling Psychologist, 16*, 69–90.

Moldovan, A. R., & David, D. (2011). Effect of obesity treatments on eating behavior: psychosocial interventions versus surgical interventions. A systematic review. *Eating behaviors, 12*, 161–167.

Mottillo, S., Filion, K. B., Belisle, P., Joseph, L., Gervais, A., O'Loughlin, J., et al. (2009). Behavioural interventions for smoking cessation: A meta-analysis of randomized controlled trials. *European Heart Journal, 30*, 718–730.

Mowrer, O. H. (1960). *Learning theory and behavior.* New York, NY: Wiley.

National Association of Social Workers. (1996). *Code of ethics.* Washington, DC: NASW. Retrieved October 17, 2013, from http://www.naswdc.org/pubs/code/code.asp.

National Association of Social Workers. (2005). *NASW standards for clinical social work in social work practice.* Washington, DC: NASW.

National Association of Social Workers. (2006). *Life's journey: Help starts here.* Washington, DC: NASW. Retrieved from http://www.socialworkers.org/pressroom/swm2006/swmToolKit2006.pdf

Norcross, J. C., Garofalo, A., & Koocher, G. P. (2006). Discredited psychological treatments and tests: A Delphi poll. *Professional Psychology: Research and Practice, 37*, 515–522.

Norton, P. J., & Price, E. C. (2007). A meta-analytic review of adult cognitive-behavioral treatment outcome across the anxiety disorders. *Journal of Nervous and Mental Disease, 195*(6), 521–531. doi:10.1097/01.nmd.0000253843.70149.9a

Ost, L. G. (2008). Efficacy of the third wave of behavioral therapies: A systematic review and meta-analysis. *Behaviour Research & Therapy, 46*, 296–321.

Pavlov, I. P. (1927). *Conditioned reflexes.* Translated by G. V. Anrep. New York, NY: Dover.

Perkins, K. A., Conklin, C. A., & Levine, M. D. (2008). *Cognitive-behavioral therapy for smoking cessation.* New York, NY: Taylor & Francis.

Pignotti, M., & Thyer, B. A. (2009). Use of novel, unsupported and empirically supported therapies by licensed clinical social workers: An exploratory study. *Social Work Research, 33*, 5–17.

Powers, M. B., Vedel, E., & Emmelkamp, P. M. G. (2008). Behavioral couples therapy (BCT) for alcohol and drug use disorders: A meta-analysis. *Clinical Psychology Review, 28*, 952–962.

Prochaska, J. O., & Norcross, J. C. (2010). *Systems of psychotherapy* (7th ed.). Belmont, CA: Cengage.

Reas, D. L., & Grilo, C. M. (2008). Review and meta-analysis of pharmacotherapy for binge-eating disorder. *Obesity, 16*(9), 2024–2038.

Reynolds, B. C. (1942). *Learning and teaching in the practice of social work.* New York, NY: Farrar & Rinehart.

Richard, D. C. S., & Lauterbach, D. L. (2007). *Handbook of exposure therapies.* Boston: Academic Press.

Rose, V., & Perz, J. (2005). Is CBT useful in vocational rehabilitation for people with a psychiatric disability? *Psychiatric Rehabilitation Journal, 29*, 56–58.

Roy-Byrne, P. P., Craske, M. G., Stein, M. B., Sullivan, G., Bystritsky, A., Katon, W., et al. (2005). A randomized effectiveness trial of cognitive-behavioral therapy and medication for primary care panic disorder. *Archives of General Psychiatry, 62*, 290.

Sackett, D. L., Straus, S. E., Richardson, W. S., Rosenberg, W., & Haynes, R. B. (2000). *Evidence-based medicine: How to practice and teach EBM.* Edinburgh: Churchill Livingstone.

Schraufnagel, T. J., Wagner, A. W., Miranda, J., & Roy-Byrne, P. P. (2006). Treating minority patients with depression and anxiety: What does the evidence tell us? *General Hospital Psychiatry, 28*, 27–36.

Scogin, F., Welsh, D., Hanson, A., Stump, J., & Coates, A. (2005). Evidence-based psychotherapies for depression in older adults. *Clinical Psychology: Science and Practice, 12*, 222–237.

Segal, Z. V., Williams, J. M. G., & Teasdale, J. D. (2002). *Mindfulness-based cognitive therapy for depression—A new approach to preventing relapse.* New York, NY: Guilford Press.

Shapiro, F. (1991). Eye movement desensitization and reprocessing procedure: From EMD to EMD/R-A, and treatment model for anxiety and related trauma. *The Behavior Therapist, 5*, 128–133.

Simpson, S. (2009). Psychotherapy via videoconferencing: A review. *British Journal of Guidance & Counselling, 37*, 271–286.

Singh, N. N., Lancioni, G. E., Wahler, R. G., Winton, A. S. W., & Singh, J. (2008). Mindfulness approaches in cognitive behavior therapy. *Behavioral and Cognitive Psychotherapy, 36*, 659–666.

Skinner, B. F. (1938). *The behavior of organisms: An experimental analysis.* Oxford: Appleton-Century.

Skinner, B. F. (1963). Operant behavior. *American Psychologist, 18*, 503–515.

Taylor, S. (1996). Meta-analysis of cognitive-behavioral treatments for social phobia. *Journal of behavior therapy and experimental psychiatry, 27*, 1–9.

Thompson-Brenner, H. J. (2003). *Implications for the treatment of bulimia nervosa: A meta-analysis of efficacy trials and a naturalistic study of treatment in the community.* Ann Arbor: University of Michigan Press.

Thyer, B. A. (2002). Principles of Evidence-based practice and treatment development. In A. Roberts & G. J. Greene (Eds.), *Social work desk reference* (pp. 739–742). New York, NY: Oxford University Press.

Thyer, B. A., & Myers, L. (2011). Behavioral and cognitive therapies. In J. Brandell (Ed.), *Theory and practice in clinical social work* (2d ed., pp. 21–40). Thousand Oaks, CA: SAGE.

van Balkom, A. J. L. M., van Oppen, P., Vermeulen, A. W. A., van Dyck, R., Nauta, M. C. E., & Vorst, H. C. M. (1994).

A meta-analysis on the treatment of obsessive-compulsive disorder: A comparison of antidepressants, behavior, and cognitive therapy. *Clinical Psychology Review, 14*, 359–381.

Vocks, S., Tuschen-Caffier, B., Pietrowsky, R., Rustenbach, S. J., Kersting, A., & Herpertz, S. (2010). Meta-analysis of the effectiveness of psychological and pharmacological treatments for binge eating disorder. *International Journal of Eating Disorders, 43*, 205–217.

Vos, T., Haby, M. M., Barendregt, J. J., Kruijshaar, M., Corry, J., & Andrews, G. (2004). The burden of major depression avoidable by longer-term treatment strategies. *Archives of General Psychiatry, 61*(11), 1097–1103.

Watson, J. B. (1925). *Behaviorism*. New York, NY: Norton.

Watson, J. B., & Rayner, R. (1920). Conditioned emotional reactions. *Journal of Experimental Psychology, 3*, 1–14.

Watson, J. P., Gaind, R., & Marks, I. M. (1971). Prolonged exposure: A rapid treatment for phobias. *British Medical Journal, 1*, 13–15.

Weissman, M. M., & Sanderson, W. C. (2002). Promises and problems in modern psychotherapy: The need for increased training in evidence-based treatments. In M. Hager (Ed.). *Modern Psychiatry: Challenges in education health professionals to meet new needs.* (pp. 132–165). New York, NY: Josiah Macy Jr. Foundation.

Weissman, M. M., Verdeli, H., Gameroff, M. J., Bledsoe, S. E., Betts, K., Mufson, L., et al. (2006). National survey of psychotherapy training in psychiatry, psychology, and social work. *Archives of General Psychiatry, 63*, 925–934.

Williams, D. A. (2003). Psychological and behavioural therapies in fibromyalgia and related syndromes. *Best Practice & Research Clinical Rheumatology, 17*, 649–665.

Wilson, C. J., & Cottone, R. R. (2013). Using Cognitive Behavior Therapy in Clinical Work With African American Children and Adolescents: A Review of the Literature. *Journal of Multicultural Counseling and Development, 41*, 130–143.

Wolpe, J. (1958). *Psychotherapy by reciprocal inhibition.* Redwood City, CA: Stanford University Press.

Wolpe, J. (1969). *The practice of behavior therapy.* New York, NY: Pergamon Press.

Wykes, T., Steel, C., Everitt, B., & Tarrier, N. (2008). Cognitive behavior therapy for schizophrenia: Effect sizes, clinical models, and methodological rigor. *Schizophrenia Bulletin, 34*(3), 523–537. doi:10.1093/schbul/sbm114

Young, J. E. (1994). *Cognitive therapy for personality disorders: A schema-focused approach.* Sarasota, FL: Professional Resource Press.

Young, J. E., Klosko, J. S., & Weishaar, M. E. (2003). *Schema therapy: A practitioner's guide.* New York, NY: Guilford Press.

FURTHER READING

Academy of Cognitive Therapy: http://www.academyofct.org

Anxiety Disorders Association of America: http://www.adaa.org/

Association for Behavioral and Cognitive Therapies: http://www.abct.org/home/

Beck Institute for Cognitive Behavior Therapy: http://www.beckinstitute.org/

Behavior Therapy Training Institute: http://www.ocfoundation.org/btti.aspx

International OCD Foundation: http://www.ocfoundation.org/

ADDIE WEAVER, JOSEPH HIMLE,
GAIL STEKETEE AND JORDANA MUROFF

COLLABORATIVE PRACTICE

ABSTRACT: Social workers are uniquely prepared to provide leadership for collaborative practice, especially when they employ intervention logic. Intervention-driven collaboration develops interdependent relationships among people. These relationships are cemented by norms of reciprocity and trust, enabling participants to organize for collective action in response to "wicked" problems characterized by uncertainty, novelty, and complexity.

Among the family of "c-words" (for example, communication, coordination), collaboration is the most difficult to develop, institutionalize, and sustain because it requires new organizational designs, including inter-organizational partnerships, as well as policy change. Notwithstanding the attendant challenges, collaborative practice is a mainstay in multiple sectors of social work practice, including mental health, substance abuse, school social work, complex change, anti-poverty initiatives, international social work, workforce development, and research. Growing collaboration with client systems connects collaborative practice with empowerment practice and facilitates the achievement of social work's mission.

KEY WORDS: collaboration; social work practice; collective action; complex change

Social workers, like other helping professionals, are encountering growing needs and opportunities for collaborative practice. For example, the limitations of industrial-age professions, organizations, and institutions are becoming apparent as a new genus of problems develops. These new problem clusters, called "wicked problems" because they encompass intractable dilemmas and defy ready solutions (Mason & Mitroff, 1981), are marked by unprecedented complexity, novelty, and uncertainty. Examples include concentrated poverty (also called social exclusion and social isolation) and the threats to global sustainability caused by pollution, food shortages, wars, ethnic hostilities, and multiple insecurities. Such wicked problems require collaborative practice, especially forms of collaborative practice led and performed by social workers who advance democracy as they promote social and economic justice for vulnerable, oppressed populations.

Social workers have made unique, significant contributions to the concept of collaborative practice and for good reason. An option for some professions, collaborative practice is an essential, defining feature of social work practice. For example, social workers, perhaps more than other helping professionals, strive to establish collaborative working relationships with their clients systems. Moreover, social workers often are instrumental in facilitating interprofessional (interdisciplinary) and interorganizational collaboration (Abramson & Rosenthal, 1995).

The following is structured to introduce relevant details. It begins with an intervention-oriented, conceptual framework for collaborative practice. Then it provides examples of social workers' collaborative practice in multiple sectors. Collaborative practice's import for social work's mission provides a fitting conclusion.

An Intervention-Oriented, Conceptual Framework

Collaborative practice arguably is a defining characteristic of "macropractice" because it cross-cuts the other kinds of practice in this category. These other kinds include community building and development, interprofessional practice, interorganizational practice, and social planning—all foci for other entries in this volume. Because collaborative practice is embedded in these other kinds of macropractice, it has the potential to unite them and provide much-needed coherence. These benefits and others depend on a research-supported, theoretically sound conceptual framework. One such framework follows.

ENHANCING THE LAY DEFINITION WITH INTERVENTION LOGIC Collaborative practice, in lay terms, means "working together." While this lay approach is fundamentally accurate, it also is both imprecise and incomplete. It conceals important distinctions among a variety of collaborative practices. This problem carries with it the threat that well-intentioned social workers will err when they elect a kind of collaborative practice that does not correspond to presenting needs, problems, and opportunities.

Intervention logic, a hallmark of sound, clinical social work practice, helps prevent collaborative practice errors. It prioritizes the correspondence, or more simply "the fit," between the practice solution (intervention) and the presenting problem, need, or opportunity. This logic requires social work professionals to make theoretically sound inquiries into "the theory of the problem" so as to determine its etiology. Such an etiology includes relevant causes, correlates, and antecedents. Three inseparable questions facilitate these inquiries:

- What is wrong that needs to be fixed?
- What is good and correct that needs to be maintained?
- How can the answers to these two questions be pieced together, producing an accurate and coherent "theory of the problem," that is, one that enables social workers to select among alternative strengths-based, solution-focused, and culturally competent interventions?

Because intervention logic helps to pinpoint the theory of the problem, it maximizes the probability that social workers will select the optimal, collaborative practice intervention.

VARIETIES OF COLLABORATIVE PRACTICE: A FRAMEWORK FOR THE FAMILY OF "C-WORDS" Owing in part to the theoretical and empirical contributions of social work researchers (Abramson & Rosenthal, 1995; Anderson-Butcher & Ashton, 2004; Briar-Lawson, Lawson, Hennon, & Jones, 2001; Bronstein, 2003; Claiborne & Lawson, 2005; Lawson, 2003, 2004), enhanced conceptual frameworks for collaborative practice now are available. Arguably intervention logic has been a facilitator for framework developments and serves as a defining characteristic of the best ones and the optimal practice alternatives they encompass.

The best frameworks make firm distinctions among a family of "c-words": communication, consultation, coordination, and collaboration. Unfortunately, all lend themselves to competing definitions, conceptual confusion, and conflicting practices. Problems like these and the errors they spawn can be prevented when each c-word is framed as a special intervention. Then each can be tailored to special needs, problems, and opportunities (Claiborne & Lawson, 2005; Lawson, 2003, 2004).

Communication. In most conceptual frameworks, communication is the easiest and most simplistic form of collaborative practice. Effective communication with other service providers and also with service users is a hallmark of collaborative practice. Only when people share information and gain consensus through it can they work together. The importance of communication is revealed when it is absent or flawed (Lawson, 2003).

Consultation. Consultation starts with the communication of information, but it also includes a more intricate and important "move" toward more sophisticated collaborative practice. In lieu of assuming automatically that one professional knows best what to do, this form of collaborative practice proceeds with the assumption that other persons offer invaluable expertise. These persons include other professionals, service users, and persons knowledgeable about service users and their surrounding social ecologies, including their family members, friends, and neighborhood communities (Lawson, 2003).

Consultation entails eliciting these persons' views on the theory of the problem and gaining their intervention recommendations. Because it draws on others' expertise, often in unique practice contexts, consultation facilitates the identification of diversity and paves the way for culturally responsive and competent practice (Lawson, 2003).

Coordination. Coordination encompasses communication and consultation, but it also introduces increasing complexity. Coordinated, collaborative practice is especially salient when multiple needs, problems, and opportunities are encountered; and when the efforts of multiple persons must be orchestrated. In this form of collaborative practice, social workers must harmonize and synchronize their assessments, interventions, and improvement-oriented practice evaluations with other persons—notably other professionals and service users. Examples include interprofessional teams, the several kinds of family-centered practice, and community-based work involving coalitions (Lawson, 2003).

Importantly, in coordinated, collaborative practice the participants remain autonomous and independent. They take turns contributing to problem-solving and opportunity maximization. Just as many sports coaches must orchestrate the multiple movements of their athletes, someone, ideally a social worker, usually is required to orchestrate, synchronize, and harmonize the respective contributions of the multiple participants involved in coordinated, collaborative practice.

Collaboration. Collaboration encompasses the other c-words. It is the most sophisticated and complex form of collaborative practice (Claiborne & Lawson, 2005; Lawson, 2003, 2004). For example, in comparison to the other c-words, collaboration requires more time, dedicated resources, and special leadership. The most costly and challenging of the various kinds of collaborative practice, it also is the most difficult to institutionalize and sustain.

Three keynote features of collaboration lend credence to these claims and others that follow. First, collaboration both develops and requires interdependent relationships. Second, collaboration is a warranted response to needs, problems, opportunities, and situations manifesting complexity, novelty, and uncertainty, especially those in which available knowledge and understanding are limited or even nonexistent. Wicked problems, identified at the outset, especially require collaboration. Third, power and authority differentials must be suspended as much as possible, enabling partner-participants to work together as much as possible as equals (Lawson, 2003, 2004).

In brief, when social workers opt for collaboration with other professionals, service users, and other needed constituencies, they do so because they cannot be successful and effective without them. In other words, interdependent relationships emblematic of collaboration develop when no one person can achieve their aims, goals, and objectives alone. Each fundamentally depends on the others, and so they often adopt common purposes (Schorr, 2006). This interdependence is especially apparent when no one knows what to do in complex, novel, and uncertain situations, and especially when vexing needs and problems nest in one another (for example, those accompanying poverty). Collaboration thus entails developing shared awareness of this interdependence and inherent complexity, developing shared goals, and then creating a feasible, warranted system of roles, rules, and social relations, which is tied to effective, collective action strategies (Bronstein, 2003).

The social relations for collaboration are cemented by norms of reciprocity and trust. Both are maximized when "the right mix" of participants is convened and organized for collective action. After all, norms of reciprocity (that is, voluntary, mutual "give and receive" relations) and trust take time to develop and require mutual familiarity. These special norms and trust relationships are easier to develop and witness when stakeholders have enjoyed prior histories of successful working relationships. Additionally, norms of reciprocity and trust are likely to develop when all of the participating stakeholders view each other as credible, dependable, competent, and legitimate. These several features reduce the risks of depending on others, and risk reduction is especially important in today's outcomes-oriented, accountability practice environments (Lawson, 2004).

Collaboration is not, however, without its challenges-as-opportunities. For example, when everyone shares responsibility for outcomes, the risk remains that no one is responsible or accountable. When outcomes improve and other benefits are evident, questions often arise as to who deserves the credit. Questions about recognition and rewards are especially likely to arise when "free riding" occurs, that is, when some participants end up contributing little or nothing to outcomes even though they are officially recognized as one of the collaborators (Lawson, 2003).

Above all, conflict is endemic in collaboration. This unavoidable feature highlights the necessity for conflict mediation and resolution mechanisms; strengths-based, solution-focused language; behavioral norms to ensure high quality, positive interactions during moments of conflict; and "barrier-busting" protocols. When these several conflict-related mechanisms are in place, the positive, generative–creative propensities of conflict and collaboration can be maximized. Among the benefits are two kinds of powerful innovations (Lawson, 2004). Collaboration routinely yields process innovations (new ways of practicing and "doing business") and product innovations (new service delivery structures, programs, and services).

In short, collaboration responds to complexity and interdependent relationships, and it also promotes them. New for many of its developers, it also creates both novelty and complexity. Furthermore, collaboration is an innovation, which incubates other innovations in response to environmental changes. Daunting complexity like this indicates why collaboration is so difficult to develop, institutionalize, and sustain. It also indicates why complexity theory is salient to collaboration's development and theoretical analysis (Warren, Franklin, & Streeter, 1998).

It follows that collaboration entails a special kind of leadership, which may be described as adaptive, shared, results-oriented, and distributed leadership. It must be adaptive to be responsive to changing needs and context. It must be shared because top–down, compliance-oriented, one-person leadership derails collaboration. It must be results-oriented because of modern accountability requirements and also because of moral imperatives for ensuring that collaboration actually helps individuals, families, communities, and the social work workforce. Additionally, this leadership must be distributed because it must span group, family, professional, organizational, and community boundaries. Fortunately, this is the kind of leadership for which social workers enjoy special preparation. Indeed, this cross-boundary, collaborative leadership

is engrained in the history of the profession (Abbott, 1995), and the future holds prospects for more of it.

THE IMPORT OF ORGANIZATIONAL SETTINGS The several forms of collaborative practice require optimal conditions. For example, the organizational environments (Abramson & Rosenthal, 1995) and community settings for these practices must be conducive to collaborative practice. Supportive policies are another practical necessity. A brief explanation follows.

Social workers and others engaged in collaborative practices typically do so under the aegis of at least one organization. When several professions are involved, the multiple organizations that employ them are also involved (Abramson & Rosenthal, 1995). These organizations provide the settings for collaborative practice. Ideally, these settings are conducive to, and facilitative of, collaborative practice. Since these setting-related features do not evolve and occur naturally, it is important to identify important examples so they can be created by design. Both intra- and interorganizational designs are needed. Interorganizational designs increasingly are called partnerships. The rationale: Reserving "partnerships" for organizations also reserves the family of c-words to refer to and depict interactions among people.

The features of supportive organizational settings start with the time, facilities, resources, supports, incentives, and rewards for collaborative practice. For example, many organizations have a preferred program and service model, and it needs to include, support, and reward collaborative practice. Other features include leadership, management, and supervisory structures that are aligned with collaborative practice, including both top-down and bottom-up mechanisms for obtaining information and feedback for learning and improvement. They include data-management systems, both intra- and inter-organizational. They also include training, technical assistance, and capacity-building mechanisms needed to advance collaborative practice (Bardach, 1998; Lawson, 2003).

THE IMPORT OF SUPPORTIVE POLICY ENVIRONMENTS Individual organizations and clusters of them are disciplined by policies and the institutional arrangements they structure. Social workers, arguably more than any other profession, are prepared to understand and to help change policies that do not support collaborative practice. Since social workers rarely change policies alone, this policy-oriented leadership comprises another kind of collaborative practice.

Social Workers and Collaborative Practice

The opportunities and sectors for collaborative practice by social workers appear to be growing rapidly. Three reasons are especially relevant. The first is a new policy environment that favors social workers over other professions (for example, psychiatry, psychology). Growing understanding about co-occurring, interlocking needs manifested by many service users, especially the most vulnerable ones, is the second reason. Concern over the lack of effectiveness of conventional, clinical-direct services by a solo professional is the third.

SECTORS FOR COLLABORATIVE PRACTICE This short article can do little more than identifying relevant sectors of practice and providing references for readers' personalized follow-up inquiries. After these sectors are identified, a pivotal distinction between two kinds of collaborative practice is amplified. This distinction is especially important to unique social work practice.

Local, State, and National Sectors. Here, then, is a starter inventory of the service sectors in which social workers engage in, and often lead, collaborative practice. These sectors are: (a) schools (Anderson-Butcher, Lawson, Bean, Boone, & Kwuatkowski, 2004); (b) hospitals (Abramson & Mizrahi, 1996); (c) mental health agencies (Hodges & Hardiman, 2006); (d) public health agencies (Roussos & Fawcett, 2000); (e) child welfare agencies (Sallee, Lawson, & Briar-Lawson, 2001; Smith & Mogro-Wilson, 2008); (f) juvenile justice agencies (Byrnes, Boyle, & Yaffe-Kjosness, 2005; Marks & Lawson, 2005); (g) welfare-to-work programs (Briar-Lawson, 1999); (h) elder-serving agencies (McCallion, Grant-Griffin, & Kolomer, 2000) and initiatives (Bronstein, McCallion, & Kramer, 2006); (i) substance abuse agencies (O'Hare, 2002); (j) domestic violence agencies; (k) youth development agencies (Anderson-Butcher, Stetler, & Midle, 2006); (l) family service agencies (Briar-Lawson et al., 2001); (m) agencies charged with leadership for community-based coalitions (Mizrahi & Rosenthal, 2001); and (n) agencies charged with disaster relief (Briar-Lawson, 2006).

International Sectors. Disaster relief in the United States points toward international needs and opportunities for collaborative practice, and a timely response to the 2004 tsunami in Indonesia serves as an example (Hardiman, Martinek, & Anderson-Butcher, 2005). This international work includes border-crossing assistance to immigrants and migrants, including the growing number of divided family systems residing in different nations (Lawson, 2001). It also includes cross-national adoptions for needy children (as documented in the *Journal of Community Practice*).

New Sectors. As workforce recruitment, retention, and optimization become priorities, and as knowledge grows about how and why organizational contexts "push out" good workers, a new sector for collaborative practice has developed. Organizational development, via organizational design and improvement teams, is one such emergent opportunity (Lawson, McCarthy, Briar-Lawson, Miraglia, Strolin, & Caring, 2006).

Moreover, as the limitations of conventional research methodologies become apparent, another sector is developing: *The research sector.* This encompasses collaborative research (as a collaborative practice), including research focused on collaborative practice. It also entails collaborative research methodologies, including community-based, participatory research, action science, and participatory action research (Greenwood & Levin, 2006; Kreuter, Lezin, & Young, 2000).

A PIVOTAL DISTINCTION AND CHOICE POINT Partly because conventional practices have enjoyed limited effectiveness, interest is growing in new forms of collaborative practice involving service users as experts and providers. For example, so-called consumer-provided mental health services are gaining considerable popularity (Hodges & Hardiman, 2006; Mancini, Hardiman, & Lawson, 2005), and so are parent-to-parent service strategies (Briar-Lawson, 2000). In these examples, the target system (client system) becomes the action system in close concert with social workers and other helping professionals. Arguably, this emergent practice paradigm provides a unique, splendid opportunity for social work leadership in service of vulnerable people, also benefiting the profession writ large.

COLLABORATIVE PRACTICE'S IMPORT FOR SOCIAL WORK'S MISSION The achievement of social work's mission—to eliminate oppression and alleviate poverty—fundamentally depends on effective, creative collaborative practice. Only when social workers engage other people in this important mission, building their capacities for collaborative practice and reinforcing their political will, can this mission be achieved. Here, collaborative practice meets empowerment practice. A technical-procedural challenge in one light, in another this kind of integrated, complex practice is a moral obligation and an ethical imperative associated with the renewal of responsive democracy. Social work's leadership for 21st-century collaborative practice begins here, and it spans local, state, regional, national, and international contexts.

Acknowledgment

Several colleagues were exemplars for collaborative practice as they generously provided materials and suggestions for improving this article. I am grateful to all of them.

REFERENCES

Abbott, A. (1995). Boundaries of social work or social work of boundaries? *Social Service Review, 68*, 545–562.

Abramson, J., & Mizrahi, T. (1996). When social workers and physicians collaborate: Positive and negative interdisciplinary experiences. *Social Work, 41*, 270–281.

Abramson, J., & Rosenthal, B. (1995). Interdisciplinary and interorganizational collaboration. In R. L. Richards (Ed.), *Encyclopedia of social work*, Vol. II (19th ed., pp. 1479–1489). Washington, DC: National Association of Social Workers Press.

Anderson-Butcher, D., & Ashton, D. (2004). Innovative models of collaboration to serve children, youth, families, and communities. *Children & Schools, 26*(1), 39–53.

Anderson-Butcher, D., Lawson, H., Bean, J., Boone, B., & Kwuatkowski, A. (2004). Implementation guide: Ohio community collaboration model for school improvement. Columbus, OH: Ohio Department of Education. Available at: http://cle.osu.edu/familycivicengagement/documents/references-and-guides/downloads/implementation-guide-combined-occmsi.pdf

Anderson-Butcher, D., Stetler, G., & Midle, T. (2006). Collaborative partnerships in schools: A case for youth development. *Children & Schools, 28*(3), 155–163.

Bardach, E. (1998). *Getting agencies to work together: The practice and theory of managerial craftsmanship.* Washington, DC: The Brookings Institution.

Briar-Lawson, K. (1999). Implications of TANF for children, youth and families: Interprofessional education and collaboration. *Teacher Education Quarterly, 26*(4), 159–172.

Briar-Lawson, K., (2000). The rainmakers. In P. Senge, N. Cambron-McCabe, T. Lucas, Kleiner, J. Dutton, & B. Smith (Eds.), *Schools that learn* (pp. 529–538). New York: Doubleday.

Briar-Lawson, K. (2006, November). *Social work and disasters.* Alliance of Universities for Democracy, Katowice, Poland.

Briar-Lawson, K., Lawson, H., & Hennon, C., & Jones, A. (2001). *Family-supportive policy practice: International perspectives.* New York: Columbia University Press.

Bronstein, L. (2003). A model for interdisciplinary collaboration. *Social Work, 48*(3), 297–306.

Bronstein, L., McCallion, P., & Kramer, E. (2006). Developing an aging prepared community: Collaboration among counties, consumers, professionals and organizations. *Journal of Gerontological Social Work, 48*(1/2), 193–202.

Byrnes, E., Boyle, S., & Yaffe-Kjosness, J. (2005). Enhancing interventions with delinquent youths: The case for specifically treating depression in juvenile justice populations. *Journal of Evidence-Based Social Work: Advances in Practice, Programming, Research, and Policy, 2*(3/4), 49–71.

Claiborne, N., & Lawson, H. (2005). An intervention framework for collaboration. *Families in Society: The Journal of Contemporary Human Services, 86*(1), 93–103.

Greenwood, D., & Levin, M. (2006). *Introduction to action research.* Thousand Oaks, CA: Sage Publishers.

Hardiman, E., Martinek, T., & Anderson-Butcher, D. (2005, February). The international workshop on addressing trauma and depression through sport. Invited workshop presented for the Indonesian National Government, Jakarta, Indonesia.

Hodges, J., & Hardiman, E. (2006). Promoting healthy organizational partnerships and collaboration between consumer-run and community mental health agencies. *Administration and Policy in Mental Health: Mental Health Services Research, 33*(3), 267–278.

Kreuter, M. W., Lezin, N. A., & Young, L. A. (2000). Evaluating community-based collaborative mechanisms: Implications for practitioners. *Health Promotion Practice, 1*(1), 49–63.

Lawson, H. (2001). Globalization, flows of culture and people, and new century frameworks for family-centered policies, practices, and development. In K. Briar-Lawson, H. Lawson, & C. Hennon (Eds.), *Family-centered policies and practices: International implications* (pp. 338–376). New York: Columbia University Press.

Lawson, H. (2003). Pursuing and securing collaboration to improve results. In M. Brabeck & M. Walsh (Eds.), *Meeting at the hyphen: Schools-universities communities-professions in collaboration for student achievement and well being* (pp. 45–73). The 102nd Yearbook of the National Society for the Study of Education Yearbook. Chicago: University of Chicago Press.

Lawson, H. (2004). The logic of collaboration in education and the human services. *The Journal of Interprofessional Care, 18*, 225–237.

Lawson, H., McCarthy, M., Briar-Lawson, K., Miraglia, P., Strolin, J., & Caringi, J. (2006). A complex partnership to optimize and stabilize the public child welfare workforce. *Professional Development: The International Journal of Continuing Social Work Education, 9*(2–3), 122–139.

Mancini, M., Hardiman, E., & Lawson, H. (2005). Making sense of it all: Consumer providers' theories about factors facilitating and impeding recovery from psychiatric disabilities. *Psychiatric Rehabilitation Journal, 29*(1), 48–55.

Marks, M., & Lawson, H. (2005). The import of co-production dynamics and time dollar programs in complex, community-based child welfare initiatives for "hard to serve" youth and their families. *Child Welfare, 84*, 209–232.

Mason, O., & Mitroff, I. (1981). *Challenging strategic planning assumptions: Theory, case, and techniques.* New York: Wiley.

McCallion, P. J., Grant-Griffin, L., & Kolomer, S. (2000). Grandparent caregivers II: Service needs and service provision issues. *Journal of Gerontological Social Work, 33*(3), 57–84.

Mizrahi, T., & Rosenthal, B. (2001). Complexities of coalition building: Leaders' successes, strategies, struggles, and solutions. *Social Work, 46*(1), 63–77.

O'Hare, T. (2002). Evidence-based social work practice with mentally ill persons who abuse alcohol and other drugs. *Social Work in Mental Health, 1*(1), 43–62.

Roussos, S., & Fawcett, S. (2000). A review of collaborative partnerships as a strategy for improving community health. *Annual Review of Public Health, 21*, 369–402.

Sallee, A., Lawson, H., & Briar-Lawson, K. (2001). *Innovative practices with vulnerable children and families.* Dubuque, IA: Eddie Bowers Publishers, Inc.

Schorr, L. (2006). *Common purpose: Sharing responsibility for child and family outcomes.* New York: National Center for Children in Poverty, Mailman School of Public Health at Columbia University.

Smith, B., & Mogro-Wilson, C. (2008). Inter-agency collaboration: Policy and practice in child welfare and substance abuse treatment. *Administration in Social Work, 32*, 5–24.

Warren, K., Franklin, C., & Streeter, C. (1998). New directions in systems theory: Chaos and complexity. *Social Work, 43*(4): 357–372.

FURTHER READING

Center for Effective Collaboration and Practice website: http://cecp.air.org/

HAL A. LAWSON

COMMON FACTORS IN PSYCHOTHERAPY

ABSTRACT: This is an examination of the common factors approach in social work and in related professions. The term "common factors" refers to a set of features that are shared across different specific models of psychotherapy and social services, but may not always be conceptualized as being curative influences. The common factors approach broadens the conceptual base of potentially curative variables for practice and research. The history of common factors, the research designs and statistical methods that have led to the approach's elaboration, the approach's empirical base, and its fit with social work's person-in-environment perspective are each explored. The intersection of the common factors approach with the evidence-based practice movement is examined. The role of common factors in the psychotherapy integration movement is also discussed.

The implications of the common factors approach for research, policy, and practice in social work are identified.

KEY WORDS: common factors; evidence-based; practice; outcomes; process; psychotherapy

Introduction

CONCEPTUALIZING WHAT CAUSES CHANGE IN PSYCHOTHERAPY IS COMPLEX Several decades of research have documented the benefits of psychotherapy (Bergin & Garfield, 1971, 1978, 1986, 1994; Lambert, 2004, 2013; U.S. Department of Health and Human Services, 1999). Lambert and Ogles (2004) and Wampold (2001) have aggregated the results of several quantitative and qualitative studies to document that over 75% of psychotherapy patients show benefits. More recently, psychotherapy outcome research has focused in detail on identifying the factors that contribute to change in psychotherapies of many kinds, regardless of duration or modality. Norcross and Lambert (2012) point out that many factors impact psychotherapy outcomes. These factors include the characteristics of the patient and of the clinician, the nature of their relationship, treatment techniques, hope, placebo effects, and context. Psychotherapy is a complex and multifaceted endeavor.

Psychotherapy and other social work interventions are best understood as socially complex phenomena. In contrast to an intervention consisting only of a course of medication of a verified dosage, psychosocial interventions involve client motivation, the client–therapist relationship, hope, expectancy, warmth, genuineness, and empathy, among other factors. These factors are shared across different models of specific interventions and are generally viewed as common among all of them. Each of these factors may be more or less important in the delivery of a specific form of therapy to a particular client. It is too simple and quite misleading just to ask, "Do treatments cure disorders or do relationships heal people?" (Norcross & Lambert, 2011, p. 3). The curative influences affecting the outcomes of psychosocial interventions are best conceptualized as being composed of many factors, some more overt and technique driven and others more implicit than explicitly recognized and emphasized.

SPECIFIC AND COMMON FACTORS IN PSYCHOTHERAPY PRACTICE In the psychotherapy and clinical social work literature, curative factors are called "specific factors" when they are unique to the techniques of an intervention. For example, the miracle question is specific to solution-focused interventions, whereas transference interpretation is specific to psychodynamic interventions. On the other hand, social workers providing any type of psychosocial intervention are likely to treat clients with respect, to be warm, and to be empathic. In their intervention processes, social workers seek to establish agreement on treatment goals, to encourage hope, and to develop a shared set of expectations about how the intervention will "work." Factors shared across intervention models and processes are known as "common factors" in the psychotherapy literature (Drisko, 2004; Rosenzweig, 1936).

Social workers and other mental health professionals are routinely educated about both specific and common factors in planning and delivering interventions. Many social work texts and social work accreditation standards identify phases of intervention including engagement and contracting that scholars view as common, or shared, across specific interventive models that draw upon different theories and techniques. Skills of active listening, providing clarifying feedback, and offering support are shared across most models of psychosocial intervention (Hepworth, Rooney, Rooney, Strom-Gottfried, & Larsen, 2010). Thus, when researchers seek to determine "what works" in a therapy or an intervention program, both specific and common factors must be accounted for as influences on client outcomes.

EVEN MEDICATION EFFECTS MAY BE CAUSED BY COMMON FACTORS Recent empirical research indicates that the impact of both active and placebo, or sham, medications is actually a socially complex phenomenon. That is, even the effectiveness of medications may vary based on socially determined factors. For example, blue sham pills have better effects than those of other colors, and clients who are told a sham pill is more expensive than another pill also demonstrate better results (Waber, Shiv, Carmon, & Ariely, 2008). This result occurs despite the fact that the manufacturers of the pills do not intend for them to have any beneficial effects. Recent research also indicates that sham medications may have actual active biological effects in some circumstances (Benedetti, 2009; Harrington, 1997). Even medication effects appear to share both specific and common components. Here, too, the biopsychosocial complexity of clearly defined interventions with people requires careful and comprehensive conceptualization and study.

WHY COMMON FACTORS MATTER The common factors model is critically important to intervention outcome research for both psychotherapy and social programs. Addressing only specific intervention components may lead to research results that falsely inflate or devalue the importance of common factors involved in client change. Including attention to a wide range of specific and common factors gives a more comprehensive and valid picture of the influences on client change (Drisko, 2004). This approach can lead to improved models for the matching of particular clients with individualized interventive models (Norcross & Wampold, 2011). The approach is also important in planning how best to educate social workers and other mental health professionals to serve their clients optimally (Cameron & Keenan, 2012).

On the other hand, much quantitative research seeks to examine just one variable in experiments used to determine whether an intervention causes a change. This ability to make cause-and-effect determinations is, of course, a major strength of experimental outcome research (Campbell & Stanley, 1963; Cook & Campbell, 1979). Removing or reducing complexity can be methodologically useful for researchers. Solely emphasizing specific factors in research, such as techniques of therapy, however, may yield misleading results if common factors are ignored. Thus, there has been an ongoing debate about the relative roles and importance of common versus specific factors in the outcome of psychosocial interventions. Specific factors are much more often addressed in research than are the many common factors that can also influence client outcomes.

The Origins and History of the Common Factors Approach

Both clinical observations and formal research evidence shaped the common factors model. Reviewing early research results, Rosenzweig (1936) observed that the outcomes of different psychotherapies were essentially equivalent. He hypothesized that this was caused in part by the operation of implicit, unspoken, and unidentified factors linked to the personality of the therapist. He also argued that the consistency of belief in a model of healing between client and therapist fostered change. Finally, he argued that different personalities interpreted psychological events in unique ways that limited the impact of specific differences among therapies. Rosenzweig's view that these universal factors are equally or more important than are the specific differences among therapies is the core of the common factors model. The common factors model is based on a broad review of research results: it is an empirically based model.

As more psychotherapy outcome studies were undertaken, several studies again reported no significant or meaningful differences in results between different types of psychotherapy for common adult disorders (for example, Luborsky, Singer, & Luborsky, 1975; Smith & Glass, 1977; Smith, Glass, & Miller, 1981). There were also claims that psychotherapy was simply not effective (Eysenck, 1952).

FRANK'S LIST OF COMMON FACTORS If different types of psychotherapy yielded similar results, the factors that led to change needed to be better identified. This led psychiatrist Jerome Frank (1971) to explore the commonalities among psychotherapies as well as other healing processes and rituals across world cultures. He concluded that several formal aspects of psychotherapy may be vital to its success and are shared with the healing practices of other cultures (Frank; Frank & Frank, 1991).

Frank (1971) identified six common factors in psychotherapy. The features common to all psychotherapies begin with (a) an emotionally charged, confiding relationship with the therapist/healer. Client and therapist must (b) share a rationale explaining the cause(s) of the person's distress and ideas about how to relieve it. During the interventive process, (c) new information about the nature and sources of the problems, as well as new ways to address them, is provided or uncovered. Frank notes that much of this new information is gained through self-discovery, but the therapist or groups (where used) are also valuable sources of knowledge. (d) The personal qualities and societal status of the therapist, as well as the setting in which the work is undertaken, strengthen the client's expectations of help. Provision of success experiences of many kinds also (e) heightens the client's sense of hope and increasing competence. Such experiences change the client's self-image in positive ways. Finally, all therapies (f) facilitate emotional arousal, which "seems to be a prerequisite to attitudinal and behavioral change" (Frank, p. 351). Frank argues that the dominant psychotherapeutic approach of an era reflects its current cultural attitudes, but that "the same techniques keep recurring under different guises, suggesting that . . . they all may be variations on a few underlying themes" (p. 358).

Although comparative studies revealed common factors across many types of healers and therapies, more and stronger research evidence has accumulated indicating that specific factors might not be as important as some had imagined. One technical research innovation that enhanced support for the common factors model was meta-analysis.

Recent Meta-analyses on Psychotherapy and the Common Factors

META-ANALYTIC STUDIES POINT TO THE IMPACT OF COMMON FACTORS IN PSYCHOTHERAPY Meta-analyses are integrative studies that combine the results of several studies on a specific topic. In studies of adult psychotherapy, meta-analyses usually draw upon carefully controlled and tightly supervised experimental efficacy studies. *Efficacy studies* are tightly controlled comparisons that seek to determine whether a carefully defined therapy is effective (Hollon, 1996). However, efficacy studies require such tight client inclusion criteria, differential diagnosis, and supervised treatment that they may not reflect real-world clients and therapies very well (Seligman, 1995). *Absolute efficacy* refers to the difference in outcome for people receiving psychotherapy compared with those who have not received psychotherapy. Researchers can also use meta-analyses to examine the relative efficacy of psychotherapies. *Relative efficacy* refers to differences in outcome between one or more different types of psychotherapy. Other meta-analyses examine the effectiveness of psychotherapy as professionals actually practice it in everyday settings. *Effectiveness studies* are done in real-world settings (Seligman). Clients are not so carefully screened and treatments are not so tightly monitored as in efficacy studies. Effectiveness studies may therefore fail to rule out comorbid conditions or treatments that differ somewhat from their intended models. They are more prone to threats to interval validity than are efficacy studies (Hollon). Social workers should note, however, that both efficacy and effectiveness studies tend to deemphasize environmental factors such as agency setting and the adequacy of client support systems as influences on client outcomes (Drisko, 2004).

RESEARCH SUPPORTING THE COMMON FACTORS MODEL Since Smith and Glass (1977) first applied meta-analysis to psychotherapy outcome studies, few enduring differences across types of psychotherapy have been demonstrated. The conclusion that there are no or very minimal differences across therapies has been a fairly common result (Ahn & Wampold, 2001; Elliot, 1996; Grawe, Caspar, & Ambuhl, 1990; Robinson, Berman, & Neimeyer, 1990; Sloan, Staples, Cristol, Yorkston, & Whipple, 1975; Smith & Glass,

1977; Smith, Glass, & Miller, 1981; Wampold, 2001; Wampold et al., 1997). These studies generally examine the relative efficacy of psychotherapies. The results are telling because the statistical methods of meta-analysis have improved over the years. In recent meta-analytic studies of psychotherapy, regression approaches have been used to control for differential reactivity in outcome measures; greater standardization of selection criteria for inclusion is evident, and the statistical methods used in meta-analysis have improved (for example, a range of statistics for effect size, enhanced understanding of the distribution of results) (Lipsey & Wilson, 2001; Wampold). If there are few significant differences in outcome by type or technique of psychotherapy, the curative factors in psychotherapy must be common factors that have not yet been carefully identified and studied by most researchers.

Then again, some meta-analyses *do* indicate differences in relative efficacy between psychotherapies. In 1982, D. A. Shapiro and Shapiro (1982) reported that cognitive therapy was superior to systematic desensitization and minimal intervention. However, a later reanalysis of this data by Berman, Miller, and Massman (1985) found only minimal difference. On child work, Weisz, Weiss, Han, Granger, and Morton (1995) found behavioral and cognitive–behavioral interventions to be more effective for certain disorders than are other therapies. In the core concerns of depression and anxiety, Dobson (1989) and Durham and Allan (1993) found cognitive interventions to be more effective than behavioral and other interventions.

In social work, Reid (1997) reviewed numerous meta-analyses on a much broader range of problems and programs than are found in psychotherapy reviews. Reid reported that across a wide range of concerns of interest to social workers with relatively large sample sizes, behavioral and cognitive interventions were often more effective than alternatives. Reid also noted that many challenges to meta-analysis exist: selection and measurement biases resulting from the "therapeutic allegiance" of the researcher are possible or even likely; behavioral measures are often more reactive than are nonbehavioral measures; and the use of "therapy analogs" rather than actual therapies may undermine the "clinical realism" of some included studies (pp. 11–14). However, Reid purposefully addressed studies of problems (such as juvenile delinquency, mental retardation, and smoking) and interventions that differ from those generally examined in meta-analyses of adult psychotherapy, more narrowly defined. Some individual studies and meta-analyses indicate differences in outcome among psychotherapies. Yet, more often, many others do not.

Recent meta-analyses report no significant differences across the results of adult psychotherapies (Ahn & Wampold, 2001; Stevens, Hynan, & Allen, 2000; Wampold et al., 1997). Wampold (2001) noted that rigorous reviews of meta-analytic findings often reveal no significant difference among the psychotherapies examined. He also noted that some reports of differences between psychotherapies are expectable by chance alone, given statistical decision-making criteria. Even where complex research designs are employed, no differences may be found. For example, Luborsky et al. (2002) did not find differences in effect sizes using an innovative method to control for researcher allegiance to specific therapeutic models. It appears that there is an extensive and often-reviewed, even deconstructed, set of meta-analytic studies in which very few enduring differences in the outcomes of different psychotherapies are reported. These meta-analyses indicate that common factors may be more important to positive outcome than are specific techniques (Ahn & Wampold; Hubble, Duncan, & Miller, 1999; Lambert & Bergin, 1994; Luborsky et al.; Norcross & Wampold, 2011; Wampold). In this sense, the common factors model has a large empirical research base or foundation.

IMPLICATIONS FOR RESEARCH, EDUCATION, AND PRACTICE Such findings have great significance for research, education, and practice. They suggest that educators should pay greater attention to common factors, including the context of therapy; the characteristics of both the client and the practitioner; the match between client, therapy, and practitioner; and their actual working alliance (Norcross, 2011). Studies that simply compare the results of different therapeutic techniques, without attention to common factors, may be reductionist and misleading. In education, these research results suggest educators should pay greater attention to educating students about common factors and the working alliance. Attention to exploring the client's motivation, social supports, and views about healing may prove more important than are specific techniques. In practice, these results suggest greater attention to the working alliance, the client's views about change, and the client's views of the therapist. They point to greater attention by practitioners to relationship factors (Norcross, 2011, 2012).

Estimating the Contribution of Factors that Generate Therapeutic Change

Lambert (1992) estimated the percentage of improvement in psychotherapy clients partitioned into four areas. He attributed 40% to extratherapeutic change including client factors, 30% to common factors in therapy, 15% to specific therapeutic techniques, and 15% to expectancy or placebo effects. These estimates were not directly derived from meta-analysis, but included extremes in research designs to represent studies with widely divergent outcomes (Lambert & Barley, 2001). Drawing on over 100 studies providing statistical analyses, the rough average influence of each factor was determined. This set of estimates has been widely reported in the common factors literature.

NORCROSS AND LAMBERT'S WEIGHTED LIST OF COMMON FACTORS In a more recent update, Norcross and Lambert (2011) revised these estimates by adding a large percentage of "unexplained variance." Because of the complexity and variation in human endeavors, most statistical research in the social sciences "explains" only a small part of the variance in outcomes. This is because factors not specifically examined in a study may also alter its outcome. Further, errors in measurement and in research methods lead to unexplained variance in outcomes (Norcross & Lambert, 2011).

In their current model, Norcross and Lambert (2011) attribute 40% of the variance in psychotherapy outcomes to unexplained variance. This large chunk of unexplained variance represents factors not included in Norcross and Lambert's model that lead to variation in client outcomes. Of the remaining 60% of explained variance in outcome, they assign 30% to "client contribution," 12% to the therapeutic relationship, 8% to specific therapeutic techniques, 7% to individual therapist characteristics, and 3% to other factors (pp. 11–14). They note that common factors are "spread across the therapeutic factors" (p. 14). Common factors pertain in part to the patient, some to the therapeutic relationship, some to the specific model of therapy, and some to the specific practitioner.

Note carefully that the largest percentage of explained change results from the client contribution. Most outcome studies on psychotherapy and social services do not include a detailed assessment of client characteristics and social situation; instead they focus on clearly defining a target disorder or problem. This effort to focus on a specific problem and a single treatment fits well with the strengths of experimental research designs. Failing to include attention to common factors, however, does not seem to be an optimal fit to the complexity of psychotherapy clients and the psychotherapeutic process. Further, this narrow research model does not fit well with social work's person-in-environment perspective.

Including Social Factors and Context in the Common Factors Model

Drisko (2004, 2008) added a social work perspective to the common factors model. He applied a broader, person-in-environment perspective to Frank's (1971) and Lambert's (1992) individually centered models of common factors. Drisko argued that factors such as the client's support system, community context, and even agency context would also affect the changes individual clients make in psychotherapy. Such factors would account for some of the unexplained variance in outcomes in Lambert's (1992) estimates, as well as for some of the client contribution variance. For example, a client who sought therapy with some ambivalence might be quite discouraged when his parent commented that "it was a stupid thing to do." On the other hand, an affirming and encouraging comment from his parent might enhance the client's motivation and could even be the basis for help in transportation to therapy or in creating a greater opportunity to reflect between sessions. In another example, a client of color who enters a clinic waiting room populated almost exclusively by white staff and clients might be affirmed by finding magazines like *Heart and Soul* or *Tu Salud* in the waiting room. The client's social support system and both the community and the agency context may be important in shaping, supporting, and sustaining the client's investment in therapy.

The magnitude of such social and setting factors is difficult to assess and is not yet part of most common factors models in psychiatry and psychology. To social workers, the importance of such broader, contextual factors is clear. This expansion of the common factors model to include greater attention to social and contextual variables—in detail—will be a step toward more fully explaining what causes change in psychotherapy.

COMMON FACTORS AND HUMAN DIVERSITY Sue and Sue (2007) note that the common factors model also has implications for the ways in which social workers and others serve people of color and from different cultural backgrounds. The impact of socially structured oppression can also be a significant factor in many therapy and social service interventions (Drisko, 2004). Social workers will note that a wide range of variables in human diversity may be vital to consider in treatment planning and delivery.

APPLYING THE COMMON FACTORS MODEL TO SOCIAL WORK PRACTICE Cameron and Keenan (2010) further elaborated the common factors model as it applies to clinical social work interventions. Drawing on the work of Lambert (1992), Grencavage and Norcross (1990), and Drisko (2004), they provide a detailed list of influences that are likely to impact client outcomes. Cameron and Keenan (2010) offer both common factors and a set of therapeutic techniques, noting that both combine synergistically to generate client change. That is, common factors may serve to enhance specific treatment models or to limit their effectiveness. The combination of attention to common factors and to specific techniques synergistically enhances client outcomes.

Cameron and Keenan (2012) further extended the common factors model to generalist social-work practice. Their text integrates evidence-based practice and evidence-based relationships that work with social work's person-in-environment perspective. Cameron and Keenan's (2012) book explores the critical practice conditions and processes that research shows lead to positive client outcomes. These conditions include attributes of the client, the social work practitioner, their working relationship, and the supporting networks that influence and enable work. They note that the common factors model fits very well with generalist social work practice and social work's core values.

Common Factors and Evidence-Based Practice

Evidence-based medicine and evidence-based practice focus on (a) integrating research evidence with intervention planning that also *equally includes* (b) the client's state and circumstances, (c) the client's own values and preferences, and (d) the clinical expertise of the practitioner (Haynes, Devereaux, & Guyatt, 2002). The practice approaches that have developed from the evidence-based medicine and evidence-based practice model give priority to research results based on large-scale, experimental research (Greenhalgh, 2010; Oxford University Centre for Evidence-Based Medicine, 2011). As noted, this type of research seeks to examine the impact of one intervention of a well-specified disorder to limit the impact of unexplained factors and error terms. In many respects, this research model examines specific techniques or intervention models as a single, consistent variable. For example, Elkin and colleagues (1989) examined whether psychotropic medication was more effective than interpersonal therapy or cognitive therapy for adults who have depression. Great care was taken to rule out any other

co-occurring disorders, to define each treatment, to provide supervision to ensure the psychotherapies were provided correctly and completely, and to use highly regarded measures of depression.

HOW COMMON FACTORS AUGMENT EVIDENCE-BASED PRACTICE RESEARCH The common factors model proposes that techniques alone are neither accurate nor sufficient descriptions of what actually happens in psychotherapy. Differences among clients, among their support systems and social circumstances, among the practitioners, and in the synergistic way in which client, practitioner, and therapy interact over time all strongly impact client outcomes. Norcross and Lambert's (2011) estimates assign just 8% of variance in outcome to specific therapeutic techniques. This percentage is less than the 30% assigned to the client contribution and the 12% assigned to the client–therapist relationship. Drisko (2004) and Cameron and Keenan (2010) argue that the 8% of variance assigned to specific therapeutic technique may well be much less than that resulting from social and contextual factors (as part of the 40% of variance left "unexplained" to other factors). This implies that a narrow focus on techniques or types of therapy alone may be too limited an evidence base for guiding practice. It also implies that research on psychotherapy must take a much broader view of factors that influence outcomes and look very carefully at client factors, practitioner factors, setting, and the client–therapist relationship.

In many respects, the evidence-based medicine/evidence-based practice hierarchy of research evidence and the common factors approach represent two very different viewpoints about disorders and treatments (Drisko & Grady, 2012). One approach highlights research designs and methods; the other starts with a broader conceptualization of disorders, therapeutic process, and acceptable types of research evidence. Within the American Psychological Association these two very different perspectives have created a split between strident advocates of techniques or specific factors and those advocating the common factors model (Carey, 2004). Advocates of specific techniques, such as Chambless (as cited in Carey), argued that they led to good results for her clients. In contrast, Gabbard (as cited in Carey) responded that

the move to worship at the altar of these scientific treatments has been destructive to patients in practice, because the methods tell you very little about how to treat the real and complex people who actually come in for therapy. (paragraph 20)

Similar views have been expressed among social work researchers. A useful resolution may be the combination of attention to both common factors and specific techniques. As Cameron and Keenan (2012) point out, it is the synergy of client and practitioner that combines to create a successful experience. "What works" for a specific client in specific circumstances may vary across specific providers of several different specific interventions.

Applying Common Factors to Direct Practice
There have been three major applications of the common factors approach to direct practice. These may be characterized as (a) the psychotherapy integration movement, (b) the empirically based relationship movement, and (c) a range of applications of common factors to specific models or modalities of therapy. The psychotherapy integration movement has a fairly lengthy history in psychology, but is less prominent in social work. The movement seeks to look for the commonalities across specific treatment models, including attention to common factors (Duncan, Miller, Wampold, & Hubble, 2010; Lampropoulous, 2000; Norcross & Goldfried, 2005). The empirically based relationship movement seeks to link the common factors approach with evidence-based practice. Using a wide range of meta-analyses, its supporters have documented an extensive database showing the importance of relationship and the therapeutic alliance to therapy and service outcomes (Norcross, 2011, 2012). Cameron and Keenan's (2012) application of the common factors to generalist social work practice combines attention to the integration of practice and to the empirical evidence base for such efforts. Further, a number of authors have emphasized the role of common factors in specific therapies and modalities. For example, Paterson (2010) applied common factors to the treatment of anxiety disorders and Sprenkle, Davis, and Lebow (2009) applied them to couple and family therapy.

THE THERAPY INTEGRATION MOVEMENT Since the 1950s, several authors have examined the similarities among therapies and have sought to integrate their strengths to make for more effective treatments. The work of Dollard and Miller (1950), Wachtel (1977), and Arkowitz and Messer (1984) shows steady interest in integrating behavioral and psychodynamic therapies. Such models sought a single, integrated approach to psychotherapy. Strickler (2010) notes that the psychotherapy integration movement ranges much further: "Psychotherapy integration includes various efforts

to look beyond the confines of single school approaches to see what can be learned from other perspectives" (p. 4). One approach is to focus on common factors. Two other approaches focus on the integration of theories and the integration of techniques. A fourth variant emphasizes the assimilative integration of various perspectives and techniques to create an encompassing but unified approach (Strickler). This assimilative integration is the core of the current psychotherapy integration movement (Norcross & Goldfried, 2005; Strickler, 2010). Both common and specific factors are combined to develop an optimal therapeutic approach for each specific client.

Contributions from practitioner theorists, such as both Bohart and Tallman's (1999) and Duncan and Miller's (2000) emphasis on the "heroic" contributions of many clients, also shaped the psychotherapy integration movement. Duncan and Miller's close look at the importance and challenge of the client's role in psychotherapy both brought renewed attention to common factors and expanded emphasis on how clients contribute to change. The expert role of the practitioner was questioned, and the contribution of the client was given central emphasis. A related development was Prochaska's stages-of-change model (Prochaska, Norcross, & DiClemente, 1994). This model addresses how the goals and roles of each client require different emphases within intervention models. For example, a mandated client who has not yet begun to view a substance abuse problem as a "problem" is likely to benefit more from efforts such as motivational interviewing prior to specific substance abuse interventions. The goal is to flexibly and purposefully "start where the client is" rather than to force the client into an ill-timed or ill-suited treatment approach. Prochaska and Norcross (2009) apply the stages-of-change approach transtheoretically, integrating common factors with specific techniques based on client needs. They note that such purposefully timed interventions appear to yield better outcomes for more clients than do "one-size-fits-all" models.

THE EMPIRICALLY BASED RELATIONSHIP MOVEMENT The current administrative and fiscal climate requires a solid evidence base for funded professional efforts. A number of common factors practitioners and researchers have worked to document that the client–practitioner relationship, also called the therapeutic alliance, is a vital component to positive therapy outcomes. Given Norcross and Lambert's (2011) estimate that 12% of therapeutic change is attributable to the client–practitioner relationship and that this contribution is larger than the 8% caused by specific therapeutic techniques, exploring how to enhance this relationship offers a way toward improved outcomes.

Works by Castonguay and Beutler (2006) and Norcross (2011) provide extensive documentation of research on variables that enhance, or detract from, the client–practitioner relationship. They identify a set of empirically supported principles based on client factors, practitioner factors, and their matching in the therapeutic relationship. Generally, client expectations play an important role in overall therapy outcomes. Further, clients with high levels of impairment, who have personality disorders, or who have had significant interpersonal problems in their early development are likely to have poorer outcomes (Castonguay & Beutler, 2006). Practitioners who are creative and flexible, who have secure attachment patterns, who are comfortable with intense emotions, and who target interventions at the client's level of assimilation are likely to have better outcomes. Practitioners who are open-minded and able to accept and support clients' religious views are also likely to have better general outcomes (Castonguay & Beutler, 2006). Interventions that are responsive to and consistent with the client's level of problem assimilation are likely to be generally more effective. Clients with high levels of impairment respond better when offered long-term intensive treatment rather than a nonintensive and brief treatment, regardless of treatment model and type of treatment. The use of treatments that do not induce client resistance is preferable, as is the use of less directive interventions with clients who are resistant. That is, interventions employed should be less directive in nature if the client displays more resistance (Castonguay & Beutler, 2006). These broad, empirically supported principles link a clear research evidence base with the common factors approach (Norcross & Lambert, 2012).

The yield of this research has led to suggestions to improve direct practice and supervision. Duncan (2012) applies this research base to guidance for becoming a better therapist. Watkins (1995) and Norcross and Halgin (1995) examine how common factors research can be applied in psychotherapy supervision. Both the actions of practitioners and the matching of clients to treatments are addressed.

COMMON FACTORS APPLIED TO SPECIFIC THERAPIES OR MODALITIES
A small but growing literature moves from general principles to the application of common factors to specific treatments. The most widely developed application is to individual therapy, followed

by couple and family therapy. Sprenkle et al. (2009) view common factors as the overlooked foundation of couple and family work. Davis (2009) examined how prominent family therapists view the importance of common factors in their practices.

There is need for further application of the common factors approach to other modalities, populations, and disorders. Clarkin, Frances, and Perry (2005) examine treatment planning at the macro and micro levels, applying an integrative approach that considers context and agency mission as key parts of treatment planning across several treatment modalities. Feldman and Powell (2005) address the strengths and limitations of psychotherapy integration in individual, family, and group modalities. J. Shapiro, Friedberg, and Bardenstein (2006) discuss the application of common factors to child therapy. As mentioned, Paterson (2010) applies the common factors approach to the treatment of anxiety disorders. Most in need of theoretical development and research are group therapy and residential treatment.

An innovative research project by Castonguay, Goldfried, Wiser, Raue, and Hayes (1996) documented that cognitive psychotherapy for depression was only effective when a strong and positive therapeutic relationship was also present. Clients who did not experience a positive therapeutic relationship generally did not improve, despite being treated with the same therapy. This research result supports the importance of the common factors approach. Similarly, Norcross and Wampold (2011) report good evidence supporting the importance of the therapist variable in most therapies, but encourage more research about the impact of both common and specific factors. Further, carefully designed research is needed to distinguish the impact of common and specific factors.

Summary
The common factors approach expands the conceptual base for psychotherapy and social service practice, research, and policy. The legacy of the pioneering work of Rosenzweig (1936) and Frank (1971) is enduring and has grown into an important way to understand therapy processes and outcomes (Alarcón & Frank, 2011). An extensive research evidence base supports the impact of common factors and their importance to treatment planning and outcomes. The common factors model has been expanded to include the social circumstances and social contexts of clients and is increasingly applied within social work. Thus, the model has utility for conceptualizing both practice and research. The evidence base supporting

common factors also has important policy-level implications for funders of optimally effective services in treatment planning and in practitioner–client matching. The common factors approach fits well with social work's core person-in-environment perspective and fully addresses the complexity of psychotherapy and social service interventions.

REFERENCES

Ahn, H., & Wampold, B. (2001). Where, oh where, are the specific ingredients? A meta-analysis of component studies in counseling and psychotherapy. *Journal of Consulting and Clinical Psychology, 48,* 251–257.

Alarcón, R., & Frank, J. B. (2011). *The psychotherapy of hope: The legacy of "Persuasion and Healing."* Baltimore, MD: Johns Hopkins University Press.

Arkowitz, H., & Messer, S. (1984). *Psychoanalytic therapy and behavior therapy: Is integration possible?* New York, NY: Plenum Press.

Benedetti, F. (2009). *Placebo effects: Understanding the mechanism behind health and disease.* New York, NY: Oxford University Press.

Bergin, A., & Garfield, S. (Eds.). (1971). *Handbook of psychotherapy and behavior change: An empirical analysis.* New York, NY: Wiley.

Bergin, A., & Garfield, S. (Eds.). (1978). *Handbook of psychotherapy and behavior change* (2nd ed.). New York, NY: Wiley.

Bergin, A., & Garfield, S. (Eds.). (1986). *Handbook of psychotherapy and behavior change* (3rd ed.). New York, NY: Wiley.

Bergin, A., & Garfield, S. (Eds.). (1994). *Handbook of psychotherapy and behavior change* (4th ed.). New York, NY: Wiley.

Berman, J., Miller, C., & Massman, P. (1985). Cognitive therapy versus systematic desensitization: Is one treatment superior? *Psychological Bulletin, 97,* 451–461.

Bohart, A., & Tallman, K. (1999). *How clients make therapy work: The process of active self-healing.* Washington, DC: American Psychological Association.

Cameron, M., & Keenan, E. K. (2010). The common factors model: Implications for transtheoretical clinical social work practice. *Social Work, 55*(1), 63–73.

Cameron, M., & Keenan, E. K. (2012). *The common factors model for generalist practice.* New York, NY: Pearson.

Campbell, D., & Stanley, J. (1963). *Experimental and quasi-experimental designs for research.* New York, NY: Wadsworth.

Carey, B. (2004, August 10). For psychotherapy's claims, skeptics demand proof. Retrieved August 12, 2004, from http://www.nytimes.com/2004/08/10/science/for-psychotherapy-s-claims-skeptics-demand-proof.html?pagewanted=all&src=pm

Castonguay, L., & Beutler, L. (2006). Common and unique principles of therapeutic change: What do we know and what do we need to know? In L. Castonguay and L. Beutler (Eds.), *Principles of therapeutic change that work* (pp. 353–369). New York, NY: Oxford University Press.

Castonguay, L., Goldfried, M., Wiser, S., Raue, P., & Hayes, A. M. (1996). Predicting the effect of cognitive therapy for depression: A study of unique and common factors. *Journal of Consulting and Clinical Psychology, 64,* 497–504.

Clarkin, J., Frances, A., & Perry, S. (2005). Differential therapeutics: Macro and micro level of treatment planning. In J. Norcross & M. Goldfried, M. (Eds.), *Handbook of psychotherapy integration* (pp. 463–502). New York, NY: Oxford University Press.

Cook, T., & Campbell, D. (1979). *Quasi-experimentation: Design & analysis issues for field settings.* New York, NY: Houghton Mifflin.

Davis, S. (2009). *What makes couples therapy work? Common factors across the practices of prominent couples therapy model developers.* Saarbrücken, Germany: VDM Verlag.

Dobson, K. (1989). A meta-analysis of the efficacy of cognitive therapy for depression. *Journal of Clinical and Consulting Psychology, 57*(3), 414–419.

Dollard, J., & Miller, N. (1950). *Personality and psychotherapy: An analysis in terms of learning, thinking and culture.* New York, NY: McGraw-Hill.

Drisko, J. (2004). Common factors in psychotherapy effectiveness: Meta-analytic findings and their implications for practice and research. *Families in Society 85*(1), 81–90.

Drisko, J. (2008). Common factors. In A. Roberts (Ed.), *The Social Worker's Desk Reference* (2nd ed., pp. 220–225). New York, NY: Oxford University Press.

Drisko, J., & Grady, M. (2012). *Evidence-based practice in clinical social work.* New York: Springer-Verlag.

Duncan, B. (2012). *On becoming a better therapist.* Washington, DC: American Psychological Association.

Duncan, B., & Miller, S. (2000). *The heroic client.* San Francisco, CA: Jossey–Bass.

Duncan, B., Miller, S., Wampold, B., & Hubble, M. (Eds.). (2010). *The heart and soul of change: Delivering what works* (2nd ed.). Washington, DC: American Psychological Association.

Durham, R., & Allan, T. (1993). Psychological treatment of generalised anxiety disorder: A review of the clinical significance of results in outcome studies since 1980. *British Journal of Psychiatry, 163,* 19–26.

Elkin, I., Shea, T., Watkins, J., Imber, S. D., Sotsky, S. M., Collins, J. F., et al. (1989). National Institute of Mental Health treatment of depression collaborative research program: General effectiveness of treatments. *Archives of General Psychiatry, 46,* 971–982.

Elliot, R. (1996). Are client centered/experiential therapies effective? A meta-analysis of outcome research. In U. Esser, H. Pbast, & G. Speierer (Eds.), *The power of the person-centered approach: New challenges–perspectives–answers* (pp. 125–138). Koln, Germany: GwG Verlag.

Eysenck, H. (1952). The effects of psychotherapy: An evaluation. *Journal of Consulting Psychology, 16,* 319–324.

Feldman, L., & Powell, S. (2005). Integrating therapeutic modalities. In J. Norcross & M. Goldfried (Eds.), *Handbook of psychotherapy integration* (pp. 503–532). New York, NY: Oxford University Press.

Frank, J. (1971). Therapeutic factors in psychotherapy. *American Journal of Psychotherapy, 25,* 350–361. A differently paginated version of this article is available online; retrieved from http://focus.psychiatryonline.org/article .aspx?articleid=50633

Frank, J. D., & Frank, J. B. (1991). *Persuasion and healing: A comparative study of psychotherapy* (3rd ed.). Baltimore, MD: Johns Hopkins University Press.

Grawe, K., Caspar, F., & Ambuhl, H. (1990). The Bernese comparative psychotherapy study. *Zeitschrift for Klinische Pscyhologie, 19*, 287–376.

Greenhalgh, T. (2010). *How to read a paper: The basics of evidence based medicine* (4th ed.). Hoboken, NJ: BMJ Books/ Wiley–Blackwell.

Grencavage, L., & Norcross, J. (1990). Where are the commonalities among the therapeutic common factors? *Professional Psychology: Research & Practice, 21*, 372–378.

Harrington, A. (Ed.). (1997). *The placebo effect: An interdisciplinary exploration.* Cambridge, MA: Harvard University Press.

Haynes, R., Devereaux, P., & Guyatt, G. (2002). Clinical expertise in the era of evidence based medicine and patient choice. *Evidence-Based Medicine, 7*, 36–38.

Hepworth, D., Rooney, R., Rooney, G., Strom-Gottfried, K., & Larsen, J. (2010). *Direct social work practice: Theory and skills* (8th ed.). Belmont, CA: Brooks/Cole.

Hollon, S. (1996). The efficacy and effectiveness of psychotherapy relative to medications. *American Psychologist, 51*(10), 1025–1030.

Hubble, M., Duncan, B., & Miller, S. (1999). Introduction. In M. Hubble, B. Duncan, & S. Miller (Eds.), *The heart and soul of change: What works in therapy* (pp. 1–19). Washington, DC: American Psychological Association.

Lambert, M. (1992). Implications for outcome research for psychotherapy integration. In J. Norcross & M. Goldstein (Eds.), *Handbook of psychotherapy integration* (pp. 94–129). New York, NY: Basic Books.

Lambert, M. (Ed.). (2004). *Bergin and Garfield's handbook of psychotherapy and behavior change* (5th ed.). New York, NY: Wiley.

Lambert, M. (2013). *Bergin and Garfield's handbook of psychotherapy and behavior change* (6th ed.). New York, NY: Wiley.

Lambert, M., & Bergin, S. (1994). The effectiveness of psychotherapy. In A. Bergin & S. Garfield (Eds.), *Handbook of psychotherapy and behavior change* (4th ed., pp. 143–189). New York, NY: Wiley.

Lambert, M., & Ogles, B. (2004). The efficacy and effectiveness of psychotherapy. In M. Lambert (Ed.), *Bergin and Garfield's handbook of psychotherapy and behavior change* (5th ed., pp. 139–193). New York, NY: Wiley.

Lampropoulous, C. (2000). Evolving psychotherapy integration. *Psychology and Psychotherapy: Theory, Research and Practice, 37*, 285–297.

Lipsey, M., & Wilson, D. (2001). *Practical meta-analysis.* Thousand Oaks, CA: Sage.

Luborsky, L., Rosenthal, R., Diguer, L., Andrusyna, T. P., Berman, J., Levitt, J., et al. (2002). The dodo bird verdict is alive and well—Mostly. *Clinical Psychology: Science and Practice, 9*, 2–12.

Luborsky, L., Singer, B., & Luborsky, L. (1975). Is it true that "everyone has won and all must have prizes"? *Archives of General Psychology 3*, 995–1008.

Norcross, J. (Ed.). (2011). *Psychotherapy relationships that work.* New York, NY: Oxford University Press.

Norcross, J., & Goldfried, M. (2005). *Handbook of psychotherapy integration.* New York, NY: Oxford University Press.

Norcross, J., & Halgin, R. (1995). Integrative approaches to psychotherapy supervision. In C. Watkins (Ed.), *Handbook of psychotherapy supervision* (pp. 203–222). Hoboken, NJ: Wiley.

Norcross, J., & Lambert, M. (2011). Evidence-based therapy relationships. In J. Norcross (Ed.), *Psychotherapy relationships that work* (pp. 3–21). New York, NY: Oxford University Press.

Norcross, J., & Lambert, M. (2012). *Evidence-based therapy relationships.* Retrieved March 1, 2012, from http://www .nrepp.samhsa.gov/Norcross.aspx

Norcross, J., & Wampold, B. (2011). Evidence-based therapy relationships: Research conclusions and clinical practices. *Psychotherapy, 48*(1), 98–102.

Oxford University Centre for Evidence-Based Medicine. (2011). *The Oxford levels of evidence 2011.* Retrieved October 3, 2011, from http://www.cebm.net/mod_product/ design/files/CEBM-Levels-of-Evidence-2.1.pdf

Paterson, C. (2010). *Great expectations: The application of common factors theory to practice in psychotherapy for anxiety.* Saarbruecken, Germany: Lambert Academic.

Prochaska, J., & Norcross, J. (2009). *Systems of psychotherapy: A transtheoretical analysis.* New York, NY: Brooks/Cole.

Prochaska, J., Norcross, J., & DiClemente, C. (1994). *Changing for good: The revolutionary program that explains the six stages of change and teaches you how to free yourself from bad habits.* New York, NY: Morrow.

Reid, W. (1997). Evaluating the dodo's verdict: Do all interventions have equivalent outcomes? *Social Work Research, 21*(7), 5–15.

Robinson, L., Berman, J., & Neimeyer, R. (1990). Psychotherapy for the treatment of depression: A comprehensive review of controlled outcome research. *Psychological Bulletin, 108*, 30–49.

Rosenzweig, S. (1936). Some implicit common factors in diverse methods of psychotherapy. *American Journal of Orthopsychiatry, 6*(3), 412–415.

Seligman, M. (1995). The effectiveness of psychotherapy: the *Consumer's Report's* study. *American Psychologist, 50*(12), 965–974.

Shapiro, D. A., & Shapiro, D. (1982). Meta-analysis of comparative therapy outcome studies: A replication and refinement. *Psychological Bulletin, 92*, 581–604.

Shapiro, J., Friedberg, R., & Bardenstein, K. (2006). *Child and adolescent therapy: Science and art.* Hoboken, NJ: Wiley.

Sloan, R., Staples, F., Cristol, A., Yorkston, N., & Whipple, K. (1975). *Psychotherapy versus behavior change.* Cambridge, MA: Harvard University Press.

Smith, M., & Glass, G. (1977). Meta-analysis of psychotherapy outcome studies. *American Psychologist, 32*, 752–760.

Smith, M., Glass, G., & Miller, T. (1981). *The benefits of psychotherapy*. Baltimore, MD: Johns Hopkins University Press.

Sprenkle, D., Davis, S., & Lebow, J. (2009). *Common factors in couple and family therapy: The overlooked foundation for effective practice*. New York, NY: Guilford Press.

Stevens, S., Hynan, M., & Allen, M. (2000). A meta-analysis of common factor and specific treatment effects across the outcome domains of the phase model of psychotherapy. *Clinical Psychology: Science and Practice, 7*, 273–290.

Strickler, G. (2010). *Psychotherapy integration*. Washington, DC: American Psychological Association.

Sue, D., & Sue, D. (2007). *Foundations of counseling and psychotherapy: Evidence-based practices for a diverse society*. Hoboken, NJ: Wiley.

U.S. Department of Health and Human Services. (1999). *Mental health: A report of the Surgeon General*. Rockville, MD: U.S. Department of Health and Human Services, Substance Abuse and Mental Health Services Administration, Center for Mental Health Services, National Institutes of Health, and National Institute of Mental Health.

Waber, R., Shiv, B., Carmon, Z., & Ariely, D. (2008). Commercial features of placebo and therapeutic efficacy. *Journal of the American Medical Association, 299*(9), 1016–1017.

Wachtel, P. (1977). *Psychoanalysis and behavior therapy*. New York, NY: Basic Books.

Wampold, B. (2001). *The great psychotherapy debate: Models, methods and findings*. Mahwah, NJ: Erlbaum.

Wampold, B., Mondin, G., Moody, M., Stich, F., Benson, K., & Ahn, H. (1997). A meta-analysis of outcome studies comparing bona fide psychotherapies: Empirically, "all must have prizes." *Psychological Bulletin, 122*, 203–215.

Watkins, C. E. (Ed.). (1995). *Handbook of psychotherapy supervision*. New York, NY: Wiley.

Weisz, J., Weiss, B., Han, S., Granger, D., & Morton, T. (1955). Effects of psychotherapy with children and adolescents revisited: A meta-analysis of treatment outcome studies. *Psychological Bulletin, 117*, 450–468.

FURTHER READING

Castonguay, L., & Beutler, L. (2006). *Principles of therapeutic change that work*. New York, NY: Oxford.

Drisko, J., & Grady, M. (2012). *Evidence based practice in clinical social work*. New York, NY: Springer.

Gallardo, M., & McNeill, B. (2009). *Intersections of multiple identities: A casebook of evidence-based practices with diverse populations*. New York, NY: Rutledge.

Lambert, M., & Barley, D. (2001). Research summary on the therapeutic relationship and psychotherapy outcome. *Psychotherapy, 38*(4), 357–361.

Littell, J., Corcoran, J., & Pillai, V. (2008). *Systematic reviews and meta-analysis*. New York, NY: Oxford University Press.

Lin, Y. (1994). *Conceptualizing common factors in counseling*. Retrieved from http://agc.ncue.edu.tw/text27.1-1.pdf (available in English and in Chinese)

Norcross, J. (Ed.). (2011). *Psychotherapy relationships that work*. New York, NY: Oxford University Press.

Norcross, J., & Halgin, R. (1995). Integrative approaches to psychotherapy supervision. In C. Watkins (Ed.), *Handbook of psychotherapy supervision* (pp. 203–222). Hoboken, NJ: Wiley.

Norcross, J. (and others) (2012). *Evidence-based therapy relationships*. Retrieved from http://www.nrepp.samhsa.gov/Norcross.aspx

Prochaska, J., & Norcross, J. (2009). *Systems of psychotherapy: A transtheoretical analysis*. New York, NY: Brooks/Cole.

JAMES DRISKO

COMMUNITY: PRACTICE INTERVENTIONS

ABSTRACT: Major social changes resulting from globalization, the increase in multicultural societies, and growing concerns for human rights, especially for women and girls, will affect all community practice in this century. Community-practice processes—organizing, planning, sustainable development, and progressive social change—are challenged by these trends and the ethical dilemmas they pose. Eight distinct models of community-practice intervention are described with examples from around the globe. The values and ethics that ground community-practice interventions are drawn from international and national literature. Model applications are identified for work with groups, urban and rural communities, organizations and coalitions, and in advocacy and leadership for social justice and human rights.

KEY WORDS: community development; community interventions; community organizing; community organization; community practice models; global practice; global social changes; human rights; macro practice; social justice; social work values; social work ethics

Introduction

Although community residents have always worked collaboratively on common needs, the evolution of formal practice interventions for community work in the United States has its origins in the late 19th century. With the formalization of social work as a profession and community organization as a recognized method of social work, increasing numbers of professionals began working with communities. Social work that emerged from this focus on community issues is now called community practice. While a parallel development of the profession of social work was ongoing in many countries, we will refer primarily to the development of community practice in North America, but we will describe its application in a global context.

HISTORY Several streams of engagement by early community researchers and practitioners were the antecedents of community-practice social work. The settlement-house and charity-organization-society movements formed the context for the development of social work as a profession, and, from its genesis, community practice has been an essential element (Abbott, 1937; Addams, 1902/1964, 1910; Garvin & Cox, 2001; McNutt, 2011). Both movements were adapted from British approaches. After spending the summer of 1877 studying the work of the Charity Organization Society (COS) in London, Stephen Gurteen returned to Buffalo, New York, to establish the first COS in America, focusing on systematically coordinating philanthropy and developing "scientific" charity services (Gurteen, 1882). Jane Addams, one of the founders of the Settlement Movement in the United States, visited and studied the work of the first settlement, Toynbee Hall in London, in 1881. After returning to Chicago, she and Ellen Gates Starr founded Hull House in 1889, focusing initially on neighborhood services, community organizing, and group work with the area's many impoverished immigrant groups, and later expanding to social research, employment and labor issues, and social-policy development (Addams, 1930; Deegan, 1990). A third stream of community work in the United States was developed through rural extension workers to help communities build cooperative electric systems, water and irrigation systems, and schools and community centers (Austin & Betten 1990; Christenson & Robinson, 1989).

These three historical streams of community intervention form the primary background for the development of community-practice social work, sometimes referred to as community organization, and the variety of intervention methods that emerged in the 1940s and 1950s (Carter, 1958; Dunham, 1940; Lurie, 1959; Ross, 1955, 1958; Sieder, 1956). In addition to these major streams of community intervention, the historical context of a developing democracy provided opportunities for social movements such as the labor, women's, and civil rights movements to explore and practice ways that people collectively organize collectively to seek reform for social problems (Betten & Austin, 1990; Brueggemann, 2013; Fisher, 1994).

Later trends in community practice have built upon social work developments as well as social movements, further elaborating theories, models of practice, and research methods. The Canadian scholar Murray Ross had a major role in defining professional social work roles in community organization and the development of theory-based literature. He envisioned community work in a range of environments, from education to agriculture to community development (Ross, 1955, 1958). Jack Rothman (1968) developed a construct of "Three Models of Community Organization," which he called *locality development, social planning,* and *social action.* Rothman continued an elaboration of his conceptualization over time to illustrate the mixing and phasing of models in actual practice and to rename the three strategies *planning and policy practice, community capacity development,* and *social advocacy* (Rothman, 2008). Saul Alinsky introduced a style of organizing currently continuing through the Industrial Areas Foundation's (IAF) grassroots work and leadership training, building a national network of multiethnic and interfaith community organizations (Alinsky, 1971; Betten & Austin, 1990; IAF, 2013). Current practice focuses on capacity building, organizing, and planning for a range of challenges that emerge at both the local and the global levels. These include continuing efforts to alleviate poverty and close the widening gap between wealthy and poor populations; migration and displacement of populations; human rights, especially for women and girls; and the need for sustainable development in the face of climate change, environmental disasters, toxic contaminants that can alter human development and other species, and food insecurity (Alzate, Andharia, Chowa, Weil, & Doernberg, 2013; Chaskin, 2013; Chowa, Masa, Sherraden, & Weil, 2013; Eade, 1997; Gamble & Hoff, 2013; Midgley & Conley, 2010; Weil, Reisch, & Ohmer, 2013b).

Community practice in the United States has also reflected the cultural contexts of different communities at different times in its history, especially relating to African American groups (Burwell, 1996; Carlton-LaNey, 2001; King, 1958), Native Americans (Bearse, 2011; LaDuke, 2005; St. Onge, 2013; Sides, 2006), Asian Americans (Balgopal, 2011; Rivera & Erlich, 1998), Hispanic communities, and labor organizations (La Raza, 2013; United Farm Workers, 2013).

Community-intervention methods continue to be refined through practice, research, and application of theory and cultural perspectives, most recently by Brown (2006); Gamble & Weil (2010); Gutierrez, Lewis, Dessel, & Spencer (2013); Hardina (2012); Homan (2011); Netting, Kettner, McMurtry, & Thomas (2011); Pyles (2009); and Rubin & Rubin (2007). *The Handbook of Community Practice* (Weil, Reisch, & Ohmer, 2013a), and the *Journal of Community Practice* sponsored by the Association of Community Organization and Social Administration (ACOSA, 2013) provide extensive literature on community practice.

Weil and Gamble's eight models of community practice presented here provide a structured comparison of community practice interventions. Models are useful in both teaching and practice settings because clarification of concepts, strategies for change, roles, and purposes can "increase insight into a problem and improve one's ability to share that insight with others" (Robards & Gillespie, 2000, p. 563). These models provide a way for community practitioners to compare and analyze "ideal" intervention types for community-problem-solving approaches (Weber, 1970). The models have been refined and updated in this entry with the introduction, in Table 1, of three major practice "lenses" that will permeate community practice throughout the world in coming decades: the effects of *globalization*; the increase in *multicultural societies* as the result of forced and voluntary migrations; and the struggles to expand *human rights*, especially rights for women and girls.

How Social Work Has Contributed to Community Practice Interventions

Community-practice interventions within social work incorporate two important qualifications: practice within a value-base founded in social justice and human rights and the use of theory and outcome research to inform practice interventions (Ohmer, Sobeck, Teixeria, Wallace, & Shapiro, 2013; Reisch, Ife, & Weil, 2013; Weil & Ohmer, 2013). Working from within an identified value base and being able to benefit from a large body of literature, research, and practice knowledge are among the major contributions social work has made to community practice.

The social work values that guide community practice are articulated in the National Association of Social Work's (NASW) (1996/2008) *Code of Ethics* and the International Federation of Social Workers' (IFSW) *Ethics in Social Work: Statement of Principles* adopted in 2004 (2013). Social workers are directed (in Section 6 of the NASW Code) toward "ethical responsibilities to the broader society," and the promotion of "social, economic, political and cultural values and institutions that are compatible with the realization of social justice."

Community-practice social workers make use of a wide range of literature in their education and practice from social work, social science, the humanities, health education, and environmental sciences, as well as indigenous and feminist knowledge and critical theory from related disciplines. Research relating to the outcomes of community-practice interventions is of particular importance (Ohmer & Korr, 2006; Ohmer et al., 2013; Minkler & Wallerstein, 2008; Raheim, Noponen, & Alter, 2005).

Eight Models of Community Practice Intervention

Eight current models of community practice intervention are described below, including several refinements from their earlier presentations (see Table 1). For each model, we define the purpose, identify the theory and conceptual understandings that ground it, provide one intervention example, and discuss the primary roles played by practitioners working within the model. These eight models are more fully described in *Community Practice Skills: Local to Global Perspectives* (Gamble & Weil, 2010) and its accompanying workbook with teaching and learning exercises, *Community Practice Skills Workbook: Local to Global Perspectives* (Weil, Gamble, & MacGuire, 2010). The examples used here are brief and classic. Many more examples are provided in *Community Practice Skills*. Models are ideal types (Weber, 1970) that provide an opportunity to analyze the goals, actions, and outcomes that help the community practitioner compare purposes of the intervention and the roles and skills needed (for example, when facilitation is more effective than formal leadership, or when advocacy is more effective than negotiation). In practice settings, models are likely to be mixed or blended, and often, communities and practitioners will progress from one model type to another as the organization develops and local circumstances change.

Neighborhood and Community Organizing

This model relates to organizing that takes place in a geographic location where face-to-face encounters occur regularly as part of community interaction. The organizing effort has a triple focus: to develop and stimulate leadership and organizations, to strengthen the organizational capacity by improving leadership and organizational functioning, and to help organizations take successful actions toward the improvement of quality-of-life conditions and opportunities for their communities.

This intervention model is grounded in personal and interpersonal, group, empowerment, organizational, community, globalization, and social-change theories. The most useful concepts from these theory streams for intervention are related to group process, facilitation, dialogue and discourse, principles of democratic participation, power and empowerment, social capital, and collective efficacy (Bandura, 1986; Couto & Guthrie, 1999; DeFilippis, Fisher, & Shragge,

TABLE 1

Models of Community Practice in 21st Century Contexts: Globalization, Increase of Multicultural Societies Worldwide, and Expansion of Rights for Women and Human Rights

COMPARATIVE CHARACTERISTICS	NEIGHBORHOOD AND COMMUNITY ORGANIZING	ORGANIZING FUNCTIONAL COMMUNITIES	SOCIAL, ECONOMIC, AND SUSTAINABLE DEVELOPMENT	INCLUSIVE PROGRAM DEVELOPMENT	SOCIAL PLANNING	COALITIONS	POLITICAL AND SOCIAL ACTION, AND POLICY PRACTICE	MOVEMENTS FOR PROGRESSIVE CHANGE
Desired outcome	Develop capacity of members to organize; direct and/or or moderate the impact of regional planning and external development	Action for social justice focused on advocacy and on changing behaviors and attitudes; may also provide service	Promote grassroots plans; prepare citizens to use social and economic resources without harming environments; expand livelihood opportunities	Expansion, redirection and new development of programs to improve service effectiveness using participatory engagement methods	Neighborhood, citywide for act, or regional proposals ion by (a) neighborhood groups (b) elected body, and/or (c) planning councils and social agencies	Build a multiorganizational power base to advocate for standards and programs, to influence program direction and draw down resources	Action for social justice focused on changing policies or policy makers	Action for social, economic, and environmental justice that provides new paradigms for the healthy development of people and the planet
Systems targeted for change	Municipal/regional government; external developers; local leadership	General public; government institutions	Banks; foundations; external developers; laws that govern wealth creation	Financial donors; boards of directors; service providers; and organized beneficiaries of services	Perspectives of (a) neighborhood planning groups (b) elected leaders (c) human services leaders	Elected officials; foundations; government policy and service organizations	Voting public; elected officials; inactive/ potential participants in public debates and elections	General public; political, social, and economic systems that are oppressive and destructive
Primary constituency	Residents of neighborhood, parish, rural community, village	Like-minded people in a community, region, nation, or across the globe	Low-wealth, marginalized, or oppressed population groups in a city or region	Agency board and administrators; community representatives	(a) neighborhood groups (b) elected leaders (c) social agencies and interagency organizations	Organizations and. people that have a stake in the particular issue	Citizens in a particular political jurisdiction	Leaders, citizens, and organizations able to create new visions and just social and economic structures

(cont.)

TABLE 1
(cont.)

COMPARATIVE CHARACTERISTICS	NEIGHBORHOOD AND COMMUNITY ORGANIZING	ORGANIZING FUNCTIONAL COMMUNITIES	SOCIAL, ECONOMIC, AND SUSTAINABLE DEVELOPMENT	INCLUSIVE PROGRAM DEVELOPMENT	SOCIAL PLANNING	COALITIONS	POLITICAL AND SOCIAL ACTION, AND POLICY PRACTICE	MOVEMENTS FOR PROGRESSIVE CHANGE
Scope of concern	Quality of life in geographic area; increased ability of grassroots leaders and organizations to improve social, economic and environmental conditions	Advocacy for particular issue or population (examples: environmental protection; women's participation in decision making)	Well-being investments (that is, income and assets, education, social support and health care); access to capital and "green" livelihoods; Employ equality, opportunity and responsibility to guide human behavior	Service development for specific populations (examples: children's access to health care; security against domestic violence; elimination of exclusion because of difference)	(a) neighborhood level planning (b) integration of social, economic, and environmental needs into public planning; (c) human services coordination	Organizational partners joining in a collaborative relationship to improve social, economic and environmental conditions and human rights	Building the level of participation in political activity; ensuring that elections are fair and not controlled by wealth	Social, economic and environmental justice within society (examples: basic human needs; basic human rights and freedoms; environmental protection and restoration)
Social work and community practice roles	Organizer Facilitator Educator Coach Trainer Bridge builder	Organizer Advocate Writer/speaker Facilitator	Negotiator Bridge builder Promoter Planner, Educator Manager Researcher Evaluator	Spokesperson Planner/evaluator Manager/Director Proposal Writer Trainer Bridge builder Visionary	Researcher Proposal writer Communicator Planner Manager Evaluator	Mediator Negotiator Spokesperson Organizer Bridge builder Leader	Advocate Organizer Researcher Candidate Leader	Advocate Facilitator Leader

Source: Adapted from Gamble and Weil (2010).

2010; Freire, 1970/1972; Gamble, 2013; Kaner, Lind, Toldi, Fisk, & Berger, 1996; Putnam, 2007; Rubin & Rubin, 2007; Toseland & Rivas, 2011; VeneKlasen & Miller, 2007).

Examples of neighborhood and community organizing are found in all parts of the world. In San Martin, Guatemala, World Neighbors' staff assisted Cakchiquel Indian communities in improving their yields of corn and beans by 300% in the first seven years of the project. They built upon local knowledge and experience (for example, indigenous knowledge of soil, climate, cultural preferences, local skills, and economic conditions), and then added external coaching (for example, methods to enrich soil, prevent erosion, and facilitating dialogue to build organizations in the Cakchiquel communities) in a process called "assisted self-reliance." Through continued collaboration, the community members also established a lending cooperative, co-constructed earthquake-proof dwellings, and improved their overall nutrition and health outcomes (Krishna & Bunch, 1997). World Neighbors continues to do community organizing and development, primarily in rural communities, in 13 countries, building "local capacity with the goal of having local people lead their development process as early as possible—ideally, from the start" (Killough, 2013, p. 701).

The roles of community-practice workers in neighborhood and community organization are primarily those of organizer, facilitator, educator, coach, trainer, and bridge builder. The community-practice worker helps community members to become advocates for their communities and to take actions on their own behalf (Staples, 2004). In this kind of intervention the social worker is not the leader and takes care to develop and facilitate leadership within the community rather than usurp leadership positions.

Organizations and resources such as the Center for Participatory Change (2013), PICO National Network (2013), and the Community Tool Box at the University of Kansas (2013) can help in conceptualizing the work of neighborhood and community organizing.

ORGANIZING FUNCTIONAL COMMUNITIES Functional communities, often referred to as communities of identity or interest, comprise people who have specific common interests but do not necessarily live in proximity. Their interests are in taking actions toward social-justice goals and expanding education and information about their issues to the wider public. These are people organizing, for example, to protect human rights, especially for groups that have been marginalized;

to respond to the needs of children with developmental disabilities; to support people with HIV/AIDS; to prevent the trafficking of women and children for slavery and sexual exploitation; to establish services for homeless teens; or to eliminate land mines. Because they are not necessarily located in proximity to one another, newsletters, telephone, and Internet sources are their primary means of communication, augmented at times by conferences or direct opportunities to engage in action together.

This practice-intervention model is grounded in theories dealing with social change, groups and empowerment, organizational development, interorganizational work (for example, networks and coalitions), and communications. Necessary conceptual understandings include a deep understanding of the social-justice and human-rights aspects of the particular issue, strategies for advocacy (including education), campaigns for or against a particular issue, collaboration, contest, direct action, and knowledge of a variety of communication methods that will be culturally effective and inclusive (Brager, Specht, & Torczyner, 1987; Finn & Jacobson, 2008; Gutierrez & Lewis, 1998; Homan, 2011; Reisch et al., 2013; Rivera & Erlich, 1998; VeneKlasen & Miller, 2007; Weil et al., 2013a).

Practice examples are found in local and global settings. Functional community organizing brings people with similar interests together so that they may learn from one another, identify and create useful resources, work to change problematic policies or practices, and benefit from the emotional connection shared because of their common concerns. In many parts of the world, organizing occurs to identify families of children with special needs. Historically, people with disabilities were often shunned and institutionalized in the United States and other societies until the middle of the 20th century (Mackelprang, 2011). Fortunately many state, national, and international organizations have formed to advocate for people with disabilities. These organizations are the result of people with similar concerns coming together to promote the needs and interests of the disabled, often facilitated by social workers. In 1990, the Americans with Disabilities Act was enacted, ensuring the rights of disabled people in most areas of society (Mackelprang, 2011). While concerns for people with disabilities still remain, organizations supporting the need to secure rights for people with disabilities have continued working on such problems as health care and adequate housing to allow for independent living. The outcome of organization by like-minded people across the planet led to the recognition of persons with disabilities by the United Nations in 1992, and the UN Convention on the rights of Persons with Disabilities, which entered into force in 2008 with an emphasis on inclusion and accessibility (United Nations International Day of Persons with Disabilities, 2012). The UN planned to hold discussions in September 2013, in order to incorporate the contributions, rights, and concerns of people with disabilities into the development agenda that will succeed the Millennium Development Goals, with a targeted ending date of 2015 (United Nations Millennium Development Goals, 2013).

The roles that are most important for social workers to assume in order to work with functional communities are organizer, advocate, writer, speaker, and facilitator. As advocates, social workers are always careful to represent appropriately the views of those who will benefit from the organizing effort, and they strive to incorporate, without exploitation, the voices of people who directly experience the condition needing to be changed.

COMMUNITY SOCIAL, ECONOMIC, AND SUSTAINABLE DEVELOPMENT The United Nations' (1948) Universal Declaration of Human Rights describes the conditions for an adequate livelihood: "...the right to work...free choice of employment...right to equal pay...a family existence worthy of human dignity...right to join trade unions...right to rest and leisure...standard of living adequate for the health and well-being of self and family...education...and right to freely participate in the cultural life of the community" (Articles 23–27). This model relates to community interventions that stimulate the development of income, assets, community economic structures and opportunities, basic and continuing education, and social support. We speak of livelihoods, rather than work or jobs, because all communities gain from both the paid and unpaid work of their members, and all families thrive primarily because of the nurturing and caring labor provided by its members for one another. The addition of "sustainable development" in this model recognizes the impact of the natural environment on a community's livelihood and the challenges future generations will encounter for livelihood development as climate change results in migrations, violent storms, and food scarcity. Having depleted extensive nonrenewable resources and fouled the soil, water, and air, we now need to rethink personal and global behaviors, policies, and investments to rescue and sustain the planet and its inhabitants (Gamble & Hoff, 2013; Gore, 2006; Lingam, 2013).

Theory streams and knowledge that inform this model are from recent human-development perspectives, especially the writings of Sen (1999) and Nus-

sbaum (2011) on the role of capabilities and freedom as necessary aspects of human development, social and economic development (Murphy & Cunningham, 2003), sustainable development, poverty alleviation, social capital, environmental reclamation, and adult education. Necessary conceptual understandings include the Human Development Index (United Nations Development Program [UNDP], 2011), the role of gender in development outcomes, opportunities for "green" livelihoods (for example, environmentally efficient construction, local farmers markets, seed preservation and trading, recycling), sustainable community indicators, and networking and mutual learning opportunities (Ellerman, 2006; Estes, 1993; Haq, 1995; Hart, 1999; Hawken, 2007; Midgley & Livermore, 2005; Prigoff, 2000; Shiva, 2005,2008; Uphoff, Esman, & Krishna, 1998).

A useful conceptual representation of how to think about community sustainable development was prepared by Oxfam International for discussion at the Rio+20 UN Conference on Development and the Environment held in June 2012 (Raworth, 2012). Oxfam proposed that development efforts must work toward the eradication of poverty by ensuring food, water, health care, and energy for all people, while at the same time protecting the biosphere from further climate change or biodiversity loss. This means living and working within "planetary boundaries" and creating a "safe and just space for humanity" within social boundaries (Raworth, 2012, p. 4).

Practice examples for social, economic, and sustainable development tend to be geographically local, but they must be connected to regional markets, support systems, education and training opportunities, and bioregional resources. One example is the Farm to Table nonprofit that was organized in Santa Fe, New Mexico, in 2001. Farm to Table started as an organization to support local small farmers by developing a successful and well-functioning farmer's market. The organization expanded its mission and now works in three broad areas:

1. Facilitating a food and agricultural policy council that brings together people from "health, social services, agriculture and [the] environment" to support programs and policies that strengthen health, agriculture and local economies.

2. Linking fresh food from farmers with school cafeterias for meals and snacks as well as initiating school gardens and healthy eating through special projects and classroom lessons.

3. Engaging farmers and ranchers in the Southwest Marketing Network (SWMN), which links the Four Corners states (New Mexico, Colorado,

Nevada, and Arizona), as well as Native Americans in the Tribal Lands, to support the economic viability of those small producers through "business management tools, marketing strategies, technical and financial assistance, crop insurance information, and peer examples" (Farm to Table New Mexico, 2013).

In addition to these projects, the organizers foresee having to devote more time to securing water resources because of expected drought conditions threatening the Southwest of the United States as the result of climate change. The wiser use of scarce water resources as well as the conservation of watersheds will be important work for all communities.

The roles useful to a community social worker in this model include negotiator, bridge builder, promoter, planner, educator, manager, and evaluator. The social- and economic-development plan for a place will be most successful if local participants are involved from the beginning to assess needs and resources, and to identify goals (Pennell, Noponen, & Weil, 2005). The most useful participatory engagement methods come from popular education (Freire, 1970/1972) and participatory appraisal (Chambers, 1997), described by Gamble (2013).

INCLUSIVE PROGRAM DEVELOPMENT This model involves the initiation or expansion of services by an agency, community-based organization, or coalition of organizations to respond to underserved populations. It would address issues such as the increase, in the early 21st century, in homeless teens and street children; HIV/AIDS survivors and their families' under- and unemployment; and food-security issues. This model involves collaboration between social workers and allies with the engagement of the community, especially potential participants, in the reinvention of services to meet existing and emerging needs, including advocacy for prevention and public education (Gamble & Weil, 2010; Motes & Hess, 2007; Weil, 2013).

Theory that informs this intervention model is drawn from organizational development and management, mutual work with clients and communities, strategic planning, program design and development, social justice, and health and human development (Netting et al., 2011; Weil, 2013). Conceptual understanding important for social workers in this model will relate to community assessments, community-based participatory research, organizational development, and resource generation (Austin, 2002; Brody,

1993; Brodkin, 2013; Finn & Jacobson, 2008; Israel, Shulz, Parker, & Becker, 1998; Mizrahi, Rosenthal, & Ivery, 2013; Netting & O'Connor, 2013).

One practice example, from southeastern Missouri, started with a clinical visit from a social worker to a woman who suffered depression after losing her baby. The visit developed into a full-scale organizing effort to respond to rural women's mental health needs (Price, 2005). In most communities, but especially in rural communities, people are supposed to be independent, strong, and never acknowledge the need for help, especially for mental health issues. As the social worker explored women's needs, local women were reluctant to identify and name their feelings as "depression." With facilitated discussion to explore how life could be better with certain changes, women were able to define their own mental health needs. Collaborating with the social worker, they developed a public-education campaign called "Mental Health Is Part of Every Woman's Wellness." The campaign not only brought needed services for women, it also transformed the region's perspective about mental health (Price, 2005). Expanding the services provided by mental health centers to reach new populations such as these rural women, military men and women returning from war with post-traumatic stress disorder, and people who have lost their jobs after economic crises are aspects of the work of inclusive program development. Identifying these new populations requires a recognition that the people themselves will be most helpful in framing the kind of services and programs from which they can benefit. Weil (2013) offers detailed planning steps for situations in which a recognized need is not being met because of inadequate resources or services. Drawing from a number of national and international sources, she includes participatory steps to gather maximum input from the people who will be served by the expanded program.

Social workers in this model are expected to engage in a variety of roles, including spokesperson, planner, manager/director, proposal writer, trainer, evaluator, visionary, and boundary spanner. In addition to having significant knowledge of the program area and service organization/network characteristics (for example, missions, funding streams, policy strengths and limitations, leadership strength), the community practitioner must also develop respectful and co-learner relationships with constituent population groups. It is especially important not to treat the constituent groups as victims or passive bystanders. When constituent or beneficiary groups are engaged in service planning—and, later, implementation, advising, and evaluation—the resulting service program has a much greater chance of actually meeting the service needs and empowering participants (Gamble & Weil, 2010).

SOCIAL PLANNING Planning requires forward-looking assessments of population characteristics and needs with an analysis of the resources and structures necessary to respond to those needs (Friedmann, 2011; Jones, 1990). Social planning is often done within a communitywide or regional social planning organization, but it can also occur within an agency or neighborhood, or at a national or international level (Sager & Weil, 2013; Wates, 2000; Weil, 2013). "Social" planning cannot effectively occur in isolation, as it is related to economic and environmental conditions, as well as available infrastructure and resources (Gamble & Weil, 2010). Planning involves the use of technical skills for assessment, data analysis, optimal future scenario development, and evaluation.

At the neighborhood or community level, community practitioners engage with community members to learn their perspective on neighborhood conditions, needs, assets, and directions. They share technical skills with community members and coach them in carrying out assessments, analyses, and community-based planning decisions (Weil, 2013).

Social planning is grounded in planning and change theory, as well as theories relating to human development, participatory planning, and research (Guyette, 1996; Hinsdale, Lewis, & Waller, 1995; Kahn, 1969; Kitchen, 2006; Kretzmann & McKnight, 1993; UNDP, 2011; Weil, 2013).

In northwestern North Carolina, an MSW student working for hospice noted that an increasing number of the hospice referrals were gay men who had earlier escaped local stigma regarding their sexual orientation and found broader work opportunities by relocating to large cities. After years in the Northeast or Midwest, they were returning home to die. Hospice responded to AIDS patients and their families by helping them to die with dignity. By the early 1990s, more effective treatments were available, enabling people with HIV/AIDS to live much longer with productive lives, but local physicians were still referring all patients living with HIV/AIDS to hospice. The student realized that this was not the service these men needed and that new service planning was necessary. He gathered men living with HIV/AIDS, hospital and health care providers, human-services staff, and representative citizen groups to talk about the kind of support that was desirable in this new reality. A coalition formed to complete needs assessments, with the interviews conducted by people with HIV/

AIDS. This process uncovered a far larger population needing support services than was previously recognized. The coalition undertook planning with the constituent group and presented its proposals to local governments and nonprofit donors. With funding, they opened a new Support Service Center for people living with HIV/AIDS and their families (Weil, 2005, pp. 235–236).

Community practitioners working in the planning model can be expected to engage in roles relating to research (assessments, evaluations, etc.), proposal writing, communication, planning, managing, and evaluating (Sager & Weil, 2013). The National Network of Planning Councils provides examples of social planning at city and regional levels. Geographic Information Systems (GIS) are increasingly used in social planning and have provided a technology that planners can share with community members. GIS programs can overlay a range of services, programs, and data about schools and other civic institutions. It provides ways of identifying the assets in communities as well as indicating demographic data and overlapping programs. GIS, whether web-based or desktop applications, can provide massive information for planning and analyzing tasks performed by community-practice planners (Hillier & Culhane, 2013) Social workers are also involved in many national social-planning efforts related to health services and prevention, domestic violence, child welfare, and mental health, among others.

COALITIONS This model brings together organizations that have a common interest in a social, civic, economic, environmental, or political concerns on a temporary or longer-term basis for the purpose of building a power base large enough to influence policy decisions, change conditions, and secure needed resources. Coalitions' actions usually include a major public-education campaign to enlarge their ranks and educate the public. Building a coalition requires attention to relationships among the organizations, the relative commitment of each organization, the comparative competence and resources of each organization, and their respective contributions toward the effort (Mizrahi & Rosenthal, 2001; Mizrahi et al., 2012).

Theories that inform this work include coalitions, interorganizational relations, collaboration, social change, social movements, power, and empowerment (Alter, 2011; Bailey & Koney, 2000; Bayne-Smith, Mizrahi, & Garcia, 2008; Jones, Cook, & Webb, 2007; Mattessich, Murray-Close, & Monsey, 2001). Social workers help build coalitions for social justice and human rights, and therefore, conceptual understanding of these value bases will be important to this work (Cohen, de la Vega, & Watson, 2001; Finn & Jacobson, 2008; Roberts-DeGennaro & Mizrahi, 2005).

While it is sometimes easier to develop and maintain a coalition in which values, perspectives on needed changes, and strategies are shared, it is also possible for coalitions to be built within small communities, bringing together geographically close but ideologically distant organizations to accomplish important social change, such as bringing ranchers, hunters, and environmentalists together to protect land and water resources. Coalitions can also span the globe, such as the International Baby Food Action Network (IBFAN, 2013), which began a campaign in 1997 and continues today to limit aggressive marketing of commercial infant formula in place of breast milk. The campaign was initiated after health research demonstrated an increase in mortality rates for babies in low-wealth neighborhoods and countries born to mothers who used only infant formula. In 2013, IBFAN coordinated more than 200 citizen groups in 95 countries that monitor the advertising of breast milk substitutes.

Although there has long been concern about gun violence in the United States and the numbers and types of guns available to residents, the December 2012 shooting of 20 elementary school children and their six teachers created new interest in efforts to curtail gun violence. The Coalition to Stop Gun Violence coordinates the efforts of 47 national organizations from public health, social services, social justice, religion, and child welfare to lobby for policies that they believe will reduce morbidity and mortality from the use of a gun (Coalition to Stop Gun Violence, 2013). The organization supports policies that will require a background check for all gun purchases, control assault weapons, and stamp serial numbers on all shell casings for identification purposes. Community-practice workers and public health organizers have come together in some communities to build coalitions that will diminish gun violence. In 2000, the National Association of Social Workers joined in a campaign to end gun violence, a campaign that involved social work students across the country (NASW, 2000).

In 1977, the U.S. group Infant Formula Action Coalition (INFAC) started a campaign to boycott the Swiss manufacturer of the infant formula, Nestlé. The campaign was based on research in low-wealth neighborhoods and countries, which showed higher mortality among infants using commercial formula in place of breast milk. Use of contaminated water and dilution of the formula to stretch the supply contributed to the higher mortality. In addition, unlike mother's milk, the formula did not contain antibodies to help build babies' immune systems to resist certain illnesses. Advertising of infant formula in hospitals and health clinics made mothers feel they were depriving their child of modern—even scientific—benefits if they did not use the formula. The boycott of Nestlé's products and the public-education campaign spread across the globe. The coalition was instrumental in persuading the World Health Assembly to adopt, in 1981, the International Code of Marketing Breast Milk Substitutes, which prohibits certain kinds of advertising and aggressive marketing. IBFAN in England in 2013 coordinated more than 200 citizens' groups in 95 countries that monitor the actions of Nestlé/Carnation and other infant-formula corporations to prevent free samples and inappropriate advertising from taking place in health clinics. The boycott was dropped for a period of time to monitor corporate responsibility, but it was resumed in 1988 when monitors found that companies were not complying.

Coalitions require a number of roles to be played by involved community-practice workers (Ray, 2002; Roberts, 2004). Important roles include leader, mediator, negotiator, spokesperson, organizer, and bridge builder. Understanding interorganizational behavior theory, strategies for social change, and employing empowerment principles in organization building all relate to effective practice for workers in this model (Jaskyte & Lee, 2006).

POLITICAL AND SOCIAL ACTION This model is focused on taking action for social justice by changing policies, laws, and policy makers. It involves research that identifies and exposes social, economic, and environmental injustice, and follows with efforts to engage in lobbying, class-action lawsuits, testimony, advocacy, and political campaigns to change oppressive and damaging policies and institutions (Hoefer, 2011; Jansson, 2013). Political and social action has a long tradition in social work. When Jane Addams found garbage a foot thick over the cobblestones in the 1890 Chicago slum neighborhoods, she lobbied for more regular garbage pick-up. When lobbying failed to achieve the needed results that she and her neighbors had identified, she campaigned to be appointed garbage inspector—and won. From that position, she was able to monitor and influence more effective garbage collection (Addams, 1910).

Theories that support this model are derived from power and empowerment theory, political economy, participatory democracy, and social-change theory

(Mondros, 2013; Schneider & Lester, 2001). Conceptual understandings for this model relate to human rights, social justice, strategy development, professional ethics, and advocacy (Couto & Guthrie, 1999; Hick & McNutt, 2002; Haynes & Mickelson, 2009; IFSW, 2004/2013; Jansson, Heidemann, McCroskey, & Fertig, 2013; Reisch, 2013; United Nations, 1948; VeneKlasen & Miller, 2007).

Examples of this model can be identified in local settings across the globe, and they can be seen in actions that may have global consequences when successful. In the U.S. Civil Rights Movement of the mid-20th century, a variety of methods were used to change laws that permitted, and even enforced, discrimination against African Americans. Direct, non-violent action was the most widely used strategy to demonstrate the inhumanity of the existing laws and practices (Anderson, 1995). In Greensboro, North Carolina, students organized a sit-in at a lunch counter where they were customarily denied service. With their success in integrating Woolworth's, they sparked actions in other parts of the country to dismantle segregation laws. In Montgomery, Alabama, after the arrest of Rosa Parks for declining to give up her seat on a public bus to a white man, African Americans refused to ride city buses as long as they were prevented from selecting a seat anywhere on the bus. The bus boycott, which involved organizing churches, student groups, and civic groups, lasted more than a year, causing enormous economic harm to the bus system and forcing an eventual settlement. The Highlander Center in New Market, Tennessee, began "literacy schools" for African Americans to overcome the "voting tests" imposed by many Southern states. The African American Mississippi Freedom Democratic Party tried to be seated at the Democratic National Convention in 1964, resulting in a major national controversy. Though it was unsuccessful in being seated, the world was made aware of the policies that kept African Americans from voting and becoming candidates for office. In that same year, the Civil Rights Act of 1964 was passed by Congress to strengthen voting rights and prevent discrimination on the basis of race, color, religion, or national origin in any program receiving funds from the federal government; additionally, the Equal Employment Opportunity Commission was established to make sure that people's rights were not denied in work situations. In 1993, social workers were actively involved in passage of the Voter Registration Act of 1993, also known as the Motor Voter Act, which facilitated the registration of people to vote when they applied for a drivers license or for social services (U.S. Department of Justice, 2013).

Since 2010, Republican-dominated state legislatures have tried, and in some cases succeeded, to pass laws restricting voting rights by requiring voter identification cards with photos, by decreasing the number of days voters have to vote prior to election day, and by making it more difficult for working people to become registered to vote (Brennen Center for Justice, 2011). The directive to social workers in this regard seems clear from the NASW's *Code of Ethics*, 6. 04, "Social workers should act to prevent and eliminate domination of, exploitation of, and discrimination against any person, group, or class on the basis of race, ethnicity, national origin, color, sex, sexual orientation, age, marital status, political belief, religion, or mental or physical disability" (NASW, 2008). In 2011, members of Congress who were social workers, friends of social work, or supporters of the clients who are served by social workers formed a Social Work Caucus led by Rep. Edolphus "Ed" Towns (D-NY). After Towns' retirement in 2013, Barbara Lee (D-CA) assumed the chairmanship. The Caucus, 60 members strong in 2013, brings social work issues to the front burner with briefings on legislation that can help social workers improve their ability to serve clients (Congressional Social Work Caucus, 2013).

The important roles for social workers engaged in political and social action are advocate, organizer, researcher, leader, and sometimes, candidate (Haynes & Mickelson, 2009; Mondros, 2013; Myers & Granstaff, 2011; Schneider, Lester, & Ochieng, 2011). In 2012, there were seven former social workers serving in the House of Representatives and two in the Senate (Manning, 2011). In 2013, more than 150 members of NASW served in state and local elected positions (NASW, 2012).

MOVEMENTS FOR PROGRESSIVE CHANGE This model includes activities to influence major social change toward measurable improvements of quality of life for vulnerable groups and individuals (Humphries, 2008). While social movements can have goals to prevent positive change for these groups, our model is grounded in action toward progressive change that will increase opportunities, human rights, and social justice in accordance with social work values (Reisch et al., 2013).

Theories that ground this model are drawn from social-change, social-movement, social-transformation, and collective-action theory (Gil, 1998; Reisch, 2013). Conceptual understandings that are useful to social workers involved in social-movement activity relate to ethical practice, collective efficacy, leadership, coalition building, gender issues, and a range of strategies for social change (Anderson, 1995; Bandura, 1986; IFSW, 2004/2013; Meyer & Staggenborg, 1996; NASW, 2008; Piven & Cloward, 1977; Reisch, 2011).

An example of a current movement that presents opportunities for social work involvement is the range of local-to-global interventions taking place to promote sustainable development. Estes (1993) describes nine related movements as the historical antecedents for sustainable development: environmental/ecological, antiwar/antinuclear, world order, world dynamics modeling, green, alternative economics, women's movement, indigenous peoples, and human rights (pp. 7–8). All of these local-to-global movements, which began in the 1960s and continue to the present, have converged into what Estes (1993) describes as "successfully uniting widely divergent theoretical and ideological perspectives into a single conceptual framework" (p. 1). For Estes (1993), Richard Falk's (1972) seven values provide a set of principles that encompass *sustainable development*: "unity of humanity and life on earth, the minimization of violence, the maintenance of environmental quality, the satisfaction of minimum world welfare standards, the primacy of human dignity, the retention of diversity and pluralism, and universal participation" (p. 12). It is a movement that has drawn social-justice, human-rights, and environmental-justice champions from around the globe (Gore, 2006; Hawken, 2007; LaDuke, 2005; Peeters, 2012; Shiva, 2005, 2008). This movement offers seven levels of intervention for social work engagement, beginning with "individual and group empowerment" through processes of conscientization, all the way to "world building," by creating new social, political, economic, and environmental institutions (Estes, 1993, pp. 16–17; Gamble & Hoff, 2013, pp. 223–224). Weil (2013) describes the merging of alternative, sustainable, and human-development perspectives into a model for development focusing on social transformation. The World Social Forum, the Arab Spring, the Spanish Indignants, and the Occupy movements that emerged in the first two decades of the 21st century may well be examples of the social-transformation perspective, because they often combine concerns for economic fairness, indigenous people's rights, environmental recovery and protection, basic human needs, and human rights and freedoms, especially for women and girls.

The 2008 financial crisis that caused economic crises for the most vulnerable populations all across the globe was in part the impetus for the "Occupy" movement that started in Zuccotti Park, in the Wall Street area, in New York City in September 2011. By October of the same year, "occupy" demonstrations had occurred in more than 600 cities and towns across the United States and in 80 countries (The Guardian, 2012; Occupy, 2013). While the goals of the Occupy movement were not always explicit, its activists identified with concerns about the growing gap between the rich and poor in the United States and across the globe. The movement's slogan became "We are the 99%," identifying with the majority of the world's population that controls the fewest assets and has the least power (Occupy, 2013; Stiglitz, 2012).

Social workers provided more leadership for social movements in the past, but social movements continue to provide stimulation for social work engagement (Reisch, 2013). Among the many social workers providing leadership for the civil rights movement were Whitney Young, who was president of NASW in 1966, and Dorothy Height, who was president of the National Council of Negro Women for 40 years. Social workers, including the authors, were also involved with the Welfare Rights Movement in the 1960s and early '70s (Piven & Cloward, 1977). The roles social workers in social movements play on many different levels can be those of advocate, facilitator, and leader. Whether society is engaged in a movement for civil rights, women's rights, children's safety, food security, elimination of sexual and child-labor trafficking, or environmental responsibility and preservation, we can benefit from the growing body of interdisciplinary research and documentation to help move the communities in which we find ourselves toward progressive social change.

CONTEXTS AND CHALLENGES FOR COMMUNITY-PRACTICE INTERVENTIONS
The effects of *globalization*, the increase in *multicultural societies* as the result of forced and voluntary migration, and the struggles to expand *human rights*, especially rights for women and girls, are challenging community-practice-intervention processes—organizing, planning, sustainable development, and progressive change—in the 21st century.

Governments make decisions about global trade regulations, development assistance, and wars. Corporate and financial institutions extract resources and create massive, complex financial arrangements that have disastrous results when they collapse. New trade rules provide temporary economic benefits for some communities and eliminate livelihoods in others. The increasing frequency of natural disasters (for example, hurricanes, earthquakes, and tsunamis) that may be the result of global warming plagues the most vulnerable populations on the planet. Civil and state-sponsored wars and cross-border incursions ravage communities, even after hostilities cease (Van Soest, 1997). Peace making has a body of knowledge easily accessible to proponents of peaceful strategies for resolving local, regional, national, and global conflicts, but its use requires willing leaders and facilitators (Elkins, 2006; McConnell & van Gelder, 2003; Moix, Smith, & Staab, 2004).

Communities are increasingly multicultural as population migration makes nearly every country and every community a host to people from different cultures and ethnicities (UNHCR, 2013). Refugees often flee their homelands because of ethnic conflicts, natural disasters, and political oppression, and millions of people are displaced within their own countries (Cox and Pawar, 2012). Numerous migrants also travel to other countries for basic economic survival. Immigrants from Mexico to the United States, for example, send approximately $13.3 billion in remittances annually to their often-destitute families and communities of origin. Social workers can work to change the conditions that force migration and can also engage in working toward integration, mutual understanding, and inclusion by facilitating dialogue among different groups and promoting inclusive economic and social development (Anderson and Carter, 2003; Dessel, Rogge, & Garlington, 2006; Fong and Furuto, 2001; Gutierrez et al., 2013).

Human rights are a primary concern of social work, as outlined in the IFSW (2004/2013), and in seven international human-rights declarations and conventions, including the Convention on the Elimination of All Forms of Discrimination Against Women and The Convention on the Rights of the Child. The framers of the Millennium Development Goals (MDG) agreed that gender equality is a central focus because "women are agents of development" (UNDP, 2003, p. 7; United Nations, 2011). Securing rights for women and girls is a major international challenge, as evidenced by the Gender Empowerment Measure (GEM) (UNDP, 2003, pp. 314–317), and the Social Institutions and Gender Index (SIGI) developed by the Organization for Economic Cooperation and Development (OECD, 2012).

The values and behaviors of community practitioners who engage in organizing, planning, sustainable development, and progressive change will determine their ability to be co-learners with members of the communities in which they work. Co-learning involves setting aside assumptions about the people with whom you are working and their environments so that one can learn from their perspectives (in their words) and through their experiences. Working with community members and organizations in this way becomes a *collaborative engagement*. This process is described by Finn and Jacobson as "action and accompaniment," a rethinking of the roles of social work as "always carried out in the context of social relationships" (1948, pp. 313–375).

Working within an ethical framework requires community-practice social workers to evaluate their actions and interventions daily. Along with specific change goals, practitioners should seek to measure advances in human rights, increased social capital that results in open and inclusive community structures, increased economic opportunity and well-being, and recovered and protected environments. Community-participant involvement in reflection on community outcomes should also be a consistent aspect of community practice evaluation.

REFERENCES

Abbott, E. (1937). *Some American pioneers in social welfare: Select documents with editorial notes.* Chicago, IL: University of Chicago Press.

Addams, J. (1902/1964). *Democracy and social ethics.* Cambridge, MA: Belknap Press of Harvard University Press.

Addams, J. (1910). *Twenty years at Hull-House.* New York: Macmillan.

Addams, J. (1930). *The second twenty years at Hull-House.* New York: Macmillan.

Alinsky, S. (1971). *Rules for radicals.* New York: Random House.

Alter, C. (2011). Interorganizational practice interventions. In T. Mizrahi & L. E. Davis (Eds.), *Encyclopedia of social work* (20th ed., Vol. 2, pp. 528–533). Washington DC/New York: NASW Press/Oxford University Press.

Alzate, M. M., Andharia, J., Chowa, G. A. N., Weil, M., & Doernberg, A. (2013). Women and leadership in development, planning, organizing, and social change. In M. Weil, M. Reisch, & M. L. Ohmer (Eds.), *The handbook of community practice* (2nd ed., pp. 553–681). Thousand Oaks, CA: Sage Publications.

Anderson, J., & Carter, R. W. (Eds.) (2003). *Diversity perspectives for social work practice.* Boston: Allyn & Bacon.

Anderson, T. H. (1995). *The movement and the sixties: Protest in America from Greensboro to Wounded Knee.* New York: Oxford University Press.

Association of Community Organization and Social Administration (ACOSA). (2013). Retrieved May 11, 2013, from http://www.acosa.org/joomla/

Austin, D. (2002). *Human services management: Organizational leadership in social work practice.* New York: Columbia University Press.

Austin, M. J., & Betten, N. (1990). Rural organizing and the agricultural extension service. In N. Betten & M. J. Austin (Eds.), *The roots of community organizing, 1917–1939* (pp. 94–105). Philadelphia, PA: Temple University Press.

Bailey, D., & Koney, K. M. (2000). *Strategic alliances among health and human services organizations: From affiliations to consolidations.* Thousand Oaks, CA: Sage Publications.

Balgopal, P. R. (2011). Asian Americans: Overview. In T. Mizrahi & L. E. Davis (Eds.), *Encyclopedia of social work* (20th ed., Vol. 1, pp. 153–160). Washington, DC/New York: NASW Press/Oxford University Press.

Bandura, A. (1986). *Social foundations of thought and action: A social cognitive theory.* Englewood Cliffs, NJ: Prentice-Hall.

Bayne-Smith, M., Mizrahi, T., & Garcia, M. L. (2008). Interdisciplinary Community Collaboration (ICC): Perspectives of community practitioners on successful strategies. *Journal of Community Practice, 16,* 249–269.

Bearse, M. (2011). Native Americans: Practice interventions. In T. Mizrahi & L. E. Davis (Eds.), *Encyclopedia of social work* (20th ed., Vol. 3, pp. 299–308). Washington DC/New York: NASW Press/Oxford University Press.

Betten, N., & Austin, M. J. (1990). *The roots of community organizing: 1917–1939.* Philadelphia, PA: Temple University Press.

Brager, G., Specht, H., & Torczyner, J. L. (1987). *Community organizing* (2nd ed.). New York: Columbia University Press.

Brennen Center for Justice. (2011, October 3). *Voting law changes in 2012.* New York University School of Law. Retrieved May 11, 2013, from http://www.brennancenter.org/publication/voting-law-changes-2012

Brodkin, M. (2013). Creating a model children's service system: Lessons from San Francisco. In M. Weil, M. Reisch, & M. L. Ohmer (Eds.), *The handbook of community practice* (2nd ed., pp. 531–546). Thousand Oaks, CA: Sage Publications.

Brody, R. (1993). *Effectively managing human service organizations.* Thousand Oaks, CA: Sage Publications.

Brown, M. J. (2006). *Building powerful community organizations.* Arlington, MA: Long Haul Press.

Brueggemann, W. G. (2013). History and context for community practice in North America. In M. Weil, M. Reisch, & M. L. Ohmer (Eds.), *The handbook of community practice* (2nd ed., pp. 27–46). Thousand Oaks, CA: Sage Publications.

Burwell, N. Y. (1996). Lawrence Oxley and locality development: Black self-help in North Carolina, 1925–1928. *The Journal of Community Practice Special Issue: African American Community Practice Models: Historical and Contemporary Responses,* 2(4), 49–69.

Carlton-LaNey, I. B. (2001). *African American leadership: An empowerment tradition in social welfare history.* Washington, DC: National Association of Social Workers Press.

Carter, G. W. (1958). Practice theory in community organization. *Social Work, 3,* 54–69.

Center for Participatory Change (CPC). (2013). Center for Participatory Change Web site. Retrieved May 11, 2013, from http://www.cpcwnc.org

Chambers, R. (1997). *Whose reality counts?: Putting the first last.* London: Intermediate Technology Publications.

Chaskin, R. J. (2013). Theories of community. In M. Weil, M. Reisch, & M. L. Ohmer (Eds.), *The handbook of community practice* (2nd ed., pp. 105–122). Thousand Oaks, CA: Sage Publications.

Chowa, G. A. N., Masa, R. De V., Sherraden, M., & Weil, M. (2013). Confronting global poverty: Building economic opportunity and social inclusion. In M. Weil, M. Reisch, & M. L. Ohmer (Eds.), *The handbook of community practice* (2nd ed., pp. 607–631). Thousand Oaks, CA: Sage Publications.

Christenson, J. A., & Robinson, J. W., Jr. (Eds.). (1989). *Community development in perspective.* Ames: Iowa State University Press.

Coalition to Stop Gun Violence. (2013). Issues and campaigns. Retrieved May 11, 2013, from http://www.csgv.org/issues-and-campaigns

Cohen, D., de la Vega, R., & Watson, G. (2001). *Advocacy for social justice: A global action and reflection guide.* Bloomfield, CT: Oxfam/Advocacy Institute and Kumarian Press.

Community Tool Box at the University of Kansas. (2013). What's inside the community toolbox: Practical resources for your work. Retrieved May 11, 2013, from http://ctb.ku.edu/en/default.aspx

Congressional Social Work Caucus. (2013, March). Membership in 113th Congress. Retrieved May 11, 2013, from http://socialworkcaucus-lee.house.gov/membership

Couto, R., & Guthrie, C. S. (1999). *Making democracy work better: Mediating structures, social capital, and the democratic prospect.* Chapel Hill: University of North Carolina Press.

Cox, D. & Pawar, M. (2012). *International social work* (2nd ed.). Thousand Oaks, CA: Sage Publications.

Deegan, M. J. (1990). *Jane Addams and the men of the Chicago school: 1892–1918.* New Brunswick, NJ: Transaction Books.

DeFilippis, J., Fisher, R., & Shragge, E. (2010). *Contesting community: The limits and potential of local organizing.* New Brunswick, NJ: Rutgers University Press.

Dessel, A., Rogge, M., & Garlington, S. (2006). Using intergroup dialogue to promote social justice and change. *Social Work,* 51(4), 303–316.

Dunham, A. (1940). The literature of community organization. In *Proceedings of the national conference of social work* (pp. 410–422). New York: Columbia University Press.

Eade, D. (1997). *Capacity-building: An approach to people-centered development.* Oxford, UK: Oxfam Publications.

Elkins, C. (2006). *Monitoring and evaluation (M&E) for development in peace-precarious situations.* Research Triangle Park, NC: Research Triangle Institute International.

Ellerman, D. (2006). *Helping people help themselves: From the World Bank to an alternative philosophy of development assistance.* Ann Arbor, MI: University of Michigan Press.

Estes, R. J. (1993). Toward sustainable development: From theory to praxis. *Social Development Issues,* 15(3), 1–29.

Falk, R. (1972). *This endangered planet: Prospects and proposals for human survival.* New York: Vintage Books.

Farm to Table New Mexico. (2013). Retrieved June 13, 2013 from http://www.farmtotablenm.org/

Finn, J. L., & Jacobson, M. (2008). *Just practice: A social justice approach to social work* (2nd ed.). Peosta, IA: Eddie Bowers Publishing.

Fisher, R. (1994). *Let the people decide: Neighborhood organizing in America.* New York: Twayne Publishers.

Fong, R., & Furuto, S. (Eds.) (2001). *Culturally competent practice: Skills, interventions, and evaluations.* Boston: Allyn & Bacon.

Freire, P. (1970/1972). *Pedagogy of the oppressed.* Middlesex, England: Penguin Books, Ltd.

Friedmann, J. (2011). *Insurgencies: Essays in planning theory.* New York: Routledge.

Gamble, D. N. (2013). Participatory methods in community practice. In M. Weil, M. Reisch, & M. L. Ohmer (Eds.), *The handbook of community practice* (2nd ed., pp. 325–344). Thousand Oaks, CA: Sage Publications.

Gamble, D. N., & Hoff, M. (2013). Sustainable community development. In M. Weil, M. Reisch, & M. L. Ohmer (Eds.), *The handbook of community practice* (2nd ed., pp. 215–232). Thousand Oaks, CA: Sage Publications.

Gamble, D. N., & Weil, M. (2010). *Community practice skills: Local to global perspectives.* New York: Columbia University Press.

Garvin, C. D., & Cox, F. (2001). A history of community organizing since the Civil War with special reference to oppressed communities. In J. Rothman, J. L. Erlich, & J. E. Tropman (Eds.), *Strategies of community intervention* (6th ed., pp. 65–100). Itasca, IL: F. E. Peacock Publishers.

Gil, D. (1998). *Confronting injustice and oppression: Concepts and strategies for social workers.* New York: Columbia University Press.

Gore, A. (2006). *An inconvenient truth: The planetary emergency of global warming and what we can do about it.* New York: Rodale Books.

The Guardian. (2012). On the occupy movement, November 28, 2012. Retrieved May 11, 2013, from http://www.guardian.co.uk/world/occupy-movement

Gurteen, S. H. (1882). *Handbook of charity organizations.* Buffalo, NY: Charity Organization Society.

Gutierrez, L. M., & Lewis, E. A. (1998). A feminist perspective on organizing with women of color. In F. G. Rivera & J. L. Erlich (Eds.), *Community organizing in a diverse society* (3rd ed., pp. 97–116). Needham Heights, MA: Allyn & Bacon.

Gutierrez, L. M., Lewis, E. A., Dessel, A., & Spencer, M. (2013). Principles, skills, and practice strategies for promoting multicultural communication and collaboration. In M. Weil, M. Reisch, & M. L. Ohmer (Eds.), *The handbook of community practice* (2nd ed., pp. 445–460). Thousand Oaks, CA: Sage Publications.

Guyette, S. (1996). *Planning for balanced development: A guide for Native American and rural communities.* Santa Fe, NM: Clear Light.

Haq, M. ul. (1995). *Reflections on human development.* New York: Oxford University Press.

Hardina, D. (2012). *Interpersonal social work skills for community practice.* New York: Springer Publishing.

Hart, M. (1999). *Guide to sustainable community indicators* (2nd ed.). North Andover, MA: Hart Environmental Data.

Hawken, P. (2007). *Blessed unrest: How the largest movement in the world came into being and why no one saw it coming.* New York: Viking.

Haynes, K., & Mickelson, J. (2009). *Affecting change: Social workers in the political arena* (7th ed.). Boston: Allyn & Bacon.

Hick, S., & McNutt, J. (Eds.). (2002). *Advocacy, activism and the Internet: Community organization and social policy.* Chicago, IL: Lyceum Books.

Hillier, A. & Culhane, D. (2013). GIS applications and administrative data to support community change. In M. Weil, M. Reisch, & M. L. Ohmer (Eds.), *The handbook of community practice* (2nd ed., pp. 827–844). Thousand Oaks, CA: Sage Publications.

Hinsdale, M. A., Lewis, H. M., & Waller, S. M. (1995). *It comes from the people: Community development and local theology.* Philadelphia, PA: Temple University Press.

Hoefer, R. (2011). Highly effective human services interest groups. *Journal of Community Practice, 9*(2), 1–14.

Homan, M. S. (2011). *Promoting community change: Making it happen in the real world* (5th ed.). Belmont, CA: Wadsworth/Thomson Learning, Brooks/Cole.

Humphries, B. (2008). *Social research for social justice.* Basingstoke, UK: Palgrave Macmillan

Industrial Areas Foundation (IAF). (2013). About us. Retrieved May 11, 2013, from http://www.industrialareasfoundation.org/

International Baby Food Action Network (IBFAN). (2013. All about us. Retrieved May 11, 2013, from http://www.ibfan.org/

International Federation of Social Workers (IFSW). (2004/ 2013). Ethics in social work: Statement of principles. Retrieved May 11, 2013, from http://ifsw.org/policies/statement-of-ethical-principles/

Israel, B. A., Shulz, A. J., Parker, E. A., & Becker, A. B. (1998). Review of community-based research: Assessing partnership approaches to improve public health. *Annual Review of Public Health, 19*, 173–204.

Jansson, B. S. (2013). *Becoming an effective policy advocate: From policy practice to social justice* (7th ed.). San Diego: Brooks-Cole.

Jansson, B. S., Heidemann, G., McCroskey. J., & Fertig, R. (2013). Eight models of policy practice: Local, state, national, and international arenas. In M. Weil, M. Reisch, & M. L. Ohmer (Eds.), *The handbook of community practice* (2nd ed., pp. 403–420). Thousand Oaks, CA: Sage Publications.

Jaskyte, K., & Lee, M. (2006). Interorganizational relationships: A source of innovation in nonprofit organizations? *Administration in Social Work, 20*(3), 43–54.

Jones, B. (1990). *Neighborhood planning: A guide for citizens and planners.* Chicago, IL: American Planning Association/Planners Press.

Jones, J. M., Crook, W. P., & Webb, J. R. (2007). Collaboration for the provision of services: A review of the literature. *Journal of Community Practice, 15*, 41–71.

Kahn, A. J. (1969). *The theory and practice of social planning.* New York: Russell Sage Foundation.

Kaner, S., Lind, L., Toldi, C., Fisk, S., & Berger, D. (1996). *Facilitator's guide to participatory decision-making*. Gabriola Island, BC: New Society Publishers.

Killough, S. A. (2013). Building local capacity for rural development. In M. Weil, M. Reisch, & M. L. Ohmer (Eds.), *The handbook of community practice*, (2nd ed., pp. 701–724). Thousand Oaks, CA: Sage Publications.

King, M. L., Jr. (1958). *Stride toward freedom: The Montgomery story*. New York: Ballantine Books.

Kitchen, T. (2006). *Skills for planning practice*. London: Palgrave MacMillan.

Kretzmann, J. P., & McKnight, J. L. (1993). *Building communities from the inside out*. Chicago: Acta Publications.

Krishna, A., & Bunch, R. (1997). Farmer-to-farmer experimentation and extension: Integrated rural development for smallholders in Guatemala. In A. Krishna, N. Uphoff, & M. J. Esman (Eds.), *Reasons for hope: Instructive experiences in rural development* (pp. 137–152). West Hartford, CT: Kumarian Press.

La Raza (National Council of La Raza). (2013). About us. Retrieved May 11, 2013, from http://www.nclr.org/index.php/about_us/

LaDuke, W. (2005). *Recovering the sacred: The power of naming and claiming*. Cambridge, MA: South End Press.

Lingam, L. (2013). Development theories and community development practice: Trajectory of changes. In In M. Weil, M. Reisch, & M. L. Ohmer (Eds.), *The handbook of community practice* (2nd ed., pp. 195–214). Thousand Oaks, CA: Sage Publications.

Lurie, H. L. (Ed.). (1959). The *community organization method in social work education* (Vol. IV, CSWE Curriculum Study). New York: Council on Social Work Education.

Mackelprang, R. W. (2011). Disability: Overview. In T. Mizrahi & L. E. Davis (Eds.), *Encyclopedia of Social Work* (20th ed., Vol. II, pp. 36–43). Washington DC/New York: NASW/Oxford University Press.

Manning, J. E. (2011, March 1) *Congressional Research Service: Membership of the 112th Congress*. Retrieved May 11, 2013, from http://www.senate.gov/reference/resources/pdf/R41647.pdf

Mattessich, P., Murray-Close, M., & Monsey, B. (2001). *Collaboration: What makes it work* (2nd ed.). St. Paul, MN: Amherst Wilder Foundation.

McConnell, C., & van Gelder, S. R. (2003). *Making peace: Healing a violent world*. Bainbridge Island, WA: Positive Futures Network.

McNutt, J. (2011). Social work practice: History and evolution. In T. Mizrahi & L. E. Davis (Eds.), *Encyclopedia of social work* (20th ed., Vol. 4, pp. 138–141). Washington DC/New York: NASW/Oxford University Press.

Meyer, D. S., & Staggenborg, S. (1996). Movements, counter-movements, and the structure of political opportunity. *American Journal of Sociology*, 101(6), 1628–1660.

Midgley, J., & Conley, A. (2010). *Social work and social development*. New York: Oxford University Press.

Midgley, J., & Livermore, M. (2005). Development theory and community practice. In M. Weil (Ed.), *The handbook of community practice* (pp. 153–168). Thousand Oaks, CA: Sage Publications.

Minkler, M., & Wallerstein, N. (Eds.) (2008). *Community-based participatory research for health: From processes to outcomes* (2nd ed.). San Francisco: Jossey-Bass/Wiley.

Mizrahi, T., & Rosenthal, B. (2001). Complexities of effective coalition building: A study of leaders' strategies, struggles, and solutions. *Social Work*, 46, 63–78.

Mizrahi, T., Rosenthal, B., & Ivery, J. (2013). Coalitions, collaborations and partnerships: Interorganizational approaches to social change. In M. Weil, M. S. Reisch, & M. L. Ohmer (Eds.), *The handbook of community practice* (2nd ed., pp. 383–402). Thousand Oaks, CA: Sage Publications.

Moix, B., Smith, D., & Staab, A. (2004). *Peaceful prevention of deadly conflict: Developing an alternative to war*. Washington, DC: Friends Committee on National Legislation. Retrieved June 13, 2013, from http://fcnl.org/assets/pubs/ppdc_booklet.pdf

Mondros, J. (2013). Political, social and legislative action. In M. Weil, M. Reisch, & M. L. Ohmer (Eds.), *The handbook of community practice* (2nd ed., pp. 345–360). Thousand Oaks, CA: Sage Publications.

Motes, P. S., & Hess, P. M. (2007). *Collaborating with community-based organizations through consultation and technical assistance*. New York: Columbia University Press.

Murphy, P.W., & Cunningham, J.V. (2003). *Organizing for community controlled development: Renewing civil society*. Thousand Oaks, CA: Sage Publications.

Myers, R., & Granstaff, C. (2011). Political social work. In T. Mizrahi & L. Davis (Eds.), *The encyclopedia of social work* (20th ed., Vol. 3, pp. 383–387). New York: Oxford University Press.

National Association of Social Workers (NASW). (2008). *Code of ethics*. Retrieved July, 2012, from http://www.socialworkers.org/pubs/code/code.asp

National Association of Social Workers (NASW). (2000, April 21). NASW supports end to gun violence. Retrieved February 7, 2013, from http://www.naswdc.org/pressroom/2000/042100.asp

National Association of Social Workers (NASW). (2012). NASW Members holding federal, state and local elected office. Retrieved February 7, 2013, from http://www.naswdc.org/pace/state.asp

Netting, F. E., Kettner, P. M., McMurtry, S. L., & Thomas, M. L. (2011). *Social work macro practice* (5th ed.). Boston: Pearson Education/Allyn & Bacon.

Netting, F.E., & O'Connor, M.K. (2013). Program planning and implementation: Designing responses to address community needs. In M. Weil, M. Reisch, & M. L. Ohmer (Eds.), *The handbook of community practice* (2nd ed., pp. 757–772). Thousand Oaks, CA: Sage Publications.

Nussbaum, M. (2011). *Creating capabilities: The human development approach*. Cambridge, MA: Belknap Press of Harvard University Press.

Occupy Together. (2013). Learn about occupy together, background and timeline. Retrieved May 11, 2013, from http://www.occupytogether.org/aboutoccupy/#background

Ohmer, M. L., & Korr, W. S. (2006). The effectiveness of community practice interventions: A review of the literature. *Research on Social Work Practice, 16*(2), 132–145.

Ohmer, M. L., Sobeck, J. L., Teixeria, S., Wallace, J., & Shapiro, V. B. (2013). Community-based research: Rationale, methods, roles, and considerations for community practice. In M. Weil, M. Reisch, & M. L. Ohmer (Eds.), *The handbook of community practice* (2nd ed., pp. 791–808). Thousand Oaks, CA: Sage Publications.

Organization for Economic Cooperation and Development (OECD). (2012). Social Institutions and Gender Index (SIGI). Retrieved May 11, 2013, from http://www.oecd.org/document/39/0,3746,en_2649_33935_42274663_1_1_1_1,00.html

Peeters, J. (2012). Sustainable development: A mission for social work? A normative approach. *Journal of Social Intervention: Theory and Practice, 21*(2), 5–22.

Pennell, J., Noponen, H., & Weil, M. (2005). Empowerment research. In M. Weil (Ed.), *The handbook of community practice* (pp. 620–635). Thousand Oaks, CA: Sage Publications.

PICO National Network. (2013). Unlocking the power of people. Retrieved July 7, 2013, from http://www.piconetwork.org/

Piven, F., & Cloward, R. (1977). *Poor people's movements: Why they succeed and how they fail.* New York: Pantheon.

Price, S. K. (2005). Experience as educator: The journey from clinician to practice-based researcher. *Reflections: Narratives of Professional Helping, 11*(4), 37–47.

Prigoff, A. (2000). *Economics for social workers: Social outcomes of economic globalization with strategies for community action.* Stamford, CT: Thomson Learning, Brooks/Cole.

Putnam, R. D. (2007). *Bowling alone: The collapse and revival of American community.* New York: Simon and Schuster.

Pyles, L. (2009). *Progressive community organizing: A critical approach for a globalizing world.* New York: Routledge.

Raheim, S., Noponen, H., & Alter, C. F. (2005). Supporting women's participation in community economic development: The microcredit strategy. In M. Weil (Ed.), *The handbook of community practice* (pp. 548–565). Thousand Oaks, CA: Sage Publications.

Raworth, K. (2012). A safe and just space for humanity: Can we live within the doughnut? Retrieved May 11, 2013, from http://www.oxfam.org/sites/www.oxfam.org/files/dp-a-safe-and-just-space-for-humanity-130212-en.pdf

Ray, K. (2002). *The nimble collaboration: Fine tuning your collaboration for lasting success.* St. Paul, MN: Wilder Publishing Center.

Reisch, M. (2011). Social movements. In T. Mizrahi & L. Davis (Eds.), *Encyclopedia of social work* (20th ed., Vol. 4, pp. 52–56). New York/Washington DC: Oxford University Press/NASW.

Reisch, M. (2012). Radical community organizing. In M. Weil, M. Reisch, & M. L. Ohmer (Eds.), *The handbook of community practice* (2nd ed., pp. 361–382). Thousand Oaks, CA: Sage Publications.

Reisch, M., Ife, J., & Weil, M. (2013). Social justice, human rights, values and community practice. In M. Weil, M. Reisch, & M. L. Ohmer (Eds.), *The handbook of community practice* (2nd ed., pp. 73–104). Thousand Oaks, CA: Sage Publications.

Rivera, F. G., & Erlich, J. L. (Eds.). (1998). Community organizing in a diverse society (3rd ed.). Needham Heights, MA: Allyn & Bacon.

Robards, K. J., & Gillespie, D. F. (2000). Revolutionizing the social work curriculum: Adding modeling to the systems paradigm. *Journal of Social Work Education, 36*(3), pp. 561–572).

Roberts, J. M. (2004). *Alliances, coalitions and partnerships: Building collaborative organizations.* Gabriola Island, BC, Canada: New Society.

Roberts-DeGennaro, M., & Mizrahi, T. (2005). Coalitions as social change agents. In M. Weil (Ed.), *The handbook of community practice* (pp. 305–318). Thousand Oaks, CA: Sage Publications.

Ross, M. G. (1955). *Community organization: Theory and principles.* New York: Harper & Brothers.

Ross, M. G. (1958). *Case histories in community organization.* New York: Harper & Row.

Rothman, J. (1968). Three models of community organization practice. In J. Rothman (Ed.), *Social Work Practice* (pp. 16–47). New York: Columbia University Press.

Rothman, J. (2008). Multimodes of community intervention. In J. Rothman, J. L. Erlich, & J. E. Tropman (Eds.), *Strategies of community intervention* (7th ed., pp. 141–170). Peosta, IA: Eddie Bowers.

Rubin, H. J., & Rubin, I. S. (2007). *Community organizing and development* (4th ed.). Boston: Allyn & Bacon.

Sager, J. S., & Weil, M. (2013). Larger scale social planning. In M. Weil, M. Reisch, & M. L. Ohmer (Eds.), *The handbook of community practice* (2nd ed., pp. 299–326). Thousand Oaks, CA: Sage Publications.

St. Onge, P. (2013). Cultural competency: Organizations and diverse populations. In M. Weil, M. Reisch, & M. L. Ohmer (Eds.), The handbook of community practice (2nd ed., pp. 425–444). Thousand Oaks, CA: Sage Publications.

Sen, A. (1999). *Development as freedom.* New York: Alfred A. Knopf/Random House.

Schneider, R. L., & Lester, L. (2001). *Social work advocacy.* San Diego: Brooks/Cole.

Schneider, R., Lester, L., & Ochieng, J. (2011). Advocacy. In T. Mizrahi & L. Davis (Eds.), *Encyclopedia of social work* (20th ed., Vol. 1, pp. 59–65). New York/Washington DC: Oxford University Press/NASW Press.

Shiva, V. (2005). *Earth democracy: Justice, sustainability and peace.* Cambridge, MA: South End Press.

Shiva, V. (2008). *Soil not oil: Environmental justice in a time of climate crisis.* Cambridge, MA: South End Press.

Sides, H. (2006). *Blood and thunder: An epic of the American West.* New York: Doubleday.

Sieder, V. M. (1956). What is community organization practice in social work? In *Proceedings of the national conference of social work* (pp. 76–87). New York: Columbia University Press.

Staples, L. (2004). *Roots to power: A manual for grassroots organizing* (2nd ed.). Westport, CT: Praeger.

Stiglitz, J. E. (2012). *The price of inequality: How today's divided society endangers our future.* New York: W. W. Norton.

Toseland, R. W., & Rivas, R. F. (2011). *An introduction to group work practice* (7th ed.). Boston: Pearson Education/Allyn & Bacon

United Farm Workers. (2013). About us. Retrieved July 7, 2013, from http://www.ufw.org/_page.php?menu=about&inc=about_vision.html

United Nations. (1948). Universal declaration of human rights. Retrieved from http://www.un.org/en/documents/udhr

United Nations Millennium development goals. (2013). We can end poverty: 2015 Millennium Development Goals. Retrieved May 11, 2013, from http://www.un.org/millenniumgoals/

United Nations International Day of Persons with Disabilities. (2012). On International Day of Persons with Disabilities, Ban calls for new push to improve access to society. Retrieved February 7, 2013, from http://www.un.org/apps/news/story.asp?NewsID=43663&Cr=disabilities&Cr1=#.USWTqo59m5Q

United Nations Development Program (UNDP). (2003). *Human development report, 2003.* New York: Oxford University Press.

United Nations Development Program (UNDP). (2011). *Human development report, 2011: Sustainability and equity: A better future for all.* Retrieved July 7, 2013, from http://hdr.undp.org/en/reports/global/hdr2011/

United Nations High Commission on Refugees (UNHCR). (2013). About us. Retrieved May 11, 2013, from http://www.unhcr.org/cgi-bin/texis/vtx/home

U.S. Department of Justice. (2013). On the Voter Registration Act of 1993. Retrieved May 11, 2013, from http://www.justice.gov/crt/about/vot/nvra/activ_nvra.php

Uphoff, N., Esman, M. J., & Krishna, A. (1998). *Reasons for success: Learning from instructive experiences in rural development.* West Hartford, CT: Kumarian Press.

Van Soest, D. (1997). *The global crisis of violence: Common problems, universal causes, shared solutions.* Washington, DC: NASW Press.

VeneKlasen, L., & Miller, V. (2007). *A new weave of power, people and politics: The action guide for advocacy and citizen participation.* Warwickshire, UK: Practical Action Publishers.

Wates, T. (2000). *The community planning handbook: How people can shape their cities, towns and villages in any part of the world.* London: Earthscan.

Weber, M. (1970). In J. E. T. Eldridge (Ed.), *Max Weber: The interpretation of social reality.* London: Michael Joseph.

Weil, M. (2005). Social planning with communities: Theory and practice. In M. Weil (Ed.) *The handbook of community practice* (pp. 215–243). Thousand Oaks, CA: Sage Publications.

Weil, M. (2013). Community-based social planning: Theory and practice. In M. Weil, M. Reisch, & M. L. Ohmer (Eds.), *The handbook of community practice* (2nd ed., pp. 265–298). Thousand Oaks, CA: Sage Publications.

Weil, M., Gamble, D. N., & MacGuire, E. (2010). *Community practice skills workbook: Local to global perspectives.* New York: Columbia University Press.

Weil, M., & Ohmer, M. L. (2013). Applying practice theories in community work. In M. Weil, M. Reisch, & M. L. Ohmer (Eds.). *The handbook of community practice* (2nd ed., pp. 123–161). Thousand Oaks, CA: Sage Publications.

Weil, M., Reisch, M., & Ohmer, M. L. (Eds.) (2013a). *The handbook of community practice* (2nd ed.). Thousand Oaks, CA: Sage Publications.

Weil, M., Reisch, M., & Ohmer, M L. (2013b). Introduction. In M. Weil, M. Reisch, & M. L. Ohmer (Eds.). *The handbook of community practice* (2nd ed., pp. 3–25). Thousand Oaks, CA: Sage Publications.

FURTHER READING

Addams, J. (1907). *Newer ideals of peace.* Syracuse, NY: The Mason-Henry Press.

Addams, J. (1945). *Peace and bread in time of war* (1915–1945 anniversary ed.). New York: King's Crown Press.

Association of Community Organization and Social Administration (ACOSA). (2013). Retrieved July, 2013, from http://www.acosa.org/joomla/

Axinn, J., & Stern, M. J. (2000). *Social welfare: A history of the American response to need* (5th ed.). Boston: Allyn & Bacon.

Biklen, D. P. (1983). *Community organizing theory and practice.* Englewood Cliffs, NJ: Prentice-Hall.

Brueggemann, W. G. (2006). *The practice of macro social work* (3rd ed.). Belmont, CA: Thompson Learning, Brooks Cole.

Elliott, D., & Mayadas, N. S. (1996). Social development and clinical practice in social work. *Journal of Applied Social Sciences, 21*(1), 61–68.

Elshtain, J. B. (Ed.). (2002). *The Jane Addams reader.* New York: Basic Books.

Hardcastle, D. A., Powers, P. R., & Wenocur, S. (2004). *Community practice: Theories and skills for social workers* (2nd ed.). New York: Oxford University Press.

Highlander Center. (2013). Highlander Research and Education Center. Retrieved June 13, 2013, from http://www.highlandercenter.org

Hoff, M. (Ed.). (1998). *Sustainable community development: Studies in economic, environmental and cultural revitalization.* Boca Raton, FL: Lewis Publishers.

International Federation of Social Work (IFSW). (2006). International policy statement on globalization and the environment. Retrieved May 11, 2013, from http://www.ifsw.org/en/p38000222.html

Lauffer, A. (2013). Fundraising and community practice: A stakeholder model. In M. Weil, M. Reisch, & M. L. Ohmer (Eds.). *The handbook of community practice* (2nd ed., pp. 773–788). Thousand Oaks, CA: Sage Publications.

Sytz, F. (1960). Jane Addams and social action. *Social Work, 5*(4), 62–67.

Taylor, S. H., & Roberts, R. W. (Eds.). (1985). *Theory and practice of community social work.* New York: Columbia University Press.

Weil, M. (1996). Model development in community practice: An historical perspective. In M. Weil (Ed.), *Community practice: Conceptual models* (pp. 5–67). New York: The Haworth Press.

Weil, M. (2000). Social work in the social environment: Integrated practice—an empowerment/structural approach. In P. Allen-Meares & C. Garvin (Eds.), *Handbook of social work direct practice* (pp. 373–410). Thousand Oaks, CA: Sage Publications.

World Commission on Environment and Development (WCED). (1987). *Our common future*. Oxford, UK: Oxford University Press.

DOROTHY N. GAMBLE AND MARIE WEIL

CRIMINAL JUSTICE: OVERVIEW

ABSTRACT: The criminal justice system traces its roots to ancient times. When the 13 original colonies were formed, they brought many of the laws and legal processes from England. Traditionally, the criminal justice system is viewed as including law enforcement, judiciary, and corrections. However, state legislatures and Congress must be viewed as essential components of the criminal justice system because they pass laws that influence the other three components. A number of controversial practices and policies exist within the criminal justice system. Social work, which has had a long involvement in the criminal justice system, including spearheading the creation of the juvenile justice system in the United States, is involved in all phases of the criminal justice system.

KEY WORDS: law enforcement; probation; parole; judiciary; corrections; capital punishment; restorative justice

The criminal justice system traces its roots to the Sumerian Code and the Code of Hammurabi (Allen, Latessa, & Ponder, 2013). When the American colonies formed, they transported many criminal laws and practices from England. Children and adults were dealt with similarly by the early, fledgling criminal justice system. Child-care advocates from the Progressive Era were able to initiate some separation of children from adults during the development of reformatory institutions. In Chicago in the late 19th century, social workers from Hull-House provided educational services to youth in detention centers. These settlement house workers envisioned a system just for juveniles and collaborated with the Chicago Bar Association and the Illinois Conference of Charities and Corrections to lobby successfully the Illinois legislature to create the first juvenile court in 1899 (Alexander,

1997). Demonstrating the influence of the settlement workers at Hull-House, the first juvenile court was located across the street; the first juvenile court probation officer was a settlement house worker from Hull-House (Alexander). In the 1920s settlement house workers from Cleveland, Ohio, advocated for women who were incarcerated at the Ohio Reformatory for Women, as did other social workers who were actively involved with discharge planning for adult offenders (Alexander, Butler, & Sias, 1993).

Traditionally, the criminal justice system has been envisioned as consisting of three components: law enforcement, judiciary, and corrections. Law enforcement officers, represented by the police, arrest offenders. The judiciary tries these offenders and determines whether they are guilty or not guilty. For those offenders who are adjudicated guilty, corrections manages them by probation, incarceration, and parole. Corrections may be further divided into institution-based (that is, prison or reformatories) and community-based (that is, probation, parole, home confinement, and residential program).

Another important component of the criminal justice system is the legislative arena, which includes state legislatures and Congress. State legislatures and Congress determine behaviors that are criminal in the first place and the sentences to be meted out for those found or pleading guilty. For instance, stalking, computer solicitation of sex with a minor, viewing child pornography on the Internet, and racketeering are relatively new crimes. Legislatures have passed laws that have created new categories of crime, for example, related to various forms of sexual assault and drug possession.

Some laws have been changed to decrease the number of offenders, such as possession of small amounts of marijuana and the killing of one's spouse in response to domestic abuse.

Components of the Criminal Justice System

LAW ENFORCEMENT Police officers, deputies, state troopers, border patrols, and the Federal Bureau of Investigation (FBI) make arrests and initially charge individuals. Most law enforcement officers see their jobs as to protect and serve the community. In 2011, there were 698,460 law enforcement officers (FBI, 2012). Of this total, 88.2% were male and 11.8% were female (FBI, 2012). In 2012, 48 law enforcement officers were killed feloniously in the line of duty (FBI, 2013a). Twenty-two of these officers were killed in the South (FBI, 2013a).

The best source for determining the number of crimes in the United States is data collected by the

FBI for the Uniform Crime Reports and the National Crime Victim Survey (Allen et al., 2013). These data tell us whether crime has increased or decreased over the past year. However, some crimes are not known to the police or are underreported; some do not have individual victims; and some victims may not report crimes, such as domestic assaults.

Since the 1930s, the FBI has submitted yearly reports about statistics regarding yearly arrests for various crimes. Local jurisdictions report their arrests in their jurisdictions. Although not every jurisdiction in the United States participates in this activity, most do, and the Uniform Crime Report offers the best official statistics about crimes in the United States. However, there are still some crimes that are not reported to local law enforcement. Crimes are categorized into Part I crimes, the most serious, and Part II crimes, the other serious crimes. Part I crimes are also called index crimes. These Part I or index crimes are murder/manslaughter, rape, armed robbery, aggravated assault, arson, burglary, larceny–theft, and motor vehicle theft. These crimes are further broken down into violent or personal crimes, consisting of murder, rape, armed robbery, and aggravated assault. Property crimes are grouped; this grouping entails arson, burglary, larceny–theft, and motor vehicle theft. Part II crimes are all crimes that are not considered Part I crimes. The number of crimes is presented by rate, typically per 100,000, which allows comparison of large cities with small cities.

Overall, in 2012, citizens committed 1,214,462 violent crimes, an increase of approximately 0.7% from the amount of violent crimes in 2011 (FBI, 2013b). Still, the number of crimes in 2012 was almost 13% lower than the number of crimes in 2008 and 12% lower than the number of crimes in 2003 (FBI, 2013b). In 2013, the overall violent crime rate was 386.9 violent crimes per 100,000, similar to the rate of violent crimes in 2011 (FBI, 2013b). Of violent crimes, aggravated assaults accounted for 63% reported to law enforcement in 2012; 29% were robberies, almost 7% were rape, and 1.12% were murder (FBI, 2013b). Firearms were used in approximately 70% of murders, 41% of robberies, and 22% of aggravated assaults (FBI, 2013b). In 2012, 84,376 forcible rapes were reported to law enforcement, constituting 52.9 per 100,000 females (FBI, 2013b). The number of rapes was about 0.2% higher than in 2011, 7% lower than in 2008, and 10% lower than in 2003 (FBI, 2013b).

To improve data collection regarding crime, the FBI created the National Incident-Based Reporting System. Its purpose is to improve data collection from the Uniform Crime Report. The system provides more detailed information for each single crime occurrence. Employed to its full potential at the agency level, the National Incident-Based Reporting System tells precisely when and where a crime takes place, what form it takes, and the characteristics of its victims and perpetrators. This system is better able to assess the scope of the nation's crime problem. For example, in 2012 there were 5,001,060 criminal incidents in the United States (FBI, 2013c). This total yielded 5,734,653 offenses, 6,050,049 victims, and 4,556,193 known offenders (FBI, 2013c).

On a directive from Congress, in 1992 the FBI began reporting data on hate crimes in the United States. In 2012, a total of 1,730 law enforcement agencies stated that 6,718 offenses occurred to be categorized as hate; these constituted 5,796 hate crimes (FBI, 2013d). These offenses involved 7,151 victims and 5,322 offenders (FBI, 2013c). Particularly, 49.2% of these hate crimes were racially motivated (FBI, 2013d). The second percentage, 19.2%, was motivated by sexual orientation (FBI, 2013c). Religious bias was third and represented 17.4% (FBI, 2013c). Twelve percent concerned ethnicity or national origin bias (FBI, 2013d). Racially, 66.1% represented anti-bias and 22.4% were anti-White bias (FBI, 2013c). In addition, Sandholtz, Langton, and Planty (2013) reported and compared hates crimes from 2003 to 2006 and from 2007 to 2011. The majority of hate crimes were racially based, comprising over 60% from 2003 to 2006 compared to about 55% from 2007 to 2011 (Sandholtz et al., 2013). Unlike the statistics in the previous paragraph, these researchers had a category of association hate crimes, which represented slightly less than 30% from 2003 to 2006 and slightly more than 30% from 2007 to 2011 (Sandholtz et al.). Religious-based hate crimes increased from 10% from 2003 to 2006 to slightly more than 21% from 2007 to 2011 (Sandholtz et al.). There was a slight increase in hate crimes based on sexual orientation, from 16% from 2003 to 2006 to approximately 18% from 2007 to 2011 (Sandholtz et al.).

JUDICIARY The judiciary consists of the trial process, which generally involves the judge, prosecutors, defense attorneys, and juries. However, most cases are decided by plea bargains and only a small number of cases actually go to trial. Estimates are that more than 90% of cases are decided by plea bargains or nolo contendere, that is, a plea meaning that the defendant does not wish to contest the charges (Lynch, 2003). In 2002, a total of 1,114,000 adults were convicted in federal and state courts for felonies. Approximately 94% of this total was in state courts and 69% were sentenced to incarceration either in prison or in the local jails (Bureau of Justice Statistics, 2006).

The judiciary may decide whether to try a juvenile in juvenile court or adult court. In some states the legislatures have taken this decision out of the hands of prosecutors and judges and mandated that some juveniles and children as young as 12 years be tried as adults if these children have been accused of murder or other very serious offenses (Allard & Young, 2002).

The judiciary is also involved in cases in which a convicted defendant has filed an appeal for his or her conviction or sentence. This is especially so in capital cases where the death penalty has been imposed. A capital case may be in state and federal appellate courts for 15 to 20 years before a death sentence is actually carried out. Often, the U.S. Supreme Court is the final court in a death penalty case but the Court may refuse to intervene and decide a case. Snell (2013) reported that at the end of 2011, a total of 3,082 individuals were under the death sentence. More than half of persons sentenced to death were in California, Florida, Texas, and Pennsylvania (Snell). Most persons under the death sentence were White, a total of 55%; 42% were Black and 14% were Hispanic (Snell). Only 2% of persons under the death sentence were female. From 2000 to 2011, the percentages of persons under the death sentences remained unchanged (Snell).

CORRECTIONS At the end of 2005, almost 5 million adult men and women were under the control of federal, state, and local probation and parole jurisdictions. Of this total, about 4,162,500 were on probation and about 784,400 were on parole. In terms of incarceration, at the end of 2005, a total of 2,193,798 prisoners were held in federal or state prisons or in local jails. The incarceration rates for racial groups were as follows: African American males, 3,145 per 100,000; Latino males, 1,244 per 100,000; and White males, 471 per 100,000. An analysis of trends shows that incarceration in the United States has increased significantly since the 1970s.

Glaze and Herberman (2013) documented that 6,937,600 offenders were under the supervision of the adult criminal justice system at the end of 2012. This number was the fourth consecutive decline in the correction population (Glaze & Herberman). Although Glaze and Herberman did not report race and sex data in their tables, they did provide data from 2000 to 2012 on placements in community corrections and percentages of crimes for several years.

For example, the United States had 3,060 per 100,000 adults supervised by the correctional system in 2000, but that amount decreased to 2,870 per 100,000 in 2012 (Glaze & Herberman). The United States had 2,160 per 100,000 adults under community supervision in 2000 compared to 1,980 adults per 100,000 in 2012 (Glaze & Herberman). In terms of the incarcerated population, there were 920 adults per 100,000 in 2000 compared to 920 per 100, 000 in 2012 (Glaze & Herberman). However, in 2006, 2007, and 2008, the United States had 1,000 adults per 100,000 incarcerated (Glaze & Herberman). According to traditional practice, probation constituted the most utilized sanction by the criminal justice system.

The Bureau of Justice defines probationers as offenders confined in the community in lieu of incarceration as well as those allowed to remain in their homes (often with electronic monitoring). Parolees are offenders supervised in the community after serving a prison term. Parole boards decide whether to release inmates to community-based parole supervision. The federal government and some states have abolished parole.

STATE LEGISLATURES AND CONGRESS Legislative bodies are often overlooked as part of the criminal justice system, but they make laws and decide what criminal conduct is. Prior to 1990, there was no law forbidding stalking. A police officer in Ohio was convicted of multiple counts of stalking–fourth-degree felonies (State v. Barnhardt, 2006). In addition, laws regarding computer behaviors have been enacted, and police officers are now on the lookout for cybersex predators. Also, legislatures have authorized adult trials for some children who have been accused of serious crimes, such as school shootings; adult trials have occurred for children as young as 12 years. Since the 1980s, Congress has actively persuaded states to reform some of their laws by tying the receipt of federal funds to changes in states laws. For example, most states have Megan laws, which require states to notify people when sex offenders have moved into their neighborhoods. In addition, some states have passed laws permitting civil commitment of sex offenders to prevent these offenders from being released from prison confinement. Last, some states have passed laws, such as Three Strikes, permitting the sentencing of felons who have been convicted three times to receive life sentences.

CONTROVERSIES WITHIN THE CRIMINAL JUSTICE SYSTEM A number of controversies exist within the criminal justice system, at all levels and in all components. In law enforcement, the primary criticisms are racial profiling and police brutality. Studies have been conducted on the extent to which race is a factor in police stops of minorities, particularly African Americans, both on streets and on highways. Widely publicized, brutal incidents involving African Americans or people of color and police officers, many of whom are White, make matters worse. Prominent examples include the Rodney King beating by officers in California; the Abner Louima incident, in which a Haitian was sodomized with a stick while in police custody; the Amadou Diallo incident, in which Diallo was fired at 41 times and killed; and more recently, the incident in New York when Sean Bell was shot at more than 50 times and killed after he and his friends left a bachelor party. These incidents, as well as many other incidents that do not make the news but are known within the African American community, make it difficult for law enforcement to establish a collaborative and trusting relationship with the African American community to address crime in the community (Alexander, 2005b).

RACIAL AND ETHNIC DISPARITIES EXIST IN THE CRIMINAL JUSTICE SYSTEM African Americans are overrepresented among those incarcerated (Mauer, 2006). Reports have been issued on the high number of African Americans who are under the control of prisons, probation, and parole (Mauer). The high number of African Americans in prisons cannot be viewed in isolation because it is the judiciary system that sends them to prisons and it is the law enforcement system, backed sometimes by laws passed by the legislatures, that initiates entrance into the judiciary system.

To illustrate, since the 1980s, differential, and what some characterize as discriminatory, laws punish possession of crack cocaine more seriously than possession of powder cocaine. Cocaine is an expensive drug, and many users are actors, actresses, athletes, and business executives, many of whom are White. Crack cocaine was developed to make cocaine affordable for poor people—poor Whites, Latinos, and African Americans. Crack cocaine is punished more harshly than equal amounts of powered cocaine. With the help of racial profiling, a high number of African Americans are stopped, searched, and arrested for possessing crack cocaine. Although African Americans have complained since the 1980s, most legislatures have failed to act or make the punishments more equal.

To illustrate this point, a U.S. District Court judge, who was a drug policy adviser to the first President Bush and who then advocated for tough laws for crack cocaine crimes, stated that "the policy had gone too far and was undermining faith in the judicial system" (Apuzzo, 2006, p. A7). Trafficking in 500g of powder cocaine carries a five-year sentence but it takes only 5g of crack cocaine to get a sentence of five years—a 100-to-1 disparity. Judge Reggie B. Walton noted that crack is an inner-city drug and cocaine is a suburban drug; the differences in punishment are unconscionable and "contributed to the perception within minority communities that courts are unfair" (Apuzzo, p. A7).

The Federal Sentencing Commission has asked Congress thrice to address the sentencing disparity between cocaine and crack but it had refused to do so. Congress has not even been willing to increase the punishment for cocaine (Apuzzo, 2006), although it proclaimed to have a war on drugs. This failure to increase the penalty for cocaine possession may be attributable to race because it affects mostly Whites (Alexander, 2005b).

However, in 2010, President Obama signed the Fair Sentencing Act, which reduced the disparity between powder cocaine and crack cocaine (Lee, 2010). In 2013, President Obama used this law to reduce the sentences of 8 federal prisoners and pardoned 13 others (Flatow, 2013).

Some observers point to the high number of African Americans involved in drugs, violent crimes, and weapons possession as to why there are disproportionately more African Americans than Whites in prison. Alexander (2005b) points out that Whites commit most of the violent crimes in the United States, use the most drugs, and are more likely to be arrested for possessing weapons. The FBI defines serious crimes or Part I crimes as (a) murder or manslaughter, (b) rape, (c) aggravated assault, (d) armed robbery, (e) burglary, (f) arson, and (g) theft; violent crimes include the first four. In 2003, 61% of those arrested for violent crimes were White and 37% were African American (U.S. Department of Justice, 2004). Although this pattern has been shown consistently, many Americans still believe that African Americans are responsible for the most serious crimes in the United States. As an illustration, African Americans constitute approximately 33% of persons arrested for sex crimes, but they are frequently depicted as the most common rapists, an image that has a long history in the United States. However, although Whites are more likely to be arrested for drug crimes and weapons possession, they do not go to prison in numbers comparable to their arrests. The same pattern is found among White juveniles; they too are not committed to juvenile incarceration proportionately.

Snyder (2012) presented a fairly comprehensive table on arrests. It described the number of arrests by sex, race, and perpetrator status, including whether the perpetrator was an adult or juvenile. As an illustration, in 2010, a total of 9,792,190 males were arrested compared to 3,329,920 females. Of the total number of arrests, 11,479,470 adults were arrested and 1,642,650 juveniles. By race, 9,122,010 were White and 3,655,620 were Black. The statistics involving race mirrored the statistics and arguments made by Alexander (2006). Some conservatives explain the overrepresentation of Blacks in the criminal justice system as being the result of Blacks committing more violent crimes, carrying weapons illegally, and being involved with drugs. Alexander (2006) disputes this assertion. Of the most serious crimes in 2010, the only crime in which Blacks exceed Whites was robbery, 62,020 to 48,310 (Snyder). The murder numbers were slightly higher for Whites than for Blacks, 5,540 to 5,430 (Snyder). For forcible rape, Whites outnumbered Blacks by 13,210 to 6,300 (Snyder) and Whites also outnumbered Blacks in arrests for aggravated assaults, 260,770 to 136,400 (Snyder). In terms of drugs, there were 1,093,910 Whites arrested and 519,830 Blacks (Snyder). For weapons violations, 92,630 Whites were arrested compared to 63,710 Blacks (Snyder).

It may not be well known that many African Americans are incarcerated in prisons located in rural areas; as a result, their incarceration benefits rural communities for census purposes and grants obtained at the expense of urban areas from where most prisoners come. Stinebrickner-Kauffman (2004) was one of the first to question the legality of the census bureau counting prisoners where they are incarcerated. Alexander (2005a), picking up on Stinebrickner-Kauffman's argument, explored other implications of this phenomenon, noting how additional monies have been used to help rural communities. He argued that most offenders commit their crimes in their own communities and in fact have damaged their communities. Thus, if money is generated from incarceration, then it should go to the community in which the damage has been done. In fact, this is the central argument of restorative justice, which seeks to motivate offenders to repair the harm they have done to the community (Alexander, 2006).

There is also the issue of the collateral damage done to the African American community by the get-tough-on-crime campaigns (Mauer, 2003, 2006). Convictions and imprisonment for a large number of African Americans carry considerable damage, such as loss of voting rights and employment discrimination. Pager (2003) sought to test the impact of an antidiscrimination law in Wisconsin that banned discrimination against ex-felons when the convictions had nothing to do with a job being sought. She tested for entry-level jobs requiring only a high school education. On the basis of a tactic long used to detect housing discrimination by landlords, Pager gave Whites and African Americans the same profile of drug convictions and prison sentences. She then gave another group of Whites and African Americans no criminal records when they applied for jobs in the city of Milwaukee. Her dependent variable was whether an employer called the applicant offering a job after the interview. Pager found that 34% of Whites without records received callbacks, compared with 17% of Whites with a criminal record. For African Americans, 14% of those who had no criminal records received callbacks, compared with 5% of African Americans with criminal records. Simply put, a White man with a criminal record has a better chance of getting a job than does an African American man without a criminal record. This discrimination occurred in a state with protective legislation, which means that discrimination may be worse in states without such laws.

Other controversial issues in the criminal justice system involve sex offenders and especially child molesters. Indeed, some child sex offenders have killed children in the process of assaulting and molesting them. As a result, there has been an outcry to pass legislation that protects children. The two most popular laws have been community notification and restriction of sex offenders from living too close to schools, playgrounds, and community centers (Hundley, 2007). Quoting Allison Taylor, the executive director of the Council on Sex Offender Treatment of the Texas Department of State Health Services, Hundley reported that sexual assaults cannot be stopped by passing an ordinance and there is no evidence that proximity to a school, playground, or child-care center contributed to recidivism by sex offenders. To date, no study has reported that these measures effectively protect children. Children are more likely to be sexually molested by a family member, a neighbor who is not a convicted child molester, a teacher, or a coach (Alexander, 2004). Further, the more popular laws concerning where offenders can live establish 1,000 feet as the boundary. But no research has been reported that shows that children are more likely to be molested within 1,000 feet as opposed to more than 1,000 feet away (Alexander, 2010).

Capital punishment also remains a controversial issue. Society has endeavored to find the most humane method of executing prisoners. In these endeavors, various forms of executions have been tried and subsequently abandoned, including firing squad, hanging, the gas chamber, and the electric chair. Lethal injection was believed to be the most humane method of execution, but even that has come under attack because of some botched executions in Florida and California, wherein executioners could not find veins. Moreover, the U.S. Supreme Court has ruled that executing individuals who were younger than 18 years of age at the time they committed their crimes violated the cruel and unusual clause of the Eighth Amendment to the U.S. Constitution (*Roper v. Simmons*, 2005). In addition, the U.S. Supreme Court ruled that executing someone who is mentally retarded also violated the prohibition against cruel and unusual punishment (*Atkins v. Virginia*, 2002). Advocates are seeking a further narrowing of capital punishment by arguing that it is cruel and unusual to execute individuals who were mentally ill at the time they committed their crimes.

Another issue involving capital punishment is that many prisoners have been released from death row and prison because of wrongful convictions. Much of the impetus to this movement has been generated by the Innocence Project, headed by Barry Scheck and Peter Neufeld (The Innocence Project, 2007). This project focuses on using DNA to prove that some convicted persons on death row and in prison were in fact innocent of their crimes. The Innocence Project has a web site where it keeps a running total of the persons who have been exonerated. Special issues in criminal justice and law review journals have been devoted to wrongful convictions (Alexander, 2007).

SOCIAL WORKERS' INVOLVEMENT IN THE CRIMINAL JUSTICE SYSTEM As social work was emerging as a profession in the late 19th and early 20th centuries, some social workers expressed doubts about workers being involved in the criminal justice system because of the lack of self-determination of clients and possible conflicts with social-work values (Alexander, 1997). Criminal justice is not the most popular area for practice among social-work students and professionals. Lennon (2005) reported that only 713 of 26,137 undergraduate students (2.7%) and only 798 of 37,052 postgraduate students (2.2%) were placed in field settings involving criminal justice.

Still, social workers occupy a number of positions inside and related to the criminal justice system. Social workers are employed as institutional counselors and juvenile and adult probation and parole officers. One of the more prominent positions held by social workers is victims' advocate in the legal process. As society became more responsive to victims and

their families, a number of prosecutors' offices began to employ social workers to assist and support victims and families in the courtrooms during trials, at sentencing, and at the time of parole hearings.

In prisons, social workers are typically employed in mental-health units to work with inmates with psychiatric problems. In some states, social workers have become prison wardens.

Some social workers are employed by public defenders offices to work with indigent defendants who need mental-health treatment, substance-abuse treatment, or other specialized services. Also, in the area of employee assistance programs, some social workers have contact with law enforcement officers and provide counseling to them. The counseling may help police officers address challenging issues in their personal lives or difficulty coping with a traumatic incident, such as a shooting.

Social workers must address issues of limits of confidentiality with a duty to warn. As an example, the U.S. Supreme Court case of *Jaffee v. Redmond et al.* (1996) involved the issue of whether a social worker's counseling with an officer was protected as privileged information. In this case, a police officer shot and killed a man and saw a social worker to deal with the trauma. The officer was sued by the family of the deceased, and the plaintiff's lawyer attempted to get the information from the social worker, setting up a legal issue for the U.S. Supreme Court to decide.

Social workers have been prominent in the area of restorative justice—a growing trend. One website reported the addresses of 86 organizations that embraced some aspects of restorative justice (Restorative Justice Online, 2005). Within the School of Social Work at the University of Minnesota, social workers have established the Center for Restorative Justice and Mediation. Furthermore, numerous social workers have written about restorative justice (Adams, 2004; Beck & Britto, 2006; Burford & Adams, 2004; Gumz, 2004; Holtquist, 1999; Umbreit, Coates, & Vos, 2004; van Wormer, 2003, 2006).

In conclusion, the criminal justice system has expanded considerably since the 1970s. The United States incarcerates a high number of its citizens, with minorities being overrepresented in the prison system. Furthermore, the United States executes more persons than other industrialized countries do. Social workers played a prominent role in the creation of the first juvenile court in 1899 and currently act as victims' advocates with the legal system. Recently, social workers have played a prominent role in humanizing the criminal justice system by espousing and embracing restorative justice.

REFERENCES

Adams, P. (2004). Restorative justice, responsive, regulation, and democratic governance. *Journal of Sociology and Social Welfare, 31*(1), 3–5.

Alexander, R., Jr. (1997). Juvenile delinquency and social work practice. In C. A. McNeece & A. Roberts (Eds.), *Social work policy and practices in the justice system* (pp. 181–197). Chicago, IL: Nelson–Hall.

Alexander, R., Jr. (2004). The United States Supreme Court and civil commitment of sex offenders. *Prison Journal, 84,* 361–378.

Alexander, R. Jr. (2005a). The relationship of prisoners, poverty measures, and social welfare allocations in Ohio. *Journal of Policy Journal, 4,* (2), 69–82.

Alexander, R., Jr. (2005b). *Racism, African Americans, and social justice.* Lanham, MD: Rowman & Littlefield.

Alexander, R., Jr. (2006). Restorative justice: Misunderstood and misapplied. *Journal of Policy Practice, 5*(1), 67–81.

Alexander, R., Jr. (2007). A wrongful conviction from Georgia. *Journal of the Institute of Justice and International Studies, 7,* 75–89.

Alexander, R., Jr. (2010). *Beyond micro: A macro perspective of human behavior and the social environment.* Newbury, CA: Sage.

Alexander, R., Jr., Butler, L., & Sias, P. (1993). Woman offenders incarcerated at the Ohio penitentiary for men and the Ohio reformatory for women from 1913–1923. *Journal of Sociology and Social Welfare, 20*(3), 61–79.

Allard, P., & Young, M. (2002). *Prosecuting juveniles in adult court: Perspectives for policymakers and practitioners.* Washington, DC: The Sentencing Project.

Allen, H. E., Latessa, E. J., & Ponder, B. S. (2013). *Corrections in America: An introduction.* Upper Saddle River, NJ: Prentice Hall.

Apuzzo, M. (2006, November 15). Federal judge decries disparity in cocaine sentencing. *Columbus Dispatch,* p. A7.

Atkins v. Virginia, 536 U.S. 304 (2002).

Beck, E., & Britto, S. (2006). Using feminist methods and restorative justice to interview capital offenders' family members. *Afflilia: Journal of Women and Social Work, 21*(1), 59–70.

Bureau of Justice Statistics (2006a). Probation and parole statistics. Retrieved December 27, 2006, from http://www.ojp.usdoj.gove/bjs/pandp.htm/

Burford, G., & Adams, P. (2004). Restorative justice, responsive regulation and social work. *Journal of Sociology and Social Welfare, 31*(1), 7–26.

Federal Bureau of Investigation (FBI). (2012). *Crime in the United States 2011.* Retrieved from http://www.fbi.gov/about-us/cjis/ucr/leoka/2012/officers-feloniously-killed/felonious_topic_page_-2012/

Federal Bureau of Investigation (FBI). (2013a). *Officers feloniously killed.* Retrieved from http://www.fbi.gov/about-us/cjis/ucr/leoka/2012/officers-feloniously-killed/felonious_topic_page_-2012/

Federal Bureau of Investigation (FBI). (2013b). *Crimes in the United States, 2012.* Retrieved from http://www.fbi.gov/about-us/cjis/ucr/crime-in-the-u.s/2012/crime-in-the-u.s.-2012/violent-crime/violent-crime/

Federal Bureau of Investigation (FBI). (2013c). *2012 National incident-reporting system.* Retrieved from http://www.fbi.gov/about-us/cjis/ucr/nibrs/2012/

Federal Bureau of Investigation (FBI). (2013d). *2012 hate crime statistics.* Retrieved from http://www.fbi.gov/about-us/cjis/ucr/hate-crime/2012/topic-pages/incidents-and-offenses/incidentsandoffenses_final/

Flatow, N. (2013, December 19) *Obama uses pardon power to release prisoners sentenced under draconian drug laws.* Retrieved from http://thinkprogress.org/justice/2013/12/19/3090681/obama-uses-pardon-power-release-prisoners-sentenced-draconian-drug-laws/#/

Glaze, L. E, & Herberman, E. J. (2013). *Correctional populations in the United States, 2012.* Washington, DC: Bureau of Justice Statistics.

Gumz, E. J. (2004). American social work, corrections and restorative justice: An appraisal. *International Journal of Offender Therapy and Comparative Criminology, 48*(4), 449–460.

Holtquist, S. E. (1999). Nurturing the seeds of restorative justice. *Journal of Community Practice, 6*(2), 63–77.

Hundley, W. (2007, November). Cities' residency restrictions don't move registered sex offenders. *Dallas Morning News,* Retrieved November 13, 2007, from http://www.dallasnews.com/sharedcontent/dws/news/localnews/stories/110407dnmetsexordinance.2cee065.html/

The Innocence Project. (2007). *The faces of exonerations.* Retrieved November 13, 2007, from http://www.innocenceproject.org/

Jaffee v. Redmond et al., 518 U.S. 1 (1996).

Lee, J. (2010). *President Obama signs the Fair Sentencing Act.* Retrieved from http://www.whitehouse.gov/blog/2010/08/03/president-obama-signs-fair-sentencing-act/

Lennon, T. M. (2005). *Statistics on social work education in the United States: 2003.* Alexandria, VA: Council on Social Work Education.

Lynch, T. (2003, Fall). The case against plea bargaining. *Regulation, 26,* 24–27.

Mauer, M. (2003). *Lessons of the get tough movement in the United States.* Washington, DC: The Sentencing Project.

Mauer, M. (2006). *Race to incarcerate.* New York, NY: New Press.

Pager, D. (2003). The mark of a criminal record. *American Journal of Sociology, 108,* 937–975.

Restorative Justice Online. (2005). *Restorative justice sites listed alphabetically.* Retrieved November 13, 2007, from http://www.restorativejustice.org/

Roper v. Simmons, 543 U.S. 551 (2005).

Sandholtz, N., Langton, L., & Planty, M. (2013). *Hate crime victimization, 2003–2011.* Washington, DC: Bureau of Justice Statistics.

Snell, T. L. (2013). *Capital punishment, 2011—Statistical tables.* Washington, DC: Bureau of Justice Statistics.

Snyder, H. N. (2012). *Arrest in the United States, 1990–2010.* Washington, DC: Bureau of Justice Statistics.

State v. Barnhardt, 2006 Ohio 4531; 2006 Ohio App. LEXIS 4495.

Stinebrickner-Kauffman, T. (2004). Counting matters: Prison inmates, population bases, and "one person, one vote." *Virginia Journal of Social Policy and the Law,* 11, 229–305.

Umbreit, M., Coates, R. B., & Vos, B. (2004). Restorative justice versus community justice: Clarifying a muddle or generating confusion? *Contemporary Justice Review,* 7(1), 81–89.

U.S. Department of Justice. (2004). *Crime in the United States, 2003.* Washington, DC: Author.

van Wormer, K. (2003). Restorative justice: A model for social work practice with families. *Families in Society,* 84(3), 441–448.

van Wormer, K. (2006). The case for restorative justice: A crucial adjunct to the social work curriculum. *Journal of Teaching in Social Work,* 26(3/4), 57–69.

FURTHER READING

Bureau of Labor Statistics. (2006). *Occupational outlook handbook, 2006–07 edition.* Probation officers and correctional treatment specialists. Retrieved December 29, 2006, from http://www.ait.org.tw/infousa/enus/economy/workforce/docs/OOH_2006.pdf/

RUDOLPH ALEXANDER JR.

CULTURAL COMPETENCE

ABSTRACT: Cultural competence emerged as a concept in the 1980s, took form as a set of organizational, educational, advocacy, policy, and practice constructs in the 1990s, and has since matured into a broad rubric that addresses social justice and service delivery quality, equity, access, and efficacy for people and groups of diverse backgrounds. Cultural competence has become an essential element of social work at every level of the field, from direct practice to social policy. The evolution of cultural competence and its role in social work is examined and summarized in this entry.

KEY WORDS: cultural competence; cultural competency; ethno-cultural competence; social justice; cultural relevance; cultural awareness; diversity

This is an overview of cultural competence generally with a particular focus on organizations, systems, and policy level issues. Cultural competence has been defined in social work practice as the capacity to function effectively as a helper in the context of cultural differences (Cross, 2007). It has also been defined at the organizational and systems level as a set of congruent policies, structures, procedures, and practices that together enable and empower social work service providers to work effectively in cross-cultural situations (Cross, Bazron, Dennis, & Issacs, 1989; SAHMSA, 1997).

History

Cultural competence has its roots in a rapidly changing demographic context, in a shifting political environment, in social advocacy and action (Lum, 2007), as well as in social justice theory (Van Soest & Garcia, 2003), ethnic sensitivity (Devore & Schlesinger, 1999) and cultural awareness models (Green, 1999). Cultural competence emerged as a theoretical construct in the 1980s and developed into a generally accepted framework for multicultural practice by the late 1990s. "We can trace a historical progression of related multicultural themes such as ethnic sensitivity, cultural awareness, cultural diversity, and now cultural competence. These concepts are not mutually exclusive. Rather, cultural competence serves as a rubric that embraces these areas of concern" (Lum, 2007).

In the 1950s and 1960s the civil rights movement, along with the War on Poverty and the Great Society policy initiatives, transformed the relationship between social work and people of color in the United States (Gutierrez, Zuniga, & Lum, 2004; Schram, Soss, & Fording, 2003). Prior to this period social work was almost exclusively a profession made up of White service providers. Services to communities of color, if available at all, were predominantly aimed at rescuing, assimilating, or maintaining the status quo. For example, social work was largely responsible for the assimilationist transracial adoption programs of the 1950s and 1960s that saw thousands of American Indian children separated from their families without due process or services ever being offered to families (Mallon & McCartt Hess, 2005). At the same time, social work services were virtually unavailable to most African, Hispanic, or Asian Americans (Karger & Stoesz, 2005). African Americans in some states were systematically excluded from aid to families with dependent children by race-biased eligibility rules (Kiltz & Segal, 2006; Schram, Soss, & Fording, 2003).

The important results of the 1960s civil rights struggles, policy shifts, and progressive programs were the educational rights and resources secured by people of color. Social work education opportunities for people of color expanded rapidly, from funds channeled through the National Institute for Mental Health, the Children's Bureau, and the Indian Health Service, to mention only a few. During the 1970s and into the early 1980s an entire generation of social workers of color entered the field through these opportunities only to find that even with a formal social work education, they were ill prepared to practice in their own communities. The theories, models, and practices learned in the course of their social work education proved to be ethnocentric. In addition, many people of color realized that most mainstream social workers serving communities of color were using methods and practices in these communities that were ineffective at best and at worst damaging (Gutierrez, Zuniga, & Lum 2004; Van Soest & Garcia, 2003).

Young professionals of color began to search for answers. Many began to formulate new practice models, advance new theories, advocate for their communities, and to provide cultural awareness training. Some became the social work educators who would craft a new framework for practice in a multicultural society. Social workers of color working as grassroots advocates began to hold their mainstream collogues accountable through advocacy for individual clients, or whole communities. Professional organizations, child advocacy organizations, and branches of government came under pressure to address the issues presented by professionals of color, eventually leading to the development of, or changes in, standards, codes of ethics, and policies (Lum, 2007). By 2011, cultural competence was well integrated as a cornerstone of ethical social work practice by Dolgoff, Loewenberg, and Harrington (2011) in *Ethical Decisions for Social Work Practice*.

Literature

Literature by social workers of color began producing helpful direction on working cross-culturally. At first, this literature was largely aimed at understanding ethnic culture, discussing a particular group, their life-ways, and the implications for social work. Journal articles published in the 1970s were the first to begin to address these issues. In the early 1980s books began to appear, such as *Ethnic Sensitive Social Work Practice* by Devore and Schlesinger (1981) and *Cultural Awareness in the Human Services* by Green and Associates (1982). These were important early works in the evolution of what would become the encompassing rubric known as cultural competence. Green and Associates (1982) coined the term *ethnic competence* and was the first to discuss a theoretical framework for effective cross-cultural practice that was not ethnic group specific. By the mid-1980s social workers of color were beginning to use the term *cultural competence* in training events, conference presentations, and school of social work electives. In 1988 a series of nonattributed articles on cultural competence were published in *Focal Point* (see Cross, 2007). One of these articles, "What Is a Culturally Competent Profes-

sional" (Cross, 2007), proposes five conditions for the development of culturally competent practices. These five conditions—(a) awareness and acceptance of difference, (b) cultural self-awareness, (c) understanding the dynamics of difference, (d) developing cultural knowledge, and (e) adaptation of practice skills to fit the cultural context of the client—were largely based on the work of Green and Associates (1982). They would become central to uniting several related theories and models under the rubric of cultural competence.

These articles, written by Cross and Mason (McManus, 1988), also provided much of the content for the seminal work *Toward a Culturally Competent System of Care* (Cross et al.) published in 1989. This monograph provides a definition for organizational cultural competence at the mesolevel and describes a continuum of competence evidenced by organizations (Cross et al., 1989). This work is considered the first systematic treatment of the topic (Lum, 2007). Also in 1989, Penderhughes described culturally competent practice in her book *Understanding Race, Ethnicity, and Power*: "Cultural Competence demands that clinicians develop flexibility in thinking and behavior, because they must learn to adapt professional tasks and work styles to the values, expectations, and preferences of specific clients" (Penderhughes, 1989). In Lum's 1997 hallmark work *Culturally Competent Practice* cultural competence is conceptualized as a framework for practice. Lum's first comprehensive treatment of the subject is followed up with second and third editions. Van Soest and Garcia (2003) bring cultural competence back to its roots with their social work education text *Diversity Education for Social Justice: Mastering Teaching Skills*. In it they criticize the cultural competence movement for not holding social justice as the true compass and declare that without addressing racism and discrimination there can be no cultural competence. The issue is further illuminated by Abrams and Mojo (2009), who address the challenges of extending the application of cultural competence beyond race and suggest an alternative approach. By the turn of the century, cultural competence has evolved into "a major subject area for culturally diverse social work practice and a process of individual and professional growth" (Lum, 2007). Further criticism of cultural competence has been raised by authors who judge cultural competence to be unachievable and fundamentally contrary to the social work value of self-determination and individuality (Johnson & Munch, 2009). Despite criticism and proposed alternatives, cultural competence remains the guiding rubric for the field and the leading catalyst for dialogue.

Policy Developments

During the 1990s, several professional organizations, federal agencies, and state governments began to embrace the principles of cultural competence as expressed by Cross et al. (1989). Organizations such as the Child Welfare League of America developed committees that drafted cultural competence position statements, policies, or standards. In the field of psychology and counseling, organizations such as the American Association for Counseling and Development identified competencies for multicultural counseling (Sue, Arrendondo, & McDavis, 1992). By 1993, the American Psychological Association had committed itself to multicultural competence (APA, 1993; Lum, 2007). In the mid-1990s the Substance Abuse and Mental Health Services Administration began including cultural competence as a criterion for grant applications and in 1997 published its own definition of cultural competence based on the work of Cross et al. (1989). In 1995, Mason published an organizational self-assessment for cultural competence, further advancing the field.

In 1999, the National Association of Social Workers (NASW, 2001) adopted language on cultural competence into the *NASW Code of Ethics*, for the first time making the delivery of culturally competent services an ethical issue. In 2001, the NASW "Standards for Cultural Competence in Social Work Practice" adopted a broad meaning of *cultural* "to include sociocultural experience of people of different genders, social class, religious and spiritual beliefs, sexual orientations, ages, and physical and mental abilities" (Lum, 2007; NASW, 2001). This move formally recognized the growing pressure from advocates of diverse backgrounds for the social work field to be competent across a range of differences, not just ethno-cultural. In so doing, the rubric of cultural competence gained momentum, stakeholders, and allied scholars. At the same time, expanding the definition of *culture* brought debate. Ridley (2005) discusses this debate, questioning the application of the term *cultural* to other diverse people. Lum (2007) concludes that as long as advocates for these groups make a case for application of the cultural competence framework to their experience there will be broad application.

In 2002, under pressure from advocates of color and other diverse populations within the social work education community, the Council on Social Work Education (CSWE) adopted diversity standards that encompass and advance the established frameworks for culturally competent social work. In addition, the CSWE standards on social and economic justice further address cultural diversity, reinforcing the social justice aspect of cultural competence. Although not using the term *cultural competence* directly, the standards provide clear guidelines and professional sanction for the growing movement (see Educational Policy and Accreditation Standards, 2002.) CSWE has become one of the leading publishers of cultural competence literature. With the direct involvement of diverse social work educators, it has become a key resource for social work educators to build the depth and breadth of the cultural competence in professional social work education.

Controversies

As the cultural competence movement progressed, it generated confusion regarding its definition and application. In part, this is a product of the complexity of the issues it addresss, but it is also because many authors have approached the issues from diverse perspectives. Lum (2007) outlines several levels and dimensions of cultural competence and reviews the literature addressing the issue at the micro (practice), meso (agency), and macro (system) levels. Miley, O'Melia, and Dubois (1998) also discuss cultural competence at the practitioner, agency, and community levels. Cross et al. (1989) discuss how a culturally competent system requires effective individual cross-cultural practice and appropriate organizational level values, policies, structures, and programs that are supported by system-wide policies, regulations, and funding mechanisms that empower both individual and agency multicultural service delivery. The National Center for Cultural and Linguistic Competence at Georgetown University Child Development Center provides several useful tools for organizational development of cultural competence (http://gucchd.georgetown.edu .nccc/pa.html). Nybell and Gray (2004) address the inherent conflictual nature of achieving cultural competence within organizations. In their study of several organizations they found that achieving cultural competence required a redistribution of power toward clients, programs, and communities of color, and in reality most predominantly mainstream social service agencies are reluctant to relinquish control to disenfranchised people. Further, Abrams and Mojo (2009) review several studies regarding the challenges of teaching this model in social work education, including both student readiness and instructor preparedness, but cite shortcomings of the model itself as the underlying issue.

Advancements

Among the works addressing cultural competence at the level of the professional field are those of Ponterotto, Casas, Suzuki, and Alexander (1995), Pope-Davis and

Coleman (1997), Fong and Furuto (2001), Fong (2004), Constantine and Sue (2005), and Orlandi, Weston, and Epstein (1992). Each of these authors has contributed to the advancement of cultural competence through documenting examples of implementation and providing insights into emerging efforts to advance the cross-cultural effectiveness of the field. Further, Straussner (2001) uses the term *ethnocultural competence* to describe the complex contextual issues of cross-cultural practice and provides insight into the deeper dimensions of effective cross-cultural practice. Finally, Lum (2007) provides a comprehensive look into the richness of culturally competent practice with his framework for culturally competent practice that poses four levels, each with generalist and advanced characteristics. The first is cultural awareness, both personally and professionally, of diverse people and the oppression that impacts them. The second is the acquisition of cultural knowledge that plausibly explains behavior. The third is skill development based on the awareness and acquired knowledge. The fourth is inductive learning, which is characterized by innovation and contribution of new insights to the field (Lum, 2007).

A significant paradigm shift is evidenced in these discussions. Where the early works emphasized understanding of specific cultural groups and their values and lifeways as the unit of study, the most recent works emphasize culture, culturally based experiences, and power dynamics as the units of study. This shift is away from the notion that the practitioner should simply know about a person's cultural group. The practitioner should now be able to understand and adapt to the following: the person's experience of his or her culture, the specific social and mental health challenges experienced by people of any specific group, the dynamics of power differentials, and identity and oppression and their impact on behavior. It is the complex interplay between personality and the sociocultural environment that accounts for human behavior. In this new paradigm for multicultural practice, social and economic justice are placed at the forefront of achieving competence. Lum (2007) states, "The social context of diversity, racism, sexism, homophobia, discrimination, and oppression is with us as we help people with problems. The message is that these contextual factors must be confronted and dealt with on a constant basis." Increasingly, social service systems and agencies are recognized as being part of the sociocultural environment. Cultural competence is not just about the relationship between worker and client but about creating organizations that are accountable for ensuring that their services and policy not only reach diverse populations but are relevant to their culturally based needs and to the pursuit of social justice.

Advancements in social work theory have also emerged from scholars of color whose ideas have come to light via the empowerment afforded them by the movement itself. This is particularly true among indigenous scholars. Blackstocks' "Breath of Life Theory" (2009, 2011) informs social work based on Indigenous thought. Likewise, work by Weaver (1999, 2009) on historic trauma and identity is providing social work with important and unique perspectives not heretofore available to the field.

Converging Theories

While the concepts foundational to cultural competence anchor the field, new and emerging theories continue to impact our understanding of cultural competence. The theory of social constructionism (Norton, 1993) relates to the process by which "people use the ecology of their environment to construct meaning for themselves based on their experiences" (Lum, 2007). Applied to cultural competence, this theory supports the paradigm that encourages culture as a unit of study. Identity development theory (Morton & Atkinson, 1983) also supports the notion of a complex interplay between personality and culture both of which are influenced and shaped by personal experience. Fong and Furuto (2001) in their work *Culturally Competent Practice: Skills, Interventions, and Evaluations* advance several theories of cultural competent practice in line with the paradigm shift described earlier. Theories regarding ethnicity, culture, minority status, social class, and acculturation (Devore & Schlesinger, 1999; Gordon, 1978; Green, 1999; Inglehart & Becerra, 1995; Paniagua, 2005) are essential to culturally diverse practice (see Lum, 2007, pp. 157–182, for a full discussion).

Implications for Social Work

Cultural competence is an ethical obligation, a professional standard, a defined practice framework with its own knowledge base and skill set and established principles for effective multicultural service delivery at the practice, agency, and system levels. It is about the complex interplay between the individual and the environment and the power dynamics associated with being different. As social work struggles to incorporate social justice with effective practice, it has had to align its institutions, theories, and helping approaches to respond to the growing demands of a shifting demographic and the advocates from diverse cultures that have entered and are now shaping the field. Cultural competence is now evolving through practice and dialogue and continues to be advanced by the thinking of the beneficiaries of its design.

REFERENCES

Abrams, L. S. & Mojo, J. A. (2009). Critical Race Theory and Cultural Competence. *Journal of Social Work Education*, Fall, pp. 245-249. Downloadaed August 2012, from http://164.67.121.27/files/downloads/Critical_Race_Theory_and_Cultural_Competence_Abramsand_Mojo.pdf.

American Psychological Association. [APA]. (1993). Guidelines for providers of psychological services to ethnic, linguistic, and culturally diverse populations. *American Psychologist*, 48, 45–48.

Blackstock, C. (2009). Why addressing the over-representation of First Nations children in care requires a new theoretical approach. *Journal of Social Work Values and Ethics*, 6(3).

Blackstock, C. (2011). The emergence of the breath of life theory. *Journal of Social Work Values and Ethics*, 8(1), 1–16.

Constantine, M. G., & Sue, D. W. (Eds.). (2005). The American Psychological Association's guidelines on multicultural education, training, research, practice, and organizational psychology: Initial development and summary. In M. G. Constantine & D. W. Sue (Eds.), *Strategies for building multicultural competence in mental health and educational settings* (pp. 3–15). Hoboken, NJ: Wiley.

Council on Social Work Education (CSWE), Commission on Accreditation. (2002). *Educational policy and accreditation standards*. Alexandria, VA.

Cross T. L. (2007, Spring). *What is a culturally competent professional? Pathways Practice Digest*, pp. 10–11. Portland, OR: National Indian Child Welfare Association.

Cross, T. L., Bazron, B. J., Dennis, K. W., & Issacs, M. R. (1989). *Toward a culturally competent system of care*. Washington, DC: Georgetown University Child Development Center.

Cross, T. L., & Mason, J. (1988). Services to minority populations: Cultural competence continuum. In M. C. McManus, (Ed.), *Focal point: A national bulletin on family support and children's mental health*, 3(1) pp. 1–3. Portland, OR: Portland State University, Research and Training Center on Family Support and Children's Mental Health.

Devore, W., & Schlesinger, E. G. (1981). *Ethnic-sensitive social work practice*. St. Louis, MO: Mosby.

Devore, W., & Schlesinger, E. G. (1999). *Ethnic-sensitive social work practice*. New York: Allyn & Bacon.

Dolgoff, R., Loewenberg, F. M., & Harrington, D. (2011). *Ethical decisions for social work practice*. Salt Lake City, UT: Brooks Cole Publishing, Co.

Fong, R. (Ed.). (2004). *Culturally competent practice with immigrant and refugee children and families*. New York: Guilford Press.

Fong, R., & Furuto, S. (Eds.). (2001). *Culturally competent practice: Skills, interventions, and evaluations*. Boston: Allyn & Bacon.

Gordon, M. M. (1978). *Human nature, class, and ethnicity*. New York: Oxford University Press.

Green, J. W., & Associates. (1982). *Cultural awareness in the human services*. Englewood Cliffs, NJ: Prentice-Hall.

Green, J. W. (1999). *Cultural awareness in the human services: A multiethnic approach*. Boston: Allyn & Bacon.

Gutierrez, L., Zuniga, M., & Lum, D. (2004). *Education for multicultural social work practice: Critical viewpoints and future directions*. Alexandria, VA: CSWE.

Inglehart, A. P., & Becerra, R. M. (1995). *Social services and the ethnic community*. Boston: Allyn & Bacon.

Johnson, Y. M., & Munch, S. (2009). Fundamental Contradictions in Cultural Competence. *Social Work*, 54(3), pp. 227-229. Downloadable at http://calstatela.edu/academic/hhs/sw/PDF/FE_Train/Fundamental_Contradictions_in_CC.pdf.

Karger, H. J., & Stoesz, D. (Eds.). (2005). *American social welfare policy: A pluralistic approach* (4th ed.). San Francisco: Pearson.

Kiltz, K. M., & Segal, E. A. (Eds.). (2006). *The promise of welfare reform: Political rhetoric and the reality of poverty in the 21st century*. New York: Haworth Press.

Lum, D. (Ed.). (2007). *Culturally competent practice: A framework for understanding diverse groups and justice issues* (3rd ed.). Belmont, CA: Thomson Brooks/Cole.

Mallon, G. P., & McCartt Hess, P. (2005). *Child welfare for the 21st century: A handbook of practices, policies, and programs*. New York: University Press.

Mason, J. L. (1995). *Cultural competence self-assessment questionnaire: A manual for users*. Portland, OR: Portland State University, Research and Training Center on Family Support and Children's Mental Health.

Miley, K. K., O'Melia, M., & Dubois, B. I. (1998). *Generalist social work practice: An empowering approach*. Boston: Allyn & Bacon.

Morton, G., & Atkinson, D. R. (1983). Minority identity development and preference for counselor race. *Journal of Negro Education*, 52(2), 156–161.

National Association of Social Workers. [NASW]. (2001). NASW Standards for cultural competence in social work practice. http://www.naswdc.org/pub/standards/cultural.htm

Norton, D. G. (1993). Diversity, early socialization, and temporal development: The dual perspective revisited. *Social Work*, 38(1), 82–90.

Nybell, L. M., & Gray, S. S. (2004). Race, place, space: Meanings of cultural competence in three child welfare agencies. *Social Work*, 49, 17–26.

Orlandi, M. A., Weston, R., & Epstein, L. G. (Eds.). (1992). *Cultural competence for evaluators: A guide for alcohol and other drug abuse prevention practitioners working with ethnic/racial communities*. Rockville, MD: U.S. Department of Health and Human Services, Office for Substance Abuse Prevention.

Paniagua, F. A. (2005). *Assessing and treating culturally diverse clients: A practical guide*. Thousand Oaks, CA: Sage.

Penderhughes, E. (1989). *Understanding race, ethnicity, and power: The key to efficacy in clinical practice*. New York: Free Press.

Ponterotto, J. G., Casas, J. M., Suzuki, L. A., & Alexander, C. M. (Eds.). (1995). *Handbook of multicultural counseling.* Thousands Oaks, CA: Sage.

Pope-Davis, D. B., & Coleman, H. L. K. (Eds.). (1997). *Multicultural counseling competencies: Assessment, education and training, and supervision.* Thousand Oaks, CA: Sage.

Ridley, C. R. (2005). *Overcoming unintentional racism in counseling and therapy: A practitioner guide to intentional intervention.* Thousand Oaks, CA: Sage.

Schram, S. F., Soss, J., & Fording, R. C. (2003). *Race and the politics of welfare reform.* Ann Arbor: University of Michigan Press.

Straussner, S. L. A. (2001). Ethnocultural issues in substance abuse treatment. In S. L. A. Straussner (Ed.), *Ethnocultural factors in substance abuse treatment* (pp. 3–28). New York: Guilford Press.

Sue, D. W., Arrendondo, P., & McDavis, R. J. (1992). Multicultural counseling competencies and standards: A call to the profession. *Journal of Counseling and Development, 70,* 477–486.

Van Soest, D., & Garcia, B. (2003). *Diversity education for social justice: Mastering teaching skills.* Alexandria, VA: CSWE.

Weaver, H. N. (2009). The colonial context of violence: Reflections on violence in the lives of Native American women. *Journal of Interpersonal Violence, 24*(9), 1552–1563. First published on September 3, 2008.

Weaver, H. N., & Yellow Horse Brave Heart, M. (1999). Examining two facets of American Indian identity: Exposure to other cultures and the influence of historical trauma. *Journal of Human Behavior in the Social Environment, 2*(1), 19–33.

TERRY L. CROSS

D

DISPROPORTIONALITY AND DISPARITIES

ABSTRACT: Racial disproportionality and disparities are problems affecting children and families of color in the child welfare, juvenile justice, education, mental-health, and health-care systems. The term "disproportionality" refers to the ratio between the percentage of persons in a particular racial or ethnic group at a particular decision point or experiencing an event (maltreatment, incarceration, school dropouts) compared to the percentage of the same racial or ethnic group in the overall population. This ratio could suggest underrepresentation, proportional representation, or overrepresentation of a population experiencing a particular phenomenon. The term "disparity" refers to "unequal treatment or outcomes for different groups in the same circumstance or at the same decision point." A close examination of disproportionality and disparities brings attention to differences in outcomes, often by racial group, and by social service systems. It is necessary to examine the reasons for these differences in outcomes and to be sure that culturally competent practices are upheld.

KEY WORDS: racial disproportionality; disparities; African Americans; Latinos; Native Americans; Asian Americans

Racial Disproportionality and Disparities

The term "disproportionality" refers to the ratio between the percentage of persons in a particular racial or ethnic group at a particular decision point or experiencing an event (such as maltreatment, incarceration, school dropouts) compared to the percentage of the same racial or ethnic group in the overall population (Alliance for Racial Equity, 2010; McRoy, 2005; Wells, 2011). This ratio could suggest underrepresentation, proportional representation, or overrepresentation of a population experiencing a particular phenomenon. A close examination of disproportionality brings attention to differences in outcomes, often by racial group, and it is necessary to examine the reasons for these differences.

Whereas disproportionality refers to the state of being out of proportion, "disparity" refers to a state of being unequal. In health and social service systems, disparity is typically used to describe unequal outcomes experienced by one racial or ethnic group when compared to *another* racial or ethnic group (in contrast, disproportionality compares the proportion of one racial or ethnic group to the *same* racial or ethnic group in the population). For example, an examination of disparities may look at differences by race or ethnicity at various points of entry into the child welfare or juvenile justice system, differences by county or region, or differences by age (for example, infants, adolescents) to better understand the dynamics of disparities present in a given system. In addition to disproportionality and disparities that can occur within systems, there may be overlapping challenges that can occur between systems.

Here, disproportionality and disparities will be examined by looking at various racial or ethnic population breakdowns in relation to the representation and outcomes for each of those groups in the following systems: child welfare, education, juvenile justice, mental health, and health. The causes as well as overlapping challenges and struggles between systems will be highlighted.

Review of Disproportionality and Disparities in Social Service Systems

Disproportionality and disparities manifest themselves differently across health and social service systems, yet they are present in each and share similar characteristics and causes, affecting outcomes, interventions, and policies.

DISPROPORTIONALITY AND DISPARITIES IN CHILD WELFARE Within the context of the child welfare system, disproportionality occurs when the proportion of one racial or ethnic group in the child welfare population (for example, children in foster care) is proportionately larger than the proportion of the same group in the general child population. This phenomenon has most significantly affected African American children, with estimates from 2012 indicating that African American children represented 26% of children in foster care, although they represented only 14.5% of children in the general population (U.S. Census Bureau, 2012; U.S. Department of Health and Human Services, Administration for Children and Families,

141

Administration on Children, & Youth and Families, Children's Bureau, 2013). Similarly, disproportionality has consistently been observed among American Indian or Alaska Native children. As of 2012, American Indian or Alaska Native children represented 2% of children in foster care, although they represented only 0.9% of children in the general population (U.S. Census Bureau; U.S. Department of Health and Human Services).

In contrast, Asian American and Pacific Islander children have consistently been underrepresented in foster care (Summers, Wood, & Russell, 2012). Similarly, Latino children have historically been underrepresented when examined at the national level. However, in recent years there has been growing awareness of the need to better understand disproportionality as it affects Latino children because of significant regional differences. As of 2012, Latino children represented 21% of children in foster care, whereas they represented 20.1% of children in the general population (U.S. Census Bureau, 2012; U.S. Department of Health and Human Services, 2013). However, significant statewide differences exist in which Latino children are overrepresented in some states whereas they are underrepresented in others.

One factor that is often identified as leading to disproportionality in the child welfare system is that children of color tend to suffer disproportionately from poverty. For example, in 2010, only 12.4% of White children were poor compared to 39.1% of African American children, 35% of Hispanic children, and 14.4% of Asian children (Children's Defense Fund [CDF], 2012). A related factor that may contribute to poverty is that fewer than 40% of African American children live with both of their parents (CDF, 2011). In fact, African American children are more than twice as likely as White children to live with neither parent, and African American children are more than seven times as likely as White children to have a parent in prison (CDF). Although poverty does not cause maltreatment, a large body of research has documented that maltreatment occurs disproportionately among poor families (see, for example, Drake, Lee, & Jonson-Reid, 2009; Drake & Pandey, 1996; Freisthler, Bruce, & Needell, 2007). This was confirmed in the most recent National Incidence Study of Child Abuse and Neglect, which found that children in low-socioeconomic-status households experienced some form of maltreatment at a rate more than five times the rate of other children (Sedlak et al., 2010b).

Once experiencing abuse and neglect, the availability of services can make a difference in outcomes for children. In 2009, about 40% of children who were abused and neglected received no services and many others received insufficient services to address their needs (CDF, 2011). Some have suggested individual bias on the part of child welfare workers and mandated reporters that may impact their decision making regarding the need for services. Others have identified cultural bias, cultural insensitivity, or failure to seek culturally responsive resources as impacting the likelihood of seeking and receiving appropriate services (Chibnall et al., 2003; Dettlaff & Rycraft, 2008). For example, Rivaux et al. (2011) completed a study to better understand why African American children were placed in foster care at higher rates than White children. She and her co-investigators found that even when controlling for risk, poverty, and other relevant factors, race affected the decision to provide services and to remove children from their homes.

In 2007, the U.S. Government Accountability Office (GAO) issued the findings of a study that examined the multiple causes of the overrepresentation of African American children in foster care. According to this report, cultural misunderstandings, stereotypes, assumptions, and bias all lead to disparate decision making (U.S. GAO, 2007). In addition, Sedlak, McPherson, & Das (2010a) noted that high rates of poverty in African American communities can impact longer stays in the foster-care system. Given that many children come from single mothers who are poor, live in impoverished neighborhoods and communities with few resources, experience long waiting lists to receive needed services, and may experience discrimination, they have decreased likelihood of achieving family reunification and instead remain in foster care for longer periods of time.

In response to the growing problem of disproportionality and disparities, Simmel (2011) challenged child welfare workers to avoid taking a "one size fits all approach" to service delivery and to recognize that factors such as age, gender, and ethnicity of children should be taken into consideration, calling for the assessment of "parenting practices and family characteristics with cultural sensitivity" (p. 108). Culturally competent recruitment of child welfare staff, subcontracting with minority specializing agencies, increased use of kinship adoptions, and customary adoptions within tribal communities are all culturally relevant approaches to addressing the disproportionate number of children of color in the child welfare system. There is also growing awareness of the need for efforts to be directed toward the prevention of maltreatment and the reduction of maltreatment-related risk factors among children and families of color, as well as the need to address the underlying social problems that contribute to disproportionate need. These strategies call for increased efforts by child welfare agencies to collaborate with community stakeholders to address these issues and facilitate children being maintained in their homes and reducing disproportionality.

DISPROPORTIONALITY AND DISPARITIES IN JUVENILE JUSTICE OUTCOMES

Not only are children of color overrepresented in the child welfare system, but also two-thirds of youth in the juvenile justice system are youth of color (CDF, 2011). Data indicate that youth of color are significantly more likely than their White counterparts to be arrested, detained, prosecuted, incarcerated, given probation, or transferred to adult court (Models for Change, 2011). Within the juvenile justice system, this phenomenon is referred to as disproportionate minority contact (DMC). In 2009, among the 1.5 million youth seen in juvenile courts, 34% were African American, although they represented only 16% of youth ages 10 to 17 in the population (Puzzanchera & Kang, 2011). Similarly, Latino youth represented 25% of youth who were incarcerated, although they represented only 19% of youth ages 10 to 17 (Saavedra, 2010). Statistics appear to suggest that Asian American or Pacific Islander and American Indian youth are proportionally represented within this system. However, American Indian youth are largely seen in federal courts because crimes committed on tribal lands are considered federal offenses. These contacts are not included among those with the juvenile justice system and thus affect the interpretation of those data.

Several studies have noted that many of the youth in the juvenile system are "dually involved" or "crossover youth" who have experienced both juvenile justice and child welfare system involvement (Herz et al., 2012). Therefore, many may have complex needs because of prior abuse and neglect, frequent moves, unstable situations, and lack of services to address these issues (Ryan, Herz, Hernandez, & Marshall, 2007). All of these factors may increase the likelihood of these youth entering residential or group settings and sometimes juvenile facilities.

Similar to the child welfare system, the causes of DMC are complex and include racial bias within the system, differences in the types and levels of offending behavior, legislation and policies with dispropor-

tionate impact, and the presence of other risk factors, including family economic status, family structure, and neighborhood (Huizinga et al., 2007). Further, disproportionality that exists in other systems may contribute to disproportionality within the juvenile justice system. In addition to overrepresentation in the child welfare system, youth of color are more likely than their White counterparts to have unmet mental-health needs (Kataoka, Zhang, & Wells, 2002) and experience difficulties in school (National Council of La Raza, 2011)—each of which can contribute to involvement in the juvenile justice system.

The Office of Juvenile Justice and Delinquency Prevention (OJJDP) reports that as of 2008, 25 states were engaged in programs to provide alternatives to detention as a means of addressing DMC, whereas 15 states were providing cultural competency training as part of their efforts to address this problem (OJJDP, 2009). Other approaches include early intervention programs to prevent crime and delinquency, whereas systems-change efforts focus on the use of structured decision-making models to reduce the impact of racial bias and legislative reforms to address laws and policies that may have differential impacts on youth of color (OJJDP, n.d.).

DISPROPORTIONALITY AND DISPARITIES IN EDUCATIONAL OUTCOMES

In addition to the disproportionality that is evident in the juvenile justice and child welfare systems, it also exists in the educational system, where it can manifest in a number of different ways. These include underrepresentation in gifted and talented programs and overrepresentation in special education programs. For example, White and Asian American students comprise nearly three-fourths of all students enrolled in gifted and talented programs, whereas African American, Latino, and American Indian students are disproportionately underrepresented in these opportunities (U.S. Department of Education [U.S. DOE], Office of Civil Rights, 2012). Conversely, African American children are disproportionately overrepresented among children identified with a learning disability or emotional disturbance. Further, African American students represent only 16% of sixth to eighth graders, yet comprise 42% of students in those grades who are held back one year (U.S. DOE, Office of Civil Rights).

Disproportionality can also involve overrepresentation among youth receiving disciplinary actions. For example, African American students are more than three times as likely as their White peers to be suspended or expelled (U.S. DOE, Office of Civil Rights, 2012). Additionally, Latino and African American students comprise 56% of students expelled from school under zero-tolerance policies, although they represent only 45% of the student body (U.S. DOE, Office of Civil Rights). The increasing use of zero-tolerance policies has resulted in growing awareness of what is often referred to as the "school-to-prison pipeline" because children who have been suspended are more likely to fall behind in school, be retained a grade, drop out of high school, commit crimes, and become incarcerated as adults (Advancement Project, 2000).

Root causes of disproportionality within the educational system are complex, but most discussions of these causes focus on the historical advantages that White children have benefitted from in the American educational system. Access to learning and full educational opportunities were not accessible to non-Whites for the majority of this nation's history. Institutionalized racism that remains within educational systems exacerbates this White advantage (Singleton & Linton, 2006). Further, socioeconomic conditions are frequently cited as compounding the educational barriers that students of color encounter (Robinson, 2010).

Strategies to address disproportionality vary widely across educational systems, yet most begin with identification and awareness of disproportionality as a problem. Although some districts have implemented concerted efforts to address disproportionality in their state and local systems, others have lacked a coordinated response to this problem. Beyond identification and awareness, efforts have included an emphasis on culturally responsive teaching—a pedagogy that recognizes the importance of including students' cultural references in the classroom—as well as raising awareness of the historical causes of differences in educational outcomes, efforts to create more supportive learning environments, and system-wide efforts to improve school climate, eliminate racial bias, and promote cultural competence.

DISPROPORTIONALITY AND DISPARITIES IN MENTAL-HEALTH OUTCOMES

Although mental-health disorders and the need for mental-health services are present across racial and ethnic groups, considerable disparities exist in the mental-health system. These disparities exist in access to mental-health services, the quality of services provided, and outcomes that result from services. Specifically, African Americans, Asian Americans, and Latinos in need of mental-health services are all significantly less likely to utilize mental-health services compared to Whites (Office of Minority Health and Health Disparities, 2007). For example, Garland et al. (2005) found that among youth receiving services in a large, publicly funded system of care in San Diego, 79% of non-Hispanic White youths received mental-health services compared to only 59% of Asian Americans or Pacific Islanders, 64% of African Americans, and 70% of Latino Americans. They also found that there were racial or ethnic differences by type of service used. Although outpatient mental-health services were used most frequently overall, African American and Asian American or Pacific Islander youth were less likely to use this type of service than non-Hispanic White youth.

Barriers to mental-health services include economic barriers (such as cost, lack of insurance), lack of awareness of mental-health issues, and stigma associated with mental illness. Additional barriers include a lack of culturally competent mental-health providers and prior negative experiences with the mental-health system (Yeh, McCabe, Hough, Dupuis, & Hazen, 2003). For some racial or ethnic groups, an additional barrier may include a lack of services available in their native language. Further, immigration status can serve as a barrier to accessing services because undocumented immigrants may fear being deported or prohibited from becoming naturalized if they attempt to access certain resources.

Social conditions within predominantly racial or ethnic communities may also present barriers to accessing mental-health services. Geographical segregation can restrict employment opportunities, and thus insurance, as well as access to mental-health services (Alegría, Pescosolido, Williams, & Canino, 2011). Communities with high proportions of African American and Latino residents have been found to be four times as likely as those with predominantly White residents to have a shortage of providers, regardless of community income (Putsch & Pololi, 2004). As a result, those in need of care may be more likely to seek services in the primary-care sector, where their concerns will receive considerably less attention (Tai-Seale, McGuire, Colenda, Rosen, & Cook, 2007).

Strategies to address mental-health disparities within the mental-health system include insurance reforms, particularly as they affect Medicaid eligibility criteria, and efforts to improve the cultural competence of mental-health providers to ensure appropriate diagnosis and referrals. Additional strategies include addressing the organizational climate of agencies that may serve as barriers to care for racial or ethnic minorities. Within racial or ethnic communities, strategies to reduce disparities include general education and improved health literacy, as well as increased efforts to engage with community systems to reduce stigma and mistrust that may be associated with mental-health providers. This includes ensuring access to mental-health services within racial or ethnic communities.

DISPROPORTIONALITY AND DISPARITIES IN HEALTH OUTCOMES
Health disparities include health status; access to, and utilization of, health care; and social determinants of poorer health. In each of these areas, people of color fare worse than their White counterparts. Disparities in health status are numerous and include higher rates of disease and illness, higher rates of death from disease, higher rates of chronic illness, and higher rates of infant mortality (Robert Wood Johnson Foundation, n.d.). Racial or ethnic minorities receive lower quality care than Whites—regardless of where they live, their income, or their health insurance coverage. African Americans and Hispanics receive a lower quality of care across disease areas, including cancer, HIV/AIDS, diabetes, and other chronic illnesses. For example, African Americans with coronary artery disease or who have experienced heart attacks are less likely than Whites to receive appropriate procedures or therapies. Further, African Americans are *more likely* than Whites to receive less desirable services, such as amputation (Institute of Medicine, 2003). Social determinants of health include poverty, median household income, no high school diploma, unemployment, wage gap, and incarceration rate. In each of these indicators, people of color fare worse than their White counterparts (James, Salganicoff, Ranji, Goodwin, & Duckett, 2012).

Similar to other systems, the factors contributing to these disparities are complex and at cross-system levels. Aspects of health systems—including financing, organization, and access to services—likely pose significant barriers for people of color. Shifts brought about by cost-control efforts and the movement to managed care may more negatively impact people of color as community-based care is decreased. People of color are less likely to have health insurance, which affects access to services. Even for those with insurance coverage, people of color are more likely to be enrolled in lower tiered plans and have fewer choices for health products and services (Institute of Medicine, 2003). Among providers, those who are unfamiliar with the racial or ethnic backgrounds of their patients may be vulnerable to uncertainty and misdiagnosis. Differences may also be present in the health-seeking behaviors of people of color because they may be more likely to refuse recommended services or delay seeking treatment. However, this may be the result of distrust or negative prior interactions with health-care systems.

Among children and youth, those of color are disproportionately uninsured and tend to experience more "preventable and treatable health conditions from birth through adulthood. In fact, one in five American Indian children, one in six Hispanic children, and one in eight Black children are uninsured compared to one in 14 White children" (CDF, 2011, p. E-2). This lack of insurance, coupled with disproportionate poverty, may be partly responsible for the finding that Black and Hispanic children are almost three times as likely to be in poor or fair health and more likely to have an unmet medical need than White children. Also, Hispanic children are 76% more likely and Black children are 50% more likely than White children to have an unmet health need because of cost (CDF, p. E-8).

Strategies to address health disparities begin with raising awareness of these disparities among key stakeholders, including providers, health plan purchasers, and the broader society. Health systems can make efforts to improve access to care, including ensuring interpreter services are available and expanding the use of community health workers. Systems also must take steps to ensure that financial incentives do not disproportionately impact people and communities of color. Similar to the mental-health system, efforts to improve health literacy among people and communities of color may play a role in reducing health disparities. Further, cross-cultural training and education for providers are necessary to ensure that unconscious biases or stereotypes do not interfere with the quality of patient interactions.

Challenges in Overlapping Systems
There are clearly overlapping challenges in the education, health, mental-health, child welfare, and juvenile justice systems. As these systems overlap and disproportionately impact children and families of color, policies and culturally appropriate interventions that take into account these interrelated systems are needed to address and prevent these disproportionate outcomes. Further, it is important for these overlapping social systems to provide services that address ethnically diverse contexts and are meaningful and relevant to the populations being served, resulting in increasing calls for cultural competence in all aspects of assessment, intervention, and evaluation. Services that are embedded with ideas from the majority culture can be limited by a number of factors—conceptual mismatches, language barriers, differing values, or differences in the meaning and manifestation of emotions—each of which can lead to poor outcomes.

Thus, effective assessment, intervention, and evaluation of services designed for diverse cultures require not only cultural competence, but also an increased awareness and understanding of the populations being served. Systems must understand how diverse groups perceive the services being provided, communicate their views and experiences, and respond to interventions. Further, systems working with diverse cultures must understand a number of different variables within those cultures, including diversity within an ethnic minority group or cultural contexts in help-seeking behaviors. As a result, cultural competency is not only an essential component of overlapping service systems, but also a necessary skill for service providers in those systems.

Yet the notion of cultural competence is sometimes misinterpreted to imply that service providers must know everything there is to know about a particular culture to be competent in that culture. This interpretation of cultural competence may not be practical because it is not possible to be perfectly competent in every culture for which one might provide services. Rather, service providers must have skills working cross-culturally that allow them to have an open mind, avoid making assumptions, and gather the appropriate information to make accurate assessments and intervention plans. To do this, providers must invest time learning about the history and culture of the population to understand what questions must be asked and what interventions are culturally appropriate. For overlapping systems, this will involve significant input from and collaboration with community-based stakeholders and others with expertise in the social, cultural, and historical contexts in which the social service system is based.

Overlapping challenges in the child welfare system have largely focused on the African American population. However, concerns are increasing regarding disparities that affect other children of color. Understanding how disparities and disproportionality manifest themselves for Native American and Latino children is important and strategies that address these disparities must be implemented and evaluated. Additionally, although there is a large body of research that focuses on understanding the factors that contribute to disproportionality and disparities, there is much less research on how to address or reduce them. The evidence base of strategies designed to address and reduce disproportionality and disparities must be strengthened and improved, not only through additional research, but also by ensuring that rigorous evaluation methods are employed.

Further, increased collaboration is needed across systems to more effectively meet the needs of youth involved across systems. This collaboration is necessary both to increase the understanding of the complex needs of cross-over youth and to improve service delivery. For example, youth involved in the juvenile justice system often have cross-system involvement with both the child welfare and the mental-health systems. Enhanced efforts also must be made to better understand and address the school-to-prison pipeline, whereby large disparities among youth of color in suspensions, expulsions, and school-based arrests contribute to the disparities that exist in the juvenile justice system.

In addition to collaboration among systems, increased collaboration and involvement are necessary with youth and the families involved in the juvenile justice system to ensure that their voices are heard and integrated into system improvement efforts. Efforts are also needed to improve the evidence base of interventions designed to reduce disproportionality in this system. Although promising practices have been identified, much further research is needed to strengthen the evidence base of these interventions. Further, more attention must be given to the evaluation of cross-systems efforts to reduce disproportionality and disparities, such as those that involve collaborations with the child welfare, mental-health, and educational systems.

Efforts are needed to transform the culture within schools to one that is responsive to changing demographics. Although the populations of schools reflect these changing demographics, the practices, procedures, protocols, and structures have remained the same. As part of these efforts, attention should be given to workforce development that ensures that educators are not only reflective of the populations whom they serve, but also understand the historical foundations of race and racism in the United States and how the existing structures within schools may perpetuate the inequalities that exist.

Educational systems must be equipped with culturally relevant curricula materials and resources as part of the overall process of system improvement. This is necessary not only to engage diverse students, but also to ensure that educational systems respect and value the histories, experiences, and value systems of culturally diverse groups. Increased efforts must be made to address the disparities that result from zero-tolerance policies within educational systems. These disparities contribute not only to poor educational outcomes for youth of color, but also to their involvement in other systems, particularly involvement in the juvenile justice system. Increased collaboration with the juvenile justice system is needed as part of these efforts to better understand and address the school-to-prison pipeline.

Efforts are needed that emphasize the development of a workforce of racial and ethnic minority professionals who are well trained in evidence-based mental-health and behavioral-health treatments that address the diverse needs of youth and families of color. This is important to facilitate not only culturally competent service provision, but also engagement of children and families of color in the health and mental-health systems.

Implications for Practice and Policy

At the systems level, strategies are needed to address the institutional issues that contribute to bias and inequities in social services offered in child welfare, juvenile justice, education, mental-health, and health systems. These efforts include examining and addressing the ways in which funding streams, payment methods, insurance coverage, and other institutional policies limit access to services or otherwise perpetuate existing inequities. Efforts are needed to ensure that the voices of children and families of color are included and valued in the development and delivery of mental-health services. This can be addressed through multiple methods, including enhanced community engagement with communities of color, increased use of community-based paraprofessionals, and increased involvement of service recipients in policy development and service decisions.

Because disparities in child welfare, juvenile justice, education, mental-health, and health systems are closely tied to the factors that affect the well-being of children and families of color, such as limited income and lack of health-care benefits, addressing the financial and structural barriers to social services is essential as children and families of color are disproportionately represented among the poor, the near poor, and those with insufficient services and benefits. Initiatives are needed to improve cultural competency and linguistic appropriateness within social service systems to enhance and increase engagement of people of color in preventative services. These must be extended to the engagement of communities of color through direct interaction and access to services within those communities. More attention is needed to develop strategies to improve public awareness of child welfare, juvenile justice, education, mental-health, and health disparities and to improve knowledge and literacy among racial and ethnic minorities to increase engagement in health services. These approaches must include considerable outreach to and engagement with communities of color that are most vulnerable to these disparities.

REFERENCES

Advancement Project. (2000). *Opportunities suspended: The devastating consequences of zero tolerance and school discipline.* Washington, DC: Author.

Alegría, M., Pescosolido, B., Williams, S., & Canino, G. (2011). Culture, race/ethnicity and disparities: Fleshing out the socio-cultural framework for health services disparities. In B. Pescosolido, J. Marin, J. McLeod, & A. Rogers (Eds.), *Handbook of the sociology of health, illness, and healing: A blueprint for the 21st century* (pp. 363–382). New York, NY: Springer.

Alliance for Racial Equity. (2010, July). *What does the research tell us about racial and ethnic disproportionality and disparity in the child welfare system?* Baltimore, MD: Symposium hosted by the Alliance for Racial Equity.

Chibnall, S., Dutch, N. M., Jones-Harden, B., Brown, A., Gourdine, R., Smith, J., et al. (2003). *Children of color in the child welfare system: Perspectives from the child welfare community.* Department of Health and Human Services Children's Bureau [and] Administration for Children and Families. Retrieved from http://www.childwelfare.gov/pubs/otherpubs/children/children.pdf

Children's Defense Fund (CDF). (2011). *Portrait of inequality 2011. Black children in America.* Retrieved from http://www.childrensdefense.org/programs-campaigns/black-community-crusade-for-children-II/bccc-assets/portrait-of-inequality.pdf

Children's Defense Fund (CDF). (2012). *The State of America's Children Handbook 2012.* Retrieved from http://www.childrensdefense.org/child-research-data-publications/data/soac-2012-handbook.pdf

Dettlaff, A. J., & Rycraft, J. R. (2008). Deconstructing disproportionality: Views from multiple stakeholders. *Child Welfare, 87*(2), 37–58.

Drake, B., Lee, S. M., & Jonson-Reid, M. (2009). Race and child maltreatment reporting: Are Blacks overrepresented? *Children and Youth Services Review, 31,* 309–316.

Drake, B., & Pandey, S. (1996). Understanding the relationship between neighborhood poverty and specific types of child maltreatment. *Child Abuse and Neglect, 20,* 1003–1018.

Freisthler, B., Bruce, E., & Needell, B. (2007). Understanding the geospatial relationship of neighborhood characteristics and rates of maltreatment for Black, Hispanic, and White children. *Social Work, 52,* 7–16.

Garland, A. F., Lau, A. S., Yeh, M., McCabe, K. M., Hough, R. L., & Landsverk, J. A. (2005). Racial and ethnic differences in utilization of mental health services among high-risk youths. *American Journal of Psychiatry, 162*(7), 1336–1343.

Herz, D., Lee, P., Lutz, L., Stewart, M., Tuell, J., & Wiig, J. (2012). *Addressing the needs of multisystem youth: Strengthening the connection between child welfare and juvenile justice.* Washington, DC: Center for Juvenile Justice Reform.

Huizinga, D., Thornberry, T. P., Knight, K. E., Lovegrove, P. J., Loeber, R., Hill, K., et al. (2007). *Disproportionate minority contact in the juvenile justice system: A study of differential* minority arrest/referral to court in three cities. Washington, DC: Office of Juvenile Justice and Delinquency Prevention.

Institute of Medicine. (2003). Unequal treatment: Confronting racial and ethnic disparities in health care. Washington, DC: National Academies Press.

James, C., Salganicoff, A., Ranji, U., Goodwin, A., & Duckett, P. (2012). Putting men's health care disparities on the map: Examining racial and ethnic disparities at the state level. Menlo Park, CA: Kaiser Family Foundation.

Kataoka, S. H., Zhang, L., & Wells, K. B. (2002). Unmet need for mental health care among U.S. children: Variation by ethnicity and insurance status. American Journal of Psychiatry, 159, 1548–1555.

McRoy, R. G. (2005). Overrepresentation of children and youth of color in foster care. In G. P. Mallon, & P. M. Hess (Eds.), Child welfare for the twenty-first century: A handbook of practices, policies and programs. New York, NY: Columbia University Press.

Models for Change. (2011). Knowledge brief: Are minority youths treated differently in juvenile probation? Retrieved from http://www.modelsforchange.net/publications/314

National Council of La Raza. (2011). Men in motion in the community and the Philadelphia Latino Juvenile Justice Network: Reducing disproportionate minority contact, strengthening reentry, and building community. Retrieved from http://www.modelsforchange.net/publications/327

Office of Juvenile Justice and Delinquency Prevention (OJJDP). (n.d.). DMC strategies. Retrieved from http://www.juvenilejustice-tta.org/resources/dmc/dmc-strategies

Office of Juvenile Justice and Delinquency Prevention (OJJDP). (2009). OJJDP in focus: Disproportionate minority contact. Retrieved from https://www.ncjrs.gov/pdffiles1/ojjdp/228306.pdf

Office of Minority Health and Health Disparities. (2007). Fact sheet: Eliminate disparities in mental health. Retrieved from http://www.cdc.gov/omhd/amh/factsheets/mental.htm

Putsch, R. W., & Pololi, L. (2004). Distributive justice in American healthcare: Institutions, power, and the equitable care of patients. American Journal of Managed Care, 10, 45–53.

Puzzanchera, C., & Kang, W. (2011). Easy access to juvenile court statistics: 1985–2009. Retrieved from http://www.ojjdp.gov/ojstatbb/ezajcs/

Rivaux, S. L., James, J., Wittenstrom, K., Baumann, D. J., Sheets, J., Henry, J., et al. (2011). Race, poverty, and risk: Understanding the decision to provide services and remove children. In D. K. Green, K. Belanger, R. G. McRoy, & L. Bullard (Eds.), Challenging racial disproportionality in child welfare: Research, policy, and practice (pp. 91–100). Washington, DC: CWLA Press.

Robert Wood Johnson Foundation. (n.d.). Disparities. Retrieved from http://www.rwjf.org/en/topics/rwjf-topic-areas/health-policy/disparities.html

Robinson, E. (2010). Disintegration: The splintering of Black America. New York, NY: Doubleday.

Ryan, J. P., Herz, D., Hernandez, P. M., & Marshall, J. M. (2007). Maltreatment and delinquency: Investigating child

welfare bias in juvenile justice processing. Children and Youth Services Review, 29, 1035–1050.

Saavedra, J. D. (2010). Just the facts: A snapshot of incarcerated Hispanic youth [Fact Sheet]. Washington, DC: National Council of La Raza.

Sedlak, A. J., McPherson, K., & Das, B. (2010a, March). Supplementary analyses of race differences in child maltreatment rates in the NIS-4. Washington, DC: Office of Planning, Research, and Evaluation and the Children's Bureau Administration for Children and Families of the U.S. Department of Health and Human Services. Retrieved from http://www.acf.hhs.gov/sites/default/files/opre/nis4_supp_analysis_race_diff_mar2010.pdf

Sedlak, A. J., Mettenburg, J., Basena, M., Petta, I., McPherson, K., Greene, A., et al. (2010b). Fourth National Incidence Study of Child Abuse and Neglect (NIS–4): Report to Congress. Washington, DC: U.S. Department of Health and Human Services, Administration for Children and Families.

Simmel, C. (2011). Demographic profiles of children reported to the Child Welfare System. Journal of Public Child Welfare, 5(1), 87–110.

Singleton, G. E., & Linton, C. (2006). Courageous conversations about race. Thousand Oaks, CA: Corwin.

Summers, A., Wood, S., & Russell, J. (2012). Disproportionality rates for children of color in foster care. Reno, NV: National Council of Juvenile and Family Court Judges.

Tai-Seale, M., McGuire, T., Colenda, C., Rosen, D., & Cook, M. A. (2007). Two-minute mental health care for elderly patients: Inside primary care visits. Journal of the American Geriatrics Society, 55, 1903–1911.

U.S. Census Bureau. (2012). 2010 census data [Data file]. Retrieved from http://www.census.gov/2010census/data/

U.S. Department of Education, Office of Civil Rights. (2012). The transformed civil rights data collection—March 2012 data summary. Retrieved from http://www2.ed.gov/about/offices/list/ocr/data.html

U.S. Department of Health and Human Services, Administration for Children and Families, Administration on Children, & Youth and Families, Children's Bureau. (2013). The AFCARS report: Preliminary FY 2012 estimates as of July 2013 #20. Retrieved from http://www.acf.hhs.gov/sites/default/files/cb/afcarsreport20.pdf

U.S. Government Accountability Office (GAO). (2007, July). African American children in foster care: Additional HHS assistance needed to help states reduce the proportion in care. GAO-07-816. Retrieved from http://www.gao.gov/new.items/d07816.pdf

Wells, S. J. (2011). Disproportionality and disparity in child welfare. In D. Greene, K. Belanger, R. G. McRoy, & L. Bullard (Eds.), Challenging racial disproportionality in child welfare: Research, policy, and practice (pp. 3–14). Washington, DC: Child Welfare League of America.

Yeh, M., McCabe, K., Hough, R. L., Dupuis, D., & Hazen, A. (2003). Racial/ethnic differences in parental endorsement of barriers to mental health services for youth. Mental Health Services Research, 5(2), 65–77.

ROWENA FONG, RUTH MCROY, AND ALAN DETTLAFF

E

ECOLOGICAL FRAMEWORK

ABSTRACT: Ecological concepts and principles enable social workers to keep a simultaneous focus on people and their environments and their reciprocal relationships, not only in direct practice with individuals, families and groups, but also in influencing organizations and communities and in policy practice. Ecological concepts emphasize the reciprocity of person: environment exchanges, in which each shapes and influences the other over time. Ecological concepts are reviewed.

KEY WORDS: People:Environment (P:E) fit; abuses of power; habitat and niche; life course (individual, historical, and social time); life stressor; stress and coping; resilience; deep ecology; ecofeminism

A continuing thread in the historical development of social work has been a dual concern for people and their environments, and the relationship between the two in ways that gave equal attention to both. Until the 1960s and 1970s and the advent of systems (Hearn, 1969) and ecological notions (Germain, 1973, 1976, 1978a, 1987b), the profession lacked concepts, methods, and skills to implement its equal commitment to both people and their environments. Systems and ecological ideas provided the profession with an alternative to the medical and disease metaphor rooted in simple linear etiology. Ecological ideas came to the fore because ecologists were among the first system thinkers, and their perspective was systemic; yet, it avoided the seemingly dehumanizing language of general system theorists. Coming out of the life science of Biology rather than the physical science of Physics, ecological ideas were found to be less abstract and closer to the human experience. Over time the conceptual framework of the ecological perspective was elaborated and refined (Germain, 1983, 1985, 1990, 1994; Germain & Gitterman, 1987, 1995) and operationalized by the Life Model of social work practice (Germain & Gitterman, 1979, 1980, 1996; Gitterman, 1996, 2007, 2010; Gitterman & Germain, 1976, 2008; Gitterman & Heller, 2011).

Ecological concepts enable social workers to keep a simultaneous focus on people and their environments and their reciprocal relationships, not only in direct practice with individuals, families, and groups, but also in influencing organizations and communities, and in policy practice. Ecological concepts emphasize the reciprocity of person-environment exchanges, in which each shapes and influences the other over time. Ecological thinking recognizes that (x) and (y) are in a reciprocal rather than a linear or unidirectional relation. Reciprocal relations may act in a way that leads to change in (y), whereupon that change in (y) leads to change in (x), which in turn affects (x), thus forming a continuous loop of reciprocal influences over time. Each element in the loop directly or indirectly influences every other element. As a consequence, simple linear notions of cause and effect lose their meaning. Therefore, social workers should concentrate on helping to change dysfunctional relationships between people and their environments. We should ask the questions, "What is going on?" "Why is it going on?" and "How can the 'what' be changed?" rather than "Who should be changed (or blamed)?" Werner, Altman, Oxley, and Haggard (1987) capture the complexity of these reciprocal relationships:

> Psychological phenomena are best understood as holistic events composed of inseparable and mutually defining psychological processes, physical environments and social environments, and temporal qualities. There are no separate actors in an event; the actions of one person are understood in relation to the actions of other people, and in relation to spatial, situational and temporal circumstances in which the actors are embedded. These different aspects of an event are so intermeshed that understanding one aspect requires simultaneous inclusion of other aspects in the analysis. (p. 244)

The first part of this entry briefly reviews original ecological concepts. The second part briefly introduces newer ecological concepts drawn from resilience theory, deep ecology, and ecofeminism.

Ecological Concepts

People:Environment (P:E) fit is the perceived degree of fit between an individual's or collective group's needs, aspirations, and capacities and the qualities and operations of their social and physical environments

149

within particular cultural and historical contexts. Over the life course, people strive to deal with and improve the *level of fit* with their environments. When a perceived "good" fit evolves between a people and their environment, they perceive the availability of sufficient personal and environmental resources and experience a condition of *adaptedness* (Dubos, 1968). When a "poor" fit evolves between a people's perceptions of environmental resources and their needs, aspirations, and capacities, they experience *stress*. When exchanges over time are generally negative, development, health, and social functioning might be impaired and the environment could be damaged. How overwhelming and disabling is the stress of daily life experienced by people and how effectively they manage the associated life tasks will depend largely upon *the perceived level of fit* between their personal and environmental resources. When the level of fit is perceived to be unfavorable, or simply adequate, people, alone or with professional help, may improve the level of fit by *adaptive* behaviors. Adaptive behaviors are active efforts to (a) improve oneself (for example learn new skills) or (b) influence the environment or (c) improve the person:environment transactions. Abuses of power by those economically and politically advantaged and withholding of power from vulnerable and marginalized populations lead to poor schools, chronic unemployment or underemployment of those whom the schools failed to educate, lack of affordable and safe housing, homelessness, inadequate health care, and differential rates of chronic illness and mortality rates among people of color as compared to whites. Poverty, institutional racism, sexism, homophobia, and xenophobia are created and maintained through misuses and abuses of power. Dominant groups also exploit the environment by polluting the air, food, water, and soil. Toxic materials continue to be present in dwellings, schools, and workplaces, especially in poor communities. Abuses of power reflect destructive relationships between people and their environment in which the social order permits some people to inflict grave injustice and suffering on others.

Habitat and niche delineate the nature of the social and physical environments. Physical *habitat* may be rural or urban, and include residential dwellings, physical settings of schools, hospitals, workplaces, religious structures, social agencies, and transportation systems, and amenities such as parks, recreation facilities, entertainment centers, libraries, and museums. Human habitats evoke spatial and temporal behaviors that help shape P:E transactions regulating social distance, intimacy, privacy, and other interpersonal processes in family, group, community, and organizational life. Habitats may promote or interfere with basic functions of family and community life. Habitats that do not support the growth, health, and social functioning of individuals and families, and do not provide community amenities to an optimum degree, are likely to produce isolation, disorientation, and helplessness.

Niche refers to the status occupied by an individual, family, or group in the social structure of a community. What constitutes a growth-supporting, health-promoting human niche is defined differently in various societies and in different historical eras. In the United States, a set of rights, including the right to equal opportunity, generally shapes a niche. Yet millions of children and adults occupy niches that do not support human needs, rights, and aspirations, often because of some personal or cultural characteristic such as race, ethnicity, place of birth, gender, age, sexual orientation, poverty, or physical or mental states. Stigmatized and destructive niches designate human beings as "drug addict," "borderline personality," "person with AIDS," "mentally ill," "welfare mother," and so on. These niches are shaped and sustained by society's tolerance of the misuse of power in political, social, and economic structures (Germain & Gitterman, 1987, 1995, 2008).

Life course refers to the unique pathways of development that each human being takes—from conception and birth through old age—in varied environments and to our infinitely varied life experiences. In contrast to stage models of development, which assume a fixed and predictable sequence, biopsychosocial development is conceived as consisting of non-uniform, indeterminate pathways within diverse environments, cultures, and historical eras. Human development is further placed within the context of individual, historical, and social time. "Individual time" refers to the continuity and meaning of individual life experiences, over the life course. Both are reflected in the life stories that people construct and tell to others and themselves. The constructing and sharing of life stories provide meaning and continuity in life events. Historical time refers to the formative effects of historical and social change on birth cohorts (segments of the population born at the same time point) that help account for generational and age differences in biopsychosocial development, opportunities, and social expectations. For example, cohorts of North American women born between 1990 and 2000 differ—in psychosocial development, opportunities, expectations of marriage, parenting, and work—from earlier cohorts.

Finally, *social time* refers to the timing of individual, family, and community transitions and life events as influenced by changing biological, economic, social, demographic, and cultural factors. Until the 1960s, social time consisted of sequential "timetables" that prescribed the timing of certain life transitions: the proper time to enter school, leave home, marry, have a child, retire. Such timetables are no longer viable, which is a manifestation of the accelerated rate of social change (historical time). The early childhood education movement created a new age group—preschoolers—who attend day care and nursery schools, Head Start programs, and so on. Elders go back to school for high school certificates or college degrees, grown children remain at home after finishing college, some children bear and rear children, while some adults postpone childbearing until the last possible moment. Many elders do not regard themselves as old until their late seventies or eighties. These and other life transitions are becoming age-independent. In parallel fashion, the phenomenon of gender crossover has progressively expanded. Gendered family roles and work roles have dramatically changed in regard to childrearing, household management, and careers.

The life stressor, stress, and coping paradigm fits well with the ecological perspective as it takes into account the characteristics of the person and the operations of the environment, as well as the exchanges between them (Lazarus, 1999; Lazarus & Lazarus, 2006). Life stressors, which are usually externally generated, take the form of a real or perceived harm or loss, or threat of a future harm or loss (for example illness, bereavement, job loss, difficult transition, interpersonal conflict, or countless other painful life events and traumas). Poverty and oppression create chronic and acute stressors and make other stressors more difficult to manage. The resulting *stress*, which is internally generated, may have physiological or emotional consequences. Frequently, it has both. Physiological and emotional stresses are the consequence of people's intuitive or reasoned appraisal that a difficult life transition, traumatic life event, environmental or interpersonal pressure exceeds their perceived available personal and environmental resources to deal with it. When people appraise sufficient personal and environmental resources to deal with life stressors, they experience positive feelings and anticipated mastery associated with the challenge. In dealing with stress, people use *coping measures* to deal with the demands posed by the life stressor(s). Personal resources for coping include motivation; management of feelings; problem-solving; flexibility; a hopeful outlook; and an ability to seek environmental resources and to use them effectively. Environmental resources include formal service networks such as

public and private agencies and institutions and informal networks of relatives, friends, neighbors, workmates, and coreligionists. Formal and informal networks serve as buffers against stress. Even the perception of their availability can make it easier to cope with a life stressor by altering appraisals. The natural and built physical environments (parks, oceans, transportation, dwellings) also contribute to physical and emotional well-being and support coping efforts.

Newly Added Ecological Concepts

Resilience is an ecological concept, reflecting complex person:environment transactions rather than simply attributes of a person (Gitterman, 2001a, 2001b; Gitterman & Shulman, 2005; Ungar, 2008). Some people do not succeed in spite of positive personal attributes. Yet, other people thrive, rather than simply survive, in the face of life's inhumanities and tragedies. Protective factors (biological, psychological, or environmental processes) act as a buffer against life stressors by preventing them, lessening their impact, or ameliorating them more quickly. The protective factors include: (1) temperament; (2) family patterns; (3) external supports; and (4) environmental resources (Fraser, 2004; Smith & Carlson, 1997). Temperament includes such factors as activity level, coping skills, self-esteem, and attributions. For example, feelings of self-worth emerge from positive intimate relationships, and successful task accomplishment (for example academics, sports, music, employment). In family patterns, a nourishing parent-child relationship serves as a protective factor in cushioning dysfunctional family processes as well as in increasing the child's self-esteem. The presence of a caring adult such as a grandparent leads to similar outcomes. External support from a neighbor, parents of peers, teacher, clergy, or social worker also serve as significant cushioning and protective factors. Finally, the broader social and physical environment and the opportunity structure create the conditions that influence all other factors. When social structures and institutions provide essential resources and supports, they are critical buffers, helping people cope with life transitions, environment, and interpersonal stressors.

The direction of a life trajectory is often determined by what happens at critical turning points in people's lives rather than long-standing attributes. Exercising foresight and taking active steps to cope with environmental challenges are critical factors. It is important to note that while planning and foresight are important protective factors, there is always the simple element of chance, good fortune and misfortune, or "God's will." While our efforts to be scientific may distance us from chance or spiritual beliefs and explanations, they may well enhance our understanding of and feeling for the human experience. Humor, an additional protective factor, has a profound impact on everyday interactions (Gitterman, 2003). For poor and oppressed populations, humor and laughter provide a safety valve for coping with painful realities. Religious, ethnic and racial humor help a stereotyped group to vent anger and to dismissively laugh at the dominant culture's stereotypes. Humor also helps the subtle and less visible forms of prejudice and discrimination to surface. By making the less visible more visible, oppression is challenged. To be able to laugh in the face of adversity and suffering releases tension and provides hope.

Deep ecology conceptualizes that all phenomena are interconnected and interdependent as well as dependent on the cyclical processes of nature (Greif, 2003; Ungar, 2002). Living systems are viewed as *networks* interacting and intertwined with other systems of networks. Through the processes of self-regulation and self-organization, new behaviors, patterns, and structures are spontaneously created and the networks' equilibrium constantly evolves. The interdependence of networks and the self-correcting feedback loops allow the living system to adapt to changing conditions and to survive disturbances. Thus, *interdependence of networks*, the *self-correcting feedback loops*, and the *cyclical nature of ecological processes* are three basic principles of deep ecology (Capra, 1996). Since the environment constantly changes and fluctuates, living organisms must keep themselves in a flexible state and adapt to changing conditions. Thus, *flexibility* is another ecological principle. However, living organisms have certain "tolerance limits" to how much change they can manage. If changing conditions go beyond what a network can deal with, it faces the danger and threat of collapse and disintegration. Diversity in the system will increase its potential resilience as stronger parts can replace the weaker ones. Diversity has the potential to enrich all the relationships and the system as a whole. However, if the system is *fragmented by the differences* among the parts and characterized by prejudice and discrimination, the diversity may decrease the system's resilience and its chances for survival.

Ecofeminism (or ecological feminism) challenges the culture-nature dichotomy and the sexual hierarchy. Western industrial societies assume the destructive domination of nature as their right. This destruction reinforces the subordination of women, long identified with nature. To ecofeminists, oppression of women and ecological degradation are *intertwined*. They both arise from hierarchical, male domination. For the ecofeminists, social justice cannot be achieved without the earth's well being. They took up the cause against toxic waste, animal abuse, deforestation, and nuclear disarmament. They combined ecology, feminism, and liberation for all of nature. The adage of "the personal is political" reflected an effort by feminist scholars to challenge the dualistic arrangement underlying the sexual hierarchy in Western views (Mack-Canty, 2004).

IMPLICATIONS FOR SOCIAL WORK PRACTICE AND RESEARCH The Life Model of Social Work practice operationalizes the ecological perspective. The purpose of life-modeled practice is to *improve the level of fit* between people and their environments, especially between human needs and environmental resources. In providing direct services to individuals, families, and groups, the purpose of social work is to (a) eliminate, or alleviate life stressors and the associated stress by helping people to mobilize and draw on personal and environmental resources for effective coping; and (b) influence social and physical environmental forces to be responsive to people's needs. In mediating the exchanges between people and their environments, social workers encounter daily the lack of fit between people's perceived needs and the environment. Thus the purpose of life-modeled practice also includes professional responsibility for bearing witness against social inequities and injustice. This is done by *mobilizing community resources* to influence quality of life in the community, by *influencing unresponsive organizations* to develop responsive policies and services, and by *politically influencing local, state, and federal legislation and regulations* to support social justice.

Naturalistic qualitative methods, widely used in Anthropology and Biology, are compatible with social work's ecological framework. In naturalistic explorations, the investigator is the major instrument of study. The social worker skilled in inviting and exploring clients' stories is a natural investigator into people's transactions with their social and physical environment. Constructivist researchers study the personal meanings people attribute to events in their lives. They believe that human experience cannot be studied by standing on the outside and can only be understood as a subjective reality. Subjective data must be gathered via people's narratives. Naturalistic inquiry is life-oriented and directed to context as well as people.

Acknowledgment

Carel B. Germain, my dear friend and collaborator for almost twenty-five years, died in 1995. Professor

Germain, an internationally recognized social work theoretician and historian, introduced the ecological perspective to the profession she deeply loved as a viable theoretical metaphor for social work practice (Germain, 1973).

REFERENCES

Capra, F. (1996). *The web of life*. New York: Anchor Books.

Dubos, R. (1968). *So human an animal*. New York: Scribner.

Fraser, M. (Ed.). (2004). *Risk and resilience in childhood: An ecological perspective*. Washington, DC: NASW Press.

Germain, C. B. (1973). An ecological perspective in casework. *Social Casework, 54*(6), 323–330.

Germain, C. B. (1976). Time: An ecological variable in social work practice. *Social Casework, 57*(7), 419–426.

Germain, C. B. (1978a). General systems theory and ego psychology: An ecological perspective. *Social Service Review, 52*(4), 535–550.

Germain, C. B. (1978b). Space, an ecological variable in social work practice. *Social Casework, 59*(9), 515–522.

Germain, C. B. (1983). Using social and physical environments. In A. Rosenblatt & D. Waldfogel (Eds.), *Handbook of clinical social work* (pp. 110–134). San Francisco: Jossey-Bass.

Germain, C. B. (1985). The place of community work within an ecological approach to social work practice. In S. H. Taylor & R. W. Roberts (Eds.), *Theory and practice of community social work* (pp. 30–55). New York: Columbia University Press.

Germain, C. B. (1990, March). Life forces and the anatomy of practice. *Smith College Studies in Social Work, 60*, 138–152.

Germain, C. B. (1994). Using an ecological perspective. In J. Rothman (Ed.), *Practice with highly vulnerable clients: Case management and community based service* (pp. 39–55). Englewood Cliffs, NJ: Prentice Hall.

Germain, C. B., & Gitterman, A. (1979). The life model of social work practice. In F. Turner (Ed.), *Social work treatment* (pp. 361–384). New York: Free Press.

Germain, C. B., & Gitterman, A. (1980). *The life model of social work practice*. New York: Columbia University Press.

Germain, C. B., & Gitterman, A. (1987). Ecological perspective. In A. Minahan (Ed.), *The encyclopedia of social work* (18th ed., pp. 488–499). Silver Spring, MD: National Association of Social Workers.

Germain, C. B., & Gitterman, A. (1995). Ecological perspective. In R. L. Edwards (Ed.), *Encyclopedia of social work* (19th ed., pp. 816–824). Silver Spring, MD: National Association of Social Workers.

Germain, C. B., & Gitterman, A. (1996). *The life model of social work practice: Advances in theory and practice* (2nd ed.). New York: Columbia University Press.

Gitterman, A. (1996). Advances in the life model of social work practice. In F. Turner (Ed.), *Social work treatment: Interlocking theoretical approaches* (pp. 389–408). New York: The Free Press.

Gitterman, A. (2001a). Vulnerability, resilience, and social work with groups. In T. Berman-Rossi, T. Kelly & S. Palombo (Eds.), *Strengthening resiliency through group work* (pp. 19–34). Binghamton, NY: Haworth Press.

Gitterman, A. (2001b). Social work practice with resilient and vulnerable and resilient populations. In A. Gitterman (Ed.), *Social work practice with vulnerable and resilient populations* (2nd ed., pp. 1–38). New York: Columbia University Press.

Gitterman, A. (2003). The uses of humor in social work practice. *Reflections: Narratives of Professional Helping, 9*(2), 79–84.

Gitterman, A. (2007). The life model of social work practice. In A. Roberts & G. J. Greene (Eds.), *Social work desk reference* (pp. 231–241). New York: Oxford University Press.

Gitterman, A. (2010). Advances in the life mode of social work practice. In F. Turner (Ed.), *Social work treatment: Interlocking theoretical approaches* (pp. 279–292). New York: Oxford University Press.

Gitterman, A., & Germain, C. B. (1976, December). Social work practice: A life model. *Social Service Review, 50*, 601–610.

Gitterman, A., & Germain, C. B. (2008). *The life model of social work practice: Advances in theory and practice* (3rd ed.). New York: Columbia University Press.

Gitterman, A., & Heller, N. (2011). Integrating social work perspectives and models with concepts, methods and skills with other professions' specialized approaches. *Clinical Journal of Social Work Practice, 39*(2), 204–211.

Gitterman, A., & Shulman, L. (2005). The life model, oppression, vulnerability and resilience, mutual aid, and the mediating function. In A. Gitterman & L. Shulman (Eds.), *Mutual aid groups, vulnerable and resilient populations, and the life cycle* (3rd ed., pp. 3–37). New York: Columbia University Press.

Greif, G. L. (2003). In response to Michael Ungar's "A deeper, more social ecological social work practice." *Social Service Review, 77*(2), 306–308.

Hearn, G. (Ed.). (1969). *The general systems approach: Contributions toward a holistic conception of social work*. New York: Council on Social Work Education.

Lazarus, R.S. (1999). *Stress and emotion: A new synthesis*. New York: Springer.

Lazarus, R. S., & Lazarus, B. N. (2006). *Coping with aging*. New York: Oxford University Press.

Mack-Canty, C. (2004). Third-wave feminism and the need to reweave the nature/culture duality. *NWSA Journal, 16*(3), 154–179.

Smith, C., & Carlson, B. (1997). Stress, coping and resilience in children and youth. *Social Service Review, 71*(2), 231–256.

Ungar, M. (2002). A deeper, more social ecological social work practice. *Social Service Review, 76*(3), 480–497.

Ungar, M. (2008). Resilience across cultures. *The British Journal of Social Work, 38*(2), 218–235.

Werner, C., Altman, I., Oxley, D., & Haggard, L. (1987). People, place, and time: A transactional analysis of neighborhoods.

In W. Jones & D. Perlman (Eds.), *Advances in personal relationships* (pp. 243–275). New York: JAI Press.

ALEX GITTERMAN AND CAREL B. GERMAIN

ETHICS AND VALUES

ABSTRACT: Social workers' understanding of professional values and ethics has matured considerably. During the earliest years of the profession's history, social workers' attention was focused primarily on cultivating a set of values upon which the mission of the profession could be based. More recently, social workers have developed comprehensive ethical standards to guide practitioners and decision-making frameworks that are useful when practitioners face difficult ethical dilemmas. Today's social workers also have a better understanding of the relationship between their ethical decisions and potential malpractice risks.

KEY WORDS: ethical theory; ethical decision making; ethical dilemmas; ethics; *NASW Code of Ethics*; risk management; values

Ethics and values are at the heart of the social work profession. Although there has been considerable stability in the core values of the profession, the day-to-day ethical issues that social workers encounter have not remained static. On the contrary, applications of core values in social work have undergone substantial change over the years in response to social, political, and economic developments.

The Evolution of Social Work Ethics and Values

Social workers' thinking about values and ethics has evolved during four major periods (Reamer, 1998, 2013a). The first stage, the *morality period*, began in the late 19th century, when social work was formally introduced as a profession. During this period social work was much more concerned about the morality of the client than about the morality or ethics of the profession or its practitioners. Over time, particularly during the Settlement House movement and Progressive era in the early 20th century, social workers' attitudes began to shift from concern about the morality, or immorality, of the poor to the need for significant social reform designed to ameliorate a wide range of social problems, for example, those related to housing, health care, sanitation, employment, poverty, and education. During the Great Depression and New Deal years, social workers promoted social reforms to address structural problems.

During the second stage, the *values period*, concern about the morality of the client continued to recede. During the next several decades, especially during the 1960s and 1970s, a group of social workers engaged in ambitious attempts to develop a consensus about the profession's core values (Biestek, 1957; Gordon, 1962; Keith-Lucas, 1977; Levy, 1973, 1976; McDermott, 1975; Pumphrey, 1959; Teicher, 1967; Timms, 1983). It was during this period that the National Association of Social Workers (NASW; 1960) adopted its first formal code of ethics.

In addition to exploring the core values of social work, some of the literature during this period also reflects practitioners' efforts to examine and clarify the relationship between their own personal values and the profession's values (for example, Hardiman, 1975; Varley, 1968). Not surprisingly, given the widespread social challenges and turbulence in the 1960s and 1970s, social workers engaged in complex debates about values concerning the core constructs of social justice and rights (welfare rights, clients' rights, prisoners' rights, women's rights, patients' rights, and so on).

Until the late 1970s, social work focused primarily on the profession's core values and value base. In the third stage, the *ethical theory and decision-making period*, social work underwent another significant transition in its concern about values and ethical issues (Banks, 2012; Barsky, 2009, Beckett & Maynard, 2005; Dolgoff, Harrington, & Loewenberg, 2012; Gray & Webb, 2010; Reamer, 2009, 2012a). During the mid- and late 1970s a number of professions (medicine, law, business, journalism, engineering, nursing, social work, psychology, psychiatry, criminal justice, and others) began to explore ethical issues in depth (Callahan & Bok, 1980). During this period the new academic field of applied and professional ethics (also known as practical ethics) emerged. Led especially by developments in the bioethics field, various professions engaged in ambitious attempts to identify key ethical dilemmas, formulate ethical decision-making protocols, and develop guidelines for ethics consultation. During this period the NASW *Encyclopedia of Social Work* included, for the first time, an article directly exploring the relevance of philosophical and ethical concepts to social work ethics (Reamer, 1987). Unlike social work's earlier literature, publications on social work ethics in the 1980s began to explore the relevance of moral philosophy and ethical theory (for example, theories of metaethics, normative ethics, deontology, and utilitarianism) to ethical dilemmas faced by practitioners.

The most recent stage in the evolution of social work ethics in the United States, the *ethical standards and risk-management period*, reflects the dramatic maturation of social workers' understanding of ethical issues. This stage is characterized by the significant expansion of ethical standards to guide practitioners' conduct and by increased knowledge concerning ethics-related negligence and professional malpractice. More specifically, this period includes the development of a comprehensive code of ethics for the profession, the emergence of a significant body of literature focusing on ethics-related malpractice and liability risks, and practical risk-management strategies designed to protect clients and prevent ethics complaints and ethics-related lawsuits (Barker & Branson, 2000; Houston-Vega, Nuehring, & Daguio, 1997; Reamer, 2003, 2006).

Current thinking about social work ethics and values is broad in scope. In general, it encompasses three distinguishable, though related, sets of issues. The first concerns the nature of the profession's core values and their relevance to the overall mission, goals, and priorities of social work, especially as reflected in the *NASW Code of Ethics* (NASW, 2008). The second issue pertains to ethical dilemmas and decisions that social workers encounter as they carry out their professional duties and obligations, particularly their efforts to meet clients' needs and protect them and relevant third parties from harm. The third issue relates to ethics risk management, that is, practical steps that social workers can take to protect clients and prevent ethics-related litigation and ethics complaints filed with state licensing boards and professional associations.

Value Base of Social Work

The subject of social work values has always been central to the profession. Values have several important attributes and perform several important functions: They are generalized, emotionally charged conceptions of what is desirable; historically created and derived from experience; shared by a population or a group within it; and provide the means for organizing and structuring patterns of behavior (Williams, 1968).

Values have been important in social work in several key respects, with regard to (1) the nature of social work's mission; (2) the relationships that social workers have with clients, colleagues, and members of the broader society; (3) the methods of intervention that social workers use in their work; and (4) the resolution of ethical dilemmas in practice.

Social work's fundamental aims and mission are rooted in deep-seated beliefs among the profession's founders and contemporary practitioners concerning the values of helping, aiding, and assisting people who experience problems in living (Reid, 1992). Social work is not mere technology; rather, it is a value-based and value-inspired effort designed to help vulnerable people through the use of sophisticated methods of intervention (Timms, 1983).

Social workers' values influence the kinds of relationships they have with clients, colleagues, and members of the broader society (Hamilton, 1940; Mattison, 2000; Younghusband, 1967). Social workers make choices about the people with whom they want to work. For example, some practitioners devote their careers to clients they perceive as victims, such as abused children and individuals born with severe physical disabilities. Others choose to work with people living in poverty or clients perceived by many to be perpetrators, such as prison inmates convicted of serious sex offenses.

Social workers' values also influence their decisions about the intervention methods they will use in their work with clients—whether individuals, families, groups, communities, or organizations (Banks, 2012; McDermott, 1975; Varley, 1968). For example, some social workers prefer to use confrontational techniques in their work with juvenile delinquents and people struggling with addictions, believing that these are the most effective means for bringing about behavior change. Other practitioners who work with these same populations may be critical of confrontational methods that seem dehumanizing and, because of their values, may prefer forms of counseling that emphasize clients' strengths, clients' right to self-determination, and the building of therapeutic alliances.

Or a social worker who is an advocate for low-income housing in a poor neighborhood may prefer direct confrontation with public officials—in the form of demonstrations, rallies, and harassment—in an effort to promote affordable housing. For this practitioner the value of providing basic shelter for poor people is paramount, and direct confrontation may be necessary to bring it about. Another practitioner may reject such tactics because of his belief in the value of collaboration and respectful exploration of differences.

This leads to another way in which values are central to social work: They are key to efforts to resolve ethical dilemmas that involve conflicts of professional duties and obligations. Ethical dilemmas ordinarily involve values that clash, for example, when a client's right to confidentiality conflicts with the social worker's duty to disclose confidential information, without a client's consent, to protect a third party from harm.

When faced with ethical dilemmas, social workers ultimately base their decisions on their beliefs about the nature of social work values—particularly as they are translated into specific professional duties and obligations—and which values take precedence when they conflict.

As social work has evolved, it has continually stressed the need to attend both to the needs of individual clients and to the ways that the community and society create and respond to those needs. Thus, there has always been a simultaneous concern in social work for individual well-being and the environmental factors that affect it. This unique perspective—which reflects the evolution of scholarly thinking in the profession about the nature of its core values and the professional mission based on them—is stated clearly in the preamble to the *NASW Code of Ethics* (2008):

> The primary mission of the social work profession is to enhance human well-being and help meet the basic human needs of all people, with particular attention to the needs and empowerment of people who are vulnerable, oppressed, and living in poverty. A historic and defining feature of social work is the profession's focus on individual well-being in a social context and the well-being of society. Fundamental to social work is attention to the environmental forces that create, contribute to, and address problems in living. . . .
>
> The mission of the social work profession is rooted in a set of core values. These core values, embraced by social workers throughout the profession's history, are the foundation of social work's unique purpose and perspective: service; social justice; dignity and worth of the person; importance of human relationships; integrity; and competence. (p. 1)

Social workers' values often shape their professional actions and ethical decisions. Some moral philosophers argue that professionals' own moral virtues and character are at the heart of ethical decisions (MacIntyre, 1984). From the point of view of *virtue ethics*, an ethical person has virtuous values and character traits—such as integrity, truthfulness, generosity, loyalty, sincerity, kindness, compassion, and trustworthiness—and acts in a manner consistent with them. These core virtues provide the foundation that leads to professionals' deep respect for clients' fundamental right to autonomy and self-determination, commitment to helping people in need and avoiding harming others, and pursuit of justice (Beauchamp & Childress, 2012).

The most visible contemporary typology of social work values appears in the current *NASW Code of Ethics* (2008). The NASW Code of Ethics Revision Committee decided to include in this version of the code, for the first time in social work's history, a list of core values for the profession. After systematically reviewing many historical and contemporary discussions of social work values in an effort to identify key themes and patterns, the committee generated a list of six core values and developed a broadly worded, value-based ethical principle and brief annotation for each of these values (pp. 5–6):

1. Value: *Service*

   Ethical Principle: *Social workers' primary goal is to help people in need and to address social problems.* Social workers elevate service to others above self-interest. Social workers draw on their knowledge, values, and skills to help people in need and to address social problems. Social workers are encouraged to volunteer some portion of their professional skills with no expectation of significant financial return (pro bono service).

2. Value: *Social Justice*

   Ethical Principle: *Social workers challenge social injustice.* Social workers pursue social change, particularly with and on behalf of vulnerable and oppressed individuals and groups of people. Social workers' social change efforts are focused primarily on issues of poverty, unemployment, discrimination, and others forms of social injustice. These activities seek to promote sensitivity to and knowledge about oppression and cultural and ethnic diversity. Social workers strive to ensure access to needed information, services, and resources; equality of opportunity; and meaningful participation in decision making for all people.

3. Value: *Dignity and Worth of the Person*

   Ethical Principle: *Social workers respect the inherent dignity and worth of the person.* Social workers treat each person in a caring and respectful fashion, mindful of individual differences and cultural and ethnic diversity. Social workers promote clients' socially responsible self-determination. Social workers seek to enhance clients' capacity and opportunity to change and to address their own needs. Social workers are cognizant of their dual responsibility to clients and to the broader society. They seek to resolve conflicts between clients' interests and the broader society's interests in a socially responsible manner consistent with the values, ethical principles, and ethical standards of the profession.

4. Value: *Importance of Human Relationships*

Ethical Principle: *Social workers recognize the central importance of human relationships.* Social workers understand that relationships between and among people are an important vehicle for change. Social workers engage people as partners in the helping process. Social workers seek to strengthen relationships among people in a purposeful effort to promote, restore, maintain, and enhance the well-being of individuals, families, social groups, organizations, and communities.

5. Value: *Integrity*

Ethical Principle: *Social workers behave in a trustworthy manner.* Social workers are continually aware of the profession's mission, values, ethical principles, and ethical standards and practice in a manner consistent with them. Social workers act honestly and responsibly and promote ethical practices on the part of the organizations with which they are affiliated.

6. Value: *Competence*

Ethical Principle: *Social workers practice within their areas of competence and develop and enhance their professional expertise.* Social workers continually strive to increase their professional knowledge and skills and to apply them in practice. Social workers should aspire to contribute to the knowledge base of the profession.

Ethical Dilemmas and Decisions

Social workers encounter a wide range of ethical dilemmas. Ethical dilemmas occur when social workers must choose among conflicting professional values, duties, and rights that arise sometimes due to their competing obligations to clients, employers, colleagues, the social work profession, and society at large. Moral philosophers and ethicists often refer to these situations as "hard cases." These are cases that require a difficult choice between conflicting duties, or what the philosopher W. D. Ross (1930) referred to as conflicting "prima facie duties"—duties that, when considered by themselves, social workers are inclined to perform. Eventually, social workers must choose what Ross called an "actual" duty from among conflicting prima facie duties.

In social work many ethical decisions are routine, such as obtaining clients' consent before releasing confidential information and avoiding sexual contact with clients. These prima facie duties are clear. In some instances, however, prima facie duties are unclear and ethical decisions are much more complex and troubling.

Ethical dilemmas in social work occur in three domains: relationships with clients in direct-practice settings (delivery of services to individuals, families, and small groups); social work involving "macro" practice, such as community practice (community organizing and advocacy or social action), administration, management, and policy development and implementation; and relationships among professional colleagues. Examples of challenging ethical dilemmas include the following:

- Privacy, confidentiality, and privileged communication: Under what circumstances do clients forfeit their rights, particularly if the client threatens to harm himself or others, has abused or neglected a child or vulnerable adult, or if a court of law orders social workers to disclose information? How do social workers protect client confidentiality when they communicate using email and store clinical records electronically?
- Client self-determination and professional paternalism: What are the limits to clients' right to self-determination, particularly when they engage in self-harming behavior or threaten others? Is it ever justifiable to lie to clients or withhold information from them, paternalistically, "for their own good"?
- Boundaries and dual relationships: How should social workers handle, for example, personal relationships with former clients, self-disclosure to clients, electronic communications with clients (for example, on social networking sites and via email), bartering for services, relationships in small and rural communities, gifts offered by clients, and clients' invitations to attend life-cycle events?
- Adhering to laws, policies, and regulations: Is it ethically permissible for social workers to violate laws, policies, and regulations that they consider to be unjust or harmful to clients (for example, unusually strict eligibility standards and policies that discriminate against undocumented immigrants)?
- Whistle-blowing: Under what circumstances are social workers obligated to disclose ethical misconduct engaged in by colleagues or agency administrators?
- Distribution of limited resources: What is the most ethical way to allocate scarce resources, such as agency funds or subsidized housing units? Should social workers distribute resources based on need, the principle of equality (in the form of a lottery; first come, first served; or, when possible, equal shares), affirmative action criteria,

cost-benefit considerations, or clients' ability to pay?

- Conflicts between personal and professional values: How should social workers resolve clashes between their deeply held personal beliefs and their professional duties (for example, with respect to clients' reproductive rights or end-of-life decisions)?

Ethical Decision Making and Standards

There is no simple, tidy formula for resolving ethical dilemmas. By definition, ethical dilemmas are complex. Reasonable, thoughtful social workers can disagree about the ethical principles and standards that ought to guide ethical decisions in any given case. But ethicists generally agree that it is important to approach ethical decisions systematically, to follow a series of steps to ensure that all aspects of the ethical dilemma are addressed. By following a series of clearly formulated steps, social workers can enhance the quality of the ethical decisions they make and the likelihood that they will protect clients, third parties, and themselves. Typically these steps involve the following: (1) identifying the ethical issues, including the social work values and conflicting duties; (2) identifying the individuals, groups, and organizations likely to be affected by the ethical decision; (3) tentatively identifying all viable courses of action and the participants involved in each, along with the potential benefits and risks for each; (4) thoroughly examining the reasons in favor of and opposed to each course of action, considering relevant ethical theories, principles, and guidelines; codes of ethics and legal principles; social work practice theory and principles; and personal values (including religious, cultural, and ethnic values and political ideology); (5) consulting with colleagues and appropriate experts (such as agency staff, supervisors, agency administrators, agency ethics committee, attorneys, ethics scholars); (6) making the decision and documenting the decision-making process; and (7) monitoring, evaluating, and documenting the decision (Barsky, 2009; Congress, 1999; Dolgoff, Harrington, & Loewenberg, 2012; Linzer, 1999; Reamer, 2001a, 2013a).

Social workers can use several tools—including codes of ethics, ethical principles, and ethical theory—to help make ethical decisions.

CODES OF ETHICS   Nearly all professions have developed codes of ethics to assist practitioners who face ethical dilemmas; most were developed during the 20th century. Codes of ethics serve several functions

in addition to providing general guidance related to ethical dilemmas: They also protect the profession from outside regulation, establish norms related to the profession's mission and methods, and enunciate standards that can help adjudicate allegations of misconduct (Reamer, 2006).

In North America social work has had two prominent codes of ethics: the *NASW Code of Ethics* and the Code of Ethics of the Canadian Association of Social Workers. Ethics guidelines are also featured in the Code of Ethics of the National Association of Black Social Workers and the Code of Ethics of the Clinical Social Work Association. Social work organizations in many other nations have also adopted codes of ethics. Key examples include codes developed by social work associations in Australia, Denmark, Finland, France, Germany, Ireland, Israel, Italy, Japan, Luxembourg, Norway, Portugal, Russia, Singapore, Spain, Sweden, Switzerland, Turkey, and the United Kingdom. In addition, the International Federation of Social Workers (IFSW) developed a prominent code of ethics that includes important principles pertaining to human rights, human dignity, social justice, and professional conduct. The IFSW Code of Ethics focuses especially on broad ethical concepts related to clients' strengths and right to self-determination, client confidentiality, nondiscrimination, cultural and social diversity, distributive justice, social action, and professionals' competence, integrity, compassion, and self-care.

The best-known ethics code to which social workers in the United States subscribe is the *NASW Code of Ethics*. The organization has published several versions of the code, reflecting changes in the broader culture and in social work standards. The first NASW code was published in 1960, five years after the organization was formed. The 1960 Code of Ethics consisted of a series of proclamations concerning, for example, every social worker's duty to give precedence to professional responsibility over personal interests; respect the privacy of clients; give appropriate professional service in public emergencies; and contribute knowledge, skills, and support to programs of human welfare. Brief first-person statements (such as "I give precedence to my professional responsibility over my personal interests" and "I respect the privacy of the people I serve") were preceded by a preamble that set forth social workers' responsibility to uphold humanitarian ideals, maintain and improve social work service, and develop the philosophy and skills of the profession. In 1967 a principle pledging nondiscrimination was added to the proclamations.

However, over time some NASW members began to express concern about the code's vagueness, its scope and usefulness in resolving ethical dilemmas, and its provisions for handling ethics complaints about practitioners and agencies. In 1977 the NASW Delegate Assembly established a task force to revise the profession's code of ethics and to enhance its relevance to practice. The revised code, ratified in 1979, was much more detailed; it included six sections of brief principles preceded by a preamble setting forth the general purpose of the code, the enduring social work values upon which it was based, and a declaration that the code's principles provide standards for the enforcement of ethical practices among social workers. The 1979 code set forth principles related to social workers' conduct and comportment, and to ethical responsibility to clients, colleagues, employers and employing organizations, the social work profession, and society. A number of the code's principles were concrete and specific (for example, "The social worker should under no circumstances engage in sexual activities with clients," and "The social worker should respect confidences shared by colleagues in the course of their professional relationships and transactions"), whereas others were more abstract, asserting ethical ideals (for example, "The social worker should promote the general welfare of society," and "The social worker should uphold and advance the values, ethics, knowledge, and mission of the profession").

The 1979 code was revised twice. In 1990 several principles related to solicitation of clients and fee setting were modified after the Federal Trade Commission (FTC) began an inquiry in 1986 concerning the possibility that NASW policies promoted "restraint of trade." As a result of the inquiry, NASW revised principles in the code in order to remove prohibitions concerning solicitation of clients from colleagues or one's agency and to modify wording related to accepting compensation for making a referral. NASW also entered into a consent agreement with the FTC concerning the issues raised by the inquiry.

In 1992 the president of NASW appointed a national task force, chaired by this author, to suggest several specific revisions of the code. In 1993, based on the task force recommendations, the NASW Delegate Assembly voted to amend the code to include several new principles related to the problem of social worker impairment and the problem of inappropriate boundaries between social workers and clients, colleagues, students, and so on.

Because of growing dissatisfaction with the 1979 NASW code, and because of dramatic developments in the field of applied and professional ethics since the ratification of the 1979 code, the 1993 NASW Delegate Assembly also passed a resolution to establish a task force to draft an entirely new code of ethics for submission to the 1996 Delegate Assembly. The task force, chaired by this author, was established in an effort to develop a new code of ethics that would be far more comprehensive in scope and relevant to contemporary practice. Since the adoption of the 1979 code, social workers had developed a much keener grasp of a wide range of ethical issues facing practitioners, many of which were not addressed in the NASW code. Moreover, the broader field of applied and professional ethics, which had begun in the early 1970s, had matured considerably, resulting in the identification and greater understanding of novel ethical issues not cited in the 1979 code.

THE CURRENT NASW CODE OF ETHICS The current code was adopted by the 1996 Delegate Assembly. In 2008 the Delegate Assembly approved wording changes in standards related to cultural competence and social diversity, respect for colleagues, discrimination, and social and political action. The code contains the most comprehensive contemporary statement of ethical standards in social work and includes four major sections . The first section, "Preamble," summarizes the mission and core values of social work, the first ever sanctioned by NASW for its code of ethics.

The second section, "Purpose of the NASW Code of Ethics," provides an overview of the code's main functions and a brief guide for dealing with ethical issues or dilemmas in social work practice. The brief guide in this section of the code to dealing with ethical issues highlights various resources social workers should consider when faced with difficult ethical decisions. Such resources include ethical theory and decision making, social work practice theory and research, laws, regulations, agency policies, and other relevant codes of ethics. The guide encourages social workers to obtain ethics consultation when appropriate, perhaps from an agency-based or social work organization's ethics committee, regulatory bodies (for example, a state licensing board), knowledgeable colleagues, supervisors, or legal counsel.

An important feature of this section of the code is its explicit acknowledgment that instances sometimes arise in social work in which the code's values, principles, and standards conflict. Moreover, at times the code's provisions can conflict with agency policies, relevant laws or regulations, and ethical standards in allied professions (such as psychology and counseling). The code does not provide a formula for resolving such conflicts and "does not specify which values, principles, and standards are most important and ought to outweigh others in instances when they conflict." (NASW, 2008, p. 3)

The code's third section, "Ethical Principles," presents six broad ethical principles that inform social work practice, one for each of the six core values cited in the preamble. The principles are presented at a fairly high level of abstraction to provide a conceptual base for the profession's more specific ethical standards. The code also includes a brief annotation for each of the principles.

The code's final section, "Ethical Standards," includes 155 specific ethical standards to guide social workers' conduct and provide a basis for adjudication of ethics complaints filed against NASW members. The standards fall into six categories concerning social workers' ethical responsibilities to clients, to colleagues, in practice settings, as professionals, to the profession, and to society at large. The introduction to this section of the code states explicitly that some standards are enforceable guidelines for professional conduct and some are standards to which social workers should aspire. Furthermore, the code states, "The extent to which each standard is enforceable is a matter of professional judgment to be exercised by those responsible for reviewing alleged violations of ethical standards" (NASW, 2008, p. 7).

ETHICAL THEORY One key trend in professional education and training is to introduce students and practitioners to ethical theories and principles that may help them analyze and resolve ethical dilemmas (Congress, Black, & Strom-Gottfried, 2009; Reamer, 1990). These include theories and principles of what moral philosophers call *metaethics*, *normative ethics*, and *practical* (or *applied*) ethics. Briefly, metaethics concerns the meaning of ethical terms or language and the derivation of ethical principles and guidelines. Typical metaethical questions concern the meaning of the terms *right* and *wrong* and *good* and *bad*. What criteria should we use to judge whether someone has engaged in unethical conduct? How should we go about formulating ethical principles to guide individuals who struggle with moral choices? Normative ethics attempts to answer the question, "Which general moral norms for the guidance and evaluation of conduct should we accept and why?"

In contrast to metaethics, which is often abstract, normative ethics tends to be of special concern to social workers because of its immediate relevance to practice. Normative ethics consists of attempts to apply ethical theories and principles to actual ethical dilemmas. Practical (or applied) ethics is the attempt to apply ethical norms and theories of normative ethics to specific problems and contexts, such as professions, organizations, and public policy. Such guidance is especially useful when social workers face conflicts among duties they are ordinarily inclined to perform.

Theories of normative ethics are generally grouped under two main headings. Deontological theories (from the Greek *deontos*, "of the obligatory") are those that claim that certain actions are inherently right or wrong, or good and bad, without regard for their consequences. Thus a deontologist might argue that telling the truth is inherently right, and therefore social workers should never lie to clients, even if it appears that lying might be more beneficial to the parties involved. The same might be said about keeping promises made to colleagues, upholding contracts with managed care organizations and insurance companies, obeying a mandatory reporting law, and so on. For deontologists, rules, rights, and principles are sacred and inviolable. The ends do not necessarily justify the means, particularly if they require violating some important rule, right, principle, or law.

The second major group of theories, *teleological* theories (from the Greek *teleios*, 'brought to its end or purpose'), takes a different approach to ethical choices. From this point of view, the rightness of any action is determined by the goodness of its consequences. Teleologists think it is naive to make ethical choices without weighing potential consequences. To do otherwise is to engage in what the philosopher Smart (Smart & Williams, 1973) referred to as "rule worship." Therefore, from this perspective (also known as *utilitarianism* and *consequentialism*), the responsible strategy entails an attempt to anticipate the outcomes of various courses of action and to weigh their relative merits.

A noteworthy problem with utilitarianism is that different people are likely to consider different factors and weigh them differently, as a result of their different life experiences, values, education, political ideologies, and so on. In addition, when taken to the extreme, classic utilitarianism can justify trampling on the rights of a vulnerable minority in order to benefit the majority, an outcome that is anathema to social workers.

Two other ethical theories have important implications for social workers: *communitarianism* (also known as community-based theory) and the *ethics of care*. According to communitarianism, ethical decisions should be based primarily on what is best for the community and communal values (the common good, social goals, and cooperative virtues) as opposed to individual self-interest. The ethics of care, in contrast, reflects a collection of moral perspectives rather than a single moral principle. This view emphasizes the importance in ethics and moral decision making of the need to care for, and willingness to act on behalf of, persons with whom one has a significant relationship (Spano & Koenig, 2003). For social workers this perspective emphasizes the critical importance of commitment to their clients.

Ethics Enforcement and Risk Management
Sometimes ethics complaints and lawsuits are filed against social workers. Members of NASW, for example, may be named in ethics complaints alleging violation of standards in the association's *Code of Ethics*. In addition, social workers can be named in complaints filed with a state licensing board. Also, disgruntled parties may file lawsuits against social workers alleging they were harmed as a result of practitioners' ethics-related professional negligence (for example, as a result of an inappropriate dual relationship, incompetent service delivery, or unauthorized disclosure of confidential information). Social workers can prevent lawsuits and ethics complaints by conducting an ethics audit, which is designed to assess the adequacy of practitioners' and agencies' ethics-related policies, practices, and procedures (Reamer, 2001b).

NASW and state licensing boards follow very strict procedures when they process complaints filed against social workers to ensure that all parties receive a fair hearing consistent with due process standards. NASW members who are named in ethics complaints have the opportunity to testify, present witnesses, and challenge any evidence that is presented against them. Using a peer review process, an NASW committee decides whether there is sufficient evidence to conclude that a member has violated the NASW *Code of Ethics*. NASW may impose sanctions or require various forms of corrective action when there is evidence of ethical misconduct, such as suspension from NASW; mandated supervision or consultation; censure in the form of a letter; or instructions to send the complainant a letter of apology. In some cases the sanction may be publicized.

In contrast to NASW ethics proceedings, state licensing boards must determine whether social workers have violated provisions in state licensing laws or regulations. State licensing boards that find evidence of violation can impose a range of sanctions or require various forms of corrective action, such as license suspension or revocation; mandated supervision, consultation, or continuing education; and censure in the form of a letter. Some sanctions are publicized, for example, in local newspapers or the licensing board's website.

Lawsuits filed against social workers alleging ethics-related negligence are processed according to legal procedures for civil litigation and related standards of proof (Reamer, 2003). The process may include subpoenas of records, depositions, interrogatories, expert witness testimony, and trial before a judge or jury. Most lawsuits are settled pretrial, often for dollar amounts agreed to by the parties. Cases that go to trial may result in monetary awards.

In a very small percentage of cases social workers are indicted on criminal charges that allege ethical misconduct. Examples include instances when a social worker has submitted fraudulent bills to clients' insurance companies, embezzled funds from an employer, or engaged in sexual misconduct with a client who is a minor.

In some instances social workers involved in ethical misconduct are impaired. Impairment involves problems in a social worker's functioning reflected in an inability or unwillingness to follow professional standards; an inability or unwillingness to acquire professional skills in order to reach an acceptable level of competency; and an inability or unwillingness to control personal stress and emotional problems that interfere with professional functioning (Reamer, 1992; Zur, 2007). Impairment may involve failure to provide competent care or violation of the profession's ethical standards. It may also take such forms as providing flawed or inferior counseling to a client, sexual involvement with a client, or failure to carry out professional duties as a result of substance abuse or mental illness.

It is important for social workers to design ways to prevent impairment and respond to impaired colleagues. They must be knowledgeable about the indicators and causes of impairment so that they can recognize problems that colleagues may be experiencing. Social workers must also be willing to confront impaired colleagues, offer assistance and consultation, and, if necessary, as a last resort, refer the colleague to a supervisor or local regulatory or disciplinary body.

Social workers who become aware of a colleague's impairment or unethical conduct may have to make a difficult ethical decision about whether to "blow the whistle." In these instances social workers should consult colleagues, supervisors, ethics experts, and guidelines in the *NASW Code of Ethics* (sections 2.09, 2.10, 2.11) for guidance and support.

In an effort to prevent ethical misconduct and enhance social workers' ethical judgment, NASW chapters and NASW's national office, state licensing boards, social work education programs, and continuing education organizations sponsor ethics education programs throughout the United States. Many states require licensed social workers to take continuing education courses on ethics.

The Future of Social Work Ethics

Social workers have been concerned about ethics and values since the profession began. Social work has a long-standing history of commitment to issues of social justice and to the dignified, fair treatment of people in need of assistance. Although many of the ethical issues of current concern in the profession have been the focus of attention for decades, others have emerged only recently. Future changes in the profession will no doubt lead to new ethical issues and questions.

There is no way to know with certainty what issues are likely to emerge in the future, but several trends are worth noting. First, it will be important for social workers to pay close attention to ethical issues created by technological advances that affect the profession. For example, developments in computer, digital, and other electronic technology will continue to lead to difficult issues related to privacy and confidentiality. The proliferation and widespread use of digital and electronic technology has created novel and unprecedented ethical challenges for social workers, especially related to informed consent, privacy, confidentiality, and boundaries. The popularity of Facebook, LinkedIn, Twitter, email, mobile and smartphones, videoconferencing, and telephone and Web-based therapies has created a wide range of challenging ethical issues that did not exist when many contemporary practitioners concluded their formal education (Gutheil & Simon, 2005; Lamendola, 2010; Menon & Miller-Cribbs, 2002; Reamer, 2012b, 2013b; Zur, 2012). Practitioners who use Facebook must decide whether to accept clients' requests for friend status. Similarly, practitioners must decide whether they are willing to exchange email and text messages with clients and, if so, under what circumstances; share their personal mobile telephone numbers with clients; or offer clinical services by means of videoconferencing or other cybertherapy options, such as those that allow clients to represent themselves using graphical avatars rather than real-life images.

Considerable controversy surrounds social workers' use of online interventions, social media, and electronic communications. Some practitioners are enthusiastic supporters of these technologies as therapeutic tools. Others are harsh critics or skeptics, arguing that heavy reliance on online interventions and social media compromises the quality of social work services and could endanger clients who are clinically vulnerable and who would be better served by in-person care. In addition, critics argue that widespread delivery of services using electronic and digital technology may interfere with social workers' ability to serve people living in poverty and other oppressed people who may have no or very limited access to this technology. Social work licensing boards and regulatory bodies are developing new ethics guidelines for social workers who use digital and other electronic technology.

In addition, developments in medical technology will raise new ethical questions related to the allocation of health care, end-of-life decisions, and the use of novel medical interventions. In response to these advances, many social work agencies have formed ethics committees to consult on difficult decisions, educate staff about ethical issues, and formulate ethics-related policies (Hester, 2007; Reamer, 1987).

Another critical issue concerns employment patterns among social workers themselves. Some social workers resist entering the public social service sector that serves particularly vulnerable, oppressed, and low-income people. This raises important ethical questions about the mission of social work and its value base. To what extent should social work place primary emphasis on the poor and oppressed as opposed to more affluent clients who have ample assets or insurance coverage to pay for services? What portion of the profession's resources should be devoted to clinical issues as opposed to social action, such as advocacy on behalf of the least advantaged?

In addition, as social work develops new specialties, novel questions of ethics and values are likely to emerge. For example, some practitioners are pursuing dual careers as social workers and as lawyers, clergy, and life coaches. These combinations pose unique ethical challenges related to professional–client boundaries, informed consent, confidentiality, and privacy. Practitioners who are both social workers and lawyers or clergy, for example, are accountable to very different, sometimes conflicting, ethical standards pertaining to confidentiality and privileged communication. Social workers who function as life coaches may face complex challenges concerning professional boundaries, particularly if the coaching services involve clients' disclosure of deeply personal information, home visits, and casual meetings in social settings, such as restaurants. Also, as social workers' involvement in managed care organizations has grown, so too have ethical issues concerning the allocation of limited health care resources.

The future of social work cannot be predicted with precision, but it is certain that ethical and value issues will continue to permeate the profession. Although some of these issues will change in response to new trends and developments, the fundamental issues related to ethics and values in social work will persist, such as the nature of social work's core mission and values, the balance between public and private sector responsibility for social welfare, practitioners' moral duty to aid those most in need, the nature and limits of clients' right to confidentiality and self-determination, management of professional boundaries, and challenges involving the allocation of limited social services resources. Hence, it will always be essential for social workers to examine these issues, which in the end form the very foundation of the profession.

REFERENCES

Banks, S. (2012). *Ethics and values in social work* (4th ed.). Basingstoke, UK: Palgrave Macmillan.

Barker, R. L., & Branson, D. M. (2000). *Forensic social work* (2nd ed.). New York: Haworth Press.

Barsky, A. E. (2009). *Ethics and values in social work: An integrated approach for a comprehensive curriculum.* New York: Oxford University Press.

Beauchamp, T., & Childress, J. (2012). *Principles of biomedical ethics* (7th ed.). New York: Oxford University Press.

Beckett, C., & Maynard, A. (2005). *Values and ethics in social work: An introduction.* London: Sage.

Biestek, F. P. (1957). *The casework relationship.* Chicago, IL: Loyola University Press.

Callahan, D., & Bok, S. (Eds.) (1980). *Ethics teaching in higher education.* New York: Plenum Press.

Congress, E. (1999). *Social work values and ethics.* Belmont, CA: Wadsworth.

Congress, E., Black, P., & Strom-Gottfried, K. (2009). *Teaching social work values and ethics: A curriculum resource* (2nd ed.). Alexandria, VA: Council on Social Work Education.

Dolgoff, R., Harrington, D., & Loewenberg, F. (2012). *Ethical decisions for social work practice* (9th ed.). Belmont CA: Brooks/Cole.

Gordon, W. E. (1962). A critique of the working definition. *Social Work, 7*(4), 3–13.

Gray, M., & Webb, S. (Eds.). (2010). *Ethics and value perspectives in social work.* Basingstoke, UK: Palgrave Macmillan.

Gutheil, T., & Simon, R. (2005). E-mails, extra-therapeutic contact, and early boundary problems: The internet as a "slippery slope." *Psychiatric Annals, 35,* 952–960.

Hamilton, G. (1940). *Theory and practice of social casework.* New York: Columbia University Press.

Hardiman, D. G. (1975). Not with my daughter, you don't! *Social Work, 20*(4), 278–285.

Hester, D. M. (Ed.) (2007). *Ethics by committee: A textbook on consultation, organization, and education for hospital ethics committees.* Lanham, MD: Rowman & Littlefield.

Houston-Vega, M. K., Nuehring, E. M. & Daguio, E. R. (1997). *Prudent practice: A guide for managing malpractice risk.* Washington, DC: NASW Press.

Keith-Lucas, A. (1977). Ethics in social work. In J. B. Turner (Ed.), *Encyclopedia of social work* (17th ed., Vol. 1, pp. 350–355). Washington, DC: National Association of Social Workers.

Lamendola, W. (2010). Social work and social presence in an online world. *Journal of Technology in the Human Services, 28,* 108–119.

Levy, C. S. (1973). The value base of social work. *Journal of Education for Social Work, 9*(1), 34–42.

Levy, C. S. (1976). *Social work ethics.* New York: Human Sciences Press.

Linzer, N. (1999). *Resolving ethical dilemmas in social work practice.* Boston, MA: Allyn & Bacon.

MacIntyre, A. (1984). *After virtue* (2nd ed.). Notre Dame, IN: University of Notre Dame Press.

Mattison, M. (2000). Ethical decision-making: The person in the process. *Social Work, 45*(3), 201–212.

McDermott, F. E. (Ed.). (1975). *Self-determination in social work.* London: Routledge & Kegan Paul.

Menon, G. M., & Miller-Cribbs, J. (2002). Online social work practice: Issues and guidelines for the profession. *Advances in Social Work, 3,* 104–116.

National Association of Social Workers [NASW]. (1960). *NASW code of ethics.* Washington, DC: Author.

National Association of Social Workers. (2008). *NASW code of ethics.* Washington, DC: Author.

Pumphrey, M. W. (1959). *The teaching of values and ethics in social work education.* New York: Council on Social Work Education.

Reamer, F. G. (1987). Values and ethics. In A. Minahan (Ed.), *Encyclopedia of social work* (18th ed., Vol. 2, pp. 801–809). Silver Spring, MD: National Association of Social Workers.

Reamer, F. G. (1990). *Ethical dilemmas in social service* (2nd ed.). New York: Columbia University Press.

Reamer, F. G. (1992). The impaired social worker. *Social Work, 37*(2), 165–170.

Reamer, F. G. (1998). The evolution of social work ethics. *Social Work, 43*(6), 488–500.

Reamer, F. G. (2001a). *Tangled relationships: Managing boundary issues in the human services*. New York: Columbia University Press.

Reamer, F. G. (2001b). *The social work ethics audit: A risk management tool*. Washington, DC: NASW Press.

Reamer, F. G. (2003). *Social work malpractice and liability: Strategies for prevention* (2nd ed.). New York: Columbia University Press.

Reamer, F. G. (2006). *Ethical standards in social work: A review of the NASW code of ethics* (2nd ed.). Washington, DC: NASW Press.

Reamer, F. G. (2009). *The social work ethics casebook: Cases and commentary*. Washington, DC: NASW Press.

Reamer, F. G. (2012a). *Boundary issues and dual relationships in the human services*. New York: Columbia University Press.

Reamer, F. G. (2012b). The digital and electronic revolution in social work: Rethinking the meaning of ethical practice. *Ethics and Social Welfare*, ePub ahead of print. doi: 10.1080/17496535.2012.738694.

Reamer, F. G. (2013a). *Social work values and ethics* (4th ed.). New York: Columbia University Press.

Reamer, F. G. (2013b). Social work in a digital age: Ethical and risk-management challenges. *Social Work*. doi: 10.1093/sw/swt003. Available at http://sw.oxfordjournals.org/content/early/2013/03/24/sw.swt003.full.pdf+html

Reid, P. (1992). The social function and social morality of social work: A utilitarian perspective. In P. N. Reid & P. R. Popple (Eds.), *The moral purposes of social work* (pp. 34–50). Chicago, IL: Nelson-Hall.

Ross, W. D. (1930). *The right and the good*. Oxford, UK: Clarendon.

Smart, J. J. C., & Williams, B. (1973). *Utilitarianism: For and against*. Cambridge, UK: Cambridge University Press.

Spano, R., & Koenig, T. (2003). Moral dialogue: An interactional approach to ethical decision making. *Social Thought, 22*, 91–103.

Teicher, M. (1967). *Values in social work: A re-examination*. New York: National Association of Social Workers.

Timms, N. (1983). *Social work values: An enquiry*. London: Routledge/Kegan Paul.

Varley, B. (1968). Social work values: Changes in value commitments from admission to MSW graduation. *Journal of Education for Social Work, 4*, 67–85.

Williams, R. M., Jr. (1968). The concept of values. In D. L. Sills (Ed.), *International encyclopedia of the social sciences* (Vol. 16, pp. 283–287). New York: Macmillan/Free Press.

Younghusband, E. (1967). *Social work and social values*. London: Allen and Unwin.

Zur, O. (2007). *Boundaries in psychotherapy: Ethical and clinical explorations*. Washington, DC: American Psychological Association.

Zur, O. (2012). TelePsychology or TeleMentalHealth in the digital age: The future is here. *California Psychologist, 45*, 13–15.

FREDERIC G. REAMER

ETHICS IN RESEARCH

ABSTRACT: Social work researchers hold themselves to general ethical standards for biomedical and social science research and to the values specific to social work. This article describes (a) the general ethical principles guiding research involving human beings, (b) mechanisms for the ethical review of studies involving human beings, (c) ethical issues in research on vulnerable populations such as children and adolescents, recipients of care, and other socially marginalized groups, and (d) plagiarism, authorship, and conflict of interest. Current topics in the responsible conduct of research include the use of clinical and audio or video data, participatory action research, and Internet-based studies.

KEY WORDS: ethics; research; research ethics; responsible conduct of research; informed consent; confidentiality; IRB; vulnerable populations

As research activity in social work has increased, so has attention to ethics in research. Ethical standards and practices in research guide the relationship between researcher(s) and research participant(s), guide relationships among researchers and scholars, guide how researchers relate to the organizations and communities in which their studies are conducted, and safeguard the integrity of the scientific enterprise as a whole. Vulnerable groups in the United States—non-Whites, women, prisoners, and people with disabilities—have in the past been harmed by biomedical and social science research. The *responsible conduct of research* (RCR) considers the ethics of research on many levels—individual research participants, researchers, groups and communities studied, the scientific and scholarly enterprise, and society as a whole.

Current standards for RCR trace their origins to the 1947 Code of Nuremberg that emerged from international trials addressing war crimes committed by the Nazi regime in the mid-20th century, including crimes carried out in the name of research (Steneck, 2007; Israel & Hay, 2006). The World Medical Association's Declaration of Helsinki followed in 1964. In 1979, based on these codes and in part in reaction to the infamous Tuskegee Experiment (Jones, 1993), the Report of the National Commission on the Protection of Human Subjects of Biomedical and Behavioral Research, known as the Belmont Report, set forth ethical standards and regulatory mechanisms to be used in all government-funded research and research settings in the United States—standards that continue to guide the design and conduct of research studies in medicine, the social sciences, and the helping professions. International Ethical Guidelines for Biomedical Research Involving Human Beings, called "CIOMS" after its authoring organization, The Council for International Organizations of Medical Sciences, were adopted in 1982 and revised in 2002. However, as societies, research funding mechanisms, and research technologies change, best practices in the ethics of research and scholarship continually evolve.

Social work research must also reflect the professional and ethical aims of all social work activities (Antle & Regehr, 2003; Butler, 2002; Barsky, 2010; Hugman, 2010; Nichols-Casebolt, 2012). Social workers have ethical responsibilities to clients and others with whom they work, including research participants; to the practice settings and other organizations in which they function; to colleagues and to the profession itself; and to the broader society, commitments that all must be reflected in the conduct of research.

Beneficence, Justice, and Respect

Although there are differing philosophical bases for research ethics (Christians, 2005; Fuchs & Macrina, 2005; Israel & Hay, 2006; Shamoo & Resnik, 2009), codes of ethical conduct for research are based on three major principles: *beneficence, justice,* and *respect*. Because no specific code of conduct can ever address all possible situations, one must understand the principles that underlie specific standards of practice (Butler, 2002; Israel & Hay, 2006; Sieber, 1992; Steneck, 2007). While these principles are widely accepted, risks and benefits are not always easy to reconcile, and differences of judgment about the risks and benefits of a study commonly arise.

Non-malfeasance, or the injunction to do no harm, is subsumed in the United States under the principle of beneficence. In some other national and organizational codes, this fourth principle, also traced to the Nuremberg Code, is separately mentioned (Butler, 2002). In the most infamous example of malfeasance in medical research in the United States, the Tuskegee Experiment, which ended only in 1972 (Jones, 1993), poor and mostly illiterate African American sharecroppers with syphilis were studied without consent, without information about the true nature of their disease, and without effective treatment even when it became available—practices that are no longer permissible in treatment research.

It has been argued that for social work, *justice* means that research activities and findings should promote social justice and equity in society (Antle & Regehr, 2003) and empower research participants.

Justice also drives the relatively recent requirement of researchers seeking federal funding that exclusion of participants of either gender or of any racial or ethnic group must be specifically justified. This measure seeks to correct past practice in which women and non-Whites were routinely excluded from medical and other studies, leading to a systematic lack of data on their health and well-being and on treatments that do and do not work for them.

The Basic Principles of Research Ethics Defined

Beneficence means that no undue harm shall be done to research participants and that some demonstrable benefit must possibly derive from any proposed research, if not to the research participants themselves, then at least to others like them in the future or to society as a whole. Adherence to this principle means that any possible risks to research participants must be anticipated and steps taken to minimize them (see below). In social work, it means that research must address goals such as improving social work services, enhancing our understanding of client problems, and informing the participants of policies, financing, and regulatory systems that affect social workers and the people they serve. It also means that research must be methodologically sound so that any findings from it will have scientific credibility. The way social work research is conducted should affirm, respect, and unite study participants and colleagues and give something back to those studied.

"*Justice* in research focuses on the fair distribution of burden and benefit" (Antle & Regehr, 2003, p. 138), meaning that all involved, those who are studied and those who do the studying, are treated with fairness, and this also applies to traditionally understudied groups and communities. The most recent Council for International Organizations of Medical Sciences (CIOMS) guidelines (2002) address this issue as it relates to biomedical research in disadvantaged nations and communities: "the sponsor and the investigator must make every effort to ensure that the research is responsive to the health needs and priorities of the population or community in which it is carried out; and any intervention or product developed, or knowledge generated, will be made reasonably available for the benefit of that population or country" (p. 34).

Respect means that the autonomy and self-determination of those who participate in research must be safeguarded. Anyone who is part of a study must consent to do so voluntarily and after being fully informed of what will be required of them, including any risks they might incur during the conduct of the study or from the dissemination of its findings. Respect must also be extended to the organizations and communities in which research is carried out as well as to all of those involved in the conduct of the research.

Institutional Review Boards

In the United States, the 1979 Belmont Report began a system of overseeing biomedical and behavioral research: the use of Institutional Review Boards (IRBs) at all institutions and organizations that receive any form of government financial support (Grigsby & Roof, 1993; Shore & West, 2005; Bankert & Amdur, 2006). Similar regulatory mechanisms now exist in many other nations as well (Israel & Hay, 2006). Any social worker who conducts research with people or who uses information about them that would otherwise be private must apply to one of these boards for permission to conduct their research. (What constitutes a "human subject" in research, what is considered a "no risk" or "minimal risk" study, and what is acceptable training in research ethics are all spelled out in federal regulations, guidelines for IRBs, and the specific policies of each individual IRB. Who should and must serve on IRB review panels is also specified in the CIOMS standards and elsewhere.) Anyone proposing to conduct research under IRB supervision must document that they have been trained in the ethical conduct of research with human participants.

Practitioners often question the ethics of research designs that withold or delay ("lagged") promising interventions, but these risks can be minimized (Noble, Gelfand & DeRubeis, 2005). Even when the risks of participation in a study are minimal, as in most social work research, studies must be conducted in such a way as to minimize risks. However, no level of risk is acceptable unless there is a real potential for a study to advance knowledge based on the scientific soundness of its methodology. There have been specific concerns about how fairly such bodies may view qualitative, oral history, or participatory action studies, for example, since IRBs often appear to be oriented to the value of the experimental and quantitative methods used in biomedical studies (CSWE, 2007; Lincoln, 2005). The most common IRB feedback to social work researchers concerns strengthening procedures (data collection, sample recruitment, data storage) to protect the autonomy of participants or the confidentiality of data. Most have concluded that routine outside review of the ethical safeguards employed in proposed studies involving human beings is a worthwhile protective mechanism for researcher and researched alike.

An issue that has been discussed since the original Belmont Report is the boundary between practice, especially the evaluation of practice and programs, and research (Grigsby & Roof, 1993; Shore & West, 2005; Holosko, Thyer & Danner, 2009). Often it is the intent to publish (suggesting that generalizable knowledge will be generated from a study and that information about service recipients will be shared with people not involved in their care) that differentiates research from practice evaluation and triggers IRB review. International standards and procedures also vary (International Compilation of Human Research Standards, n.d.).

Code of Ethics Content on Research and Scholarship

The content in the *NASW Code of Ethics* (NASW, 1999) that specifically addresses research ethics is in Section 5.02, although other sections are relevant as well. These guidelines are necessary, but not sufficient to ensure that research is conducted responsibly, and social work researchers commonly encounter ethical dilemmas in their work (Apgar & Congress, 2005b, p. 73). As Butler (2002) states, "At all stages of the research process, from inception, resourcing, design, investigation, and dissemination, social work … researchers have a duty to maintain an active, personal and disciplinary ethical awareness and to take practical and moral responsibility for their work" (p. 245). The Council on Social Work Education (CSWE) has also developed a national Statement on Research Integrity in Social Work (2007), and others have written comprehensively on the topic (MacFarlane, 2009; Nichols-Casebolt, 2012).

Minimizing Risks to Research Participants

Many of the ethical dilemmas that occur in research stem from the power differential between researchers and research participants who are the "objects" of the research (Halse & Honey, 2005). Involvement in research studies is based in part on the participants' views of the research enterprise itself as benign (or not), which can be influenced by the history that a group or community, including indigenous people, has had with biomedical or social research in the past (Barata, Gucciardi, Ahmad, & Stewart, 2006; Fisher et al., 2002; Martin & Meezan, 2009; Schinke, Enosse, Peletier & Lightfoot, 2010; Hugman, Pittaway & Batolomei, 2011). Cultural competence must therefore infuse all parts of the research process (Oliver, 2003). Enhancing benefits to participants is also important (Bay Cheng, 2009).

Informed Consent. There are two vital dimensions to informed consent: that research participation is *voluntary* and that consent is given in *full knowledge* about the nature of the study and of what will be required of study participants. Models of consent forms can be obtained from individual IRBs and from the website of the federal Office for Human Research Protection (OHRP) (see Suggested Links). The nature, probability, and likely severity of any risks of research participation should be described (Boothroyd & Best, 2003). However, initial consent to participate leaves participants free not to answer specific questions or take part in specific procedures and to withdraw their consent at any point in the conduct of the study—rights that must also be made clear.

Social work research often involves service users, and assurance must be given to them that declining to participate in or withdrawing from a study will not compromise the services or care they are getting in any way. Usually it is someone other than a treating professional involved in their care who must request research consent so that the service user will feel more free to decline. In addition, the practice of offering research participants some compensation for the time and effort they contribute to a study is common, and such rewards must not constitute an *undue inducement* to volunteer (Ripley, Macrina, Markowitz & Gennings, 2010). Some believe that a cash gift to drug-using study participants, for example, may be riskier to their well-being than a gift or a gift certificate, although Festinger et al. (2005) did not find this to be true. An emerging practice in participant compensation is offering a lottery award to participants, but there is debate about its ethical use (Brown, Schonfeld, & Gordon, 2006). Careful attention to any effects of the power differential between researcher and potential study participants conveys a respect that can actually enhance the data that is obtained (Sieber, 1992).

Consent forms and the opportunity to discuss research participation must take into account the language of the participant and their abilities (for example, any vision problems affecting the reading of forms, level of literacy). Hence one area of concern involves how much information to convey about a study in the consent process. Perhaps to avoid litigation, the tendency over time has been to give ever more detailed information, but this trend can result in long and detailed consent documents that are hard for potential participants to read and understand. Because peoples' motivations to enroll or not enroll in a study are complex (Stone, 2004), how much to

say in a consent form as well as where and how to say it for the most effective communication is currently being studied and debated (Boothroyd & Best, 2003; Fisher et al., 2002; Lynöe & Hoeyer, 2005).

Confidentiality. Social workers usually know how to protect the confidentiality of client information and therefore understand the need for secure storage of research data. Identifiable data on research participants, including signed consent forms and lists linking names to research codes, must be stored separately from the research data itself, which is identified only by a code number or pseudonym. Data stored electronically must also be secure, that is, password-protected. When and how data will be destroyed must also be specified.

Although laws vary from state to state, the confidentiality of data collected by social workers for research rather than for clinical purposes is less well-protected. In certain sensitive areas, such as the mandated reporting of child or elder abuse, there are clear limits to the confidentiality that a social work researcher can offer, limits that must be made clear to research participants. If data on illegal activities, drug use, or other sensitive information is being collected, it may be desirable to obtain a Certificate of Confidentiality (Wolf & Zandecki, 2006), although such certificates may not include all relevant areas like domestic abuse (Hofman, 2004; Wolf & Zandecki, 2006).

The 1996 Health Insurance Portability and Accountability Act (HIPAA) has imposed some additional regulatory constraints on research information derived from medical and other covered settings and from some kinds of patient records. However, data from affected records can still be used for research if it is de-identified. A link to further information on HIPAA and its effects on research activities is given later (see Suggested Links).

Vulnerable Populations

All negotiations of consent for participation in research depend on the "presumption of the universalized subject" who can act freely and rationally in forming a social contract (Halse & Honey, 2005, p. 2152). While the implications of this assumption have not been fully addressed, it is well understood that some potential research participants are vulnerable in the consent process for a variety of reasons, many of them of interest to social work researchers. Cognitive or communicative vulnerability, institutional vulnerability, deferential vulnerability, medical vulnerability, economic vulnerability, and social vulnerability must all be considered (Anderson & Dubois, 2007). CIOMS (2002) guidelines (pp. 49–51) and federal regulations (see the OHRP website) also give special attention to studies involving pregnant women, fetuses, and neonates.

Children and adolescents are not legally able to represent themselves in consenting to participation in research, although the age(s) and circumstances, like being an emancipated minor, at which adolescents are considered able to consent, vary across jurisdictions. The consent of a parent or guardian must be sought when children are to participate in research, unless it can be demonstrated to an IRB that seeking such consent could in fact endanger the child, as can be the case, for example, if youth who are gay, lesbian, bisexual or questioning are to be studied and if they have not disclosed their sexual identities to their parents for fear of rejection or abuse. In such cases, a waiver of parental consent can be granted and an advocate appointed to assist each participating young person (Martin & Meezan, 2009). Children and adolescents who are wards of the state also present a special circumstance, and each state has its own method of assisting them with an advocate for research consent purposes. To respect the autonomy and dignity of adolescents and older children, it is desirable also to seek formal *assent* for research participation from them and to proceed only if both parental consent and participant assent are obtained (see the OHRP website for information on involving children and adolescents as participants in research, including models for assent documents).

Prisoners, people who live in institutions, or others in need of services are considered vulnerable in the consent process either because they may feel undue inducement to enroll in studies (for example, prisoners may volunteer to demonstrate good conduct when applying for parole) or because there will be negative consequences if they decline (Arboleda-Flórez, 2005). Similar concerns about power issues arise in research with both immigrant and indigenous groups (Schinke, Enosse, Peletier & Lightfoot, 2010; Hugman, Pittaway & Batolomei, 2011). In addition, anyone who might have *diminished capacity* to understand what is being asked of them as a research participant or to make decisions in their own best interest is also considered vulnerable. This group includes those with some forms of mental illness, those with intellectual deficits or age-related cognitive impairments, some who abuse drugs, and some of those with life-threatening or serious medical illnesses (APA, 2006; Anderson & Dubois, 2007; Boothroyd & Best, 2003; Fisher et al., 2002; Roberts, 2002; Dunn & Misra, 2009). Only when a person has been legally determined to be incompetent is incapacity to consent clear-cut,

and overprotection can restrict research on important problems, especially studies in which the perspectives of those with any of these conditions are included.

Most people who have disorders or disabilities can, in fact, consent to participation in research if communication in the consent process is adapted to their needs, as in reading the consent form aloud for the visually impaired or communication in American Sign Language (ASL) for those who are deaf, although issues of confidentiality can be magnified in their relatively small social networks (Eckhardt & Anastas, 2007). Social work research often involves people considered vulnerable because they may be at risk of painful emotional reactions consequent to speaking of sensitive personal and emotional issues (Boothroyd & Best, 2003), such as in research on those who are bereaved (Stroebe, Stroebe, & Schut, 2003) or who have experienced trauma (Mudaly & Goddard, 2009; Newman & Kaloupek, 2009). When and how to approach such potential participants must be carefully considered, and it is common to build in safeguards, as offering referral for professional assistance to any participant who seems to be distressed. In these situations, to avoid potential conflicts of interest or dual roles (Congress, 2001; Landau, 2008; Lunt & Fouché, 2010), any assistance offered must be from an independent source.

Clinical and video or audio data. Anyone who is observed or interviewed in person can be offered confidentiality protection but is by definition not anonymous. Similarly, individual clinical or case study data can include enough detail that inferred identification of the participants can be made by someone who may know them; as in case reports used in education and training, alteration and disguise of selected information is the usual remedy for this problem. However, when audiotaped or videotaped information is collected, these data pose special challenges in safeguarding participant, provider, family, and community privacy (IVSA, 2009). Separate and specific consent to the collection of such data and especially to any sharing of data in these forms, as in conference presentations of findings, should be obtained (see APA, 2002, 8.03, p. 11 and the OHRP website).

Minimizing Risks to Scholarship and Knowledge Development

There is no benefit to the conduct of social work research unless there is confidence in the integrity of the profession's knowledge-generating and dissemination activities as a whole. The Office of Research Integrity (ORI) describes four key values in this area:

honesty, "conveying information truthfully and honoring commitments"; *accuracy*, "reporting findings precisely and taking care to avoid errors"; *efficiency*, "using resources wisely and avoiding waste"; and *objectivity*, meaning "letting the facts speak for themselves and avoiding...bias" (Steneck, 2007, p. 10).

Although there are few well-known examples of questionable ethical conduct in social work research and scholarship, the kinds of problems that can arise are known from related fields (Gibelman & Gelman, 2001). The most common kinds of research misconduct are the fabrication of data, the falsification of data, and plagiarism (Gibelman & Gelman, 2001; Steneck, 2007, p. 21). While the last is known to occur in social work and in social work education, there is little or no systematic information available about plagiarism or the kinds of sanctions imposed when it occurs. The APA has a very useful and succinct statement about how to avoid plagiarism: "...do not present portions of another's work or data as one's own, even if the other work or data source is cited occasionally" (APA, 2002, p. 12).

Conflicts of interest. Collaboration is common in social work research, and people involved in research occupy different positions and have differing access to power and resources, differences that occur among those conducting the research as well as between researchers and participants. Researchers' sources of funding are coming under increasing scrutiny for the effects they may have on findings and their dissemination (Oliver, 2003). In program evaluation, it may be difficult to draw conclusions that are critical of the agency studied or that may compromise program funding. Agency employees who are study informants may be vulnerable to unintended harms, which must be minimized (Hilton, 2006). Different stakeholders in the research may have conflicting needs and desires concerning intellectual property, publication, and the ownership of the data collected. Open discussion of all matters such as the ownership of data, copyright (as for any data collection instrument developed), authorship (including those with students), supervision of findings, and their dissemination is recommended at the inception of the study and periodically throughout (CSWE, 2007; Macrina, 2005; Netting & Nichols-Casebolt, 1997; Oliver, 2003; Shamoo & Resnik, 2009; Smith, 2003; Steneck, 2007).

Authorship. Although the principle of not taking credit for the work of others is clear, there are no social-work specific guidelines for addressing authorship issues; in fact considerable variation in beliefs exists even among social work educators (Apgar &

Congress, 2005a; Gibelman & Gelman, 1999). In addition, there is evidence that many social work researchers, especially when students, have had adverse experiences with authorship (Netting & Nichols-Casebolt, 1997). Social workers' beliefs about the weight that should be given to some tasks when determining authorship credit, such as data analysis (Apgar & Congress, 2005a), is at variance with that in other fields (see, for example, chapter 2 in Shamoo & Resnik, 2009), and more study and discussion of authorship issues and practices are needed. Resources from other fields should be consulted (e.g., Street, Rogers, Israel & Braunack-Mayer, 2010; Welfare & Sackett, 2010).

Current Issues and Future Trends in the Responsible Conduct of Research

Qualitative methods. Perhaps because the researcher is seen as an instrument of the research in qualitative studies (Haverkamp, 2005), more has recently been published about ethical dilemmas faced by researchers in this area than in others. Face-to-face encounters with participants discussing emotionally laden experiences and prolonged engagement with them can evoke strong emotional reactions in researchers or even a conflict between the "helping" and the "studying" roles (see for example, Davison, 2004). Qualitative researchers have been more ready than some others to consider power differentials in the relationships between researchers and study participants; to call for researcher reflexivity, reciprocity, and participant empowerment; and to consider the implications of all these factors for research ethics (Christians, 2005; Haverkamp, 2005; Lincoln, 2005).

Participatory action research. Social work researchers concerned with the social justice aims of research are embracing an investigational model most commonly called *participatory action research* (PAR) that seeks maximal power-sharing between researchers and those being studied, individually and collectively (see Community-Based Participatory Research). In PAR procedures and findings are generated collaboratively over the course of a study, making it difficult to comply with what IRBs require in an application for approval of a study, since sampling plans, data-gathering procedures, data analysis plans, and even the nature of anticipated findings are not pre-determined. Articulating the risks and benefits of PAR and explicating how protections can be offered within different assumptions and procedures are essential (Brydon-Miller, Greenwood, & Eikeland, 2006; Khanlou & Peter, 2005).

Internet-based studies. Research using the World Wide Web is becoming more common, and ethical issues in Internet research is an emerging area of discussion (Buchanan, 2004; Ess & AoIR, 2002; Rhodes, Bowie, & Hergenrather, 2005; Whitehead, 2007; Enyon, Schroeder & Fry, 2009). Internet research can involve simply recruiting participants for conventional forms of data-gathering, analyzing content on existing sites such as chat rooms, or gathering data via Web-based surveys. Ethnographic and qualitative research can also be done in cyberspace (Buchanan, 2004). Informed consent can be compromised without face-to-face interaction, as when a child represents himself or herself as an adult and parental consent is therefore not obtained. Even special measures may not ensure anonymity or the privacy of data collected: "encryption…can protect responses to an online questionnaire but cannot protect the respondent's IP address" (Rhodes et al., 2005, p. 71), a limitation that must be acknowledged. In addition, again because there is no face-to-face interaction, it is difficult to determine if a study has produced distress in a participant. Doing Internet-based research therefore requires staying current with emerging best practices in the ethical conduct of such studies.

REFERENCES

American Psychiatric Association's Task Force on Research Ethics. (2006). Ethical principles and practices for research involving human participants with mental illness. *Psychiatric Services, 57,* 4 552–557.

American Psychological Association (APA). (2002). *APA Ethics Code 2002.* Retrieved January 3, 2007, from http://www.apa.org/ethics/code2002.pdf

Anderson, E. E., & Dubois, J. M. (2007). The need for evidence-based research ethics: A review of the substance abuse literature. *Drug & Alcohol Dependence, 86,* 95–105.

Antle, B. J., & Regehr, C. (2003). Beyond individual rights and freedoms: Metaethics in social work research. *Social Work, 48*(1), 135–143.

Apgar, D. H., & Congress, E. (2005a). Authorship credit: A national study of social work educators' beliefs. *Journal of Social Work Education, 41*(1), 101–112.

Apgar, D. H., & Congress, E. (2005b). Ethical beliefs of social work researchers: Results of a national study. *Journal of Social Service Research, 32*(2), 61–80.

Arboleda-Flórez, J. (2005). The ethics of research on prisoners. *Current Opinion in Psychiatry, 18,* 514–517.

Barata, P. C., Gucciardi, E., Ahmad, F., & Stewart, D. E. (2006). Cross-cultural perspectives on research participation and informed consent. *Social Science & Medicine, 62*(2), 479–490.

Barsky, A. E. (2010). The virtuous social work researcher: Metaethics in social work research. *Social Work, 48*(1), 135–143.

Bay-Cheng, L. Y. (2009). Research note: Beyond trickle-down benefits to research participants. *Social Work Research, 33*(4), 243–247.

Boothroyd, R. A., & Best, K. A. (2003). Emotional reactions to research participation and the relationship to understanding of informed consent disclosure. *Social Work Research, 27*(4), 242–251.

Brown, J. S., Schonfeld, T. L., & Gordon, B. G. (2006). "You may have already won…": An examination of the use of lottery payments in research. *IRB: Ethics & Human Research, 28*(1), 12–16.

Brydon-Miller, M., Greenwood, D., & Eikeland, O. (2006). Conclusion: Strategies for addressing ethical concerns in action research. *Action Research, 4*(1), 129–131.

Buchanan, E. A., (Ed.). (2004). *Readings in virtual research ethics: Issues and controversies.* Hershey, PA: Information Science Publishers.

Butler, I. (2002). A code of ethics for social work and social care research. *British Journal of Social Work, 32,* 349–248.

Christians, C. G. (2005). Ethics and politics in qualitative research. In N. K. Denzin & Y. S. Lincoln (Eds.), *The SAGE handbook of qualitative research* (3rd ed., pp. 139–164). Thousand Oaks, CA: Sage Publications.

Congress, E. (2001). Dual relationships in social work education: Report on a national survey. *Journal of Social Work Education, 37*(2), 255–266.

Council for International Organizations of Medical Sciences (CIOMS). (2002). *International ethical guidelines for biomedical research involving human subjects.* Geneva, Switzerland. Author, World Health organization (WHO). Retrieved February 2, 2007, from http://www.cioms.ch/frame_guidelines_nov_2002.htm

Council on Social Work Education (CSWE). (2007). *National Statement on Research Integrity in Social Work.* Alexandria, VA: Author. Retrieved February 15, 2007, from http://cswe.org/home/!Final%20National%20Statement%20%201-31-2007.pdf

Davison, J. (2004). Dilemmas in research: Issues of vulnerability and disempowerment for the social worker/researcher. *Journal of Social Work Practice, 18*(3), 379–393.

Dunn, L. B. & Misra, S. (2009). Research ethics issues in geriatric psychiatry. *Psychiatric Clinics of North America, 32,* 395–411.

Eckhardt, E. A., & Anastas, J. W. (2007). *Journal of Social Work and Disability Research* (May, 2007), vol. 6, issues 1 & 2. Simultaneously published as a chapter in F. Yuen (Ed.), *Disability and social work education: Practice and policy issues* (pp. 233–250). West Hazelton, PA: Haworth Press.

Enosse, L., Peltier, D., Watson, J., & Lightfoot, N. (2010). Cultural missteps and ethical considerations with indigenous populations: Preliminary reflections from Northeastern Ontario, Canada. *Journal of Academic Ethics, 8,* 233–242.

Enyon, R., Schroeder, R., & Fry, J. (2009). New techniques in online research: Challenges for research ethics. *21st Century Society, 4*(2), 187–199.

Ess, C., & the Association of Internet Researchers (AoIR) Ethics Working Committee. (2002). *Ethical decision-making and Internet research.* Approved by AoIR, November 27, 2002. Available online at http://www.aoir.org/reports/ethics.pdf

Festinger, D. S., Marlowe, D. B., Croft, J. R., Dugosh, K. L., Mastro, N. K., Lee, P. A., et al. (2005). Do research payments precipitate drug use or coerce participation? *Drug and Alcohol Dependence, 78*, 275–281.

Fuchs, B. A., & Macrina, F. L. (2005). Ethics and the scientist. In F. L. Macrina, *Scientific integrity: Text and cases in responsible conduct of research* (3rd. ed., pp. 19–37). Washington, DC: ASM Press.

Fisher, C. B., Hoagwood, K., Boyce, C., Duster, T., Frank, D., Grisso, T., et al. (2002). Research ethics for mental health science involving ethic minority children and youths. *American Psychologist, 57*(12), 1024–1040.

Gibelman, M., & Gelman, S. R. (2001). Learning from the mistakes of others: A look at scientific misconduct in research. *Journal of Social Work Education, 37*(2), 241–254.

Gibelman, M., & Gelman, S. (1999). Who's the author? Ethical issues in publishing. *Arete, 23*(1), 77–88.

Grigsby, R. K., & Roof, H. L. (1993). Federal policy for the protection of human subjects: Applications to research on social work practice. *Research on Social Work Practice, 3*(4), 448–461.

Halse, C., & Honey, A. (2005). Unraveling ethics: Illuminating the moral dilemmas of research ethics. *Signs, 30*(4), 2141–2162.

Haverkamp, B. E. (2005). Ethical perspectives on qualitative research in applied psychology. *Journal of Counseling Psychology, 52*(2), 146–155.

Hilton, T. F. (2006). Staff members are human subjects, too. *Journal of Substance Abuse Treatment, 31*, 9–15.

Holosko, M. J., Thyer, B., & Danner, J. E. H. (2009). Ethical guidelines for designing and conducting evaluations of social work practice. *Journal of Evidence-Based Social Work, 6*, 348–360.

Hugman, R. (2010). Social work research and ethics. In Shaw, I., Briar-Lawson, K., Orme, J., & Ruckdeschel, R. (Eds.), *The Sage handbook of social work research* (pp. 149–163). Los Angeles, CA: Sage Publications.

Hugman, R., Pittaway, E., & Batolomei, L. (2011). When "do no harm" is not enough: The ethics of research with refugees and other vulnerable groups. *British Journal of Social Work*, 1–17.

Israel, M., & Hay, I. (2006). *Research ethics for social sciences: Between ethical conduct and regulatory compliance.* London: Sage Publications.

IVSA Code of Research Ethics and Guidelines. (2009). *Visual Studies, 24*(3), 250–257.

Jones, J. H. (1993). *Bad blood: The Tuskegee Syphilis Experiment* (2nd ed). New York: Free Press.

Khanlou, N., & Peter, E. (2005). Participatory action research: Considerations for ethical review. *Social Science & Medicine, 60*, 2333–2340.

Landau, R. (2008). Social work research ethics: Dual roles and boundary issues. *Families in Society: The Journal of Contemporary Social Services, 689*(4), 571–577.

Lincoln, Y. S. (2005) Institutional Review Boards (IRBs), methodological conservatism, and academic freedom: The challenge to and from phenomenological paradigms. In N. K. Denzin & Y. S. Lincoln (Eds.), *The SAGE handbook of qualitative research* (3rd ed., pp. 165–181). Thousand Oaks, CA: Sage Publications.

Lunt, N. & Fouché, C. (2010). Practitioner research, ethics, and research governance. *Ethics and Social Welfare, 4*(3), 219–235.

Lynöe, N., & Hoeyer, K. (2005). Quantitative aspects of informed consent: Considering the dose response curve when estimating quantity of information. *Journal of Medical Ethics, 31*, 736–738.

Macfarlane, B. (2009). *Researching with integrity: The ethics of academic inquiry.* New York and London: Routledge.

Macrina, F. L. (2005). *Scientific integrity: Text and cases in responsible conduct of research* (3rd ed). Washington, DC: ASM Press. http://www.scientificintegrity.net

Martin, J. I. & Meezan, W. (2009). Applying ethical standards to research and evaluation involving lesbian, gay, bisexual, and transgender populations. In Meezan, W. & Martin, J.I. (Eds.), *Handbook of research with lesbian, gay, bisexual, and transgender populations* (pp. 19–39). Routledge.

Mudaly, N., & Goddard, C. (2009). The ethics of involving children who have been abused in child abuse research. *International Journal of Children's Rights, 17*, 261–281.

National Association of Social Workers. (1999). *Code of Ethics of the National Association of Social Workers.* Washington, DC: NASW Press.

National Commission for the Protection of Human Subjects of Biomedical and Behavioral Research. (1979). *The Belmont Report.* Retrieved January 2, 2006, from http://www.dhhs.gov/ohrp/humansubjects/guidance/belmont.htm

Netting, F., & Nichols-Casebolt, A. (1997). Authorship and collaboration: Preparing the next generation of social work scholars. *Journal of Social Work Education, 33*, 555–564.

Newman, E., & Kaloupek, D. (2009). Overview of research addressing ethical dimensions of participation in traumatic stress studies: Autonomy and beneficence. *Journal of Traumatic Stress, 22*(6), 595–602.

Nichols-Casebolt, A. (2012). *Research integrity and responsible conduct of research.* New York: Oxford University Press.

Noble, R. S., Gelfand, L. A., & DeRubeis, R. J. (2005). Reducing exposure of clinical research subjects to placebo treatments. *Journal of Clinical Psychology, 61*(7), 881–892.

Oliver, P. (2003). *The student's guide to research ethics.* Philadelphia: Open University Press.

Ripley, E., Macrina, F., Markowitz, M., & Gennings, C. (2010). Why do we pay? A national survey of investigators and IRB chairpersons. *Journal of Empirical Research on Human Research Ethics, 5*(3), 43–56.

Roberts, L. W. (2002). Ethics and mental illness research. *Psychiatric Clinics of North America, 25*, 525–545.

Shamoo, A. E., & Resnik, D. B. (2009). *Responsible conduct of research* (2nd ed.). New York: Oxford University Press.

Shore, N., & West, P. (2005, September 14). Social worker researchers and the Institutional Review Board: Benefits, challenges, and ideas for support. *Journal of Social Work Values and Ethics, 2*(2). Retrieved December 28, 2006, from http://www.socialworker.com/jswve/content/view/22/37/.

Sieber, J. E. (1992). *Planning ethically responsible research: A guide for students and internal review boards.* Newbury Park, CA: Sage Publications.

Smith, D. (2003, January). Five principles of research ethics. *APA Monitor, 34*(1), 56–60. Retrieved January 3, 2007, from http://www.apa.org/monitor/jan03/principles.html.

Steneck, N. H. (2007). *ORI introduction to the responsible conduct of research* (rev. ed.). Rockville, MD: U.S. Dept. of Health and Human Services, Office of Research Integrity.

Stone, T. J. (2004). Making the decision about enrollment in a randomized control trial. In M. Smythe & E. Williamson (Eds.), *Researchers and their "subjects:" Ethics, power, knowledge and consent* (pp. 35–54). Bristol, England: Policy Press.

Street, J. M., Rogers, W. A., Israel, M., & Braunack-Mayer, A. (2010). Credit where credit is due? Regulation, research integrity and the attribution of authorship in the health sciences. *Social Science & Medicine, 70,* 1458–1465.

Stroebe, M., Stroebe, W., & Schut, H. (2003). Bereavement research: Methodological issues and ethical concerns. *Palliative Medicine, 17,* 235–240.

Welfare, L. E., & Sackett, C. R. (2010). Authorship in student-faculty collaborative research: Perceptions of current and best practices. *Journal of Academic Ethics, 8,* 199–215.

Whitehead, L. C. (2007). Methodological and ethical issues in Internet-mediated research in the field of health: An integrated review of the literature. *Social Science & Medicine, 65,* 782–791.

Wolf, L. E., & Zandecki, J. (2006). Sleeping better at night: Investigators' experiences with Certificates of Confidentiality. *IRB: Ethics & Human Research, 28*(6), 1–7.

FURTHER READING

http://www.socialworkers.org/pubs/code/default.asp
The National Association of Social Workers' (NASW) *Code of Ethics* online.

http://www.socialworkers.org/research/naswResearch /1006Ethics/default.asp
This web page, developed and maintained by NASW, has principles of research ethics, a bibliography, and links to other useful resources.

http://cswe.org/home/!Final%20National%20Statement%20 -%201-31-2007.pdf
The Council on Social Work Education convened a work group that developed this CSWE National Statement on Research Integrity in Social Work.

http://www.dhhs.gov/ohrp
This is the homepage of the Office for Human Research Protections (OHRP), the federal office that ensures adherence to federal regulations for the conduct of research studies and for the Institutional Review Boards that oversee individual studies at a local level within these

guidelines. Online training in research ethics and information about dealing with vulnerable populations in research (e.g., children, prisoners).

http://ori.dhhs.gov/documents/rcrintro.pdf
The Department of Health and Human Services' Office of Research Integrity has a publication entitled "ORI Introduction to the Responsible Conduct of Research." The office's newsletter is also available on their website.

http://privacyruleandresearch.nih.gov/pr_02.asp
The 1996 Health Insurance Portability and Accountability Act (HIPAA) has imposed new restrictions on some research activities, including clinical and health services research. Information and links to additional topics within this area, including a summary booklet about the regulations for researchers, are provided.

http://grants.nih.gov/grants/policy/coc/
This NIH site is the "kiosk," or entry point, for further information on Certificates of Confidentiality and how to apply for one.

http://www.research.utoronto.ca/ethics/pdf/human/nonspecific/ Internet%20Research%20Ethics.pdf
In 2002, the Association of Internet Researchers (AoIR) membership, which is transdisciplinary and international, approved a set of ethical guidelines for researchers using the Internet. These are intended to supplement, not supplant, any profession-specific standards, and the site also includes links to other useful resources.

http://www.dhhs.gov/ohrp/humansubjects/guidance/belmont .htm
This is the link to a copy of the 1979 Belmont Report codifying ethical standards for research in the United States.

http://www.cioms.ch/frame_guidelines_nov_2002.htm
This site contains the complete text of the CIOMS *International Ethical Guidelines for Biomedical Research Involving Human Subjects.*

http://www.hhs.gov/ohrp/references/nurcode.htm
The complete text of the Nuremberg Code can be found here.

http://www.cirp.org/library/ethics/helsinki/
This site has the complete text of the 1964 Declaration of Helsinki as reproduced in the British Medical Journal, No 7070, Volume 313, 7 December 1996.

http://www.hhs.gov/ohrp/international/intlcompilation/ intlcompilation.html
International Compilation of Human Research Standards. Office of Human Research Protections, U. S. Dept. of Health of Health and Human Services. This website links to a lengthy document detailing ethical standards for the conduct of research with human beings by region and nation, including international standards, compiled by OHRP.

JEANE W. ANASTAS

EVIDENCE-BASED PRACTICE

ABSTRACT: Evidence-based practice (EBP) is an educational and practice paradigm that includes a series of predetermined steps aimed at helping practitioners and agency administrators identify, select, and implement efficacious interventions for clients. This entry identifies definitions of EBP and trace the evolution of EBP from its origins in the medical profession to its current application in social work. Essential steps in the process of EBP and challenges associated with applying EBP to social work practice, education, and research are noted.

KEY WORDS: evidence-based practice; social work education

Evidence-based practice (EBP) is a five-step process used to select, deliver, and evaluate individual and social interventions aimed at preventing or ameliorating client problems and social conditions. At its most basic level, EBP seeks to systematically integrate evidence about the efficacy of interventions in clinical decision-making. Adhering to EBP, however, is a complex process that requires practitioners to be skilled at posing practice-relevant questions and proficient at accessing evidence that answers these questions. Importantly, practitioners must have the requisite methodological skills to evaluate evidence about the efficacy of interventions from clinical trials, systematic reviews, and meta-analyses. Finally, to teach the process of EBP, social work educators must be competent in tasks associated with information retrieval and interpretation of evidence.

A recent surge of interest in EBP is raising awareness about the importance of considering empirical evidence in selecting interventions among practitioners who may not have considered such evidence in the past. At the same time, the sudden growth of EBP gives rise to a cautionary note about the many different ways that EBP is being defined in published works and taught in the classroom. A consistent definition of EBP and an educational commitment to the process steps required in EBP are critical at this juncture to prevent the misuse or misunderstanding of this new paradigm.

Definitions and Evolution of EBP

EBP appeared in the medical profession in the 1990s as a process to help physicians select effective treatments for their patients. The introduction of EBP in medicine was viewed by many scholars and practitioners as an effective way to bring research findings to medical practice decisions. The rapid diffusion of EBP since then has been attributed to advances in knowledge about the prevention and treatment of medial conditions and to economic forces that emphasize the selection of efficacious treatments as a strategy to reduce health care costs (Gray, 2001).

The growth of EBP in medicine has also been a product of an increasingly active and well-informed patient population. Unlike prior generations, a significant portion of today's patients are well educated about their medical problems and demand that they receive the most optimal treatments for their conditions. The sophistication of medical consumers has required physicians to become more skilled at evaluating and applying evidence to medical practice decisions (Gambrill, 2006; Gray, 2001; Wennberg, 2002).

Definitions and perceptions of what EBP is—and what it is not—vary widely. In what is arguably the most widely accepted definition of EBP, Sackett and colleagues (Sackett, Straus, Richardson, Rosenberg, & Haynes, 2000) state that EBP is "the integration of best research evidence with clinical expertise and [client] values" (p. 1). In this definition, EBP is implied to be a process characterized by specific steps and actions. In an earlier publication, Sackett, Richardson, Rosenberg, and Haynes (1997) had defined EBP as "the conscientious, explicit, judicious, use of current best evidence in making decisions about the care of individual [clients]" (p. 2).

The introduction of EBP in medicine has created considerable interest in the process of applying evidence to medical practice decision-making. Importantly, scholars also believe that EBP has moved the medical profession away from its long-standing reliance on authority-based decision-making processes that fail to adequately consider empirical evidence (Gambrill, 1999, 2005).

Essential Steps of EBP

As the above definitions imply, EBP is both a philosophy of practice and a process that implies a series of structured steps. Sackett et al. (2000) have been credited with developing the five essential steps of EBP.

STEP 1: CONVERTING PRACTICE INFORMATION NEEDS INTO ANSWERABLE QUESTIONS An important first step in the process of EBP requires practitioners to define information needs about a particular client problem. Sackett et al. (2000) suggest that this information needs to be framed in the form of answerable questions. Further, they recommend that questions identify the client population, intervention type, and anticipated outcomes.

Several scholars have brought elements of this first step in the EBP process to social work. In an important book on the subject of EBP, Gibbs (2003) identified a framework for posing questions that emphasizes the need for practicality. According to Gibbs, questions must be client-oriented and they must be specific enough to guide a search for evidence using electronic resources. Gambrill (2005) summarized effectively the types of questions that are generally posed in EBP processes. Her synopsis includes the following question types: 1) effectiveness, 2) prevention, 3) assessment, 4) description, 5) prediction, 6) harm, and 7) cost-benefit.

Framing practice-relevant questions is the foundation of the EBP process. Questions must be specific and posed in terms that lead to a rational search for evidence. An illustration of an effectiveness question may be helpful in understanding the importance of this point. Suppose a practitioner in a substance abuse program is interested in knowing whether a cognitive-behavioral intervention is more effective than a 12-step treatment program for addressing alcohol abuse in adults. In this case, a logical practice question might be: Is a structured cognitive-behavioral intervention more effective than a self-help program in treating alcohol abuse in adults? In a second example, suppose practitioners and teachers in a local elementary school are concerned about the negative effects of bullying behaviors in the classroom. In this example, a school social worker might pose a question about the best way to address aggression. A typical question might be: Is a universal prevention approach aimed at changing social norms about aggression more effective than a skills training approach that seeks to reduce aggression by targeting only high-risk youth?

Posing answerable questions requires precision and practice. Students and practitioners must be trained to pose different types of practice-relevant questions and learn ways to retrieve evidence that is critical in answering such questions.

STEP 2: LOCATING EVIDENCE TO ANSWER QUESTIONS
Step 2 requires practitioners to search for and locate evidence pertaining to the questions they pose. At least four sources are available currently to search for empirical evidence: 1) books and journals, 2) systematic reviews organized by client problem or treatment approach that detail the effects of interventions on specified outcomes, 3) published "lists" of effective programs by federal entities and research centers, and 4) practice guidelines that offer treatment protocols based on empirical evidence.

Books and Journals. Books and journals represent a traditional approach to answering practice-relevant questions identified in step 1. Printed books and journal articles are readily available and have traditionally been helpful information sources. However, practitioners must also be aware of the limitations inherent in books and journals. For example, there is often a significant time lag between the submission and subsequent publication of a book or journal article. Practitioners must also have the skills to identify and discern published findings that pertain to their questions. This requires knowing how to select and search appropriate databases for information. In addition, practitioners must be trained to recognize that findings reported in book chapters and other outlets are quite likely not subject to peer review processes.

A final limitation of books and journals as information sources relates to the types of articles commonly published in social work. For example, at least one investigation has revealed that relatively few intervention outcome studies are published in social work literature (Rosen, Proctor, & Staudt, 1999). The lack of outcome studies poses a limitation to practitioners searching for evidence pertaining to the efficacy of interventions.

Systematic Reviews. Systematic reviews are comprehensive evaluations that examine evidence about the effectiveness of interventions targeted to a range of client populations and problems. Leadership in disseminating knowledge of effective prevention and treatment approaches through the publication of systematic treatment outcome reviews has come from international interdisciplinary teams organized under the Campbell Collaboration (2007, http://www.campbellcollaboration.org) and the Cochrane Collaboration (2007, http://www.cochrane.org). Each of these groups disseminates the results of systematic reviews to inform practitioners about the effects of interventions in health, behavioral, and educational settings. Importantly, systematic reviews of treatment outcomes are also becoming more available in social science literature (Vaughn & Howard, 2004).

Lists of Efficacious Programs. A third dissemination approach has been organized by federal entities and independent research centers such as the Substance Abuse and Mental Health Services Administration (SAMHSA) and the Center for the Study and Prevention of Violence (CSPV) at the University of Colorado. For example, SAMHSA (2007, http://www.modelprograms.samhsa.gov) publishes a list of efficacious substance abuse prevention and treatment programs in the National Registry of Evidence-Based

Programs and Practices. The agency identifies promising, effective, and model programs on the basis of methodological rigor and client outcomes. CSPV (2007, http://www.colorado.edu/cspv/) identifies effective violence prevention programs as part of its Blueprints for Violence Prevention dissemination effort. At least one group concerned with the effects of school-based educational programs for high-risk youth has also published lists of effective interventions (Collaborative for Academic, Social, and Emotional Learning, 2003).

In psychology, concern about the failure of many therapists to use empirically supported treatments led to the establishment of the American Psychological Association (APA) Task Force on the Promotion and Dissemination of Psychological Procedures in 1993 (Barlow, Levitt, & Bufka, 1999). The Task Force was established by the APA Society of Clinical Psychology (Division 12) to identify efficacious treatments across a range of mental health disorders and problems. Task Force members with expertise in diverse therapeutic approaches and populations developed criteria for treatments deemed to be well established and empirically validated and for treatments considered to be probably efficacious. Well-established treatments were those therapies that evidenced efficacy in at least two independent and rigorous experimental studies. Probably efficacious treatments were therapies in which only one study supported a treatment's efficacy, or therapies that had been tested by a single investigator (Task Force on the Promotion and Dissemination of Psychological Procedures, 1995).

The Task Force recognized randomized clinical trials as the most rigorous and acceptable method of producing empirically supported treatments. In lieu of randomized trials, findings from a large series of single case design experiments were accepted as criteria. The Task Force initiated a search for efficacious and probably efficacious treatments in 1993 (Task Force on the Promotion and Dissemination of Psychological Procedures, 1995). The subsequent list of efficacious therapies has since been updated twice (Chambless et al., 1996; Chambless et al., 1998).

Compilations of effective programs allow practitioners to access considerable information about the efficacy of interventions targeted to a wide range of client groups and problems. Credible lists such as those identified above use rigorous selection criteria to identify effective programs. For example, to be included on the program list compiled by the CSPV at the University of Colorado, intervention studies must use strong research designs and demonstrate sustained effects. Replication of effects is also required

to meet criteria for the highest level of evidence. Similarly, APA criteria clearly identify the levels of research rigor that are necessary to meet standards for efficacious or probably efficacious treatments.

Lists of EBPs lead practitioners to potentially effective interventions. However, such lists cannot simply be accepted uncritically. In all cases, practitioners should scrutinize the criteria used to identify effective programs and interventions when they consider selecting and implementing programs from lists of EBPs.

Practice Guidelines. Practice guidelines are a fourth method of disseminating knowledge of efficacious interventions to practitioners. Proctor and Rosen (2003) defined practice guidelines as "a set of systematically compiled and organized knowledge statements designed to enable practitioners to find, select, and use appropriately the interventions that are most effective for a given task" (p. 108). Guidelines offer specific treatment protocols for practitioners that, when followed, mirror the strategies used in efficacious interventions with similar types of clients. Clinical practice guidelines were introduced in medicine and have recently spread to psychology and social work. Guidelines in social work have been met with mixed reaction and their development and application have been limited to date (see Howard & Jenson, 1999a, 1999b, 2003 and Rosen & Proctor, 2003 for a discussion of practice guidelines in social work).

Summary. Sources of information and evidence have proliferated widely in recent years. Practitioners must possess a range of information retrieval skills to identify appropriate sources of credible evidence. The appraisal of such evidence, discussed next, is a critical next step in the EBP process.

STEPS 3 & 4: APPRAISING AND APPLYING EVIDENCE TO PRACTICE AND POLICY DECISIONS EBP requires practitioners to use their knowledge of research design and methodology to evaluate and apply evidence to practice situations. These steps require familiarity with research methodology and the ability to draw conclusions about the utility of information on the basis of levels of evidence. The scientific community recognizes findings produced by randomized controlled trials as the most rigorous and acceptable level of evidence. However, results from studies using correlation, single-subject, quasi-experimental, experimental, and meta-analytic designs must also be considered and evaluated in steps 3 and 4 (Thyer, 2004).

Evaluating the rigor of studies and selecting interventions that meet high research standards require advanced training in methodology and intervention research. Unfortunately, current standards for research training in most Master of Social Work programs fall short of assuring the advanced skills necessary to critically evaluate the validity and applicability of research reports. Additional course work in evaluating evidence should be included in the graduate social work curriculum.

A second concern in appraising and applying evidence to practice situations comes from studies suggesting that practitioners fail to routinely consult research evidence when selecting interventions. For example, several studies show that practitioners often choose interventions for reasons other than empirical evidence (Elliott & Mihalic, 2004; Rosen, Proctor, Morrow-Howell, & Staudt, 1995). In addition, agency and organizational policies that limit the choice of intervention approaches available to practitioners often constrain practitioners' ability to use EBP.

The flurry of activity associated with EBP is not confined to selecting and implementing well-tested programs. To develop new knowledge about the effects of interventions, a small but increasing number of social work researchers are testing the effects of interventions across different problem areas in controlled efficacy trials (Reid & Fortune, 2003). This is a promising development in view of findings suggesting there is a dearth of intervention studies in social work (Fraser, 2003; Jenson, 2005; Rosen et al., 1995). More intervention research by social work investigators is needed to contribute to the knowledge base of efficacious prevention and treatment approaches.

STEP 5: EVALUATING THE PROCESS   The steps in EBP appear deceptively simple at first glance. However, the process of EBP requires knowledge of current literature about the onset, prevention, and treatment of client or social problems, the ability to search for relevant information and data, and skills to evaluate and apply knowledge obtained in systematic searches. The complexity involved in steps one to four demands an ongoing evaluation of one's knowledge of current literature, familiarity with constantly changing electronic databases, and skills in drawing conclusions based on methodological rigor.

Gibbs (2003) summarizes effectively the process of EBP: "Placing the client's benefits first, evidence-based practitioners adopt a process of lifelong learning that involves continually posing specific questions of direct and practical importance to clients, searching effectively for the current best evidence to each question, and taking appropriate action guided by evidence" (p. 6). Most scholars would agree that the social work profession is in the beginning stage of implementing the process defined by Gibbs in practice, and education and research settings.

CHALLENGES AND IMPLICATIONS   The promotion of EBP in social work was attributed initially to individual scholars and small groups of researchers (e.g., Gambrill, 1999, 2003; Howard & Jenson, 1999a; Proctor & Rosen, 2003; Thyer, 2004). These early efforts were aimed largely at exposing social workers to definitions of EBP and to concurrent developments in evidence-based medicine. Discussion of the process of applying EBP principles to social work practice and policy soon followed (for example, Bilson, 2005; Gambrill, 2003, 2006; Gibbs, 2003).

A significant number of social work researchers and educators have since acknowledged the importance of EBP. Support is evident in the exponential growth in the number of books and articles on EBP since 2003 (see Gambrill, 2005, 2007; Howard, Himle, Jenson, & Vaughn, 2009; Rosenthal, 2004 for reviews). Sessions on EBP have increased significantly at recent national social work conferences sponsored by the Society for Social Work and Research and the Council on Social Work Education. Further, a 2006 University of Texas at Austin symposium on EBP signaled an increasing recognition of the importance of teaching EBP in the social work curriculum. The Austin conference led to the publication of a 2007 special issue of *Research on Social Work Practice* that summarized the viewpoints of presenters at the symposium. Transparency in the use of EBP in practice and education (Gambrill, 2007), steps required to teach EBP (Mullen, Bellamy, Bledsoe, & Francois, 2007), and structural curricular reforms consistent with EBP (Howard & Allen-Meares, 2007; Jenson, 2007) are among the topics discussed in that issue.

An increase in attention to EBP by social work educators is indisputable. However, EBP is not without its critics. There have been voices of skepticism (Taylor & White, 2002) and even rejection (Webb, 2001) characterized by claims that EBP offers nothing new to the field. Others point to the lack of an effective knowledge base for certain client problems and populations, which hinders the advancement of EBP in the field.

EBP is at an important turning point in social work. To some, it reflects a new and revolutionary practice approach that holds great promise for building stronger bridges between science and social work

(Gambrill, 2007; Jenson, 2005). Others view EBP as a repackaged attempt to integrate research and practice that is fraught with educational and implementation problems (Webb, 2001). Regardless, the challenges of EBP to social work education, practice, and research are varied and complex.

EBP AND SOCIAL WORK EDUCATION

The Challenge of Educational Reform. Rubin and Parrish (2007) reported that more than 70% of respondents from a survey of social work educators were in favor of teaching EBP in the MSW curriculum. Rapp-Paglicci (2007) noted that as many as 40 social work programs have created classes that incorporate principles of EBP. At least one school of social work—the Brown School of Social Work at Washington University—has identified EBP as the organizational framework for its graduate curriculum (Edmond, Rochman, Megivern, Howard, & Williams, 2006; Howard, McMillen, & Pollio, 2003). Importantly, the Council on Social Work Education has identified EBP as an important principle in its educational policy and accreditation documents (Council on Social Work Education, 2004). These and other examples illustrate the increasing attention being paid to EBP in the social work curriculum.

It is also clear, however, that interest in EBP has not yet resulted in the adoption or implementation of significant curriculum reform. To illustrate, Woody, D'Souza, and Dartman (2006) reported less than encouraging findings from a survey of social work deans and directors examining whether and how their programs teach empirically supported interventions. Woody et al. (2006) noted that, "only 31 programs, less than half, had endorsed teaching specific ESI [Empirically Supported Interventions] content; still fewer, 26, had designated courses to teach specific ESI content; and of the 31 programs that had endorsed teaching ESI, very small numbers required ESI training materials designed for teaching students the skills and techniques for implementing the interventions" (p. 474).

Significant structural and pedagogical changes in social work education are necessary to teach EBP. For example, a new generation of students must be exposed to the complexities involved in posing relevant practice and policy questions. Students must become experts in information retrieval and possess the methodological skills necessary to evaluate and apply evidence. New and innovative teaching approaches will be required to systematically teach EBP. Faculty will need to be trained, and in some cases retrained, to

teach EBP. Finally, the appropriate location for teaching the actual process of EBP must be determined in undergraduate and graduate curricula.

Teaching the Process of EBP. Above all, EBP is a process characterized by the five specific steps discussed above. Thus, a logical assumption is that educators should focus their efforts on teaching the actual process of conducting EBP. However, the degree to which faculty members in schools of social work are teaching the five-step process of EBP—or simply informing students of effective interventions—is unclear. Several scholars, most notably Gambrill (2007), caution that exposing students to only EBPs identified on compiled lists and national registries is inconsistent with the fundamental premise of EBP. She accurately notes that a singular focus on effective interventions, expressed through commonly used terms such as *best practices*, is taking focus away from teaching students the actual process of EBP. Gambrill (2007) further suggests that emphasizing EBPs at the cost of understanding the process of EBP is inconsistent with the original intent of EBP as an approach that fosters transparency and systematic decision-making with clients.

The importance of teaching students the actual process steps of EBP cannot be overstated. EBP is a philosophy and an approach to practice that requires students and practitioners to understand and apply its essential steps. Teaching students to identify and use lists of established EBPs to select interventions is but one small part of the EBP process. As Gambrill (2007) so eloquently states, the emphasis on EBPs "ignores the process of EBP that describes skills designed to help practitioners to integrate external findings with other vital information (e.g., concerning client characteristics and circumstances) such as posing well-structured questions, and ignores the importance of creating tools practitioners need such as access to high-speed computers with relevant databases" (p. 430).

Schools of social work must take bold steps to integrate EBP across the curriculum. Training in EBP occurs sporadically in most schools, with little consistent application across key parts of the curriculum. Therefore, discussions about the best place (e.g., practice or research courses) to teach the process of EBP in the curriculum are needed. In addition, new teaching techniques such as problem-based learning that are compatible with EBP should be examined for applicability in social work education (Gambrill, 2007; Sackett et al., 2000). Finally, structural changes in long-held traditions such as advanced standing may need to be considered in the interest of increasing students' exposure to the complexities of EBP (Jenson, 2007).

EBP AND SOCIAL WORK PRACTICE EBP is receiving considerable attention from local, state, and federal policy makers and funding sources. State and local systems of care, private foundations, and federal entities have entered the debate about the best ways to select and implement effective interventions for clients and client systems. Agency administrators and practitioners are working diligently to understand EBP in an effort to develop competitive research proposals and implement effective program components.

One significant practice challenge is how to teach principles of EBP to practitioners and agency administrators. Community agencies vary widely with respect to their awareness, understanding, and acceptance of EBP. Community partnerships and collaborative research projects such as those being developed at the University of Toronto (Regehr, Stern, & Shlonksy, 2007) are needed to help practitioners apply EBP principles in a wide variety of practice settings. At Toronto, the faculty of social work at the University of Toronto has created an institute for evidence-based social work that aims to develop and foster community collaborations (Regehr et al., 2007). This and similar models should be further developed and tested.

EBP AND RESEARCH EBP relies on the availability of accrued knowledge about a range of individual and social problems. Thus, it is imperative that new knowledge about the etiology, prevention, and treatment of problems be consistently developed. In this regard, rigorous research is needed across many or all substantive areas in social work. Intervention research to assess the efficacy and effectiveness of social interventions is particularly lacking. Such studies are necessary to advance the etiological and intervention knowledge bases available to practitioners who are interested in implementing EBP.

The translation of research evidence to practice and policy is a second important area of research. In many service sectors there is a considerable lag between the identification of efficacious treatments and the application of such treatments to practice and policy. Recently, entities such as the National Institute of Mental Health have emphasized the importance of translating research findings to the field (Brekke, Ell, & Palinkas, 2007). Models for translating research evidence to practice and policy in health care and adolescent service sectors have been offered by Gray (2001) and Jenson and Fraser (2006) respectively.

The careful translation of research into practice is particularly important in view of the rapid increase in practices and publications that are promoted as EBP but in reality fall short of the principles implied in EBP. For example, the sudden infusion and proliferation of terms that resemble EBP, but are not EBP, may have an adverse effect on the profession's interest in using EBP to enhance the connection between science and intervention. Phrases such as "best practices" and "exemplary programs" are frequently used for marketing clinical and community interventions. On closer examination, these terms may or may not reflect the underlying processes of EBP. In many cases, interventions packaged under such names are not based on empirical evidence and have not been subject to rigorous evaluation. Promoting untested interventions as evidence-based promotes a false sense of efficacy, erodes the basic principles of EBP, and dilutes commonly accepted definitions of EBP used in medicine and psychology.

Finally, research is needed to systematically assess the effects of implementing EBP with clients. Embedded in EBP is the notion that client outcomes will be improved significantly by using EBP. As EBP becomes more widely applied in practice, studies will be needed to assess the relationship between its use and client outcomes.

EPB offers the promise of a new approach to social work education and practice that will dramatically alter the profession for years to come. The move to EBP as a guiding educational framework will require schools of social work to include the essential elements of EBP training (e.g., posing practice-relevant questions, gaining sophisticated information retrieval skills, interpreting systematic reviews, applying clinical practice guidelines, etc.) in graduate courses. In addition, schools of social work must also assume leadership in assisting community-based and human service sectors to understand and apply EBP in practice and policy settings. The challenge and risk of such comprehensive change represents an exciting new opportunity in social work practice and education. The endorsement of EBP is a risk well worth taking.

REFERENCES

Barlow, D. H., Levitt, J. T., & Bufka, L. F. (1999). The dissemination of empirically supported treatments: A view to the future. *Behaviour Research and Therapy, 37,* 147–162.

Bilson, A. (Ed.). (2005). *Evidence-based practice in social work.* London: Whiting & Birch.

Brekke, J. S., Ell, K., & Palinkas, L. A. (2007). Translational science at the National Institute of Mental Health. Can social work take its rightful place? *Research on Social Work Practice, 17,* 123–133.

Campbell Collaboration. (2007). Retrieved April 30, 2007, from http://www.campbellcollaboration.org

Center for the Study and Prevention of Violence. (2007). *Blueprints for violence prevention.* Retrieved April 30, 2007, from the University of Colorado Web site: http://www.colorado.edu/cspv/.

Chambless, D. L., et al. (1996). An update on empirically validated therapies. *The Clinical Psychologist, 49,* 5–18.

Chambless, D. L., et al. (1998). Update on empirically validated therapies. II. *The Clinical Psychologist, 51,* 3–15.

Cochrane Collaboration. (2007). Retrieved May 1, 2007, from http://www.cochrane.org

Collaborative for Academic, Social, and Emotional Learning. (2003). *Safe and sound: An educational leader's guide to evidence-based social and emotional learning.* Chicago: Author.

Council on Social Work Education. (2004). *Educational policy and curriculum policy standards.* Washington, DC: Author.

Edmond, T., Rochman, E., Mcgivern, D., Howard, M., & Williams, C. (2006). Integrating evidence-based practice and social work field education. *Journal of Social Work Education, 42,* 377–396.

Elliott, D. S., & Mihalic, S. (2004). Issues in disseminating and replicating effective prevention programs. *Prevention Science, 5,* 47–52.

Fraser, M. W. (2003). Intervention research in social work: A basis for evidence-based practice and practice guidelines. In A. Rosen & E. K. Proctor (Eds.), *Developing practice guidelines for social work intervention: Issues, methods, and research agenda* (pp. 17–36). New York: Columbia University Press.

Gambrill, E. (1999). Evidence-based practice: An alternative to authority-based practice. *Families in Society, 80,* 341–350.

Gambrill, E. (2003). Evidence-based practice: Implications for knowledge development and use in social work. In A. Rosen & E. K. Proctor (Eds.), *Developing practice guidelines for social work intervention: Issues, methods, and research agenda* (pp. 37–58). New York: Columbia University Press.

Gambrill, E. (2005). *Critical thinking in clinical practice* (2nd ed). Hoboken, NJ: John Wiley and Sons.

Gambrill, E. (2006). Evidence-based practice and policy: Choices ahead. *Research on Social Work Practice, 16,* 338–357.

Gambrill, E. (2007). To be or not to be: Will five-step be used by clinicians? *Research on Social Work Practice, 17,* 428–434. A review of J. C. Norcross, L. E. Beutler & R. F. Levant (Eds.), *Evidence-based practices in mental health: Debate and dialogue on the fundamental questions.* Washington, DC: American Psychological Association.

Gambrill, E. (2007). Transparency as the route to evidence-informed professional education. *Research on Social Work Practice, 17,* 553–560.

Gibbs, L. (2003). *Evidence-based practice for the helping professions.* Pacific Grove, CA: Brooks/Cole.

Gray, J. A. M. (2001). *Evidence-based health care: How to make health policy and management decisions* (2nd ed.). New York: Churchill Livingstone.

Howard, M. O., Allen-Meares, P., & Ruffolo, M.C. (2007). Teaching evidence-based practice: Strategic and pedagogical recommendations for schools of social work. *Research on Social Work Practice, 17,* 561–568.

Howard, M. O., Himle, J., Jenson, J. M., & Vaughn, M. G. (2009). Revisioning social work clinical education: Recent developments in relation to evidence-based practice. *Journal of Evidence-Based Social Work, 6,* 256–273.

Howard, M. O., & Jenson, J. M. (1999a). Clinical practice guidelines: Should social work develop them? *Research on Social Work Practice, 9,* 283–301.

Howard, M. O., & Jenson, J. M. (1999b). Barriers to development, utilization, and evaluation of social work practice guidelines: Toward an action plan for social work research. *Research on Social Work Practice, 9,* 347–364.

Howard, M. O., & Jenson, J. M. (2003). Clinical practice guidelines and evidence-based practice in medicine, psychology, and allied professions. In E. Proctor, & A. Rosen (Eds.), *Developing practice guidelines for social work intervention: Issues, methods, and research agenda* (pp. 83–107). New York: Columbia University Press.

Howard, M. O., McMillen, J. C., & Pollio, D. (2003). Teaching evidence-based practice: Toward a new paradigm for social work education. *Research on Social Work Practice, 13,* 234–259.

Jenson, J. M. (2005). Connecting science to intervention: Advances, challenges, and the promise of evidence-based practice. *Social Work Research, 29,* 131–135.

Jenson, J. M. (2007). Evidence-based practice and the reform of social work education: A response to Gambrill and Howard and Allen-Meares. *Research on Social Work Practice, 17,* 569–573.

Jenson, J. M., & Fraser, M. W. (2006). *Social policy for children and families: A risk and resilience perspective.* Thousand Oaks, CA: Sage.

Mullen, E. J., Bellamy, J. L., Bledsoe, S. E., & Francois, J. J. (2007). Teaching evidence-based practice. *Research on Social Work Practice, 17,* 574–582.

Proctor, E. K., & Rosen, A. (2003). The structure and function of social work practice guidelines. In A. Rosen & E. K. Proctor (Eds.), *Developing practice guidelines for social work intervention: Issues, methods, and research agenda* (pp. 108–127). New York: Columbia University Press.

Rapp-Paglicci, L. (2007). To be or not to be: Will evidence-based practice be used by clinicians? *Research on Social Work Practice, 17,* 427–428. A review of A. R. Roberts & K. R. Yeager (Eds.), *Evidence-based practice manual: Research and outcome measures in health and human services.* New York: Oxford University Press.

Regehr, C., Stern, S., & Shlonsky, A. (2007). Operationalizing evidence-based practice: The development of an institute for evidence-based social work. *Research on Social Work Practice, 17,* 408–416.

Reid, W. J., & Fortune, A. E. (2003). Empirical foundations for practice guidelines in current social work knowledge. In A. Rosen & E. K. Proctor (Eds.), *Developing practice guidelines for social work intervention: Issues, methods, and research agenda* (pp. 59–79). New York: Columbia University Press.

Rosen, A., & Proctor, E. K. (Eds.). (2003). *Developing practice guidelines for social work intervention: Issues, methods, and research agenda.* New York: Columbia University Press.

Rosen, A., Proctor, E. K., Morrow-Howell, N., & Staudt, M. M. (1995). Rationales for practice decisions: Variations in knowledge use by decision task and social work service. *Research on Social Work Practice, 5,* 501–523.

Rosen, A., Proctor, E. K., & Staudt, M. (1999). Social work research and the quest for effective practice. *Social Work Research, 23,* 4–14.

Rosenthal, R. N. (2004). Overview of evidence-based practice. In A. R. Roberts & K. R. Yeager (Eds.), *Evidence-based practice manual. Research and outcome measures in health and human services* (pp. 20–29). New York: Oxford University Press.

Rubin, A., & Parrish, D. (2007). Views of evidence-based practice among faculty in master of social work programs: A national survey. *Research on Social Work Practice, 17,* 110–122.

Sackett, D. L., Rosenberg, W., Gray, J. A. M., Haynes, R. B., & Richardson, W. S. (1997). Evidence-based medicine: What it is and what it isn't. *British Medical Journal, 312,* 71–72.

Sackett, D. L., Straus, S. E., Richardson, W. S., Rosenberg, W., & Haynes, R. B. (2000). *Evidence-based medicine: How to practice and teach EBM* (2nd ed.). New York: Churchill Livingstone.

Substance Abuse and Mental Health Services Administration. (2007). *National Registry of Evidence-Based Programs and Practices.* Retrieved April 29, 2007, from http://nrepp .samhsa.gov/

Task Force on Promotion and Dissemination of Psychological Procedures (1995). Training in and dissemination of empirically-validated psychological treatments. *The Clinical Psychologist, 48,* 3–23.

Taylor, C., & White, S. (2002). What works about what works? Fashion, fad, and EBP. *Social Work and Social Sciences Review, 10,* 63–81.

Thyer, B. A. (2004). What is evidence-based practice? *Brief Treatment and Crisis Intervention, 4,* 167–176.

Vaughn, M. G., & Howard, M. O. (2004). Integrated psychosocial and opioid-antagonist treatment for alcohol dependence: A systematic review of controlled evaluations. *Social Work Research, 28,* 41–55.

Webb, S. (2001). Some considerations on the validity of evidence-based practice in social work. *British Journal of Social Work, 31,* 57–79.

Wennberg, J. E. (2002). Unwanted variations in healthcare delivery: Implications for academic medical centers. *British Medical Journal, 325,* 961–964.

Woody, J. D., D'Souza, H. J., & Dartman, R. (2006). Do Master's in social work programs teach empirically-supported interventions? *Research in Social Work Practice, 16,* 469–479.

JEFFREY M. JENSON AND MATTHEW O. HOWARD

F

FAMILY: OVERVIEW

ABSTRACT: Families in almost all societies are viewed as the basic unit for coordinating personal reproduction and the redistribution of goals within the larger societal context of production and exchange. They are vulnerable to the rapidly changing economics of the environments in which they live. Universals regarding families worldwide include a delay in marriage, an increase in divorce rates, a decrease in household size and fertility rates, and nontraditional living arrangements. The most studied aspect of families continues to be family diversity, with greater emphasis on an interdisciplinary framework. There is also a movement toward more effective ways of treating families. Placing families in an historical context, this entry discusses evidence-based family interventions, the latest research on families, family diversity, and implications for social work practice and education.

KEY WORDS: demographics; interdisciplinarity; best practices

Introduction

It is generally believed that the family, however it's defined, has been the foundation of every civilization in human history. In other words, families in almost all societies are viewed as the basic unit for coordinating personal reproduction and redistribution within the larger societal context of production exchange. It is important to note, however, that across these basic units are several different types of families. It is critical that these different types of families be viewed and understood as alternative family systems, not as a deviation from some ideal structure created by groups with different positions or power in the societal structure (McGoldrick, Carter, & Garcia-Preto, 2011). Some of the more prevalent alternative family systems currently experienced in the United States had its origin in the destructive impact of European colonization. The impact of these destructive influences can be seen on the Native American kinship societies and the family system and social support networks of the enslaved Africans (Coontz, 1988; Franklin, 1997; Gutman, 1976; Logan, 2001; Logan, Freeman, & McRoy, 1990; Mintz & Kellogg, 1988; Stevenson, 1997).

Historical Perspectives on Families

The emergence of the Industrial Revolution, the influx of immigrants from Europe, and the westward expansion called attention to the influence of ethnic traditions and class relations on family dynamics. It was noted that these developments led to the emergence of "whiteness" as a category the European immigrants could use to differentiate themselves from ethnic groups of color or other groups near or at the bottom of the economic hierarchy (Jones, 1998; Roediger, 2007).

The period following the Civil War was marked by rapid industrialization and urbanization. It was during this period that American families took on characteristics associated with the so-called modern family. For example, families became smaller, had lower fertility rates, became less extended and more focused on the nuclear core; parents became more emotionally involved in rearing their children; and the separation between home and work increased. These changes, however, held different meanings for families, depending on the level of income, ethnicity, and the country of origin. The divergent and sometimes contradictory responses of the masses to the impact of industrialization and urbanization on family organization eventually led to the production of the six trends associated with the Industrial Revolution (Coontz, 2000; Katz, Doucet, & Stern, 1982):

1. The separation of the home and workplace (started among the working class and among the wage-earning segment of the business class)
2. The increased nuclearity of household structure (started among the working class and among the wage-earning segment of the business class)
3. The decline in marital fertility (started among the business class, particularly among its least affluent, most specialized, and most mobile sectors)
4. The prolonged residence of children in the home of their parents (began at about the same time in both working and business class, though the children of the former usually went to work and the latter to school)
5. The lengthened period in which husbands and wives live together after their children have left home (did not occur until the 20th century and represented a reversal of 19th century trends)

6. The reintegration of women into productive work, especially the entry of mothers into paid work outside the home and the immediate neighborhood (represents a reversal of 19th-century or older trends).

These six trends capture the differences as well as similarities among American families. They also highlight how life has changed in one significant way for all families: women of color no longer have significantly higher rates of labor force participation than do white women. According to Spain and Bianchi (1996), a growing number of women from all social and racial and ethnic groups now combine motherhood with paid employment, and fewer women are quitting work for prolonged periods while their children are young.

Overall, this historical overview highlights the diversity within families as well as the vulnerability of families to the external forces such as the rapidly changing economics of the environments in which they live.

Demographics

It is increasingly evident that the demographic structures of families in the United States are very diverse. Available research suggests that this increased diversity seen in the structure of family life reflects the changing landscape of the economy and related social factors. The following factors support this contention (Teachman, 2000):

1. That the average family has shown little, if any, economic progress since the mid-1970s;
2. That the number of American families with poor labor market skills and little education, which impede economic growth, is significantly high;
3. That most American families are duel career families out of necessity. Women in general are now a more critical source of economic support for their families. Men are simply no longer the sole wage earners in families.

Families of diverse types, structures, cultural, and ethnic experiences exist within the above context. This diversity among families seems to suggest a changing trend in family demography. For example, it can no longer be assumed that a family will consist of partners of the opposite sex, and that women will marry young, bear children, not work outside the home, and live with the same partners. Instead, evidence suggests that there has been a retreat from traditional early marriage, and among some groups, particularly African Americans, there has been a reversal of a long-time trend of being married by ages 20–24.

African Americans are now marrying at a much later age (35–39) than are persons of other ethnic groups. Additionally, African American men and women spend fewer years in their first marriages and are slower to remarry than in decades past. It is important to place this noticeable issue of marriage decline in context, but for purposes of this discussion the changing family structure will only be considered from the perspective of the children and their overall well-being (Taylor, 2000; Taylor, Chatters, Tucker, & Lewis, 1990). Data still suggest that the number of children younger than 18 years in the United States living in poverty continues to increase (Duncan & Brooks-Gunn, 1999; U.S. Department of Health and Human Service, 2003). Further, these children are living in female-headed households where the median income continues to be very low. Research supports the notion that the economic well-being of children is linked to family structure. For example, children who live with a single mother are more likely to live in poverty than are children who live with two parents. Available evidence suggests that those children younger than 18 years living in a mother-headed household are at a greater risk for a variety of negative outcomes. In other words, poverty experienced before age 6 is particularly destructive to positive development. These children experience behavioral problems, lower cognitive and academic achievements, and a greater likelihood of out-of-wedlock pregnancy (Duncan & Brooks-Gunn, 1999). It is, however, not the intention to oversimplify the complex dynamics reflected in this proposition. The intent is to underscore the continuing detrimental impact of poverty on children's well-being and family structure. There is increasing consensus that the delay in marriages, the rise in divorce rates, the rapidly changing economy, and the renegotiation of the division of economic and household labor are some of the important factors influencing current family demography.

INTERDISCIPLINARY CONNECTIONS There is an increasing recognition of the complexity inherent in studying, researching, and understanding contemporary family life. In part, this recognition is grounded in the awareness that there is no one type of family and also that there is no one way of viewing families. Multiple perspectives on families are emerging in undergraduate and graduate programs through the creation of special courses to expose students to inquiry-based learning and methods of data collection and analysis (Allen, 2001; Allen, Floyd-Thomas, & Gillman, 2001). Additionally, scholars on family life are being encouraged through a variety of forums to incorporate the issues and practices of other disciplines in their teaching and research (Tools for Transformation, 2000). Given that many family scholars are interdisciplinary in their training, it is only natural that linkages would occur between such disciplines as social work, history, sociology, religion, and psychology. The bottom line, however, is that interdisciplinary goes beyond the adding-on approach through a few select readings on families. Available data suggest that effective interdisciplinary connections for understanding families involve collaboration, partnerships, and teamwork (Adams, 2004). With the expanding diversity among families, it is imperative that family researchers, educators, and students learn new and expanded methodologies, both to understand how one field applies a concept in a different or similar way to the same situation under study. It is this complementary relationship between different disciplines that supports transformative teaching, learning, and research.

THEORETICAL PERSPECTIVES No single theory is preeminent in guiding practice and research on family life and dynamics. This is especially true when attempting to understand family dynamics with different gender, socioeconomic status, sexual orientation, age, and ethnic racial groups as well as different family types. Theories that support a better understanding of the interactions are still being conceptualized.

Queer theory and oppression theory are two theories that are available for supporting an understanding of intersectionality. According to Kumashiro (2004), *queer theory* focuses on the production of queerness. For example, he says that something could not be normal (like opposite-sex attraction) if other things were not already abnormal (like same-sex attraction). Therefore, queerness is produced as a contrast against which normalcy is established. In other words, queer theory tells us that these standards of normalcy actually produce queerness. By saying that this is what it means to be beautiful, we are simultaneously saying that other images of beauty are pretty queer. Oppression theory flows out of the type of reasoning undergirding queer theory. Collins (2008) conceptualizes oppression theory as interlocking systems of race, class, and gender. She contends that although these three systems have historically impacted the lives of African American women, they are not necessarily the most critical oppressions for other oppressed groups in society. She believed that research would reveal the particular "matrix of domination" for other groups in society.

Other perspectives and theoretical approaches fit the traditional and emergent categories. Most practitioners, educators, and researchers tend to practice, teach, and do research based on multiple and interrelated theories. These theories may be grouped into two broad categories with some overlap (Compton, Galaway, & Cournoyer, 2005): prescriptive theories and descriptive theories. Prescriptive theories are used to prescribe how problems should be resolved or needs should be met and are said to operate in concert with underlying descriptive theories. The prescriptive theories are those theories that include cognitive development theory, ecological theories, family systems theory, personality theory, risk, and resilience theory, social exchange theory, social role theory, and sociological theory. Descriptive theories are bodies of knowledge and related assumptions about human behavior. They explain such behavioral phenomena as how individuals grow and develop the dynamics and causes involved in organizations and communities. The descriptive theories include cognitive development theory, Bowenian family theory, psychodynamic theory, structural family theory, functional family theory, and general systems theory.

The 1990s and early 2000s witnessed several new or emergent theories for working with and understanding families. These theories and treatment approaches are grouped under the umbrella of postmodernism, a reaction to the widespread belief that the truth could be revealed through observation and movement. Advancing technology, globalization, and greater exposure to other cultures forced the recognition that more than one way exists for viewing and living in the world. Michael Foucault was a leading proponent in helping to construct our accepted truths handed down by the various disciplines: education, literature, religion, psychology, political science, social work, and medicine. He saw these constructed truths as principles or stories developed by these disciplines to protect the group's interest and existence and to subjugate alternative points of view (Foucault, 1965, 1980). One of the most influential critiques against these so-called truths was the feminist critique. As a theory and therapy, feminist family treatment gained increased recognition, and issues related to gender increased along with the emphasis on gender-sensitive issues in family treatment, and other theories continue to emerge world wide (Nicholas, 2010). In the West, de Shazer (1994) and Berg (1994), along with O'Hanlon and Weiner-Davis (1989) and several others, were developing solution-focused therapy. Meanwhile, White (1995) in Australia and Epston (1994) in New Zealand were developing narrative therapy. Interestingly, the emergent theories differed markedly from the traditional theories in that they were based on social constructionism, a philosophy that states that our experiences are a function of how we think about them instead of objective entities (Gergen, 1985). Other theories for the treatment of families that emerged in 1990s and early 2000s included the following:

1. The reflecting team approach (Andersen, 1991)
2. The therapeutic conversation model (Anderson, 1997)
3. The improvisational therapy model (Keeney, 1990)
4. The psychoeducational model (Anderson, Reiss, & Hogarty, 1986)
5. The internal family systems model (Schwartz, 1994)
6. Community family therapy (Rojano, 2004).

The theories and therapies discussed here are not intended to be an exhaustive representation of what exists in that different strategies for working with families are constantly emerging, which may not be as well recognized as those discussed here.

Latest Research and Best Practices

The literature on families suggests that there are multiple ways of studying families and that perhaps the most studied aspects of families continue to be family diversity. Researchers are examining the compelling differences within and among families from the perspective of social stratification such as race and ethnicity, class/socioeconomic status, gender, age, and sexual orientation. Obviously this approach to examining families will occur until it is a natural recognition that families are diverse, that they view and experience their worlds differently and are treated differently based on how they are viewed and thought of in the larger societal context. Coupled with the increasing recognition of family variation and structure is the movement toward more effective ways of treating families. The most effective ways of treating families are grouped under the umbrella term of best practices. A "best practice" can be thought of as a practice that best meets the needs and supports the healing process of the family being served within the human, technical, and financial resources of the provider. Further, it is expected that in these instances where family interventions are based on outcome studies and other reliable empirical evidence, the "best practice" should be as close to interventions based on outcome studies or evidence-based models as circumstances permit. Evidence-based practices may be de-

fined as interventions for which there is consistent scientific evidence showing that the interventions improve client outcomes. An evidence-based practice has been studied using appropriate scientific methodology and meets the following criteria (Ganju, 2001):

1. It has been replicated in more than one geographic or practice setting with consistent results.
2. It has been recognized in scientific journals by one or more published articles.
3. It is manualized.
4. It produces specific outcomes.

Corcoran (2003), in the first book on this, included eight evidence-based family interventions in her book on clinical application of evidence-based family interventions. These evidence-based interventions included the following:

• Cognitive–behavioral interventions
• Behavioral interventions
• Multisystemic treatment
• Multiple family psychoeducation
• Psychoeducation
• Reinforcement training
• Solution-focused therapy
• Structural family therapy.

Despite the usefulness of having available the evidence that supports the traditional and emergent theories that are available for working with families, the evidenced-based approach to practice with families is not without controversy. On the one hand, it is questionable whether the search for evidence-based intervention is more to satisfy the push of managed care requirements of accountable practice or to better serve families. According to Yalom (2009), there is no evidence that practitioners' adherence to manuals positively correlates to recovery consistent in practices.

Diversity and Multicultural Context

The extent or amount of diversity in American families today is probably no greater than in most periods in the past. However, what is different today is that so many different family types have found their voices and are demanding social recognition and support for their evidence (Demo, Allen, & Fine, 2000). Although the professional literature continues to expand on this topic, there continues to be ambiguity and confusion about the conceptualization and meaning of diversity (Logan, 2003). However, several lessons about family diversity have emerged from teaching practice and research since the mid-1980s. Perhaps the most important of these lessons is the need to not allow the racial/ethnic category that a family occupies to become the defining characteristic in appreciating the impact of diversity on family life. In addition to race/ethnicity, attention must be given to the multiple dimensions of family life, which include the social context, financial challenges, sexual orientation, and other important factors that intersect family life.

Despite the expansion of literature on family diversity, the treatment literature has not kept pace. Additionally, there is still a lack of familiarity with the beliefs and customs of culturally diverse families, coupled with the tendency to look for dysfunction. This approach to understanding diversity has led to errors in clinical assessment and interventions (Hardy & Laszloffy, 1992; Kurilla, 1998; Jenicus & Duba, 2002). Essentially, treatment approaches have not been expanded or refined to address the diversity that has been recognized in and across family groups. It is evident that the available theories continue to emphasize white, heterosexual, middle-income, married couples with children. This recognition serves to highlight a gap in teaching, service, and research. Hopefully, this awareness will serve to encourage experiential learning and research that will propel the profession toward expanding our current knowledge base to include fuller explanations of diverse family life forms and effective culturally responsive strategies for intervening in diverse family life (Almeida, Dolan-Del Vecchio, & Parker, 2008; Freeman, 2011).

International and Comparative Perspective
As indicated earlier, the world in which all families exist today is one of economic globalization and rapid technological and social change. It is a world of racial, religious, domestic, and economic violence. It is a world of involuntary and voluntary migration. It is also a world in which many people are attempting to resolve conflict and work for peace and change. Within this context, family scholars are providing knowledge about families. Despite the progress being made toward understanding families within a cultural context, the literature suggests that at least two examples of truly comparative international family studies exist (Kamerman & Kahn, 1998; Walters, Warzywoda, & Gurko, 2003). The literature that does exist identifies several universal issues as well as the apparent gaps in international family studies.

The first set of issues in international family studies are regional limitations. It is not surprising that some countries are more represented by family research and scholarship. The reasons for their omissions from the

literature include the lack of communication between scholars of the various countries (Adams, 2004). Although e-mail and the Internet provide greater access to and information about these countries, current contacts are limited or nonexistent. Regional limitation is also impacted by lack of funds to implement research projects as well as strong conservative values that do not support value free analysis of families and family problems.

At least six factors have been identified to support collaborative cross-cultural family research. These factors include a host coprincipal investigator, clearance from host country to carry out the research, sensitivity to local conditions such as wars, ethnic instability, or natural disasters. Additionally, sampling, translating, and consideration of the value of the research to the host country are important. Of equal importance is the need to engage interviewers who may be found among local teachers or university students (Adams, 2004).

The gaps in knowledge about the world's families include groups such as refugees, the oppressed, nomads, rural residents, poor urbanites, and the very rich. These are groups that are usually omitted by research designs because of governmental isolation, inaccessibility, or social exclusiveness. Among these groups, the gaps in knowledge are illustrated by the changing dynamics surrounding inheritance and property, the varied responses to child and elders abuse, domestic violence, and hesitancy in discussing intimate family issues such as marital satisfaction (Adams, 2004; Logan, 2006).

The universals regarding the world's families include changes in family patterns such as decreases in household size and fertility rates, increases in divorce, and nontraditional living arrangements. Much of these changes are attributed to the increase in women's education and employment outside the home (Logan, 2007). However, it is important to note that these changes have not resulted in gender equality. It is clear from the literature that women in the world's nations are still struggling to change the unequal basis for marriage and divorce, still seeking legislation to prevent abuse of all kinds, still lack access to land and financial security, still working to end discrimination and sexual harassment in the workplace and in educational settings, and still working to raise men's consciousness about gender equality (Adams, 2004; Logan, 2007).

TRENDS, CHALLENGES, AND FUTURE DIRECTION
Speculation abounds about what we can expect with regard to family meaning change and politics in this

century and beyond. What does seem clear in the early 21st century is that "the family" system has been or is being transformed globally. Demographers are recording worldwide the rising rates of divorce and unwed motherhood, declining birth rates, the feminization of poverty, and the increasing number of women attempting to raise their families without the emotional or financial support of their children's father. Although the challenges, debates, and ethical issues are implicit in the trends that have been addressed throughout this overview on families, perhaps the most pervasive of the ever widening scope of challenges and ethical issues are related to managing mental health care and technology.

Defining families. There is general consensus that scholars interested in the study of family life must go beyond the U.S. Bureau of Census' definition of families. However, it is becoming increasingly clear that we must encourage families to define themselves. The family definitions of themselves have implications of how families live their lives on a day-to-day basis, but also for the type of services provided, and for financial and policy matters. Finally, the depth and breadth of the challenges inherent in how same-gender couples define themselves as family and the effects of marriages, civil unions, and domestic partnership on the health and well-being of the children are virtually unknown to the general public and perhaps to many social workers (Pawelski et al., 2006). Defining families must also take into consideration the intersections of race, ethnicity, class, gender, age, and sexual orientation.

Researching and understanding families. It was very popular and trendy in the 1990s to forge multidisciplinary collaborations (researchers from more than one discipline are involved in a particular field but tend to conduct their work separately from one another). The language of the 2000s, to date, has been interdisciplinary collaboration. There is more dialogue among researchers, but researchers are holding steadfast to their root discipline and accompanying methodologies. The question, therefore, is whether it is possible for researchers to be transdisciplinary, to let go of disciplinary roots and boundaries on the questions and concerns about family life that is informed by knowledge and skills derived from the root discipline and beyond. This integrative, critical consciousness about families suggests a parallel to exploring and understanding the dynamics of family life.

Some scholars and researchers on family life are proposing a more flexible, postpositivist approach to family research (Allen, Floyd-Thomas, & Gillman,

2001). This approach suggests that there are many ways of viewing, knowing, and understanding families. Similarly, there are a variety of healthy, adaptive, and successful ways for families to live and be in the world. Moreover, a more flexible integrative approach to studying families is needed. Such an approach would not only address the structural variables that impact family life, but will also address processes, interactions, and behaviors within families. Mixed methodologies involving both quantitative and qualitative methods would be required to effectively address family life from within as well as externally.

Role and Implications for Social Work

According to McGoldrick, Carter, & Garcia-Preto (2011, p. 1), "we are born into families. Our first relationships, our first group, our first experience of the world are with and through our families." In short, families are at the center of our existence as individuals and as practitioners, educators, and researchers.

As a mode of intervention, family-based treatment approaches have expanded greatly since the mid-1990s. Practitioners and researchers have confirmed the effectiveness of treatment when including parents and extended family members in the helping process. However, opportunities have been limited not only to institute effective treatment models in practice settings but to create experiences so as to expand educators, students, and practitioners' knowledge about diverse family beliefs and customs. Given the proven usefulness of ethnographic research and instituting effective treatment models in practice settings, it is important that opportunities be made available for exploring and testing new and expanded ways of working with families and understanding and appreciating family diversity.

It is expected that the social work profession would bring to the forefront explicit statements and discussions regarding social policy and its effect on families. Current examples of social policies that impact family functioning and that should be included in these discussions are welfare reform, universal health care, affirmative action, the effect of marriage, civil unions, and domestic partnering laws on the health and well-being of children, and immigration policies. Additionally, these should also be included as a part of the required curriculum in schools of social work. As a profession, we must continue to ask new and challenging questions about families as well as learn to suspend the impositions of our beliefs about families in all their diversities.

REFERENCES

Adams, B. N. (2004). Families and family study in international perspective. *Journal of Marriage and Family, 66,* 1076–1088.

Allen, K. (2001). Finding new paths to family scholarship: A response to James White and Sheila Marshall. *Journal of Marriage and Family, 63,* 899–901.

Allen, K. R., Floyd-Thomas, S. M., & Gillman, L. (2001). Teaching to transform: From volatility to solidarity in an interdisciplinary family studies classroom. *Family Relations, 50,* 317–323.

Almeida, R. V., Dolan-Del Vecchio, K., & Parker, L. (2008). *Transformative family therapy: Just families in a just society.* Boston: Allyn & Bacon.

Andersen, T. (1991). *The reflecting team: Dialogues and dialogues about the dialogues.* New York: W. W. Norton & Company.

Anderson, H. (1997). *Conversation language and possibilities: A postmodern approach to therapy.* New York: Basic Books.

Anderson, C. M., Reiss, D. J., & Hogarty, G. E. (1986). *Schizophrenia and the family: A practitioner's guide to psychoeducation and management.* New York: Guilford Press.

Berg, I. K. (1994). *Family-based services: A solution-focused approach.* New York: Norton.

Compton, B. R., Galaway, B., & Cournoyer, B. R. (Eds.). (2005). *Social work processes* (7th ed.). Upper Saddle River, NJ: Prentice-Hall.

Coontz, S. (1988). *The social origins of private life: A history of American families, 1600–1900.* London: Verso.

Coontz, S. (2000). Historical perspectives on family diversity. In D. H. Demo, K. R. Allen, & M. A. Fine (Eds.), *Handbook of family diversity* (pp. 15–31). New York: Oxford University Press.

Corcoran, J. (2003). *Clinical applications of evidence-based family interventions.* New York: Oxford University Press.

de Shazer, S. (1994). *Words were originally magic.* New York: Norton.

Demo, D. H., Allen, K. R., & Fine, M. A. (Eds.). (2000). *Handbook of family diversity.* New York: Oxford University Press.

Duncan, G., & Brooks-Gunn, J. (Eds.) (1999). *Consequences of growing up poor.* New York: Russell Sage Foundations.

Epston, D. (1994). Extending the conversation. *Family Therapy Networker, 18,* 30–17, 62.

Foucault, M. (1965). *Madness and civilization: A history of insanity in the age of reason.* New York: Random House.

Foucault, M. (1980). *Power/knowledge: Selected interviews and other writings.* New York: Pantheon.

Franklin, D. (1997). *Ensuring inequality: The structural transformation of the African American family.* New York: Oxford University Press.

Freeman, E. M. (2011). *Narrative approaches in social work practice: A life span, culturally centered, strengths perspective.* Springfield, IL: Charles C. Thomas Publisher.

Ganju, V. (2001). *Bridging the gap between research and service with evidenced-based practices.* Alexandria, VA: National Technical Assistance Center for State Mental Health Planning.

Gergen, K. (1985). The social constructionist movement in modern psychology. *American Psychologist, 40,* 266–275.

Gutman, H. (1976). *The black family in slavery and freedom, 1750–1925.* New York: Pantheon.

Hardy, K. V., & Laszloffy, T. A. (1992). Training racially sensitive family therapists: Context, content, and contact. *Families in Society, 73,* 364–370.

Jenicus M., & Duba, J. D. (2002). Creating a multicultural family practice. *The Family Journal,* 410–414.

Jones, J. (1998). *American work: Four centuries of black and white labor.* New York: Norton.

Kamerman, S. B., & Kahn, A. J. (Eds). (1998). *Family change and family policies in Great Britain, Canada, New Zealand and the Unites States.* New York: Oxford University Press.

Katz, M., Doucet, M., & Stern, M. (1982). *The social organization of early industrial capitalism.* Cambridge, MA: Harvard University Press.

Keeney, B. P. (1990). *Improvisational therapy: A practical guide for creative clinical strategies.* New York: Guilford Press.

Kumashiro, K. K. (2004). *Against common sense: Teaching and learning toward social justice.* New York: Routlege Falmer.

Kurilla, V. (1998). Multicultural counseling perspectives: Culture specificity and implications in family therapy. *Family Counseling: Counseling and Therapy for Couples and Families, 6,* 207–211.

Logan, S. L. (2001). *The black family: Building strength, self-help, and positive change* (2nd ed.). Boulder, CO: Westview Press.

Logan, S. L. (2003). Issues of multiculturalism: Multicultural practice, cultural diversity and competency. In R. English (Ed.), *Encyclopedia of social work and supplement* (19th ed., pp. 95–105). Washington, DC: NASW.

Logan, S. L. (2006). The changing role of Ghanaian women. Paper presented at University of South Carolina Women Studies Annual National Conference, Columbia, SC.

Logan, S. L., Freeman, E. M., & McRoy, R. G. (1990). *Social work practice with black families: A culturally specific perspective.* New York: Longman.

McGoldrick, M., Carter, B., & Garcia-Preto, N. (Eds.). (2011). *The expanded family life cycle: Individual, family, and social perspectives* (4th ed.). New York: Allyn & Bacon Classics.

Mintz, S., & Kellogg, S. (1988). *Domestic revolutions: A social history of American family life.* New York, NY: Free Press.

Nicholas, M. P. (2010). *The essentials of family therapy* (5th ed.). Upper Saddle River, NJ: Prentice-Hall.

O'Hanlon, W. H., & Weiner-Davis, M. (1989). *In search of solutions: A new direction in psychotherapy.* New York: Norton.

Pawelski, J. G., Perrin, E. C., Foy, J. M., Allen, C. E., Crawford, J. E., Monte, Del M., et al. (2006). The effects of Marriage Civil Union, and Domestic Partnership

Laws on the health and well-being of children. *Pediatrics*, *118*, 349–364.

Roediger, D. (2007). *The wages of whiteness: Race and the making of the American working class*. London: Verso.

Rojano, R. (2004). The practice of community family therapy. *Family Process, 43*, 59–77.

Schwartz, R. C. (1994). *Internal family systems therapy*. New York: Guilford Press.

Spain, D., & Bianchi, S. (1996). *Balancing act: Motherhood, marriage, and employment among American women*. New York: Russell Sage Foundation.

Stevenson, B. E. (1997). *Life in black and white: Family and community in the slave south*. New York: Oxford University Press.

Taylor, R. L. (2000). Diversity within African American family. In D. H. Demo, K. R. Allen, & M. A. Fine (Eds.), *Handbook of family diversity* (pp. 232–251). New York: Oxford University Press.

Taylor, R. L., Chatters, L., Tucker, M. B., & Lewis, E. (1990). Development in research on black families: A decade review. *Journal of Marriage and the Family, 52*, 993–1014.

Teachman, J. D. (2000). Diversity of family structure: Economic and social influence. In D. H. Demo, K. R. Allen, & M. A. Fine (Eds.), *Handbook of family diversity* (pp. 32–58). New York: Oxford University Press.

Tools for Transformation. (2000). *Interdisciplinary Core Social Science courses*. University of Washington.

U.S. Department of Health and Human Services. (2003). *Trends in the well-being of America's children and youth*: (8th ed.). Washington, DC: Office of the Assistant Secretary for Planning and Evaluation.

Walters, L. H., Warzywoda, W., & Gurko, T. (2003). Cross cultural studies of families: Hidden differences. *Journal of Comparative Family Studies, 33*, 433–449.

White, M. (1995). *Re-authoring lives: Interview and essays*. Adelaide, South Australia: Dulwich Center Publications.

Yalom, I. (2009). CBT is not what it's cracked up to be . . . or, Don't be afraid of the EVT bogeyman. In I. Yalom (Ed.), *The gift of therapy. An open letter to a new generation of therapists and their patients* (pp. 222–224). New York: Harper Collins.

FURTHER READING

Bonnington, S. B., McGrath, P., & Martinck, S. A. (1996). The fax of the matter: The electronic transfer of confidential material. *Family Journal: Counseling and Therapy for Couples and Families, 4*, 155–156.

Caudell, O. B., Jr. (1999). The technology trap. *Family Therapy News, 30*, 20, 22.

Cohen, J. A. (2003). Managed care and the evolving role of the clinical social worker in mental health. *Social Work, 48*(1), 34–42.

Foos, J. A., Ottens, A. J., & Hill, L. K. (1991). Managed mental health: A primer for Counselor. *Journal of Counseling and Development, 69*, 332–336.

Haas, L. J., & Malouf, J. L. (2005). *Keeping up the good work: A practitioner's guide to mental health ethics* (4th ed.). Sarasota, FL: Professional Resource Exchange.

FAMILY THERAPY

ABSTRACT: Family intervention has become an important tool for social work practitioners. This introduction provides a brief history of family intervention and important influences as well as a synopsis of current research. Although these interventions require more research to better understand the populations for whom they are most effective, the evidence supports their usefulness in addressing such issues as aggression, substance use, and depression, among others.

KEY WORDS: evidence-based research; family intervention; history; systems theory; research

History

Family intervention became an important treatment approach in the 1950s following a period in which practitioners worked primarily with individuals (Janzen, Harris, Jordan, & Franklin, 2006). Practitioners began to define presenting problems in terms of family dynamics, and goals for treatment focused on changing patterns of family interaction. Early contributors to family therapy pioneered interventions based on systems theories. Family interventions in social work practice are guided by systems theory and are, therefore, concerned with structure and interactions within the family as well as interactions among the family members and larger systems (Franklin & Jordan, 1999). The Ecomap, for example, is a popular family assessment tool developed within social work; it helps social workers to map family communication and relationships between the family and other systems (Hartman & Laird, 1983). Family assessment approaches, such as Bowen's Genogram, are also used in practice. Family interventions aim to remove problematic patterns of family interaction rather than focusing on changing the behavior of an individual. Changing the structure and patterns of interaction within a family results in changes in the behavior of each family member (Franklin & Jordan, 1999). In addition to working with the family, practitioners consider the environmental factors affecting the family and may work to improve family connections with larger systems, such as schools and community service organizations (Hartman & Laird, 1983).

Family-therapy models that have particularly influenced social work practice include structural family therapy, developed by Salvador Minuchin; the Gestalt approach, developed by Kempler; the Communicative-Interactive approach, developed by Satir (Janzen et al., 2006); and the multigenerational model, developed by Murray Bowen. Later models that influenced family practice include social-learning approaches such as parent management, solution-focused brief therapy, narrative therapy, and feminist and post-modern perspectives, although from the vantage point of practice interventions, the feminist and post-modern perspectives served mostly as philosophical frameworks to help examine and critique the traditional family-therapy models and further aid the practitioners' work with important family dynamics and change. Family interventions have been used primarily to address child and adolescent behavioral and mental-health issues. These include conduct problems such as oppositional behavior and aggression, drug abuse, anxiety, and depression. The most well-researched family approaches are parent-management training programs that address opposition and aggression (Kazdin & Whitley, 2003; Larner, 2004). Meta-analyses and systematic reviews of research indicate that family interventions are more effective than no treatment (Larner, 2004; Shadish, Montgomery, Wilson, Bright, & Okwumabua, 1993; Shadish, Ragsdale, Glass, & Montgomery, 1995).

Evidence-Based Family Interventions

The research on family therapy has made advances over the last decade, and several family-therapy interventions now have considerable empirical support. As research has advanced in family therapy, these interventions were evaluated in clinical trials and quasi-experiments, and different family therapies were found to work well with a variety of clients. In particular, family therapies have been effective in reducing problem behaviors in adolescents. Family therapies with the best research employ similar techniques. These approaches typically have foundations in cognitive, behavioral, structural, or strategic therapy. They provide opportunities to develop communication and problem-solving skills as well as instructional components. Practitioners intervene on multiple ecological levels by working with the individual, family, school staff, and community-service providers, for example. Families have opportunities to practice new skills and are provided with regular feedback about their behavior. Practitioners work with families to develop behavioral goals that define treatment success (Roans & Hoagwood, 2000; Schinke, Brounstein, & Gardner, 2002).

Although research on family-therapy approaches is continuously evolving, the following have research support for their effectiveness. Brief Strategic Family Therapy, developed by Jose Szapocznik, has been shown to reduce adolescent conduct and behavior problems, and drug use, in controlled research trials (Robbins et al., 2011; Santisteban et al., 2003). Multisystemic Therapy, developed by Scott Henggeler, is another well-researched family intervention. Multiple well-controlled studies evaluating this home-based intervention demonstrate that it is effective in reducing substance use and antisocial behavior among juvenile offenders between the ages of 12 and 17. (Randall & Cunningham, 2003). Multidimensional Family Therapy, developed by Howard Liddle, has effectively reduced marijuana use, delinquent behavior, and symptoms of depression and anxiety (Dennis et al., 2002; Henderson, Dakof, Greenbaum, & Liddle, 2010; Liddle et al., 2001; Liddle et al., 2002; Rowe, Liddle, & Dakof, 2001). Functional Family Therapy (FFT) is another intervention used successfully with adolescents to reduce substance use and behaviors associated with conduct disorder, oppositional defiant disorder, and disruptive behavior disorder (Alexander et al., 1998; Center for the Study and Prevention of Violence, 2006; Sexton & Turner, 2010). Solution-focused, brief therapy is also a promising, strengths-based, intervention that is being more widely researched within schools and in community agencies, and it has been found to be effective in several studies (Franklin, Kim, & Tripodi, 2006; Gingerich, Kim, Stams, & MacDonald, 2012; Kim & Franklin, 2009).

The Incredible Years, an intervention for families with younger children developed by Carolyn Webster-Stratton, reduces conduct problems and behaviors associated with oppositional defiant disorder (Foster, Olchowski, & Webster-Stratton, 2007; SAMHSA Center for Substance Abuse Prevention, 2005). Parent–Child Interaction Therapy, developed by Eyeberg and colleagues, has resulted in improved family interaction and fewer behavior problems for children with conduct disorder (Eyberg & Robinson, 1982; Foote, Eyberg & Schuhmann, 1998; The Child Anxiety Network, 2006). Parent Management Training (PMT) has also resulted in fewer behavior problems, such as opposition and aggression, and more prosocial behaviors (Feldman & Kazdin, 1995; Hautman et al., 2011; Hoagwood, 2005; Kazdin & Whitley, 2003; Ogden & Amlund Hagen, 2008).

Family interventions have demonstrated positive outcomes for adults as well as children. Family Psychoeducation, for example, has demonstrated positive outcomes for families caring for an individual diagnosed with depression, bipolar disorder, and/or schizophrenia (Anderson et al., 1986; Brennan, 1995; Holden & Anderson, 1990; Schwartz & Schwartz, 1993). The family learns about the diagnosis, symptoms, and treatment, as well as skills for coping and maintaining support networks (Franklin & Jordan, 1999). Multifamily psychoeducational groups include the members of multiple families and effectively helps them manage negative symptoms of schizophrenia (Breitborde, Woods, & Srihari, 2009; Katsuki et al., 2011; Voss, 2003). Behavioral Couples Therapy is one of the most extensively researched family interventions and has also demonstrated positive outcomes for families of individuals diagnosed with schizophrenia, depression and alcoholism. It has also effectively reduced behavior problems in children (Campbell, 1997; Larner, 2004; Pinsoff & Wynne, 2000; Shadish & Baldwin, 2005). Emotion-focused therapy is also gaining a body of experimental research on its effectiveness with couples (Jantzen et al., 2006).

As with any evidence-based practice, the body of research supporting the above family interventions is continuously developing, and researchers may have disagreements about whether they should be classified as evidence based. The "evidence-based" status of Multisystemic Therapy, for example, has been recently called into question by some researchers who assert that the intervention may not be any more effective than alternative treatments (Littell, Popa, & Forsythe, 2005). It is, therefore, important to stay abreast of developments in research on family interventions, because research developments change, other promising family-based interventions exist, and the research on these interventions is always progressing, as well. For example, The Parenting with Love and Limits model that is used in juvenile-justice settings has been discussed as a promising model by the Office of Juvenile Justice and continues to gain more research studies (Difficult. Net). The family-therapy field appears to be active with many other promising approaches and interventions, and the models that were once discussed as unique approaches are also currently being integrated or blended (for example, structural, strategic, behavioral, solution-focused) as the field makes new strides toward discovering common factors across approaches. For family interventions to advance further, they will require more well-controlled outcome studies demonstrating their effectiveness and more manualized treatment protocols. Research is still needed, for example, to determine the populations, presenting problems, and contexts for which family interventions are most effective (Larner, 2004).

Summary

Family interventions are supported by a growing body of research that demonstrates their effectiveness in addressing many issues, from childhood behavior problems to adult depression, couples problems, and substance abuse. Practitioners provide instruction and feedback and apply cognitive and behavioral techniques in helping families develop new patterns of interaction. By changing the patterns of interactions, family interventions effectively address the presenting problems of individual family members. Family Interventions have made progress in developing evidence, and the field is active with many effective and promising interventions. Current trends suggest that the future of family therapy may include continued integration of perspectives to create more effective therapeutic interventions, as well as the blending of family-practice perspectives with individual approaches. The adaptation and usefulness of family therapy with diverse families from different cultural backgrounds will also become better known. As a widely used clinical approach, family therapy has come of age, and current approaches provide many useful techniques to be considered in helping clients. Future research may further elucidate common factors and core ingredients that make family practice effective with a wide range of clients.

REFERENCES

Alexander, J., Barton, C., Gordon, D., Grotpeter, J., Hansson, K., Harrison, R., et al. (1998). Functional family therapy: Blueprints for violence prevention. Book 3. In D. S. Elliott (Ed.), *Blueprints for violence prevention* series. Boulder, CO: Center for the Study and Prevention of Violence, Institute of Behavioral Science, University of Colorado.

Anderson, C., Reiss, D., & Hogarty, G. (1986). *Schizophrenia and the family*. New York: Guilford Press.

Breitborde, N. J. K., Woods, S. W., & Srihari, V. H. (2009). Multifamily psychoeducation for first-episode psychosis: A cost-effectiveness analysis. *Psychiatric Services, 60*, 1477–1483.

Brennan, J. (1995). A short term psycho educational multiple family group for bipolar clients and their families. *Social Work, 40*(6), 737–743.

Campbell, T. L. (1997). Research reports: Effectiveness of family therapy. *Family Systems and Health, 15*, 123–129.

Center for the Study and Prevention of Violence. (2006). Blueprints model programs: Functional family therapy. Retrieved September 29, 2006 from http://www.colorado.edu/cspv/blueprints/modelprograms/FFT.html

Dennis, M., Titus, J. C., Diamond, G., Donaldson, J., Godley, S. H., Tims, F. M., et al. (2002). The Cannabis Youth Treatment (CYT) experiment: Rationale, study design and analysis plans. *Addiction*, Suppl. 1, 16–34.

Eyberg, S. M., & Robinson, E. A. (1982). Parent–child interaction training: Effects on family functioning. *Journal of Clinical Child Psychology, 11*, 130–137.

Feldman, J., & Kazdin, A. E. (1995). Parent management training for oppositional and conduct problem children. *The Clinical Psychologist, 48*(4), 3–5.

Foote, R., Eyberg, S. M., & Schuhmann, E. (1998). Parent–child interaction approaches to the treatment of child behavior disorders. In T. H. Ollendick & R. J. Prinz (Eds.), *Advances in clinical child psychology*, Volume 20. New York: Plenum Press.

Foster, E. M., Olchowski, A. E., & Webster-Stratton, C. H. (2007). Is stacking intervention components cost-effective? An analysis of the incredible years program. *Journal of the American Academy of Child & Adolescent Psychiatry*, 46(11), 1414–1424.

Franklin, C., & Jordan, C. (1999). *Family practice: Brief systems methods for social work*. Pacific Grove, CA: Brooks Cole Publishing Co.

Franklin, C., Kim, J. S., & Tripodi, S. (2006). Solution-focused, brief therapy intervention for students at-risk to dropout. In C. Franklin, M. B. Harris, & P. Allen-Meares (Eds.), *The school services sourcebook: A guide for school-based professionals* (pp. 691–704). New York: Oxford University Press.

Gingerich, W. J., Kim, J. S, Stams, Gert, J .J. M., & MacDonald, A. J. (2012). Solution focused brief therapy outcome research. In C. Franklin, T. S. Trepper, W. J. Gingerich, & E. E. McCollum (Eds.), *Solution-focused brief therapy: A handbook of evidence-based practice* (pp. 3–19). New York: Oxford University Press.

Hartman, A., & Laird, J. (1983). *Family centered social work practice*. New York: Free Press.

Hautmann, C., Stein, P., Eichelberger, I., Hanisch, C., Plück, J., Walter, D., & Döpfner, M. (2011). The severely impaired do profit most: Differential effectiveness of a parent management training for children with externalizing behavior problems in a natural setting. *Journal of Child & Family Studies*, 20(4), 424–435.

Henderson, C. E., Dakof, G. A., Greenbaum, P. E., & Liddle, H. A. (2010). Effectiveness of multidimensional family therapy with higher severity substance-abusing adolescents: Report from two randomized controlled trials. *Journal of Consulting & Clinical Psychology*, 78(6), 885–897.

Hoagwood, K. E. (2005). Family-based services in children's mental health: A research review and synthesis. *Journal of Child and Family Psychiatry*, 46(7), 690–713.

Holden, D., & Anderson, C. M. (1990). Psychoeducational family intervention for depressed clients and their families. In G. I. Keitner (Ed.), *Depression and families: Impact and treatment* (pp. 57–84). Washington, DC: American Psychiatric Press.

Janzen, C., Harris, O., Jordan, C., & Franklin, C. (2006). *Family treatment: Evidence-based practice with populations at risk* (4th Ed.). Pacific Grove, CA: Brooks/Cole.

Katsuki, F., Takeuchi, H., Konishi, M., Sasaki, M., Murase, Y., Naito, et al. (2011). Pre-post changes in psychosocial functioning among relatives of patients with depressive disorders after Brief Multifamily Psychoeducation: A pilot study. *BMC Psychiatry*, 11(1), 56–62.

Kazdin, A. E, & Whitley, M. K. (2003). Treatment of parental stress to enhance therapeutic change among children referred for aggressive and antisocial behavior. *Journal of Consulting and Clinical Psychology*, 71, 504–515.

Kim. J. S., & Franklin, C. (2009). Solution-focused brief therapy in schools: A review of the literature. *Children and Youth Services Review*, 3(4), 464–470.

Larner, G. (2004). Family therapy and the politics of evidence. *Journal of Family Therapy*, 26, 17–39.

Liddle, H. A., Dakof, G. A., Parker, K., Diamond, G. S., Barrett, K., & Tejeda, M. (2001). Multidimensional family therapy for adolescent drug abuse: Results of a randomized clinical trial. *American Journal of Drug and Alcohol Abuse*, 27(4), 651–688.

Liddle, H. A., Rowe, C. L., Quille, T., Dakof, G., Sakran, E., & Biaggi, H. (2002). Transporting a research-developed adolescent drug abuse treatment into practice. *Journal of Substance Abuse Treatment*, special edition on transferring research to practice, 22, 231–243.

Littell, J., Popa, J. H., & Forsythe, B. (2005). Multi-systemic therapy for social, emotional, and behavioral problems in youth aged 10–17, *Campbell Collaboration Review*, 2. Retrieved November 10, 2006 from http://www .campbellcollaboration.org/lib/download/23/

Ogden, T., & Amlund Hagen, K. (2008). Treatment effectiveness of parent management training in Norway: A randomized controlled trial of children with conduct problems. *Journal of Consulting & Clinical Psychology*, 76(4), 607–621.

Pinsoff, W. M., & Wynne, L. C. (2000). Towards progress research: closing the gap between family therapy practice and research. *Journal of Marital and Family Therapy*, 26, 1–8.

Randall, J., & Cunningham, P. B. (2003). Multisystemic therapy: A treatment for violent substance-abusing and substance-dependent juvenile offenders. *Addictive Behaviors*, 28, 1731–1739.

Roans, M., & Hoagwood, K. (2000). School-based mental health services: a research review. *Clinical Child and Family Psychology Review*, 3(4), 223–241.

Robbins, M. S., Feaster, D. J., Horigian, V. E., Bachrach, K., Burlew, K., Carrion, I., et al. (2011). Brief strategic family therapy versus treatment as usual: Results of a multisite randomized trial for substance using adolescents. *Journal of Consulting & Clinical Psychology*, 79(6), 713–727.

Rowe, C. L., Liddle, H. A., & Dakof, G. A. (2001). Classifying adolescent substance abusers by level of externalizing and internalizing symptoms. *Journal of Child and Adolescent Substance Abuse*, 11(2), 41–66.

Santisteban, D. A., Coatsworth, D., Perez-Vidal, A., Kurtines, W. M., Schwanz, S. J., LaPerriere, A., et al. (2003). The efficacy of brief strategic family therapy in modifying Hispanic adolescent behavior problems and substance use. *Journal of Family Psychology*, 17, 121–133.

Schinke, S., Brounstein, P., & Gardner, S. (2002). *Science-based prevention programs and principles*. Rockville, MD: U.S. Department of Health and Human Services.

Schwartz, A., & Schwartz, R. (1993). *Depression: Theories and treatments*. New York: Columbia University Press.

Sexton, T., & Turner, C. W. (2010). The effectiveness of functional family therapy for youth with behavioral problems in a community practice setting. *Journal of Family Psychology, 24*(3), 339–348.

Shadish, W. R., & Baldwin, S. A. (2005). Effects of behavioral marital therapy: A meta-analysis of randomized controlled trials. *Journal of Consulting and Clinical Psychology, 73*(1), 6–14.

Shadish, W. R., Montgomery, L. M., Wilson, P., Bright, I., & Okwumabua, T. (1993). Effects of family and marital psychotherapies. *Journal of Consulting and Clinical Psychology, 61*(6), 992–1002.

Shadish, W. R., Ragsdale, K., Glass, R. R., & Montgomery, L. M. (1995). The efficacy and effectiveness of marital and family therapy: a perspective from meta-analysis. *Journal of Marital and Family Therapy, 21*, 345–360.

Substance Abuse and Mental Health Services Administration (SAMHSA) Center for Substance Abuse Prevention. (2005). SAMHSA model programs. Retrieved December 10, 2005 from http://www.nrepp.samhsa.gov/

The Child Anxiety Network. (2006). Specialized programs: Parent–child interaction therapy. Retrieved September 29, 2006 from http://www.childanxiety.net/Specialty_Programs.htm

Voss, W. D. (2003). Multiple family group (MFG) treatment and negative symptoms in schizophrenia: Two-year outcomes. Dissertation Abstracts International: Sciences and Engineering, 63(11B), 5541.

FURTHER READING

American Association of Marriage and Family Therapy, www.aamft.org

Savannah Family Institute, www.difficult.net/

SAMHSA's National Registry of Evidence-Based Programs and Practices www.nrepp.samhsa.gov

The Institute for the Study of Therapeutic Change (ISTC) and Partners for Change www.talkingcure.com/

U.S. Department of Health and Human Services Administration for Children and Families: Child Welfare Information Gateway, www.childwelfare.gov/

CYNTHIA FRANKLIN AND LAURA HOPSON

FINANCIAL SOCIAL WORK

ABSTRACT: Financial well-being is an individual responsibility in 21st century America, even though research reveals a serious inability for many Americans to attain it. Social workers have the education and training to help people modify behavior and a history of working with low-income and minority families, as well as the skills to engage and empower clients, making them the best professionals to help Americans take control of their money and their lives. This article explains how incorporating financial-literacy skills and models of financial behavioral change into the social work curriculum would benefit both social

workers and their clients. It describes the financial social work model and an understanding of its relevance to the social work profession.

KEY WORDS: financial social work; financial literacy; financial well-being; social work curriculum; financial behavioral change

The Growing Need for Financial Knowledge

In today's times, individuals are required to have both greater financial knowledge and investment skills. The need for greater financial sophistication stems from a variety of factors: (a) the financial deregulation process that started in the 1970s that has led to a wider variety of financial products; (b) the greater complexity involved and degree of self-reliance expected in terms of retirement planning due to changes that have taken place with the proportion of retirement income being covered by Social Security and defined benefit employer pension plans, and the shift to defined contribution 401(k) type plans; and (c) the increase in financial responsibility in other areas, such as college-tuition costs and insurance costs for health, long-term care, and disability (Boshara, 2010). For example, 40% of employed adults who have benefits packages report seeing a decrease and/or elimination of their benefits (such as health care, retirement savings, insurance, or training) (NEFE, 2012).

Aside from individuals needing to take greater charge of their financial well-being, the cost for attaining many components of the American dream (such as purchasing a home or funding a child's college education) has increased since the 1980s and 1990s and is expected to continue to rise throughout the 21st century (FINRA Investor Education Foundation, 2009). As a result of the increased costs of living, and the changes in the financial landscape, the consequences of not having the necessary skills to make sound financial decisions have become much more serious. This is particularly true in the case of an economic downturn, when there is a greater risk of job loss or decrease in income. According to several academics, think tanks, and others, the current economic slump is expected to continue for several years (Boshara, 2010).

Unfortunately, despite the necessity of financial know-how, Americans repeatedly demonstrate, in study after study, little knowledge about financial concepts and products (Boshara, 2010) and rather poor financial capability (FINRA Investor Education Foundation, 2009). To illustrate, according to the first National Financial Capability Study (FINRA Investor Education Foundation, 2009) conducted in the United

States by the Financial Industry Regulatory Authority (FINRA) in consultation with the Treasury Department, nearly half of survey respondents reported facing difficulties in covering monthly expenses and paying bills. In addition, half of American adults (49%) do not have "rainy-day" funds set aside for unanticipated financial emergencies and, similarly, do not plan for predictable life events, such as their children's college education or their own retirement. Also, more than one in five respondents reported engaging in high-cost, alternative borrowing methods, such as payday loans and pawn shops (FINRA Investor Education Foundation, 2009).

Furthermore, according to the National Foundation for Credit Counseling's (NFCC) survey on financial literacy (2012), 40% of U.S. adults gave themselves a grade of a "C," "D," or "F" on their knowledge of personal finance, and more than half (56%) admit that they do not have a budget.

While some of the results from the NFCC survey (2012) differ from those of the FINRA Investor Education Foundation (2009), the overall trends are identical and highlight the struggle that so many men and women experience in the management of their day-to-day expenses. One third do not pay their bills on time, and 39% are carrying credit card debt month to month (NFCC, 2012). In addition, 39% of U.S. adults report no retirement savings, and a quarter of those indicate that if they were to begin saving, they would keep their savings at home in cash (NFCC, 2012).

TODAY'S FINANCIAL CRISIS Today, more and more Americans are experiencing some form of financial crisis. There were a total of 1,362,847 personal bankruptcies filed in 2011 (ABI, n.d.); 23% of the roughly 50 million residential mortgages in the United States are currently "underwater," that is, the amount owed exceeds the value of the underlying home, and about 8 million consumers have faced a new foreclosure filing since 2007 (Dynan, 2012); the average credit card debt is $6,503 (CardTrak.com, 2012).

In addition to struggles with credit card debt, many Americans face student-loan debt: two-thirds (66%) of college seniors who graduated in 2011 had student-loan debt, with an average of $26,600 (TICAS, 2012). The difficult job market poses particular challenges for those college graduates who need to begin paying back student loans; the unemployment rate for this group was at 8.8% in 2012, and many graduates are underemployed—either working part time but wanting a full-time position, or working at a position that does not require a college degree (TICAS, 2012).

While research continues to show strong economic returns on investments in college degrees, graduating with high debt is a serious and growing concern in the United States. It can limit career options and make it difficult to save for a home, family retirement, or one's own children's education (TICAS, 2012).

In the past, home ownership was perceived as achieving the American Dream. In the early 21st century, the most important financial goal for nearly half of American adults (47%) is being able to save enough money for retirement (NEFE, 2011). In marked contrast, only 17% felt home ownership was their top goal (NEFE, 2011).

THE OVERALL POVERTY RATE IS INCREASING In 2011, median household income was $50,054, a 1.5% decline in real terms from 2010. Real median household income was 8.1% lower than in 2007, the year before the most recent recession, and it was 8.9% lower than the median household income peak that occurred in 1999 (U.S. Census Bureau, 2012a).

The overall poverty rate in 2011 was 15%, representing 46.2 million people living in poverty. While this poverty rate was statistically unchanged from 15.1% in 2010, it had risen significantly in seven of the prior ten years, from a low of 11.3% in 2000 (U.S. Census Bureau, 2012a).

In addition, 6.6% of all people, or 20.4 million people, lived in deep poverty—that is, they had income below one-half the poverty threshold, or $11,511 for a family of four. Minorities were hit the hardest. African American children experienced the highest poverty rate, at 37.4%, and Hispanics were close, at 34%. For non-Hispanic Caucasian children, the rate was 12.5%, giving an overall child poverty rate of 21.9%, or 16.1 million children living in poverty (U.S. Census Bureau, 2012a).

Furthermore, the official poverty threshold does not take into account costs such as health insurance, transportation, or housing, nor does it factor in income from transfer programs such as food stamps. Hence, the U.S. Census Bureau has developed a supplemental poverty measure to address these shortcomings (U.S. Census Bureau, 2012b).

When looking at the overall supplemental poverty rate, it is higher at 16.1% vs. the official measure at 15% for 2011. That said, for some groups, it is lower [for children under 18 and blacks] and for others, it is higher [seniors—15.1% supplemental vs. 8.7% official; Asian Americans—16.9% supplemental vs. 12.3% official, and slightly higher for those 18–64, Hispanics, and non-Hispanic whites] (U.S. Census Bureau, 2012b).

Most notably, the Supplemental Poverty Measure data show that out-of-pocket medical costs are the main expense contributor of poverty, followed by work-related expenses (such as transportation), while Social Security is by far the most critical program for reducing poverty, followed by tax credits such as the Earned Income Tax Credit (EITC) or the child tax credit (CTC) (Boteach, 2012; U.S. Census Bureau, 2012b).

Specifically, the refundable tax credits for working families, such as earned income and child tax credits, was successful at raising 8.7 million people out of poverty in 2011. Similarly, the Supplemental Nutrition Assistance Program (which replaced the Food Stamps Program) raised 4.7 million people out of poverty in 2011 (Boteach, 2012).

Financial Capability

Restoring economic security for all families is one of the U.S. government's priorities (President's Advisory Council on Financial Capability, 2012). Hence, the Barack Obama administration set a goal to improve the financial capability of every American, that is, to empower "every individual with the knowledge, skills and access to tools to manage their finances effectively for long-term well-being (p. 4)." To this end, as of 2013, it stressed the critical role community involvement via public-private and private-private partnerships will need to play in equipping consumers with needed financial skills and put together a resource guide for this very purpose, "Every American Financially Empowered: A Guide to Increasing Financial Capability Among Students, Workers and Residents in Communities" (President's Advisory Council on Financial Capability, 2012).

DETERMINANTS OF FINANCIAL BEHAVIOR Financial behavior is defined as any human behavior related to money management, that is, spending, borrowing, saving, investing, budgeting, and risk managing (Xiao, 2008). There are many internal and external influences on an individual's financial behavior. Internal factors include personality, individual psychology and cognition, family history. and environment (Shim, Xiao, Barber, & Lyons, 2009; Nyhus & Webley, 2001; Xiao et al., 2010).

Parents impact financial behaviors by influencing children's and adolescents' norms and values with respect to how much they believe in the importance of saving vs. spending and overall materialism (Hira, 2010; Nyhus & Webley, 2001; Shim et al., 2009; Webley & Nyhus, 2006; Xiao et al., 2010). According to Webley & Nyhus (2006), modeling and discussion may be the dominant mechanisms by which the fundamental approach to money matters is transmitted from parents to children.

Parental factors such as income, wealth, education, and race also influence the financial socialization process (Xiao et al., 2010). Parents who have greater economic resources at their disposal are able to make significant investments in their children that lead to an increase in their children's human, social, and financial capital (Conger, Conger & Martin, 2010; Xiao et al., 2010).

External elements consist of influences such as media, markets, and peers (Hira, 2010; Xiao et al., 2010). In addition, factors such as culture, herding (following the crowd's behavior), and social mood impact financial behavior (Hira, 2010; Xiao et al., 2010). Another potential influence on financial behavior is moral hazard, or the tendency to take more risk when it is perceived that losses incurred as a result of risky behavior will be insured or subsidized (Hira, 2010; Xiao et al., 2010). As per Grochulski (2010), in the event of financial hardship, individuals may consider taking on more debt in anticipation of being discharged of their liabilities via bankruptcy laws.

Last, there is the simultaneous impact of self-worth, net worth. and social signaling on shopping behavior. In a world that too often measures success in financial terms, people often confuse their self-worth with their net worth. As a result, individuals who are impoverished (or who struggle to keep up with their neighbors' purchases) experience low self-esteem and poor sense of self (Sivanathan & Pettit, 2010; Wolfsohn, 2012a). This lower self-worth often manifests itself in feeling undeserving of a better financial future and actualizing that outcome by engaging in self-sabotaging behaviors, such as indulging in high-status items that one can ill-afford (Sivanathan & Pettit, 2010; Wolfsohn, 2012a). As per Arnold and Reynolds (2009), spending behavior is a form of mood repair and affect regulation with the goal of hedonic gratification that drives consumption behavior.

In fact, the persistence of poverty may be in part due to the "conspicuous consumption" that takes place as the poor try to distinguish themselves from the very poor, according to Moav and Neeman's (2010) economic model. Low-income individuals increase their consumption of luxury goods in order to send a social signal of a change in their financial circumstances, despite the fact that this action may reverse their economic gain by increasing their debt and maintaining their status of poverty (Moav & Neeman, 2010).

FEELINGS OF DISCONNECT FROM MONEY Individuals may also spend more than what they would like as a result of their feelings of disconnect from their money. Consumers today can choose from a wide variety of payment options such as: cash, check, credit card, debit card, bank drafts, money orders, traveler's checks, gift certificates, gift cards, stored-value cards such as those used in mass transit and tolls, and more (Raghubir & Srivastava, 2008). As a result of engaging in these payment methods and employing various direct-deposit methods for income and benefits, consumers are living in an increasingly cashless society. The increasingly cashless society, in turn, is leading individuals to experience feelings of disconnect from their money (Wolfsohn, 2004). This financial disconnect is expressed through the difficulties that consumers experience in knowing how much money they have and understanding the impact that their spending has on their financial circumstances (Raghubir & Srivastava, 2008; Soman, 2003; Wolfsohn, 2004).

With regards to the use of credit cards vs. cash, for example, people tend to spend more (Chatterjee & Rose, 2012; Pettit & Sivanathan, 2011; Raghubir & Srivastava, 2008; Sivanathan & Pettit, 2010; Soman, 2003). This is primarily the result of the "pain of paying" and the transparency effect (Soman, 2003). The closer a form of payment is to cash, the more an individual will feel its potency, or the "pain of paying," and the less the individual will spend (Chatterjee & Rose, 2012). Conversely, the more a person is able to psychologically decouple the payments from the consumption by buying on credit, the less pain the individual will feel, and the more positive perceived overall assessment of the value of the transaction the consumer will have, and therefore, the more the consumer will spend.

The transparency effect of cash refers to the ability of individuals to remember spending it due to its physical form (bills/coins) and the amount of payment (it needs to be counted) (Soman, 2003). This transparency, in turn, makes it easy for consumers to see the money they are spending, and therefore, they tend to spend less of it. Conversely, consumers tend to be less aware of their credit card payments, and therefore, they spend more (Soman, 2003).

Social Workers and Financial Literacy

While it would be beneficial for many front-line professionals who work with the public (such as case managers, employee-assistance counselors, and family and community advocates) to seek training in financial capability, social workers are particularly well suited for the role of helping consumers achieve behavioral change in the financial arena. This is because they have the education, training, and experience to help people modify their behavior, and they also have a long tradition of working with many struggling, financially low-income and minority families (Birkenmaier, 2012; Birkenmaier & Curley, 2009; Hawkins & Kim, 2012; Sherraden, Laux, & Kaufman, 2007; Wolfsohn, 2012b).

Furthermore, social workers are likely to already be involved in providing some assistance on financial matters via employment training, providing material needs (such as housing, food, and utility assistance) to families undergoing crises, and asset-development programs (Individual Development Account [IDA] programs). Social workers are also federal- and state-policy advocates regarding the Earned Income State Tax Credit (EITC) and other matters that affect the financial well-being of low-income Americans (Birkenmaier, 2012; Birkenmaier & Curley, 2009).

SOCIAL WORKERS COULD BENEFIT FROM ADDITIONAL TRAINING That said, despite the National Association of Social Workers (2008) ethical mandate that social workers "enhance human well-being and help meet the basic human needs of all people, with particular attention to the needs and empowerment of people who are vulnerable, oppressed, and living in poverty," students in schools of social work receive little or no practical training in helping families manage household finances (Sherraden et al., 2007). Hence, social workers tend to lack the necessary skills and expertise to provide financial assistance in spite of the high likelihood that they will confront financial issues on a daily basis in their work (Birkenmaier, 2012; Birkenmaier & Curley, 2009; Despard & Chowa, 2010; Sherraden et al., 2007).

Social workers need to increase their financial knowledge of financial institutions and their products and services (Birkenmaier, 2012), as well as the public policies and benefits that affect their clients (Romich, Simmelink, & Holt, 2007). It is important for social workers to become educated about mainstream financial institutions and alternative financial providers so as to be able to serve as a conduit for their clients in this regard (Birkenmaier, 2012). This is because low-income families comprise a large proportion of the unbanked population (those who do not have a savings or checking account); 83% of unbanked households earn under $25,000 (Barr, 2004). In order to conduct their financial business, the "unbanked" often resort to relying upon local high-cost, nonbank providers such as check cashers, payday lenders, and tax-refund-anticipation lenders. To illustrate the high cost of these alternative financial providers, the range of fees for check cashing is about 1.5 to 3.5% of the face value of a check, and payday loans carry high implicit annual interest rates, with an average APR of over 470% (Barr, 2004).

Beyond the low-income population of the unbanked, there are the "underbanked," that is, is a broader group of low-to middle-income families who have bank accounts but still rely on high-cost, nonbank providers to conduct most of their financial transactions (Barr, 2004). It is only by having an understanding of the various financial institutions that social workers will be able to help low-income families connect to mainstream financial institutions, so that they will retain more of their income and spend less on costly services provided by high-cost, nonbank providers (Birkenmaier, 2012).

Aside from knowledge about our financial institutions, social workers need to be familiar with the public policies that result in benefit reductions and/or ineligibility and tax increases when their clients' earnings increase (Romich et al., 2007). This is because under some conditions, due to the late 20th century/early 21st century reforms to policies that affect the working poor, greater earnings can trigger reductions in several benefits. It is only after social workers understand what an earnings change may trigger for a particular client that they may be able to communicate this information in such a way that helps their clients achieve their financial objectives, despite the impending changes in benefits and taxes (Romich et al., 2007).

To be adequately prepared for their roles with clients, social workers would benefit from a financial social work curriculum to help them understand their own relationship to their money and then be able to serve as role models and guides to their respective clients (Birkenmaier & Curley, 2009; Gillen & Loeffler, 2012; Wolfsohn, 2012b). While interest and recognition in the need for a financial-empowerment approach is slowly growing among social workers and social services organizations, the number of social workers who routinely engage clients in financial management is small relative to other areas of social work practice and could be greatly expanded (Birkenmaier & Curley, 2009; Gillen & Loeffler, 2012; Sherraden et al., 2007).

In addition to empowering clients to be able to take more control of their financial lives through the employment of a financial-empowerment model

(Birkenmaier et al., 2013; Kent & Sun, 2012; Wolfsohn, 2012a), social workers may ask new clients a number of financial-related questions as part of the intake process (whether they have a checking account or savings account, or use payday loans/check-cashing outlets, and other factors to get a picture of their financial practices) (Chang, Wagner, & Herr, 2010), provide their clients with information about financial institutions, and suggest questions for unbanked/underbanked clients to ask of banks in order to facilitate a banked relationship (Birkenmaier, 2012).

THE CENTER FOR FINANCIAL SOCIAL WORK   Financial Social Work is a transformative learning model that was first developed by Reeta Wolfsohn, CMSW at the Center for Financial Social Work (Wolfsohn, 2012b). The changes that result from a transformative model are deep and long-lasting (Garvett, 2004; Lusardi, Clark, Fox, Grable, & Taylor, 2010; Mezirow, 2000). While it is an approach that leads to positive financial outcomes for recipients of diverse backgrounds, it originated from "Femonomics," a term Wolfsohn created while working exclusively with the female population back in 1997. "Femonomics" broadened into an applicable methodology for both men and women in 2005 (Wolfsohn, 2012a).

This model is multidisciplinary and strengths-based; it incorporates a psychosocial focus on the thoughts, feelings, and attitudes that determine each person's relationship and behavior with money. It expands self-awareness and sense of self, and provides financial knowledge. It also helps people integrate better decision-making and self-assessment into their daily lives (Wolfsohn, 2012b).

Individuals' relationship with their money drives their financial behavior, and it's their financial behavior that determines their financial circumstances (Vitt, 2009; Wolfsohn, 2012a). One of the underlying tenets of Financial Social Work is to help individuals gain control over their money to ultimately attain [better] control of their lives (Wolfsohn, 2012a). Diener, Weiting, Harter, and Arora (2010) found that economic wealth (income and ability to purchase luxury goods) and social-psychological prosperity (relative power and autonomy) were the best predictors of well-being in their deep dive of data gathered from a World Gallup poll (Diener et al., 2010).

Improved financial circumstances require increased self-awareness. Often more unconscious than conscious, an individual's thoughts, feelings, and attitudes about money are reflected in every financial decision an individual makes and in how he or she chooses to spend and save (or not to save) (Vitt, 2009; Wolfsohn, 2012a). The more insight a person has about where, why, when, and how thoughts, feelings, and attitudes came to be so ingrained in his or her belief system, the more likely the person is to make financial choices that will improve his or her financial future (Vitt, 2009; Wolfsohn, 2012a).

Within the framework of Financial Social Work, the uniqueness of each individual's personal journey to a better financial future is respected. Consumers are encouraged to choose their own paths by engaging with what resonates most to them based on where they currently are in their life cycle and in their readiness and willingness to change, as per the Transtheoretical Model of Behavior Change (TTM) (Ozmete & Hira, 2011; Xiao et al., 2004; Xiao et al., 2010). In addition, as indicated in TTM (Ozmete & Hira, 2011; Xiao et al., 2004), ongoing education, motivation, and support are critical components of the work, to ensure optimal results (Wolfsohn, 2012a).

Financial Social Work is taught by the Center for Financial Social Work via a self-study online process (Wolfsohn, 2012a). The model, as of 2013, was being extensively researched for efficacy using a carefully crafted logic model in Erie, Pennsylvania (the city suffering the highest poverty rate of any major city in that state) under the auspices of United Way (Bates, 2012). The program's goal is to create sustainable, long-term financial behavioral change that supports self-sufficiency and financial stability in individuals and families via education, motivation and support. Research findings were expected to be available in early 2015.

Assessment

While the field of financial capability is still in its early stages of development (Collins and Birkenmaier, 2013); the importance of including financial literacy as a component of social work education is slowly becoming recognized as demonstrated by the recent endeavors of a number of higher education institutions and other organizations attempting to train BSW- and MSW-level students, alumni, as well as other human resource staff in this capacity (Birkenmaier et al., 2013).

Among some professional circles, there is the recognition that adults are most likely to learn and establish long-lasting financial skills within a Transformative Learning framework (Lusardi et al., 2010; Mezirow, 2000), such as the Financial Social Work model developed by Wolfsohn (2012a). This is because financial behavior is a function of our values, attitudes, and thoughts, and a model that is going to lead to long-term financial changes requires an evaluation of those conscious and previously unconscious socialization factors (Schuchardt et al., 2009; Vitt, 2009; Wolfsohn, 2012b). Positive correlations have been demonstrated between increased financial knowledge and positive financial behaviors, attitudes, and thoughts; research has been unable to definitively establish that financial education leads to more improved financial behavior, however (Hira, 2010; Lusardi et al., 2010; Schuchardt et al., 2009; U.S. Government Accountability Office, 2011) the evaluation of financial-capability programs remains a challenge to overcome in terms of developing a common set of reliable measures (Collins & O'Rourke, 2010; Schuchardt et al., 2009; Vitt et al., 2010).

Finally, social work advocacy on a macro level to ensure equal access is critical. To increase the range of available opportunities to the low-income and most oppressed populations, we need to try to reduce the growing wage inequality by: (a) joining political organizations that seek to limit the political power of wealth so as to facilitate the election of officials less indebted to economic elites and permitted to support measures to reduce inequality, (b) lobbying for direct job creation by the government, (c) engaging in living-wage campaigns to raise the minimum wage and Earned Income Tax Credit, (d) joining unions and advocate for labor's commitment to reforms on behalf of all workers (not just union members), (e) pressing for an improved measure of poverty to increase the potential number of beneficiaries and constituencies for reform, and (f) pressing for implementation of consumer protection laws (Goldberg, 2012).

Additional ways in which social workers could assist the impoverished on a macro level include: (a) seeking governmental funding to enable supportive financial social work services to be extended to larger numbers of low-income people (Anderson, Zhan, & Scott, 2007), (b) lobbying for increased access to financial services and institutions in low-income neighborhoods (Anderson et al., 2007; Sherraden et al., 2007), and (c) engaging with bankers and other community partners to help discourage predatory financial practices (Anderson et al., 2007).

REFERENCES

American Bankruptcy Institute (ABI). (n.d.). *Annual business and non-business filings by year* (1980–2011). Retrieved Feb 1, 2013 from http://www.abiworld.org/AM/AMTemplate.cfm?Section=Home&TEMPLATE=/CM/ContentDisplay.cfm&CONTENTID=65139.

Anderson, S., Zhan, M., & Scott, J. (2007). Improving the knowledge and attitudes of low-income families about banking and predatory financial practices. *Families in Society*, 88(3), 443–452.

Arnold, M. J., & Reynolds, K. E. (2009). Affect and retail shopping behavior: Understanding the role of mood regulation and regulatory focus. *Journal of Retailing*, 85(3), 308–320.

Barr, M. S. (2004). *Banking the poor: Policies to bring low-income Americans into the financial mainstream*. Washington, DC: Brookings Institution.

Bates, C. (2012). *Evidence-based research and evaluation of financial social work e- book*. Retrieved February 25, 2013 from http://www.financialsocialwork.com/about/financial-social-work-evidence

Birkenmaier, J. (2012). Promoting bank accounts to low-income households: Implications for social work practice. *Journal of Community Practice*, 20(4), 414–431.

Birkenmaier, J., & Curley, J. (2009). Financial credit: Social work's role in empowering low-income families. *Journal of Community Practice*, 17(3), 251–268.

Birkenmaier, J., et al. (2013). The role of social work in financial capability: Shaping curricular approaches. In Birkenmaier, Curley & Sherraden (Eds.), *Financial capability and asset development: Research, education, policy and practice* (pp. 278–301). New York, NY: Oxford University Press.

Boshara, R. (2010). *The NEFE quarter-century project: 25 years of research in financial education: Theme 4: Consumer trends in the public, private and nonprofit sector*. Retrieved October 4, 2012 from www.nefe.org/quartercenturyproject

Boteach, M. (2012). *New poverty data provide key insights into fiscal cliff negotiations*. Center for American Progress. Retrieved January 7, 2013 from http://www.americanprogress.org/issues/poverty/news/2012/11/14/44898/new-poverty-data-provide-key-insights-into-fiscal-cliff-negotiations/

CardTrak.com. (2012, 9 January). *Credit Card Debit*. Retrieved Feb 1, 2013 from http://cardtrak.com/data/38365/credit-card-debit/

Chang, C., Wagner, S. L., & Herr, T. (2010, September). *Surprising diversity in financial stability: A cluster analysis of Center for Working Families clients in 12 low-income Chicago communities*. Chicago, IL: Project Match.

Chatterjee, P., & Rose, R. L. (2012). Do payment mechanisms change the way consumers perceive products? *Journal of Consumer Research*, 38(6), 1129–1139.

Collins, J. M., & Birkenmaier, J. (2013). Building the capacity of social workers to enhance financial capability and asset development. In Birkenmaier, Curley, & Sherraden (Eds.), *Financial capability and asset development: Research, education, policy and practice* (pp. 302–322). New York, NY: Oxford University Press.

Collins, J. M., & O'Rourke, C. M. (2010). Financial education and counseling—Still holding promise. *The Journal of Consumer Affairs*, 44(3), 483–498.

Conger, R. D., Conger, K. J., & Martin, M. J. (2010). Socio-economic status, family processes, and individual development. *Journal of Marriage and Family*, 72(3), 685–704.

Despard, M., & Chowa, G. A. N. (2010). Social workers' interest in building individuals' financial capabilities. *Journal of Financial Therapy*, 1(1), 23–41.

Diener, E., Weiting, N., Harter, J., & Arora, R. (2010). Wealth and happiness across the world: Material prosperity predicts life evaluation, whereas psychosocial prosperity predicts positive feeling. *Journal of Personality and Social Psychology*, 99, 52–61.

Dynan, K. (2012). *Addressing the problems in the U.S. housing market*. The Brookings Institution. Retrieved February 1, 2013 from http://www.brookings.edu/research/papers/2012/03/07-econgrowth-housing-dynan

FINRA Investor Education Foundation. (2009). *Financial capability in the United States national survey: Executive summary*. Washington, DC: Author.

Garvett, S. (2004). Action learning and transformative learning in teaching development. *Educational Action Research*, 12, 259–271.

Gillen, M., & Loeffler, D. (2012). Financial literacy and social work students: Knowledge is power. *Journal of Financial Therapy*, 3(2), 28–38.

Goldberg, G. S. (2012). Economic inequality and economic crisis: A challenge for social workers. *Social Work*, 57(3), 211–224.

Grochulski, B. (2010). Optimal personal bankruptcy design under moral hazard. *Review of Economic Dynamics, 13*, 350–378.

Hawkins, R. L., & Kim, E. J. (2012). The Socio-economic empowerment assessment: Addressing poverty and economic distress in clients. *Clinical Social Work Journal*, 40(2), 194–202.

Hira, T. K. (2010). *The NEFE quarter century project: Implications for researchers, educators, and policy makers from a quarter century of financial education*. Denver: National Endowment for Financial Education. Retrieved October 4, 2013 from www.nefe.org/quartercenturyproject

The Institute for College Access & Success (TICAS). (2012, October). *Student debt and the class of 2011*. Retrieved March 11, 2013 from http://projectonstudentdebt.org/files/pub/classof2011.pdf

Kent, M., & Sun, I-H. (2012). Taking financial education to the next level. *Bridges*, Fall, 2012. Federal Reserve Bank of St. Louis. Retrieved February 2, 2013 from http://www.stls.frb.org/publications/br/articles/?id=2302

Lusardi, A., Clark, R. L., Fox, J., Grable, J., & Taylor, E. (2010). The NEFE quarter century project: 25 years of research in financial education: *Theme 1: Promising learning strategies, interventions, and delivery methods in financial literacy education*. Denver: National Endowment for Financial Education. Retrieved October 4, 2012 from www.nefe.org/quartercenturyproject

Mezirow, J. (2000). Learning to think like an adult: Core concepts of transformation theory. In J. Mezirow & Associates (2000). *Learning as transformation* (pp. 3–34). San Francisco, CA: Jossey-Bass.

Moav, O., & Neeman, Z. (2010). Status and poverty. *Journal of the European Economic Association*, 8(2–3), 413–420.

National Association of Social Workers (NASW). (2008). *Code of ethics of the National Association of Social Workers: Ethical principles*. Washington, DC: Author. Retrieved February 7, 2013 from http://www.socialworkers.org/pubs/code/default.asp

National Endowment for Financial Education (NEFE). (2011). *Nearly half of U.S. adults say top financial goal is retirement.* Retrieved January 25, 2013 from http://www.nefe.org/press-room/news/american-dream.aspx

National Endowment for Financial Education (NEFE). (2012). *The benefits blues: A growing epidemic among U.S. workers.* Retrieved January 25, 2013 from http://www.nefe.org/press-room/news/the-benefits-blues.aspx

National Foundation for Credit Counseling, Inc. (NFCC). (2012). *Financial literacy survey exposes significant gaps in grasp of personal finance skills.* Retrieved January 29, 2013 from http://www.nfcc.org/newsroom/newsreleases/SIGNIFICANT_GAPS.cfm

Nyhus, E. K., & Webley, P. (2001). The role of personality in household saving and borrowing behaviour. *European Journal of Personality, 15,* s85–s103.

Ozmete, E., & Hira, T. K. (2011). Conceptual analysis of behavioral theories: Application to financial behavior. *European Journal of Social Sciences, 18*(3), 386–404.

Pettit, N. C., & Sivanathan, N. (2011). The plastic trap. *Social Psychological and Personality Science, 2*(2), 146–153.

President's Advisory Council on Financial Capability. (2012, May). *Every American financially empowered: A guide to increasing financial capability among students, workers and residents in communities.* Retrieved October 5, 2012 from http://www.whitehouse.gov/sites/default/files/financial_capability_toolkit_5.10.2012.pdf

Raghubir, P., & Srivastava, J. (2008). Monopoly money: The effect of payment coupling and form on spending behavior. *Journal of Experimental Psychology: Applied, 14*(3), 213–225.

Romich, J. L., Simmelink, J., & Holt, S. D. (2007). When working harder does not pay: Low-income working families, tax liabilities, and benefit reductions. *Families in Society, 88*(3), 418–426.

Schuchardt, J., Hanna, S. D., Hira, T. K., Lyons, A. C., Palmer, L., & Xiao, J. J. (2009). Financial literacy and education research priorities. *Journal of Financial Counseling and Planning, 20,* 84–95.

Sherraden, M., Laux, S., & Kaufman, C. (2007). Financial education for social workers. *Journal of Community Practice, 15*(3), 9–36.

Shim, S., Xiao, J. J., Barber, B. L., & Lyons, A. C. (2009). Pathways to life success: A conceptual model of financial well-being for young adults. *Journal of Applied Developmental Psychology, 30,* 708–723.

Sivanathan, N., & Pettit, N. C. (2010). Protecting the self through consumption: Status goods as affirmational commodities. *Journal of Experimental Social Psychology, 46,* 564–570.

Soman, D. (2003). The effect of payment transparency on consumption: Quasi experiments from the field. *Marketing Letters, 14,* 173–183.

U.S. Census Bureau. (2012a, 14 November). *Census bureau releases 2011 new supplemental poverty measure research findings.* Retrieved January 14, 2013 from http://www.census.gov/newsroom/releases/archives/poverty/cb12-215.html

U.S. Census Bureau. (2012b). *Income, poverty, and health insurance coverage in the United States: 2011.* Retrieved January 14, 2013 from www.census.gov/prod/2012pubs/p60-243.pdf

U.S. Government Accountability Office. (2011). *Financial literacy: The federal government's role in empowering Americans to make sound financial choices* (GAO-11-504T). Washington, DC: Author. Retrieved October 4, 2012 from http://www.gao.gov/assets/130/125996.pdf

Vitt, L. (2009). *Values centered financial education: Understanding cultural influences on learners' financial behaviors.* Denver: National Endowment for Financial Education. Retrieved October 4, 2012 from http://www.smartaboutmoney.org/Portals/0/lifevalue/financialeducation.pdf

Vitt, L.A., et al. (2010). The NEFE quarter century project: 25 years of research in financial education: *Theme 3: Evaluation and measurement of learner outcomes in financial education.* Denver: National Endowment for Financial Education. Retrieved October 4, 2012 from www.nefe.org/quartercenturyproject

Webley, P., & Nyhus, E. K. (2006). Parent's influence on children's future orientation and saving. *Journal of Economic Psychology, 27,* 140–164.

Wolfsohn, R. (2004). *Financial social work certification program.* Asheville, NC: Center for Financial Social Work, Inc. Retrieved November 8, 2012 from http://www.financialsocialwork.com

Wolfsohn, R. (2012a). *Financial social work basics and best practices.* Retrieved November 8, 2012 from http://www.financialsocialwork.com/tools/financial-social-work-ebook#.UI66hELJDzI

Wolfsohn, R. (2012b). Linking policy and practice. In E. F. Hoffler & E. J. Clark (Eds.), *Social Work Matters: Power of Linking Policy and Practice* (pp. 219–223). Washington, DC: NASW Press.

Xiao, J. J. (2008). Applying behavior science theories in financial behaviors. In J. J. Xiao (Ed.), *Handbook of consumer finance research* (pp. 69–81). New York: Springer.

Xiao, J. J., Collins, M., Ford, M., Keller, P., Kim, J., & Robles, B. (2010). The NEFE quarter century project: 25 Years of research in financial education: *Theme 2: A Review of financial behavior research: Implications for financial education.* Denver: National Endowment for Financial Education. Retrieved October 4, 2012 from www.nefe.org/quartercenturyproject

Xiao, J. J., Newman, B. M., Prochaska, J. M., Leon, B., Bassett, R. L., & Johnson, J. (2004). Applying the transtheoretical model of change to debt reducing behavior. *Journal of Financial Counseling and Planning, 15*(2), 89–100.

Reeta Wolfsohn and Dorlee Michaeli

GENERALIST AND ADVANCED GENERALIST PRACTICE

ABSTRACT: Generalist and advanced generalist practice evolved out of a century-long debate about what constitutes social work practice. Generalist practice currently refers to the practice of a bachelor-level social worker who demonstrates basic competencies in multi-level, multimethod approaches. Advanced generalist practice refers to the practice of a master-level social worker who possesses advanced competencies in multilevel, multimethod approaches and is equipped to work in complex environments that may require specialized skill sets. The definition and educational content of generalist and advanced generalist practice are poised to be influenced by national debate once again, as the profession examines the merits of evidence-based practice and its implications for social work education.

KEY WORDS: generalist; advanced generalist; evidence-based practice; EBP; practitioners; pedagogy

Defining generalist practice and advanced generalist practice marks an important passage in the development of the social work profession. These definitions evolved in the background of nearly a half century of debate about the nature of social work practice. A paramount question in these discussions was how to educate and prepare social workers for practice. Debates about the elements, scope, and focus of social work practice continue today in discussions about evidence-based practice (EBP). EBP proposes that practitioners and students will benefit from a rigorous approach to evaluating proposed outcomes, best practices in the field, and the risks and benefits associated with social work interventions. Therefore, it is important to understand the distinctions between generalist practice and advanced generalist practice and how they evolved in order to assist the profession in gaining clarity about the appropriateness and currency of its value base, theoretical orientations, practice methods, and movements such as EBP.

Historical Context
BACKGROUND The profession of social work initially emerged as a response to human suffering and community disorganization in the latter part of the 19th century. The earliest forms of social work practice were typified by the activities of the leaders within the Charitable Organization Society and the Settlement House Movement. During the first part of the 20th century, the philosophical orientations and values attached to these activities were debated, resulting in the earliest definitions of social work practice. Mary Richmond focused on the assessment of factors that contributed to or detracted from the social functioning of a person, including one's state of mind and behavior, the influences of one's family and social environment, and the personal strengths of the person. Assessing the interactions of an individual with his or her social environment was a key element of Richmond's model (1917, 1922). Jane Addams's orientation differed from that of Richmond. Her experiences in settlement houses such as England's Toynbee Hall influenced her thinking about the origin of social problems, and community-based responses to them. Addams's early essays (1902) reflect her focus on social, political, and economic influences that produce human suffering and community disorganization. Addams also wrote about the shortcomings of the scientific charity movement. She did not dismiss the efforts that came out of this movement; rather she maintained that a broader orientation was primary to understanding how social problems present at the individual level.

These value orientations competed with each other in the early part of the 20th century, until 1929 when the American Association of Social Workers (AASW) labored over a four-year period to define social work practice under the rubric of social case work. The Milford Conference underscored the importance of giving social workers a generic foundation of knowledge that they could use to address the needs of communities and organizations, as well as individuals, and upon which they could build specialized practice. The content required for generic social case work was stated to include:

1. Knowledge of typical deviations from accepted standards of social life.
2. The use of norms for human life and relationships.
3. The significance of a social history as the basis of particularizing the human being in need.

4. Established methods of study and treatment of human beings in need.

5. The use of established, community resources in social treatment.

6. The adaptation of scientific knowledge and formulations of experience to the requirements of social case work.

7. The consciousness of a philosophy, which determines the purposes, ethics, and obligations of social case work.

8. The blending of the foregoing elements into social treatment (American Association of Social Workers [AASW], 1929, p. 15).

This content comprised the first formal set of standards for generic social case work, a precursor to generalist practice. These standards also helped to define the essential foundational knowledge required to conduct case work and set a precedent for a form of practice that "superseded agency-specific specializations based on a particular problem or practice" (Schatz, Jenkins, & Sheafor, 1990, p. 218).

A national report by Hollis and Taylor (1951) was also instrumental in defining standards for social work practice during the first half of the 20th century. This report was an outcome of a project commissioned by the AASW with the assistance of the Carnegie Foundation and occurred at a time when the majority of persons employed as social workers did not have the level of education desired by professional social work organizations. The charge of the project was to assess the professional development and educational needs of practicing social workers. This report achieved several important objectives. First, the authors demonstrated the need for basic and advanced forms of training for a workforce that was primarily composed of technicians or volunteers. Second, they identified an expanded role for social work in contemporary society, reinforcing the ongoing need for professional education. Third, the authors defined preparatory content for undergraduate and graduate social work education, proposing that social work education should be anchored in the arts and sciences, maintain a generic orientation, and allow for specialization at the advanced graduate level. The Hollis and Taylor report offered a rationale for professionalizing social work and a contemporary framework for delivering social work content in classrooms. It also underscored the point that the manner in which the profession defines itself has strong implications for how social workers are prepared to practice.

CONCEPTUALIZATIONS OF SOCIAL WORK PRACTICE AND EDUCATION The merging of seven professional social work organizations during the mid-1950s helped to unify national discussion about social work practice, and eventually, social work education. In 1955, the American Association of Social Work, the Association for the Study of Community Organization, the American Association of Medical Social Workers, the American Association of Psychiatric Social Work, the National Association of Group Workers, and the Social Work Research Group merged with the National Association of Social Workers (NASW). This newly defined organization charged its Commission on Practice to study and develop a common definition of social work practice that all parties could support.

In 1958, the Commission released *Working Definition of Social Work Practice* under the authorship of its chairperson, Bartlett. In this seminal piece, Bartlett characterized social work practice as a "constellation of value, purpose, sanction, knowledge and methods." *Value* reflected the philosophical orientation of social work practice and its concern for the well-being and uniqueness of individuals, as well as the mutual responsibility and interdependence they share with society. The *purpose* of social work practice was to assist individuals, groups, and communities with identifying, resolving, and preventing problems that could interfere with a person's functioning. Closely related to purpose was *sanction* or what Bartlett referred to as the permission granted to the profession by governmental agencies, voluntary agencies, and the profession itself to help address the basic needs of individuals. Bartlett considered *knowledge* of human development and human behavior as essential for being able to respond to spontaneous and unpredictable situations. She placed specific emphasis on understanding the reciprocal influences of one's social environment, social and economic circumstance, human psychology, communication, group process, cultural and religious and spiritual heritage, and relationships as essential elements of knowledge required by social workers. Finally, Bartlett acknowledged the importance of the methods employed by social workers to convey its value, purpose, sanction, and knowledge in practice situations. She defined *method* as "an orderly systematic mode of procedure" that included techniques and skills to facilitate interactions between an individual and his or her environment, observe and assess the effects of these interactions, and evaluate one's practice for the sake of improving it. Bartlett did not consider her definition of social work practice as definitive. Rather, she considered it a work in progress to be debated and refined by the profession over time.

During the same time period, efforts to define social work practice content for educational purposes were conducted by the Council on Social Work Education (CSWE). The CSWE came into being as a result of a merger between the American Association of Schools of Social Work (AASSW), and the National Association of Schools of Social Administration (NASSA) in 1952. The AASSW had focused on professional development and graduate education for social workers, while the NASSA promoted undergraduate-level social work education. The CSWE focused its efforts on curriculum development and enlisted Werner Boehm to specify content for a contemporary form of social work education. Similar to Bartlett, Boehm (1959) envisioned social work practice as addressing multiple systems and using multiple methods to enhance social functioning. Boehm's study resulted in specific objectives for a social work curriculum. They included foundational knowledge in human growth and behavior, social welfare policy and services, values and ethics; methods designed to address the needs of individuals, groups and communities; and field instruction. He also distinguished the learning needs of an undergraduate social worker from that of a master's level social worker. Boehm's work was contemporary for his time. It reflected the profession's concerns about a common definition for social work practice and the need to strengthen social work education. His contributions are still reflected in present day social work educational standards that define generalist and advanced generalist education.

Bartlett was succeeded as chair of the NASW Commission on Social Work Practice by William Gordon, a social work educator who is noted for his critique of the working definition. Gordon's conception of social work practice was more dynamic than Bartlett's. He proposed that social work was a dynamic process primarily fueled by the *integration* of value, purpose, knowledge, sanction, and methods. He advocated for a person-in-environment perspective and envisioned social work practice as an "interventive action" framework that addressed social dysfunction and should be guided by theoretical structures and the principles of scientific inquiry. Gordon (1969) elaborated further on his conceptualization of social work practice in *The general systems approach: Contributions toward an holistic conception of social work* (Hearn, 1969). He discussed how systems theory could be used to support social work's interventive framework. Gordon was enthusiastic

about this theoretical perspective, and saw it as a logical conceptual framework for social work to adopt. He encouraged the profession to concern itself with exchanges between person and environment because they revealed human coping behavior and possible points of intervention. Gordon's perspective on the nature of social work practice was quickly adopted as a primary theoretical orientation for teaching social workers about human behavior and the social environment and how to conduct practice.

Release of *The Common Base of Social Work Practice* in 1970 also helped to further define social work practice (Bartlett, 1970). Building on responses to the working definition, Bartlett defined core concepts of social work practice, including task, coping, social environment, and environmental demand, all of which were eventually incorporated into social work curriculum. She also advocated for a systematic approach to knowledge building and theory development, using as much rigor and objectivity as possible. Bartlett helped to broaden the conceptualization and mission of social work practice even further in this writing. She also challenged the profession to move beyond the boundaries of just doing to "thinking about doing" in order to forge a clearer theoretical framework for social work practice.

The outcomes of the Milford Conference, the Hollis and Taylor report, the mergers of national organizations to seek common ground, Bartlett's treatises, Boehm's study, Gordon's contributions, and the ongoing discourse about a working definition for social work practice all helped to specify the need for professional social work education. They also represented convergent agreement that more specific standards for educating social workers were needed.

Translating the Practice Framework Into Pedagogy

An operational definition for generalist practice emerged in the mid-1970s and was embraced by practitioners and educators alike, in spite of continued debate about the purpose and objectives of social work practice (Landon, 1995; Minahan, 1981). Early definitions of generalist practice framed it as a multilevel, multimethod approach that used an eclectic theory base and maintained a dual focus on both the personal matters of a client and issues of social justice. Yet there still were concerns about the level of education required of undergraduate and graduate students of social work and how to make distinctions between undergraduate education versus graduate content. Prior to the formation of national educational standards for social work, only persons holding a master's degree were considered professional social workers. Case workers who did not hold this degree were labeled nonprofessionals. This distinction promoted a sense of inferiority among members of the latter group, many of whom performed valuable case work activities for public and private agencies. This dilemma, along with a forecasted social worker shortage, prompted the NASW and CSWE to support the institution of a bachelor degree in social work and to develop educational content for this degree using a generalist perspective (Brieland, 1995).

CSWE published its first educational standards for baccalaureate degree programs in 1974. An inconsistency in how generalist practice was being taught in classrooms was quickly identified, however. Ripple (1974) reported that some schools taught generalist practice as a multimethod approach involving the mastery of specific methods or treatment modalities that could be used in specific or specialized client settings. Others taught generalist practice from a more skills-oriented perspective, to produce a "utility worker" (p. 28) who understood the elements of human behavior, social situations, and resource acquisition, and had sound communication, observational, and problem-solving skills that could be used across multiple settings or problem areas. By the mid-1980s, and after a second iteration of the CSWE standards, the profession finally arrived at a clearer consensus about what generalist practice entailed and where it should be placed in the curriculum. This milestone was authenticated by the first entry on the generalist perspective in the 18th edition of the *Encyclopedia of Social Work*.

Sheafor and Landon (1987) described the history and evolution of the generalist perspective. Their entry included discussion about the generalist framework as a valid practice orientation and foundation for specialization, specification of the generic foundation knowledge that all social workers need, and prerequisite practice principles upon which generalist and specialist practice rest. One of the major contributions of this entry is found in their description of the components of generalist practice. The first component involved a perspective that assists a social worker to envision "all possibilities for intervention" when approaching a practice situation (p. 666). The second component consisted of a requisite knowledge of four theoretical approaches to inform generalist practice, including the systems framework, the structural framework, the ecological framework, and the social learning framework. The third component

of generalist practice, the planned change process, included classical steps of the helping process: (a) intake and engagement, (b) assessment, (c) planning and contracting, (d) intervention, (e) monitoring and evaluation, and (f) termination, as well as a description of essential activities required to execute the tasks of the planned change process. The features of the planned change process represent a classical model of the helping process that is still taught in classrooms today. Sheafor and Landon close their entry by stating that the future of the generalist perspective should include "its refinement into a solid conceptual framework" addressing the "appropriate breadth and depth for each level of generalist practice" (p. 668).

Refining the Generalist Framework

Sheafor moved forward with colleagues to refine the conceptualization of generalist social work practice. Their work is featured in *Milford Redefined: A Model of Initial and Advanced Generalist Social Work* (Schatz et al., 1990), a qualitative report on the Delphi Study, which involved 42 authors and educators from schools of social work across the nation. The proposed model that emerged from the Delphi Study contained three distinct levels of learning: a generic foundation, content for initial generalist practice, and advanced generalist practice. The generic foundation was visioned to support the education and development of initial generalist education, and eventually, advanced generalist education, including specializations in practice. It rested on a liberal arts base, the biological and social sciences, basic understanding of the person-in-environment paradigm, basic knowledge of the profession and its role and sanction in society, basic communication and helping skills, ethnic or diversity sensitivity, and basic understanding of problem resolution, the process of change, and human relationships.

The initial generalist perspective included knowledge of sociobehavioral and ecosystems concepts, the ideologies of democracy, humanism, and empowerment, methods of social intervention that were "open" or not highly defined by either theory or precise method, forms of direct and indirect interventions, a client-centered, problem-focused approach, and research to inform practice. Initial generalist content also included knowledge gain in specific competencies. These initial competencies included being able to engage in interpersonal helping, managing the change process, using multilevel intervention modes with individuals, families, groups, communities and institutions, being able to perform varied practice roles (for example, broker, advocate, mediator, educator, social actionist, and clinician), being able to assess and examine one's own practice, and knowing how to function within a social agency (Schatz, et al., 1990).

Advanced generalist content reflected greater breadth and depth of social work knowledge, values and the application of generalist practice methods in both direct and indirect services. The advanced generalist was expected to function more independently in practice situations and demonstrate increased skills in indirect practice, including supervision, administration, social policy, research, and evaluation. Advanced generalists were expected to conduct an eclectic practice and synthesize and refine knowledge and competencies gained at the generic and initial generalist levels. This conceptual model also reflected that specialist practice could occur at either the initial generalist or advanced generalist level of practice (Schatz et al., 1990).

The Delphi Study helped to forge a conceptual model and pedagogical foundation for generalist and advanced generalist practice at a time when more clarity about the content of social work knowledge was needed. The results helped to create a template for social work education that resembled a continuum of learning. It left room for specialization at both initial and advanced levels and seemed to address long-standing needs for a systematic approach to formal preparation of social workers for practice in diverse settings. Although the authors of Milford redefined acknowledge that the model they described did not seamlessly match the NASW's classification system for BSW and MSW education and experience at that time, it was anticipated that a level of agreement between the education and professional communities over the definitions of initial generalist and advanced generalist could be resolved over time.

Generalist practice currently is defined similarly by authors of widely adopted social work practice texts (DuBois & Miley, 2010; Johnson & Yanca, 2010; Kirst-Ashman & Hull, 2009; Landon & Feit, 1999; Pilonis, 2007; Poulin, 2005; Suppes & Wells, 2003; Turner, 2005). The authors' definitions of general practice, by and large, converge on the concepts of systems, multiple methods, problem solving, and partnership with client. The definitions emphasize the purpose and values of social work, the various roles or capacities in which social workers serve, and the use of a planned change process to address social problems and restore social functioning. These concepts are similar to those found in Bartlett's working definition and the "stuff of practice" to which Gordon (1962) referred over half a century ago.

These descriptions also align with the most current definition of generalist practice published by the Association of Baccalaureate Program Directors (BPD) (2012). The BPD defines generalist practice as follows:

Generalist social work practitioners work with individuals, families, groups, communities, and organizations in a variety of social work and host settings. Generalist practitioners view clients and client systems from a strengths perspective in order to recognize, support, and build upon the innate capabilities of all human beings. They use a professional problem solving process to engage, assess, broker services, advocate, counsel, educate, and organize with and on behalf of client and client systems. In addition, generalist practitioners engage in community and organizational development. Finally, generalist practitioners evaluate service outcomes in order to continually improve the provision and quality of services most appropriate to client needs. Generalist social work practice is guided by the NASW Code of Ethics and is committed to improving the well being of individuals, families, groups, communities and organizations and furthering the goals of social justice.

Debate About the Advanced Generalist Framework

In 1984, the generalist model became the preferred framework for baccalaureate social work education, and was deemed analogous to the foundation year of the master's degree by CSWE (Landon, 1995). The last year of a master's degree program was reserved for building knowledge and skills in advanced forms of practice. Soon thereafter, Hernández, Jorgensen, Judd, Gould, and Parsons (1985) described the development of an advanced generalist curriculum designed to prepare social workers as "social problem specialists." These authors viewed their curriculum as an answer to the call for a new type of social worker, one equipped to respond to the growing complexities of social problems, as defined in the 1960s and 1970s. The authors sought to develop a curriculum that integrated elements of "a broad range of interventive techniques across micro and macro systems based on the specific needs of a problem situation" (p. 30). The curriculum emphasized six professional roles for advanced generalists—conferee, enabler, broker, mediator, advocate and guardian—to address needs across five client systems—individual, family, small group, organization, and community. This conceptual framework also integrated concepts of empowerment and social competency, viewing people as fundamentally healthy and able to meet the demands of their social environments. It viewed social work students as capable of fulfilling various roles and intervening in a manner that placed the focus of intervention on the desired outcome, as opposed to the stated problem (Parsons, Jorgensen, & Hernández, 1994). This model attempted to address the merits of specialist versus generalist content at the graduate level and was an exemplar of how to configure advanced generalist content during the last year of graduate education.

Gibbs, Locke, and Lohman (1990) attempted to address the debate about advanced generalist practice by reframing baccalaureate and master's educational content as a continuum of learning, where workers take on progressively challenging roles and content through the last year of graduate education. Similar to Hernández et al. (1985), these authors agreed that social workers needed to be equipped for situations for which insufficient knowledge existed. They argued that a curriculum that promotes generalist practice at all levels supports work in traditionally unserved areas, such as rural and small town communities and communities that have limited resources. The authors argued that the depth and breadth of advanced social work practice allowed the practitioner greater latitude to address such conditions and also equipped them to engage in "higher level organizational positions . . . and independent practice" (p. 236).

The conceptual models presented by Hernández et al. (1985), Parsons et al. (1994), and Gibbs et al. (1990) were intended to respond to increasingly complex practice settings and practice situations where access to resources and specialists was limited. They also attempted to address how advanced forms of social work practice could be conducted without resorting to specialties or tracks that encourage narrow theoretical perspectives about personal and social problems. These models provided a counterargument for debates in the profession about the merits of preparing social workers for generalist versus specialist practice. Brieland and Korr (2000) characterized these debates as representative of the "sharp division" between parties that viewed specialization "as inevitable and desirable," and others who were concerned about fragmentation of services and "the need to bring fragmented resources together to meet the needs . . . of the whole person" (p. 130).

Maguire (2002) has proposed a contemporary approach to advanced clinical practice that shares many of the principles of advanced generalist practice. Similar to Hernández et al., Gibbs et al., and Parsons et al., he believes that it is not enough for an advanced practitioner to use just a basic generalist approach to clients. Nor is it suitable to view every case through the lens of a narrowly defined theoretical orientation. Rather, it is both logical and appropriate for an advanced practitioner to maintain a generalist, systems-oriented perspective in order to adequately respond to complex practice situations. Maguire states that the viewpoint of a highly skilled clinical social worker is synonymous with that of an advanced generalist. First, they share the same systems-oriented base. They apply "higher levels of knowledge, skills and expertise," recognize the effects of the "interacting social environment," employ strategies that build from "broad to specific methods," utilize "rigorous practice research as a basis for practice," and use "a variety of major, validated theories and subsequent interventionist methods drawn from commonly accepted human behavioral perspectives" (pp. 36–37). Maguire encourages clinical social workers to think like an advanced generalist because "no single theory adequately explains human behavior except those that rely upon a broad systemic orientation" (p. 40). He provides a convincing argument that integrating a systemic, generalist perspective with appropriate clinical strategies is a form of advanced generalist practice that more fully equips clinical social work to address diverse forms of human need in increasingly complex environments.

The 2008 CSWE accreditation standards do not specify the content of advanced curriculum (CSWE, 2010). Rather, practice is expected to incorporate, build upon, and apply ten core competencies taught at the foundation in one or more areas of concentration. This policy has its advantages and disadvantages. It is advantageous in that it has given programs leverage to develop conceptual frameworks for teaching advanced content that responds to regional need and postmodernist perspectives. In fall 2011, 46 of the 208 master's degree programs that responded to a survey of CSWE-accredited master's programs reported offering an advanced generalist concentration (CSWE, 2012). A cursory visit to the websites of programs with the largest programs (serving 300 or more MSW students) featured advanced generalist content in transcultural perspectives, practice designed to address regional needs, practice with a range of diverse and vulnerable populations, leadership at institutional, organization, and community levels, policy development and analysis, and multilevel practice. The Council's stance on advanced content curriculum is disadvantageous, though, in that the development of a more unified conceptualization of advanced generalist practice has expanded beyond the discussion of integrative models proposed in the early 1990s.

Landon (1995) acknowledged that the generalist perspective was "embedded in the profession, both in practice and education," but she warned that "the perception that generalist programming is for bachelor's level education only must be put to rest." She urged the profession to explore how the generalist perspective could be integrated further into advanced generalist content, by principally exploring the various levels and competencies of generalist practice (p. 1106). Roy & Vecchiola (2004) responded to this concern by featuring six advanced generalist models and curriculums in the U.S. and applying them to several areas of social work practice. More recently, Lavitt (2009) proposed advanced generalist practice entails three key elements: multidimensional problem setting, leadership and self-reflection, and ethical advocacy. A number of articles can be also found in *Social Work Abstracts* that discuss implications for advanced generalist practice in schools, groups, health care, rural settings, and with older adults. However, discussion about the elements of advanced generalist practice in social work and how it is distinct from bachelor's level generalist practice is left for programs to decide on their own. Given the number of accredited programs that offer advanced generalist concentrations, it appears these discussions are taking place but are not being published. The challenge of studying the differences between levels and competencies in generalist practice, however, is being brought to bear in current discussions about EBP.

The EBP Movement

The term evidence-based practice (EBP) entered the national discourse of social work practice and social work education almost two decades ago and has implications for social work practice and how to prepare students for generalist practice and advanced generalist practice. These implications are primarily related to the value orientations of social workers, the identification and implementation of best practices in the field, and measuring the effects and outcomes of interventions. Utilizing EBP requires a practitioner to take three essential elements into consideration: the practitioner's individual expertise, the client's values and expectations about the intervention, and the best external evidence available about a condition or situation and is considered both a philosophy and a process (Gambrill, 2005). The philosophy of EBP in social work calls into question the evidentiary nature

of social work interventions, using a process of critical appraisal of current research about a given intervention. Its process involves specific steps a practitioner should take to evaluate the efficacy and effectiveness of an intervention before using it in a client situation. The EBP process includes five steps. First, a practitioner must formulate an answerable question related to the client situation at hand. Second, the practitioner must engage in an efficient strategy for locating evidence that will help answer the questions posed. The "hierarchy" of credible sources of evidence includes (in descending order) randomized controlled trials (RCTs), systematic reviews and meta-analyses of RCTs, well-controlled quasi-experimental studies, pretest and posttest studies, case studies, observational studies, and descriptive reports and qualitative studies. Third, the practitioner is expected to conduct a critical appraisal of the evidence for its validity, objectivity, effect size, and usefulness. Fourth, the practitioner must determine if the evidence can be applied to the client situation, and apprise the client of the findings, taking into consideration the client's values and preferences in making a practice decision. Finally, the practitioners must evaluate the "effectiveness and efficiency" of this process, as a means of improving it (Gambrill, 2005; Rubin & Parrish, 2007). The benefits of using an EBP approach are threefold. First, it helps the practitioner determine the outcomes, as well as the benefits and risks associated with an intervention. Second, EBP helps the practitioner keep abreast about best practices in the field. Third, it encourages ethical practice. The philosophy and process of EBP is not restricted to micro-level interventions with individuals; it is also applicable to mezzo and macro practice situations (Howard, McMillen, & Pollio, 2003). Gibbs (2003) has also demonstrated how EBP can be used in social work classrooms to support adherence to the CSWE educational policy and accreditation standards for diversity, and promote the use of a strengths-based orientation in practice.

EBP currently is being embraced by segments of the social work practice and social work education communities for several reasons. First, it emphasizes the use of scientific evidence to guide decision-making in practice. Second, it encourages rigorous, critical thinking, and inquiry about practice interventions. Third, it addresses current demands for accountability, benchmarks, and outcomes for social work practice and education. Fourth, it holds promise for enhancing the credibility of the profession. Fifth, EBP supports the ethical standards of research and evaluation in the Code of Ethics (Gambrill, 2003; Howard et al., 2003; NASW, 1999). EBP is not without its critics. Gibbs and Gambrill (2002) identified 27 objections to EBP. They propose that these objections are based on ignorance about EBP or one of a series of arguments either appealing to tradition, an *ad hominem* basis (appealing to personal considerations rather than to logic or reason), confusion and disagreement about educational practices, ethical grounds, and philosophy. The authors provide cogent and persuasive counterarguments to each of the 27 objections, concluding that they "have not yet heard an objection to EBP based on concerns about clients" (p. 471). These authors' counterarguments are not intended to quell criticisms of EBP, as much as to demonstrate what EBP has to offer the profession. Gibbs and Gambrill state that "criticism is essential to the growth of knowledge" (p. 458). Criticism, objections, and counterargument to objections can lead to insights that can feasibly reduce barriers to adopting EBP principles, address skepticism about the rigorous evidentiary standards of EBP, enhance the way in which EBP is taught, and identify other forms of critical inquiry that can be brought to bear in making well-informed decisions about the effects of interventions by generalist and advanced generalist practitioners. EBP is a response to three essential questions posed by the Campbell Collaboration that should concern social work (American Institutes for Research, 2007): What helps? What harms? Based on what evidence? Incorporating the principles of EBP into generalist and advanced generalist practice curriculums could help to strengthen this content and produce new models for addressing the complexities and ambiguities of modern day practice settings, using a continuum of multilevel, multimethod approaches.

REFERENCES

Addams, J. (1902). *Democracy and social ethics*. New York: Macmillan.

American Association of Social Workers, Studies in the Practice of Social Work (Ed.). (1929). *Social case work: Generic and specific: A report of the Milford Conference*. New York: American Association of Social Workers.

American Institutes for Research. (2007). *Campbell Collaboration*. Retrieved February 12, 2007, from http://www.campbellcollaboration.org/index.asp

Association of Baccalaureate Program Directors. (2012). *Definition of generalist social work practice*. Retrieved from http://www.bpdonline.org/

Bartlett, H. M. (1958). Toward clarification and improvement of social work practice. *Social Work*, 3(2), 3–9.

Bartlett, H. M. (1970). *The common base of social work practice*. New York: National Association of Social Workers.

Boehm, W. W. (1959). *Objectives of the social work curriculum of the future*. New York: Council on Social Work Education.

Brieland, D. (1995). Social work practice: History and evolution. In R. L. Edwards (Ed.), *Encyclopedia of social work*. Washington, DC: NASW Press.

Brieland, D., & Korr, W. S. (2000). *Social work at the millennium: Critical reflection on the future of the profession*. New York: Free Press.

Council on Social Work Education. (2012). *2011 Statistics on social work education in the United States*. Alexandria, VA: Author.

Council on Social Work Education, Commission on Accreditation. *2008 EPAS Handbook* (revised March 27th, 2010). Alexandria, VA: Author.Retrieved from http://www.cswe.org/Accreditation/2008EPASHandbook.aspx

DuBois, B., & Miley, K. K. (2010). *Social work: An empowering profession* (7th ed.). Boston: Allyn & Bacon.

Gambrill, E. (2003). A client-focused definition of social work practice. *Research on Social Work Practice*, 13(2), 310–323.

Gambrill, E. (2005). *Critical thinking in clinical practice: Improving the quality of judgments and decisions* (2nd ed.). Hoboken, NJ: Wiley.

Gibbs, L. E. (2003). *Evidence-based practice for the helping professions*. Pacific Grove, CA: Brooks/Cole-Thomson Learning.

Gibbs, L., & Gambrill, E. (2002). Evidence based practice: Counterarguments to objections. *Research on Social Work Practice*, 12(3), 452–476.

Gibbs, P., Locke, G. L., & Lohman, R. (1990). Paradigm for the generalist-advanced generalist continuum. *Journal of Social Work Education*, 26(3), 232–243.

Gordon, W. E. (1962). A critique of the working definition. *Social Work*, 7(4), 3–13.

Gordon, W. E. (1969). Basic construct for an integrative and generative conception of social work. In G. Hearn (Ed.), *The general systems approach: Contribution toward an holistic conception of social work*. New York: Council on Social Work Education.

Hearn, G. (1969). *The general systems approach: Contributions toward an holistic conception of social work*. New York: Council on Social Work Education.

Hernández, S. H., Jorgensen, J. D., Judd, P., Gould, M. S., & Parsons, R. J. (1985). Integrated practice: An advanced generalist curriculum to prepare social problem specialists. *Journal of Social Work Education*, 3, 28–35.

Hollis, E. V., & Taylor, A. L. (1951). *Social work education in the United States: The report of a study made for the national council on social work education*. New York: Columbia University Press.

Howard, M. O., McMillen, C. J., & Pollio, D. E. (2003). Teaching evidence-based practice: Toward a new paradigm for social work education. *Research on Social Work Practice*, 13(2), 234–259. doi: 10.1177/1049731502250404.

Johnson, L. C., & Yanca, S. J. (2010). *Social work practice: A generalist approach*. Boston: Allyn & Bacon.

Kirst-Ashman, K. K., & Hull, G. H., Jr. (2009). *Understanding generalist practice*. Belmont, CA: Brooks/Cole.

Landon, P. (1995). *Generalist and advanced generalist practice*. Washington, DC: National Association of Social Workers.

Landon, P. S., & Feit, M. (1999). *Generalist social work practice: A functional approach*. Dubuque, IA: Eddie Bowers.

Lavitt, M. R. (2009). What is advanced in generalist practice? A conceptual discussion. *Journal of Teaching in Social Work, 29*(4), 461–473. doi: 10.1080/08841230903253267.

Maguire, L. (2002). *Clinical social work: Beyond generalist practice with individuals, groups, and families*. Pacific Grove, CA: Brooks/Cole.

Minahan, A. (1981). Purpose and objectives of social work revisited. *Social Work, 26*(1), 5–6.

National Association of Social Work. (1999). *NASW code of ethics*. Washington, DC: NASW Press.

Parsons, R. J., Jorgensen, J. D., & Hernández, S. H. (1994). *The integration of social work practice*. Pacific Grove, CA: Brooks/Cole.

Pilonis, E. M. (2007). *Competency in generalist practice: A guide to theory and evidence-based decision making*. New York: Oxford University Press.

Poulin, J. (2005). *Strengths-based generalist practice: A collaborative approach* (2nd ed.). Belmont, CA: Brooks/Cole.

Roy, A. W. & Vecchiolla, F. J. (2004). *Thoughts on an advanced generalist education: Models, readings and essays*. Dubuque, IA: Eddie Bowers.

Richmond, M. (1917). *Social diagnosis*. New York: Russell Sage Foundation.

Richmond, M. (1922). *What is social case work?* New York: Russell Sage Foundation.

Ripple, L. (1974). *Structure and quality of social work education*. New York: Council on Social Work Education.

Rubin, A., & Parrish, D. (2007). Views of evidence-based practice among faculty in master of social work programs: A national survey. *Research on Social Work Practice, 17*(1), 110–122.

Schatz, M. S., Jenkins, L. E., & Sheafor, B. W. (1990). Milford redefined: A model of initial and advanced generalist social work. *Journal of Social Work Education, 26*(3), 217–231.

Sheafor, B. W., & Landon, P. S. (1987). Generalist perspective. In A. Minahan (Ed.), *Encyclopedia of social work*. Silver Spring, MD: National Association of Social Workers.

Suppes, M. A., & Wells, C. C. (2003). *The social work experience: An introduction to social work and social welfare* (4th ed.). New York: McGraw-Hill.

Turner, F. J. (2005). *Social work diagnosis in contemporary practice*. New York: Oxford University Press.

VIRGINIA RONDERO HERNANDEZ

GROUP WORK

ABSTRACT: This entry begins with a brief history of group work in the United States. Next, there is a description of the wide range of treatment and task groups used by social workers. This is followed by a discussion of group dynamics, diversity, and social justice issues. Then, there is a brief overview of the developmental stages that groups go through and widely used practice models. The chapter concludes with a brief review of the evidence base for the effectiveness of group work practice.

KEY WORDS: group work; group dynamics; group development; history of group work; task groups; treatment groups; evidenced-based group work

Along with casework and community organization, group work is one of the three major modalities of social work practice. Group work can be defined as goal-directed activity that brings together people for a common purpose or goal. Group work is aimed at meeting members' socioemotional needs and accomplishing tasks. Group work may be directed at individual members, the group as a whole, or the environment in which the group works. Groups are found in almost all settings where social work is practiced.

The Historic Roots of Group Work

Unlike casework that came about in England and the United States as a part of the charity house movement in the late 1800s, group work grew up mostly in settlement houses. While charity organizations were focused primarily on identifying the worthy poor and determining who should receive aid, settlement houses focused on socializing new citizens to democratic values and the American way of life. It gave ordinary citizens opportunities for education, recreation, social support, and community involvement. Historically, group work focused on enlightened collective action and democratic participation (Follett, 1926; Slavson, 1939). The contrast between casework and group work can be seen in the early writing of Mary Richmond who in 1917 wrote the first textbook on social casework, called *Social Diagnosis* (Richmond, 1917). Richmond used legalistic proceedings to carefully study and diagnose the needs of the poor in order to determine if they were worthy of aid. In contrast, the first book written about group work by Grace Coyle, *Social Processes in Organized Groups* (1930), focused on the processes that occurred during group meetings. The early history of group work focused heavily on adult education, social action, social justice, and social change (Coyle, 1935, 1938). This was in part due to the Great Depression and the emphasis on the struggle for workers' rights and the unions that were forming during the 1920s and the 1930s.

Gradually, during the 1940s and 1950s, group work began to be used more frequently to provide therapy in child guidance clinics and inpatient and outpatient mental health settings.

Fritz Redl (1944) and Giesela Konopka (1949) helped make group services an integral part of child guidance clinics. The interest in groups for therapy was also spurred on by psychoanalysis and ego psychology (Schilder, 1937; Slavson, 1940; Wender, 1936) and the severe shortage of trained workers to deal with the mentally disabled war veterans returning from World War II (Trecker, 1956). Gradually, group workers who had their roots in many different disciplines, such as adult education and recreation, began to align themselves with social work. The American Association of Group Workers, formed in 1946, was a part of the National Conference on Social Work, but it was not until 1955 that group workers formally joined with other social workers to form the National Association of Social Work.

During the 1960s and 1970s interest in group work declined somewhat because there was a movement away from specializations in casework, group work, and community organization to a curriculum in schools of social work that emphasized generic social work practice. Although generic social work practice was supposed to emphasize casework, group work, and community organization, in practice, casework became the dominant mode of intervention. To increase awareness of the importance of group work, in 1978 social workers came together to establish the journal *Social Work with Groups*, and in 1979 group workers throughout the United States and Canada came together for the First Annual Symposium for the Advancement of Group Work, and this Annual Symposium has grown into an international organization, with chapters throughout the world.

The Range of Group Work Practice

Today, group work is practiced with a wide range of groups. Two major types of groups can be distinguished in group work practice: treatment groups and task groups. Treatment groups are focused on the needs of individual members whereas task groups are focused on the task or the work to be accomplished. Treatment groups can be distinguished from task groups because their focus is always on the needs of the members of the group. In contrast, the work of task groups may or may not affect the members of the group themselves. The work of task groups is focused on a goal or an objective that goes beyond the members of the group. According to Toseland and Rivas (2005) there are five broad types of treatment groups: (1) support groups, (2) educational groups, (3) growth groups, (4) therapy groups, and (5) socialization, recreation, and activity groups.

There are also three main types of task groups: those that meet client needs, those that meet organizational needs, and those that meet community needs. Groups that meet member needs include teams, treatment conferences, and staff development groups. Task groups that meet organizational needs include (1) committees, (2) cabinets, and (3) boards of directors. Task groups that meet community needs include (1) social action groups, (2) coalitions, and (3) delegate councils.

Diversity and Social Justice in Group Work Practice

When social workers hear the word "diversity" with regard to group work, they may think of a mixed group of Black and White Americans. Diversity, however, comprises not just racial differences, but ethnic, gender, sexual, age, intellectual, and physical diversity among others. It is important to understand how diversity influences group cohesiveness and the effectiveness of group work practice. Indeed, the essence of group work is to create an environment that is sensitive to and respectful of all differences, and help individuals thrive within that group environment (Fluhr, 2004). Gender, race, disability status, and other forms of diversity have a profound effect on group processes (Brown & Mistry, 1994; Davis & Proctor, 1989; Garvin & Reed, 1983). Groups are a microcosm of the wider society and any group process will replicate the sociopolitical status and power relationships evident in the relevant society (Brown & Mistry, 1994).

There is an ongoing discussion in group work literature regarding the advantages of groups that are homogenous versus those that are heterogeneous. Some support the idea that a group's composition should be homogenous (Richards, Burlingame, & Fuhriman, 1990; Tajfel & Turner, 1986), especially when group tasks are associated with issues relevant to the particular groups' common characteristic. For example, there is evidence that same-sex groups are advantageous for women, when the group task relates to personal identity, social oppression, and empowerment (Brown & Mistry, 1994). Similarly, groups designed to meet the needs of people who are lesbian, gay, or transgendered do not afford the benefits of group membership to "out-group" members.

The use of homogenous groups in agencies, treatment centers, and counseling centers has been endorsed because it is believed that sameness will expedite treatment. That is, group cohesion will be fostered more quickly and the group bond will be stronger if the group members have more in common (Fluhr, 2004). Kruglankski et al. (2002) suggest the commonality of experience will allow for shared opinions and therefore a more satisfying group experience. Social identity theory supports this point of view (Perrone, 2000) because it posits that people classify themselves and others into various social categories (e.g., racial, gender, and age cohorts) as part of the process of social identification (Tajfel & Turner, 1986). The sharing of common characteristics facilitates a perceived sense of oneness with a group of people.

Similar to same-sex groups, an ethnic- or race-specific group is often preferred by members and is more productive when issues of racial identity, racism, and culture are central to the task (Brown & Mistry, 1994; Davis, 1979, 1984). The concept of "support" is sometimes emphasized as a reason for employing racially homogeneous groups (Boyd-Franklin, 1991; Brayboy, 1971, 1974; Curtis & Hodge, 1994; Davis, 1979, 1984; Denton, 1990; Fenster & Fenster, 1998; Frances-Spence, 1994; Jones & Hodges, 2001; McKay, Gonzales, Quintana, Kim, & Abdul-Adil, 1999). These authors suggest that self-disclosure in situations of trust and mutual support is beneficial to group members with homogeneous backgrounds, and this need for support is one reason many Black men and women prefer a racially homogenous form of group treatment.

Perhaps the most convincing argument for the use of homogenous groups concerns the empirically supported idea that the structurally determined oppression of racism, sexism, and homophobia are replicated as a powerful dynamic in small groups of mixed membership (Brown & Mistry, 1994). Few would question the salience of race in the therapeutic relationship and indeed, literature exists which addresses its importance (Banks, 1971; Beckett, 1980; Dana, 1981; Davis, 1984; Goodman, 1969; Green, 1982; Sue, 1977, 1981). Clearly, people enter groups with their own personal and social frame of reference and as such, bring their experiences with racism, sexism, and homophobia with them into the group experience. The group worker's responsibility is to understand the way in which larger society is an "in-group" experience, and, at the same time, work to counteract the replication of social oppression and facilitate the empowerment of all group members (Brown & Mistry, 2005).

Although there is empirical evidence for the use of homogenous groups in certain situations, heterogeneous groups are much more representative of the reality experienced by practitioners working in the field. Fluhr (2004) states, "[e]mbedded in social work ethics is a dedication to serve a multitude of people from every background, life experience, developmental stage and value structure. This service is expected to be delivered without bias and without judgment.... Group work with a heterogeneous membership embraces that code of ethics and promotes its realization" (p. 39).

Multiethnic groups are increasingly common as ethnic diversity widens in American cities. School social workers, particularly those in urban areas, see the changing multicultural face of America firsthand and must strive to encourage acceptance of differences so that bridges can be built between multiple cultures, languages, and worldviews. Making connections across multiple worldviews involves considerations of dimensions such as individualism–collectivism, masculinity–femininity, power–distance, and uncertainty–avoidance (Hofstede, 1980). Perhaps the most salient issue for group workers is to become aware of their own issues with sexism, homophobia, and racism. The dynamics, which often occur between members and workers of heterogeneous groups, include the deep-rooted feelings and reactions to these issues. Anti-oppressive practice demands not only specific actions toward equalizing the power and position of group members, but "constant awareness and vigilance to ensure a consistent approach to all aspects of the group work process" (Brown & Mistry, 2005, p. 140).

Social justice is an ideal condition in which all members of a society have the same basic rights, protection, opportunities, obligations, and social benefits (Barker, 1995). One of the principles upon which group work as a method rests is its conviction that group work can and should prepare individuals for democratic participation in their communities (Breton, 2004). Groups geared toward social action (i.e., collective action directed toward a shared goal) demonstrate the way in which social justice is operationalized.

In recent years there has been a resurgence of interest in social action group work. Such work couples internal group processes of empowerment with an external agenda of collective social action. In social action groups, the learning goals as well as the learning tools employed are creative and flexible. For example, participants with an interest in social justice typically desire to be challenged about their own biases. Thus, goals might include a thorough examination of personal resistance, being critiqued on communication skills, and learning how to educate others about prejudice. Some of the techniques used to promote social change include experiential learning (for example, cultural tour of a city or cultural immersion experiences), readings, dialogue, and the use of media images. The learning that takes place in action groups typically extends beyond the group itself to the creation of agendas and plans for promoting social change in the larger community.

Linking personal change with social change is clearly part of the process in a social action group. However, a common misconception is the belief that engaging in social change cannot lead to personal healing and that personal healing cannot lead to social change (see Breton, 2006). Donaldson (2004) and others, however, make it clear that therapeutic benefits can be gained, including increased self-esteem, self-efficacy, and confidence. There is little research documenting the therapeutic effects of social action groups. However, there is consensus regarding the idea that an empowerment approach to social work practice is both a "clinical and community oriented approach" (Lee, 2001, p. 30).

A focus on diversity in group work is becoming increasingly salient in the United States, especially in urban centers. Decisions about group composition (for example, homogeneous versus heterogeneous membership) should be made based on the purpose of the group, its goals, and the skill of the worker(s). Likewise, the number, race, and sex of group leaders should be carefully considered. More than one group leader may be recommended in certain situations (for example, when social modeling is being used as a group learning technique). Group workers should expect that members seeking treatment will enter groups unequal in power, both structurally and interpersonally (Brown & Mistry, 1994) and overt and subtle forms of oppression will call for different responses from minority versus majority group leaders (p. 143).

Social action group work is a vehicle through which diversity is recognized and valued. For the worker, the emphasis is on the understanding and use of group processes and the ways members help one another to accomplish the purposes of the group (Abels & Garvin, 2005). Positive group processes have the potential to effect social change. Understanding the occurrence and use of differences within groups is the cornerstone of effecting such change.

The Phases of Group Development

No matter what type of group is used in practice, groups go through a series of developmental steps or phases during their lives. These steps can be divided into planning, beginning, middle, and ending phases. The first step in planning a group is to develop the group's purpose. The group leader needs to think carefully about the goals of the group and its intended purpose. In the planning phase, the worker also needs to consider the best sponsor for the group,

and which members should attend. Although the workers may think of their own agency or organization as the most likely sponsor for the group, there are times when they may want to think of a different sponsor, or having joint sponsors. For example, if a worker is trying to reach out to a group of African-Americans, a church in an African-American community or a community center located near where the members live may be the best sponsor. Once a sponsor is identified, the worker can go about recruiting members, carefully considering the composition of the group and how the members will fit together. As members are selected they can be oriented to the purpose of the group and contracted for the duration and nature of their participation in the group. The planning phase should also take into consideration practical issues such as where the group will meet and any resources the group will need to conduct its meetings.

The beginning phase of group activity is often characterized by tentativeness as members get to know each other and begin to work together. The worker's job is to help members to learn about one another and begin to work together on shared goals. There is a period of assessment when the needs of members, the tasks to be accomplished, and the goals of the group are decided upon. As the beginning phase progresses and norms begin to be established, some group theorists suggest that there is a period of conflict when members test norms or challenge the existing status quo. Garland, Jones, and Kolodny (1976), for example, suggested that after a pre-affiliation phase there is a stage of power and control when members vie for their place in a group, and challenge initial norms. The beginning phase is also characterized by assessment when the worker and the members decide upon the needs of the group and its members and formulate goals to be accomplished in later sessions.

The middle phase of group work is a time when the majority of the work of the group gets accomplished. During the middle phase the worker structures the group's work, making sure that individual and group goals are the focus of the work. One of the worker's major tasks is to involve and empower members so that they feel a part of the group and their psychosocial needs and task needs are being met. The worker also engages reluctant and resistant group members so that they take part in the life of the group. During the middle phase the worker also monitors and evaluates the group's progress, trying to help the group accomplish individual and group goals while keeping in mind the overall goals of the sponsoring organization.

The ending phase of group work is the time to consolidate the work of the group. Members should be helped to finish their work on goals set earlier. The ending phase is also a time to help members maintain and generalize the changes they have already made and to plan for the future. Endings should help members plan for independent functioning when they leave the group. Referrals to additional services or resources may be made, and members should be helped to consider obstacles that may interfere with goal achievement once the group breaks up. Ending sessions are also a time to help members with any feelings they have about ending their participation in a group, and to recount and take stock of what they have achieved and what has been accomplished in the group.

In task groups, ending meetings start by making sure there is an agenda and the group keeps to it. The group worker's job is to make sure that members keep to the topic. In such groups, the worker may be a member, the chair, or a staff member assigned to the group. Each member should be given the opportunity to speak, but at the same time, the worker has to consider the time for each topic, and limit the time that any one member can speak on the topic. The worker should summarize frequently and try to summarize each topic as it is discussed. If more time is needed, the worker can note that and at the end of the agenda for the meeting, discuss with the members the need to return to certain points during the next meeting. The worker should also make sure that any assignments to be completed by members after a meeting are clear and consider forming subgroups to do some of the work between meetings that can then be reported to the larger group the next time everyone meets. In the ending phase of task groups the major tasks are to review the decisions and plans for action, and to make sure that there is a plan for follow through so that members know their role in helping to solve the problem or accomplish the task after the group ends. The ending of task group meetings is also a time for self-critique when the members of the group discuss what was done well and what needs to be improved or done differently the next time (Schwarz, 2002). This can be done collectively, by asking each member what he or she did well and would like to improve on the next time.

Models of Group Work

In 1962, Papell and Rothman described three historically relevant models of group work practice that are still relevant today. These models include (1) the social goals model, (2) the remedial model, and (3) the reciprocal model. In addition to these three models a task group model can be added.

The social goals model is focused on social responsibility, social action, and informed democratic participation. It is used in community development agencies, community centers, and youth organizations for the purpose of introducing members to democratic values and empowering them to achieve goals set by themselves rather than by the worker. At its core is the value of social justice where members take on the responsibility for changing oppressive social structures for their own betterment and for the welfare of the larger community. The leader is available to help empower members and to guide them as they take the necessary steps to help themselves and to change the systems that affect their daily lives. Some of the early pioneers of the social goals model, such as Klein (1953, 1970, 1972) and Tropp (1968, 1976), emphasized the autonomy of the members of the group and the need for the worker to empower members so that they could establish and pursue their own goals. More recently, Breton (1994, 1995, 1999), Lee (1991), Nosko and Breton (1997–1998), and Pernell (1986) are some of the many group workers who have made contributions to the empowerment strategies embodied in the social goals model. The social goals model can also be seen as a task group model because although its focus in on helping members of the group, the goals of reducing repression, improving social justice, and empowerment can also help individuals who are not part of the group.

The remedial model is focused on restoring the functioning of individual group members. First promulgated by Vinter (1967) the remedial model grew out of the principles of deviance, social role theory, and ego psychology. The focus of the remedial model is on helping members with problems to change their behavior and restore their functioning. The remedial model views the worker as an expert who helps to structure the group and set up the necessary conditions so that members can learn new ways of behaving and coping with problems. Focusing on problem solving (Sundel, Glasser, Sarri, & Vinter, 1985), social learning theory (Rose, 1998), and task-centered social work (Garvin, 1997), the remedial model emphasizes structured, time limited, goal directed activity to solve specific problems.

The reciprocal model focuses on the interaction of members with society. The worker is a mediator helping members find common ground between their own needs and that of the larger society. The emphasis in the group is on mutual aid, and for the worker to foster a therapeutic environment in the group to help the group as a whole to achieve its objectives. The worker's role is not only to foster mutual aid and to help the group as a whole to achieve its goals but also for the sponsoring agency and the larger social environment to better meet members' needs. Schwartz (1976) was one of the early pioneers of the reciprocal model, but Gitterman and Shulman (1994) are also known for this approach to group work practice.

Blending Group Work Practice Models

In 1980 Papell and Rothman (1980) proposed a mainstream model of group work practice that incorporated elements of three previously described models. The mainstream model that they proposed was characterized by common goals, mutual aid, and the creation of a group structure that increased the autonomy of members as the group developed. Allisi (2001) pointed out that mainstream group work models included five common elements: (1) a commitment to democratic values, voluntary association, collective decision making and action, and individual liberty and freedom with the responsibility to promote the common good, (2) a focus on the welfare of the individual group member and the society as a whole, (3) an emphasis on program activities that take into consideration the needs, aspirations, and interests of members, (4) an emphasis on small group processes as the medium through which the group operates and achieves its goals, and (5) the worker as a guide working with rather than for the members of the group.

Because social workers work with task groups as well as treatment groups, the task group model can be added to the three historically relevant models and the mainstream model described by Pappell and Rothman. In the task group model the focus is on problem solving, making decisions, and achieving mutually agreed-on goals based on a shared understanding of the problem or task facing the group. The major distinction between treatment and task groups is the focus of the work. Unlike treatment groups where the members are the primary target of the work of the group, the primary target of a task group's work is a larger constituency outside the group who will be affected by the group's work. The goal of the task group model is to help members work effectively and efficiently together on the tasks facing the group. In a classic text Ivan Steiner (1972) made the point that actual productivity in solving a problem equals potential productivity minus process losses. This way of thinking about task groups has been followed up by more recent writers such as Richard Hackman (2002). Thus, the main thrust of the task group model is to help members to work together in a cooperative fashion so that process losses from a lack of cohesion and disagreements about goals will not interfere with the productivity of the group. The core values of the task group model are a creation of shared purpose and meaning. Although there is room for individual initiative, creativity, and input, and all opinions are welcome and valued, the focus is on collective choice of the solution to the problem, based on a sharing of all relevant information. Therefore, the leader is a facilitator of group processes helping the group make the best use of the contributions of individual members. The group facilitator strives to maintain and enhance interpersonal, intergroup, and interorganizational relationships. The facilitator is always striving to point out the value of an individual's input to the group process and at the same time the collective wisdom of the group. The facilitator strives for collaborative interaction that builds consensus and produces meaningful outcomes endorsed and shared by all members of the group. The facilitator tries to set aside his or her own personal opinions, supporting instead the group's right to make its own choices about how to solve the problem or complete the task facing the group. In *The Skilled Facilitator*, Schwarz (2002) discusses the unilateral control model and the give-up-control model as two models of group facilitation that do not work over the long run. Instead, he suggests the mutual learning model. In this model each member of the group has information and perspectives that should be respected. Each member of the group may see things that others do not. In fact, I may be contributing to the problem and not seeing it or knowing it. My feelings or positions may be getting in the way. Therefore, differences of opinion should be viewed as opportunities for learning.

Schwarz (2002) suggests testing assumptions and inferences, sharing all relevant information, giving examples and defining terms to clarify what an individual group member is saying, explaining the reasoning and intent behind information or opinions, combining advocacy with inquiry by explaining your position and the reasoning you used to get there while at the same time asking others about their point of view, and inviting others to ask questions about your point of view. Schwarz (2002) also advocates focusing on interests, not positions, jointly defining the approach to the problem or task, discussing any un-discussible or taboo subjects, discussing next steps and ways to test any disagreements in members' positions, and using a decision making rule that generates consensus building and the commitment needed to solve the problem or get the task accomplished.

The goal in these steps is to reduce process losses by helping everyone's opinions to be heard and valued and to get members to listen to each others' points of view. Then what follows is working out disagreements by testing assumptions, or collecting additional data, and coming up with decision rules that will generate consensus and help everyone feel that they had a part in coming up with the solution or contributing to the accomplishment of the task facing the group.

Recent Practice Models

Despite the focus on a single mainstream model of group work practice, there remain several distinct approaches to group work practice within the current literature. Breton (2006) and Knight (2006), for example, continue to champion the social goals model and social action in groups. Similarly, there continues to be a strong emphasis on the reciprocal model of group work and its focus on mutual aid for vulnerable yet resilient populations (Shulman & Gitterman, 2005). Perhaps the greatest growth in group work models, however, has come in the area of remedial models of group work practice, particularly those that are focused on cognitive behavior therapy in groups. For example, White and Freeman (2000) focus on the use of cognitive-behavioral therapy for a variety of different problems and populations. Similarly, Bieling, McCabe, and Antony (2006) focus on the general principles and practice of cognitive-behavioral therapy in groups. Both books then go on to describe the use of cognitive-behavior therapy for specific types of problems. There has also been a recent focus on group work with specific sub-populations. For example, Malekoff (2004) has prepared a book on group work with adolescents and Salmon and Graziano (2004) have focused on group work with the aging. In the task group arena there has been an increased attention given to team work practice and the facilitation of task groups (see for example, Levi, 2007; Schwarz, 2002).

Technological Innovations in Group Work Practice

In recent years there has been a growing interest in the use of technology to enable individuals to meet together in virtual groups when they are unable to meet in person. There are many reasons why people may not be able to meet face-to-face in groups. A lack of transportation or living in a remote location may make it impossible for members to join a group. Members with debilitating illnesses, or those caring for someone with a severe illness, may not be able to leave their home in order to attend a group meeting. There may also not be enough members with rare diseases to form a group in a small geographic area. There are also some individuals who simply prefer not to attend face-to-face groups because it is too time-consuming, or because they are shy or find face-to-face meetings stigmatizing.

The two most common forms of virtual groups are telephone groups and Internet groups. Telephone groups are made possible through teleconferencing equipment. Although still relatively expensive the cost of telephone conferencing has gone down in recent years with the use of voice-over Internet providers. It is also possible for social service agencies to purchase the equipment to enable them to conduct telephone groups at low cost. Contrary to what might be expected, there is a high level of self-disclosure in telephone groups, possibly because of the lack of verbal cues to distract members from the central focus of the group (McKenna & Green, 2002). We have found that members can stay on the telephone for one to one and a half hours without getting fatigued and that they enjoy the benefit from the experience (Smith & Toseland, 2006; Toseland, Naccarato, & Wray, 2007).

Internet groups have also become much more popular in recent years. Communication in Internet groups may be synchronous or asynchronous, that is, members may all be present and communicating at the same time, or members may log on to sites that allow them to communicate with each other over an extended period of time. According to Santhiveeran (1998), there are four forms of internet groups: (1) chat rooms where members communicate at the same time for a designated period of time, (2) bulletin boards where members can post messages, (3) e-mail generally between two or a few members, and (4) list-serves which go out to many members. Like telephone groups, Internet groups offer support and education to members who may not want to attend in-person groups, or who may be unable to attend them. They offer a kind of anonymity similar to telephone groups but they may particularly appeal to those who enjoy written communication or who value 24-hour access. There has not been a great deal of research on the effectiveness of telephone or Internet groups, and we are aware of no comparisons of the effectiveness of the two modalities. More research will be needed as they grow in popularity in future.

There are also software programs for facilitating decision making in task groups. Multiattribute Utility Analysis (MAU) is a decision making approach that has members of the task group decide on the attributes of a problem, the utility function associated with each attribute, and the weight that should be assigned to each problem attribute. Using a statistical procedure called multiple regression, a worker using MAU can compute the weights and the functional forms that the group members appear to be using to make their judgments about the cases under review. For more about this approach see Jessup and Valacich (1993), Toseland and Rivas (2005), or Reagan-Cirincione (1994).

The Future of Group Work Practice: Evidence-based Approaches

About twenty years ago Feldman (1987) did a review of two decades of social work research. This was followed in 1994 by an article by Tolman and Molidor (1994) that examined a decade of group work research. Both these articles concluded that there was increasing but limited evidence for the effectiveness of social work with groups. However, Brower, Arndt, and Ketterhagen (2004), Garvin (2001), and Hoyle, Georgesen, and Webster (2001) were more positive as they found that group work research is increasing. Unfortunately, there have not been any new systematic reviews of group work in social work literature in recent years. A more recent review of group counseling literature (Burlingame, Fuhriman, & Johnson, 2004) revealed that there is some limited evidence for the effectiveness of group counseling with certain specific problems. This evidence is largely limited to social-skills, cognitive-behavioral, and psychoeducational group approaches, although interpersonal group work approaches have shown some effectiveness (Burlingame et al., 2004). There is also a chapter by Gant (2004) on the evaluation of social group work effectiveness that attempts to look at some of the recent outcome-related studies, but this chapter is a selected review of the contents of specific journals, not a comprehensive review of the recent outcome literature on social group work. Overall, it appears that the situation has not changed appreciably in recent years. Although there has been a recent push within social work to increase the use of evidenced-based practice (see, for example, Roberts & Yeager, 2006), there is still not a great deal of knowledge about the effectiveness of group work practice within social work. Therefore, in future, more attention should be paid to examining the outcomes of group work practice. There is even a striking lack of knowledge about the therapeutic factors that make group work effective. Many of the group work studies that have been conducted have looked at outcomes for individual members, but there has been little effort to look at the therapeutic factors that have made these outcomes possible. We know very little, for example, about what makes for effective leaders, or what types of group dynamics lead to more effective outcomes. These studies are difficult to conduct because they require multiple groups led by multiple leaders and measures of group processes as well as group outcomes. Still, to advance the field in future years, these are the types of studies that are needed.

A Research Agenda for Group Work

As we move forward in the 21st century, there should be a dual focus on evidence-based practice approaches, and more studies focused on the group work processes that help us to achieve desired outcomes. Over the years, there has been a focus on evidence-based practices for a few mental health disorders such as depression, and for other problems such as men who use violence, chronic health conditions such as cancer, and the stress associated with caregiving. Typically, however, there is very little emphasis on the fact that these problems are addressed in groups. The emphasis is on the techniques or the curriculum used to address the problems rather than the group processes that occurred while the problems were being addressed. Thus, one research agenda for the future is making sure that group processes are described even when the intervention focus is on a particular mental or physical health problem. Instead of focusing on the notion of individual treatment within a group context, more weight should be given to group processes and the group context and how these can be used to help individual members and the group as a whole to achieve its goals. There is also a need for more studies on the group work processes that lead to successful outcomes. Although there have been a few articles on the group processes that can lead to detrimental or favorable outcomes in groups (Bedner & Kaul, 1994; Smkowoski, Rose, & Bacallao; 2001; Smkowoski, Rose, Todar, & Reardon, 1999), additional work that identifies helpful and detrimental group processes would be welcome. To this end it would be helpful to have additional measures of group process that would allow us to quickly assess the dynamics of a group as it unfolds. Magen (2004) identifies some measurement issues and measures, but additional work is needed in this area as well.

We also need to continue to focus on the power of groups to address specific problems and to address the effectiveness of these efforts using randomized controlled designs that can add to the evidence-based effectiveness of group work practice for specific mental health, social, and health problems. Although there is a growing base of studies on groups for specific problems (see Bieling, McCabe, & Antony, 2006; Garvin, Gutierrez, & Galinsky, 2004), there is still much more that can be done in social work. For example, the book by Bieling and colleagues is not focused on social work groups. Finally, additional research is needed on virtual groups such as those conducted by telephone, over the Internet, and through videoconferencing, because these media will become more popular as technology progresses and more and more work is done through the Internet. These groups are receiving additional attention in the literature (Meier, 2004; Smith & Toseland, 2006), but more work is needed.

REFERENCES

Abels, P. A., & Garvin, C. D. (2005). *Standards for social work practice with groups* (2nd ed.). Alexandria, VA: Association for Advancement of Social Work with Groups (AASWG), Inc.

Allisi, A. S. (2001). The social group work tradition: toward social justice in a free society. *Social Group Work Foundation Occasional Papers*, 1–25.

Banks, G. (1971). The effects of race on one to one helping interviews. *Social Service Review, 45*, 137–146.

Barker, R. L. (1995). *The social work dictionary* (3rd ed.). Washington, DC: NASW.

Beckett, J. (1980). Perspectives on social work intervention and treatment with black clients: A bibliography. *Black Caucus Journal, 11*, 24–32.

Bedner, K., & Kaul, T. (1994). Experimental group research: Can the cannon fire? In A. Bergin & S. Garfield (Eds.), *Handbook of psychotherapy and behavior change* (4th ed., pp. 631–662). New York: John Wiley and Sons.

Bieling, P. J., McCabe, R. E., & Antony, M. M. (2006). *Cognitive-behavioral therapy in groups*. New York: The Guilford Press.

Boyd-Franklin, N. (1991). Recurrent themes in the treatment of African-American women in group therapy. *Women and Therapy, 11*, 25–40.

Brayboy, T. (1971). The Black patient in group therapy. *International Journal of Group Psychotherapy, 21*, 288–293.

Brayboy, T. (1974). Black and White groups and therapists. In D. Milham & G. Goldman (Eds.), *Group process today: Evaluation and perspective* (pp. 288–293). Springfield, Ill: Charles C. Thomas.

Breton, M. (1994). On meaning of empowerment and empowerment-oriented social work practice. *Social Work with Groups, 12*, 75–88.

Breton, M. (1995). The potential for social action in groups. *Social Work with Groups, 18*, 5–13.

Breton, M. (1999). The relevance of structural approach to group work with immigrant and refugee women. *Social Work with Groups, 22*, 11–29.

Breton, M. (2004). An empowerment perspective. In C. D. Garvin, L. M. Gutierrez, & M. J. Galinsky (Eds.), *Handbook of Social Work with Groups* (pp. 58–75). New York: Guilford Press.

Breton, M. (2006). Path dependence and the place of social action in social work practice. *Social Work with Groups, 29*, 25–44.

Brower, A., Arndt, R., & Ketterhagen, A. (2004). Very good solutions really do exist for group work research design problems. In C. D. Garvin, L. M. Gutierrez, & M. J. Galinsky (Eds.), *Handbook of social work with groups*. New York: Guilford Press.

Brown, A., & Mistry, T. (1994). Group work with "mixed membership" groups: Issues of race and gender. *Social Work with Groups, 17*, 5–21.

Brown, A., & Mistry, T. (2005). Group work with "mixed membership" groups: Issues of race and gender. *Social Work with Groups, 28(3/4)*, 133–148.

Burlingame, G. M., Fuhriman, A., Johnson, J. E. (2004). Process and outcome in group psychotherapy: A perspective. In J. L. DeLucia-Waack, C. Kalodner, & M. Riva (Eds.), *Handbook of group counseling and psychotherapy* (pp. 49–62). Thousand Oaks, CA: Sage Publications.

Coyle, G. (1930). *Group work and social change*. New York: Richard Smith.

Coyle, G. (1935). Education for social action. In *Proceedings of the National Conference of Social Work*, 393. Chicago: University of Chicago Press.

Coyle, G. (1938). Education for social action. In J. Lieberman (Ed.), *New trends in group work* (pp. 1–14). New York: Association Press.

Curtis, L., & Hodge, M. (1994). Old standards, new dilemmas: Ethics and boundaries in community support services. *Psychosocial Rehabilitation Journal, 18*, 13–33.

Dana, D. (1981). *Human services for cultural minorities*. Baltimore: Baltimore University Park Press.

Davis, L. E. (1979). Racial composition of groups. *Social Work, 24*, 208–213.

Davis, L. E. (1984). Essential components of group work with Black Americans. *Social Work with Groups, 7*, 87–109.

Davis, L., & Proctor, E. (1989). *Race, gender, and class: Guidelines for individuals, families, and groups*. Englewood Cliffs, NJ: Prentice Hall.

Denton, T. (1990). Bonding and supportive relationships among Black professional women: Rituals of restoration. *Journal of Organizational Behavior, 11*, 447–457.

Donaldson, L. P. (2004). Toward validating the therapeutic benefits of empowerment-oriented social groups. *Social Work with Groups, 27*, 159–175.

Feldman, R. A. (1987). Group work knowledge and research: A two decade comparison. In S. D. Rose & R. A. Feldman (Eds.), *Research in Social Group Work* (pp. 7–14). New York: Haworth Press.

Fenster, A., & Fenster, J. (1998). Diagnosing deficits in basic trust in multiracial and multicultural groups: Individual or social pathology? *Group Work, 22*, 81–93.

Fluhr, T. (2004). Transcending differences: Using concrete subject matter in heterogeneous groups. *Social Work with Groups, 27(2/3)*.

Follett, M. P. (1926). *The new state: Group organization, the solution of popular government*. New York: Longman, Green.

Frances-Spence, M. (1994). Group work and Black women viewing networks as groups: Black women meeting together for affirmation and empowerment. *Group Work, 7,* 109–116.

Garland, J., Jones, H., & Kolodny, R. (1976). A model of stages of group development in social work groups. In S. Bernstein (Ed.), *Explorations in group work.* Boston: Charles River Books.

Garvin, C. D. (1997). *Contemporary group work.* (3rd ed.). Boston: Allyn and Bacon.

Garvin, C. D. (2001). The potential impact of small-group research on social work practice. In T. Kelly, T. Berman-Rossi, & S. Polombo (Eds.), *Group work: Strategies for strengthening resiliency* (pp. 51–70). New York: Haworth Press.

Garvin, C., Gutierrez, L., & Galinsky, M. (Eds.). (2004). *Handbook of social work with groups.* New York: Guilford Press.

Garvin, C. D., & Reed, B. (Eds.). (1983). Group work with women/group work with men (Special issue). *Social Work with Groups, 6(3/4).*

Gitterman, A., & Shulman, L. (Eds.). (1994). *Mutual aid groups, vulnerable populations and the life cycle* (2nd ed.). New York: Columbia University Press.

Gitterman, A., & Shulman, L. (Eds.). (2005). *Mutual aid groups, vulnerable and resilient populations, and the life cycle.* New York: Columbia University Press.

Goodman, J. (Ed.). (1969). *Dynamics of racism in social work practice.* Washington, DC: NASW.

Gant, L. (2004). Evaluation of Group Work. In C. Garvin, L. Gutierrez, & M. Galinsky (Eds.), *Handbook of social work with groups.* New York: Guilford Press.

Green, J. (1982). *Cultural awareness in the human services.* Englewood Cliffs, NJ: Prentice-Hall.

Hackman, R. (2002). *Leading teams: Settings the stage for great performances.* Boston: Harvard Business School Press.

Hofstede, G. (1980). *Culture's consequences.* Beverly Hills, CA: Sage.

Jessup, L., & Valacich, J. (1993). Support group systems (Special issue). *Small Group Research, 24,* 427–592.

Hoyle, R. H., Georgesen, J. C., & Webster, J. M. (2001). Analyzing data from individuals in groups: The past, the present, and the future. *Group Dynamics, 5(1),* 41–47.

Jones, L. V., & Hodges, V. G. (2001). Enhancing psychosocial competence among Black women: A psycho-educational group model approach. *Social Work with Groups, 24,* 33–52.

Klein, A. (1953). *Society, Democracy and the Group.* New York: Whiteside.

Klein, A. (1970). *Social work through group process.* Albany: School of Social Welfare, State University of New York at Albany.

Klein, A. (1972). *Effective group work.* New York: Associated Press.

Knight, C. (2006). Groups for individuals with traumatic histories: Practice considerations for social workers. *Social Work, 51,* 20–30.

Konopka, G. (1949). *Therapeutic group work with children.* Minneapolis: University of Minnesota Press.

Kruglankski, A., Shah, J., Pierro, A., & Mannetti, L. (2002). When similarity breeds content: Need for closure and the allure of homogeneous and self-resembling groups. *Journal of Personality and Social Psychology, 83,* 648–662.

Lee, J. (2001). *The empowerment approach to social work practice: Building the beloved community.* New York: Columbia University Press.

Levi, D. (2007). *Group dynamics for teams* (2nd ed.). Thousand Oaks, CA: Sage Publications.

Magen, R. (2004). Measurement issues. In C. Garvin, L. Gutierrez, & M. Galinsky (Eds.), *Handbook of social work with groups.* New York: Guilford Press.

Malekoff, A. (2004). *Group work with adolescents: Principles and practice* (2nd ed.). New York: Guilford Press.

McKay, M. M., Gonzales, J., Quintana, E., Kim, L., & Abdul-Adil, J. (1999). Multiple family groups: An alternative for reducing disruptive behavioral difficulties of urban children. *Research on Social Work Practice, 9(5),* 593–607.

McKenna, K. Y. A., & Green, A. S. (2002). Virtual group dynamics. *Group Dynamics: Theory, Research, and Practice, 6,* 116–127.

Meier, A. (2004). Technology Mediated Groups. In C. Garvin, L. Gutierrez, & M. Galinsky (Eds.), *Handbook of social work with groups.* New York: Guilford Press.

Nosko, A., & Breton, M. (1997–98). Applying strengths, competence and empowerment model. *Groupwork, 10,* 55–69.

Papell, C., & Rothman, B. (1962). Social group work models: Possession and heritage. *Journal of Education for Social Work, 2,* 66–77.

Papell, C., & Rothman, B. (1980). Relating the mainstream model of social work with group to group psychotherapy and the structure group approach. *Social Work with Groups, 3,* 5–23.

Pernell, R. (1986). Empowerment and social group work. In M. Parnes (Ed.), *Innovations in social group work* (pp. 107–118). New York: Haworth Press.

Perrone, K. (2000). A comparison of group cohesiveness and client satisfaction in homogenous and heterogeneous groups. *Journal for Specialists in Group Work, 25,* 243–251.

Reagan-Cirincione, P. (1994). Improving the accuracy of group judgment: A process intervention combining group facilitation, social judgment analysis, and information technology. *Organizational Behavior and the Human Decision Making Process, 58,* 246–270.

Redl, F. (1944). Diagnostic group work. *American Journal of Orthopsychiatry, 14(1),* 53–67.

Richards, R. L., Burlingame, G. M., & Fuhriman, A. (1990). Theme-oriented group counseling. *The Counseling Psychologist, 18,* 80–92.

Richmond, M. (1917). *Social diagnosis.* New York: Russell Sage Foundation.

Roberts, A. R., & Yeager, K. R. (Eds.). (2006). *Foundations of evidence-based social work practice.* New York: Oxford University Press.

Rose, S. (1998). *Group therapy with troubled youth.* Newbury Park, CA: Sage.

Salmon, R., & Graziano, R. (Eds.). (2004). *Group work and aging: Issues in practice research and education*. New York: Haworth Press.

Schilder, P. (1937). The analysis of ideologies as a psychotherapeutic method, especially in group treatment. *American Journal of Psychiatry, 93*, 601–615.

Schwartz, W. (1976). Between client and system: The mediating function. In R. Roberts & H. Northen (Eds.), *Theories of Social Work with Groups* (pp. 171–197). New York: Columbia University Press.

Schwarz, R. (2002). *The skilled facilitator: New and revised*. San Francisco: Jossey Bass.

Slavson, S. (1939). *Character education in a democracy*. New York: Association Press.

Slavson, S. (1940). Group psychotherapy. *Mental Hygiene, 24*, 36–49.

Smith, T. L., & Toseland, R. W. (2006). The effectiveness of a telephone support program for caregivers of frail older adults. *The Gerontologist, 46*, 420–629.

Smkowoski, P., Rose, S., Todar, K., & Reardon, K. (1999). Postgroup-casualty status, group events, and leader behavior: An early look into the dynamics of damaging group experiences. *Research on Social Work Practice, 9*(5), 555–574.

Smkowoski, P., Rose, S., & Bacallao, M. (2001). Damaging experiences in groups: how vulnerable consumers become group casulties. *Small Group Research, 32*(2), 223–251.

Steiner, I. (1972). *Group process and productivity*. New York: Academic Press.

Sue, D. (1977). Counseling the culturally different: A conceptual analysis. *Personnel and Guidance Journal, 55*, 422–425.

Sue, D. (1981). *Counseling the culturally different: Theory and practice*. New York: John Wiley.

Sundel, M., Glasser, P., Sarri, R., & Vinter, R. (1985). *Individual change through small groups* (2nd ed.). New York: Free Press.

Tajfel, H., & Turner, J. C. (1986). The social identity theory of intergroup behavior. In S. Worchel & W. G. Austin (Eds.), *Psychology of intergroup relations* (2nd ed., pp. 7–24). Chicago: Nelson-Hall.

Tolman, R., & Molidor, C. (1994). A decade of social group work research: Trends in methodology, theory and program development. *Research on Social Work Practice, 4*, 142–59.

Toseland, R., Naccarrato, T., & Wray, L. (2007). Telephone groups for older persons and family caregivers. *Clinical Gerontologist, 31*, 59–76.

Toseland, R., & Rivas, R. (2005). *An introduction to group work practice*. Boston: Allyn & Bacon.

Trecker, H. (1956). *Group work in the psychiatric setting*. New York: William Morrow.

Tropp, E. (1968). The group in life and in social work. *Social Casework, 49*, 267–274.

Tropp, E. (1976). A development theory. In R. Roberts & H. Northern (Eds.), *Theories of social work with groups* (pp. 198–237). New York: Free Press.

Vinter, R. (Ed.). (1967). *Readings in group practice*. Ann Arbor, MI: Campus Publishing.

Wender, L. (1936). The dynamics of group psychotherapy and its application. *Journal of Nervous & Mental Disorders, 84*, 54–60.

White, J., & Freeman, A. (Eds.). (2000). *Cognitive behavioral group therapy for specific problems and populations*. Washington, DC: American Psychology Association.

RONALD W. TOSELAND AND HEATHER HORTON

H

HEALTH CARE: PRACTICE INTERVENTIONS

ABSTRACT: Social work in health care emerged with immigration and urbanization associated with industrialization, and the resultant shift from physician visits to the patient's home and workplace to hospital-centered care. This change is alleged to have resulted in a loss of the doctor's perspective of the psychosocial influences on physical health. Originally, some nurses were assigned the function of addressing this loss. But eventually, the function became recognized as that of a social worker. From its beginnings in the general hospital setting in the late 1800s, social work in health care, that is, medical social work, has expanded into multiple settings of health care, and the role of the social worker from being a nurse to requiring a Master's Degree in Social Work (MSW) from a university. However, the broad function of social work in health care remains much the same, that is, "to remove the obstacles in the patient's surroundings or in his mental attitude that interfere with successful treatment, thus freeing him to aid in his own recovery" (Cannon, 1923. p 15). Health care social workers are trained to work across the range of "methods," that is, work with individuals, small groups, and communities (social work "methods" are called "casework," "group work," and "community organization"). They work to assist the patient, using a broad range of interventions, including, when indicated, speaking on behalf of the client (advocacy), helping clients to assert themselves, to modify undesirable behaviors, to link with needed resources, to face their challenges, to cope with crises, to develop improved understanding of their health-related thought processes and habits, to build needed self-confidence to do what is required to help themselves deal with their health problem, to gain insight and support from others who are in a similar situation, to gain strength from humor, or from a supportive environment, and through spiritual experience, and from practicing tasks that are needed to deal with their health-related problems or from joining forces with others in the community to modify it in the interest of improved health status for all, or to gradually restore a sense of stability and normalcy after a traumatic experience. Most important of all, perhaps, is the "helping relationship" between client and social worker, which needs to be one of total understanding and acceptance of the client as a person. A sizable portion of the U.S. population lacks financial access to health care, where health care is regarded as a privilege rather than a right, as it is seen in all other industrial nations (except South Africa). Current trends in the U.S. health care system reflect efforts to control rising health care costs without dealing with the "real problems," which are: (1) the lack of a single-payer health care system and (2) the lack of focus on "public health."

KEY WORDS: psychosocial; biopsychosocial

Overview

Health care social workers provide services across the continuum of care and in various settings. Social workers are present in public health, acute and chronic care settings, long-term care, rehabilitation, and hospice. They provide a range of services to patients and families, including health education, crisis intervention, supportive counseling, and case management. They also perform group, community, advocacy, and management functions. In response to critical incidents that are both global and national, health care social workers are increasingly trained to provide interventions to prepare for and respond to traumatic events and disasters.

Social workers implement intervention and treatment plans that promote client well-being and a continuum of care. Planning shall be based on a comprehensive, culturally competent assessment with interdisciplinary input. The function, basis, flexibility, and scope of social work intervention in health care is described in *NASW Standards for Social Work Practice in Health Care Settings* (2005): The 'client' of the social work intervention may be an individual, all or part of a family or any other small group of people, or another larger sector of the community or society—such as the people in a neighborhood, a population of people concerned with a particular health problem, all residents of a treatment center, rehabilitation center, or halfway house, or all patients in a day treatment, day care, or other outpatient program. The client is the person or group that requests and, or, will benefit from the social work intervention.

"Intervention and treatment plans are steps identified by the health care social worker in collaboration

221

with the client and with other members of the team, to achieve the objectives identified during assessment. Health care social workers adapt practice techniques to best meet client needs within their health care setting to work effectively with individuals across their life-span, across different ethnicities, cultures, religions, socioeconomic and educational backgrounds, and across the range of mental health and disability conditions."

HISTORICAL BACKGROUND Social work first emerged in the United States around the late 1800s, when its early practitioners were engaged in home visiting to address the problems of individual families, providing direct casework services. They also focused on early community organization and advocacy efforts to address the health-related problems of workplace hazards, poverty, overcrowding, lack of proper water and sewage systems that accompanied urbanization, immigration, industrialization, and ignorance or lack of acceptance of the dawning germ theory of disease (Cowles, 2003, p. 87).

The specialty field of "medical social work" began with the emergence of the general hospital. It is traced to 1905, when Richard C. Cabot, M.D., Chief of the Massachusetts General Hospital Internal Medicine Clinic, appointed a nurse, Garnet I. Pelton, to fill the first hospital social work position. Ida Cannon, who soon replaced Pelton, wrote a book about her experiences (Cannon, 1923). Cannon claimed that social work in hospitals evolved as a result of the shift of medical practice from being centered in the community, where the physicians had been in touch with the patient's home and workplace, to the hospital, resulting in the physician's loss of perspective of the bio-psycho-social context of the patient's health problems. As Ida Cannon stated, "The social worker seeks to remove those obstacles in the patient's surroundings or in his mental attitude that interfere with successful treatment, thus freeing him to aid in his own recovery" (Cannon, 1923, p. 15).

Over the years since then, medical social work has gradually extended from general hospitals into specialty hospitals, as well as other community-based programs— such as public health agencies, neighborhood primary care clinics, group medical practices, family medical practice residency programs, health maintenance organizations, employee assistance programs, suicide prevention programs, school and college based health clinics, emergency rooms, and free clinics. Furthermore, medical social workers are now employed in home health care agencies, hospice programs, rehabilitation programs, nursing homes, and other residential care facilities.

Settings Across the Care Continuum

To some extent, the "settings" of medical social work intervention, that is, (1) public health, (2) primary care (out-patient care), (3) hospital care, (4) home care, (5) nursing home or other residential care facility, and (6) hospice care, reflect the stages of development of the health problem. The associated role of the social worker can move from (a) helping to promote health and prevent the onset and development of health problems to (b) enhancing the cure process and helping health and other associated human problems from further compounding to (c) maximizing comfort and function when health problems have become chronic or terminal, and preventing "secondary disabilities," that is, undesirable "side effects" of the health problem. Sometimes this is referred to as the "continuum of health care"—from *prevention* and *health promotion* to *curing* of already developed health problems to *caring* for patients with chronic and terminal health problems.

Currently, the role of the social worker also extends to community-based programs, such as public health agencies, neighborhood primary care clinics, group medical practices, health maintenance organizations, employee assistance programs, suicide prevention programs, school and college-based health clinics, emergency rooms, and free clinics. In addition, currently, medical social workers are employed in home health-care agencies, hospice programs, rehabilitation programs, nursing homes, and other residential care facilities.

Since early 2000 the National Association of Social Workers (NASW) has established credentials for social workers, depending on their field of practice and qualifications. The credential for social work in health care is entitled "Certified Social Worker in Health Care" (C-SWHC). The requirements relate to professional association membership, academic degree in social work, credentials of the school from which the degree was earned, and post-degree relevant practice experience.

METHODS Intervention methods of social work in health care, as in other fields of social work practice, include the range of micro-, mezzo-, and macro-level interventions, including casework, group work, community organization, and administration and management, depending on such variables as whether the "client" is an individual, couple, small group, all or part of a community, or an organization, as well as the practice setting, the location of the problem and its solution, available resources, and the training and function of the social worker.

Social Work Interventions

Social work intervention may occur at any stage of the helping process. By "intervention" we refer to what the social worker does in an effort to address the client's health-related psychosocial problems and needs. However, the intervention may involve variations in any stage of the helping process, such as "how" the social worker (1) engages the client, (2) collects the data, (3) assesses relevant information, (4) plans the intervention, (5) conducts the treatment or intervention, (6) evaluates the intervention effect, or later (7) terminates the relationship with the client. The client may be impacted by his or her interaction with the social worker, not only by what the social worker intended to do to help the client, but also by what actually happens at any stage of the helping relationship.

Kerson (1997) has identified the following social work interventions in health care: advocacy, assertiveness training, behavior modification, caring confrontation, care management, cognitive-behavioral therapy, concrete services (for example, community resource linkage), crisis intervention, critical incident stress debriefing, education and information, ego-building oriented casework, family therapy, grief counseling, group therapy, humor, milieu therapy, modeling, psychoanalysis, relaxation therapy, reminiscence therapy, skills training, solution-focused therapy, spiritual beliefs exploration, supportive counseling, supportive environment development, and task-oriented counseling.

The latest *Standards for Social Work Practice in Health Care Settings* (2005) defines 'Intervention or Treatment Plans' as "Strategies to address needs identified in the assessment; information, referral, and education; individual, family, or group counseling; vocational, educational, and supportive counseling; psycho-educational support groups; financial counseling; case management; discharge planning; interdisciplinary care planning and collaboration; client and systems advocacy; and identification of goals and objectives."

A review of social work in health care journals (*Social Work in Health Care*, 2007; *Health and Social Work*, 2003; *National Association of Social Workers*, 2003) over the past few years finds continued use of many traditional social work interventions, but with some apparent variations, for example, from work with groups of individuals to groups of families; various combinations of modalities; assistance with decision making concerning matters such as advance directives;

use of story-telling to engage "hard to reach" clients; therapy with groups of clients whose health is impacted by a common source of personal stress; from "cure" efforts to "harm reduction"; from acute to chronic disease-management; and to addressing communities with high rates of certain health problems; crisis intervention with individual and community victims of terrorism; and outreach to newly diagnosed groups of people to offer counseling and support.

Two challenges the social worker faces are finding affordable resources for clients without health insurance to cover those needs, or personal resources to afford them; and brief contacts with clients, making it difficult to accomplish all that the social worker sees is needed.

ORGANIZATION AND FINANCING OF HEALTH CARE: CURRENT TRENDS

1. Increased cost of health care since 2000, in spite of the introduction of "managed care" in 1983.
2. Continued shortened hospital stays with focus on rapid discharge planning.
3. Reduction in tax funding for public health programs and services (Garrett, 2000) right at the time when the nation is threatened with terrorism, bird flu, HIV and AIDS, as well as nationwide epidemics of depression and obesity with secondary Type II diabetes, heart disease, and functional impairment.
4. The obesity epidemic, coronary artery disease, depression, and Type II diabetes are sometimes interdependent, and may reflect such conditions as lack of education about nutrition and preparation of healthy meals at low cost, lack of regulation of the commercial food industry which promotes a lot of "junk," lack of regular physical exercise, a lack of social supports, and a generalized sense of powerlessness.
5. Growing awareness of the need for more health promotion and disease prevention programs to address population-wide, health-related conditions and associated behavior.
6. There is also increased longevity with associated increase in age-related chronic health conditions, at the same time that many traditional family caregivers work outside the home.
7. Increasing numbers of immigrants (especially Mexican), and changing demographics, which require increased recognition of the importance of culturally appropriate social worker interventions to enhance their effectiveness.

8. Increased participation of social workers on bi-oethics committees to make hard decisions concerning medical interventions to prolong life.

9. Less extensive or prolonged counseling and more "solution-focused therapy" and evidence-based practice as well as linkage of the client with coordinated community-based services and resources, referred to as "case (or care) management."

10. Growing awareness of the need for more health-promotion and disease-prevention programs to address population-wide health-related conditions and associated behavior.

11. Developing public awareness of the greater efficiency and cost savings of a single-payer health care financing system, such as the Medicare system, and, alternatively, the inefficiency of multiple, profit-oriented, health insurance company payers, each with multimillion-dollar executives whose salaries and bonuses are financed through the cost of health care. In addition, the public is also developing awareness of the relationship between the price of pharmaceuticals and the entertainment and gift expenses of those companies in their product promotion efforts to health care providers. Finally, one wonders why the very same medications manufactured in the United States are sold in most foreign countries, including Mexico and Canada, for a fraction of their purchase price in the United States (http://www.pnhp.org).

12. A currently expanding grassroots movement throughout the United States to develop a tax-supported, single-payer health insurance plan, as many working-class citizens find themselves unemployed as a result of their former company employers no longer being able to compete with the lower cost of products manufactured in other industrial nations, where health care is financed through pooled payroll taxes rather than by the employer (http://www.pnhp.org). An increase in primary and ambulatory care neighborhood-clinics funded by the federal government or staffed by volunteer medical and ancillary health care professionals, such as nurses, social workers, and dietitians, for people with no health insurance, many of whom relied most of their lives on factory work, and now lack the education and skills to obtain other kinds of employment, and who now manifest a variety of health problems, mental and physical, often associated with prolonged unemployment and "giving up" (http://www.pnhp.org). (Note: the author works in such a clinic.)

13. Increased community-centered medical care in hospital-affiliated medical group practices.

REFERENCES

Cannon, I. M. (1923). *Social work in hospitals* (p. 15). New York: Russell Sage.

Cowles, L. A. F. (2003). *Social work in the health field: A care perspective*. Binghamton, NY: Haworth Press.

Garrett, L. (2000). *Betrayal of trust: The collapse of global public health*. New York: The Hyperion Press.

Kerson, T. S. (1997). *Social work in health settings: Practice in context* (2nd ed.). Binghamton, NY: The Haworth Press.

FURTHER READING

Health Care Social Work. (2007). Credentials. http://www.socialworkers.org/credentials/default.asp

Health United States. (2003). *Health care expenditures* (p. 10). Hyattsville, MD: National Center for Health Statistics.

Johnson, J. L., & Grant, G., Jr. *Medical social work (casebook series)*. Boston: Allyn & Bacon.

National Center for Health Statistics. Health, United States, 2003 (Table 111, p. 305). Washington, DC: U.S. Government Printing Office.

Poland, B. D., Green, L. W., & Rootman, I. (Eds.). (2000). *Settings for health promotion: Linking theory and practice*. Thousand Oaks, CA. Sage.

Raphael, D. (Ed.). (2004). *Social Determinants of Health: Canadian Perspectives*. Ontario: Canadian Scholars Press.

A comprehensive nine-page list of websites for social workers in health care: http://www.library.wisc.edu/libraries/SOCIALWORK/healthcare.html

Physicians for a National Health Program http:www.pnhp.org

A history of early social work in health care; Massachusetts General Hospital Social Work. http://www.mghsocialwork.org/history.html

Health Insurance Coverage 2005. Highlights. http://www.U.S.Census.Gov

LOIS F. COWLES

HOUSING

ABSTRACT: Housing, especially homeownership and affordable housing, remains essential to the American Dream but also among our most challenging social issues, particularly given the collapse of the housing market in the early 21st century. Housing and affordable housing are inextricably linked to both our national economic crisis and our wavering social policies. Housing is both symptomatic of and a catalyst for overarching social and economic issues, such as poverty, economic and educational inequality, and racial disparities, and it remains an unmet need for a significant portion of our population, such as the elderly, disabled, victims of abuse, those aging out of child welfare, veterans, ex-offenders, and others who encounter unique difficulties and lack of supportive services and service coordination. Advancing comprehensive and coordinated housing policies and programs remains important for social work and in the struggle for decent and affordable housing for all.

KEY WORDS: affordable housing; aging out; community development corporation; cooperative housing; disability; discrimination; disinvestment; economic crisis; fair housing; foreclosure; gentrification; homelessness; homeownership; HOPE IV; housing bubble; housing choice; housing cost burden; individual development accounts; mixed-income housing; mortgage default; New Urbanism; predatory lending; public housing; redlining; rental assistance; rental vouchers; Section 8; smart growth; sprawl; subprime lending; underwater; working poor

Among the myriad problems that beset our society, few have proven as stubborn and challenging as our nation's affordable housing dilemma. Social work, from the Progressive Era through the decades of varying housing and human service policies, has remained a strong advocate for adequate shelter and affordable housing as a basic human need. For the social-work profession, housing problems remain at once a symptom of and a catalyst for other overarching issues, such as poverty, income inequality, racial disparities, and discrimination. Long-standing shelter and housing issues must now be viewed in the wake of the "housing bubble" that collapsed, along with our economy, in 2007 and the resultant economic crisis, often referred to as the "Great Recession." Housing is also reflective of other social problems, such as domestic violence, substance abuse, mental illness, and other conditions, that put citizens at risk of homelessness and in search of affordable housing. Housing remains a significant private trouble and public issue, but one to which fewer resources and less public policy are being devoted.

Elizabeth Mulroy (1995), in the entry "Housing," noted that housing is a key issue for social workers in the 1990s because it reflects a continued failure of policy and programs that have fallen short of our national goals and weakened the American Dream for many. Almost two decades later, with a housing crisis that has only deepened in the wake of our economic crisis, social work's voice seems even weaker in the housing arena. Housing, however, continues as a major social issue for compelling reasons:

- The collapse of the housing bubble and housing market in the financial crisis of 2007 resulted in plummeting home values and a skyrocketing number of mortgage foreclosures; foreclosure rates climbed to a high of one every 13 seconds in 2009 and, while declining through 2013, continue to be problematic in many states (Center for Responsible Lending, 2012).
- Housing remains our largest household expense, at over 25% of one's income, but over 20 million people—most renters—are "cost overburdened," paying more than 50% of their income (Joint Center for Housing Studies, 2012).
- A total of 95 million people, or a third of the nation, have housing problems, whereas 41 million people, 14.6% of the U.S. population, lacked health insurance, and 33.6 million or 12% lack food security (America's Neighbors, 2004).
- Housing and location choice continue to contribute greatly to the condition and quality of one's life, including opportunities for a good education (Schwartz, 2010).

As income and other social indicators document a growing socioeconomic divide in our country, housing problems only further accentuate the class divide in America between the "haves" and the growing number of "have nots" and "used to haves"—those with mortgage foreclosures. Our nation's housing ills are symptomatic of and contributors to other problems in poverty, education, employment, racial segregation, and other forms of discrimination, subtle or overt. Homeownership, the hallmark of the American Dream, has faltered:

- By the fourth quarter of 2011, the homeownership rate dropped to 66%, the lowest since 1998 (Braave, Bolton, Couch, & Crowley, 2012).
- Housing demand has slowed dramatically since the recession, with fewer net new households formed each year between 2007 and 2011—the lowest levels since the 1940s. The largest declines were among the under-25 and 25- to 34-year-old populations, which contributed about equally to the slowdown as many more members of these two groups lived with their parents rather than on their own (Joint Center for Housing Studies, 2012).
- Subprime lending rose from near zero in the early 1990s to 20.1% in 2006, which led to mortgage foreclosures (Joint Center for Housing Studies, 2007) and helped precipitate our national housing and economic collapse (Joint Center for Housing Studies, 2012).

Since the start of the 21st century, our nation's housing crisis has continued under the faltering policies and programs from the 1980s and 1990s, with the following results:

- Between 2007 and 2010, the number of U.S. households paying more than half of their incomes for housing rose by an astounding 2.3 million, bringing the total to 20.2 million households (Joint Center for Housing Studies, 2012, p. 5).
- A total of 42 million households (37%) pay more than 30% of their income for housing (moderate burden), whereas 20.2 million (18%) pay more than half (severe burden). Between 2001 and 2010, the number of severely cost-burdened households climbed by a staggering 6.4 million (Joint Center for Housing Studies, 2012, p. 27).
- The number of poor households spending more than 50% of their incomes on rent increased by 6%, from 5.9 million in 2009 to 6.2 million in 2010, with 75% of all poor renter households having severe housing cost burdens (National Alliance to End Homelessness, 2012).
- The year 2009 saw a shortage of 3.4 million affordable housing units (Braave, DeCrappeo, Pelletiere, & Crowley, 2011).
- On any given day, about three quarters of a million people are homeless (Joint Center for Housing Studies, 2007), a trend that continued until 2011–2012, which finally saw a drop in the homeless rate of 1%, largely attributed to federal rapid rehousing under the "stimulus program" (Joint Center for Housing Studies, 2012).
- Even when the minimum wage is fully implemented, households with an individual minimum wage earner will still be unable to rent a basic two-bedroom unit anywhere in America (Joint Center for Housing Studies, 2007). In 20 states, even households with two minimum wage earners cannot afford a fair-market-rate two-bedroom rental unit (Braave et al., 2012).

In their State of the Nation's Housing 2007 report, the Joint Center for Housing Studies of Harvard University concluded that "affordability" continues to be the most pressing housing challenge into the 21st century and that the heaviest burden falls on the shoulders of the working poor, the disabled, and retirees (Joint Center for Housing Studies, 2007); the situation has fared no better in the 2012 report (Joint Center for Housing Studies, 2012). The housing crisis in America can be seen in the levels of homelessness, the greater share of household incomes dedicated to meeting housing needs, and the increasing levels of mortgage foreclosures in the wake of the recent housing and economic crisis. Social work must reengage in the

housing arena to better connect to the range of social and community needs that contribute to this crisis.

Housing Policies Past and Present

Early housing issues, largely from the Progressive Era, focused on concerns of health, sanitation, and overcrowded conditions, especially in urban areas. The Depression saw rampant unemployment, homelessness, and overcrowded conditions, but out of this economic disaster emerged a range of emergency relief and housing acts to address these shortages of adequate housing and to shore up the weakened housing finance industry, such as the Federal Home Loan Bank System (1937); the National Housing Act of 1934 that established the Federal Savings and Loan Insurance Corporation and the Federal Housing Administration to insure mortgages; the U.S. Housing Act of 1937 that promoted slum clearance for building public housing; and even the Servicemen's Readjustment Act of 1944 (the "GI Bill") that provided guaranteed loans and led to major home building, especially in the new "suburbs."

In the middle of the 20th century, the U.S. government, with the Housing Act of 1949 (1949), declared that the nation's health and living standards required "the realization as soon as feasible of the goal of a decent home and suitable living environment for every American family" (Section 2.63 Stat. 413).

All subsequent housing policies and programs have built upon and sought to address this core goal of decent and suitable shelter for its citizenry, to various degrees of success and failure. However, it is important to recognize that even the 1949 act's major public housing unit goal targeted for 1955 was not realized until more than 2 decades later (Oberlecke, as cited in Lang & Sohmer, 2000).

The construction of public housing, which began in the Roosevelt era, continued through the postwar years, especially through the Housing Act of 1954 and with the creation of the Department of Housing and Urban Development in 1965 as a cabinet position. These urban policies escalated in the 1960s, spurred by domestic unrest and, with the Demonstration Cities and Metropolitan Development Act of 1966 or "Model Cities" Act, supported various programs for urban renewal, such as slum clearance, infrastructure improvements, rental subsidies, and especially mortgage support toward homeownership that underscored the "Great Society" programs of President Lyndon Johnson. Although these efforts did help reduce the shortage of housing and improved housing conditions, they also increased homeownership along with a significant out-migration from city to suburb that has continued into the 21st century, leaving behind in many cities an older and poorer population and fomenting in new ones "suburban sprawl."

The Housing Moratorium in 1974 under the Nixon administration halted this frenzy of housing-related programs and, with the Housing and Community Development Act of 1974, consolidated many programs within HUD and advanced new strategies of revenue sharing and other housing initiatives, including a rental assistance program, Section 8 under this act. These and other federal initiatives under Nixon began devolving housing and other social policies and programs from federal to more state and local levels.

The last 2 decades of the 20th century saw housing policies and programs draw attention to aging and deteriorating housing stock, promote community development strategies, address issues of affordability, and extol the virtues of homeownership. All this occurred while housing was undergoing a substantial federal retrenchment, especially under the Reagan presidency, when HUD's subsidized housing programs fell from their $32.2 billion peak (1978) to merely $9.8 billion by 1988. While programs like the project-based development subsidy of Section 8 for constructing low-income, affordable housing were being phased out and rental subsidies fell by nearly three quarters annually from 1978 (Bratt, 1997), greater emphasis was given to the mainstay of U.S. housing subsidies (that is, income tax credits), such as the Low-Income Housing Tax Credit program under the Tax Reform Act of 1986, as well as enhanced focus on the Housing Choice Voucher Program under Section 8 of the 1974 act. These low-income tax incentives built upon the country's long-standing and largest housing subsidy, the "homeownership tax deduction" established with the Personal Income Tax in 1915.

Despite the Clinton administration's Housing Opportunities for People Everywhere (HOPE VI) initiative, which was more an effort to change the face of public housing communities from low- to "mixed-income" communities than to generate additional housing, housing programs and HUD itself have struggled for survival. The HUD budget at the close of the Bush administration stood at $35.2 billion (HUD, 2007), roughly equivalent to its peak budget of $32.2 billion (HUD Archives/Budgets 1978, 2007). The 2012 HUD budget showed a 9% reduction, mostly in community development block grants to states and other housing rehabilitation programs that, unfortunately, are significant employment generators. Federal subsidies and renewals for Section 8 project-based developments and Section 8 voucher programs have been threatened at a time when waiting lists in most cities numbered in the thousands. Although many new communities replaced aging, deteriorating, and dangerous public housing communities to the satisfaction of the modest number of returning residents, serious questions remain regarding the fate of tenants, especially at-risk families, displaced under HOPE VI (Popkin et al., 2004) without adequate case management, resources, and follow-up for effective transition. Public housing demolition has continued in many cities; however, now relocation, support services, and management of subsidized housing are largely nonexistent.

The focus on community development strategies in housing policy programs reflected a further step in the devolution of policies and programs from the federal to state to local levels, notably to county and city authorities, as well as to community and faith-based nonprofit organizations (Swanstrom, 1999). Programs such as Habitat for Humanity have demonstrated the importance of local, voluntary support and sweat equity; however, despite their noble efforts, they are too modest in scope to make a major impact on either housing supply or community development. Community development corporations—community-based organizations that engage in housing and commercial revitalization—have assumed significantly greater responsibility for low-income housing construction, rehabilitation, preservation/reuse, and homeownership programs in cities across America. However, in the wake of the housing and budgetary crisis, many community development corporations and their intermediary funding and technical support agencies are fading from the urban landscape.

Much of the nation's housing development strategies came to a screeching halt in the wake of the housing and economic collapse that began in the waning years of the Bush administration in 2007 and has continued with only modest relief during the Obama administration. Blame was initially heaped on those who took advantage of predatory lending practices and easy-to-get mortgages to become homeowners—moving households from renting to homeowning was a major Bush housing strategy. However, the deeper realities of economic collapse in 2007 revealed how a largely deregulated financial industry had manipulated and grown the housing bubble as an engine of financial, not housing, growth, until it burst (Krugman, 2012). Even government-backed housing lenders Freddie Mac and Fannie Mae succumbed to this mortgage crisis that fueled the nation's economic collapse. Unfortunately, the Housing and Economic Recovery Act of 2008 was one of the few federal initiatives, and the impact of policy in this crisis has been limited, with national mortgage relief programs' response for individual homeowner refinancing was seen as constrained by overly cautious bureaucrats and lenders (Applebaum, 2012). However, the disparity between the government's massive financial bailouts for the banking industry and modest and constrained aid extended to "underwater" homeowners whose mortgages now outstrip their homes value has not gone without criticism (Krugman, 2012). How America's policy response in this housing and financial crisis will be judged eventually is a matter for future analysts, but aid to individual homeowners in distress has not seemed a priority.

Housing Discrimination and Fair Housing

Housing discrimination laws enacted through congressional acts and presidential orders have powerfully influenced housing opportunities and redressed glaring inequalities and disparities in housing. Among the better known of these are Title VI of the Civil Rights Act of 1964, which prohibits discrimination on the basis of race, color, or national origin and discrimination in housing; and Title VIII of the Civil Rights Act of 1968—better known as the Fair Housing Act—which prohibits discrimination in the sale, rental, and financing of dwellings and in other housing-related transactions based on race, color, national origin, religion, sex, familial status, and disability.

Several subsequent policies from the Architectural Barriers Act of 1968 to Section 504 of the Rehabilitation Act of 1973 and Title II of the Americans with Disabilities Act of 1990 further address housing-related discrimination based on disability in any program or construction supported with federal funds. Fair housing has also been the focus of several presidential orders, which are used to clarify national policy through their programmatic implementation, notably Executive Order 11063, which addresses discrimination in properties and facilities owned or operated by the federal government or with federal funds, and especially Executive Order 12892, which requires federal agencies and their grantees to "affirmatively further fair housing."

Many of these laws and regulations addressed discrimination in the housing sector relative to federal programs and funding; however, the private financial and real-estate sector became a growing concern in the late 1960s and early 1970s over issues of "redlining"—marking off areas where housing lending would not be encouraged and to which certain racial groups would be steered. Whereas the Fair Housing Act addressed racial steering, the Community Reinvestment Act of 1977 enforced financial institution investment in otherwise "disinvested" communities.

Even successful housing strategies, such as the cooperative housing movement, which spurred urban housing markets between World War I and World War II, especially in the 1950s and 1960s, did more to advance the housing needs for those of middle and upper income (Seigler & Levy, 1986). Although envisioned as a housing movement to address the needs of those of low and moderate income, more often cooperative housing served to further discrimination in housing through exclusionary housing practices by cooperative ownership boards and managers.

The HUD and its local governmental agencies were also the targets of legal actions in the 1990s through consent decrees around issues of discrimination in housing choice, racial composition of housing, and lack of affordable housing or other housing resources (Popkin et al., 2003). Despite legislated reduction in glaring discrimination, inequality of opportunity by race continues, often fueled by the limited social safety net, a lack of coordination in social policies and programs (Popkin et al., 2003), growing disparities in income and housing affordability (Burchell & Listokin, 1995), and an ongoing not-in-my-backyard mentality.

The current economic and housing climate has seen a drop in homeownership and a drastic rise in housing foreclosure (Bravve et al., 2012), leading more households to become renters. In this challenging housing landscape, issues of housing affordability and the difficulties of economically distressed homeowners to secure mortgage relief have somewhat blurred racial and ethnic distinctions in a growing mix of economically distressed households. Instead, this economic and housing crisis has placed a brighter spotlight on economic disparity and the growing inequality between the haves and the have nots.

Further Considerations: Trends, Issues, and Program Implications

As the 21st century unfolds, housing policies, programs, and practices must consider social and economic trends and issues that will continue to shape our housing and social policies, programs, and practices for decades to come. Unfortunately, the economic crisis has set a somber tone for homeownership and affordable housing policy, and as the ranks of renters have grown (Braave et al., 2012), the concern regarding affordable housing has also increased.

Economic restructuring in the growing global marketplace, which saw huge declines in U.S. industries and jobs (Mulroy, 1995), especially middle-class jobs (Krugman, 2002), is fueling the rise of low-wage jobs that has resulted in a new class of "working poor" in America that is the subject of government reports

(U.S. Department of Labor, 2005) and books (Ehren-reich, 2001; Shipler, 2005). That this situation has worsened with the 2007 housing collapse and economic recession is not surprising. With a middle class ever more at risk of job loss by outsourcing in the global community or their increasing debt load, greater housing costs, and rising health-insurance dilemma (Warren, 2006), the faltering of this American economic cornerstone can only foreshadow even greater difficulties for those most at risk, the poor and the working poor. For these populations, affordable housing remains an economic enigma (Harkness & Newman, 2004).

Beyond the growing inequality in socioeconomic status, we must be cognizant of essential demographic changes in the United States (Joint Center for Housing Studies, 2006, 2007; U.S. Census, 2010) and how they shape housing consumption (Masnick, 2002). Ethnically and racially, the United States is experiencing a significant shift as the White population ages and declines and minority populations, largely from both legal and illegal immigration, continue to swell until, as predicted, by the mid-21st century Whites will be in the minority. In addition to ethnic and racial make-up, the composition of households is changing, with traditional family households waning, whereas other household configurations show continued increase. Demographics on a growing aging population, as well as aging disabled populations with longer term chronic needs and housing needs, are another disconcerting trend. Although "who we are" is radically changing, "where we are" is equally in flux with migration to the South and West, along with sizeable immigration to these regions, marking major populations shifts away from the East and Midwest's older, industrial cities to new and growing urban cores in warmer regions of the country. This shift has resulted in housing shortages and extreme cost increases in new population zones, whereas older locales have seen increased vacancy and aging housing stock.

The base of homeownership has also shifted, from older White homeowners to younger Whites, as well as a growing minority homeownership, particularly from immigrant groups (Joint Center for Housing Studies, 2007). However, in this time of growing economic uncertainty, there is a drop in young homeownership because young, unemployed adults (18 to 25 years old) are returning to live with their parents and those in the 24- to 35-year-old group are finding it difficult to secure home financing, especially when they are already saddled with student loans, which is swelling the rental ranks (Joint Center for Housing Studies, 2012). In many economically strong regions

with expanding urban housing markets, low-income residents are being squeezed out of their own neighborhoods by increased housing costs and the movement back to cities. This process of "gentrification," although advantageous to rebuilding local communities, exacerbates the lack of availability and affordability of housing for those on lower and fixed incomes (Kennedy & Leonard, 2001).

The community development struggle to balance social and environmental goals, a focus of the New Urbanism (Talen, 2002), underscores competition among urban, suburban, and rural development, especially poorly planned and densely concentrated commercial and housing growth often called *sprawl* (Bruegmann, 2005/2006). Extending urban and suburban growth into rural landscapes has raised health and environmental concerns, along with concerns that inner-city poor residents are being further cut off from commercial and housing growth areas, prompting an increased focus on "sustainable development" or "smart growth" that seeks a balance of social, economic, and environmental goals. In many urban areas, the first-ring suburbs are now older and more economically, racially, and ethnically aligned with the urban core than the outer suburbs, and many are facing declines in homeownership and housing values (Puentes & Warren, 2006).

The cost of housing and of homeownership continued to rise (Joint Center for Housing Studies, 2007), fueled by housing and lending markets that, as predictions and stock market volatility portend, were overextended and at risk of serious retrenchment, if not collapse, bringing even deeper economic impact (Wilson, 2007), and came to a disastrous reality in 2007. A major issue for the then-unstable housing market was "subprime" lending—higher and variable-rate loans for those with higher risks of default—which has served more as a catalyst for just such loan defaults (Renuart, 2004). The growing concern had been with "predatory lending," especially among those of low and moderate income, whose purpose seems to be to move citizens ever deeper in debt while generating profits for loan providers (Wilson, 2007). The toll from this subprime lending, among other financial debacles, was the collapse of both the nation's housing market and the economy. Adding to the high cost of housing and the lack of affordable housing amid growing economic disparity is the rise in personal bankruptcies, which had already reached record rates in 2003 and continued at a high level (Weller, 2005). Now, with millions of homeowners "underwater" on their mortgage and many just walking away from their homes, personal bankruptcies have become almost commonplace. Home sales were already down 10% in 2006 and housing starts were down even more (Joint Center for Housing Studies, 2007) before ominous economic predictions hit home. Since 2007, housing sales have fallen precipitously; however, in 2012, the first glimmer of growth in home sales began to offer some hope of eventual recovery (Joint Center for Housing Studies, 2012).

Unfortunately, as homeownership has declined and rental housing has increased, the number of Americans spending more than half their income on housing is rising rapidly, and "cost-burdened" Americans represent nearly one in seven households (Joint Center for Housing Studies, 2007). According to the National Low Income Housing Coalition's Report, *America's Neighbors* (2004), and its current report, *Out of Reach 2012* (Braave et al., 2012), well over one third of the nation is experiencing housing problems, and two thirds of those are low-income, of whom nearly 90% are severely cost burdened. Whether renting or owning, the incidence of cost-burdened housing remains high for those on low and fixed incomes. This problem is particularly daunting for low-wage workers with limited government subsidies (Joint Center for Housing Studies, 2007). The nearly 70 million Americans facing housing cost burden are both a result of poverty and a major contributor to it. When more than 30% of one's income must be used for housing costs, less is left for other life essentials, which greatly reduces the quality of life for these households.

As the federal government has reduced its support for many social programs, including housing, it has devolved policies and programs down to the state and local levels. The mainstay for addressing these issues as they impact housing rests on an ever more fragile social safety net and the efforts of state and local agencies, along with a network of community-based organizations (Swanstrom, 1999). Housing development within a broader framework of community revitalization continues to face challenges, from lack of federal funding to local government constraints, including local attitudes against subsidized or Section 8 developments. Any limits in the supply mean higher prices and less housing available for those of lower income (Quigley, 2006), as has been the case with fewer middle-income households able to purchase or retain homes and hence becoming renters.

Some groups are more at risk in this housing market, not only because of poverty, but also because of other characteristics and needs. These groups include the elderly; the mentally, physically, and developmentally disabled; youth aging out of the child welfare system; victims of domestic and other abuse; veterans experiencing transitional issues; substance abusers; ex-offenders; and others with behavioral risks, as well as the swelling ranks of illegal immigrants and the longer term homeless populations (Pelletiere, Treskon, & Crowley, 2005). It is with these populations that social work is particularly focused within the housing arena, but these groups are also now caught up in these larger trends, issues, and challenges of this economic recession, which should also be of concern to our profession.

Moving Forward: Goals, Strategies, and Roles for Social Work

Critics of our housing policies and programs on all sides of the political spectrum (Bratt, 1997; Hockett, McElwee, Pelletiere, Schwartz, & Trekson, 2005; Redburn, 2006) note that the federal government routinely subsidizes substandard housing and offers subsidies to families in locations where they are in constant fear of violence, poorly educated in the worst schools, and isolated from economic opportunity. Moreover, our housing programs have provided little solid evidence as to who benefits, under what circumstances, and in relation to what other forms of assistance. For our country to pursue a more progressive path in response to housing needs, we must be cognizant of key trends and issues, assess where needs are greatest, and develop stronger guidelines and practices that consider housing within the larger context of poverty, community development, and social needs. We also must recover from the dire economic circumstances that have put our nation and much of our population back on its heels, if not on its knees. Sadly, it has proved hard to chart a progressive path in response to this crisis, and it is hard to find social-work leaders leading progressive initiatives in this "Great Recession" as Harry Hopkins and Frances Perkins did for the Roosevelt administration during the Great Depression.

The first step now must be developing or even implementing current policies that help foreclosed homeowners and "cost-burdened" renters survive this economic crisis. Although home buying is beginning to start up (Joint Center for Housing Studies, 2012), the Center for Responsible Lending's foreclosure ticker shows foreclosure rates are still climbing. Advocacy is needed to ensure that the Housing and Economic Recovery Act of 2008 provides meaningful help to the many households in foreclosure, even those at financial risk who were victims of predatory lending practices that helped put our nation underwater. Rapid rehousing programs that were once part of the Stimulus Bill should also be renewed, especially as targeted efforts for at-risk veterans helped reduce homelessness by 1% between 2011 and 2012 (Joint Center for Housing Studies, 2012; National Alliance to End Homelessness, 2012). In this weakened economy, supported housing programs that help move low-income households out of poverty to self-sufficiency are more critical than ever. However, much of this challenge is economic and stems from the mismatch between earned wages and fair-market housing rates. When the working poor on minimum wage cannot afford to rent a two-bedroom unit at fair-market rental rates in any state, and even two minimum wage earners are unable to jointly afford a fair-market rental in dozens of states, then the issue is one of a "liveable wage" (the Living Wage Campaign) to ensure that the working poor can afford decent and safe housing without an extreme cost burden.

Once we are able to restore our economic and housing equilibrium, developing a more balanced national housing policy that invests in both people and property would be an essential next step. In responding to the trends and issues previously discussed, future federal, state, and local housing policies and regulations must tackle difficult challenges, including the following:

- Developing housing for growing and shifting populations while meeting the nation's need for affordable housing;
- Housing those populations that are difficult to house (for example, multiproblem families, ex-offenders, public housing evictees, and the mentally and physically disabled who require greater social support or more expensive housing to accommodate their needs);
- Overcoming regulatory barriers (such as zoning, building codes, and land use) that entail both benefits and pitfalls from gentrification and restricted accessibility and housing choice;
- Addressing the competition between urban reuse—smart growth—and easy suburb new growth that can lead to "sprawl."

In reflecting on past policies and programs, a former director of HUD's Office of Policy and Research and her colleague have offered several principles that should guide housing policy in the new millennium (Schill & Wachter, 2001), including linking housing policy with other social policies, such as education, and making housing vouchers the mainstay of housing assistance programs.

Social workers should be particularly engaged in helping connect social welfare reform and housing policy. Current welfare policies at some times pose barriers and at other times fail to provide incentives for moving families and households to self-sufficiency, including affordable housing (Swartz & Miller, 2002). Coordinating housing assistance and services at one-stop job centers and expanding individual development accounts to encourage family savings for homeownership (Schreiner & Sherraden, 2006) are important approaches in an affordable housing strategy. In addition, domestic violence often presents serious housing issues for abused children and spouses, in terms of not only shelter needs, but also welfare regulations and limitations. Moreover, the issue of housing affordability for the working poor and the need for livable wages should be issues for further social-work advocacy.

Social work's domain also finds housing connected to a myriad of social needs and groups, particularly children, the elderly, and the disabled, who are most vulnerable in the housing arena and, at times, at risk of homelessness. It is within this venue of broader social-service needs and coordination, rather than in housing policy and advocacy, that social work has been engaged during the past several decades and must be focused in the decades ahead.

The Child Welfare League of America recognizes that thousands of children each year are separated from their families or unable to leave foster care because their parents are homeless, live in inadequate housing, or are displaced because of domestic violence. Young people preparing to age out of the foster-care system are also facing homelessness and critical housing needs upon their discharge (White & Rog, 2004). Although the affordable housing crisis is placing a growing burden on the child welfare system, child welfare professionals are rarely trained to assist youth and families with the difficult tasks of finding adequate housing.

Scarce affordable housing for the elderly is a problem that is only getting worse, including a lack of subsidized apartments compounded by the need for subsidized housing for the poor elderly and those who are increasingly frail and in need of services. Subsidized buildings are often the main settings where these seniors can get help. Although it is a tribute to our medical technology and humanity that we can extend life for those with chronic conditions, housing options have not kept pace, as media reports abound. Similarly, the growing number of elderly caring for aging developmentally, mentally, and physically disabled children or siblings of the "baby boom" or from the height of deinstitutionalization in the 1960s and after presents a unique social-work challenge in years ahead.

The challenge of building inclusive communities certainly raises concerns for the housing plight of people with disabilities. Although housing programs and Fair Housing requirements specify addressing the needs and access of the disabled for housing, affordable housing remains problematic (O'Hara & Miller, 2000). *Going It Alone: The Struggle to Expand Housing Opportunities for People With Disabilities* notes that discrimination remains a barrier despite the Americans with Disabilities Act, housing for the disabled remains a low priority among state and local housing officials, and the lack of collaboration between most public housing agencies and disability organizations furthers these difficulties (O'Hara & Miller, 2000). The issue of the aging disabled populations, especially those aging in group homes or other supported-living facilities that are not targeted for maintenance or new-construction funding, will become an even greater concern as younger disabled populations seek these limited resources.

The H.R. 558—100th Congress: Stewart B. McKinney Homeless Assistance Act (1987) defines a homeless person as one who "lacks a fixed, regular, and adequate night-time residence." The National Coalition for the Homeless recognizes that only 20–25% of the single, adult homeless have some form of serious mental illness or disability (National Coalition for the Homeless, 2006), with children under 18 comprising the largest percentage (39%) of a broad range of other homelessness that includes elderly, families, ex-offenders, substance abusers, veterans, and victims of domestic violence (National Coalition for the Homeless, 2007). Homelessness in the early 21st century is not merely the result of deinstitutionalization from the middle of the 20th century, but a combination of limited income/poverty and affordable housing options mixed with a lack of community support services and failed managed-care systems that put more people at risk (National Coalition for the Homeless, 2006). A growing concern is that when affordable housing options are limited, care for the mentally ill and others with cooccurring disorders, such as substance abuse, is shrinking while the homeless population is rising, and the only significant residential institutional growth in America is within the prison system. Developing supportive community services and housing resources for those in housing crisis should be a critical concern for social work.

As federal housing strategies continued a community development approach that moved away from mass public housing to redeveloping mixed-income communities, initiatives such as HOPE IV and HUD's own Office of University Partnership sought to engage higher education institutions in these revitalization and housing efforts. Many schools of social work and social-work professionals were involved in HUD's HOPE IV housing relocation initiatives, as well as the dozens of Community Outreach Partnership Centers that sought to mobilize university resources to address community-identified problems (Soska & Johnson-Butterfield, 2004), such as that in Newark, New Jersey (Newman & Anglin, 2005), where university–community partnerships are aiding in local revitalization. Many schools of social work have engaged in these university–community partnerships and assumed significant roles in connecting social services to those in housing transition, such as the Campus Affiliates Program at Tulane University, which provided HOPE VI relocation case management for residents in one New Orleans neighborhood (Kreutziger, Ager, Harrell, & Wright, 1999).

Similar to these community partnership revitalization efforts under HUD, community development corporations and other community planning interests are important allies for social workers in connecting social services to housing and community development initiatives. The social-work profession could find a strong affiliation with those advancing New Urbanism and "smart growth" strategies that see social and environmental needs being addressed in tandem (Talen, 2002). All of these efforts have at their core participatory planning, civic engagement, and equality of access to resources, interaction, and interconnectedness, which resonate well with the social-work profession.

Finally, despite policies to safeguard housing choices, America must also ensure fair and equal housing opportunities for all and overcome discriminatory practices that continue to plague the housing market. Housing inequality is tied to other disparities, most notably educational opportunity, which is often a matter of where one lives (Schwartz, 2010). Policy makers, officials, and community leaders will need to address the goals espoused in the Housing Act of 1949, which, despite real improvements since the 1960s in how we house people, seemingly remain beyond the reach of many Americans (Lang & Sohmer, 2000). Social work must embrace the affordable housing challenge within its national agenda. Social work has a major role to play in this continuing economic crisis and in connecting housing to other social services and issues, as well as in advocating on the larger issue of poverty and racism impacting affordable and adequate housing in our country, which continues to keep us from realizing our Housing Act of 1949 vision of "a decent home and a suitable living environment for every American family as soon as feasible" (Section 2.63 Stat. 413).

REFERENCES

America's neighbors: *The affordable housing crisis and the people it affects*. (2004, February). Washington, DC: National Low Income Housing Coalition. Retrieved May 9, 2013, from http://nlihc.org/sites/default/files/neighbors.pdf

Applebaum, B. (2012, August 19). *Cautious moves on foreclosures haunting Obama*. New York Times. Retrieved May 9, 2013, from http://www.nytimes.com/2012/08/20/business/economy/slow-response-to-housing-crisis-now-weighs-on-obama.html?pagewanted=all&_r=0

Bratt, R. G. (1997, July/August). *A withering commitment. Shelterforce Online*. Montclair, NJ: National Housing Institute. Retrieved from http://www.nhi.org/online/issues/94/bratt.html

Bravve, E., Bolton, M., Couch, L., & Crowley, S. (2012). *Out of Reach 2012: America's Forgotten Housing Crisis*. Washington, DC: National Low Income Housing Coalition.

Bravve, E., DeCrappeo, M., Pelletiere, D., & Crowley, S. (2011). *Out of Reach 2011: Renters Await Recovery*. Washington, DC: National Low Income Housing Coalition.

Bruegmann, R. (2005/2006). *Sprawl: A compact history*. Chicago, IL: University of Chicago Press.

Burchell, R., & Listokin, D. (1995). Influences on United States housing policy. *Housing Policy Debate, 6*(3), 559–617.

Center for Responsible Lending. (2012). *Solutions for the economy*. Retrieved May 9, 2013, from http://www.responsiblelending.org/solutions-for-the-economy.html

Ehrenreich, B. (2001). *Nickel and Dimed in America: On (not) getting by in America*. New York, NY: Holt.

Joint Center for Housing Studies. (2006). *State of the nation's housing 2006*. Cambridge, MA: Joint Center for Housing Studies of Harvard University. Retrieved May 9, 2013, from http://www.jchs.harvard.edu/research/publications/state-nations-housing-2006

Joint Center for Housing Studies. (2007). *State of the nation's housing 2007*. Cambridge, MA: Joint Center for Housing Studies of Harvard University. Retrieved May 9, 2013, from http://www.jchs.harvard.edu/research/publications/state-nations-housing-2007

Joint Center for Housing Studies. (2012). *State of the nation's housing 2012*. Cambridge, MA: Joint Center for Housing Studies of Harvard University. Retrieved May 9, 2013, from http://www.jchs.harvard.edu/sites/jchs.harvard.edu/files/son2012.pdf

Harkness, J., & Newman, S. (2004, April). *Housing problems of the working poor*. Washington DC: Center for Housing Policy of the National Housing Conference

Hockett, D., McElwee, P., Pelletiere, D. Schwartz, D., & Treskon, M. (2005). *The crisis in America's housing: Confronting myths and promoting a balanced housing policy*. Retrieved May 9, 2013, from http://nlihc.org/sites/default/files/housingmyths.pdf

Housing Act of 1949. Pub. L. No. 81–171. Section 2.63 State. 413 (1949).

H.R. 558—100th Congress: Stewart B. McKinney Homeless Assistance Act. (1987). Retrieved June 14, 2013, from http://www.govtrack.us/congress/bills/100/hr558

Kennedy, M., & Leonard, P. (2001, April). *Dealing with neighborhood change: A primer on gentrification and policy choice*. Washington, DC: Brookings Institution and PolicyLink.

Krugman, P. (2002, October 10). *For richer*. New York Times Magazine. Retrieved from http://www.nytimes.com/2002/10/20/magazine/20INEQUALITY.html

Krugman, P. (2012). *End this depression now!* New York, NY: Norton.

Kreutziger, S. S., Ager, R., Harrell, E., & Wright, J. (1999). The campus affiliates program. *American Behavioral Scientist, 42*(5), 827–839.

Lang, R., & Sohmer, R. (2000). Legacy of the Housing Act of 1949: The past, present, and future of federal housing policy. *Housing Policy Debate, 11*(2), 291–198.

Masnick, G. S. (2002). The new demographics of housing. *Housing Policy Debate, 13*(2), 275–321.

Mulroy, E. A. (1995). Housing. In R. L. Richard (Ed.), *Encyclopedia of Social Work* (19th ed.). New York, NY: NASW Press.

National Alliance to End Homelessness. (2012, January). *The state of homelessness 2012*. Washington, DC: Author.

National Coalition for the Homeless. (2006). *Fact sheet #5: Mental illness and homelessness*. Washington, DC: Author. Retrieved from http://www.nationalhomeless.org/factsheets/Mental_Illness.html

National Coalition for the Homeless. (2007). *Fact sheet #3: Who is homeless*. Washington, DC: Author. Retrieved from http://www.nationalhomeless.org/factsheets/who.html

Newman, K., & Anglin, D. (2005, January/February). *Building a university—community partnership in Newark*. Shelterforce Online, 139. Retrieved May 9, 2013, from http://www.nhi.org/online/issues/139/partnerships.html

O'Hara, A., & Miller, E. (2000). *Going it alone: The struggle to expand housing opportunities for people with disabilities*. Boston, MA/Washington, DC: Technical Assistance Collaborative/Consortium for Citizens with Disabilities Housing Task Force.

Pelletiere, D., Treskon, M., & Crowley, S. (2005, August). *Who's bearing the burden? Severely unaffordable housing: An examination of national and state affordable housing needs from the 2003 American Community Survey*. Washington, DC: National Low Income Housing Coalition.

Popkin, S. J., Levy, D. K., Harris, L. E., Comey, J., Cunningham, M. K., & Buron, L. F. (2004). The Hope VI program: What about the residents? *Housing Policy Debate, 15*(2), 385–414.

Popkin, S., Galster, G., Temkin, K., Herbig, C., Levy, D. K., & Richer, E. K. (2003). Obstacles to desegregating public housing: Lessons learned from implementing eight consent decrees. *Journal of Policy Analysis and Management, 22*(2), 179–199.

Puentes, R., & Warren, D. (2006, February). *One-fifth of America: A comprehensive guide to America's first suburbs*.

Washington, DC: Brookings Institution. Retrieved September 9, 2012, from http://www.brookings.edu/~/media/research/files/reports/2006/2/metropolitanpolicy%20puentes/20060215_firstsuburbs

Quigley, J. (2006, March). *Housing policy in the United States (Working Paper No. W06-001).* Berkeley, CA: University of California, Program on Housing and Urban Policy, Institute of Business and Economic Research.

Redburn, S. F. (2006, October). *Rethinking federal low-income housing policies.* Washington, DC: Asset Building Program, New America Foundation.

Renuart, E. (2004). An overview of the predatory mortgage lending process. *Housing Policy Debate, 13*(2), 467–502.

Schill, M., & Wachter, S. (2001). Principles to guide housing policy at the beginning of the millenium. *Cityscape: A Journal of Policy Development and Research, 5*(2), 5–19. Retrieved from http://www.huduser.org/Periodicals/CITYSCPE/VOL5NUM2/schill.pdf

Schreiner, M., & Sherraden, M. (2006). *Can the poor save? Savings and asset building in individual development accounts* (p. 372).Piscataway, NJ: Aldine Transaction.

Schwartz, H. (2010). *Housing policy is school policy: Economically integrative housing promotes academic success in Montgomery County, Maryland.* New York, NY: Century Foundation.

Seigler, R., & Levy, H. (1986). *Brief history of cooperative housing.* Washington, DC: National Association of Housing Cooperatives.

Shipler, D. (2005). *The worker poor: Invisible in America.* New York, NY: Vintage Press.

Soska, T., & Johnson-Butterfield, A. (Eds.). (2004). *University–community partnerships: Universities in civic engagement.* New York, NY: Haworth Press. Published simultaneously as *Journal of Community Practice, 12*(3/4).

Swanstrom, T. (1999). The nonprofitization of United States housing policy: Dilemmas of community development. *Community Development Journal, 34*(1), 28–37.

Swartz, R., & Miller, B. (2002, March). *Welfare reform and housing (WR&B. Brief No. 16).* Washington, DC: Brookings Institution.

Talen, E. (2002). The social goals of the New Urbanism. *Housing Policy Debate, 13*(1), 165–188.

U.S. Census. (2010). Retrieved May 9, 2013, from http://www.census.gov

U.S. Department of Housing and Urban Development (HUD) Archives/Budgets. (1978). Retrieved May 9, 2013, from http://archives.hud.gov/

U.S. Department of Housing and Urban Development (HUD) Archives/Budgets. (2007). Retrieved May 9, 2013, from http://archives.hud.gov/

U.S. Department of Labor. (2005, March). A profile of the working poor 2003 (Report No. 983). Washington, DC: U.S. Department of Labor and U.S. Bureau of Labor Statistics.

Warren, E. (2006, January/February). The middle class on the precipice: Rising financial risks for American families. *Harvard Magazine.* Retrieved from http://www.harvardmagazine.com/on-line/010682.html

Weller, C. (2005, February 18). *Rising personal bankruptcies.* Center for American Progress. Retrieved from http://www.americanprogress.org/issues/2005/02/b369011.html

White, R. A., & Rog, D. (Eds.). (2004, September/October). Housing and homelessness. *Child Welfare: Journal of Policy, Practice, and Research, 83*(5), 389–392.

Wilson, D. (2007, February 17). Around the markets: Subprime lenders and builders expose risks in U.S. stock and bond markets. *International Herald Tribune/Bloomberg News.*

FURTHER READING

Child Welfare League of America: http://www.cwla.org/programs/housing/housingaboutpage.htm

National Alliance to End Homelessness: http://www.endhomelessness.org/

National Coalition for the Homeless: http://www.nationalhomeless.org/

National Housing Institute, Shelterforce Online: http://www.nhi.org/online/

PolicyLink: http://www.policylink.org/

Smart Growth: http://www.smartgrowth.org/

State of the Nation's Housing 2007 fact sheet: http://www.jchs.harvard.edu/research/publications/state-nations-housing-2007

Sustainable Communities: http://www.sustainable.org/

Universal Living Wage Campaign: http://www.universallivingwage.org

Urban Institute, *Housing America's Low Income Families:* http://www.urban.org/housing/index.cfm

U.S. Department of Housing and Urban Development (HUD): http://www.hud.gov/

U.S. Department of Housing and Urban Development Office of University Partnerships: http://www.oup.org/

TRACY M. SOSKA

HUMAN TRAFFICKING: OVERVIEW

ABSTRACT: Human trafficking (HT), also known as modern-day slavery, has received significant emphasis during the last decade. Globalization and transnational migration trends continue to amplify economic disparities and increase the vulnerability of oppressed populations to HT. The three major types of HT are labor trafficking, sex trafficking, and war slavery. Victims of HT are exploited for their labor or services and are typically forced to work in inhumane conditions. The majority of these victims are from marginalized populations throughout the world. Although both men and women are victims of HT, women and children are heavily targeted. Interdisciplinary and multilevel approaches are necessary to effectively combat HT. Combating HT is particularly relevant to the profession of social work with its mission of social justice. To address the needs of the most vulnerable of society, implications for social workers are discussed.

KEY WORDS: human trafficking; labor trafficking; sex trafficking; war slavery; social work education & practice; social work

Introduction

Human trafficking (HT), also known as modern-day slavery, has recently received significant consideration in global circles. Globalization and transnational migration trends continue to amplify economic disparities and increase the vulnerability of oppressed populations to different forms of HT. Most victims of HT are generally exploited for labor or sexual purposes. A smaller proportion are victims of organ removal or unethical adoption processes (Roby & Bergquist, 2014). Persons most vulnerable to HT are generally the poor, the marginalized, and individuals seeking employment opportunities. Three major types of HT today are labor trafficking, sex trafficking, and war slavery. In the United States, The Victims of Trafficking and Violence Victim Protection Act (TVPA) of 2000 (P.L. 106-386) provided the following definition of HT:

(a) sex trafficking in which a commercial sex act is induced by force, fraud, or coercion, or in which the person induced to perform such an act has not attained 18 years of age; or

(b) the recruitment, harboring, transportation, provision, or obtaining of a person for labor or services, through the use of force, fraud, or coercion for the purpose of subjection to involuntary servitude, peonage, debt bondage, or slavery. (United States Department of State, 2000, p. 8)

Global estimates of HT are difficult to gather due to the secretive nature of contemporary slavery, and there is some discrepancy between figures. Bales (2004), an expert on HT, reports an estimated 27 million people exist in some form of modern-day slavery throughout the world. The International Labour Office (2013) estimates there are approximately 21 million people victims of human trafficking throughout the world. In the United States, roughly 17,000 people are trafficked into slavery each year (Bales, 2009).

Labor Trafficking

The International Labour Office (2013) estimates there are currently approximately 14.2 million victims of labor trafficking worldwide. Labor trafficking can be found in virtually every industry throughout the world. Victims of labor trafficking are forced to work without payment or without sufficient payment often in horrible conditions. Individuals are exploited for labor within their own country or across international borders, with migrants being particularly susceptible to this form of trafficking (United States Department of State, 2013). Debt bondage is the provision of services for personal debt and is recognized as the most prevalent type of labor trafficking. This type of trafficking exists mostly in India, Pakistan, Bangladesh, and Nepal (Bales, 2004).

Within the United States, common forms of labor trafficking are domestic servitude, agricultural or farming work, and factory work (Polaris Project, 2013a). Labor trafficking has also been discovered in strip clubs, in peddling and begging rings, and in the hospitality industry (Polaris Project, 2013a). Traveling sales crews that sell magazines or other items have been identified as being particularly exploitive of young adults between ages 16 and 28 (Polaris Project, 2013b). Both male and female victims are recruited with promises of opportunities to travel and earn a high income (Polaris Project, 2013b). Victims typically have limited formal education and low incomes (Polaris Project, 2013b). After an initial "honeymoon" period where the victims are treated well, they are isolated and removed from familiar territory (Polaris Project, 2013b). They may experience physical abuse, emotional abuse, or threat of abandonment (Polaris Project, 2013b).

Sex Trafficking

The International Labour Office (2013) estimates that there are 4.5 million victims of sex trafficking worldwide. Victims and their families are often misinformed regarding employment opportunities and/or the nature of the sex trade (Roby, 2005). In Thailand, impoverished families in rural areas are offered between $200 and $2000 for the contractual work of their daughter in factories or restaurants (Lusk & Lucas, 2009). When these young girls arrive in the city they are sold to brothels and forced to work in the sex industry (Bales, 2004). A brothel owner can earn up to $80,000 a month if twenty victims have sex with fourteen clients per day (Bales, 2004).

In the United States, sex traffickers generally prey upon the most vulnerable of society, often targeting individuals that have a history of mental, physical, or sexual abuse (Polaris Project, 2013c). Sex trafficking occurs in the following settings: residential brothels, hostess clubs, online escort services, fake massage businesses, strip clubs, and street prostitution (Polaris

Project, 2013c). The Internet has been identified as the primary strategic tool of sex traffickers and perpetrators to sell and purchase sexual services in the United States (Polaris Project, 2013c). Pornography, chat rooms, personal ads, and fake massage parlors are advertised on various websites, such as Backpage .com (Polaris Project, 2013c). Online predators seek out the emotionally vulnerable in cyberspace and attempt to lure individuals into the sex industry with fraudulent information (Polaris Project, 2013c). Recent studies suggest that minors are the most susceptible population to become victims of sex trafficking in America (Kotrla, 2010) The sex trafficking of youth in the United States is known as domestic minor sex trafficking (DMST).

War Slavery

Around the world, about 2.2 million people experience war slavery (International Labour Office, 2013). War slavery may be perpetrated by rebel groups or enforced by state authorities in the form of forced labor. War slavery, also referred to as state-imposed forced labor, is sometimes government sanctioned. For example, the dictatorship of Burma has enslaved tens of thousands of civilians for military campaigns and construction projects (Bales, 2004). The United Nations has reported the recruitment of child soldiers in 55 countries including: Afghanistan, Burma, Chad, the Democratic Republic of the Congo, Somalia, South Sudan, Sudan, Syria, and Yemen (as cited in Schlein, 2014). Globally there are between 250,000 and 300,000 child soldiers under the age of 18 (as cited in Schlein, 2014).

Special Groups of HT Victims

Present estimates and data indicate that the majority of HT victims today are women and girls (United States Department of State, 2013). A global study completed by the United Nations Office on Drugs and Crime (UNODC) demonstrated that women and children are more vulnerable to HT (United Nations Office on Drugs and Crime, 2012). Women are particularly vulnerable to HT in the domestic service industry where informal employment is not usually regulated by government labor laws (United States Department of State, 2013). The feminization of poverty and gender-biased cultural norms that encourage the subjugation of women increase their vulnerability to HT.

Worldwide, approximately 5.5 million victims of human trafficking are under the age of 18 (International Labour Office, 2013). Approximately 1.2 million children are trafficked annually worldwide (Blumhofer,

Shah, Grodin, & Crosby, 2011). The UNODC noted a general trend of increased child trafficking throughout the world, which was most prevalent in Africa (United Nations Office of Drugs and Crime, 2012). Armed conflict leaves children particularly vulnerable to trafficking, especially when children are refugees or are internally displaced (United States Department of State, 2013). Children are also trafficked for sexual exploitation, construction, begging, petty theft, domestic work, sweat shop work, and organ harvesting (Kara, 2009).

When women are trafficked the children they leave behind are especially vulnerable to exploitation (Faulkner, Mahapatra, Heffron, Nsonwu, & Busch-Armendariz, 2013). Although current estimates of trafficked parents and their children are unavailable, the impact of trafficking on the family unit cannot be overlooked (Faulkner et al., 2013). The effects of separation of trafficked individuals from their families is similar to the disruption that occurs in transnational families (Faulkner et al., 2013). Both groups experience many challenges which lead to an unstable family unit. Children born into trafficking situations are another extremely vulnerable group. Further research is necessary to document and understand the experiences of second generation victims of HT.

Key Determinants of HT

The key determinants of HT are related to "push and pull factors" and theories of migration. The "push" factors which contribute to the possibility of being trafficked are: poverty, limited employment, economic and political instability, environment decay, natural disasters, conflict-related displacement, limited educational opportunities, and family violence (Bryant-Davis, Tillman, Marks, & Smith, 2009). Examples of the "pull" factors that increase the probability of entering situations of HT are: demand for cheap labor and services, higher wages, and increased life opportunities. Vulnerable populations that reside in areas where several "push" factors are present have increased likelihood of entering the trafficking process.

Global Policy

In 2000, the United Nations implemented the Palermo Protocol or The Protocol to Prevent, Suppress and Punish Trafficking in Persons, Especially Women and Children (United States Department of State, 2013). The Palermo Protocol provides guidance for governments to prevent HT, protect victims of HT, and prosecute traffickers (United States Department of State, 2013). This protocol has since been adopted by over 150 countries (United States Department of State, 2013). The practical implementation of these laws and punishment of human traffickers' remains problematic as relatively few traffickers are prosecuted (United States Department of State, 2013). Identification of victims continues to be challenging with only approximately 40,000 victims identified worldwide in 2012 (United States Department of State, 2013).

The legislative discourse on HT has largely ignored the poor societal conditions that support labor trafficking (Alvarez & Alessi, 2012). Political activists and popular media have mostly focused on the sex trafficking of women and children (Alvarez & Alessi, 2012). Due to this narrow lens regarding HT, men trafficked for labor are often overlooked and may not receive support (Alvarez & Alessi, 2012). Alvarez and Alessi (2012) assert the importance of creating policies which address the societal conditions that support global labor exploitation in all its forms. High numerical estimates of labor trafficking victims, approximately 14.2 million worldwide, indicate the need for greater attention to labor exploitation in political arenas.

The pervasiveness of labor trafficking in virtually every formal and informal industry cannot be battled by labor laws and policies alone (Jägers & Rijken, 2014). Multinational corporations can have a significant impact on the reduction of labor trafficking by following fair labor practices that do not violate human rights (Jägers & Rijken, 2014). In 2011, the Human Rights Council of the United Nations adopted the U.N. Guiding Principles on Business and Human Rights Framework (Human Rights Council, 2011). This resolution encourages corporations to voluntarily accept responsibility for protecting human rights in the workplace. Without legal obligation, the adoption of these principles within corporations offers a transparency to labor practices (Jägers & Rijken, 2014). Multinational corporations that neglect to embrace these principles are subject to societal pressure and public scrutiny.

Although some may doubt the capability of public opinion and societal forces to curtail labor trafficking, the strength of corporate responsibility is gaining support. Fair trade labeling has met some success in curtailing child labor and unfair labor practices (Baradaran & Barclay, 2011). To obtain a fair trade label, companies voluntarily participate in private monitoring to ensure safe working conditions, adequate compensation, and healthy labor practices (Baradaran & Barclay, 2011). Fair trade labels certify that products have been manufactured and traded without child labor and meet standards for quality economic, social, and environmental conditions (Baradaran & Barclay, 2011). Fair trade labeling organizations, such as Transfair USA and Fairtrade Labelling Organization (FLO), promote greater transparency among businesses and ethical trading practices (Baradaran & Barclay, 2011). Fair trade organizations have had a significant impact on reducing child labor in the production of tea, coffee, and cocoa in various countries worldwide (Baradaran & Barclay, 2011). Creating governmental policies that support validated fair trade organizations could generate needed awareness necessary to effectively combat labor trafficking.

Policy regarding sex trafficking remains controversial due to discord regarding the varying approaches toward the regulation of the commercial sex industry. Sex worker advocates view the criminalization of prostitution as disrespecting the agency of women and limiting their ability to work (Berger, 2012). Sex worker advocates push for the legalization and regulation of prostitution to improve their ability to negotiate terms within the commercial sex industry (Marinova & James, 2012). Berger (2012) claims that emphasis on ending demand, which criminalizes buyers of sexual services, only drives commercial sex activity farther underground where potential for violence increases. Pro-worker advocates also contend that the legalization of prostitution would actually improve health services for sex workers and enhance their safety (Berger, 2012). If sex workers are lawfully engaged in the commercial sex industry, the probability of violent acts committed against them would be reduced (Berger, 2012). However, feminist and human rights advocates adamantly oppose these policies.

Varying policy approaches to sex trafficking have been implemented throughout the world. The legalization of sex work in the Netherlands and Greece has been found to actually increase the number of HT victims (Marinova & James, 2012). In the Netherlands the reported number of HT victims was 228 in 1998 (Marinova & James, 2012). By 2008, the number of HT victims had jumped to 826 (Marinova & James, 2012). Some take an abolitionist approach which views sexual exploitation, including trafficking and purchasing of sexual services, as acts of violence against a person's dignity (Marinova & James, 2012). Within this abolitionist concept individuals that engage in prostitution are viewed as victims of subjugation and objectification (Marinova & James, 2012). Qualitative evidence in Sweden suggests that the abolitionist approach decreases the purchase of sexual services (Marinova & James, 2012). Sweden applied criminalization policies that targeted the purchaser of sexual services, rather than the provider, and the trafficker (Marinova & James, 2012). In Sweden prevention measures of education and awareness campaigns were implemented to inform citizens and combat HT (Marinova & James, 2012). Although many nations have adopted the Palermo Protocol, the success of HT policies worldwide is largely dependent upon the actual implementation within each nation.

U.S. Policy

In the United States, HT has become a domestic problem with transnational dimensions. The passing of the Victims of Trafficking and Violence Protection Act (TVPA) in 2000 was a significant hurdle in the fight against HT (Polaris Project, 2014b). This legislation was similar to the Palermo Protocol in its approach to HT, with its focus on prevention of HT, prosecution of human traffickers, and protection for HT victims (Polaris Project, 2014b). This legislation mandated that HT be considered a federal crime. Under the direction of the Office of Refugee Resettlement, the Anti-trafficking in Persons Program (ATIP) was initiated in response to the TVPA. This program collaborates with several agencies nationwide to raise awareness and support victims of HT. For example, the National Human Trafficking Resource Center established a national hotline for trafficking victims and is supported by ATIP. The Office to Monitor and Combat Trafficking in Persons was also established with this legislation. Various adjustments and improvements have been made to the TVPA of 2000 with subsequent legislation. The act was reauthorized as the Trafficking Victims Protection Reauthorization Act in 2003, 2005, 2008, and 2013 (Polaris Project, 2014b). The TVPA has had a significant impact upon trafficking activity with reauthorized funding for federal anti-trafficking programs and specialized services to victims.

Challenges and Consequences of Human Trafficking

Even with strong policies to combat HT, the challenges of adequately addressing this complex issue can seem insurmountable within the context of globalization. The impact of global markets and technological advances including mechanization processes amplifies the gap between rich and poor. Multinational corporations make market decisions in the best interest of their companies without much consideration for labor opportunities, working conditions, environmental consequences, or the social costs to the surrounding community (Ross-Sheriff, 2007). Although these organizations are attempting to increase corporate responsibility related to these human and environmental factors, economic disparities continue to grow ever wider (Ross-Sheriff, 2007). As a result, low-skilled individuals living in economically developing nations become more vulnerable to HT. People searching for greater life opportunities and chances for financial stability become ensnared in precarious situations that may threaten their lives.

The accurate identification of traffickers and victims eludes law enforcement authorities and health professionals. Victims of HT may be linguistically, culturally, and geographically isolated from the community without legal documentation. The use of the Internet to conduct illicit business transactions, such as solicitation for labor or sexual services, further obscures victims from the public eye. The actual apprehension of traffickers is also impaired by HT conducted via the Internet where computer IP addresses rarely lead to an arrest. If the human trafficker can be found, victims of HT may not be interested in prosecuting their trafficker, due to fear of retaliation or possibility of deportation.

Moreover, the consequences of prolonged exposure to traumatic experiences severely impacts victims' physical and mental health. According to Oram, Stöckl, Busza, Howard, and Zimmerman (2012), possible physical consequences of HT include: headaches, fatigue, back and stomach pain, memory problems, traumatic brain injury, and sexually transmitted infections. The mental health disorders of HT victims may be similar to those that have lived in an active war zone or experienced torture (Williamson, Dutch, & Clawson, 2008). Prevalent mental health symptoms of HT victims include: anxiety, depression, suicidal ideation, and PTSD (Dovydaitis, 2010). These health consequences indicate the life-altering cost to victims of HT. Despite traumatic experiences, some victims of HT exhibit resilience and hope for the future (Faulkner et al., 2013).

To assist HT victims along the path to recovery multidisciplinary efforts are required. Law enforcement officials, medical personnel, border patrol security officers, legal professionals, community organization representatives, faith-based leaders, and mental health counselors must collaborate to confront this problem collectively. Social workers can fill the role of coordinator in arranging treatment for HT victims in the following settings: police stations, law offices, hospitals, court rooms, and mental health clinics (Busch-Armendariz, Nsonwu, & Heffron, 2014). With a mission of social justice and advocacy, social workers should be at the forefront in combating HT with a focus on interdisciplinary collaboration.

Implications for Social Work, Education, and Practice

To address the multidimensional dilemma of HT, social workers should utilize a multisystemic approach of prevention, intervention, education, training, and advocacy. Social workers should be involved in prevention programming to minimize the risk factors that increase the probability of trafficking activity. Empirically relevant interventions that are trauma-informed and culturally competent are essential components to addressing HT. As professionals, social workers should be at the forefront, educating youth and communities regarding the nature of HT and its consequences. HT must be added to social work curricula in institutions of higher learning. Human service programs will look to social workers to provide training for professionals who assist in identifying victims, making proper referrals, and providing clinical treatment. Finally, social workers need to be involved in advocating for legislation and encouraging faith-based initiatives that reduce HT.

Prevention of Human Trafficking

The precursor to eliminating HT begins with fulfilling the needs of vulnerable populations worldwide. Human traffickers generally seek to enslave those persons that are excluded from society, i.e. marginalized ethnic minorities, undocumented immigrants, the indigenous, the poor, and persons with disabilities (United States Department of State, 2013). Victims are often fraudulently lured into HT with promises of employment and a better life (Hodge & Lietz, 2007). Less frequently, recruiters approach families of those who live in poverty and purchase children with promises to their caregivers for improved opportunities for them in another country (Hodge & Lietz, 2007). In the United States, Fong and Cardoso (2010) report that "runaway, homeless, kidnapped children or children in or leaving foster care are at elevated risk of forced prostitution and trafficking" (p. 311).

The discussion for prevention of HT has rarely acknowledged the breakdown of the traditional family as a "push" factor. Strengthening the family unit through micro-credit, education, health prevention, and faith-based initiatives could significantly reduce the vulnerability of persons to HT. There are several evidence-based programs which have proven to curtail high-risk behavior of children and youth (United Nations Office on Drugs and Crime, 2013b). The implementation of these programs among vulnerable populations could have a dramatic effect on HT activity. Improving family bonds can provide protection for potential victims and diminish the propensity of adults to turn to the HT "business" for income or personal pleasure.

Creating awareness among vulnerable populations is another key to the prevention of HT. Awareness campaigns that target marginalized populations could limit the ability of traffickers to draw people into dangerous conditions. Culturally sensitive campaigns should access the most vulnerable of society, specifically reaching out to impoverished communities and rural areas. For example, within the United States January has been designated as National Slavery and HT Awareness Month (Obama, 2013).

Faith-based communities can also assist in educating their members about the prevalence and the prevention of HT. Awareness regarding signs of labor and sexual exploitation within these communities can aid in identification of victims. Faith-based leaders can work with health professionals, social service providers, and law enforcement representatives to combat HT within their local communities. Faith-based initiatives can help reduce the risk of individuals to exploitation by educating their members regarding tactics of traffickers and online safety.

Services to Victims

Proper victim identification has been a major barrier to provision of services to HT victims (United States Department of State, 2013). Victims of HT are sometimes identified as illegal immigrants or criminals and may be subject to arrest, detention, deportation, or prosecution (United States Department of State, 2013). In the United States, law enforcement officers are most likely to come across victims of HT in their line of work (Wilson et al., 2006). The call for increased victim identification training among government officials has been heard. The *Anti-Human Trafficking Manual for Criminal Justice Practitioners* identifies common experiences of HT victims and procedures to follow upon discovery of an HT victim (United Nations Office on Drugs and Crime, 2013a). The manual encourages criminal justice practitioners to refer the victim for counseling services for stabilization if deemed necessary. Social workers can liaison with law enforcement to coordinate multidimensional care that includes: medical services, counseling services, case management, housing services, legal services, income support, and employment services (United Nations Office on Drugs and Crime, 2013a).

According to Busch-Armendariz et al. (2014), using an Ecological Systems Perspective to guide service delivery for HT victims has demonstrated effectiveness. Social workers that were designated as the single point-of-contact for HT victims were able to provide "improved consistency, efficiency, and effective delivery of services that ultimately resulted in better services to survivors" (Busch-Armendariz et al., 2014, p. 13). Using this model, social workers are able to advocate for HT victims in accessing services and navigating legal processes (Busch-Armendariz et al., 2014).

During the first encounter with HT victims, social workers may utilize the *Comprehensive Human Trafficking Assessment* developed by the Polaris Project (Polaris Project, 2013d). This assessment provides a wide-range of questions for service professionals to help identify a HT victim which includes: general trafficking questions, sex trafficking questions, and labor trafficking questions (Polaris Project, 2013d). Social workers should attempt to make adjustments to the assessment for cultural sensitivity (Polaris Project, 2013d). Social workers should also be prepared to deal with multiple clinical issues of an HT victim, that is, psychological abuse, physical abuse, sexual abuse, forced or coerced use of drugs or alcohol, social restriction and emotional manipulation, economic exploitation and debt bondage, legal insecurity, and high-risk abusive working conditions (Zimmerman et al., 2011).

Currently, there are limited evidence-based interventions for the clinical treatment of HT victims. Williamson, Dutch, and Clawson (2008) report that post-traumatic stress disorder (PTSD) is the most commonly cited disorder in scholarly research on HT victims. Anxiety disorders, mood disorders, dissociative disorders, and substance-related disorders have also been identified as prevalent disorders among HT victims (Williamson, Dutch, & Clawson, 2008). Until appropriate treatments have been established researchers suggest utilizing treatments that have proven effective with similar populations, that is, migrant laborers, victims of sexual abuse and violence, and victims of torture (Williamson, Dutch, & Clawson, 2008).

Clawson, Salomon, and Grace (2008) recommend using trauma-informed services with victims of HT. Trauma-informed care includes having knowledge of the traumatic experiences of victims (Clawson, Salomon, & Grace, 2008). Trauma-informed services also provide a therapeutic framework for understanding the vulnerability of victims and the impact of multiple traumatic events (Williamson, Dutch, & Clawson, 2008). Busch-Armendariz et al. (2014) report that a victim-centered approach has enhanced services to HT victims and improved professional competency.

Fong and Cardoso (2010) suggest utilizing trauma-focused cognitive behavioral therapy (TF-CBT) with child trafficking victims. TF-CBT has been tested in random clinical trials with child sexual abuse victims for the treatment of symptoms of PTSD, depression, anxiety, and behavioral problems (Fong & Cardoso, 2010). The TF-CBT model centers on educating the client about sexual abuse and trauma during individual sessions and joint parent-child therapy sessions (Fong

& Cardoso, 2010). Relaxation skills, emotional regulation, coping skills, and safety planning are reviewed (Fong & Cardoso, 2010). TF-CBT could be extremely beneficial to child trafficking victims with modifications, for example, excluding a parental figure in sessions due to absence of one nearby (Fong & Cardoso, 2010). Further exploration regarding effectiveness with adult sex-trafficking victims and trafficked victims is warranted.

For the treatment of PTSD, there is empirical evidence for the use of cognitive-behavioral therapy (CBT) that integrates cognitive restructuring and exposure therapy (Williamson, Dutch, & Clawson, 2008). CBT has also been found effective in treatment for anxiety disorders and mood disorders (Williamson, Dutch, & Clawson, 2008). Major depressive disorder is a frequent diagnosis of HT victims (Williamson, Dutch, & Clawson, 2008). Further exploration on empirically based treatment for victims of HT is necessary.

Using empirically relevant modalities, although important, is not enough for the treatment of this especially vulnerable population. Due to the complex trauma that victims of HT have likely experienced, the use of a trauma-informed response is necessary for all service providers that may come into contact with HT victims. This involves recognizing the possible distrust and fear a victim may have of authority figures and being particularly sensitive to past experiences of trauma. Giving the victim time to process and make important life decisions (for example, regarding prosecution or self-deportation) directly after a traumatic experience is critical to obtaining relevant information. Also, the transnational nature that sometimes occurs with HT compels service providers to utilize cultural humility. The goal of the service provider should be to establish a foundation of trust and mutual respect. With this in place, victims of HT will likely experience greater success in therapeutic treatment.

Agency-Based Responses

There are few organizations that deal specifically with trafficking victims within the United States. The Salvation Army STOP-IT program is a faith-based agency that serves victims of HT in Chicago, Illinois (Knowles Wirsing, 2012). This agency uses a comprehensive model to provide crisis intervention, victim identification, training, and service coordination to victims of HT. The STOP-IT program serves male and female victims of labor and sex trafficking. In 2011, the STOP-IT program actively assisted 79 people and they continue to receive regular referrals (Knowles

Wirsing, 2012). Using a comprehensive model of treatment, that liaison with an array of community services is undoubtedly the most effective approach to intervention with victims of HT.

The Girls Educational & Mentoring Services program (GEMS) has also met some success with providing services to sexually exploited youth and children in New York City. The GEMS program provides direct intervention through short-term and crisis care, transitional and supportive housing, court advocacy, and holistic case management (GEMS, 2013). The case management services include trauma-based therapy and individual support sessions (GEMS, 2013). In addition, they provide an educational program, a youth development program, and a youth leadership program (GEMS, 2013). As part of the youth outreach program, members conduct peer-led facility outreach workshops within residential facilities and detention facilities (GEMS, 2013). Peer-led trainings are dynamic in their approach to HT. Evaluation of peer-led trainings vis-à-vis adult-led trainings might generate significant results for agency-based responses.

Education in Schools
Educational and outreach programs should be implemented in school systems to increase awareness among youth. These programs must include information about online predators and false advertisement for employment. As Internet access becomes ever more accessible, guarding against masquerading predators becomes more challenging. Seemingly legitimate job postings online can lead to entrapment. Traffickers may groom their victims over time with luxurious gifts or promises of high-paying jobs (Kotrla, 2010). Youth need to be educated regarding the sophisticated tactics that traffickers might use to lure them into possible HT or exploitation.

A harm reduction program completed in Minnesota demonstrated that educational efforts were successful in reducing the risk of girls being sexually exploited (Pierce, 2012). In combination with multilevel interventions, healthy sexuality education and peer support groups were provided (Pierce, 2012). Implementing psycho-education programs regarding HT within public school systems can inform youth of their rights. With a special emphasis on educating marginalized groups, outreach programs can enlighten individuals and help to curb HT.

Education in Institutions of Higher Learning
The topic of HT must be included in social work curricula. Thus far, the literature for health professionals

on HT has covered the following topics: trafficking definition and scope, health consequences, victim identification, appropriate treatment, referral to services, legal issues, security, and prevention (Ahn et al., 2013). These topics set the groundwork for the development of curriculum on trafficking (Ahn et al., 2013). Theoretical approaches to trafficking are also necessary. Ahn et al. (2013) suggest using the Social-Ecological Model to address this multisystemic problem. This model encourages prevention strategies be used at the individual, relationship, community, and societal levels (Centers for Disease Control and Prevention, 2009).

Social workers must be educated in trauma-informed care to provide services to victims of HT. High rates of physical and sexual violence experienced by trafficking victims (Oram et al., 2012) indicate the need for trauma-informed services. Addressing the possible multiple victimizations that trafficking victims may have experienced requires a special sensitivity to trauma.

Furthermore, social workers should receive cultural competence training to effectively work with victims of HT. Although it is impossible to learn every culture, social workers can be educated in sociocultural anthropology to limit ethnocentric perspectives. Becoming familiar with socioeconomic conditions of the HT victim prior to entrapment and cultural norms regarding labor practices, gender roles, and migration patterns would assist the social worker in better understanding victims of HT. Adding a second language component to social work curricula could also assist social workers in meeting the needs of diverse populations.

Due to the possible millions of sex addicts in America and a dearth of certified addiction counselors, sexual addiction counseling should be included in graduate and post-graduate education (Hagedorn, 2009). Hagedorn (2009), an expert in addiction treatment, suggests more institutions offer an empirical-based training protocol on sexual addiction counseling. The United States has been identified as a destination country, importing thousands of people for sexual purposes (United States Department of State, 2013; Landesman, 2003). The growth of the commercial sex industry calls for a greater therapeutic treatment response.

Training
Due to the hidden nature of HT, social workers must be trained in victim identification. The 2013 TIP Report calls for social workers to be informed "because children who have been abused at home, have

run away, are alcohol- or drug-dependent, or are in the care of child-welfare agencies are at high risk for HT" (United States Department of State, 2013). The Rescue and Restore Victims of Human Trafficking Campaign offers a list of possible clues that someone may be a victim of trafficking: "evidence of being controlled; evidence of inability to move or leave a job; bruises or other signs of battering; fear or depression; non-English speaking; recently brought to this country; and lack of passport, immigration, or identification documents (Administration for Children and Families, 2013; Dovydaitis, 2010, p. 464). Social workers must also be prepared to recognize the common health problems of victims, for example, anxiety, chronic pain, cigarette burns, complications with unsafe abortion, contusions, depression, fractures, gastrointestinal problems, headaches, oral health problems, pelvic pain, post-traumatic stress disorder, sexually transmitted infections, suicidal ideation, unhealthy weight loss, unwanted pregnancy, and vaginal pain (Dovydaitis, 2010).

Advocacy for HT Victims

Social workers and health professionals can advocate for legislation that gives stiffer penalties to traffickers and purchasers of sex. Generating awareness of HT in local communities and agencies with the use of awareness materials can help to inform victims and advocates (Polaris Project, 2014a). Social workers must be change agents at the state, national, and international levels. On an international level, the United States has taken the lead in combating HT with the creation of the Office to Monitor and Combat Trafficking in Persons (Polaris Project, 2014b). This office compiles the global Trafficking in Persons (TIP) report yearly which is an effective tool for monitoring and measuring HT throughout the world.

Conclusion

With increased globalization and mobility, HT is an expanding global health issue that largely affects marginalized populations, especially women and children. Modern day slavery is primarily driven by a lack of legal employment opportunities and unchecked capitalism. Improved employment policies in both the country of origin and the destination country would destroy the profit motive for HT. Challenging the societal conditions that support the exploitation of human beings will require a multidisciplinary approach. Collaborative efforts among law enforcement officials, medical personnel, border patrol security officers, legal professionals, community organization representatives, faith-based leaders, and mental health counselors can help to effectively address the needs of HT victims.

Social workers can serve as a point of contact among health professionals in coordinating treatment and assisting HT victims in navigating their alternatives in health care and legal systems. Social work professionals, with a mandate of social justice, should be at the forefront of prevention efforts, policy reform, educational campaigns, and empirically relevant therapeutic interventions to combat HT. By combining disciplinary efforts and multilevel approaches HT can become a phenomenon of the past.

References

Administration for Children and Families. (2013). National Human Trafficking Resource Center. Identifying and interacting with victims of human trafficking. Retrieved October 4, 2013, from http://www.acf.hhs.gov/sites/default/files/orr/tips_for_identifying_and_helping_victims_of_human_trafficking.pdf.

Ahn, R., Alpert, E. J., Purceli, G., Konstantopoulos, W. M., McGahan, A., Cafferty, E., et al. (2013). Human trafficking: Review of educational resources for health professionals. *American Journal of Preventive Medicine, 44*(3), 283–289.

Alvarez, M. B., & Alessi, E. J. (2012). Human trafficking is more than sex trafficking and prostitution: Implications for social work. *Affilia: Journal of Women & Social Work, 27*(2), 142–152. doi:10.1177/0886109912443763

Bales, K. (2004). *Disposable people: New slavery in the global economy.* Los Angeles: University of California Press.

Bales, K. (2009). Winning the fight. *Harvard International Review, 31*(1), 14–17.

Baradaran, S., & Barclay, S. (2011). Fair trade and child labor. *Columbia Human Rights Law Review, 43*(1), 1–63.

Berger, S. M. (2012). Why the "end demand" movement is the wrong focus for efforts to eliminate trafficking. *Harvard Journal of Law & Gender, 35*(2).

Blumhofer, R., Shah, N., Grodin, M., & Crosby, S. (2011). Clinical issues in caring for former chattel slaves. *Journal of Immigrant & Minority Health, 13*(2), 323–332. doi:10.1007/s10903-008-9217-4

Bryant-Davis, T., Tillman, S., Marks, A., & Smith, K. (2009). Millennium abolitionists: Addressing the sexual trafficking of African women. *Beliefs & Values 1*(1), 69–78. doi:10.1891/1942-0617.1.1.69

Busch-Armendariz, N., Nsonwu, M. B., & Heffron, L. C. (2014). A kaleidoscope: The role of the social work practitioner and the strength of social work theories and practice in meeting the complex needs of people trafficked and the professionals that work with them. *International Social Work, 57*(1), 7–18. doi:10.1177/0020872813505630.

Centers for Disease Control and Prevention. (2009). The social-ecological model: a framework for prevention. Retrieved July 23, 2014, from www.cdc.gov/ViolencePrevention/overview/social-ecologicalmodel.html.

Clawson, H. J., Salomon, A., & Grace, L. G. (2008). *Treating the hidden wounds: Trauma treatment and mental health recovery for victims of human trafficking*. Washington, DC: Office of the Assistant Secretary for Planning and Evaluation, U.S. Department of Health and Human Services. Retrieved February 26, 2014, from http://aspe.hhs.gov/hsp/07/humantrafficking/Treating/ib.htm

Dovydaitis, T. (2010). Human trafficking: The role of the health care provider. *Journal of Midwifery & Women's Health, 55*(5). doi:10.1016/j.jmwh.2009.12.017.

Faulkner, M., Mahapatra, N., Heffron, L. C., Nsonwu, M. B., & Busch-Armendariz, N. (2013). Moving past victimization and trauma toward restoration: Mother survivors of sex trafficking share their inspiration. *International Perspectives in Victimology, 7*(2), 46–55. doi:10.5364/ipiv.7.2.46.

Fong, R., & Cardoso, J. B. (2010). Child human trafficking victims: Challenges for the child welfare system. *Evaluation and Program Planning, 33*(3), 311–316. doi: 10.1016/j.evalprogplan.2009.06.018

Girl's Education & Mentoring Services (GEMS). (2013). Retrieved September 25, 2013, from http://www.gems-girls.org

Hagedorn, W. B. (2009). Sexual addiction counseling competencies: empirically-based tools for preparing clinicians to recognize, assess, and treat sexual addiction. *Sexual Addiction & Compulsivity, 16*(3), 190–209. doi:10.1080/10720160903202604.

Hodge, D. R., & Lietz, C. A. (2007). The international sexual trafficking of women and children. A review of the literature. *Affilia: Journal of Women and Social Work, 22*(2), 163–174.

Human Rights Council. (2011). Guiding principles on business and human rights: Implementing the United Nations "Protect, Respect and Remedy" framework. Retrieved July 15, 2013, from http://businesshumanrights.org/sites/default/files/media/documents/ruggie/ruggie-guiding-principles-21-mar-2011.pdf

International Labour Office. (2013). Victims of forced labour by region. Retrieved January 1, 2014, from http://www.ilo.org/global/about-the-ilo/newsroom/news/WCMS_181961/lang–en/index.htm

Jägers, N., & Rijken, C. (2014). Prevention of human trafficking for labor exploitation: The role of corporations. *Journal of International Human Rights, 12*(1), 47–73.

Kara, S. (2009). *Sex trafficking: Inside the business of modern slavery*. Chichester, NY: Columbia University Press.

Knowles Wirsing, E. (2012). Outreach, collaboration and services to survivors of human trafficking: The Salvation Army STOP-IT Program's work in Chicago, Illinois. *Social Work & Christianity, 39*(4), 466–480.

Kotrla, K. (2010). Domestic minor sex trafficking in the United States. *Social Work, 55*(2), 181–187. doi:10.1093/sw/55.2.181

Landesman, P. (2003). Collaborations: The key to combating human trafficking. *The Police Chief, 70*(2), 28–74.

Lusk, M., & Lucas, F. (2009). The challenge of human trafficking and contemporary slavery. *Journal of Comparative Social Welfare, 25*(1), 49–57. doi:10.1080/17486830802514049

Marinova, N. K., & James, P. (2012). The tragedy of human trafficking: Competing theories and European evidence. *Foreign Policy Analysis, 8*(3), 231–253. doi:10.1111/j.1743-8594.2011.00162.x

Obama, B. (2013). Presidential proclamation—National slavery and human trafficking prevention month, 2014. Retrieved January 13, 2014, from http://www.whitehouse.gov/the-press-office/2013/12/31/presidential-proclamation-national-slavery-and-human-trafficking-prevent

Oram, S., Stöckl, H., Busza, J., Howard, L. M., & Zimmerman, C. (2012). Prevalence of risk and violence and the physical, mental, and sexual health problems associated with human trafficking: systematic review. *PLoS Med., 9*(5). doi:10.1371/journal.pmed.1001224

Pierce, A. S. (2012). American Indian adolescent girls: Vulnerability to sex trafficking, intervention strategies. *American Indian and Alaska Native Mental Health Research (Online), 19*(1), 37–56.

Polaris Project. (2013a). Labor trafficking in the United States. Retrieved January 1, 2014, from http://www.polarisproject.org/human-trafficking/labor-trafficking-in-the-us.

Polaris Project. (2013b). Labor trafficking: traveling sales crews at-a-glance. Retrieved January 18, 2014, from http://www.polarisproject.org/resources/resources-by-topic/labor-trafficking.

Polaris Project. (2013c). Sex trafficking in the U.S. Retrieved January 18, 2014, from http://www.polarisproject.org/human-trafficking/sex-trafficking-in-the-us.

Polaris Project. (2013d). *Comprehensive human trafficking assessment*. Retrieved October 9, 2013, from http://www.polarisproject.org/resources/tools-for-service-providers-and-law-enforcement

Polaris Project. (2014a). Outreach and awareness materials. Retrieved January 13, 2014, from http://www.polarisproject.org/resources/outreach-and-awareness-materials.

Polaris Project. (2014b). Current federal laws. Retrieved January 14, 2014, from http://www.polarisproject.org/what-we-do/policy-advocacy/national-policy/current-federal-laws

Roby, J. L. (2005). Women and children in the global sex trade: Toward more effective policy. *International Social Work, 48*(2), 136–147.

Roby, J., & Bergquist, K. (2014). Editorial. *International Social Work, 57*(1), 3–6. doi:10.1177/0020872813506357.

Ross-Sheriff, F. (2007). Globalization as a women's issue revisited. *Affilia: Journal of Women & Social Work*, 133–137.

Schlein, L. (2014, March 13). UN campaigns to end recruitment of child soldiers. Retrieved from http://www.voanews.com/content/un-campaigns-to-end-recruitment-of-child-soldiers/1870550.html

United Nations Office on Drugs and Crime. (2012). *Global report on trafficking in persons 2012*. Retrieved October 8, 2014, from http://www.unodc.org/documents/data-and-analysis/glotip/Trafficking_in_Persons_2012_web.pdf

United Nations Office on Drugs and Crime. (2013a). *Anti-human trafficking manual for criminal justice practitioners*. Retrieved October 8, 2013, from http://www.unodc.org/documents/human-trafficking/TIP_module3_Ebook.pdf

United Nations Office on Drugs and Crime. (2013b). *Compilation of evidence-based family skills training programmes.* Retrieved September 18, 2013, from http://www.coe.int/t/dg3/children/corporalpunishment/positive%20parenting/UNODCFamilySkillsTrainingProgrammes.pdf.

United States Department of State. (2000). Victims of trafficking and violence protection act of 2000. Public law 106–386, 28 October 2000. Retrieved January 1, 2014, from http://www.state.gov/documents/organization/10492.pdf

United States Department of State. (2013). *Trafficking in persons report.* Retrieved September 21, 2013, from http://www.state.gov/j/tip/rls/tiprpt/2013/index.htm.

Victims of Trafficking and Violence Protection Act of 2000, P.L. 106–386, 114 Stat. 1464 (2000).

Williamson, E., Dutch, N. M., & Clawson, H. J. (2008). *Evidence-based mental health treatment for victims of human trafficking.* Washington, DC: Office of the Assistant Secretary for Planning and Evaluation, U.S. Department of Health and Human Services. Retrieved October 9, 2013, from http://aspe.hhs.gov/hsp/07/humantrafficking/mentalhealth/index.pdf

Wilson, D. G., Walsh, W. F., & Kleuber, S. (2006). Trafficking in human beings: Training and services among US law enforcement agencies. *Police Practice and Research, 7*(2), 149–160.

Zimmerman, C., Hossain, M., & Watts, C. (2011). Human trafficking and health: A conceptual model to inform policy, intervention, and research. *Social Science and Medicine, 73,* 327–335.

FARIYAL ROSS-SHERIFF AND JULIE ORME

I

IMMIGRATION POLICY

ABSTRACT: Individuals and families from around the globe form a continuous stream of immigrants to the United States, with waiting lists for entry stretching to several years. Reasons for this ongoing influx are readily apparent, because the United States is one of the most attractive nations in the world, regardless of its problems. There is much in the United States that native-born Americans take for granted and that is not available in most other countries, and there are several amenities, opportunities, possibilities, lifestyles, and freedoms in the United States (U.S.) that are not found together in any other nation. In theory, and often in reality, the U.S. is a land of freedom, of equality, of opportunity, of a superior quality of life, of easy access to education, and of relatively few human rights violations. The focus here is on immigration policy through legislative history and its impact, demographic trends, the economic impact, the immigrant workforce, educational and social service systems, ethical issues, and roles for social workers.

KEY WORDS: demographic trends; economics; ethics; immigration policy; service systems; social capital; workforce

Overview of Immigration to the United States

Individuals and families from around the globe form a continuous stream of immigrants to the United States, with waiting lists for entry stretching to several years. Unauthorized immigrants abound, and refugees and asylees arrive in record numbers. People of color from Asia, Africa, and Central and South America have been disproportionately represented in recent years, and an overwhelming majority remains despite encountering a series of barriers. Reasons for this ongoing influx are readily apparent, because the United States is one of the most attractive nations in the world, regardless of its problems. There is much in the United States that native-born Americans take for granted that is not available in most other countries, and there are many amenities, opportunities, possibilities, lifestyles, and freedoms in the United States that are not found together in any other nation. In theory, and often in reality, the U.S. is a land of freedom, equality,

opportunity, a superior quality of life, easy access to education, and relatively few human rights violations. It is a land that, in the early 21st century, is struggling toward multiculturalism and pluralism in its institutions and social outlook. It is a land that, compared to others, offers newcomers a relatively easy path through which to become integrated into its largesse.

Although individuals may wish to emigrate, immigration is highly contingent on the receptiveness of the potential host nation to immigrants in general, and immigrants from specific countries in particular. Most governments now have strict immigration laws; this was not always the case and people were relatively free to live where they chose. U.S. immigration history, since the mid-18th century, has been impacted by legislation that has substantially colored the face of immigration in the last two and a half centuries.

Legislative History and Its Impact

U.S. immigration history may be divided into seven periods during which legal measures allowed or controlled the categories of people allowed to immigrate (Kim, 1994, pp. 8–9).

1. *The colonial period (1609–1775)*: Most immigrants were from the British Isles, and the colonies had little control over immigration.
2. *The American Revolutionary period (1776–1840)*: European immigration slowed because of war; there were general anti-foreign feelings.
3. *The "old" immigration period (1841–1882)*: Local governments recruited people from Northern Europe. Chinese could also immigrate.
4. *The regulation period (1882–1920)*: Chinese were prevented from immigrating. Immigrants that were admitted were primarily from Central, Eastern, and Southern Europe.
5. *The restriction and exclusion period (1921–1952)*: A quota system restricted immigration from Central, Eastern, and Southern Europe; all Asians were excluded.
6. *The partial liberalization period (1952–1965)*: Asia had the same quota as Central, Eastern, and Southern Europe, and all were allowed naturalization.
7. *The liberalized policy period (1965 to present)*: The quota policy was repealed, allowing entry to immigrants from developing countries.

Given below are brief sketches of immigration-related legislation or action (USCIS, 2012) that, since the beginning of the liberalization period, have affected diverse populations in a variety of ways, from entry into the U.S. itself to access to fundamental rights.

Since 2007, there have been a series of unsuccessful attempts to pass additional federal immigration legislation that would limit entry, particularly that of unauthorized migrants, and that would make it more difficult for family reunification entries. Proposals for the abolition of employer-sponsored visas in lieu of a merit-based point system, such as those used by Canada and Australia, have also failed to receive sufficient legislative support. Hence, despite the years of discussion and deliberation between 2007 and 2012, the Comprehensive Immigration Reform Act of 2007 is the last piece of viable federal immigration legislation.

The DREAM Act (Development, Relief and Education for Alien Minors Act) was proposed in 2001 and was expected to provide a path to citizenship for children brought to the country illegally; it has been forestalled in deliberations for over a decade. In an attempt to recognize the lack of culpability of minors who were brought into the nation without requisite papers, President Barack Obama announced some relief for unauthorized immigrant children in June 2012. The Obama administration announced that it would not deport unauthorized immigrants that were brought to the United States as children before the age of 16, had no criminal record, and had lived in the U.S. for at least five years; further, such immigrants would receive a two-year work permit and would be permitted to enroll in institutions of higher learning. Although this policy provides relief to approximately 1.7 million unauthorized young people (National Conference of State Legislators [NCSL], 2012b), it does not allow a path to citizenship, and the DREAM Act has yet to pass the House and the Senate.

Most promising, in 2013, is the Bipartisan Framework for Comprehensive Immigration Reform drafted by the "Gang of 8" that proposes four basic pillars of legislation (Preston, 2013): 1. Creating a path to citizenship for unauthorized immigrants already living in the United States; 2. Reforming the legal immigration system to attract and keep the world's brightest and best workers; 3. Strengthening the employment verification system; and 4. Improving the process for admitting new workers and protecting their rights.

While details will need to be drafted, the bipartisan "Gang," which is composed of Republican Senators John McCain (Arizona), Lindsey Graham (South Carolina), Marco Rubio (Florida), and Jeff Flake (Arizona) and Democratic Senators Richard Durbin (Illinois), Charles Schumer (New York), Robert Menendez (New Jersey), and Michael Bennet (Colorado), suggests that this framework may be more palatable to both Democrats and Republicans. The proposal aims to address the failings of the immigration system in a comprehensive manner, rather than piecemeal (see *http://s3.documentcloud.org/documents/562528/reform0128principlessenatefinal.pdf*).

1965	*The Immigration and Nationality Act (INA)* liberalized immigration and repealed legal discrimination on the basis of race, gender, nationality, place of birth, or place of residence. While this act has been amended several times, it remains essentially unchanged.
1980	*The Refugee Act* removed refugees as a preference category. The president and Congress determined the annual ceiling and country distributions (ceilings have ranged from 50,000–90,000 immigrants per year).
1986	*The Immigration Reform and Control Act (IRCA)* legalized many unauthorized immigrants but made it unlawful to hire unauthorized workers.
1990	*The Immigration Act of 1990* increased the number of annual immigrants to 700,000 and established the Immigrant Investor Program, which was the most major change to the INA of 1965.
1996	*Welfare Reform* ended many cash and medical assistance programs for most legal immigrants.
1996	*The Illegal Immigration Reform and Immigrant Responsibility Act (IIRIRA)* expanded enforcement operations of the Immigration and Naturalization Service (INS).
2001	*The USA Patriot Act*, in response to the September 11, 2001, terror attacks on New York and Washington, DC, gave federal officials greater power to intercept national and international communications.
2007	*Comprehensive Immigration Reform Act of 2007* attempted to curtail and address the presence of unauthorized immigrants.

Implications of the Immigration and Nationality Act of 1965

The 1965 Immigration and Nationality Act had a major and permanent impact on U.S. immigration, dramatically altering the traditional immigrant origins and numbers. Prior to 1965 and the amendments of October 3rd to the Immigration Act of 1924 and the Immigration and Nationality Act of 1952, which resulted in the liberalization of immigration laws, the majority of entrants into the United States were from European countries. The 1965 amendments (i) abolished national origins quota; (ii) established preferences for relatives of citizens and permanent residents; (iii) exempted immediate relatives of citizens and some special groups (for example, certain ministers of religion, former employees of U.S. government abroad); and (iv) expanded limits of world coverage to a 20,000 per country limit, the influx of newcomers from non-European countries was and continues to be unprecedented.

Although with frequent minor modifications, the Immigration Act of October 1, 1965, directs U.S. immigration. More significantly, while INA, ACT 202, identifies the numerical limitation for foreign states, it includes in it a non-discrimination clause, stating, "no person shall receive any preference or priority or be discriminated against in the issuance of an immigrant visa because of the person's race, sex, nationality, place of birth, or place of residence" (USCIS, 2012).

The numbers of immigrants admitted legally are (a) fixed by law; (b) limited only by demands for those considered eligible; and (c) restricted by processing constraints (Gordon, 2005). The INA Act specifies between 416,000 and 675,000 immigrant annual limits. The limits for each fiscal year can be found at the website of the U.S. Department of State and fall into the three categories of family-sponsored immigrants (226,000), employment-based immigrants (144,951), and diversity immigrants (55,000) (U.S. Department of State, 2012).

A substantial number of legal immigrants include those who are not subject to these numerical limits, such as parents, spouses, and children of U.S. citizens and children born abroad to permanent residents. In 2011, 453,158 parents, spouses, and children of U.S. citizens were granted immigration, and in the same year, another 633 immigrant visas were given to children who were born to permanent residents who were living abroad when the children were born (Monger & Yankay, 2012). A unique addition to the immigration quota is the "investor program" that issues approximately 10,000 visas annually to those who are willing to invest one million dollars in urban areas or $500,000 in rural areas of the United States.

Immigration-related State Laws

In an interesting twist, the United States is seeing unique and multiple interpretations of immigration law. Immigration to a country is defined and circumscribed by federal or national policies. Immigration laws identify who can enter a country and under what conditions. Once immigrants are in the host country, immigrant policies (which sometimes vary among states) determine what resources the immigrants may access and what programs and services are available as they integrate themselves with the host culture. Approximately twice a year, the NCSL releases reports on immigration-related laws introduced or enacted by states; some laws apply to legal immigrants and refugees, while others attempt to manage the unauthorized immigrant population. In the first half of 2012, the state legislatures sponsored 948 bills and resolutions and enacted 206; nevertheless, this was a 40% drop in proposed legislation compared to the number of bills introduced during the same period in 2011, and a 20% drop in enacted legislation. The legislation covered a variety of areas, including budgets, education, employment, health, human trafficking, IDs/driver's license, law enforcement, public benefits, and voting, among others (NCSL, 2012a).

The Arizona Immigration Law SB 1070 (NYT, 2012), which aimed to discourage or keep unauthorized immigrants from the state, was among the most significant and controversial of state immigration-related laws. This law expanded the authority of state police to investigate immigration status and required individuals to carry immigration papers at all times and be subject to detention as deemed appropriate by police officers. In April 2012, the Supreme Court overturned most of the law but declined to reject the provision that authorized police officers ask for immigration papers if they believed there was reason for suspicion.

Five states—Alabama, Georgia, Indiana, South Carolina, and Utah—have enacted laws similar to that of Arizona. These states, along with Arizona, currently are facing class action suits regarding the constitutionality of these laws and the authority of states to enforce immigration laws, which should be the exclusive jurisdiction of the federal government.

Demographic Trends

Newcomers to the United States enter under a variety of conditions. Early migrants of the 18th and 19th centuries came as volunteer immigrants, indentured laborers, or slaves; most migrants of the early 20th century were volunteer immigrants—most were considered "legal immigrants," particularly in the absence of any legislation. Present-day immigrants may be categorized as voluntary immigrants (legal or unauthorized) or as refugees (and asylees). Many legal immigrants, after a minimum length of residence in the country, choose to apply for U.S. citizenship.

The U.S. Census Bureau indicated that in 2011, of the approximately 311.5 million residents of the country, 40.4 million (13%) were foreign born. On October 17, 2006, the population of the United States reached the 300 million mark, and this increase was a result of immigration in addition to birthrate. Of the 40.4 million foreign born individuals in the U.S. in 2011, 21.1% were from Europe, 28.6% were from Asia, 52.6% were from Latin America, and 6.7% were from other regions, including Africa. The largest number of migrants from any one country is from Mexico, but this still accounts for less than a quarter of the total entrants. Hence, it is essential that, while recognizing the strong Mexican presence in the United States, one remain cognizant of the diversity of immigrants.

Among those who voluntarily migrate to the United States are immigrants without the requisite papers, who are known as unauthorized (often used interchangeably with "undocumented" and "illegal") immigrants. While there is no valid method of counting unauthorized immigrants, estimates suggest numbers of about 11.2 million (Passel & Cohn, 2011). These immigrants are people who are in the United States without governmental approval and are sometimes described as economic refugees, although they are not so recognized by the United Nations High Commissioner for Refugees. Although unauthorized immigrants lack the legal documentation to continue residing in the United States, they may have entered the country either legally or illegally. Despite perceptions of unauthorized immigrants as migrants who slip across borders without appropriate documentation, a large proportion (between 40% and 50% of all unauthorized immigrants, particularly from Asian countries) are "overstays" who fail to leave when the period of their visas expires; in 2011, the Department of Homeland Security (DHS) reported that it was in the process of dealing with the backlog of 1.6 million overstayed visas (Department of Homeland Security, 2011), and this number refers only to the overstays about which DHS is aware.

Refugees and asylees, unlike immigrants, are usually involuntary migrants. The United States has always been a refuge for those fleeing from persecution and accommodates the largest number of the world's refugees (Mayadas & Segal, 2000; Segal, 2010). The 1951 convention and the 1967 protocol setting forth the mandate of the United Nations High Commission for Refugees identifies refugees as persons outside their homelands who are unable to return because of fear of persecution. The U.S. president, in consultation with Congress, establishes annual numbers and allocations of refugees based on the current political climate of the world. In recent years, these annual numbers have varied from 70,000 to 91,000. The 70,000 refugee ceiling for 2013 is allocated as follows: Africa, 12,000; East Asia, 17,000; Europe and Central Asia, 2,000; Latin America and the Caribbean, 5,000; Near East and South Asia, 31,000; and the unallocated reserve, 3,000 (Obama, 2012).

Asylees differ from refugees in that they usually enter the United States on their own volition without prior approval. Once within the United States, they apply for asylum and are detained until a determination is made regarding their legal admission as refugees or repatriation to their homelands. If refugees are legally admitted, then they may apply for a status adjustment to that of permanent resident after a year. In throwback fashion to earlier migration periods of the early 20th century, the U.S. is beginning to see three additional groups of migrants—victims of human smuggling, victims of human trafficking, and mail-order brides.

The guest worker program was part of the 2007 Immigration Reform Bill that permitted temporary workers to enter the country for a period of up to six years to assume jobs for which U.S. employers were unable to find native employees. It has been subject to a variety of interpretations and continues to be a pawn in the political arena. In reality, a "guest worker" program has unofficially long been in existence. This pattern of immigration is known as circular migration (Miller, 2009; Zuniga, 2006); however, the difference now, increasingly, is that seasonal workers are choosing to remain in the United States because cross-border movement has become extremely dangerous (Zuniga, 2006), as any daily news report will reveal. Furthermore, migration (both authorized and otherwise) from Mexico is waning, with a net migration rate of zero (Stephens, 2012), as dangers increase and economic opportunities in the United States decline. As economic opportunities increase in traditionally sending countries, migration researchers report two phenomena that are evidencing themselves more frequently—return migration as immigrants return permanently to their homelands several years, or even decades, after emigrating, and transnational migration, where individuals and families divide their time between their countries of origin and the United States.

Regardless of the process and reasons for immigration to the United States, for most, a primary impetus is economic opportunity. Few rarely sever ties with their homelands, and a significant number sends remittances to support family members, organizations, or communities.

Economic Impact of Immigration

Many deliberations in the United States surround migration's economic impact. The ongoing immigration debate juggles arguments regarding assets newcomers bring with those about drains they place on the infrastructure. The country is divided on the current net worth of immigration in the 21st century.

The Immigrant Workforce

The continuing focus on immigration reform and the guest worker program has drawn overwhelming focus toward unauthorized workers. However, of the 40+ million documented immigrants in the United States, over 23 million are employed, and approximately 15 million are children, or in the armed forces, or not in the labor force; only 2.2 million are unemployed. They are found across the occupational structure. While legal immigrants constituted 13% of the population in 2011 and were 15.7% of the labor force, 16.4% lived in poverty (U.S. Census Bureau, 2011). Between 2009 and 2010, foreign-born workers gained 657,000 jobs and native-born workers gained 685,000 jobs, with unemployment rates falling for both groups; the former reported an unemployment rate of 9.9%, while the latter indicated one of 9.0% (Kochhar, 2011). Many big businesses, construction companies, agriculturists, and employers in service industries contend that the absence of immigrant workers would cause a major catastrophe in the U.S. economy. These groups specifically refer to the absence of the unauthorized workforce (Caulfield, 2006). Unauthorized workers are estimated to fill 25% of all agricultural jobs, 17% of office and house cleaning jobs, 14% of construction jobs, and 12% of food preparation jobs. Estimates suggest that about an average of 280,000 unauthorized immigrants have entered the U.S. annually, between 2000 and 2011. The majority (73%) is believed to be from Latin America, 59% from Mexico, 16% from other countries in Central America and South America, and 10% from Asian countries (Hoefer, Rytina & Baker, 2012).

The United States is severely divided about the presence of unauthorized immigrants. Border enforcement has been heightened consistently since 1990, and especially so since 2007. Despite laws regarding workplace immigration enforcement, it still appears to have relatively low priority. Nevertheless, the Office of Homeland Security has been attempting to increase vigilance, and reported that it made 520 criminal arrests related to worksite enforcement investigations in 2012 (ICE, 2013). This is a change from 2004, when only three companies received penalty notices, down from 417 in 1999 (Portes, 2006).

While business leaders and immigration advocates believe deportation of unauthorized workers would cause a collapse in the U.S. economy (Ohlemacher, 2006), other experts suggest that more U.S. citizens would apply for some jobs filled by migrant workers if wage exploitation was less prevalent and if higher wages were offered. Low wages for immigrants are not limited to blue-collar occupations. Immigrants that enter the United States on the "high-tech" H-1B visa are usually at the bottom of the pay scale for their positions. Despite the Department of Labor's (DOL) legal equity requirements (Department of Labor, 2012), H-1B immigrants have been known to earn $13,000 less than their American counterparts (Miano, 2005).

Brain Gain Versus Brain Drain

Contrary to Emma Lazarus's wonderfully touching poem etched upon the Statue of Liberty, the majority of individuals who undertake the challenge of migration to an alien land are rarely those without substantial human capital, at least in terms of psychological, intellectual, and physical capabilities. Most immigrants move to enhance their opportunities, often coming to study and eventually adjusting to immigrant visa status, thus bringing resources that are beneficial to the United States. This process, long known as the "brain drain," is now recognized as a "brain gain" for host countries. The 2010 census indicates that college educated individuals account for 26.8% of the foreign-born population in the United States, suggesting a fairly substantial drain from countries of emigration to add to the resources of the United States. Recent lists of Nobel Prize winners reveal a disproportionate number were born outside the United States.

The brain drain indirectly helps build capacity in the country of origin as expatriates remit money to family members and communities in the homeland, helping to offset poverty for poorer or less-educated family members and communities (IOM, 2009), thus adding to economic movement in the homeland. These remittances can be quite substantial; for example, in 2011, worldwide remittances were over 370 billion dollars, and remittances to Mexico, primarily from the United States, topped 23 billion dollars (Diaz & Ng, 2012). Furthermore, recently a "reverse brain drain" is causing concern as both native-born and first-generation (immigrant) Americans are taking their college degrees and experience and moving to better opportunities outside the United States (Lee, 2011).

Less is known about the extent of "brain waste" and about a very new and emerging idea that has burgeoned with the ease of international mobility and communications, "brain circulation." When individuals occupy positions that are not commensurate with their education, training, and expertise, it reflects a wastage of talent, hence, the concept of "brain waste." Some entry barriers prevent individuals from accessing the professional stature that they may have achieved in their home countries. For example, if there is no reciprocity in credentialing or if credentials, such as licenses, are not transferable, immigrants may be unable to invest the time and money to re-credential themselves in the U.S. while earning enough to sustain themselves and their families. Literature suggests that educated immigrants from Latin America and Eastern Europe are more likely to find themselves in low skill occupations than are those from Asia and industrialized nations (Mattoo, Neagu & Özden, 2008). With economic changes around the globe, enterprising young professionals are seeing fit to utilize opportunities in several nations to augment their entrepreneurial endeavors Teferra (2005), in fact, suggests that to presume "brain drain" versus "brain gain" is outmoded, because the information superhighway "has conquered barriers of time and space" (p. 229), thus allowing nations to avail themselves of migrant knowledge and skills regardless of the country in which these individuals reside.

Impact of Migration Policies: Implications for Social Work

IMMIGRANT INFLUENCES ON THE UNITED STATES AND THE NATIVE-BORN As immigrants enter and adapt to life in the United States, they bring with them a diversity of cultures and norms. The nation influences these New Americans, but it is also influenced by their social norms, family patterns, art, music, dance, cuisine, and businesses that sometimes challenge American traditions. In addition, immigrants affect social work and human services, both as service providers and users, so focusing solely on immigrant adaptation provides a partial picture (Fong & Greene, 2009; Elliott, Segal & Mayadas, 2010).

Impact on Health, Education, and Social Service Systems

HEALTH SYSTEMS U.S. health policy and health coverage have particular implications for those in poverty, those who are near poverty, and those of low socioeconomic status and income who are self-employed. The last group is the least likely to be able to afford private insurance coverage, yet it is ineligible for means-tested coverage such as Medicaid, and the non-coverage rate is higher for minorities. Large segments

of the immigrant population are self-employed, and the exorbitant costs of private insurance correlates with low insurance coverage. Furthermore, certain segments of the new immigrant populations are likely to be poor and remain poor because they have higher levels of unemployment, less education, and larger families than do native-born groups (Haniffa, 1999), groups in other socioeconomic segments, and those who have been in the U.S. for longer periods of time (Segal, 2010). U.S. healthcare policy, hotly contested at present and labeled the "Affordable Care Act," may have important implications for immigrants, particularly for those who are underemployed.

Implications of health policy for immigrants are not limited to issues of coverage; several other cultural and educational concerns confound access to health-care services. Health policy also should address service utilization. General health-care access is fraught with problems for many immigrant groups, and these are exacerbated by the implementation of the 1995 Federal Welfare Reform law (H. R. 3734). Even immigrants that have good health-care coverage may be less knowledgeable about the availability of programs and services, more suspicious of different treatment methods, uncomfortable with interaction patterns with health-care providers, confused by insurance programs and reimbursement procedures, and less likely to utilize preventive measures. Thus, when a large segment of the immigrant population finally does access health-care services, it may be through the already overburdened emergency rooms or through practitioners who are unprepared to communicate with them, either because of language differences or because of cultural barriers. Social work, with its focus on cultural sensitivity and competence, is particularly well placed to mediate between immigrant patients, their families, and the health-care system, by interpreting the process and helping to lessen cross-cultural difficulties.

EDUCATIONAL SYSTEMS The national policy (20 USCS, Sec. 1221–1 [1999]) states that "every citizen is entitled to an education...without financial barriers" (p. 10).

Referring to federal immigration policies, Congress noted in 20 USCS, Sec. 7402–1 (1999) that the population of language-minority Americans in the United States speak almost all the world's languages and that many children and young people have limited English proficiency. In the 1960s, the debate surrounding bilingual education resulted in the Bilingual Education Act of 1968, which was a result of federal acknowledgement that there are several limited English proficiency children in the United States; it was believed that if these children were offered education also in their own languages, it would ease their transition into the U.S. educational system and allow them to gradually acquire the English language (Stewner-Manzanares, 1988). Congress recommended that elementary and secondary schools be strengthened with bilingual education, language-enhancement, and language-acquisition programs; however, recent immigrant backlash has resulted in "English only" resolutions in a number of states. Congress also proposed an emergency immigrant education policy to help immigrant children who lack English language skills to make the transition. Free public education to the secondary level is available to all U.S. residents, and schooling is mandated for all children under the age of 16 years. This mandate (and access) applies to all immigrant children, regardless of immigration status. Social work practitioners must determine how they will address the English language issue for non-English speaking clients. Becoming functional in a new language in adulthood is difficult, and as social workers provide services to those with poor English skills, they must assess their positions in the language debate, because it affects intervention.

SOCIAL SERVICE SYSTEMS While some immigrants have benefited from the Social Security Act, changes in eligibility mandated by Congress in 1996 specifically limited access, particularly to cash assistance and medical benefits, until immigrants have been in the country a certain length of time. The Personal Responsibility and Work Opportunity Reconciliation Act (PRWORA) of August 22, 1996 (10 Statutes-at-Large 2105), lists the following restrictions for "qualified" immigrants who entered the United States after that date.

Barred from SSI and food stamps. In 1996, when President Clinton signed the PRWORA, most immigrants became ineligible for several governmental programs for the first five years following their migration to the country. Thus, most immigrants are subject to a five-year bar on non-emergency Medicaid, the Child Health Insurance Program (CHIP), Temporary Assistance for Needy Families (TANF), Social Security Supplemental Security Income (SSI), and food stamps. Exemption for one year is offered for some battered spouses and children, and for those at risk of going hungry or becoming homeless. After the five-year bar, states still retain the option to determine immigrant eligibility for TANF, Medicaid, and social service block grants.

The changes mandated through PRWORA effectively bar qualified needy families, the elderly, and women with dependent children from applying for assistance. Census figures suggest that the number of needy families and elderly is sizable, and that the laws have resulted in both economic and psychological difficulties for them (Clarke, 2004). While there is some literature that indicates that, in general, social welfare services are minimally accessed by immigrants (Kretsedemas, 2003) for a number of cultural reasons, among them shame in seeking assistance from outside the family and fear and distrust of governmental authority, other studies have found that use of food stamps and Medicaid is proportionately higher among immigrant groups than the native-born population (Camarota, 2011). Thus, the social services often maintain the misconception that immigrants have few needs or that the family or immigrant community can address their needs. It may be necessary for social workers to take the lead in outreach efforts, recognizing that invisibility may not be synonymous with absence of need.

Readiness of Receiving Country for Immigrants: Social Capital

Immigration policies (that is, the laws that determine who is eligible to enter the country) and immigrant policies (that is, the laws and programs that reflect how immigrants are received once they are in the country) should be differentiated. The former are federally regulated and apply across the nation, while the latter are highly dependent on state and local programs and local public perceptions and can show a great deal of variability. Many immigrant policies are instrumental in determining how well human capital is nurtured and developed.

The readiness of a receiving country to accept immigrants in general or an immigrant group in particular is a complex matter. When immigration is viewed as inextricably bound to a nation's political, economic, and social well being, as well as to its future security interests, it is likely to be welcomed. Nevertheless, the immigration policies of many countries are temporal, reflecting what is believed to be of benefit at a particular moment. Nations also fulfill international agreements in the resettlement or provision of asylum to large numbers of refugees, to facilitate government action, and for humanitarian reasons. Policies that allow immigration often are coupled with those that permit the expulsion or deportation of foreign nationals.

Social capital, "the internal social and cultural coherence of society, the norms and values that govern interactions among people and the institutions in which they are embedded" (Serageldin, 1999, Elliott et al., 2010), is essential in ensuring that opportunities within a nation are strong and viable. It is a necessity in the creation of human capital (Coleman, 1988), and immigrants' adjustment is often linked to the social capital available to them. For successful integration, the nation's welfare policies should guarantee that all immigrants have access to appropriate public welfare services and subsidies, and that they are connected to private welfare programs as necessary.

Availability of and accessibility to social capital are paramount in the successful settlement of immigrants in their country of adoption. In addition to providing new arrivals with economic subsidies, housing, and health care, community-based educational programs and training can provide the components for new immigrants to move away from dependency on society's support programs (Lobo & Mayadas, 1997). Hence, immigrants' knowledge about disease prevention, their ability to function through society's institutional structures, and their earning capacity in the legitimate economy of the country will enhance their likelihood of self-sufficiency. Social and mental health services that recognize the difficulties associated with the immigration experience can assist immigrants in their adjustment to the receiving country. Resistance, communication barriers, personal and family background, and ethnic community identity (Lum, 2004) are exacerbated by the experience of many immigrants and refugees, who closely guard information because of fear (perhaps unfounded) of exposure, past experience with oppression, and mistrust of authority. A number of immigrants and most refugees arrive from nations in turmoil in which they do not have the freedom of speech or of choice, and many continue to fear deportation from the United States.

Ethical Issues
In addition to the several ethical issues that confront social workers on a regular basis, the major issue that they must resolve for themselves is where they stand on the debate on unauthorized immigrants. It is expected that social workers uphold U.S. laws and support both immigration and immigrant policies. As such, social workers should deny services to unauthorized immigrants, they must report them, and they ought to intervene when others allow them access to resources. On the other hand, social workers are expected to uphold the dignity of individuals, provide opportunities, and strive for social and economic

justice. Even when immigrants are documented, social workers must address ethical conflicts associated with English-only policies and face differences in cross-cultural values and behaviors. To what extent should the United States, which invites, or accepts, newcomers, adapt to them, and to what extent should the New Americans adapt? Immigrants and the country must constantly juggle what in the host country and what from the home country should be valued, and what should be discarded. These issues will continue to face social work policymakers and practitioners when they focus on immigration and immigrants.

The Role of Social Capital
It is safe to say that the flow of immigrants can strain the receiving country's support service systems. It behooves policy makers and service providers to be cognizant of the experience of immigrants so that they can appropriately meet their voiced, or unvoiced, needs and ensure that the nation's social capital is available to this group in enhancing their human capital. Receiving countries must recognize that migration across their borders will persist with improvements in transportation and with further emerging reasons for relocating. In admitting immigrants, the United States makes a commitment to them. Unless the country is willing to help immigrants through the transitional period of adjustment, the immigrants' unmet economic, social, health, and mental health needs can, in both the short and the long term, drain the country's resources. On the other hand, early attention to these very immigrants may accelerate their entry as contributors to the society (Mayadas & Elliott, 2003). While some experiences are unique to a particular immigrant group or to a specific individual, much in the immigrant experience is shared—from emigration to immigration, including reactions to and by the receiving country.

A framework that views the totality of the immigration experience, from the impetus to leave the home country to resettlement and adaptation in the host country (Segal, 2002), can provide a foundation for the interpretation of the events that influence both particular groups and individuals in those groups, specifically within the context of the receiving country's readiness to accept them. As immigration accelerates, it will be imperative for policy makers and service providers to become more sensitive to the unique needs of new arrivals and to assess the degree to which programs and services are inclusive and supportive or xenophobic and discriminatory. Such assessments may ensure that programs are modified to manage a mutually satisfactory adjustment between both the immigrant group and the host country.

Concluding Comments

Substantial changes in immigration and immigrant policies in the United States are slow to evolve; however, they do change over time. More importantly, changes in political and social attitudes affect the interpretation of these policies, at the national, state, and local levels, and even at the client contact level. This article presents a very general overview of immigration and immigrant policies and their implications. Social workers must remember that while the lives of these populations alter dramatically when they enter the country, their lives do not begin here. Many factors influenced their decisions to move to the United States, and U.S. immigration policies affected the ease of process. All immigrants and refugees have in common the newcomer experience in this land of opportunity and the experience of loss of that which they have left in their homelands. However, there the similarity ends. A close inspection of the Census data, available on the government website *http://www.census.gov*, should be made by any practitioner interested in this population. It is abundantly clear that there is no single profile of immigrants or refugees. They range in age from infancy to old age. They may be single, married, divorced, or widowed; they may come with families, without families, or as part of an extended family. They may be white, black, brown, yellow, red, or any other color under which the human species is categorized. They may be living in the United States legally or illegally. They may be professionally trained and highly skilled, or they may be laborers with skills that cannot be transferred to the U.S. economy. They may be extremely wealthy or very poor. They may be fluent in the English language and speak several other languages, or they may speak only their mother tongue, which may not be English, and they may be illiterate even in their own language. They may be from cultures that are highly hierarchical and autocratic, or they may be from cultures where there is greater equality.

Underlying difficulties in working with immigrants and refugees is a far-reaching xenophobia—both of the immigrants and by them. It is difficult to assess who should be responsible for crossing this bridge—is it the host or is it the self-invited newcomer? Should the host country accommodate immigrants and refugees, or should immigrants and refugees adapt to the host country? The United States has policies to allow 700,000 immigrants annually and, often, almost a tenth as many refugees and half as many "exempt" family members for a total yearly entry rate of well over one million. Therefore, should this host country not attempt to accommodate the immigrants that it allows to enter? Should immigrants not make attempts to adjust? With whom does the responsibility lie?

For immigrants, as for all people, much is dependent on their personal resources. More significant, however, is the readiness of the receiving country to accept immigrants and their American-born descendants. Immigration policies and programs may reflect the interests of the nation in allowing entry to certain groups of people; however, it is the opportunities and obstacles that immigrants and their offspring encounter on a daily basis that affect the ease of adjustment and mutual acceptance. Immigrants and the host nation must make a conscious attempt to adapt to each other—it is neither the exclusive responsibility of the host nation nor of the immigrant. With increasing transnational movement, countries struggle with designing, developing, and implementing immigration and immigrant policies that meet the economic, social, and political goals. The most significant issue that appears to be facing the United States is the management of unauthorized immigrants. However, the nation must also constantly assess the implications of its immigration policies and effectively manage legal migration to meet its economic needs, allow family reunification, and fulfill humanitarian expectations. Policies cannot be limited to who is allowed into the country and under what circumstances; immigrant policies and immigrant access to programs and services should enhance the social, economic, and political integration of newcomers into the society and maximize the benefits of their human capital.

For any immigrant community, it is a long road from its country of origin. The physical distance may be great, but the social, psychological, and emotional distance of immigrant travel is often greater. Nevertheless, the human condition and its similarities bind peoples together to a much greater extent than one tends to accept, regardless of social norms, culture, religion, or language. As a land of immigrants, if the United States is to be truly multicultural, as it claims to be, it must also be pluralistic and recognize, accept, and laud the diversity of people as a national asset. The United States does not have the corner on cultural diversity and immigration struggles, and in this increasingly interdependent world, it may seek to explore effective policies, programs, and services from other nations to inform its own practices (see Segal, Elliott & Mayadas, 2010).

REFERENCES

Borjas, G. (2001). *Heaven's door.* Princeton, NJ: Princeton University Press.

Borjas, G., Grogger, J., & Hanson, G. H. (2006). Immigration and African-American employment opportunities: The response of wages, employment, and incarceration to labor supply shocks. Retrieved October 7, 2006, from http://www.nber.org/papers/w12518

Camarota, S.A. (2011) Welfare use by immigrant households with children: A look at cash, Medicaid, housing, and food programs. *Backgrounder.* Center Immigration Studies. Retrieved October 5, 2012 from http://www.cis.org/articles/2011/immigrant-welfare-use-4-11.pdf.

Carrington, W. J., & Detragiache, E. (1999). How extensive is the brain drain? *Finance & Development, 36*(2). Retrieved October 7, 2006, from http://www.imf.org/external/pubs/ft/fandd/1999/06/carringt.htm

Caulfield, J. (2006). Line in the sand. *Builder, 29*(9), 90–97. Retrieved October 7, 2006, from http://www.builderonline.com/business/line-in-the-sand.aspx

Castles, S. & Miller, M.J. (2009). *The age of migration: International population movements in the modern world,* 4th Edition. New York, NY: The Guildford Press.

Chiswick, B. R., & DebBurman, N. (2004). Educational attainment: Analysis by immigrant generation. *Economics of Education Review, 23*(4), 361–379.

Clarke, V. (2004). Impact of the 1996 welfare reform and illegal immigration reform and immigrant responsibility acts on Caribbean immigrants. *Journal of Immigrant & Refugee Services, 2*(3/4), 147–166.

Coleman, J. S. (1988). Social capital in the creation of human capital. *American Journal of Sociology, 94* (supplement), S95–S120.

Department of Homeland Security. (2011). DHS' progress in 2011: Screening and vetting. Retrieved October 3, 2012, from http://www.dhs.gov/dhs-progress-2011-screening-and-vetting.

Diaz, J. L. O. & Ng, J. J. L. (2012). In 2011, remittances to Mexico recorded its highest annual growth from the last 5 years, *BBVA Research Migration Flash, BBVA Bancomer Economic Analysis,* Retrieved October 5, 2012 from http://www.bbvaresearch.com/KETD/fbin/mult/120201_FlashMigracionMexico_07_eng_tcm348-285523.pdf?ts=542012.

Department of Labor. (2012). *Labor Condition Application for H-1B Nonimmigrants, United States* Department of Labor. Retrieved on October 5, 2012 from http://www.doleta.gov/regions/reg05/Documents/eta-9035.pdf.

Donato, K. M., Stainback, M., & Bankston III, C. L. (2005). In V. Zuniga, & R. Hernandez-Leon (Eds.), *New destinations: Mexican immigration in the United States* (pp. 76–102). New York: Russell Sage Foundation.

Drake, J. (2006, February 22). Survey finds many Mexican immigrants well-educated, own cars. *Associated Press.*

(Section: State and Regional). Retrieved March 28, 2006, from http://www.banderasnews.com/0602/edatmeximmigrants.htm

Elliott, D., Segal, U.A. & Mayadas, N.S. (2010). Emerging themes and implications. In U. A. Segal, D. Elliott, & N. S. Mayadas (Eds.), *Immigration worldwide.* New York: Oxford University Press, 451–464.

Fong, R. & Greene, R. R. (2009). Risk, resilience, and resettlement. In R.R. Greene (Ed.), *Human behavior theory: A diversity framework.* New Brunswick, NH: Transaction Publishers, 147–166.

Geller, A. (2007 January 7). Dr. Jacinto's choice. *St. Louis Post-Dispatch, Associated Press,* B9.

Grieco, E. M. (2005). Temporary admissions of nonimmigrants to the United States in 2004. *Annual Flow Report,* Office of Homeland Security, Office of Immigration Statistics. Retrieved May 26, 2006, from http://www.uscis.gov/graphics/shared/statistics/publications/FlowRptTempAdmis2004.pdf

Haniffa, A. (1999, September 17). New immigrants likely to be poor and stay poor, says study. *India Abroad,* 39.

Hoefer, M., Rytina, N. & Baker, B. (2012). Estimates of the Unauthorized Immigrant Population Residing in the United States: January 2011. *Population Estimates,* DHS Office of Immigration Statistics. Retrieved October 5, 2012, from http://www.dhs.gov/xlibrary/assets/statistics/publications/ois_ill_pe_2011.pdf.

ICE (2013). *Fact sheet: Worksite enforcement.* Retrieved on April 9, 2013 from http://www.ice.gov/news/library/factsheets/worksite.htm.

IOM (2009). *IOM and remittances.* International Organization for Migration. Retrieved October 5, 2012 from http://publications.iom.int/bookstore/free/iom_and_remittances.pdf.

INS (2000). *Illegal alien resident population.* Retrieved January 25, 2006, from http://www.cestim.it/14clandestino_usa.htm

Karger, H. J., & Stoesz, D. (1998). *American social welfare policy: A pluralist approach* (3rd ed.). New York, NY: Longman.

Kim, H. C. (1994). *A legal history of Asian Americans, 1790–1990.* Westport, CT: Greenwood Press.

Kochhar, R. (2011). New jobs in recession and recovery: Who are getting them and who are not. Pew Research Center Publications. Retrieved October 5, 2012, from http://pewresearch.org/pubs/1922/congress-testimony-new-jobs-recession-recovery-who-are-getting-them-and-who-are-not.

Kochhar, R. (2005). *Survey of Mexican migrants, part three.* Pew Hispanic Center, Washington, DC. Retrieved May 31, 2006, from http://pewhispanic.org/reports/report.php?ReportID=58

Kretsedemas, P. (2003). Immigrant households and hardships after welfare reform: A case study of the Miami-Dade Haitian community. *International Journal of Social Welfare, 12*(4), 314–325.

Lee, B. (2011). "Reverse brain drain" in the U.S. *The Daily Need.* Retrieved October 5, 2012 from http://www.pbs

.org/wnet/need-to-know/the-daily-need/reverse-brain-drain-in-the-u-s/11027/

Lobo, M., & Mayadas, N. S. (1997). International social work practice: A refugee perspective. In N. S. Mayadas, T. D. Watts, & D. Elliott (Eds.), *International handbook on social work theory and practice* (pp. 411–428). Westport, CT: Greenwood Press.

Lum, D. (2004). Cultural competence, practice stages, client intersectional systems, and case studies. In D. Lum (Ed.), *Cultural competence, practice stages, and client systems*, Belmont, CA: Thomson/Brooks/Cole, 1–31.

Massey, D. S. (2005). Five myths about immigration: Common misconceptions underlying U.S. border-enforcement policy. *Immigration Policy in Focus*, 4(6). Retrieved June 4, 2006, from http://www.ilw.com/articles/2005,1207-massey.shtm

Mattoo, A., Neagu, I.C. & Özden, C. (2008). Brainwaste? Educated immigrants in the US labor market. *Journal of Development Economics*, 87(2), 255–269.

Mayadas, N. S., & Elliott, D. (2003). Social work's response to refugee issues. In *Madras School of Social Work: 50th Anniversary Publication*, Tamil Nadu, India.

Mayadas, N. S., & Segal, U. (2000). Refugees in the 1990s: A U.S. perspective. In B. Pallassana (Ed.), *Social work practice with immigrants and refugees* (pp. 167–197). New York: Columbia University Press.

Miano, J. (2005). The bottom of the pay scale: Wages for H-1B computer programmers. Center for Migration Studies. Retrieved October 7, 2006, from http://www.cis.org/articles/2005/back1305.pdf

Monger, R. & Yankay, J. (2012). U.S. legal permanent residents: 2011. *Annual flow report*. Retrieved October 3, 2012, from http://www.dhs.gov/xlibrary/assets/statistics/publications/lpr_fr_2011.pdf.

Mooney, M. (2004). Migrants' social capital and investing remittances in Mexico. In J. Durand & D. S. Massey (Eds.), *Crossing the border: Research from the Mexican Migration Project* (pp. 45–62). New York: Russell Sage Foundation.

NCSL (National Conference of State Legislators) (2012a). Immigrant Policy Project: 2012 immigration-related laws and resolutions in the states. Website: http://www.ncsl.org/Portals/1/Documents/immig/2012ImmigrationReportJuly.pdf. Retrieved October 3, 2012.

NCSL (2012b). Use of prosecutorial discretion for young unauthorized immigrants. Retrieved October 3, 2012, from http://www.ncsl.org/issues-research/immig/deferred-action.aspx/

New York Times (2012, June 25). Arizona Immigration Law (SB 107). *New York Times*, Retrieved October 3, 2012, from http://topics.nytimes.com/top/reference/timestopics/subjects/i/immigration-and-emigration/arizona-immigration-law-sb-1070/index.html

Obama, B. (2012). Presidential memorandum ~ annual refugee admissions numbers, The White House, Office of the Press Secretary. Retrieved October 3, 2012, from http://www.whitehouse.gov/the-press-office/2012/09/28/presidential-memorandum-annual-refugee-admissions-numbers

Ohlemacher, S. (2006, March 7). Number of illegal immigrants hits 12M. *Associated Press*. Retrieved March 8, 2006, from http://www.breitbart.com/news/2006/03/07/D8G6U2KO8.html

Orum, A. (2005). Circles of influence and chains of command: The social processes whereby ethnic communities influence host societies. *Social Forces*, 84(2), 921–939.

Özden, C., & Schiff, M. (Eds). (2006). *International migration, remittances, and the brain drain*. Washington, DC: The World Bank & Palgrave Macmillan.

Passel, J. S. & Cohn. D. (2011). *Unauthorized immigrant population: National and state trends, 2010*. Pew Hispanic Center. Retrieved October 3, 2012, from http://www.pewhispanic.org/2011/02/01/unauthorized-immigrant-population-brnational-and-state-trends-2010/

Portes, A. (2006, April 18). Alejandro Portes advocates enlightened programs for immigrants. *UNC School of Education: SOC News*. Retrieved October 7, 2006, from http://soe.unc.edu/news_events/news/2006/portes_alejandro.php

Preston, J. (2013, January 28). Senators offer a bipartisan blueprint for immigration. *New York Times*. Retrieved February 5, 2013, from http://www.nytimes.com/2013/01/28/us/politics/senators-agree-on-blueprint-for-immigration.html?nl=todaysheadlines&emc=edit_th_20130128&_r=0.

Saxenian, A. (2005). From brain drain to brain circulation: Transnational communities and regional upgrading in India and China, *Studies in Comparative International Development*, 40(2), 35 – 61.

Segal, U. A. (2002). *A framework for immigration: Asians in the United States*. New York: Columbia University Press.

Segal, U.A. (2010). The changing face of the United States of America. In U.A. Segal, D. Elliott, & N. S. Mayadas (Eds), *Immigration worldwide*. New York: Oxford University Press, 29–46.

Segal, U.A., Elliott, D. & Mayadas, N. S. (Eds.). (2010). *Immigration worldwide*. New York: Oxford University Press.

Serageldin, I. (1999). Foreword. In T. R. Feldman & S. Assaf (Eds.), *Social capital: Conceptual frameworks and empirical evidence (working paper #5)*. Social Capital Initiative, The World Bank. Studies in Comparative International Development (SCID), 40(2), 35–61.

Sriskandarajah, D. (2005). Reassessing the impacts of brain drain on developing countries. *Migration Information Source*. Retrieved October 7, 2006, from http://www.migrationinformation.org/Feature/display.cfm?ID=324

Stephens, B. (2012, September 28). The Paradoxes of Felipe Calderón. *Wall Street Journal*, Retrieved October 5, 2012, from http://online.wsj.com/article/SB10000872396390443916104578022440624610104.html.

Stewner-Manzanares, G. (1988). The Bilingual Education Act: Twenty years later. *NCBE, Number 6, Occasional papers in bilingual education*. The National Clearing House on Bilingual Education. Retrieved April 9, 2013 from http://www.ncela.gwu.edu/files/rcd/BE021037/Fall88_6.pdf.

Sum, A., Harrington, P., & Khatiwada, I. (2006). *The impact of new immigrants on young native-born workers, 2000–2005*.

Center for Immigration Studies. Retrieved October 7, 2006, from http://www.cis.org/articles/2006/back806.pdf

Teferra, D. (2005). Brain circulation: Unparalleled opportunities, underlying challenges, and outmoded presumptions. *Journal of Studies in International Education, 9*(3), 229–250.

United Nations High Commissioner for Refugees. Retrieved October 25, 2006, from http://www.unhcr.org.

U.S. Census Bureau. (2011). *Current populations survey (CPS)*. Retrieved October 5, 2012, from http://www.census.gov/cps/.

USCIS. (2012). *Laws*. Retrieved October 5, 2012, from http://www.uscis.gov/portal/site/uscis/menuitem.eb1d4c2a3e-5b9ac89243c6a7543f6d1a/?vgnextoid=02729c7755cb9010VgnVCM10000045f3d6a1RCRD&vgnextchannel=02729c7755cb9010VgnVCM10000045f3d6a1RCRD

U.S. Code Collection. (1999). *National policy with respect to equal educational opportunity*. Retrieved October 24, 2006, from http://uscode.house.gov/download/pls/20C31.txt

U.S. Department of Homeland Security, Office of Immigration Statistics. (2006). *2004 yearbook of immigration statistics*. Retrieved May 30, 2006, from http://uscis.gov/graphics/shared/statistics/yearbook/index.htm

U.S. Department of State. (2012). *Visa Bulletin, 48*(9). Retrieved October 3, 2012, from http://www.travel.state.gov/visa/bulletin/bulletin_5759.html

U.S. Department of State. (2012). *Proposed refugee admissions for fiscal year 2013 report to the Congress*. Retrieved February 14, 2013, from http://www.state.gov/documents/organization/198157.pdf

U.S. Department of State. (2007). *Trafficking in Person Report 2007*.http://www.state.gov/documents/organization/82902.pdf

Weber, A. M. (2004, February 23). Reverse brain drain threatens U.S. economy. *USA Today*. Retrieved October 7, 2006, from http://www.usatoday.com/news/opinion/editorials/2004-02-23-economy-edit_x.htm

Wu, H.H. (2005, Fall). Silent numbers: The economic benefits of migrant labor. *Boise State University Idaho Issues Online*. Retrieved June 3, 2006, from http://web1.boisestate.edu/research/history/issuesonline/fall2005_issues/5f_numbers_mex.html

Zohlberg, A. R. (2006). *A nation by design: Immigration policy in the fashioning of America*. Cambridge MA: Harvard University Press.

Zuniga, V. (2006, April 5). *New destinations*. Presentation at the University of Missouri-St. Louis.

FURTHER READING

Balgopal, P. (Ed.). (2000). *Social work practice with immigrants and refugees*. New York: Columbia University Press.

Bayefsky, A. F. (Ed.). (2006). *Human rights and refugees, internally displaced persons and migrant workers: Essays in memory of Joan Fitzpatrick and Arthur Helton*. Boston: M. Nijhoff.

Bernstein, N. (2006, May 21). 100 years in the back door, out the front. *New York Times* 4, 4. Retrieved March 3, 2013, from http://www.nytimes.com/2006/05/21/weekinreview/21bernstein.html?pagewanted=all.

Borjas, G.J. (2011). *Heaven's door: Immigration policy and the American economy*. Princeton, NJ: Princeton University Press.

Brettell, C. B., & Hollifield, J. F. (2000). *Migration theory: Talking across disciplines*. New York: Routledge.

Cohen, R. (Ed.). (1996). *Theories of migration*. Cheltenham, UK: Edward Elgar.

Faini, R., de Melo, J., & Zimmermann, K. F. (Eds.). (1999). *Migration: The controversies and the evidence*. Cambridge, UK: Cambridge University Press.

Flora, C. B., & Maldonado, M. (2006, June 1). Immigrants as assets for Midwestern communities. *Changing Face: Migration News*. University of California, Davis. Retrieved June 9, 2006, from http://migration.ucdavis.edu/cf/comments.php?id=190_0_2_0.

Gordon, L. W. (2005). Trends in the gender ratio of immigrants to the United States. *International Migration Review, 39*(4), 796–818.

Gouveia, L., Carranza, M. A., & Cogua, J. (2005). The Great Plains migration: Mexicanos and Latinos in Nebraska. In V. Zuniga & R. Hernandez-Leon (Eds.), *New destinations: Mexican immigration in the United States*. New York: Russell Sage Foundation, 23–49.

Immigration Timeline. Retrieved September 28, 2006, from http://library.thinkquest.org/20619/Timelinex.html.

Juss, S. S. (2006). *International migration and global justice*. Hampshire, UK: Ashgate.

Massey, D. S. (2005, October 18). Testimony of Douglas S. Massey to the United States Senate committee on the judiciary, comprehensive immigration reform II. Retrieved June 8, 2006, from http://www.judiciary.senate.gov/hearings/testimony.cfm?id=e655f9e2809e5476862f735da149ad69&wit_id=e655f9e2809e5476862f735da149ad69-2-4.

Massey, D. S., & Taylor, J. E. (Eds.). (2004). *International migration: Prospects and policies in a global market*. New York: Oxford University Press.

Migration Information Source. (2012). Retrieved October 5, 2012, from http://www.migrationinformation.org.

Office of Immigration Statistics. (2006). *2004 Yearbook of immigration statistics*. Washington, DC: Office of Homeland Security.

Peacock, J. L., Watson, H. L., & Matthews, C. R. (Eds.). (2005). *The American South in a global world*. Chapel Hill, NC: University of North Carolina Press.

Population Reference Bureau. (2010). *Immigration in America, 2010*. Retrieved October 5, 2012 from http://www.prb.org/Articles/2010/immigrationupdatehome.aspx

Portes, A., & Zhou, M. (1993). The new second generation: Segmented assimilation and its variants. *The ANNALS of the Academy of Political and Social Science, 530*, 74–96.

Potocky-Tripodi, M. (2002). *Best practices for social work with refugees and immigrants*. New York: Columbia University Press.

Rumbaut, R. G. (1997). Assimilation and its discontents: Between rhetoric and reality. *International Migration Review, 31*(4), 923–960.

Segal, U.A., Elliott, D. & Mayadas, N.S. (Eds.). (2010). *Immigration worldwide*. New York: Oxford University Press.

U.S. Census Bureau. (2006). Statistical abstract of the United States: 2006. *The national data book* (125th ed.). Washington, DC: U.S. Department of Commerce, Economics and Statistics Administration.

Zohlberg, A. R. (2006). *A nation by design: Immigration policy in the fashioning of America.* Cambridge, MA: Harvard University Press.

Zuniga, V., & Hernandez-Leon, R. (Eds.). (2005). Introduction. *New destinations: Mexican immigration in the United States.* New York: Russell Sage Foundation, xi–xxix.

UMA A. SEGAL

INTERNATIONAL SOCIAL WORK: OVERVIEW

ABSTRACT: This article presents an overview of definitions of international social work, relevant theories, history, and current practice roles. The conclusion highlights some of the current challenges facing the field: developing relevant career tracks in international social work, strengthening representation of the profession at the global level, specifying the universal elements of social work, and continuing to clarify the concept of international social work.

KEY WORDS: international social work; globalization; international history; United Nations; International Federation of Social Workers; International Association of Schools of Social Work

International social work is a concept that has evolved over the past 80 years, and now there is a significant literature on the subject. Although globalization has increased attention to international social work, the international involvements of the profession date back almost to its founding.

Definition

At times viewed as a perspective, international social work is increasingly defined as an area of social work practice. Authors differ as to how broadly the arena of practice should be drawn. Some argue that it should be relatively open: "international social work means those social work activities and concerns that transcend national and cultural boundaries" (Sanders & Pederson, 1984, p. xiv); others have advocated a narrow definition as reflected in the conclusion reached by a Council on Social Work Education (CSWE) committee in the 1950s that international social work should be restricted to the international work of the United Nations and international nongovernmental organizations (NGOs) (Stein, 1957).

In the predecessor to the *Encyclopedia*, the *Social Work Yearbook*, Warren (1939) provided a clear but complex definition. He wrote that international social work included four dimensions: international social casework (case situations involving two or more countries), international relief and assistance to suffering populations, including victims of disaster or war, international cooperation through organizations such as the International Labour Organization (ILO) and League of Nations to address social and health problems and promote peace, and the international conferences on social work and the international exchange they facilitated.

Conceptual clarity retreated in the later decades of the 20th century; as recently as 1999, Lyons summarized the definitional complexity and vagueness of international social work: international social work "is a nebulous concept, with elements of cross-national comparison and application of international perspectives to local practice, as well as participation in policy and practice activities which are more overtly cross-national or supra-national in character" (p. 12). Renewed attention in the early 21st century has enhanced understanding. Healy (2001) defined international social work as "international professional action" with four main dimensions: internationally related domestic practice and advocacy; international professional exchange; international practice in relief and development; and international policy development and advocacy. Another dimension—that of building the profession globally—was added by Cox & Pawar (2006). Others have called for a strong emphasis on human rights and social justice as the core of international social work and defined it as a field of practice (Haug, 2005; Lyons, Manion, & Carlsen, 2006).

Many years ago, Goldman (1962) called for international social work to become the fourth method of social work in addition to casework, group work, and community organization. "International social work has moved one step further outward in a series of concentric circles from casework, group work and community organization in that order in seeking international solutions to international problems as the other methods seek individual, group, community (or national) solutions to problems in their respective frame of reference" (Goldman, 1962, pp. 1–2). Nagy and Falk (2000) argued that practice with refugees and immigrants should not be included in the definition of international social work, as it is inter- or multicultural, but not international; others disagree and emphasize both the importance of international knowledge and the new emphasis on transnationalism as the rationale for including work with international populations as part of international social work practice (Healy, 2004; Lyons et al., 2006; Xu, 2006).

Thus, as defined today, international social work is a multifaceted concept. At a minimum, it involves practice and policy beyond the level of the nation or that require international knowledge for competence. It is often global in scope. Although the terms *international* and *global* are often used interchangeably, *global* connotes a worldwide scope when differentiated.

Relevant Theories

International social work is often interdisciplinary, but builds upon the core knowledge of social work. The person-in-environment framework underscores the importance of culture and can be extended to include the impact of the global context. Emphases (of social work) on social justice and cultural competence are also highly relevant in international work. More specific theoretical foundations for contemporary international social work are theories of globalization, human rights, development, and transnationalism.

The intensification of the forces of globalization since the early 1990s has been a driving force in increased attention to international social work. Globalization is defined as "a package of transnational flows of people, production, investment, information, ideas and authority" (Brysk, 2002, p. 1) or "a shared awareness of the world as a single place" (Midgley, 1997, p. 21). Knowledge of theories of globalization and its economic, social, security, cultural, and environmental impacts are essential (Dominelli, 2004; Midgley, 2004; Mishra, 1999; Tan & Rowlands, 2004). The counterbalancing concept of indigenization—the effort to adapt and innovate theory and practice to be locally specific—is also important.

Along with globalization, theories of human rights, development, and transnationalism are relevant. Driven by the initiatives of the major international intergovernmental organizations such as the United Nations and the World Bank Group, development and human rights are the two dominant foci. Knowledge of human rights philosophy and principles and of the expression of those principles in international laws are fundamental to all aspects of international social work (Ife, 2001; Reichert, 2003; UN Centre for Human Rights, 1994; Wronka, 1995). Development theories that explore and explain the causes of poverty and strategies for poverty alleviation are essential for social work in international relief, development, or disaster response (Isbister, 2003; Midgley, 1995, 1999). Social work practice with international populations requires

familiarity with migration theories, including the contemporary emphasis on transnationalism (Drachman & Paulino, 2004). There are additional useful concepts such as sustainability, social exclusion, and human security that can be adapted from international work to social work practice in all contexts.

History of International Social Work

The history of international social work practice and action reflects all the elements of the definitions outlined earlier and is instructive in thinking about the future. The use of the term *international social work* dates back to at least 1928 when Jebb (1929) discussed the necessary conditions for such work in her speech written for the First International Conference of Social Work held in Paris. Recent research indicates that American social work education was based on adaptation of ideas borrowed from Europe (Kendall, 2000). Social workers had been internationally active early in the 20th century in movements for women's rights, world peace, and improved labor conditions. Founding social work leaders Jane Addams and Alice Salomon (first president of the International Committee of Schools of Social Work and founder of social work in Germany), for example, met at a meeting of the International Council of Women in 1909 and were among the founders of the Women's International League for Peace and Freedom. They continued to work together for several decades to advance peace and social work. Eglantyne Jebb, a Charity Organization Society worker in England, founded the Save the Children Fund and wrote a Children's Charter adopted by the League of Nations in 1924; this Charter was the precursor to the United Nations Convention on the Rights of the Child. Although the United States did not join the League of Nations, Grace Abbott was named the chair of the League's Committee on the Traffic in Women and Children; Sophonisba Breckinridge was treasurer of the Women's Peace Party and participated in many international meetings on child welfare and corrections (Abbott, 1947; Branscombe, 1948). Among others, these social work leaders were practitioners of international social work in the beginning decades of the profession.

With the founding of the international social work organizations, the International Association of Schools of Social Work (IASSW), the International Council of Social Welfare (ICSW), and the International Federation of Social Workers (IFSW) in 1928, the profession became involved on an organizational level with the League of Nations and the ILO. The ILO, for example, established a documentation center on social work education in collaboration with the IASSW.

Direct social work services were provided to persons displaced by World War I and its aftermath through the International Migration Services, later renamed International Social Service. New opportunities for social work arose after World War II. War devastation generated a huge need for international relief and reconstruction work, including refugee resettlement, family reunification, work with orphaned and separated children, and the reconstruction of social services throughout Europe and East Asia. As Kendall noted, "For social work and social welfare, the restoration period following World War II can be described as a rich cornucopia filled with international programs, projects and opportunities" (1978, p. 178). Much was done under the auspices of the United Nations Relief and Rehabilitation Administration (UNRRA), an agency that gave many social workers an opportunity for international work throughout Europe and China. Howard (1946) estimated that at least 100 American social workers provided general relief, work relief projects, and services in child welfare, work with the aged, and refugees in China alone. These experiences stimulated a life-long career interest in international social work in many who were involved.

Other postwar developments also created opportunities in international social work. The United Nations took an interest in social work training as an essential element of capacity building in developing countries. From 1950 to 1971, the UN conducted and published five major surveys of social work education around the world (Healy, 1995).

In 1959, the Economic and Social Council (ECOSOC) requested the UN Secretary General to "do everything possible to obtain the participation of social workers in the preparation and application of programs for underdeveloped countries" (Garigue, 1961, p. 21). Efforts included international exchanges of students and scholars and provision of technical assistance for development of both services and training programs throughout Asia and Africa. A unique but short-lived experiment in international social work was the placement of Social Welfare Attachés in the U.S. embassies in France and India in 1948 and again in Brazil and India in 1960s. Although the contributions of social workers to the work of the State Department were valued, the positions fell victim to budget-cutting.

The role of social work inside the United Nations diminished after the 1970s as the organization turned away from its specific interest in social welfare. The profession was seemingly unable to define a clear role in the new focus on development (Healy, 2001; Kendall, 1978). Disenchantment with Western influ-ence and anti-Americanism externally and isolationism internally as a result of the Vietnam War contributed to distrust of international social work within the profession. However, international action did not cease. Individual social workers played significant roles in the global efforts against the HIV/AIDS epidemic. The professional organizations intensified their external influence at the UN through NGO activities and collaborated with the UN Centre for Human Rights in publishing a manual, *Human Rights and Social Work* (UN, 1994).

The dissolution of the Soviet empire created new opportunities for the expansion of social work education and international consultation. Growth in international migration during the 1990s and early 21st century increased the international populations of historically multicultural countries and changed the make-up of previously homogeneous nations, creating additional opportunities for an international focus. These developments, combined with the impact of accelerating globalization, contributed to the recent rise in attention to international social work.

Practice Roles in International Social Work

Currently, social workers take on many roles as international social workers. The major ones are as follows:

1. Relief and disaster intervention (micro and macro)
2. Development (macro)
3. International adoption and cross-country casework (micro)
4. Work with immigrants and refugees (micro and macro)
5. Representation of the profession and policy work on global problems
6. Building the global profession through the professional organizations

These roles fall into three major groups. The first group comprises roles in international practice providing relief and development assistance to developing and transition countries. Most such work is macropractice in planning, evaluating, and managing, although there are community-level project-organizing roles. Some direct service opportunities exist in situations of disaster relief and recovery and work with internally displaced populations in emergencies. Although development practitioners are drawn from many fields, social workers bring useful knowledge of participatory strategies and people-focused approaches to needs assessment that often enhance success. For example, the World Bank hired a social worker to assist when its projects on disability failed to engage people with disabilities.

The second group of roles is largely practiced domestically; these roles focus on international populations and require knowledge of diverse cultures, migration theory, international law, and laws of multiple countries (Drachman, 1992). These international social workers practice in international adoption, refugee resettlement, services to immigrant populations, and cross-border work on cases or service planning (Drachman & Paolino, 2004; Padilla & Daigle, 1996). Such areas of practice have become increasingly international in nature; transnational families (families with constant interactions between several countries) are now the norm among immigrants, and international adoption agencies are expanding into efforts to improve child welfare services in source countries (Stiles, Dhamaraksa, dela Rosa, Goldner, & Kalyanvala, 2001). Thus, practice demands more sophisticated global knowledge and cross-cultural communications and practice skills.

The final group of international social work roles focuses on action by and for the organized profession. These roles include international policy development and advocacy, representation of the profession on the global level, and work to build the profession globally. They can be performed on either a voluntary or paid basis, and include representing social work at the United Nations and with other intergovernmental agencies; developing global standards for the profession through the IFSW and IASSW; and working on global problems at the policy level. Some also consider the processes of international knowledge sharing that takes place through exchanges, international professional conferences, and technology transfer efforts to be components of international social work practice.

SKILLS REQUIRED FOR INTERNATIONAL SOCIAL WORK The skills required for international work include many of the skills taught in social work programs. A study of United Nations agencies and international NGOs found that planning, management, and community organization skills are highly valued, along with strong interpersonal skills and demonstrated ability to live in developing country situations (Healy, 1987); a recent survey by the National Association of Social Workers (NASW) validated these findings (NASW, 2003). The range of issues that make up the substance of international social work include HIV and AIDS, poverty, ethnic conflict, natural disaster, women's status, street children, adoption, human trafficking, child labor, orphans, family violence, and trauma. Substantive expertise in an area such as HIV prevention, poverty alleviation strategies, disaster

response, or programming for orphans and vulnerable children is valuable for international work and is held by many social workers. Advocacy roles require knowledge of international organizations and international law, knowledge of the profession as it is operationalized around the world, and skills in representing and negotiating.

Future Challenges and Trends

There are many current and future challenges for international social work. They include identifying and promoting relevant career tracks for social workers, strengthening the profession globally, and expanding social work representation in the global arena, additional attention to identify what is universal and to address the legacies of the export model that led to uncritical transfer of Western theory and practice, and ongoing work to specify the nature of international social work.

Identifying clear career tracks for international social work is essential to support the growing interest among professionals. NASW examined job requirements and responsibilities for 55 positions in international development and concluded that "social workers are qualified to carry out most of the responsibilities of the development jobs that were reviewed" (2003, p. 2). However, few international organizations advertise specifically for social work training and may not recognize its relevance for international work. Further, a recent study revealed weak engagement in international aspects of practice by agencies in one highly diverse community in the United States (Xu, 2006). Both suggest the need to more clearly explicate the contributions of social work to international practice.

Changes in the external environment will also shape the practice of international social work. The shift of emphasis in UNICEF from child survival to child protection, for example, may create new roles for social work, as child protection is an arena identified with the profession. The United Nations is also showing a renewed interest in social services and both UN and NGO agencies stress human rights, another window of opportunity for social work.

There are many global social problems that intersect with social work expertise in addition to child protection. The IASSW and IFSW are making efforts to strengthen their representation of social work at the United Nations through their consultative status as NGOs. NASW is now a member of Interaction, a coalition of more than 150 U.S.-based development agencies that engages in advocacy on global issues. Expanding representation of the profession and enhancing the contribution of social work knowledge to addressing global problems are important areas for further work.

In building the profession globally, there is a need for continued examination of what is universal and what is locally specific (Weiss, 2005). Profession-building took significant forward steps in the early years of the 21st century as agreement was reached by the IFSW and the IASSW on a revised Global Definition of Social Work (Hare, 2004; IFSW/IASSW, 2000), a revised set of ethical principles (IFSW/IASSW, 2004), and Global Standards for Social Work Education and Training, a comprehensive set of guidelines for social work education around the world (IASSW/IFSW, 2004). Gray and Fook refer to these developments as a "quest for universalism in social work" (2004, p. 625). They note that this universalism is contested by debates on globalization–localization, Westernization–indigenization, as well as the capacity of universalism to accommodate and facilitate the needed diversity in the profession. Fueling these tensions is the legacy of the export model of uncritical transfer of Western theory and practice; future efforts must ensure mutuality in international interactions (Healy, Asamoah, & Hokenstad, 2003).

As work proceeds on this ambitious agenda, the concept of international social work will gain clarity. The profession can draw from its extensive history in international work to reclaim early gains and expand its contributions to address the social impacts of globalization. In the context of globalization, it could be argued that all social work is international social work; at present, however, it is imperative to advance the practice of international social work as an identifiable component of the profession in the United States and worldwide.

REFERENCES

Abbott, E. (1947). Three American pioneers in international social welfare. *The Compass* 28(4), 3–7, 36.

Branscombe, M. (1948). A friend of international welfare. *Social Service Review,* 22(4), 436–441.

Brysk, A. (Ed.). (2002). *Globalization and human rights.* Berkeley: University of California Press.

Cox, D., & Pawar, M. (2006). *International Social work: Issues, strategies, and programs.* Thousand Oaks, CA: Sage.

Drachman, D. (1992). A stage of migration framework for service to immigrant populations. *Social Work,* 37, 68–72.

Drachman, D., & Paulino, A. (Eds.). (2004). *Immigrants and social work: Thinking beyond the borders of the United States.* Binghamton, NY: Haworth.

Garigue, P. (1961). *Challenge of cultural variations to social work. In Education for social work* (pp. 9–22) [Proceedings]. Council on Social Work Education (Ninth Annual Program Meeting).

Goldman, B. W. (1962). International social work as a professional function. *International Social Work,* 5(3), 1–8.

Gray, M., & Fook, J. (2004). The quest for a universal social work: Some issues and implications. *Social Work Education,* 23, 625–644.

Hare, I. (2004). Defining social work for the 21st century: The international federation of social workers' revised definition of social work. *International Social Work,* 47, 407–424.

Haug, E. (2005). Critical reflections on the emerging discourse of international social work. *International Social Work,* 48, 126–135.

Healy, L. M. (1987). International agencies as social work settings: Opportunity, capability and commitment. *Social Work,* 32(5), 405–409.

Healy, L. M. (2001). *International social work: Professional action in an interdependent world.* New York: Oxford University Press.

Healy, L. M. (2004). Strengthening the link: Social work with immigrants and refugees and international social work. In D. Drachman & A. Paulino, (Eds.), *Immigrants and social work: Thinking beyond the borders of the United States* (pp. 49–67). Binghamton, NY: Haworth.

Healy, L. M., Asamoah, Y. A., & Hokenstad, M. C. (2003). *Models of international collaboration in social work education.* Alexandria, VA: Council on Social Work Education.

Howard, D. S. (1946). Emergency relief needs and measures in China. *Social Service Review,* 20, 300–311.

IASSW/IFSW. (2004). Global standards for social work education and training. Retrieved February 26, 2007, from http://www.iassw-aiets.org

Ife, J. (2001). *Human rights and social work: Towards rights-based practice.* Cambridge: Cambridge University Press.

IFSW/IASSW. (2000). Definition of social work. Retrieved March 1, 2007, from http://www.ifsw.org

IFSW/IASSW. (2004). Ethics in social work: Statement of principle. Retrieved February 26, 2007, from http://www.ifsw.org

Isbister, J. (2003). *Promises not kept: Poverty and the betrayal of third world development* (6th ed.). Bloomfield, CT: Kumarian.

Jebb, E. (1929). International social service. In *First international conference of social work (Paris, July 8 –13, 1928): Proceedings* (3 vols. Vol. 1, pp. 637–655).

Kendall, K. (1978). The IASSW 1928–1978: A journey of remembrance. In K. Kendall (Ed.), *Reflections on social work education* (pp. 170–191). New York: IASSW.

Kendall, K. (2000). *Social work education: Its origins in Europe.* Alexandria, VA: Council on Social Work Education.

Lyons, K. (1999). *International social work: Themes and perspectives.* Aldershot, Hampshire: Ashgate.

Lyons, K., Manion, K., & Carlsen, M. (2006). *International perspectives on social work.* Houndmills: Palgrave Macmillan.

Midgley, J. (1995). Social development. London: Sage.

Midgley, J. (1997). *Social welfare in the global context.* Thousand Oaks, CA: Sage.

Midgley, J. (1999). Social development in social work: Learning from global dialogue. In C. S. Ramanathan & R. J. Link

(Eds.), *All our futures: Principles and resources for social work practice in a global era* (pp. 193–205). Belmont, CA: Brooks-Cole.

Midgley, J. (2004). The complexities of globalization: Challenges to social work. In N.-T. Tan & A. Rowlands (Eds.), *Social work around the world III: Globalization, social welfare and social work* (pp. 13–29). Berne: IFSW Press.

Mishra, R. (1999). *Globalisation and the welfare state.* Cheltenham, UK: Edward Elgar.

Nagy, G., & Falk, D. (2000). Dilemmas in international and cross-cultural social work education. *International Social Work, 43,* 49–60.

NASW. (2003). *Social work career opportunities in international development.* International Practice Update, 2(2).

Padilla, Y., & Daigle, L. (1996). Social and economic interdependence in the United States-Mexico border region: Critical implications for social welfare. New Global Development: *Journal of International and Comparative Social Welfare, 12,* 65–77.

Reichert, E. (2003). *Social work and human rights: A foundation for policy and practice.* New York: Columbia University Press.

Sanders, D. S., & Pederson, P. (1984). *Education for international social welfare.* Manoa, Hawaii: University of Hawaii School of Social Work.

Stein, H. (January, 1957). An international perspective in the social work curriculum. Paper presented at the Annual Meeting of the Council on Social Work Education, Los Angeles, CA.

Stiles, C. F., Dhamaraksa, D., dela Rosa, R., Goldner, T., & Kalyanvala, R. (2001). Families for children: International strategies to build in-country capacity in the Philippines, Thailand, Romania, and India. *Child Welfare, LXXX(5),* 645–655.

Tan, N.-T., & Rowlands, A. (Eds.). (2004). *Social work around the world III: Globalization, social welfare and social work.* Berne: IFSW Press.

U. N. (1994). *Human rights and social work: A manual for schools of social work and the social work profession.* Geneva: UN Centre for Human Rights with IFSW and IASSW.

Warren, G. (1939). International social work. In R. Kurtz (Ed.), *Social work yearbook 1939* (pp. 192–196). New York: Russell Sage Foundation.

Weiss, I. (2005). Is there a global common core to social work? A cross-national comparative study of BSW graduate students. *Social Work, 50(2),* 101–110.

Wronka, J. (1995). Human rights. In R. Edwards (Ed.), *Encyclopedia of social work* (19th ed., pp. 1405–1418). Washington, DC: NASW Press.

Xu, Q. (2006). Defining international social work: A social service agency perspective. *International Social Work, 49(6),* 679–692.

FURTHER READING

Hokenstad, M. C., & Midgley, J. (Eds.). (1997). *Issues in international social work: Global challenges in a new era.* Washington, DC: NASW Press.

Hokenstad, M. C., & Midgley, J. (Eds.). (2004). *Lessons from abroad: Adapting international social welfare innovations.* Washington, DC: NASW Press.

Hokenstad, M. C., Khinduka, S. K., & Midgley, J. (Eds.). (1992). *Profiles in international social work.* Washington, DC: NASW Press.

Weiss, I., Gal, J. & Dixon, J. (Eds.). (2003). *Professional ideologies and preferences in social work: A global study.* Westport, CT: Praeger.

IASSW: http://www.iassw-aiets.org
IFSW: http://www.ifsw.org
ICSW: http://www.icsw.org
Interaction: http://www.interaction.org
UN: http://www.un.org

LYNNE M. HEALY

INTERVENTION RESEARCH

ABSTRACT: This entry regards intervention research as an essential part of social work as a profession and research discipline. A brief history of intervention research reveals that use of intervention research for the betterment of human conditions is contemporary with the genesis of modern social science. Advances in intervention research are attributed to the comprehensive social programs launched during the 1960s in the United States. A contemporary and generic model of intervention research is described. It is argued that it is ethical to use intervention research and unethical not to use it. Assessment of some of the recent advances in policy making and science gives an optimistic picture of the future of intervention research.

KEY WORDS: history; essence; operational model; ethics; experiments

A Definition of Intervention Research

A very general definition of "intervention" would be any interference that would modify a process or situation. A widely used definition of social intervention was suggested by Seidman (1983) as actions that change intra-societal relationships, planned or unplanned, intended or unintended. In social work, the purpose of intervention is to induce change in order to block or eradicate risk factors, activate and mobilize protective factors, reduce or eradicate harm, or introduce betterment beyond harm eradication. Intervention research occupies a very specific place in the social work profession; we may say that social work is social intervention by its very nature. Intervention research refers to the scientific study of interventions for social and health problems.

Brief History

The notion of the betterment of conditions of individuals and societies by using modern science in the sense we understand science today is some four centuries old. During the sixteenth century, a number of books were published about Utopia, Greek for "the land which is nowhere" (Soydan, 1999), to propagate the idea of a better life and a better society. These ideas were generated to elevate human beings and communities from the poverty and misery that overwhelmed people's lives during those times. A growing number of intellectuals, among them Sir Francis Bacon, Lord Chancellor of England, emphasized that thinkers' theories and practitioners' tested experiences could and must be used by the natural sciences to control the material world (Soydan, 1999).

Much later, in the mid-eighteenth century, the analysis of society and human behavior was put on a scientific foundation by Scottish scientists, Adam Smith being the most eminent of them. It took another half a century or so before the first prototype agenda for social change by using social science was in place. The Frenchman Claude Henri de Rouvroy, mostly known as Comte de Saint-Simon, formulated an explicit program of action to induce change on the basis of scientific methods. There might be good reason to call Saint-Simon the father of intervention research (Soydan, 1999).

Intervention research in social work, in a more modern sense, was shaped during the post-World War II era. Presidents Kennedy and Johnson, and later to some extent Nixon, launched nationwide programs to improve the conditions of the most needy and underserved cross-sections of the American population (Davis et al., 2006). Such social reforms to induce change constitute an important backdrop to what later came to be defined as intervention research. Sponsors of social programs wanted to understand whether the programs they funded had any positive and intended outcomes.

One single person, the American psychologist and methodologist, Donald T. Campbell, stands as the most eminent and prominent scientist, whose legacy in intervention research is unmatched. Campbell introduced the concept of "the experimenting society," meaning that eradication of societal problems should be based on the scientific principle of experimentation and evaluation of intervention outcomes. However, social experiment—the foundation of intervention research—is not an easy enterprise. It is surrounded by methodological, practical, and ethical issues. In Donald Campbell's experimental society, the social scientist is responsible for ascertaining the effectiveness of social interventions. Much of Campbell's scientific work was focused on the study of the scientific criteria by which experimental interventions were to be studied (Campbell, 1988).

In the early 21st century, literature on intervention research became more focused after the publication of the pivotal book, *Intervention research:–Design and development for human service*, edited by Rothman and Thomas (1994). In this book, the editors and their numerous colleagues elaborate on multiple aspects of intervention research and develop an agenda for the coming decade and perhaps beyond.

An Integrative Approach to Intervention Research

Thomas and Rothman's (1994) integrative perspective on intervention research is broad and captures the endeavors of human services researchers to develop approaches to research generating knowledge pertinent to end-users such as practitioners, policymakers, and administrators. The types of research that aim at practice relevance include the following: "Intervention Knowledge Development," which refers to empirical investigations of human behavior in the context of human services intervention; "Intervention Knowledge Utilization," referring to utilization of practical knowledge in human services; and "Intervention Design and Development," which aims to develop innovative interventions. One common aspect of all of these types of research is their ultimate purpose of contributing to problem solving and problem eradication by supporting human services with practice-pertinent knowledge. This broader perspective was crafted into a practical method by narrowing it to a Design and Development issue. They formulated six main steps of intervention design and development are: a) problem analysis and project planning; b) information gathering and synthesis; c) intervention design; d) early development and pilot testing; e) evaluation and advanced development; and f) dissemination (Thomas and Rothman, 1994).

The Essence of Intervention Research as Scientific Vehicle in Social Work

The essence of intervention research in social work is to generate knowledge on whether social work interventions and programs work. Since the goal of social work interventions is the betterment of human beings and solving societal problems, it is of great importance to understand the effectiveness of these interventions. Furthermore, it is certainly of vital importance to understand whether a given intervention is harmful. The benchmark of any social work intervention is to avoid harm to the client and others who are exposed to the intervention. For instance, a Campbell Collaboration systematic review demonstrated that the very popular and widely implemented Scared Straight programs designed for juvenile crime prevention were not only not effective, but sometimes shockingly harmful (Petrosino et al., 2002). This systematic review was based on all known scientifically qualified intervention research results. Besides generating information about effectiveness and potential harm, intervention research also delivers information about whether an intervention is promising. In the absence of enough numbers of high quality intervention research studies, the few studies at hand can indicate whether a given social work intervention is promising. In such cases, social workers might like to use those interventions, but with great caution, and the intervention researchers should further study their effectiveness.

An Operational Model of Intervention Research

A useful operational model of intervention research is described by Mark Fraser (2004), who identifies the following steps of the model: Explanatory research, conceptualization, program design, efficacy testing, effectiveness testing and dissemination. Fraser, Richman, Galinsky, and Day (2009) further expanded this framework in an intervention research guidebook.

Explanatory research is the first phase of intervention research to identify and analyze the problem, as well as gather information that might be necessary for the preparation of the intervention itself. The ultimate purpose of this phase is to specify and develop a program theory or a model that can define the structure and procedures of the intervention. Explanatory research might be conducted by the intervention researchers who will be responsible for the following steps. But, in many cases, useful explanatory research results would already be at hand, thanks to previous research done by others. Observational studies such as surveys and cross-sectional and longitudinal studies are very useful in identifying and assessing risk factors and protective factors that might be involved. Knowing about risk factors and protective factors is important because they are used in the conceptualization and the design of the program that will be used as the intervention. Conceptualization and program design are two steps that define and operationalize concepts into actions to be taken as a part of the intervention. Examples of such actions are those that may generate awareness, mobilize key agents, provide support, develop skills, and provide cash support, housing, etc.

Programs are then tested for efficacy and effectiveness. Efficacy testing involves program intervention in well-controlled environments where the program is delivered with high fidelity and outcomes are measured so as to compare results of the experimental group with the control group(s). Efficacy trials that yield positive results mean that the intervention is promising and should be tested for effectiveness. Effectiveness testing takes place in sites where the clients are under less controlled but realistic conditions. Extensive effectiveness testing generates rich information about whether the intervention works and to what extent and under what circumstances. It should be kept in mind that many scholars and practitioners keep asking whether successful interventions tested in a given society can be implemented in countries with different cultural and social contexts. This is usually called external validity. There is no direct guarantee that they would work. However, successful interventions can and should be tested under diverse cultural and societal circumstances. Further, sustainability of interventions needs to be emphasized. Traditionally, successfully implemented interventions after the completion of favorable effectiveness studies would weaken in the long run because of measures for long-term sustainability. Especially with the growing awareness about the vital role of organizational settings as a seat for interventions, the issue of sustainability has come to the forefront (Palinkas & Soydan, 2012).

Once the effectiveness testing is done it is time for dissemination. Dissemination of effective interventions has historically been a difficult problem to handle. A successful dissemination requires appropriate format, a language that is understood by the users, well-identified end-users, and a high degree of transparency to secure end-users' confidence.

Traditionally, dissemination has been the last step of intervention research. During the late 1990s and early 2000s the "implementation" of social interventions became more prominent on the agendas of scholars and practitioners (Bhattacharyya et al., 2007; Kerner, 2007). Rather recently, the concept of "translation" has also been introduced. Implementation of social interventions involves organizational, client-related, and intervention-technical issues to make the implementation of an intervention as successful as possible. Translation of social interventions takes an active stand in terms of "transferring" a social intervention to new and untested sites as to make sure that the intervention is adapted to local circumstances.

The Context of Intervention Research

The context of intervention research occurs in real life situations and is either about efficiency (controlled environments) or effectiveness (loosely controlled or uncontrolled environments) studies. Interventions involve real life situations with real people and real social entities. In this sense, the context of intervention research is a web of political, moral, fiscal, and scientific issues. Thus, a number of stakeholders are always present; these may include clients, their families, social workers, social agency managers, and researchers. Smyer and Gatz (1986) suggest that three sets of questions emerge when planning intervention research: 1) Stakeholders: Who are the stakeholders? Do they support the intervention in question? What is their stake? 2) The purpose of the intervention: What is the problem to be solved? Who are the potential recipients of the intervention, and how can they be identified? What kind of interventions may be introduced? What are the unintentional effects of the intervention? Are there alternative ways of solving the problem? 3) The research: Who is seeking the answers and for what reason?

Future Trends

The use of intervention research has been relatively modest in social work (Rosen et al., 1999; Reid & Fortune, 2003). However, the use of intervention research with experimental designs in the social sciences in general has expanded during recent decades (Boruch et al., 2002). The driving motor of this development has been multiple and concurrent factors: a growing awareness about accountability and transparency issues among the public, decision makers, and professionals; the further professionalization of social work and other human services professions; and the emergence of the Cochrane and Campbell Collaborations that develop systematic and high quality syntheses of intervention studies available in plain language to end-users.

Frazer (2004, p. 212) gives examples of other advances that might positively impact the future of intervention research. These include the growing use of a risk-factor approach, the emergence of practice-relevant micro-social theories and the increased acceptance of manual-based interventions, as well as methodological advances.

It Is Ethical to Conduct Intervention Research

The code of ethics of the National Association of Social Workers prescribes the following regarding social workers' competence:

"Social workers should provide services in substantive areas or use intervention techniques or approaches that are new to them only after engaging in appropriate study, training, consultation, and supervision from people who are competent in those techniques" (NASW, 2007, p. 6).

The definition of social work adopted by the International Federation of Social Workers reads:

"Social work bases its methodology on a systematic body of evidence-based knowledge derived from research and practice evaluation" (IFSW, 2000, p. 1).

Thus, it is obvious that social workers' universal professional standards prescribe high quality scientific knowledge and training in terms of understanding whether social work interventions avoid harm to the client, and most desirably, are effective in the betterment of the client's problem. A scientifically sound social work profession has to make use of intervention research. In other words, practice of intervention research is one of the fundamentals of ethical and transparent social work practice.

It is equally true that social work interventions must be planned and executed in a responsible way and with full consent of the clients who are exposed to them. Additionally, the most apt scientific design used to measure the effects of social interventions, that is, the experimental design, must be used responsibly, only when it is appropriate, and with full transparency and the consent of the clients. Oddly, opponents of experimental studies argue that it is unethical to experiment when it comes to human behavior and especially with those human beings who are most dependent on the services of social workers. This is a fallacy, and an unethical stand: consider the case that when social workers do not base their professional practice on sound and strong scientific evidence, they in fact are "experimenting" with their clients every time they intervene and attempt to treat them; because they do not know anything about the potential harm of the intervention and techniques used, such experimentation is clearly unethical.

REFERENCES

Bhattacharyya, O., Reeves, S., Zwarenstein, M. (2007). *What is implementation research? Rationale, concepts and practices.* Stockholm: Institute for evidence-based social work practice. 2007 Stockholm Implementation and Translational Research Conference. This paper will be published in Research on Social Work Research 2008.

Boruch, R., De Moya, D., & Snyder, B. (2002). The importance of randomized field trials in education and related areas. In M. Frederick & B. Robert (Eds.), *Evidence matters* (pp. 50–79). Washington, DC: Brookings Institute Press.

Campbell, D. T. (1988). The experimenting society. In E. S. Overman (Ed.), *Methodology and epistemology for social science: Selected papers* (pp. 290–314). Chicago: University of Chicago Press.

Davis, P., Newcomer, K. & Soydan, H. (2006). Government as structural context for evaluation. In I. Shaw, J. Greene, & M. Mark (2006). *The SAGE Handbook of evaluation.* London, UK: Sage.

Fraser, M. W., Richman, M. W., Galinsky, M. J., & Day, S. H. (2009). *Intervention research: Developing social programs.* New York and Oxford: Oxford University Press.

Frazer, M. (2004). Intervention research in social work: Recent advances and continuing challenges. *Research on Social Work Practice, 14*(3), 210–222.

IFSW (2000). Definition of social work. Retrieved February 17, 2007, from http://www.ifsw.org/en/p38000208.html

Kerner, F. J. (2007). *Research dissemination & diffusion: Translation within science and society.* Stockholm: Institute for evidence-based social work practice. 2007 Stockholm Implementation and Translational Research Conference.

NASW (2007). Code of ethics. Retrieved February 17, 2007, http://www.socialworkers.org/pubs/codenew/code.asp

Palinkas, L. A. & Soydan. H. (2012). *Translational and implementation research of evidence-based practice.* New York and Oxford: Oxford University Press.

Petrosino, A., Turpin-Petrosino, C., & Buehler, J. (2002). Scared Straight and other prison tour programs for preventing juvenile delinquency. Retrieved February 15, 2007, from http://www.campbellcollaboration.org/lib/download/12/

Reid, W., & Anne, F. (2003). Empirical foundations for practice guidelines in current social work knowledge. In R. Aaron & E. Proctor (Eds.), *Developing practice guidelines for social work interventions: Issues, methods, and research agenda* (pp. 59–79). New York: Columbia University Press.

Rosen, A., Proctor, E., Staudt, M. (1999). Social work research and the quest for effective practice. *Research on social work practice, 23,* 4–14.

Rothman, J., & Thomas, E. (Eds.). (1994). *Intervention research: Design and development for human services.* New York: The Haworth Press.

Seidman, E. (1983). Introduction. In E Seidman (Ed.), *Handbook of social intervention* (pp. 11–17). Beverly Hills: Sage.

Smyer, M., & Gatz, M. (1986). Intervention research approaches. *Research on Aging, 8*(4), 536–558.

Soydan, H. (1999). *The history of ideas in social work.* Birmingham: Venture Press.

Thomas, E., & Rothman, J. (1994). An integrative perspective on intervention research. In R. Jack & T. Edwin (Eds.), (1994). *Intervention research: Design and development for human services.* New York: The Haworth Press.

FURTHER READING

The Campbell Collaboration: http://www.campbellcollaboration.org

The Cochrane Collaboration: http://www.cochrane.org

HALUK SOYDAN

INTERVIEWING

ABSTRACT: Social work interviews are purposeful conversations between practitioners and clients, involving verbal and nonverbal communication. The basic skills are regularly used by social workers and reflect the field's major practice principles and the model of change employed by the practitioner. Competency-based forms of interviewing such as motivational and solution-focused interviewing are increasingly being used in direct and indirect practice. Additional research is needed on the outcomes of specific interviewing skills and how they are learned and transferred into practice.

KEY WORDS: interviewing; skills; practice principles; strengths perspective; competency-based interviewing; related research

Social work interviews are purposeful conversations between practitioners and clients in which verbal and nonverbal communication occurs through questions and answers, listening and responding, gestures, body position, and facial expressions. The purpose of these interviews is to help clients by developing cooperative working relationships between practitioners and clients and by focusing on clients' needs, problems, strengths, resources, and solutions (Benjamin, 1987; De Jong & Berg, 2013; Kadushin, 1997).

Social workers spend more time at interviewing than at any other professional activity (Kadushin, 1997, 1996). They interview individuals, couples, families, and small groups in all fields of direct practice. Social workers also use their interviewing skills in indirect practice activities such as supervision, organizational task groups, and contacts with collaterals.

Structure and Diversity Awareness

An interview is generally thought to have beginning, middle, and ending phases that broadly parallel the overall stages of work with clients (Kadushin, 1997). In the beginning phase, worker and client get acquainted, develop a cooperative working relationship, and establish a beginning sense of the client's problem and goals. In the middle phase, the problem is assessed, goals are developed, and interventions are designed. In the ending phase, client progress is evaluated and decisions are made about the need for additional work together. With the field's growing attention to diversity, there are now several sources exploring how to adapt each phase of the interview to the norms, beliefs, values, and interactional styles of different racial and ethnic groups (Devore & Schlesinger, 1999; Lum, 2004; 2011; Sue & Sue, 1999).

Skills and Principles

Basic interviewing skills include attending and active listening, using open questions, seeking clarification and details, paraphrasing and summarizing, reflecting feelings and client perceptions, use of silence, empathizing, noticing client's nonverbal behaviors, exploring client meanings, encouraging and complimenting, providing information, setting goals, reframing, educating, challenging, and providing feedback and making suggestions. These skills are explained and illustrated at length in textbooks about interviewing skills and are taught as foundational skills in accredited bachelor's and master's social work programs (Bogo, 2006; De Jong & Berg, 2013; Ivey, Ivey, & Zalaquett, 2010; Kadushin, 1997).

The manner in which these skills are used with clients reflects the field's ethical principles. Biestek (1957), for example, offers one well-known formulation of these principles, identifying them as individualization of services, purposeful expression of feelings, controlled emotional involvement by the practitioner, acceptance of clients, nonjudgmental attitude toward clients, fostering client self determination, and respecting client confidentiality. Certain interviewing skills are employed to bring each of these principles to life in work with clients. For example, Biestek (1957, p. 25) writes that individualization of services involves treating each client "not just as a human being but as this human being with his personal differences." Respecting this principle in interaction with a client requires frequent use of several skills, including attending and active listening, using open questions, paraphrasing and summarizing, and exploring client meanings.

Emergence of Competency-Based Interviewing

In the early 1990s, the strengths perspective began challenging social work's overemphasis on pathologies and problems. Its principles called for more attention to client strengths and successes as the way to create client change and empowerment (Saleebey, 1992; Weick, 1992). At the same time, the field was recognizing that social work practitioners were working more and more with involuntary clients while the skills taught to new practitioners were still those originally developed for work with voluntary clients (Ivanoff, Blythe, & Tripodi, 1994; Rooney, 1992). Prominent among the interviewing skills typically employed were empathy, client education, and confrontation, all of which are of questionable value with involuntary clients, especially early in a social work relationship.

These two developments contributed to the increased interest in more collaborative, competency-based interviewing such as motivational and solution-focused interviewing (Berg, 1994; De Jong & Miller, 1995; de Shazer, 1985, 1988; Miller & Rollnick, 2002). Both approaches employ interviewing techniques devoted directly to fostering client change rather than first assessing problems and then intervening to reduce or resolve the problems. Motivational interviewing, developed in work with substance abusing clients, is known for refusing to confront clients about the consequences of their substance use. Instead, the interviewer reflects back any ambivalence about substance use heard in the client's beliefs, past behaviors, or future actions as a strategy to increase client motivation to make changes (Miller & Rollnick, 2002). Solution-focused interviewing, through taking a "not knowing" and accepting perspective of the client's perceptions about his situation (Goolishian & Anderson, 1991), works in the client's frame of reference and invites the client to build a clearer conception of what he wants different in his life; the client is also invited to draw on past successes, personal strengths, and resources in his own social networks and in the broader community in order to achieve the goals. By building solutions within the client's frame of reference, solution-focused interviewers find client resistance is no longer an issue, the need for educational interventions is reduced, and diversity competency as the need for foreknowledge of the beliefs and values of diverse groups is dramatically lessened (De Jong & Berg, 2013).

The strengths perspective and the skills of collaborative, competency-based interviewing are now reflected in major social-work-practice textbooks (Compton, Galaway, & Cournoyer, 2005; Kirst-Ashman & Hull, 2006; Miley, O'Melia, & DuBois, 2011; Sheafor & Horejsi, 2008). While these texts for the most part remain organized around problem assessment and intervention, they also encourage social workers to incorporate more collaborative, competency-based skills into their practice, thus giving more attention to what clients want, their related successes and strengths, and their resources in order to create solutions more meaningful to them.

Need for Research

Meta-analyses of controlled research indicate that relationship factors account for a substantially larger proportion of the variation in positive client change than specific practice models employed (Lambert, 2006). Yet, while interviewing skill is the key component defining how the professional social work relationship is conducted, it is this author's impression that far less research in social work, as in psychology, (Lambert, 2006) has been devoted to relationship skills in interviewing than to the efficacy of one practice model or intervention program versus another. More research is needed on relationship factors and skills that cut across practice models such as empathy, reflection of feelings, asking open and not knowing questions, and complimenting client strengths and successes. The field needs to learn more about the influence of these factors on building cooperative, working relationships with clients and client outcomes. More investigation of how practitioners learn interview skills and transfer that learning into work with clients also is needed (Carrillo, Gallant, & Thyer, 1993; De Jong & Cronkright, 2011; Dickson & Bamford, 1995).

Conclusion

Competency in interviewing continues to be regarded as essential for being a professional social worker. While no less fundamental to effective practice than ever before, interviewing skills are evolving along with the profession's shift in practice philosophy toward more collaborative and strengths-based ways of relating to clients, coworkers, and collaterals. More research exploring the relationship of interviewing principles and skills to practice outcomes is important to promoting the mission of social work.

REFERENCES

Benjamin, A. (1987). *The helping interview with case illustrations.* Boston: Houghton Mifflin.

Berg, I. K. (1994). *Family based services: A solution-focused approach.* New York: Norton.

Biestek, F. P. (1957). *The casework relationship.* Chicago: Loyola University Press.

Bogo, M. (2006). *Social work practice: Concepts, processes, and interviewing.* New York: Columbia University Press.

Carrillo, D. F., Gallant, J. P., & Thyer, B. A. (1993). Training MSW students in interviewing skills: An empirical assessment. *Arete, 18,* 12–19.

Compton, B. R., Galaway, B., & Cournoyer, B. R. (2005). *Social work processes* (7th ed.). Belmont, CA: Thomson Brooks/Cole.

De Jong, P., & Berg, I. K. (2013). *Interviewing for solutions* (4th ed.). Belmont, CA: Brooks/Cole.

De Jong, P., & Cronkright, A. (2011). Learning solution-focused interviewing skills: BSW student voices. *Journal of Teaching in Social Work, 31,* 21–37.

De Jong, P., & Miller, S. D. (1995). How to interview for client strengths. *Social Work, 40,* 729–736.

de Shazer, S. (1985). *Keys to solution in brief therapy.* New York: Norton.

de Shazer, S. (1988). *Clues: Investigating solutions in brief therapy.* New York: Norton.

Devore, W., & Schlesinger, E. G. (1999). *Ethnic-sensitive social work practice* (5th ed.). Boston: Allyn & Bacon.

Dickson, D., & Bamford, D. (1995). Improving the interpersonal skills of social work students: The problem of transfer of training and what to do about it. *British Journal of Social Work, 25,* 85–105.

Goolishian, H. A., & Anderson, H. (1991). An essay on changing theory and changing ethics: Some historical and post structural views. *American Family Therapy Association Newsletter, 46,* 6–10.

Ivanoff, A., Blythe, B. J., & Tripodi, T. (1994). *Involuntary clients in social work practice: A research-based approach.* New York: Aldine De Gruyter.

Ivey, A. E., Ivey, M. B. & Zalaquett, C. P. (2010). *Intentional interviewing and counseling: Facilitating client development in a multicultural society* (7th ed.). Belmont, CA: Brooks/Cole.

Kadushin, A. (1996). Interviewing. In L. Beebe & N. A. Winchester (Eds.), *Encyclopedia of social work* (19th ed., pp. 1527–1537). Washington, DC: NASW Press.

Kadushin, A. (1997). *The social work interview* (4th ed.). New York: Columbia University Press.

Kirst-Ashman, K. K., Hull, G. H. (2006). *Understanding generalist practice* (4th ed.). Belmont, CA: Thomson Brooks/Cole.

Lambert, M. J. (Ed.). (2006). *Bergin and Garfield's handbook of psychotherapy and behavior change* (5th ed.). New York: Wiley.

Lum, D. (2004). *Social work practice and people of color: A process-stage approach* (5th ed.). Pacific Grove, CA: Brooks/Cole.

Lum, D. (2011). *Culturally competent practice: A framework for understanding diverse groups and justice issues* (4th ed.). Belmont, CA: Brooks/Cole.

Miley, K. K., O'Melia, M., & DuBois, B. (2011). *Generalist social work practice: An empowering approach* (updated 6th ed.). Boston: Allyn & Bacon.

Miller, W. R., & Rollnick, S. (2002). *Motivational interviewing* (2nd ed.). New York: Guilford.

Rooney, R. H. (1992). *Strategies for work with involuntary clients.* New York: Columbia University Press.

Saleebey, D. (Ed.). (1992). *The strengths perspective in social work practice.* New York: Longman.

Sheafor, B. W., & Horejsi, C. R. (2008). *Techniques and guidelines for social work practice* (8th ed.). Boston: Allyn and Bacon.

Sue, D. W., & Sue, D. (1999). *Counseling the culturally different: Theory and practice* (3rd ed.). New York: Wiley.

Weick, A. (1992). Building a strengths perspective for social work. In D. Saleebey (Ed.), *The strengths perspective in social work practice* (pp. 18–26). New York: Longman.

FURTHER READING

European Brief Therapy Association: http://ebta.eu/

Motivational Interviewing: http://www.motivationalinterviewing.org/

Solution-Focused Brief Therapy Association: http://www.sfbta.org/

PETER DE JONG

INTIMATE PARTNER VIOLENCE

ABSTRACT: Intimate partner violence—physical, emotional, or sexual abuse experienced in both heterosexual and same-sex relationships—has emerged as a significant and complex social problem warranting the attention of social workers. Numerous risk factors have been identified in individual perpetrators and victims, as well as at the level of the relationship, community, and society. Partner violence has diverse consequences for female victims, as well as for perpetrators and children who are exposed to it. Although many female victims do seek help and end abusive relationships, seeking help from professionals such as social workers is often a last resort.

KEY WORDS: domestic violence; battering; physical abuse; emotional abuse; sexual abuse

Introduction

Feminist advocates and scholars first identified intimate partner violence (IPV), also called domestic violence or wife abuse, as a social problem during the 1970s. Initially, physically victimized wives were the focus of concern, based on the assumption that patriarchy and the institution of marriage itself established the right for husbands to use physical violence to control their wives. Over time, however, both scholars and advocates for women have learned that it is not just legally married women but women in all types of intimate relationships—dating and cohabiting as well as separated and divorced, heterosexual, and homosexual—who can experience violence and abuse by their partners.

Definitions

IPV consists of physical, sexual, and emotional or psychological abuse or violence perpetrated by intimate partners or acquaintances, including persons who are current or former spouses, cohabiting partners, boyfriends or girlfriends, and dating partners. It includes abuse in the context of same-sex as well as heterosexual intimate relationships. Regardless of how it is socially or legally defined, women are most likely to be victimized by perpetrators they know, generally men they know well (Browne & Williams, 1993; Tjaden & Thoennes, 1998). *Physical violence* is defined to include acts of physical aggression intended to harm one's partner, such as pushing, grabbing, and shoving; kicking, biting, and hitting (with fists or objects); beating up and choking; and threatening or using a knife or gun. Legal definitions of *rape* and *sexual assault* differ from state to state, although

their common element is the lack of victim consent to sexual acts. Although many states have ceased to use the term "rape" in their criminal codes, rape is generally understood to mean forced or coerced vaginal, anal, or oral penetration; sexual abuse involves either threats of sexual behavior, coerced sexual behavior that does not involve penetration, or engaging in other sexual acts with a person who cannot give consent. *Emotional* or *psychological abuse* can be defined as acts intended to denigrate, isolate, or dominate an intimate partner. Emotional abuse might include verbal attacks (including harassment, insults, ridicule, or name calling); social isolation of the victim; denying access to resources such as family income; extreme jealousy and possessiveness, monitoring of behavior, or unwarranted accusations of infidelity; threats to harm the victim's family, children, friends, or pets; threats of abandonment or infidelity; or damage or destruction of personal property (Marshall, 1999).

Prevalence

Estimating the extent of partner violence is challenging because of historical stigma, victim fear of retaliation from perpetrators, and other safety concerns. National survey studies of IPV have found widely varying estimates of its prevalence, ranging from about 1% per year (Tjaden & Thoennes, 2000) to 12% (Straus & Gelles, 1990); about one in five women are estimated to have been physically abused by a male partner in their lifetime (Tjaden & Thoennes, 2000). The National Crime Victimization Survey, an ongoing general victimization survey begun in 1972, suggests that around 5 million victimizations are experienced by females over age 12 each year, the majority perpetrated by males known to the victim, such as romantic partners (Bachman & Saltzman, 1995). These studies indicate that over their lifetimes women are more likely to be assaulted by someone they know than by a stranger.

Although there is less research about abuse in same-sex relationships, it appears that gay men and lesbians are about as likely to be abused by a romantic partner as are heterosexual women. Abuse can be physical, emotional, or sexual, but in addition, "outing" a partner, that is revealing his or her sexual orientation without consent, is a special form of abuse to which gay men and lesbians are vulnerable. Gay men and lesbians face special challenges in disclosing abuse and obtaining help because of homophobia and discrimination as well as a dearth of services sensitive to their needs. For example, seeking help from the formal service system may require disclosing one's sexual orientation, with potentially adverse consequences (Carlson & Maciol, 1997).

Risk Factors

There is no single cause of IPV. Rather, there are multiple factors that elevate the risk for IPV that exist within perpetrators and victims, in relationships and family systems, at the community level, and in society.

PERPETRATORS Risk factors affecting perpetrators have been studied extensively. Young age is among the best documented risk factors for physical and sexual violence for both victims and perpetrators (Bachman & Saltzman, 1995; Tjaden & Thoennes, 1998). Abuse of alcohol and drugs has also been found to be associated with partner violence (Aldarondo & Kantor, 1997; Leonard & Senchak, 1996) and sexual assault (Ullman, Karabatsos, & Koss, 1999). Low income (Bachman & Saltzman; Greenfeld et al., 1998) and unemployment of the male partner (Straus & Gelles, 1986) are risk factors for perpetration of abuse, perhaps because of the stress associated with insufficient income.

Although perpetrator personality characteristics or traits have been studied as possible antecedents of physical or sexual abuse, research has shown that there is no single male personality type that distinguishes men who use sexual or physical violence toward women. One research review found the following personality risk markers for male partner abuse: emotional dependence and insecurity; low self-esteem, empathy, and impulse control; poor communication and social skills; aggressive, narcissistic, and antisocial personality types; and anxiety and depression (Kaufman Kantor & Jasinski, 1998). Attempts to identify different types of batterers have concluded that there may be at least two different types of abusive men—one type that is violent only toward intimates and another that is more generally violent toward others—who may require different types of interventions (Holtzworth-Munroe & Stuart, 1994).

Because emotional or psychological abuse typically precedes as well as accompanies physical abuse (O'Leary, Malone, & Tyree, 1994), the presence of emotional abuse should be considered a risk factor for physical abuse. Some studies have found that a history of violence in the family of origin, witnessing violence between parents, or being the recipient of violent punishment are risk factors for violence toward intimates as an adult (Aldarondo & Kantor, 1997; Leonard & Senchak, 1996).

VICTIMS Many studies have found that earlier victimization, especially childhood physical and sexual abuse and witnessing violence between parents, elevates risk

for being sexually or physically assaulted by a partner (Gidycz & Koss, 1991; Maker, Kemmelmeier, & Peterson, 1998; Weaver, Kilpatrick, Resnick, Best, & Saunders, 1997). Studies have documented the association between alcohol or drug abuse and physical (Hilbert, Kolia, & VanLeeuwen, 1997; Plichta, 1996) and sexual victimization (Miller & Downs, 1993). Substance abuse may be both a cause and effect of IPV, affecting young women and women of color in particular (Kilpatrick, Acierno, Resnick, Saunders, & Best, 1997).

Social isolation is also associated with victimization and can both precede and follow partner violence (Nielsen, Endo, & Ellington, 1992). Although it can be a consequence of abuse, it may also serve as a risk factor. Much anecdotal evidence indicates that abusive men commonly attempt to control their partners by cutting them off from meaningful social contact. Having social support may be protective by lowering the risk of becoming abused, or buffering women from the adverse effects of being abused. Finally, poverty is associated with victimization, and economic dependency on the abuser can also be a barrier to women being able to terminate an abusive relationship (Horton & Johnson, 1993; Sullivan, Campbell, Angelique, Eby, & Davidson, 1994).

RELATIONSHIP TYPE Relationship status is a risk factor. Among intimates, separated and cohabiting couples are at higher risk for partner violence than are married or dating couples (Bachman & Saltzman, 1995).

COMMUNITY Two factors at the community level have been found to increase risk for IPV. IPV rates are highest in urban areas (Greenfeld et al., 1998). In addition, when services are lacking for either victims or perpetrators, as may be the case in rural areas for example, there is increased risk of being unable to exit an abusive relationship, continuing to engage in abusive behavior, or being unable to get help for the consequences of abuse.

CULTURE AND SOCIETY Sociocultural risk factors establish a broad context that has made many forms of IPV socially acceptable historically. Many agree that sexism in American society and sex-role stereotyping are risk factors for victimization of women. Rates of marital violence are highest in states where there is the most economic, educational, political, and legal inequality (Yllo & Straus, 1990). There continues to be stigma associated with being an abused woman or rape victim, and many victims feel criticized for not immediately terminating an abusive relationship.

Research on the role of race and ethnicity as possible risk factors for IPV is inconclusive. Some studies show that, compared with white women, African American women and Native American women experience higher rates of physical violence (Tjaden & Thoennes, 1998; Zlotnick, Kohn, Peterson, & Pearlstein, 1998), whereas others find higher rates for whites compared with Latino women (Sorenson, 1996), find no racial or ethnic differences, or find higher rates for Latinos (Straus & Smith, 1990). Some studies fail to take differences in socioeconomic status into consideration, possibly confounding the effects of ethnicity with poverty.

Consequences

IPV may have adverse implications for all members of a family in which it is occurring, including offenders and children. Although not all female victims of IPV report adverse consequences, those who do can experience several different types of consequences. One obvious effect is physical injury; one large, national study found that 42% of physical assault victims reported injuries, most commonly scratches, welts, and bruises (Tjaden & Thoennes, 2000). However, other adverse health effects are more likely to occur than injuries. Abused women tend to have poorer physical health than nonabused women and report more symptoms and health problems of all kinds (McCauley et al., 1995). These include gastrointestinal disorders, chronic pain, fatigue, dizziness, appetite problems, and gynecological problems such as sexually transmitted diseases (Carlson, 2007). Emotional distress also commonly occurs as a consequence of IPV, including depression, suicide attempts, posttraumatic stress, fear and anxiety, and drug and alcohol abuse (Campbell, Sullivan, & Davidson, 1995; Gelles & Straus, 1990; Kilpatrick et al., 1997; Saunders, 1994). The more severe the abuse, the greater the likelihood of experiencing symptoms. Self-blame, shame, and guilt are also common in the aftermath of abuse. For many women, cessation of the abuse is sufficient for emotional distress to subside, but other victims require professional intervention, even after an abusive relationship has ended (Zlotnick, Johnson, & Kohn, 2006).

There is the perception that many abused women remain in abusive relationships, or wait too long before they leave. In fact, many abused women do leave, nearly half within two to five years in one community sample (Zlotnick et al., 2006). However,

numerous practical and emotional barriers prevent abused women from leaving. Practical barriers include being unable to find safe, affordable housing or to financially support oneself and one's children, a problem made worse when TANF (Temporary Assistance for Needy Families) legislation imposed limits on the length of time a woman can receive public assistance. Emotional attachments to the abusive partner, lack of social support, and fear also entrap some victims (Barnett, 2001a, 2001b).

Perpetrators, too, can experience adverse consequences of abusing their partners. First, they can be injured or killed by victims who respond to long-term abuse or use violence in self-defense (Saunders, 1986). Sanctions such as arrest and incarceration are increasingly common as society comes to accept that IPV is a crime (Carlson & Worden, 2005). Batterers also risk temporary or permanent loss of their partners and children, which can lead to loss of self-esteem and self-respect.

Children can also be affected in negative ways, manifesting problems across all areas of development. Some "internalize" their responses to living in an abusive home by withdrawing; becoming passive, fearful, or insecure; or depressed. More common is a pattern of "externalizing behavior problems" such as anger, aggression, and other acting out behavior problems, and noncompliance; such children learn aggression as a way of approaching problems. Children can also be injured, intentionally or accidentally, if they are in the proximity of a violent disagreement in their homes (Carlson, 2000). An ongoing controversy is whether and under what circumstances exposing children to IPV should be considered child maltreatment, and if so, what types of interventions should be made.

Interventions

Society has increasingly accepted responsibility for the complex social problem of IPV, and domestic violence services for both victims and perpetrators are now available in most communities (Roberts, 1998).

The most commonly used formal services tend to be criminal justice, social service agencies, medical services, crisis counseling, mental health services, clergy, and women's groups (Gordon, 1996).

Research shows that abused women are not passive victims of violence in their homes but are active help-seekers (Gondolf & Fisher, 1988). Most abused women who seek help go first to informal sources such as family and friends and are satisfied with the assistance they receive (Davis & Srinivasan, 1995; Horton & Johnson, 1993; Pakieser, Lenaghan, & Muelleman, 1998). When such informal assistance is unavailable or inadequate, abused women tend to seek assistance from professionals. Abused women generally evaluate domestic violence services quite positively, despite their relatively low rates of utilization (Davis & Srinivasan, 1995; Gordon, 1996; Horton & Johnson, 1993). Although IPV services have increased dramatically since the 1980s, some victims have been dissatisfied with the help they have received from community agencies (Gondolf & Fisher, 1988).

Trends and Challenges

A continuing controversy within the IPV advocacy community is provision of mental health services for victims, due to the widespread belief that professional counselors do not adequately understand the nature of IPV and "pathologize" victims. Social workers are perceived to be among the most helpful service providers (Gordon, 1996), and IPV survivors have recommended counseling to other abused women (Horton & Johnson, 1993). Helpful strategies for professional helpers include listening and taking survivors seriously, believing their stories, being knowledgeable about abuse and understanding the circumstances of abused women, and helping survivors to see their strengths (Hamilton & Coates, 1993; Horton & Johnson, 1993).

Services for abusive men have proliferated and remain controversial for several reasons, including skepticism about their effectiveness. Most men receiving such services are mandated to do so by the justice system. In general, psycho-educational and cognitive-behavioral group approaches have been employed to help such men alter their attitudes and beliefs about women and eliminate physically and emotionally abusive behaviors.

REFERENCES

Aldarondo, E., & Kantor, G. K. (1997). Social predictors of wife assault cessation. In G. K. Kantor & J. L. Jasinki (Eds.), *Out of darkness: Contemporary perspectives on family violence* (pp. 183–193). Thousand Oaks, CA: Sage.

Bachman, R., & Saltzman, L. E. (1995). *Violence against women: Estimates from the redesigned survey.* Washington, DC: Bureau of Justice Statistics, U.S. Department of Justice.

Barnett, O. W. (2001a). Why battered women do not leave, part 1: External inhibiting factors within society. *Trauma, Violence, & Abuse, 1,* 343–372.

Barnett, O. W. (2001b). Why battered women do not leave, part 2: External inhibiting factors—social support and internal inhibiting factors. *Trauma, Violence, & Abuse, 2,* 3–35.

Browne, A., & Williams, K. (1993). Gender, intimacy, and lethal violence: Trends from 1976 through 1987. *Gender and Society, 7,* 78–98.

Campbell, R., Sullivan, C., & Davidson, W. S. (1995). Women who use domestic violence shelters: Changes in depression over time. *Psychology of Women Quarterly, 19,* 237–255.

Carlson, B. E. (2000). Children exposed to intimate partner violence: Research findings and implications for intervention. *Trauma, Violence, & Abuse, 4,* 321–342.

Carlson, B. E. (2007). Intimate partner abuse in health care settings. In K. Kendall-Tackett & S. Giacomoni (Eds.), *Intimate partner violence.*

Carlson, B. E., & Maciol, K. (1997). Domestic violence: Gay men and lesbians. In R. Edwards (Ed.), *Encyclopedia of social work, 1997 Supplement* (19th ed.). Washington, DC: National Association of Social Workers.

Carlson, B. E., & Worden, A. P. (2005). Attitudes and beliefs about domestic violence: Results of a public opinion survey. *Journal of Interpersonal Violence, 20,* 1197–1218.

Davis, L. V., & Srinivasan, M. (1995). Listening to the voices of battered women: What helps them escape violence. *Affilia, 10,* 49–69.

Gelles, R. J., & Straus, M. A. (Eds.). (1990). *The medical and psychological costs of family violence. In Physical violence in American families: Risk factors and adaptations to violence in 8,145 families.* New Brunswick, NJ: Transaction Publishers.

Gidycz, C. A., & Koss, M. P. (1991). Predictors of long-term sexual assault trauma among a national sample of victimized college women. *Violence and Victims, 6*(3), 176–190.

Gondolf, E. W., & Fisher, E. R. (1988). *Battered women as survivors.* Lexington, MA: Lexington Books.

Gordon, J. S. (1996). Community services for abused women: A review of perceived usefulness and efficacy. *Journal of Family Violence, 11,* 315–329.

Greenfeld, L. A., Rand, M. R., Craven, D., Klaus, P. A., Perkins, C. A., Ringel, C., et al. (1998). *Violence by intimates: Analysis of data on crimes by current or former spouses, boyfriends, and girlfriends.* Washington, DC: Bureau of Justice Statistics, U.S. Department of Justice.

Hilbert, J. C., Kolia, R., & VanLeeuwen, D. M. (1997). Abused women in New Mexico shelters: Factors that influence independence on discharge. *Affilia, 12*(4), 391–407.

Holtzworth-Munroe, A., & Stuart, G. L. (1994). Typologies of male batterers: Three subtypes and the differences among them. *Psychological Bulletin, 116*(3), 476–497.

Horton, A. L., & Johnson, B. L. (1993). Profile and strategies of women who have ended abuse. *Families in Society, 74,* 481–492.

Jasinski, J. L., & Williams, L. M. (1998). *Partner violence: A comprehensive review of 20 years of research.* Thousand Oaks, CA: Sage.

Kaufman Kantor, G., & Jasinski, J. L. (1998). Dynamics and risk factors in partner violence. In J. L. Jasinski & L. M. Williams (Eds.), *Partner violence: A comprehensive review of 20 years of research* (pp. 1–43). Thousand Oaks, CA: Sage.

Kilpatrick, D. G., Acierno, R., Resnick, H. S., Saunders, B. E., & Best, C. L. (1997). A 2-year longitudinal analysis of the relationships between violent assault and substance use in women. *Journal of Consulting and Clinical Psychology, 65,* 834–847.

Leonard, K. E., & Senchak, M. (1996). Prospective prediction of husband marital aggression within newlywed couples. *Journal of Abnormal Psychology, 105,* 369–380.

Maker, A. H., Kemmelmeier, M., & Peterson, C. (1998). Long-term psychological consequences in women of witnessing parental physical conflict and experiencing abuse in childhood. *Journal of Interpersonal Violence, 13,* 574–589.

Marshall, L. L. (1999). Effects of men's subtle and overt psychological abuse on low-income women. *Violence and Victims, 14*(1), 69–88.

McCauley, J., Kern, D. E., Kolodner, K., Dill, L., Schroeder, A. F., DeChant, H. K., et al. (1995). The "battering syndrome": Prevalence and clinical characteristics of domestic violence in primary care internal medicine practices. *Annals of Internal Medicine, 123*(10), 737–746.

Miller, B. A., & Downs, W. R. (1993). The impact of family violence on the use of alcohol by women. *Alcohol Health and Research World, 17,* 137–143.

Nielsen, J. M., Endo, R. K., & Ellington, B. L. (1992). Social isolation and wife abuse: A research report. In E. C. Viano (Ed.), *Intimate violence interdisciplinary perspectives* (pp. 49–59). Washington, DC: Hemisphere.

O'Leary, K. D., Malone, J., & Tyree, A. (1994). Physical aggression in early marriage: Prerelationship and relationship effects. *Journal of Consulting and Clinical Psychology, 62,* 594–602.

Pakieser, R. A., Lenaghan, P. A., & Muelleman, R. L. (1998). Battered women: Where do they go for help? *Journal of Emergency Nursing, 24*(1), 16–19.

Plichta, S. B. (1996). Violence and abuse: Implications for women's health. In M. M. Falik & K. S. Collins (Eds.), *Women's health: The Commonwealth fund study* (pp. 237–272). Baltimore, MD: The Johns Hopkins University Press.

Roberts, A. R. (1998). The organizational structure and function of shelters for battered women and their children: A national survey. In A. R. Roberts (Ed.), *Battered women and their families: Intervention strategies and treatment programs* (2nd ed., pp. 58–75). New York: Springer.

Saunders, D. G. (1986). When battered women use violence: Husband-abuse or self-defense? *Victims and Violence, 1*(1), 47–60.

Saunders, D. G. (1994). Posttraumatic stress symptom profiles of battered women: A comparison of survivors in two settings. *Violence and Victims, 9,* 31–44.

Sorenson, S. B. (1996). Violence against women: Examining ethnic differences and commonalities. *Evaluation Review, 20,* 123–145.

Straus, M. A., & Gelles, R. J. (1986). Societal change and change in family violence from 1975 to 1985 as revealed by two national surveys. *Journal of Marriage and the Family, 48,* 465–478.

Straus, M. A., & Smith, C. (1990). Violence in Hispanic families in the United States: Incidence rates and structural interpretations. In M. A. Straus & R. J. Gelles (Eds.), *Physical violence in American families: Risk factors and adaptations to violence in 8,145 families* (pp. 341–368). New Brunswick, NJ: Transaction Press.

Straus, M. S., & Gelles, R. J. (1990). How violent are American families? Estimates from the national family violence resurvey and other studies. In M. A. Straus & R. J. Gelles (Eds.), *Physical violence in American families: Risk* (pp. 95–112). New Brunswick, NJ: Transaction.

Sullivan, C. M., Campbell, R., Angelique, H., Eby, K. K., & Davidson, W. S. (1994). An advocacy intervention program for women with abusive partners: Six-month follow-up. *American Journal of Community Psychology, 22,* 101–122.

Tjaden, P., & Thoennes, N. (1998). *Prevalence, incidence and consequences of violence against women: Findings from the national violence against women survey.* Washington, DC: National Institute of Justice and Centers for Disease Control and Prevention.

Tjaden, P., & Thoennes, N. (2000). *Extent, nature, and consequences of intimate partner violence (NCJ 181867).* Washington, DC: Office of Justice Programs, U. S. Department of Justice.

Ullman, S. E., Karabatsos, G., & Koss, M. P. (1999). Alcohol and sexual assault in a national sample of college women. *Journal of Interpersonal Violence, 14*(6), 603–625.

Weaver, T. L., Kilpatrick, D. G., Resnick, H. S., Best, C. L., & Saunders, B. E. (1997). An examination of physical assault and childhood victimization histories within a national probability sample of women. In G. K. Kantor & J. L. Jasinski (Eds.), *Out of darkness: Contemporary perspectives on family violence* (pp. 35–46). Thousand Oaks, CA: Sage.

Yllo, K. A., & Straus, M. A. (1990). Patriarchy and violence against wives: The impact of structural and normative factors. In M. A. Straus & R. J. Gelles (Eds.), *Physical violence in American families: Risk factors and adaptations in 8,145 American families* (pp. 383–399). New Brunswick, NJ: Transaction Publishers.

Zlotnick, C., Johnson, D. M., & Kohn, R. (2006). Intimate partner violence and long-term psychosocial functioning in a national sample of American women. *Journal of Interpersonal Violence, 21,* 262–275.

Zlotnick, C., Kohn, R., Peterson, J., & Pearlstein, T. (1998). Partner physical victimization in a national sample of American families. *Journal of Interpersonal Violence, 13,* 156–166.

FURTHER READING

National Center for Injury Prevention and Control: http://www.cdc.gov/ncipc/factsheets/ipvfacts.htm

Bureau of Justice Statistics: http://www.bjs.gov/index.cfm?ty=pbse&sid=78

National Online Resource Center on Violence Against Women: http://www.vawnet.org

University of New Hampshire Sexual Harassment and Rape Prevention Program: http://www.unh.edu/sharpp/

Minnesota Center Against Violence and Abuse: http://www.mincava.umn.edu

BONNIE E. CARLSON

J

JUVENILE JUSTICE: OVERVIEW

ABSTRACT: The juvenile justice system was established with the 1899 founding in Chicago of the Juvenile Court, an institution that spread to all the states in a short period of time. The history, organization, structure, and operations of the system are described along with its growth. Among the key issues examined are: gender, overrepresentation of children of color, placement of mentally ill and abused or neglected children, human rights, and re-integration of juvenile offenders after their returning home.

KEY WORDS: history; court processing; disposition and placement; gender; overrepresentation; social justice issues

The establishment of the juvenile court in Illinois in 1899 led to the development of the United States juvenile justice system, which was mandated to provide for the processing, adjudication, and rehabilitation of juveniles charged with criminal violations, as well as for the care and treatment of abused and neglected children. Social advocates such as Jane Addams, as well as crusading judges such as Ben Lindsey (Tanenhaus, 2002) established the system, emphasizing care and treatment rather than punishment and control. The response to this new social invention was rapid, and the juvenile court spread throughout the United States in less than twenty-five years. Since that time, it has become a model for the legal processing of children in much of the developed world. Although the juvenile court still retains jurisdiction over the processing of abuse and neglect cases, most of the processing care and supervision of those cases lie within the child welfare system, while the juvenile justice system focuses primarily on youths charged with delinquency or status offenses. As of 2009, more than 2.8 million youths are under juvenile court supervision annually with around 1.65 million new cases processed each year (Puzzanchera, Adams, & Sickmund, 2012).

History

The principles underlying the creation of this social institution were that children are developmentally immature and required protection, they are malleable and can be habilitated or rehabilitated, and the court should aid children suffering from a broad range of problems different from those of adults. Children were assumed to be dependent, developing physically and psychologically, and in need of care and nurturance. They differed from adults by having lesser capacity for reasoning and moral judgment; thus they were less culpable for their behavior (Tanenhaus, 2002). Because the focus was on the rehabilitation of offenders, its development had an impact on court procedures and resulted in a theory of state responsibility for children as represented in the concept of *parens patriae*.

Prior to the establishment of the juvenile court, juveniles charged with delinquent acts were primarily tried in the criminal justice system, but even then age played a role in presumptions of guilt, because juveniles below the age of fourteen were presumed not to possess sufficient criminal responsibility to commit a crime. The creation of the juvenile court altered this presumption in part, providing almost exclusive jurisdiction over individuals below the age of eighteen who were charged with violating criminal laws in most states. Hearings were to be informal, private, "in the best interest of the child," and civil rather than criminal. These tenets constituted a separate system of justice that recognized the differences between children and adults (Zimring, 2002).

State legislation permitted judges to use their discretion in conducting hearings and prescribing interventions. To meet their statutory goals, the juvenile justice system employed a range of programs and services—including prevention, diversion, detention, probation, community services, and residential treatment (Rosenheim, 2002). For most of the 20th century, judges heard juvenile cases and then diverted most of them to community services outside the court, but substantial numbers were institutionalized, even for extended periods.

1960–1980. In many communities, the court failed to meet the goals of its founders to be responsible for the provision of rehabilitation. Beginning in the 1960s, the human rights movement influenced developments in juvenile justice because of growing concern that juveniles receive due process and protection of their civil liberties. Decisions of the Supreme Court in cases such as *Kent v. U.S. 383 U.S. 541 (1966)*, *In re Gault 387 U.S.1 (1967)*, and *In re Winship 397 U.S.*

352 (1970) led to many new social policy initiatives to protect children's rights to challenge arbitrary dispositions. A series of national commission reports (Presidential Commission on Law Enforcement and Criminal Justice and the Task Force on Juvenile Delinquency and Youth Crime, 1974) had positive effects, extending human rights along with policies of decriminalization, deinstitutionalization, and diversion. By the 1970s, passage of the first federal juvenile justice legislation, the Juvenile Justice and Delinquency Act of 1974, funded state efforts to reduce institutionalization and increase local community-based programming.

1980–2000. The progress of the 1960s and 1970s was dramatically reversed in the 1980s and 1990s, with the passage of federal and state legislation that emphasized incarceration and punishment, along with withdrawal of the distinction between juveniles and adults as far as certain criminal behavior was concerned. As a century of the juvenile court was celebrated in 2000, laws and philosophy had returned to many practices in place before the invention of the juvenile court. Thousands of juveniles were held in adult prisons and jails, often under very punitive conditions (Lerman, 2002). Feld (1999) argues that judicial, administrative, and legislative decisions transformed the court into a second-class criminal court that did not serve the interests of children. Much of the transformation appeared to be "justified" by the increase in juvenile crime between 1985 and 1995 (Bishop, 2000). After 1995, however, there was a dramatic decline in juvenile crime that continued through 2009, especially serious violent crime, but there has not been a corresponding reduction in the numbers of juveniles processed (Puzzanchera et al., 2012).

Since 2000. Much of the discussion about the juvenile justice system in the early twenty-first century neglects the changes in the societal context in which it operates. Garland (2001) and Beckett and Western (2000) point to the increasing culture of control and the declining provision of social welfare benefits for the population at risk for involvement in the justice system. Family structure has undergone and is undergoing substantial changes that affect children because single parents are unable to provide the necessary supervision and support, especially in the critical adolescent years. The increasing rates of poverty, the decline of public school education, the lack of physical and mental health care, and the changing economic structure, in which well-paying blue collar jobs are unavailable for young adults, have had a pronounced effect on these vulnerable youths since the mid-1990s (Holzer, 2010). Millions of dollars are spent on incarceration and control, but few resources are available

to prepare the middle- and working-class youth population for successful adulthood (Osgood, Foster, Flanagan, & Ruth, 2005; Setterstein, Furstenberg, & Rumbaut, 2005). All these factors affect juvenile crime in society and thereby the operation of the juvenile justice system. Two decisions of the U.S. Supreme Court extended human rights to juveniles: the *Roper v. Simmons* decision declared the execution of juveniles to be unconstitutional, and *Graham v. Florida* (2010) eliminated "life without parole" sentences for nonhomicidal cases. In 2012, the Supreme Court declared the sentence of life without parole unconstitutional for juveniles convicted of homicide (*Miller v. Alabama*, 2012).

Organization and Structure

The juvenile justice system comprises the statutes and policies, as well as organizations, charged with responsibility for the processing of juveniles who violate state laws and local ordinances (Ross and Miller, 2011). The legal definition of delinquency and crime varies from state to state as to the ages of youths under juvenile court jurisdiction and the roles of the various court officials responsible for the processing of juveniles into and through the court. The system varies widely among the states, because most criminal law is under state jurisdiction, but the law is administered locally. As in many other sectors, federalism characterizes the organizational structures of the courts in the United States, in contrast to many other countries.

The processing typically includes:

1. Arrest and referral of a juvenile to the court for a law violation; some police may have warning and diversion alternatives that may precede or follow initial court referral.

2. Juvenile court intake includes referral for trial, diversion of minor offenders, detention, and preliminary assessment.

3. Filing of a formal petition and deciding to try the youth in juvenile court or transfer the youth to adult court for criminal processing.

4. Hearing or trial by the court and determination of innocence or guilt.

5. Disposition decision-making by the judge and placement in a program for those adjudicated as delinquent for an indeterminate or specific period of time, depending upon state laws or judicial discretion, and release or special sanctions for the others.

6. Re-integration or reentry programming, which is formalized as parole but may also be informally and unevenly provided.

Demographics

There are many inter-state variations in the number of juveniles processed at different stages in court processing.

More than 1.91 million youths below the age of eighteen were arrested in 2009, but only 26% were arrested for serious person or property crimes or "index" crimes as these are defined (Puzzanchera, 2011). The remaining offenses were misdemeanors, drug offenses, and public order or status offenses. Juvenile crime increased substantially in the late 1980s, but by 2003, most violent crime had fallen below that observed in 1980 (Snyder, 2012). Of those arrested 1.653 million cases were referred to the juvenile court in 2008. Cases not referred—particularly "status offenses;" those behaviors that are included in the jurisdiction of the juvenile court in many states but are not classified as crimes—may be diverted to other agencies. Status offenses include running away, incorrigibility, truancy, and liquor-law violations.

Fifty-five percent of all cases are formally petitioned, and 45% are dismissed or referred to a variety of social agencies for services. If petitioned, 67% can be expected to be adjudicated delinquent, and subsequently, 62% of those are placed on probation and 22% receive an out-of-the-home placement, most often in a residential institution. Even at the final disposition stage, some juvenile cases are dismissed, and youths are released or given other sanctions outside the formal justice system. Waiver to adult court will result for about 1% of the cases, but that number has declined since 2002 (Griffin, Addie, Adams, & Firestone, 2011). Those numbers vary widely among the states, however, reflecting the differences in state statutes. Overall, fewer than 10% of the youths who enter the court system ultimately end up in a correctional institution.

Delinquency-case rates overall were 40.7 per 1,000 youth aged ten to seventeen years in 2008, but there were marked variations by age, from 4.6 per 1,000 for ten-year-olds to 109.1 per 1,000 for those seventeen years old. The overall rate was far lower than the rate of 81.6 in 1994, a reflection of the decline in crime by juveniles during a period of substantial population growth (Snyder & Sickmund, 2006). There are sex differences by age, in that female crime peaks at sixteen years while the peak age for males is seventeen.

As Table 1 indicates, most youths held in custody out of their homes are held in detention. The rate of 8.5 per 1,000 youth is nearly three times the rate of those in placement following adjudication. Placement in detention is important, because it is predictive of subsequent adjudication and referral to an institution.

TABLE 1
Youth Population and Processing Rates

	NUMBER	RATE
Population, 10–17 years (2009)	40,607,537	
Juvenile arrests (2008)	1,906,200	46.9
Referrals to juvenile court—delinquency	1,653,300	40.7
Petitions to juvenile court	924,400	22.7
Detention	347,000	8.5
Adjudications	563,900	13.8
Assigned to probation	398,700	9.6
Placed out of home	157,700	3.2
Waived to adult criminal court	8,900	0.24

Rates are calculated at the numbers per 1,000 youths processed during the year 2008.

The numbers in detention increased substantially after 1985, with drug cases explaining most of the increase (140%). Frequently arrested for drug violations, African American males are 41% of all detainees, and their detention is a key factor in their overall disproportionate representation in the juvenile justice system (Puzzanchera et al., 2012).

In the decade between 1990 and 2000, formal handling of juvenile court cases increased from 49.8% to 57.7% (McNeece & Jackson, 2004). Not surprisingly, there were subsequent increases in adjudications, waivers, and placements as formalization increased.

DISPOSITIONS On a given day in 2004, 96,655 youths were held in public and private correctional facilities (Snyder & Sickmund, 2006). Annually, more than 145,000 youths adjudicated for delinquency are sent to an out-of-home placement for a specified period or an indefinite stay. This is a small percentage of the more than 2.2 million youths arrested, and the numbers in placement declined after 2000, following the increases in most states during the 1990s, when the juvenile crime rate was substantially higher.

On February 22, 2010, there were a total of 79,165 youths in 2,259 facilities in the United States, a decline of more than one-third since 1997. The average number of days incarcerated for youths committed to residential programs was 106 in public facilities and 127 in private ones. This length of stay is considerably longer than the average of nineteen days for which youths are held in detention. (Hockenberry, 2013). The percentage of youths held in custody, both in detention and post-adjudication placement, is far less than the nearly 2 million annually arrested.

Youths charged with person crimes have a higher probability of post-adjudication placement than those

TABLE 2
Delinquency Offense, 2002

TYPE OF CRIME	REFERRAL TO COURT		POSTADJUDICATION PLACEMENT			
	%MALE	%FEMALE	%MALE	%FEMALE	%Public	%Private
Person	24	26	35	14	35	32
Property	37	38	29	12	28	27
Drugs	12	7	8	7	8	10
Public Order	27	28	10	12	26	20

From *Court Statistics, 2012*, by Puzzanchera, Adams, & Hockenberry, Washington, DC: OJJDP, Office of Justice Programs, U.S. Department of Justice. Copyright 2012 by the U.S. Department of Justice. Reprinted with permission.

charged with property or public-order crimes, as indicated in Table 2. Among the person crimes, there has been a substantial increase in processing and institutionalization of juveniles as sexual offenders for extended periods followed by placement of their names on a public registry. Zimring (2004) strongly criticizes the punitiveness of some of these practices. Although a relatively small percentage of youths are charged with drug crimes, they are likely to be placed out of the home because of the lack of drug-treatment facilities in many communities or because of parental drug abuse. The profile of offenders in public versus private facilities does not vary significantly, but offenders placed for the most serious crimes are more often found in public facilities. Out-of-home placement rose by 44% during the late 1990s, but since 2000, it has declined by 33%, primarily among property and person offenders.

Gender

Young females' rising rates of involvement with the juvenile justice system have received increased attention. Their rate of arrest rose to 30% of total juvenile arrests in 2008, and the involvement of young women in certain crimes (larceny, drugs, and simple assault) has risen more sharply than that of males (Puzzanchera et al., 2012). Because the number of male offenders is so much larger, percentage comparisons are misleading. It is less clear that female crime has increased commensurate to their involvement in the justice system—for example, their detention and placement in residential programs for status offenses, primarily involving family conflict. The rising rate of their involvement may be partly the result of changes in the roles and responsibilities of women as well as changing policies and practices that serve to bring more young women under the care and control of the justice system—for example, the referral of girls in need of mental health services to the justice system. It has been noted that 60–70% of the youths in juvenile justice have a diagnosable mental health problem,

with more females than males so diagnosed (Zahn, 2009; Kempf-Leonard, 2012). Of growing concern regarding juveniles in placement is the sexual victimization of residents by both staff and peers. In a survey completed in 2008–2009, Beck and Harrison (2010) reported that 10.3% of residents reported being sexually victimized by staff and 2.3% by another offender.

EVIDENCE-BASED MODELS OF INTERVENTION Because it has been shown that there is a wide range of factors that cause or are associated with delinquency, it is not surprising that there are many programs for prevention, early intervention, alternatives to incarceration, community-based intervention, and residential treatment. Using meta-analysis techniques, Lipsey and Wilson (1998) found the following characteristics to be associated with greater effectiveness:

- The integrity of the treatment model implementation.
- Longer duration of treatment produces better results.
- Results from well-established programs exceed new programs.
- Treatment administered by mental health professionals.
- Emphasis on interpersonal-skills training.
- Use of the teaching of family home methods.

Overall, they found community-based programs to be more effective than programs in custodial settings, so the context for the treatment is important. Voluntary participation was shown to be more effective than that which is coerced, and there are ways by which voluntary assent can be achieved. Greenwood (2006) shows that balanced and restorative justice (BARJ) programs can integrate restitution and community service by which an offender can repair the harm he or she may have caused. A report of the U.S. Surgeon General on Youth Violence (2001) concurs that many programs are effective with delinquent youths, but the report emphasizes the importance of the quality of implementation.

Elliot and his colleagues at the Center for the Study and Prevention of Youth Violence have developed "Blueprints" of ten programs meeting rigorous criteria that include demonstrated positive outcomes on problem behavior that persists beyond a youth's involvement in a program. They can be consulted at *http://www.colorado.edu/cspu/blueprints/*, for technical assistance regarding the programs that they regard as effective (Michalic, Fagan, Irwin, Ballard, & Elliot, 2002).

Greenwood (2006) has identified a large number of programs that have been shown to be effective for working with youths from preschool age through adolescence. For example, the Perry School Pre-School program was shown to reduce delinquency when the participants reached adulthood, in contrast with a comparable control group. Programs targeting a youth and his or her family have been shown to be effective, including functional family therapy, multisystemic therapy, the Seattle Social Development Program, and Big Brothers/Big Sisters. An extensive review of evidence-based models for more effective intervention is presented by (Greenwood & Turner, 2011).

Because of the lack of systematic evaluation, the effectiveness of most juvenile justice programs is unknown. Residential programs that include only delinquent youths are seldom effective in reducing recidivism, however. Other popular programs that have been shown not to be effective include boot camps, substance-abuse programs such as DARE, and "scared straight" programs.

Social Justice Issues

Some important social justice issues include overrepresentation of youths of color, prosecution of juveniles as adults, child welfare and juvenile justice, mental health of offenders, re-integration, and human rights.

OVERREPRESENTATION OF YOUTHS OF COLOR One of the most critical issues facing the entire justice system in the United States is the disproportionate representation of persons of color in all phases of the system, despite the fact that the United States has ratified the UN Convention on the Elimination of all Forms of Racial Discrimination. The juvenile justice system is not an exception, in that youths of color are disproportionately represented in all phases of the justice, child welfare, and public assistance systems, particularly African American youths. Ward (2012) highlights in *The Black Child Savers* how

extensive the discrimination has been toward African American youth throughout U.S. history. The Juvenile Justice and Delinquency Prevention Act of 1974 was amended in 1988 to mandate that states that participate in its programs make "every effort" to achieve proportional representation of youths of color in the juvenile justice system, but little has been accomplished in 15 years. As of 2008, white youths represented 53% of white youth cases petitioned in juvenile court, with 61% for African American and Native American youths and 58% Asian (Sickmund, Sladky, & Kang, 2011).

The overrepresentation of youths of color in the early stages of processing has profound effects, because if a youth is detained, there is an increased probability of being found guilty and sentenced to an out-of-home placement. As youths of color move through the justice system, there are amplification effects in the subsequent processing that add to the overrepresentation (Hawkins & Kempf-Leonard, 2005; Feld & Bishop, 2012). Unfortunately, we do not have adequate information about the Hispanic youths, as almost all are grouped with whites, but that can be expected to change with the growing Hispanic population in the United States. The overrepresentation of African American youths is most evident in the rate of placement in residential facilities, and for this we have data about Hispanic youths as well as Native American and Asian youths (Hockenberry, 2013). It is difficult not to ascribe racial discrimination to the fact that African American youths are five times more likely to be incarcerated than white youths, since the difference in being petitioned by the court is relatively small, as Table 3 indicates.

A variety of factors have been identified as causes of this disproportionality, including:

- Crime rates are higher in neighborhoods with high levels of deterioration and segregation, where youths of color reside and where police are likely to do more surveillance (Sampson, Morenoff, & Raudenbush, 2005).
- Juvenile justice agencies treat youths of color more severely than white youths, particularly early in processing (Bishop & Frazier, 2000; Bridges & Steen, 1998).
- Nunn (2002) argues that the oppression of African American youths (especially males) appears normal, because decision-makers have been socialized to undervalue the lives of these youths.
- Diversion and other alternatives to incarceration are more available in suburban areas with lower proportions of youths of color (Sarri, Shook, & Ward, 2001).

TABLE 3
Juvenile Justice Case Processing

	WHITE	AFRICAN AMERICAN	HISPANIC AMERICAN	NATIVE AMERICAN	ASIAN AMERICAN
% Rep. in Population	77.2	16.2	16.1	1.5	5.2
Petitioned in Juvenile Court	53	61	–	61	58
Rate Incarcerated per 100,000	120	606	224	369	47

Data Sources: U.S. Census, 2010
Sickmund, Sladky & Kang (2011) Easy Access to Juvenile Court Statistics, 2011. Online at http:www.ojjdp.gov/ojstatbb/azajjcsl/.
Hockenberry, S. (2013) Juveniles in Residential Placement, 2010. Online at http://www.ojjdp.gov/publications/index.html.

Discrimination against African American youths is most evident in rates of incarceration, as Table 3 indicates, and that is influenced by the disproportionate processing of them at every step in the juvenile justice process (Mulvey, 2011).

The highest rates of incarceration of youths of color are found in public residential facilities, reaching 90% in some states (Snyder & Sickmund, 2006). Overall, as of 2004, 754 African American, 496 American Indian/Native American, 348 Hispanic, 190 white, and 113 Asian youths per 100,000 were incarcerated.

PROSECUTING AND INCARCERATING JUVENILES AS ADULTS The shift toward the punitive handling of children and youths in the justice systems is best exemplified by the increased transfer of juveniles to adult criminal courts and their subsequent incarceration in adult prisons. During the 1990s, there was a proliferation of transfer legislation: forty-four states and the District of Columbia enacted at least one change easing the processing of juveniles as adults (Griffin, Addie, Adams, & Firestone, 2011). By the end of the decade, all fifty states permitted the transfer to adult courts. Although the legislative changes were made to address growing youth violence, by 2000, the majority of youths sentenced to the adult system were there for property, drug, and public order offenses. This legislation also decreased the power of the juvenile court judge and expanded that of the prosecutor. This change represented a significant shift in the role of the judge that had existed since 1900, when the court was founded.

There are three procedures by which juveniles are transferred for trial as adults: judicial discretion, prosecutorial discretion, and statutory exclusion of certain youths from the juvenile court based on offense and age. Some states do not maintain minimum age limits for trying juveniles as adults, while other states set the lower age limit between ten and sixteen years. Some states allow for a case to be designated for trial in the juvenile court with adult court rules.

The juvenile may receive a "blended sentence" that permits a youth to remain in the juvenile system, provided he or she commits no subsequent crime (Shook & Sarri, 2008).

Accurate information on the numbers of youths processed as adults is not available. Bishop (2000) reviewed a large number of studies and was unable to arrive at a sound estimate. As of 2008, 8,900 youths were waived to the adult court for processing (Griffin, et al., 2011). There has been a decline since 2000 because of the dramatic decline in serious and violent crime by juveniles, but the amount of the decline remains unknown. The U.S. Justice Department reported that as of 2004, there were 2,800 youth under 18 in adult prisons; however, this number excludes adults who were sentenced as juveniles, often with long sentences, so nationally the number may well exceed 100,000 individuals (Harrison & Beck, 2006). In 1997, there were 7,400 juveniles below the age of eighteen in state and federal prisons. As of 2011 there were 1790 youth below 18 years in adult prisons (USDOJ, 2012). The largest number of youth below 18 years were 5900 who were held in adult jails in 2011 although this practice is prohibited by the Juvenile Justice and Delinquency Prevention Act since 1974.

Juveniles of color and males are the majority of those tried as adults (Hawkins & Kempf-Leonard, 2005). Most youths in adult prisons will be released in their mid-twenties, but they will be ill-equipped to meet the demands of society for successful adulthood and parenting because of the stigma of incarceration and because of the lack of education, health care, and social services while incarcerated. Moreover, charges of human rights violations have been and are being made with respect to the conditions of incarceration (Human Rights Watch, 2005). Studies of recidivism indicate that juveniles released from adult facilities have higher rates of recidivism than similar youths released from juvenile facilities (Bishop & Frazier, 2000; Fagan, 1996). Decisions by the Supreme Court have reduced the incarceration of juveniles in adult facilities. In *Roper v. Simmons* (2005), the Court ruled that it was unconstitutional to execute a juvenile.

CHILD WELFARE AND JUVENILE JUSTICE The juvenile court serves abused and neglected children as well as those charged with delinquency, but it was expected that the two areas would be separately addressed since child welfare clients are initially victims of parental abuse or neglect, while juvenile delinquents are viewed as primarily responsible for their behavior as perpetrators of crimes. This distinction has become increasingly ambiguous as studies have shown the "drift" of child welfare clients to the juvenile justice system (Jonson-Reid & Barth, 2000; Kelly, 2002; Ryan, Hong, & Hernandez, 2010). In the Cook County, Illinois, juvenile court, it was observed that more than a third of maltreated children ended up in the juvenile justice system as delinquents.

Overall, African American and Hispanic youths with experience in foster care have been shown to be at high risk for subsequent transfer to the justice system. Most of those who "drift" into the justice system are reported to be male, and many are committed to adult prisons shortly after they "age out" of the child welfare system at eighteen years. With a large sample in California, Jonson-Reid and Barth (2000) followed youths from child welfare to entrance into the California Youth Authority. They observed that if youths were transferred to probation, the risk for subsequent transfer to the CYA for a serious felony increased significantly. Having multiple placements was correlated with transfer to the justice system.

A recent study in Michigan of adolescents who aged out of foster care reported several negative outcomes: homelessness, inadequate education, lack of employment, mental health problems, substance abuse, and experience in the justice system (Fowler & Toro, 2006). These youths also reported being physically and sexually abused. To delineate the process by which child-welfare youths "drift" into the justice system, youths frequently run away from placements, more often from congregate care than individual foster care or kin care. Some of them may engage in delinquent behavior as they attempt to survive "on the street." When they are apprehended by police, they may be taken to a detention facility pending a hearing by the court. Depending upon the outcome of that hearing, a juvenile may then be moved to juvenile-justice-system status, and the child welfare system may cease involvement with the case. Because a youth may be an older adolescent at this point, there is a tendency to view him or her more as a delinquent than as a victim of abuse or neglect.

MENTAL HEALTH AND JUVENILE COMPETENCY The collapse of the mental health system serving children and youths in the 1990s resulted in a gradual movement of mentally ill juveniles into the justice system. The inappropriateness of these placements was exacerbated by the lack of adequate legislation in many states for the assessment of competency for trial as a delinquent or as an adult. Prior to the 1990s, issues of juvenile competence were seldom raised, but findings from research on brain development and developmental maturity, as well as concerns about due process protection of youth, raised concerns in both the mental health and legal professions (Scott & Grisso, 1997). Findings from brain-development research are directly relevant to the criminal-justice processing of juveniles for both the individual's culpability and his or her ability to participate effectively in his or her defense. Recent neuroimaging studies indicate that the brain, specifically the pre-frontal lobe (PFC), continues to grow and change throughout adolescence and into the twenties. The PFC controls higher-order cognitive processes, which include motivation, inhibition, logical decision-making, risk taking, problem solving, planning, emotional regulation, sexual urges, and anticipation of consequences (Spear, 2000). Past and current trauma and stress have detrimental effects on adolescent brain functioning, and delinquent adolescents are significantly more at risk for limited cognitive development (Arnsten & Shansky, 2004; Feld & Bishop, 2012).

In trying to estimate the number of juveniles with a diagnosable mental disorder, Grisso (2004) reported that findings from several studies indicated that 60–70% of juveniles in correctional facilities have at least one disorder. Relatively few receive professional evaluations or treatment in most settings. Grisso suggests reasons for attention to these youths: (a) agencies have a legal and moral responsibility to attend to the mental health needs of juveniles; (b) juveniles are entitled to due process and equal protection under the law, including determination of their competency to participate in their own defense; and (c) protection of the public requires that juveniles with mental disorders be treated and managed in ways that maintain protection.

RE-INTEGRATION AND AFTERCARE Each year, nearly 100,000 juvenile offenders in correctional facilities are returned to their home communities, and an even larger number are released from probation, but re-integration services are poorly developed and reach a small proportion of returning youths (Griffin, 2005). In many states juveniles are released from correctional facilities under state-supervised parole, and so there is little adaptation to the circumstances of the youth or the community.

Griffin (2005) describes three court-directed programs for aftercare and reintegration—in Pennsylvania, West Virginia, and Indiana—that offered comprehensive services for education, employment, and treatment as needed along with mentoring and monitoring. Spencer and Jones-Walker (2004) offer a theory-based re-integration model that focuses on identity formation, recognizing that being in a correctional program is a life-changing experience. They present a cognitive behavioral approach that addresses the individual's environment as well as his or her personal characteristics. Their research and that of Barton (2006) found very low rates of recidivism among youths who completed programs that promoted competency, a positive sense of self, and transition programming with strong social support necessary for the youth to achieve success and stability. In a longitudinal study of 1,354 youths for seven years after conviction of a serious crime, Mulvey (2011a) observed that 91.5% decreased their criminal activity, especially if they received community-based supervision, substance-abuse treatment, and greater stability in their living arrangements, school and work.

HUMAN RIGHTS   The United States strongly advocates for the extension of human rights enforcement throughout the world, but when it relates directly to the United States, there is resistance not only to the adoption but also to the enforcement of those rights by United Nations agencies. Nowhere are the principles of human rights more at risk than in the U.S. processing of juveniles in the justice system. The International Convention on the Rights of the Child has not been ratified by the United States, and several of its provisions have been ignored. The United States has signed and ratified four other conventions, which are often negated by its practices of processing juveniles as adults, in the conditions of confinement in many facilities, in the incarceration of juveniles when community services would be more effective, and in the over-representation of youths of color in all levels of the juvenile justice system. The four other conventions include: the Convention on the Elimination of All Forms of Racism, the Covenant on Civil and Political Rights, the Convention against Torture, and the Convention on Human Rights. The relevance and importance of international law and customs was acknowledged by Justice Anthony Kennedy of the U.S. Supreme Court in his decision in *Roper v. Simmons*, in which the Court acknowledged that the juvenile death penalty was unconstitutional. In 2005, writing for the majority, Kennedy stated that international law

provided guidance for the Supreme Court, because execution of juveniles was prohibited in many Western countries many years prior to 2005. In 2010, the Court further addressed the incarceration of juveniles in *Graham v. Florida* (2010), in which it ruled that it was unconstitutional to incarcerate a youth for life for an offense that was less than a capital crime.

Human rights conventions set limits on state punishment and control, specify what is required in legal representation of children in the justice systems, reject the transferring of children to the adult justice system, mandate states to make "every effort" to achieve proportional representation of youths of color in the juvenile justice system, and specify appropriate conditions of confinement (Sarri & Shook, 2005). Attention to international law and custom is increasingly recognized in the United States, as are the more humane policies and practices in other countries (Amnesty International, 1998). Human rights frameworks provide powerful tools for effecting the processing of juveniles in the United States. It is probable that in the near future we will see a challenge to the "life without parole" sentences of juveniles, using international law as a conceptual framework for the complaint.

Future Trends and Directions

Greater attention to community-based intervention is essential if juvenile justice in the United States is to increase in effectiveness (Greenwood & Turner, 2011; Tyler, Zeidenberg, & Lotke, 2006). The efforts of the founders of the juvenile court, along with those who advocated for juvenile rights in the 1960s and 1970s need reexamination, including the goals of the Juvenile Justice and Delinquency Prevention Act, which strongly asserted that juveniles were to be primarily treated in the community. Moreover, that Act has emphasized priorities to reduce overrepresentation of youths of color, achieve gender equity, and increase community-based intervention. Edelman's presentation of the four circles for intervention in a comprehensive approach to youth policy comes the closest to recognition of the earlier priorities—reduction of poverty, universalistic approaches to youth development, education and after-school programming, and parsimony in punitive intervention (Edelman, 2002). He argues for approaches that "do no harm" as a minimum requirement.

Public opinion surveys report that a majority of the public (91%) believe that rehabilitative services and treatment for incarcerated youths can help prevent future crimes (Krisberg & Marchionna, 2007). The public also thinks that spending on rehabilitative services will save tax dollars in the long run. These attitudes suggest that in the future we may see a return to the goals of the original juvenile court, as Mears, Hay, Gertz, and Mancini (2007) suggest.

The character of the justice system is shaped by the attitudes and behavior of local communities. The newly developing programs of restorative justice, community service, and conflict resolution may provide the mechanisms for restoring community values regarding children and youths. In 2013 the National Research Council proposed a developmental strategy for juvenile justice reform which focuses on addressing the needs and characteristics of at-risk youth. Implementing such a strategy would advance the goals of the original juvenile court and of the provisions of the Juvenile Justice and Delinquency Act of 1974.

REFERENCES

Amnesty International. (1998). *Betraying the young: Human rights violations against children in the U.S. justice system.* New York: Amnesty International.

Arnsten, A., & Shansky, R. (2004). Adolescence: Vulnerable period for stress-induced prefrontal cortical function. *Annals of the New York Academy of Sciences, 1021* (Adolescent brain development: Vulnerabilities and opportunities), 143–147.

Barton, W. (2006). Incorporating the strengths perspective into intensive juvenile aftercare. *Western Criminology Review, 7*(2) 48–61.

Beck, A. & Harrison, P. (2010) *Sexual victimization in juvenile facilities reported to youth, 2008–2009.* Washington, DC: U.S. Department of Justice, Office of Justice Programs, OJJDP, BCJ228426.

Beckett, K., & Western, B. (2000). *The institutional sources of incarceration: Deviance, regulation and the transformation of state policy.* Paper presented at the American Criminology Society Annual Meeting, Toronto, Ontario, Canada.

Bishop, D. (2000). Juvenile offenders in the adult criminal justice system. In M. Tonry (Ed.). *Crime and justice: A review of research.* Chicago: University of Chicago Press.

Bishop, D., & Frazier, C. (2000). Consequences of transfer. In J. Fagan & F. Zimring (Eds.), *The changing borders of juvenile justice* (pp. 227–276). Chicago: University of Chicago Press.

Bridges, G. S., & Steen, S. (1998). Racial disparities in official assessment of juvenile offenders; Attributional stereotypes as mediating mechanisms. *American Sociological Review, 63*(4), 554–570.

Edelman, P. (2002). American government and the politics of youth. In M. Rosenheim (Eds.), *A century of juvenile justice* (pp. 310–339). Chicago: University of Chicago Press.

Fagan, J. (1996). The comparative advantage of juvenile versus criminal court sanction among adolescent felony offenders. *Law and Society, 18*(1), 77–114.

Feld, B., & Bishop, D. (2012). *Oxford handbook of juvenile justice.* New York: Oxford Univ. Press.

Fowler, P., & Toro, P. (2006). *Youth aging out of foster care in southeast Michigan.* Detroit, MI: Dept. of Psychology, Wayne State University.

Garland, D. (2001). *The culture of control.* Chicago: University of Chicago Press.

Greenwood, P. (2006). *Changing lives: Delinquency prevention as crime-control policy.* Chicago: University of Chicago Press.

Greenwood, P., & Turner, S. (2011) Establishing effective community-based care in juvenile justice. In F. Sherman & F. Jacobs, (Eds.), *Juvenile justice: Advancing research, policy and practice* (pp. 471–504). New York: Wiley.

Griffin, P. (2005). *Juvenile court-controlled reentry: Three practice models.* Special Project Bulletin. Pittsburgh, PA: Office of Juvenile Justice and Delinquency Prevention, National Center for Juvenile Justice.

Griffin, P., Addie, S. Adams, B., & Firestone, K. (2011). *Trying juveniles as adults: An analysis of state transfer laws and reporting.* Washington, DC: U.S. Department of Justice, Office of Justice Programs, OJJDP.

Grisso, T. (2004). *Double jeopardy: Adolescent offenders with mental disorders.* Chicago: University of Chicago Press.

Harrison, P., & Beck, A. (2006). *Prisoners in 2005.* Washington, DC: U.S. Dept. of Justice, Bureau of Justice Statistics. NCJ 215092.

Hawkins, D., & Kempf-Leonard. (2005). *Our children, their children.* Chicago: University of Chicago Press.

Hockenberry, S., Sickmund, M., & Sladky, A. (2011) *Juvenile residential facility census, 2008: Selected findings.* Washington, DC: U.S. Department of Justice, Office of Justice Programs OJJDP.

Hockenberry, S. (2013). *Juveniles in Residential Placement, 2010.* Washington, DC: U.S. Dept. of Justice, Office of Juvenile Justice and Delinquency.

Holzer, H. (2010) *Avoiding a lost generation: How to minimize the impact of the Great Recession on young workers.* Testimony Before the Joint Economic Committee of the U.S. Congress, May 28.

Human Rights Watch. (2005). *The rest of their lives: Life without parole for child offenders in the U.S.* New York: Author & Amnesty International.

Jonson-Reid, M., & Barth, R. (2000). From treatment report to juvenile incarceration. The role of child welfare services. *Children and Youth Services Review, 22*(7), 493–516.

Kelly, K. (2002). *Abuse/neglect and delinquency: Dually involved minors in the juvenile court.* Paper presented at the American Society of Criminology Annual Meeting, Chicago.

Kempf-Leonard, K. (2012). The conundrum of girls and juvenile justice processing. In B.C. Feld & D. Bishop (Eds.), *The Oxford history of juvenile crime and juvenile justice* (pp. 485–525). New York: Oxford University Press.

Krisberg, B., & Marchionna, S. (2007, February). *Attitudes of US voters toward youth crime and the justice system. Focus.* San Francisco: National Council on Crime and Delinquency.

Lerman, P. (2002). Twentieth century developments in America's institutional system for youth in trouble. In M. Rosenheim (Ed.), *A century of juvenile justice* (pp. 74–110). Chicago: University of Chicago Press.

Lipsey, M., & Wilson, D. (1998). Effective intervention for serious delinquency in adolescence and early adulthood. In R. Loeber & D. Farrington (Eds.), *Serious and violent juvenile offenders*. Thousand Oaks, CA: SAGE.

McNeece, C. A., & Jackson, S. (2004). Juvenile justice policy: Current trends and 21st century issues. In A. Roberts (Ed.), *Juvenile Justice Sourcebook* (pp. 41–68). New York: Oxford University Press.

Mears, D., Hay, C., Gertz, M., & Mancini, C. (2007). Public opinion and the foundation of the juvenile court. *Criminology*, 45(1), 223–258.

Michalic, S., Fagan, A., Irwin, K., Ballard, D., & Elliot, D. (2002). *Blueprints for violence prevention replications: Factors for implementation success*. Boulder, CO: Center for the Study and Prevention of Violence, Institute of Behavioral Science, University of Colorado.

Mulvey, E. (2011a). *Highlights from pathways to desistance: A longitudinal study of serious adolescent offenders*. Washington, DC: U.S. Department of Justice, Office of Justice Programs, OJJDP.

Mulvey, E. (2011b). *No place for kids: The case for reducing juvenile incarceration*. Baltimore: Annie E. Casey Foundation.

National Research Council. (2013). *Reforming juvenile justice: A developmental approach*. Washington, DC: National Academies Press, 2013.

Nunn, K. (2002). The child as other: Race and differential treatment in the juvenile justice system. *DePaul Law Review*, 51(Spring), 134–146.

Osgood, D. W., Foster, M., Flanagan, C., & Ruth, G. (2005). *On your own without a net: The transition to adulthood for vulnerable populations*. Chicago: University of Chicago Press.

Presidential Commission on Law Enforcement and the Administration of Justice. (1967). *Task Force Report*. Washington, DC: U.S. Govt. Printing Office.

Puzzanchera, C. (2011). *Juvenile Arrests, 2009*. Washington, DC: U.S. Department of Justice, Office of Justice Programs. OJJDP.

Puzzanchera, C., Adams, B., & Hockenberry, S. (2012). *Juvenile court statistics 2009*. Washington, DC: U.S. Department of Justice, Bureau of Justice Statistics, OJJDP.

Rosenheim, M. (2002). The modern American juvenile court. In M. Rosenheim, F. Zimring, D. Tanenhaus, & B. Dohrn (Eds.), *A century of juvenile justice* (pp. 341–360). Chicago: University of Chicago Press.

Ross, T., & Miller, J. (2011). How American government frames youth problems. In Sherman, F., & Jacobs, F. (Eds.), *Advancing research, policy and practice* (pp. 352–368). New York: Wiley.

Ryan, J., Hong, J., & Hernandez, P. (2010) Kinship foster care and the risk of juvenile delinquency. *Children and Youth Services Review*, 32(2), 1823–1830.

Sampson, R., Morenoff, J., & Raudenbush, S. (2005). Social anatomy of racial and ethnic disparities in violence. *American Journal of Public Health*, 95(2), 224–232.

Sarri, R., & Shook, J. (2005). Human rights and juvenile justice in the United States: Challenges and opportunities. In M. Ensalaco & L. Majka (Eds.), *Children's Human Rights* (pp. 197–228). New York: Rowman and Littlefield.

Sarri, R., Shook, J., & Ward, G. (2001). *Decision making in juvenile justice: A comparative study of four states*. Ann Arbor: Institute for Social Research, University of Michigan.

Scott, E., & Grisso, T. (1997). The evolutions of the adolescence: A developmental perspective on juvenile justice. *Journal of Criminal Law and Criminology*, 88, 137–138.

Setterstein, R., Furstenberg, F., & Rumbaut, R. (2005). *On the frontier of young adulthood: Theory, research and public policy*. Chicago: University of Chicago Press.

Shook, J., & Sarri, R. (2008), Trends in the commitment of juveniles to adult prisons: Toward an increased willingness to treat juveniles as adults. *The Wayne Law Review*, 54(4), 1725–1765.

Sickmund, M., Sladky, T. J., & Kang, W. (2011). *Easy Access to the Census of Juveniles in Residential Placement*. Retrieved from www.ojjdp.gov/ojstatbb/ezacjrp/

Snyder, H. N. (2012). Juvenile delinquents and juvenile justice clientele: Trends and patterns in crime and justice. In B. Feld & D. Bishop (Eds.), *Oxford handbook of juvenile justice* (pp. 3–30). New York: Oxford University Press.

Snyder, H. N., & Sickmund, M. (2006). *Juvenile offenders and victims: 2006 national report*. Washington, DC: OJJDP, Office of Justice Programs, U.S. Department of Justice.

Spear, L. (2000). The adolescent brain and age-related behavioral manifestations. *Neuroscience Biobehavior*, 24, 417–463.

Spencer, M. B., & Jones-Walker, C. (2004). Interventions and services offered to former juvenile offenders reentering their communities: An analysis of program effectiveness. *Youth Violence and Juvenile Justice*, 2(1), 88–89.

Tanenhaus, D. (2002). The evolution of the juvenile court in the early twentieth century. In M. Rosenheim, F. Zimring, D. Tanenhaus, & B. Dohrn (Eds.), *A century of juvenile justice* (pp. 42–74). Chicago: University of Chicago Press.

Task Force Report on Juvenile Crime and Juvenile Justice. (1974). Washington, DC: Office of Juvenile Justice and Delinquency Prevention.

Tyler, J., Zeidenberg, J., & Lotke, E. (2006). *Cost effective youth corrections: The fiscal architecture of rational juvenile justice systems*. Washington, DC: Justice Policy Institute.

U.S. Dept. of Justice, Bureau of Justice Statistics. (2012). *Census of Juveniles Below the Age of 18 in Prisons and Jails*. Retrieved from http://bjs.ojp.usdoj.gov/content/pub/pdf/p11/pdf

U.S. Surgeon General. (2001). *Delinquency prevention programs that do not work*. Washington, DC: U.S. Department of Health and Human Services.

Ward, G. (2012). *The black child-savers: Racial democracy and juvenile justice*. Chicago: University of Chicago Press.

Zimring, F. E. (2002). The common thread: Diversion in the jurisprudence of juvenile courts. In M. Rosenheim, F. Zimring, D. Tanenhaus, & B. Dohrn (Eds.), *A century of juvenile justice* (pp. 142–158). Chicago: University of Chicago Press.

Zahn, M. (2009). *The delinquent girl*. Philadelphia: Temple University Press.

Zimring, F. E. (2004). *An American travesty*. Chicago: University of Chicago Press.

ROSEMARY C. SARRI

L

LEADERSHIP, FOUNDATIONS OF

ABSTRACT: The concept of leadership has evolved from focusing on innate abilities, to learned skills, to recognition that leadership is composed of both skills and abilities. Recently, theorists and practitioners have identified core elements of leadership for social-work organizations. These elements encourage social-work leaders to understand their organizations as living systems within an interdependent world and aid them in connecting humanistic intentions with effects. Acknowledgment and enactment of these competencies secure skills of communication and guidance needed for engagement in dialog and action. Social-work students and leaders can learn and hone these qualities in social-work programs, schools, and professional development opportunities for effective leadership in the field.

KEY WORDS: leader; leadership; leadership competencies; leadership skills; leadership theory; spirituality; social-work managers

Leadership—Historical Background

Although the question "what makes a leader?" has been asked, in different iterations, since ancient Greece, formal leadership theory did not develop until the early part of the 20th century. Since that time, a number of paradigms have been proposed, the first of which was the trait approach, which corresponded with the scientific management school of organizational thought (Holland, 1959, 1962, 1966; Taylor, 1911). Members of this school sought to discover and describe the elemental characteristics of leaders and believed that leadership was an inherent ability, rather than something that could be learned and honed. Research in the 1940s and 1950s by Stogdill (1948) and Mann (1959) indicated inconsistencies in the trait approach, although more recent investigation has demonstrated a link between personality and leadership, creating renewed interest in traits (Arvey, Rotundo, Johnson, Zhang, & McGue, 2006; Bargal, 2000). The emergence of the human relations school of management in the 1930s and 1940s provided the basis for a study by Bowers and Seashore (1966) that revealed two basic leadership patterns: *consideration*, or concern for understanding employees as individuals, and *initiating structure*, or clear delineation of and monitoring of tasks. Theory "Y" Management through the 1960s encouraged leaders to balance autonomy with mutual objective setting in their organizations and to focus on goals, planning, and rational thinking (McGregor, 1960). As broad-spectrum theories broke down in the 1960s across all fields, however, the contingency leadership approach emerged, which acknowledged the unfixed face of leadership, primarily dependent upon the various contexts and situations in which an individual finds oneself (Fielder, 1967).

In the 1970s, others joined the conversation, building on the past, yet adding new perspectives on effective leadership. Paradigms that were experienced as radical quickly evoked a following, especially in the corporate boardrooms across the United States. Most notable was the concept of "servant leadership," as coined and developed by Robert K. Greenleaf (1977). Grounded in the dimensions of moral authority or conscience, Greenleaf proposed that the most effective leader (and, he would say, all who desire to live a "full life") is embodied in one who understands her or himself as a servant first and then chooses to lead. Servant leaders create effective serving organizations for which the personal growth of clients and employees is among the highest priority.

This values-based style of leadership was expanded upon and modified in the 1980s with new approaches that "revealed a conception of the leader as someone who defines organizational reality through the articulation of a vision, which is a reflection of how he or she defines an organization's mission and the values that will support it" (Bryman, 1997, p. 280). By the 1990s, the discourse returned to the interactional nature of leadership. Bass (1990) proposed that transactional and transformational leadership styles were two ends of a behavioral continuum, rather than "either/or" types. Transactional leadership involves an exchange relationship between "leaders" and "followers"; adherence to rules and standards; actions exerted solely to correct problems; and a laissez-faire leadership approach. In contrast, transformational leadership emphasizes the relationship between leaders and followers, using power to serve others, learning from criticism, open dialogue, shared recognition, and encouragement of free thinking. Transformational leadership builds a sense of vision, pride, respect, and trust; clearly communicates high expectations; encourages problem solving; and explicitly values each individual employee.

Consistent with concurrent social trends, feminist and ethnic leadership theories also emerged during this time, challenging the white, masculine culture upon which most organizations had been constructed. Feminist theory argued that women tended to lead with a more cooperative, collaborative, and empathetic style and that women leaders often used intuition, in addition to rational thought, to solve problems (Loden, 1985). Some scholars suggested that the feminist leadership approach was not exclusive to women, but rather could be used by men as a complementary approach to the traditional, masculine model. Afrocentric theory, which strongly valued interpersonal relationships and spirituality, conceptualized the leader as one who strives to encourage and nourish these relationships and the well-being of people in society. Although a potential weakness of this approach was the risk of reducing efficiency (Hasenfeld, 1983), Afrocentric leadership also values transparency, approachability, and clear communication (McFarlin, Coster, & Mogale-Pretorius, 1999), which encourage organizational productivity.

Since the 1970s, leadership scholars have incorporated and expanded the feminist and ethnic approaches to offer an ecological view of leadership (Wheatley, 1994). Inspired by theory from quantum physics, this holistic conception of leadership values interconnected networks and fluid information channels, and it recognizes that both the organization and the world beyond consist of emerging, self-organizing structures and interdependent relationships among individuals from multiple cultures. Instead of exerting command and control, leaders are encouraged to make meaning in the midst of chaos, trusting that organizations will evolve healthfully and freely if guided with self-consistency and authenticity.

Most recently, leadership scholars have developed upon the interconnected, holistic nature of life described by the ecological approach to articulate a spiritual leadership approach (Bailey, 1997, 2006; Heifetz, 1994; Owen, 1999; Scharmer, 2007). In this context, spirit is separate from political or religious doctrine, and it serves as the connecting force throughout all life (Owen; Palmer, 1998). This approach attends to the health of the organization and the people within it. Leaders with spirit recognize and cultivate softer process skills and attributes in their organizations, breathing life and inspiration into them.

Social-Work Leadership: Context and Development

Over the 20th century, social work has produced numerous well-known leaders; however, many primarily served as personnel administrators and facilitators who linked agency boards and staff members, especially in the profession's earliest years. The field itself has focused more on developing social-work administration and management, which overlaps with, but is different from, social-work leadership. This has resulted in a dearth of professional literature (Brilliant, as cited in Patti, 2003; Rank & Hutchison, 2000). Nevertheless, Mary Parker Follett, a major contributor to the scientific management theory, was a social worker.

In the 1960s, as the civil rights movement developed, social-work leaders began to challenge biased service patterns and actively forge new conceptions and processes in their organizations (Austin, 2000). In 1969, Whitney Young became the first African American president of the National Association of Social Workers (NASW). Although social-work organizations were some of the earliest to address institutionalized prejudices, this activity did not ultimately result in a new definition of social-work leadership. The competing-values framework, described by organizational behaviorist Quinn (1988), provided guiding principles for social-work leaders, which included maintaining internal stability, developing human resources, adapting to opportunities and threats in the environment, and productively and effectively reaching the organization's goals. Additionally, social workers have looked toward total quality management, which emphasizes organizational success through customer satisfaction (Abrahamson, 1996; Boettecher, 1998; Gummer & McCallion, 1995; Reeves & Bednar, 1994).

In short, while also importing theories from other fields, leadership education in social work has largely encouraged individuals in these positions to be visionary, proactive, and responsible for the development of their organizations. In the early 21st century, it remains particularly critical that social-work leaders consider how they can help their organizations reach performance goals in all areas of function to improve social-work service (Patti, 2000).

As the field of social work continues to evolve, it becomes more diverse, market driven, and research oriented. It has also become more political, with multiple social workers in the U.S. Congress and hundreds serving across the United States in local and state legislatures. Nonetheless, the field of social work receives little positive acknowledgment by contemporary society, and as a result, many social workers express the need to increase its status and access to power.

Leadership is still not a core component of social-work education, and often, leaders of social-work organizations cross over from other disciplines (Patti, 2000). Some scholars have recommended that the human services field develop a unique theoretical perspective on leadership that can be introduced into mainstream management theory and education, rather than human services simply adopting models from other fields; others have suggested that social workers need not hesitate to follow successful leadership training models from other fields, such as business and public administration (Drucker, 1993; Patti, 2003; Perlmutter, 2006; Rank & Hutchison, 2000).

Perlmutter's (2006) interviews of chief executive officers and executive directors of social services agencies revealed that many of these leaders expressed a need for highly developed analytic skills, commitment to outcome-based practice, data-driven decision making, and effective oral and written communication abilities. They noted that these skills are more often found among MBAs, MPAs, and urban planners, rather than social-work graduates. Additionally, they suggested that social-work leaders engage in preparation that extends beyond the clinical approach and addresses societal needs.

A survey of 75 deans and directors for 460 social-work programs accredited by the Council on Social Work Education and 75 executive directors and presidents of 56 chapters of the NASW conducted by Rank and Hutchison (2000) indicated that leaders in the social-work profession tend to distinguish their leadership from that in other professions because of five common elements: (a) committing to the NASW's *Code of Ethics*, (b) maintaining a systemic perspective, (c) employing a participatory leadership style, (d) advocating altruism, and (e) focusing on the public image of the profession.

This group of leaders also identified nine leadership skills specifically necessary for social workers in the 21st century, including the following:

1. Community development, or the "efforts made by professional and community residents to enhance the social bonds among members of the community, motivate the citizens for self-help, develop responsible local leadership, and create or revitalize local institutions" (Barker, as cited in Rank & Hutchison, 2000, pp. 495–496).
2. Communication or interpersonal skills, or "the verbal and nonverbal exchange of information, including all the ways in which knowledge is transmitted and received" (Rank & Hutchison).

Communication and interpersonal skills also include the ability to work with others to accomplish specific objectives through clear speaking and writing, proper allocation of time and resources, and consideration of diverse stakeholder perspectives.

3. Analytic skills, or the "systematic consideration of anything in its respective parts and their relationship to one another" (Rank & Hutchison; Hardina, 2002).
4. Technological skills, or the ability to apply knowledge and engage with computers and related technology (Meenaghan, Gibbons, & McNutt, 2005). In the field of social work, relevant technologies may include using electronic medical records, engaging in computer-assisted therapy for clients who experience physical barriers to treatment, and utilizing social networking for marketing and donation solicitations.
5. Political skills, or the coordination of "efforts to influence legislation, election of candidates, and social causes" and "running for elective office, organizing campaigns in support of other candidates or issues, fundraising, and mobilizing voters and public opinion" (Barker, as cited in Rank & Hutchison, pp. 495–496), in addition to understanding the connection between local practice and the global context (Mary, 1997).
6. Visioning skills, or the ability to conceptualize objectives for a cohort, institution, constituency, community, employees, or clients, as well as expressing this vision through verbal and written communication (Mizrahi & Rosenthal, 2001).
7. Risk-taking skills, or the attributes that enable a leader to demonstrate courage when faced with confrontation so as to improve the human condition for a cohort, institution, constituency, community, employees, or clients and that engender "tenacity and courage in employees" (Kets De Vries, Vringnaud, & Florent-Treacy, 2004, p. 479). Social-work leaders may need to take calculated risks to keep their agency relevant in changing times or in envisioning long-term organizational change processes.
8. Ethical reasoning, or the faithful reference to the values outlined by the NASW's *Code of Ethics* during decision making, including integrity, trust, credibility, and accountability.
9. Cultural competency or diversity, or "the set of academic and interpersonal skills that allow individuals to increase their understanding and appreciation of cultural differences and similarities, within, among, and between groups to reflect

the needs of all...(that is, not just the majority cultural group) with all systems" (Bailey & Aronoff, 2004, p. 136). For example, social-work leaders should consider whether an agency's staffing, communication processes, and setting (both exterior location and interior décor) reflect multicultural values.

Certainly, these abilities—among other general skills, such as strategic planning and collaboration, which are necessary for leaders in any field—are critical for leaders within the social-work profession (Mizrahi & Berger, 2005; Mizrahi & Rosenthal, 2001).

Leadership Competencies for the 21st Century

Yet, to most effectively develop, use, and sustain these skills and ourselves as leaders, we must recognize and draw upon another group of what are frequently referred to as "softer" skills. Often defined as process skills, these are competencies of "heart and head" that are implicit to our profession. To most effectively address the numerous complex challenges facing the organizations of the 21st century necessitates that these traits and skills now be made explicit and publicly reclaimed (Bailey, 1997, 2006; Bolman & Deal, 1995). Able to be taught and learned, this set of core competencies—authenticity, humility, empathy, courage and compassion, faith, patience, and love—composes the essence of life, or "spirit" (Bailey, 2006). Although only recently discussed in the literature, these elements offer a framework within which to support the nine leadership skills cited above and address the central and increasingly complex leadership demands while greatly benefiting our organizations. In fact, recent studies have shown that organizations that seek to recognize the spirit and even attempt to align their goals with the spirit outperform those that do not (for example, Mitroff & Denton, as cited in Pink, 2006). These seven components of spirit encourage social-work leaders to understand their organizations as living systems within an interconnected world (Mulroy, 2004), rather than as independent entities, and "aid them in collectively creating systems designed to enhance the human condition and co-construct cultures of inclusion" (Bailey, 2006, p. 299).

1. Authenticity: As noted earlier, the demands on leaders are increasing in amount and complexity. To meet these demands and maintain well-being, leaders must take the time to become fully aware of themselves, continuously assessing their abilities, values, and areas needing development. All leaders are different, and consequently, when leading authentically and consistently according to their character, all leaders practice slightly different styles (George, 2003). Through authentic self-knowledge, leaders develop the strength to use their abilities to full potential and with integrity, living what they believe at all times and through all choices (Bailey, 1997).

2. Humility: A derivative of the word "humus," or earth, "humility is the understanding of what one believes in; it is transcending ego to resist the lure of the trappings of authority" (Bailey, 2006, p. 299). Leadership requires one to be grounded and centered to comprehend that individuals' inherent value extends beyond title and place in society. Humble leaders acknowledge that criticism and praise are part of the holistic quest for understanding, and they recognize the unique nature of each person and acknowledge the necessity of everyone in the organization as an important part of this interconnected web (Freire, 1981). Humble leaders foster collaboration and cocreation because they understand their own limits and seek out people who bring complementary skills and perspectives.

3. Empathy: It is "the self-knowledge that comes from being able to 'hold' the perceptions and the emotions of another" (Bailey, 2006, p. 300). Being empathetic requires a mindfulness "unfolding" and moment-to-moment awareness when leaders remain grounded and true to themselves, continuously growing personally and professionally, and at the same time opening their minds and hearts to learn and know others more deeply (Kabat-Zinn, 2005). Social neuroscience has recently demonstrated that human beings possess mirror neurons, which recreate in one person's brain the neural activity that is occurring in another's brain during focused social exchanges (Goleman, 2006). These neurons actually help to establish an empathic rapport between people that strengthens interactions and relationships.

4. Courage and Compassion: Although these states of emotion and action are usually thought of as separate, the values of courage and compassion complement and strengthen each other. With both courage and compassion, leaders can make purposeful, definite, and strategic decisions while at the same time respecting the joys and struggles of others. Furthermore, courage and compassion embolden leaders to embrace the more challenging paradoxes of life, and together, they enable leaders to contemplate creative possibilities through opposition and appreciate the bigger

picture, the realities of the larger context in which both strengths and challenges coexist. For example, when a leader faces the need to downsize her organization, the balance of these two attributes can help guide her decision making. Courage alone would not allow her to take into account the full implications of eliminating positions for her employees; on the other hand, compassion alone would not necessarily suffice to maintain the organization's financial stability; however, the balance of these two skills would allow her to approach these difficult conversations with empathy, bravery, and integrity.

5. Faith: As described by Bailey (2006), "the faith of leadership is about living with uncertainty and trusting that all that happens serves a higher good; that there is a lesson to be learned in every pleasure and every pain" (p. 300). Dispelling popular misconnotations of the word, faith is not about religion; it is not contrary to reason; it does not ignore people and situations that are dishonest or dangerous; and it does not inhibit human beings from asking questions and developing new knowledge. Faith can serve as the origin of inspiration as well as the energy for continuing efforts. It encourages leaders to think beyond the known into the realm of opportunities not yet conceived. Often, the source of organizations' most effective vision statements is faith, as visions extend beyond the present into future possibilities. Although most organizations develop and tout vision statements rather easily, faith is one of the most difficult competencies to maintain because fear often replaces it, especially with constant changes and ambiguity in the world. Although elements of fear will always be present, leaders must embrace faith and extend it to the others in their organizations as they move forward in the complexities of life (Morris, 2007). Faith is particularly crucial during processes of organizational change, as it is during times of upheaval and transformation when employees turn to the agency leadership for guidance, support, and insight. A leader who demonstrates faith models how to live in times of turbulence and helps create a culture of trust and hope.

6. Patience: The patience of leadership applies to both self and to others. It is the willingness to attend to the needs and growth of all by partaking in deep listening, acknowledging the context and circumstances of each situation, and cultivating the capacity to "restore . . . and counter the destructive efforts of power stress" (Boyatzis & McKee, 2005, p. 72). Patience allows leaders to know how and when to conserve and to prune, both in their organizations and in their individual lives, trusting in the process.

7. Love: In the realm of leadership, the love that one must nurture and share is best defined as "agape." Agape goes beyond romantic and familial love; it is a love for all simply because they exist, regardless of their identities, actions, or associations (Bailey, 2006). Indeed, agape is the form of love that engenders freedom (Freire, 1981), as demonstrated through the lives of people that many consider heroes. Agape love is the culmination of all of the core competencies of leaders; it requires that leaders have invested themselves in the process to live lives as authentic, humble, empathic, courageous, compassionate, faithful, and patient beings.

In sum, the spiritual components of leadership find their roots in social work's earliest theories of expansive, collective, process-oriented engagement with others. Collectively, they form the requisite base upon which other critically important areas of knowledge and skills can be well honed and most effectively used. Social-work leadership education offers a strong example of multidisciplinary attention to relationships—between and among organizations, structures, cultures, and individual people; yet in the current era of growing accountability demands and downsizing, it must also consistently focus on building morale and improving organizational outcomes (Mizrahi & Berger, 2005; Patti, 2003). Social-work schools and departments must continue to develop macro theories and practices that will educate and support leaders for many years to come (Rothman, 2013). Attending to "leading from the spirit" advances these processes of creation and resilience while recognizing that there will always be much to learn about leadership from other fields and disciplines to enhance our service to the world.

References

Abrahamson, E. (1996). Management fashion. *Academy of Management Review, 21*(1), 254–285.

Arvey, R. D., Rotundo, M., Johnson, W., Zhang, Z., & McGue, M. (2006). The determinants of leadership role occupancy: Genetic and personality factors. *The Leadership Quarterly, 17*, 1–20.

Austin, D. M. (2000). Social work and social welfare administration: A historical perspective. In R. Patti (Ed.), *The handbook of social welfare management* (pp. 27–54). Thousand Oaks, CA: Sage.

Bailey, D. (1997). *Proceedings from Advanced Leadership Institute for Catholic Charities Directors*. Tampa, FL: Franciscan Center.

Bailey, D. (2006). Leading from the spirit. In F. Hesselbein & M. Goldsmith (Eds.), *The leader of the future 2: visions, strategies, and practices for a new era* (pp. 297–302). San Francisco, CA: Jossey-Bass.

Bailey, D., & Aronoff, N. (2004). The integration of multicultural competency and organizational practice in social work education: Recommendations for the future. In L. Gutierrez, M. Zuniga, & D. Lum (Eds.), *Education for multicultural social work practice: Critical viewpoints and future directions* (pp. 135–144). Alexandria, VA: CSWE Press.

Bargal, D. (2000). The manager as leader. In R. Patti (Ed.), *The handbook of social welfare management* (pp. 303–320). Thousand Oaks, CA: Sage.

Bass, B. M. (1990). From transactional to transformational leadership: Learning to share the vision. *Organizational Dynamics, 18*(3), 19–31.

Boettcher, R. E. (1998). A study of quality managed human service organizations. *Administration in Social Work, 22*(2), 41–56.

Bolman, L. G., & Deal, T. E. (1995). *Leading with soul*. San Francisco, CA: Jossey-Bass.

Bowers, D., & Seashore, S. (1966). Predicting organizational effectiveness with a four-factor theory of leadership. *Administrative Science Quarterly, 11*, 238–263.

Boyatzis, R. E., & McKee, A. (2005). *Resonant leadership*. Boston, MA: Harvard Business School Press.

Bryman, A. (1997). Leadership in organizations. In S. R. Clegg, C. Hardy, & W. R. Nord (Eds.), *Handbook of organization studies* (pp. 276–292). Thousand Oaks, CA: Sage.

Drucker, P. (1993). *Managing the non-profit organization: Principles and practices*. New York, NY: Harper Collins.

Fielder, F. (1967). *A theory of leadership effectiveness*. New York, NY: McGraw-Hill.

Freire, P. (1981). *Pedagogy of the oppressed*. New York, NY: Continuum.

George, B. (2003). *Authentic leadership: rediscovering the secrets to creating lasting value*. San Francisco, CA: Jossey-Bass.

Goleman, D. (2006). *Social intelligence: The new science of social relationships*. New York, NY: Bantam.

Greenleaf, R. K. (1977). *Servant leadership: A journey in the nature of legitimate power and greatness*. Mahwah, NJ: Paulist Press.

Gummer, B., & McCallion, P. (Eds.). (1995). *Total quality management in the social services*. Albany, NY: State University of New York at Albany.

Hardina, D. (2002). *Analytical skills for community organization practice*. New York, NY: Columbia University Press.

Hasenfeld, Y. (1983). *Human service organizations*. Englewood Cliffs, NJ: Prentice Hall.

Heifetz, R. A. (1994). *Leadership without easy answers*. Cambridge, MA: Belknap Press of Harvard University Press.

Holland, J. (1959). A theory of vocational choice. *Journal of Counseling Psychology, 6*, 35–45.

Holland, J. (1962). Some explorations of a theory of vocational choice. *Psychological Monographs, 76*(26), 1–545.

Holland, J. (1966). *The psychology of vocational choice*. Waltham, MA: Blaisdell.

Kabat-Zinn, J. (2005). *Coming to our senses: Healing ourselves and the world through mindfulness*. New York, NY: Hyperion.

Kets De Vries, M. F. R., Vringnaud, P., & Florent-Treacy, E. (2004). The global leadership life inventory. *International Journal of Human Resource Management, 15*(3), 475–492.

Loden, M. (1985). *Feminine leadership, or how to succeed in business without being one of the boys*. New York, NY: Times Books.

Mann, R. D. (1959). A review of the relationship between personality and performance in small groups. *Psychological Bulletin, 56*, 241–270.

Mary, N. L. (1997). Linking social welfare policy and global problems: Lessons learned from an advanced seminar. *Journal of Social Work Education, 33*(3), 587–598.

McFarlin, D. B., Coster, E. A., & Mogale-Pretorius, C. (1999). South African management development in the twenty-first century: moving toward an Africanized model. *Journal of Management Development, 18*(1), 63–78.

McGregor, D. (1960). *The human side of enterprise*. New York, NY: McGraw-Hill.

Meenaghan, T. M., Gibbons, W. E., & McNutt, J. G. (2005). *Generalist practice in larger settings: Knowledge and skill concepts*. Chicago, IL: Lyceum.

Mizrahi, T., & Berger, C. S. (2005). A longitudinal look at social work leadership in hospitals: The impact of a changing health care system. *Health and Social Work, 30*(2), 155–165.

Mizrahi, T., & Rosenthal, B. B. (2001). Complexities of coalition building: Leaders' successes, strategies, struggles, and solutions. *Social Work, 46*(1), 63–78.

Morris, J. (2007). The current leadership crisis and thoughts on solutions. In Mack, T. C. (Ed.), *Hopes and visions for the 21st century* (pp. 250–263). Bethesda, MD: World Future Society.

Mulroy, E. (2004). The context of group work: Organizational and community factors. In G. L. Greif & P. H. Ephross (Eds.), *Group work with populations at risk* (2nd ed.). New York, NY: Oxford University Press.

Owen, H. (1999). *The spirit of leadership: Liberating the leader in each of us*. San Francisco, CA: Berrett-Koehler.

Palmer, P. (1998). *The courage to teach: Exploring the inner landscape of a teacher's life*. San Francisco, CA: Jossey-Bass.

Patti, R. (2000). The landscape of social welfare management. In R. Patti (Ed.), *The handbook of social welfare management* (pp. 3–25). Thousand Oaks, CA: Sage.

Patti, R. (2003). Reflections on the state of management in social work. *Administration in Social Work, 27*(2), 1–11.

Perlmutter, F. D. (2006). Ensuring social work administration. *Administration in Social Work, 30*(2), 3–10.

Pink, D. H. (2006). *A whole new mind*. New York, NY: Berkeley.

Quinn, R. E. (1988). *Beyond rational management: Mastering the paradoxes and competing demands of high performance*. San Francisco, CA: Jossey-Bass.

Rank, M. G., & Hutchison, W. S. (2000). An analysis of leadership within the social work profession. *Journal of Social Work Education, 36*(3), 487–502.

Reeves, C., & Bednar, D. (1994). Defining quality: Alternatives and implications. *Academy of Management Review*, 19, 419–445.

Rothman, J. (2013). *Education for macro intervention: A survey of problems and prospects.* Association for Community Organization and Social Administration. Retrieved June, 2013, from https://www.acosa.org/joomla/pdf/Rothman ReportRevisedJune2013.pdf

Scharmer, O. C. (2007). *Theory U: Leading from the future as it emerges.* Cambridge, MA: Society for Organizational Learning.

Stogdill, R. M. (1948). Personal factors associated with leadership: A survey of the literature. *Journal of Psychology*, 25, 35–71.

Taylor, F. W. (1911). *The principles of scientific management.* New York, NY: Harper & Brothers.

Wheatley, M. (1994). *Leadership and the new science.* San Francisco, CA: Berrett-Koehler.

Further Reading

Cuddy, A. J. C., Kohut, M., & Neffinger, J. (2013). Connect, then lead. *Harvard Business Review*, 91(7/8), 55–61.

Ezell, M. (1991). Administrators as advocates. *Administration in Social Work*, 15(40), 1–18.

Fisher, E. A. (2005). Facing the challenges of outcomes measurement: The role of transformational leadership. *Administration in social work*, 29(4), 35–49.

Garrett, M. T., Borders, L. D., Crutchfield, L. B., Torres-Rivera, E., Brotherton, A., & Curtis, R. (2001). Multicultural SuperVISION: A paradigm of cultural responsiveness for supervisors. *Journal of Multicultural Counseling and Development*, 29, 147–158.

Mizrahi, T., & Berger, C. S. (2001). Effect of a changing health care environment on social work leaders: Obstacles and opportunities in hospital social work. *Social Work*, 46(2), 170–182.

Mulroy, E. A. (2004). Theoretical perspectives on the social environment to guide management and community practice: An organization—in-environment approach. *Administration in Social Work*, 28(1), 77–96.

Sapolsky, R. M. (2004). *Why zebras don't get ulcers* (3rd ed.). New York, NY: Henry Holt.

Slavin, S. (Ed.). (1985). *An introduction to human services management* (2nd ed.). New York, NY: Haworth Press.

Darlyne Bailey, Katrina M. Uhly, and Jessica Schaffner Wilen

LESBIAN, GAY, BISEXUAL, AND TRANSGENDER (LGBT) FAMILIES AND PARENTING

Abstract: According to U.S. census data, an estimated 270,313 American children were living in households headed by same-sex couples in 2005, and nearly twice that number had a single lesbian or gay parent. Since the 1990s, a quiet revolution has been blooming in the lesbian, gay, bisexual, and transgender (LGBT) community. More and more lesbians and gay men from all walks of life are becoming parents. LGBT people become parents for some of the same reasons that heterosexual people do. Some pursue parenting as single people and others seek to create a family as a couple; still other LGBT people became parents in a heterosexual relationship. Although there are many common themes between LGBT parenting and heterosexual parenting, there are also some unique features. Unlike their heterosexual counterparts, who couple, get pregnant, and give birth, most LGBT individuals and couples who wish to parent must consider many other variables in deciding whether to become parents because the birth option is not the only option.

Key Words: bisexual; families; gay; lesbian; LGBT; parenting; parents; adoption; gay families; transgender

Definitions

Lesbian, gay, bisexual, and transgender (LGBT) individuals and couples who wish to parent must give more careful consideration to how they will become parents and, at the outset, must be open to different ways of becoming a family and parenting children. Although many LGBT individuals and couples become parents through the birth of a child, they have also become parents through a number of additional avenues:

- Adoption
- Foster care
- Kinship care
- Surrogacy
- Donor insemination
- Birth from a heterosexual union
- Shared parenting from a custody agreement between lesbians and gay men
- Shared parenting with gay men and a heterosexual mother.

Some LGBT people choose to parent as a couple and some parent as single persons. The stresses faced by single parents will have more to do with single parenting than with their sexuality. Those individuals who parent as a couple will also face challenges to their status as a couple or a family. LGBT people who choose to create families have the advantage of redefining and reinventing their own meaning of family and parenting, precisely because they exist outside of the traditionally defined "family." They have the unique opportunity to break out of preconceived gender roles and be a new kind of parent to a child. Most LGBT people who parent are not invested in raising LGBT children, as suggested by some, but in raising children who will be authentic, happy, and self-confident and have the ability to support themselves regardless of their expression of gender or sexual orientation.

It is important to recognize that although many similarities exist, LGBT parented families also differ from heterosexually parented families. The conventional notion of a family presumes there will be two parents, one of each gender, that they will share a loving relationship and live under one roof, that they will both be biologically related to the children they raise, and that they will be recognized legally as a family. This mom-and-dad nuclear family is the baseline model in Western culture against which all other models of family are measured, and it is assumed by most to be the optimal family environment for child development; in comparison, all other types of families are viewed as deficient in some way (Mallon, 2004).

This model, however, does not apply to most families with LGBT parents. In families involving an LGBT couple, typically at least one parent has no biological relation to the child. In such cases the parent–child relationship nearly always goes unrecognized or unprotected by the law (Mallon, 2006).

Demographics

It is inaccurate to talk about the LGBT community as if it is uniform or easily identifiable. As with all communities, the LGBT community is diverse in terms of how individuals wish to define themselves and live their lives. LGBT individuals are as diverse as any other subgroup of the general population, and they are part of every race, culture, ethnic group, religious group, socioeconomic affiliation, and family in the United States in the early 21st century (Mallon, 2006).

Although in recent years they have received greater visibility, LGBT people are frequently socialized to hide their sexual orientation, and therefore, many still form part of an invisible population. According to an Urban Institute Report (Smith & Gates, 2001), the 2000 U.S. Census Bureau figures for same-sex unmarried partner households provide researchers and policy makers with a wealth of information about LGBT-headed families. Revised estimates from the 2010 Census (U.S. Census Bureau, 2011) indicate that there were 131,729 same-sex married-couple households and 514,735 same-sex unmarried partner households in the United States. The results of the

2010 Census revised estimates are closer to the results of the 2010 American Community Survey (ACS) for same-sex married and unmarried partners. The 2010 ACS estimated same-sex married couples at 152,335 and same-sex unmarried partners at 440,989 (U.S. Census Bureau, 2010).

According to analysis by Gates (2011b), demographic data indicate substantial diversity among same-sex couples with children. These families live throughout the country: of same-sex couples by region, 26% in the South, 24% in New England, and 21% in the Pacific states are raising children. Childrearing is substantially higher among racial/ethnic minorities; African Americans in particular are 2.4 times more likely than their White counterparts to be raising children. Further, among individuals in same-sex couples who did not finish high school, 43% are raising children and 20% of children raised by same-sex couples live in poverty. These data provide policy makers at every level of government with compelling arguments for why they must fulfill the policy needs of LGBT families, who live in nearly every corner of every county in America. The geographical diversity of LGBT families is striking. From big cities to small farming towns, from the Deep South to the Pacific Northwest, LGBT families are part of every American landscape. These facts will help us dispel stereotypes and present a fuller, more accurate picture of the LGBT family in America.

Interestingly, Gates (2011b) points out in his analysis that the proportion of same-sex couples raising children has begun to decline. In the 2000 Census, more than 17% of same-sex couples were raising children. That proportion peaked at 19% in 2006 and had declined to 16% in 2009. Despite the decline, the number of same-sex couples raising children is still much higher in the second decade of the 21st century than 10 years ago because many more couples are reporting themselves in Census Bureau data. In 2000, the Census reported about 63,000 LGBT couples raising children. In 2012, the figure was greater than 110,000.

According to a Williams Institute survey conducted in April 2011, approximately 3.5% of American adults identify themselves as lesbian, gay, or bisexual, whereas 0.3% are transgender—approximately 11.7 million Americans (Gates, 2011a). However, a substantially higher percentage acknowledges having same-sex attraction without identifying as LGBT. This finding makes it difficult to accurately record the demographics of LGBT people in the United States.

Just as no one knows how many people self-identify as LGBT, no one knows exactly how many

LGBT parents are raising children in the United States. One study by Gates, Badgett, Macomber, and Chambers (2007) reported the following findings, which shed some light on the statistics associated with lesbians and gay men who parent or wish to parent:

- More than one in three lesbians has given birth and one in six gay men has fathered or adopted a child.
- More than half of gay men and 41% of lesbians want to have a child.
- An estimated 2 million LGBT people are interested in adoption.
- An estimated 65,500 adopted children are living with a lesbian or gay parent.
- More than 16,000 adopted children are living with LGBT parents in California, the highest number among the states.
- LGBT parents are raising 4% of all adopted children in the United States.
- Same-sex couples raising adopted children are older and more educated and have more economic resources than other adoptive parents.
- Adopted children with same-sex parents are younger and more likely to be foreign born.

Currently, 397,122 children and youth live in foster care in the United States and more than 101,666 foster children await adoption (U.S. Department of Health and Human Services, 2012). States must recruit parents who are interested and able to foster and adopt children. Although the majority of states no longer officially deem lesbians and gay men unfit to rear a child (only two states, Mississippi and Nebraska, currently restrict LGBT individuals or couples from adopting), each state decides independently who can adopt, and legislators, more for political reasons than for reasons having to do with child well-being, continue to introduce bills barring adoptions and foster parenting by LGBT people to state legislatures every year (Tavernise, 2011).

Theory, Research, and Best Practices

Historically, in the area of practice with LGBT parents, the social-work knowledge base has relied on theoretical applications from child development, child welfare, and psychology. LGBT history indeed is rooted in decades of hiding and secrecy, when the mere whisper that one was not a stalwart heterosexual could destroy a career or a life. The keepers of public morals sought to keep those who strayed from this position firmly in line. But we must also take note of consequential shifts over time in cultural openness to LGBT people. A trio of events including the groundbreaking work of the late Dr. Evelyn Hooker in the 1950s and 1960s, which presented rigorous scientific research to provide indisputable evidence that homosexuality is not a mental illness; the advent of the Stonewall Rebellion of 1969 in New York City, generally regarded as the birth of the LGBT liberation movement; and the elimination of homosexuality from the *Diagnostic and Statistical Manual of Mental Disorders* in 1973 caused society to begin slowly to change its perceptions of homosexuality. Concurrently, throughout the late 1970s, as social activism in LGBT communities was nurturing the growth of a new sense of dignity among lesbians and gay men, adult lesbians and gays became increasingly willing to identify themselves openly. The 1980s focused mainly on a community struggling with the realities of HIV and AIDS. The 1990s focused on issues of LGBT parenting, whereas the early 21st century spotlighted lesbian and gay marriage rights. In light of this ostensible openness, many social-work practitioners have become increasingly aware of the existence of LGBT parents.

Since the mid-1970s, the theoretical underpinnings of practice with LGBT people have shifted from the professional view that an LGBT identity was equal to a diagnosis of mental illness to the more LGBT-affirming approaches of contemporary 21st-century social-work practice. Although there has been ongoing progressive change, the social-work profession undeniably continues to grapple with the reality of LGBT parenting.

Theory and Research

The nature and scope of research studies on LGBT-headed families continue to grow. The earliest documentation on lesbian mothers and gay fathers mostly explored the context of children born in heterosexual marriages that ended in divorce. Such early studies have been replaced by those focusing on children in planned LGBT-headed families without the confounding variable of divorce and the coming-out process of the parents. As with all research, there are limitations to research in the area of LGBT parenting. Because not all LGBT persons are "out," random representative sampling of LGBT parents is a challenge to methodology. This is particularly true because no reliable data exist on the number and whereabouts of LGBT parents in the general population, in the United States or elsewhere. The existing, limited research also includes biases toward White, urban, well-educated, and mature lesbian mothers and gay fathers. The relatively small samples that do exist in the research are recruited through community networks.

One of the most consistent findings since the mid-1990s is that same-gendered couples with and without children tend to establish a more even distribution of household tasks in comparison to heterosexual couples. Without socially prescribed guidance on gendered roles, LGBT parents tend to value equality in partnership and structure an equitable division of labor in housework, in childrearing, and in work outside the home. Although this repeated finding seems to be well known in the mental-health community, it has not been discussed in the mainstream dialog about the pros and cons of lesbian and gay parenting.

Stacey and Biblarz (2001) identify parental gender as predictive of parenting skill. According to their research, all mothers (heterosexual and lesbian) are more likely than fathers to be more invested and skilled at caring for children. Therefore, when two women co-parent, gender and sexual orientation interact, with two mothers both committed to and working together toward creating an equitable and mutually caring environment that provides a loving and supportive foundation for their child's developing self-esteem.

In their follow-up study, Biblarz and Stacey found that "the argument that children need both a mother and father presumes that mothering and fathering involve mutually exclusive capacities. That is not the case. Research shows that men can perform traditional 'women's work' and women can perform 'men's work' perfectly well. As many as one in five fathers of young children are now providing their primary care. The bottom line is that committed, responsible parenting involves spending time with children, caring about what they're involved in, and providing structure, limits, guidance and affection. Good parenting is good parenting, whatever package it comes in. The gender of parents only matters in ways that shouldn't matter at all to policymakers, judges, and anyone else who cares about the welfare of children" (2010, p. 22).

The research on biological gay fathers and their children is extremely limited. Two studies (McPherson, 1993; Sbordone, 1993) show similar parenting styles and skills between gay and heterosexual fathers. Mallon's study (2004) of the parenting process in a group of 20 self-identified gay fathers found these men were more likely to endorse a nurturing role for fathers, less likely to emphasize the importance of economic support, and less likely to show affection to their partner in front of the children (Barret & Robinson, 2000). Further results indicate that gay fathers are as effective as heterosexual fathers in caring for their children. They have been shown to be more

consistent in setting limits with their children than are heterosexual fathers. They have also been found to be more emotionally expressive and nurturing with their children, less likely to prioritize their "breadwinner" functions over their parenting roles, and less interested in conventional gender-role behaviors than heterosexual fathers (McCarty, 2004).

The most recent large-scale research on lesbian parents (Gartrell & Bos, 2010) expands our understanding of psychological well-being in adolescent biological offspring of lesbian mothers and therefore has implications for the pediatric care of these adolescents and for public policies concerning same-sex parenting. The study's results showed that 17 year olds of lesbian mothers were rated significantly higher in social, school/academic, and total competence and significantly lower in social problems, rule-breaking, aggressive, and externalizing problem behavior than their age-matched counterparts. This publication prompted international media attention.

Fears about LGBT Parents

Although there has been a growing body of literature about LGBT parenting since the mid-1980s, the idea of an LGBT person as a primary nurturing figure rearing children is still remarkable to many. Many social-work professionals still hold firm to a belief system grounded in the ubiquitous, negative myths and stereotypes regarding LGBT persons. Those who oppose the idea of LGBT persons as parents base their thinking on a number of fears, including the following:

- The child will be bullied or ostracized because of having LGBT parents.
- The child may become LGBT because of having an LGBT parental role model.
- Living with or having contact with an LGBT parent may harm the child's moral well-being (these beliefs may have their foundation in religious texts that condemn relationships that are other than heterosexual).
- The child will be abused (based on the myth that all LGBT persons are sexual predators).

None of these rationales is borne out or supported by evidence (Patterson, 1996; Stacey & Biblarz, 2001). Numerous studies (Golombok & Tasker, 1996; Mallon, 2004; Wainright, Russell, & Patterson, 2004) indicate that the qualities that make good fathers or good mothers are universal and are not related to sexual orientation or gender. The need for fathers to be involved in the lives of their children has been clearly established. The ability to love and care for a child is not determined by one's sexual orientation. Furthermore, the desire to parent is not exclusive to heterosexuals, but is shared by many LGBT persons.

According to the meta-analysis of the relevant research (spanning two decades) conducted by Stacey and Biblarz (2001), none of the significant differences in parenting as reported in the research applies to children's self-esteem, psychological well-being, or social adjustment, nor were there differences in parents' self-esteem, mental health, or commitment to their children. In other words, although differences exist, they were not identified as deficits.

A few studies reported some differences that could represent advantages to lesbian parenting. For example, several studies (Patterson, 1996; Vanfraussen, Ponjaert-Kristofferson, & Brewaeys, 2002, 2003) found that lesbian co-mothers share family responsibilities more equally than heterosexual married parents, and some research hints that children benefit from egalitarian co-parenting. A few studies found that lesbians worry less than heterosexual parents about the gender conformity of their children. Perhaps this finding helps to account for the few studies reporting that sons of lesbians play less aggressively and that children of lesbians communicate their feelings more freely, aspire to a wider range of occupations, and score higher on self-esteem. Most professionals view these differences as positive elements, but some critics of these studies have misrepresented the differences as evidence that the children suffer from gender confusion.

Finally, some studies reported that lesbian mothers feel more comfortable discussing sexuality with their children and accepting their children's sexuality—whatever it may be. More to the point are data reported in a 25-year British study (Golombok & Tasker, 1996). Few of the young adults in this study identified themselves as gay or lesbian, but a larger minority of those with lesbian mothers did report that they were more open to exploring their sexuality and had at one time or another considered or actually had a same-sex relationship.

Although most research to date on LGBT parenting is based on individuals who are biological parents, researchers looking at LGBT parenting have reached the same, unequivocal conclusions. That is, the children of LGBT parents grow up as successfully as the children of heterosexuals. Since 1980, more than 20 studies conducted and published in the United States, Australia, the Netherlands, and the United Kingdom have addressed the way in which parental sexual orientation impacts the children of LGBT parents (Golombok, Perry, Burston, Murray, Mooney-Somers, & Stevens, 2003; Golombok, Spencer, &

Rutter, 1983; Vanfraussen et al., 2002, 2003; Wainright & Patterson, 2006; Wainright et al., 2004). Not one study has found that the children of LGBT parents face greater social stigma. There is no evidence to support the belief that the children of LGBT parents are more likely to be abused or to suggest that the children of these parents are more likely to be gay, lesbian, bisexual, or transgender themselves. Children will, in fact, be who they are. It is important to bear in mind that the majority of lesbian and gay persons have been raised by heterosexual parents (Mallon, 2004).

Best Practice

Social workers have a key role to play in the lives of LGBT parents. From direct practice with family systems to policy and legislative advocacy, the array of opportunities for social workers in practice with lesbian and gay parents continues to broaden. Because LGBT parents are increasingly more out and open in many geographic locations of the country, LGBT parents can no longer be viewed as an invisible population. Although heterosexual privilege continues to dominate mainstream consciousness, assuming that all children live within the context of heterosexually headed families, most social workers will encounter lesbian- or gay-headed families at some point in their practice.

Best practices suggest that social workers must accept the premise that it is quality of care, not family constellation, that determines what is optimal for children's healthy development. The ability of LGBT parents to provide for the social and emotional health of their children is equal to that of heterosexual parents. Social workers must also examine their own notions of family and further learn to identify what constitutes family based on the loving bonds of responsibility that have been both intended and fulfilled, not solely on biological, legal, or conventional definitions.

Best practices for professional social workers who work with LGBT parents involve an LGBT-affirming approach. These strategies may include working with lesbian or gay individuals to assess their desire to become parents, working to support lesbian or gay persons who are in various stages of pursuing parenting, helping those who have already become parents to deal with the everyday reality of parenting, and assisting couples and families in more traditional couple or family therapy situations.

Policy practice is the responsibility of all social workers. Within the specialization of practice with LGBT parents, professional social workers partner with or represent the interests of persons and families who request assistance in advocating for policy or legislative changes. Such activities may include advocating on the local, state, or federal levels for changes in fiscal allocations and services, speaking with legislators or bureaucrats, gathering data for policy analyses and performing such analyses, or helping a person navigate the complex delivery system. The most effective policy practice activities involve consumer advocates who are most knowledgeable regarding gaps in services, unmet needs, or solutions from their experience. Within the area of practice with LGBT persons, the lesbian or gay person or family is usually the "expert" when it comes to best practices. It is the responsibility of social workers to identify needs, assist in procuring services, navigate the maze of services, and promote policies and services to better serve this population.

Practice Implications

Discussion and debate about parenting by LGBT persons occurs frequently among child welfare policy makers, social-service agencies, and social workers. All need better information about LGBT parents and their children as they make individual and policy-level decisions about the lives of children with LGBT parents.

Recent government surveys demonstrate that many lesbians and gay men are already raising children, and many more LGBT people would like to have children at some point. A report from the Urban Institute (Gates et al., 2007) estimates that 2 million LGBT people have considered adoption as a route to parenthood. Because prior research indicates that fewer than one fifth of adoption agencies attempt to recruit adoptive parents from the LGBT community, findings of the Urban Institute Report (Gates et al.) and others (Evan B. Donaldson Adoption Institute, 2003; Mallon, 2006) suggest that LGBT people comprise an underutilized pool of potential adoptive parents.

Future trends in practice with LGBT parents will be most affected not only by the increasing numbers of LGBT couples who chose parenting, but also by the heightened self-awareness and development of LGBT-affirming practice approaches of social workers who work with these parents. In addition, legislative and legal initiatives in some states seek to limit parenting opportunities for lesbians and gay men. Social workers must balance their own personal attitudes toward lesbians and gay men as parents with the reality that research suggests LGBT people do make good parents.

Future Trends

The considerable controversy surrounding the issue of parenting by gays and lesbians seems certain to escalate in the years to come. This controversy is a critical component of the debate over whether lesbians and gay men should be permitted to marry, and it continues to divide policy makers in the United States—as well as in Canada and other countries—as they formulate laws and practices relating to workplace benefits, foster care, adoption, and an array of other important social and personal questions surrounding parenting.

Even as these discussions proliferate on the legislative and rhetorical levels, however, reality on the ground is outstripping the pace of the debate. That is, a growing number of LGBT people are becoming parents and are living as families every day, irrespective of what policy makers or practitioners do or say. Lesbians and gay men are becoming mothers and fathers in many ways, but primarily through alternative insemination, surrogacy, and adoption. The latter alternative, which is becoming increasingly popular, provides critical insights into the cultural changes taking place in two major ways: demonstrating that parenting of children by lesbians and gay men is an ongoing, unabated practice and showing that Americans' attitudes are evolving.

Solid research to help inform and shape the dialogue is increasing. Some studies, for example, have reported that LGBT couples' parenting capacity and their children's outcomes are comparable to those of heterosexuals. Further research will likely assist in dispelling myths about lesbians and gay men as parents. Numerous professional societies have provided positive statements from their membership supporting LGBT parents, including the Child Welfare League of America, the National Association of Social Workers, the American Psychological Association, the American Psychiatric Association, the American Academy of Pediatrics, the American Academy of Child & Adolescent Psychiatry; the American Medical Association, the American Bar Association, and the North American Council on Adoptable Children.

For society, the bottom line is clear: lesbians and gay men are becoming parents in growing numbers. Many avenues exist for lesbians and gay men wishing to become parents. Although stereotypes and misconceptions still perpetuate policy, legislation, and practice, from a child-centered perspective the willingness of social-services agencies to accept LGBT adults as parents means that more children will have loving and permanent families.

Social-Work Practice Implications

There may continue to be a steep learning curve for some professional social workers engaged in practice with LGBT parents. Moving toward the development of an affirming practice with LGBT parents will require intensive continuing education. As social-work practitioners working with LGBT parents, it is essential for professionals to read the research and to analyze, interpret, and discuss the findings and practice implications for effective practice with this population. It is incumbent upon the professional community to be clear about the facts and able to rebut the misinformation presented by those who may not see LGBT persons as "appropriate" resources for children in need of homes as well as nurture the narratives of truth that we have witnessed through our practice (see National Resource Center for Permanency and Family Connections, 2012a, 2012b, 2012c, 2012d). Research findings and their interpretation have enormous impact in many influential arenas, including court cases for custody and visiting rights, judges, child advocates, professionals in the health and mental-health communities, and those charged with developing and enacting legislation that guides our laws. In the midst of a politically charged environment in which negative stereotypes and ideological assertions can easily gain status as "truth," it is essential for social-work practitioners to become familiar with what is known and not known from the research studies and practice implications so that LGBT parents work with and are supported by informed and competent social-work practitioners.

REFERENCES

Barret, R., & Robinson, B. E. (2000). *Gay fathers*. New York, NY: Jossey–Bass.

Biblarz, T. J., & Stacey, J. (2010). How does the gender of parents matter? *Journal of Marriage and Family, 72*(1), 3–22.

Evan B. Donaldson Adoption Institute. (2003). *Adoption by lesbians and gays: A national survey of adoption agency policies, practices, and attitudes*. New York, NY: Author.

Gartrell, N., & Bos, H. (2010). US National Longitudinal Lesbian Family Study: Psychological adjustment of 17-year-old adolescents. *Pediatrics, 126*(1): 28–36.

Gates, G., Badgett, L. M. V., Macomber, J. E., & Chambers, K. (2007). *Adoption and foster care by lesbian and gay parents in the United States*. Washington, DC: The Urban Institute.

Gates, G. J. (2011a, April). *How many people are lesbian, gay, bisexual, and transgender?* Los Angeles, CA: Williams Institute.

Gates, G. J. (2011b). *As overall percentage of same-sex couples raising children declines, those adopting almost doubles— Significant diversity among LGBT families*. Los Angeles, CA: Williams Institute.

Golombok, S., Perry, B., Burston, A., Murray, C., Mooney-Somers, J., & Stevens, M. (2003). Children with lesbian parents: A community study. *Developmental Psychology, 29*(1), 20–33.

Golombok, S., Spencer, A., & Rutter, M. (1983). Children in lesbian and single-parent households: Psychosexual and psychiatric appraisal. *Journal of Child Psychology and Psychiatry, 24*(4), 551–572.

Golombok, S., & Tasker, F. (1996). Do parents influence the sexual orientation of their children? Findings from a longitudinal study of lesbian families. *Developmental Psychology, 32*(1), 3–11.

Mallon, G. P. (2004). *Gay men choosing parenthood*. New York, NY: Columbia University Press.

Mallon, G. P. (2006). *Lesbian and gay foster and adoptive parents: Recruiting, assessing, and supporting an untapped resource for children and youth*. Washington, DC: Child Welfare League of America.

McCarty, K. (2004). *Fatherhood for gay men: An emotional and practical guide to becoming a gay dad*. New York, NY: Haworth Press.

McPherson, D. (1993). *Gay parenting couples: Parenting arrangements, arrangement satisfaction, and relationship satisfaction*. Unpublished doctoral dissertation, Pacific Graduate School of Psychology, Palo Alto, CA.

National Resource Center for Permanency and Family Connections. (2012a). *Strategies for recruiting lesbian, gay, bisexual, and transgender foster, adoptive, and kinship families*. New York, NY: Author.

National Resource Center for Permanency and Family Connections. (2012b). *LGBT prospective foster and adoptive families: The homestudy assessment process*. New York, NY: Author.

National Resource Center for Permanency and Family Connections. (2012c). *Supporting and retaining LGBT foster and adoptive parents*. New York, NY: Author.

National Resource Center for Permanency and Family Connections. (2012d). *10 things children and youth may want their LGBT foster or adoptive parents to know*. New York, NY: Author.

Patterson, C. J. (1996). Lesbian mothers and their children: Findings from the Bay Area families study. In J. Laird & R. J. Green (Eds.), *Lesbians and gays in couples and families: A handbook for therapists* (pp. 420–438). San Francisco, CA: Jossey-Bass.

Sbordone, A. J. (1993). *Gay men choosing fatherhood*. Unpublished doctoral dissertation, Department of Psychology, City University of New York.

Smith, D. M., & Gates, G. (2001). *Gay and lesbian families in the United States*. Washington, DC: The Urban Institute.

Stacey, J., & Biblarz, T. (2001). (How) does the sexual orientation of parents matter? *American Sociological Review, 66*, 159–183.

Tavernise, S. (2011, June 13). Adoptions by gay couples rise despite barriers. *New York Times*, p. A11.

U.S. Census Bureau. (2010). *Census Bureau release estimates of same-sex married couples*. Retrieved March 24, 2014, from http://www.census.gov/newsroom/releases/archives/2010_census/cb11-cn181.html

U.S. Census Bureau. (2011). *Census Bureau release estimates of same-sex married couples*. Retrieved October 31, 2012, from http://www.census.gov/newsroom/releases/archives/2010_census/cb11-cn181.html

U.S. Department of Health and Human Services. (2012). *The AFCARS report #20*. Washington, DC: Children's Bureau.

Vanfraussen, K., Ponjaert-Kristofferson, I., & Brewaeys, A. (2002). What does it mean for youngsters to grow up in a lesbian family created by means of donor insemination? *Journal of Reproductive and Infant Psychology, 20*(4), 237–252.

Vanfraussen, K., Ponjaert-Kristofferson, I., & Brewaeys, A. (2003). Family functioning in lesbian families created by donor insemination. *American Journal of Orthopsychiatry, 73*(1), 78–90.

Wainright, J. L., & Patterson, C. J. (2006). Delinquency, victimization, and substance use among adolescents with female same-sex parents. *Journal of Family Psychology, 20*(3), 526–530.

Wainright, J., Russell, S., & Patterson, C. (2004). Psychosocial adjustment, school outcomes, and romantic relationships of adolescents with same-sex parents. *Child Development*, 75(6), 1886–1898.

GERALD P. MALLON

M

MACRO SOCIAL WORK PRACTICE

ABSTRACT: Macro social work practice includes those activities performed in organizational, community, and policy arenas. Macro practice has a diverse history that reveals conflicting ideologies and multiple theoretical perspectives. Programmatic, organizational, community, and policy dimensions of macro practice underscore the social work profession's emphasis on using a person-in-environment perspective. Thus, social workers, regardless of roles played, are expected to have sensitivity toward and engage in macro practice activities.

KEY WORDS: organization; community; practice models; large systems practice; change

Macro social work, sometimes called "community social work practice" (Austin, Coombs, & Barr, 2005), is so much a part of all social work practice that it is somewhat misleading to use the adjective "macro." For a profession that embraces a person-in-environment perspective, recognizing the larger arenas in which social work is practiced, every practitioner must be sensitive to, if not active in, performing macro roles. Thus, *macro* is an important adjective used to describe those aspects of social work that take one beyond direct or clinical individual intervention and *contextualize* practice regardless of what role is performed (Brody & Nair, 2006).

Definition and Description of Macro Practice

Macro social work includes "efforts within and outside organizational, community and policy arenas intended to sustain, change, and advocate for quality of life" (Netting, 2005, p. 51). Macro activities are typically performed in organizations, communities, and policy or decision-making arenas. Rothman, Erlich, and Tropman (2001) identify three arenas of intervention: communities, organizations, and small groups. Small groups are "a tangible collection of people who can discuss matters personally and work together in close association" (p. 13), often serving as vehicles through which macro activities take place. They may be ad hoc committees in an organization, strategic alliances among interdisciplinary colleagues, coalitions of community agencies, or founders of a budding

social movement. Thus macro social work practice by definition implies working within multiple settings.

The breadth of macro social work activities is limitless because organizations and communities (both place and nonplace) are deeply embedded in political systems and their accompanying ideologies and values. Macro social work activities, then, include what Jansson (2003) has called "policy practice" because it is within organizations and communities that policies are implemented. Macro practice involves playing roles that include planning, policy analysis, program coordination, community organizing, and managing and administering organizations (Netting, Kettner, McMurtry, & Thomas, 2012). Given this diversity of roles, Brueggemann (2006) includes topics such as social change processes, community development and organization, leadership, organizational and programmatic development, policy advocacy, and international social work in the practice of macro social work. It is important to note that some practitioners will move in and out of these various roles and activities, whereas others have positions that focus on macro roles full time (Starr, Mizrahi, & Gurzinsky, 1999).

Historical Development

Macro social work has deep roots, both in the history of the profession as well as in the larger society. Feminist historians have identified women's organizing efforts that preceded the development of the profession as those of benevolence, reform, and rights (Skocpol, 1992). Often beginning in sewing circles and cent societies in the late 1700s, it was acceptable for women to work through religious structures to form missionary societies and orphanages. These were early macro organizing activities, based on identifying needs and founding organizations to address those needs. In the 1800s reformers created organizations for causes such as abolishing slavery or eliminating brothels, followed by the mid-1800s in which women's rights organizers emerged as a third tradition. Each of these traditions brought different assumptions and strategies to the macro enterprise; benevolent women worked within the system to effect change, whereas reformers and activists worked both inside and outside existing structures (McCarthy, 2003; Scott 1993).

Immigration, industrialization, and rapid population growth led to concentrated urban areas in the

1800s, accompanied by rising crime, unemployment, and poverty. Early helping efforts were driven by conflicting ideologies, some of which were judgmental and others were more progressive. Schneider and Lester (2001) identify "three separate and distinct social work movements [that emerged] in the last 20 years of the 19th century, [each with] a different perspective about wealth and poverty as well as the responsibilities one owed to the other and to the developing social systems" (p. 10). Charity organizations focused on *community justice*, settlement houses focused on *social justice*, and the third movement out of the University of Pennsylvania Wharton School focused on *distributive justice* (p. 10).

As the profession developed in the early 1900s, a long-standing tension emerged as well. Called by different names—clinical vs. community culture, cause vs. function, or direct service vs. social welfare—"an enduring tension within social work between its social change and its individual-family change dimensions" (Austin et al., 2005, p. 11) has persisted. These tensions are highlighted by Reisch and Andrews (2002) in *The Road Not Taken*. Focusing on radical social work as an alternative approach, they give "voice to the effects of nonmainstream social service and social work organizations on the creation of U.S. social welfare and the emergence of social work theories and methods" (p. ix), revealing a complex array of strongly held beliefs about the target(s) of change, ranging from social reform within the system to direct assaults on societal structures.

In the early 1900s, multiple preexisting traditions converged as the profession emerged, reflecting different beliefs about the nature of the profession, its underlying philosophy, and the methods used to carry out strongly held assumptions, around which there is continuing disagreement. Given that histories are filtered through different lenses, some voices are more privileged than others. For example, feminist historians, advocates, and radical social workers felt the need to write their own histories so that alternative voices are heard. Tensions among strongly held beliefs about what actions are necessary in order to do social work were divergent in the beginning of the profession, just as they are divergent today (Netting, 2005).

Similarly, Reamer (1993) identifies five areas about which philosophical assumptions have influenced the profession's development and its macro models of intervention: (a) the goals of government, (b) rights of citizens in relation to the state, (c) the obligations of the state toward its citizens, (d) the nature of political or civil liberty, and (e) the nature of social justice (p. 2). Historically, these philosophical assumptions have framed different views of social work macro practice, and have resulted in value choices, dilemmas, and questions. For example, are the goals of government to maintain the status quo or to work for change? Which groups of citizens and what needs receive priority? Should service delivery be centralized or decentralized? Should planning occur from the top or from the grassroots? Should consumer-directed care be instituted or is more professional oversight needed? Can social programs be built on the principle of social and economic justice? In organizational arenas, each organization's basic assumptions, underlying values, and artifacts reveal competing values (Cameron & Quinn 1999) such as seeking standardization versus celebrating differences; or designing programs to address current needs or advocating for change in the basic structure of service provision (O'Connor & Netting, 2009). In planned change processes, macro practitioners often struggle when working inside the system is seen as "selling out" and when it is more appropriate to advocate for change from a position outside the targeted system (Netting et al., 2012). Choices among values undergird every aspect of macro work, whether it is which problems are privileged, which group is targeted, or what type of intervention is selected. The self-aware practitioner will be cognizant of the assumptions and values that guide those choices and their potential consequences.

In the latter part of the 1960s, the number of courses in community organization increased in schools of social work, fueled by an intentional effort on the part of the Council on Social Work Education (CSWE) to promote teaching in this area. However, a decade later momentum began to wane. In 1976 the inaugural issue of *Administration in Social Work* appeared, and in 1980 over 30 macro educators participated in an informal session at the annual program meeting of CSWE, vowing to have a CO Symposium at the 1981 annual meeting. Roberts-DeGennaro (2002) has written a history of key events from 1960 to 1992 that influenced the development of the Association for Community Organization and Social Administration (ACOSA), as a structure for social workers interested in macro practice. This association developed out of the symposium sessions, and by 1987 a set of bylaws was approved, a steering committee was formed, and a membership organization formed to serve as an incubator for persons interested in promoting, integrating, and advocating for macro curriculum in social work programs. Today ACOSA sponsors *The Journal of Community Practice*, an interdisciplinary journal devoted to revitalizing research about, theory construction in, and teaching of macro practice.

Theoretical and Empirical Foundations for Macro Practice

Multiple theories are often used to understand the macro aspects of social work practice. Often used to describe and analyze macro arenas is social systems theory. In systems theory there are many parts of any unit of analysis (whether they are groups, organizations, communities). These units can be understood as interconnected components engaged in an interactive process with their environments—as resources enter the system (inputs), as these resources are processed (throughputs), and as something new emerges (outputs). Outcomes are actual quality of life changes that accompany outputs. For example, human service organizations attract funding, legitimacy, staff, clients, and a variety of other inputs with the intent of performing interventions that will make a difference in the interactive process.

Warren (1978), now a classic in the community literature, built on the prevailing notions of systems theory at the time and viewed communities as systems nested within systems (groups within organizations, organizations within communities, and others). He distinguished between internal and external patterns and between vertical and horizontal community linkages. Vertical linkages connect individuals, groups, and organizations within a community; whereas horizontal linkages transcend community boundaries, connecting the community to units within the larger environment.

Closely related to systems theories are human ecology theories that also examine structural patterns and relationships within place-based communities. Emanating from the 1930s work of Robert E. Park at the University of Chicago, today ecological theories focus on resident characteristics (for example, master statuses such as race, age, gender), the use of physical space (for example, land use, housing), and the social structures within communities. Communities are seen as highly interdependent, teeming with changing relationships among populations of people and organizations. Human ecologists are particularly concerned about how place-based communities deal with processes of competition, centralization, concentration, integration, and succession (Netting et al., 2012).

Equally important to a focus on space, structure, function, and relationships among systems are issues of how people behave in communities; therefore human behavior theories help macro practitioners recognize why people act as they do in large systems. Organizational and community behavior dispels any myths that macro practice is not "direct" practice because there is ongoing interaction among people; it is just more complicated because it is not always one-on-one (Netting et al., 2012). Similarly, power dependency theory, conflict theory, and resource mobilization theories are helpful in understanding the power and politics of community settings (Hardina, 2002).

Hasenfeld (2000) reveals how multiple organizational theories are used to guide managerial and administrative roles in macro practice. Recognizing that human service organizations are "inherently indeterminate and fraught with ambiguities" (p. 90), Hasenfeld identifies nine administrative tasks (achieving goals; managing people; being efficient; mobilizing resources; founding and surviving; institutionalizing practices; integrating culture; deconstructing knowledge, power and control; and promoting social change) and theories used to perform these tasks. Macro practitioners have drawn theoretical principles from various schools of thought, everything from classical bureaucratic to post-modern and critical theories (Netting et al., 2012). There is, however, a continual need to recognize that many theories used by managers and administrators have not been empirically tested. Organizational culture theory holds great promise in this regard because of the extensive studies conducted by Cameron and Quinn (1999).

In the last decade concerns have raged about evidence-based practice (EBP) in clinical social work and its importance. The debates stem from a number of macro forces that swept the United States in the 1990s when a push for accountability led to federal legislation (Kettner, Moroney, & Martin 1999), energizing calls for outcomes-based or performance measurement (Moxley & Maneia 2001), for evidence-based management (Rousseau, 2006), for evidence-based community practice (Ohmer & Korr 2006), and for evidence-based policy (Gambrill, 2006).

EBP is viewed as having three components—research, practitioner expertise or practice wisdom, and client values. Evidence-based macro practice, then, relies on the use of research conducted in a particular arena, the expertise of the practitioner, and the values of multiple stakeholders. This interplay of factors is complicated by an ongoing debate on what constitutes good science (Woody, D'Souza, & Dartman 2006). For example, a meta-analysis of the empirically based literature on community practice revealed 58 studies, of which 20 were evaluations of actual interventions. Results indicated that practitioners are able to mobilize participants to engage in change and to positively enhance their interpersonal and political skills, but it is much more difficult to address complex physical, social, and economic problems in poor communities. Thus, the ability to engage and mobilize needs to be accompanied by enhanced efforts at capacity building. More research on community interventions, using more sophisticated research methodologies, is needed (Ohmer & Korr 2006). Similarly, case studies and program evaluations are published in the organizational literature (Mulroy, 2004b), but as helpful as these are, they are not generalizable. Macro practitioners need to be aware of the debate on what constitutes "evidence" and the privileging of different types of evidence (Netting & O'Connor, 2008) as well as where to locate the latest research in outlets such as the *Journal of Community Practice, Administration in Social Work, Families in Society, Nonprofit and Voluntary Sector Quarterly*, and *Nonprofit Management and Leadership*.

Current Modes and Patterns of Macro Practice

Since macro practice includes work across programs, organizations, communities, and policies, there are overlapping and different knowledge bases that inform current modes and patterns of activities. Social workers draw from related fields such as sociology, psychology, public administration, health administration, business, management, political science, and others on an ongoing basis. This move toward a more multidisciplinary and interdisciplinary focus is relevant to knowledge dissemination (Gutierrez, Butterfield, Alvarez, & Moxley 2006).

At the programmatic level, designing effectiveness-based programs is a current mode of macro activity. Kettner et al. (1999) and Pawlak and Vinter (2004) provide guidelines for how to develop valuable human service programs. Similarly, the use of logic models to identify inputs needed, intervention strategies, outputs, and outcomes reinforces the importance of accountability and systematic data collection in program development and implementation. At the organizational level, core skills needed to engage in social work administration and management include "leadership, planning, programming, financial management, accounting, operations, MIS, personnel management, grantsmanship and fundraising, program evaluation, coordination, marketing, computer literacy, technical writing and oral communication and supervision" (Raymond, Teare, & Atherton 1996, as cited in Barak, Travis, & Bess 2004). Mulroy (2004a) underscores the importance of these skills in her work on theoretical perspectives in human service organizations.

In terms of community practice, in recent years there has been a resurgence of community building, an emphasis on partnerships and collaboration, a focus on capacity building and the importance of sustainability, and a release from geographically bound definitions of community into virtual communities of identification made possible by technology. Practice models are updated periodically and include locality development or neighborhood and community organizing, organizing functional communities, community social and economic development, social planning, program development and community liaising, political and social action, coalitions, social movements, or social reform (Hardina, 2002; Kettner et al., 1999; Rothman et al., 2001; Weil, 2004; Weil & Gamble, 1995). Strengths, empowerment, and resiliency perspectives are also used to guide contemporary macro practice, as well as planned change models relevant to organization and community change (Netting et al., 2012).

At the policy level macro practitioners have a variety of analysis models that focus on different aspects of policy. Gilbert & Terrell (2005) provide three major and interrelated types of policy analysis: (a) process, (b) product, and (c) performance (implementation and impact). Process frameworks "focus on the dynamics of policy formulation with regard to sociopolitical and technical-methodological variables" (p. 15). A process approach may examine the planning (or lack thereof) of a policy or policies, the decision-making and political processes in the formulation, development, and movement toward becoming a product. Product frameworks focus on the results of the planning process—on what is produced as a result of "a set of policy choices" (p. 16). Thus, a product model examines policy content or issues embedded within the policy, as units of analysis. Performance is "concerned with the description and evaluation of the programmatic outcomes of policy choices" (p. 16) and research methodologies are used to determine if policy implementation *works*. Two types of questions are typically asked in performance analysis: "First, how well is the program carried out? Second, what is its impact?" (Gilbert & Terrell 2005, p. 16). The first question deals with monitoring the process of implementation (formative evaluation) and the second question deals with evaluating program outcomes (summative evaluation) (Hoeffer, 2005).

Trends and Future Directions

Since social workers perform such diverse roles, there is a tendency to dichotomize micro and macro practice, yet all accredited schools of social work require that macro content be part of their curriculum (Austin et al., 2005). Certainly, depending on the school one attends, there may be specializations or concentrations that allow students to hone certain skill sets more than others, but all social workers are educated in macro content, just as all social workers study direct practice. In practice, it is often in performing direct practice roles with multiple individuals where patterns of need begin to emerge or where policy implementation is recognized as problematic. The nature of the change needed may lead to an organizational, community, or policy intervention. At this point, the direct practitioner may identify the needed change and pursue it with the help of others or they may alert other practitioners who are in a position to pursue change. The point is that all social workers are engaged in recognizing the macro nature of their work, just as practitioners who do not provide direct service must recognize the impact their work has on individuals, families, and groups.

The recognition that social workers are macro change agents may be evident in the field, but there are persistent challenges facing both educators and practitioners. As social workers move into nontraditional jobs in which their titles are policy analysts, coordinators, supervisors, information systems analysts, and a host of others their identities as social workers may be somewhat muted. For practitioners in some states, clinical licensing laws may not include roles for persons who perform other than clinical tasks. These same requirements may influence the concentration or specialization that social work students chose in their programs of study. These and other challenges are part of the ongoing professional dialogue.

REFERENCES

Austin, M. J., Coombs, M., & Barr, B. (2005). Community-centered clinical practice: Is the integration of micro and macro social work practice possible? *Journal of Community Practice, 13*(4), 9–30.

Barak, M. E. M., Travis, D., & Bess, G. (2004). Exploring managers' and administrators' retrospective perceptions of their MSW field work experience: A national study. *Administration in Social Work, 28*(1), 21–44.

Brody, R., & Nair, M. D. (2006). *Macro practice: A generalist approach* (8th ed.). Wheaton, IL: Gregory Publishing.

Brueggemann, W. G. (2006). *The practice of macro social work* (3rd ed.). Stamford, CT: Brooks/Cole.

Cameron, K. S., & Quinn, R. E. (1999). *Diagnosing and changing organizational culture: Based on the competing values framework.* Reading, MA: Addison Wesley Longman, Inc.

Gambrill, E. (2006). Evidence-based practice and policy: Choices ahead. *Research on Social Work Research, 16*(3), 338–357.

Gilbert, N., & Terrell, P. (2005). *Dimensions of social welfare policy* (6th ed.). Boston, MA: Allyn & Bacon.

Gutierrez, L. M., Butterfield, A. K., Alvarez, A. R., & Moxley, D. P. (2006). Research for community practice. *Journal of Community Practice, 14*(4), 1–3.

Hardina, D. (2002). *Analytical skills for community organization practice.* New York: Columbia University Press.

Hasenfeld, Y. (2000). Social welfare administration and organizational theory. In R. J. Patti, *The handbook of social welfare management* (pp. 89–112). Thousand Oaks, CA: Sage.

Jansson, B. (2003). *Becoming an effective policy advocate: From policy practice to social justice* (4th ed.). Pacific Grove, CA: Brooks/Cole.

Hoeffer, R. (2005). *Cutting edge social policy research.* Binghamton, NY: Haworth Press.

Kettner, P. M., Moroney, R. M., & Martin, L. L. (1999). *Designing and managing programs: An effectiveness-based approach* (2nd ed.). Thousand Oaks, CA: Sage.

McCarthy, K. D. (2003). *American creed: Philanthropy and the rise of civil society 1700–1865.* Chicago: University of Chicago Press.

Moxley, D. P., & Maneia, R. W. (2001). Expanding the conceptual basis of outcomes and their use in the human services. *Families in Society, 82,* 569–577.

Mulroy, E. A. (2004a). Theoretical perspectives on the social environment to guide management and community practice: An organization-in-environment approach. *Administration in Social Work, 28*(1), 77–97.

Mulroy, E. A. (2004b). University civic engagement with community-based organizations: Dispersed or coordinated models? *Journal of Community Practice, 12*(3/4), 35–52.

Netting, F. E. (2005). The future of macro social work. *Advances in Social Work, 6*(1), 51–59.

Netting, F. E., Kettner, P. M., & McMurtry, S. L. (2012). *Social work macro practice* (5th ed.). Boston: Allyn & Bacon.

O'Connor, M. K. & Netting, F. E. (2009). *Organization practice.* Boston: Allyn & Bacon.

Netting, F. E., & O'Connor, M. K. (2008). Recognizing the need for evidence-based practices in organizational and community settings. *Journal of Empirical Social Work Practice, 5*(3/4), 473–479.

Ohmer, M. L., & Korr, W. S. (2006). The effectiveness of community practice interventions: A review of the literature. *Research on Social Work Practice, 16*(2), 132–145.

Pawlak, E. J., & Vinter, R. D. (2004). *Designing and planning programs for nonprofit and government organizations.* Indianapolis, IN: Wiley.

Roberts-DeGennaro, M. (2002). History of ACOSA: Chronology of evolving structure and key events from the 1960s to 1992. Retrieved October 2, 2007, from http://www.acosa.org/joomla/about-acosa/history-acosa

Reisch, M., & Andrews, J. (2002). *The road not taken: A history of radical social work in the United States.* Philadelphia, PA: Brunner-Routledge.

Rothman, J., Erlich, J. L., & Tropman, J. E. (2001). *Strategies of community intervention* (6th ed.). Itasca, IL: F. E. Peacock.

Rousseau, D. M. (2006). Is there such a thing as "evidence-based management?" *Academy of Management Review*, *31*, 256–269.

Schneider, R. L., & Lester, L. (2001). *Social work advocacy: A new framework for action*. Belmont, CA: Brooks/Cole.

Scott, A. F. (1993). *Natural allies: Women's associations in American history*. Chicago: University of Chicago Press.

Skocpol, T. (1992). *Protecting soldiers and mothers*. Cambridge, MA: Harvard University Press.

Starr, R., Mizrahi, T., & Gurzinsky, E. (1999). Where have all the organizers gone? A study of Hunter CO & P Alumni. *Journal of Community Practice*, *6*(3), 23–48.

Warren, R. L. (1978). *The community in America* (3rd ed.). Chicago: Rand McNally.

Weil, M. (Ed.). (2004). *The handbook of community practice*. Thousand Oaks, CA: Sage.

Weil, M., & Gamble, D. N. (1995). Community practice models. In *The encyclopedia of social work* (19th ed., Vol. 1: pp. 577–593). Washington, DC: National Association of Social Workers.

Woody, J. D., D'Souza, H. J., & Dartman, R. (2006). Do master's in social work programs teach empirically supported interventions? A survey of deans and directors. *Research on Social Work*, *16*(5), 469–479.

FLORENCE ELLEN NETTING

MAJOR DEPRESSIVE DISORDER AND BIPOLAR MOOD DISORDERS

ABSTRACT: Depression and bipolar mood disorders are mental disorders that are characterized by mood disturbance combined with decreased functioning of the affected individuals. The focus here is on major depressive disorder and bipolar I and II disorders among adults in the United States. Bipolar disorder has unique clinical features and intervention options, and so it is discussed in a separate section after depression. Diagnosis, prevalence, comorbidity, risk factors, course, assessment, treatment, service utilization, and international perspectives are reviewed for each disorder. Finally, the implications for social work are briefly addressed.

KEY WORDS: adults; bipolar; depression; diagnosis; mental illness; mood disorders; treatment

Major Depressive Disorder

The term *depression* frequently refers to low mood states ranging from feeling down to clinical disorders known as depressive disorders. Depressive disorders adversely affect important aspects of one's life, such as interpersonal relationships, employment, and legal matters. Depression also burdens the economy: The annual economic cost of depression, which includes medical expenses, loss of productivity and other associated costs, exceeds $70 billion in the United States (Greenberg, Stiglin, Finkelstein, and Berndt, 1993; Philip, Gregory, and Ronald, 2003).

DIAGNOSIS According to the *Diagnostic and Statistical Manual of Mental Disorders* (5th ed.; *DSM-5*; American Psychiatric Association [APA], 2013), which provides a base for diagnosis of mental disorders in the United States, depression is actually diagnosed as eight disorders: disruptive mood dysregulation disorder, major depressive disorder, persistent depressive disorder (dysthymia), premenstrual dysphoric disorder, substance/medication-induced depression disorder, depressive disorder due to another condition, other specified depressive disorder, and unspecified depressive disorder. While depressive disorders share common characteristics of depressed mood, and physical and cognitive changes that significantly impact an individual's functioning, they differ in terms of duration, timing, or assumed etiology. This article addresses issues related to major depressive disorder. Complete descriptions for other depressive disorders, including their full diagnostic criteria, are available in *DSM-5* (APA, 2013).

The central feature of a major depressive disorder (MDD) is either depressed mood or loss of interest or pleasure in usual activities that persists at least two weeks. An individual is diagnosed as experiencing MDD in the presence of five or more of the following nine symptoms: persistent sadness, inability to experience pleasure, changes in sleep and appetite, psychomotor agitation or retardation, feelings of worthlessness and or guilt, difficulty with concentration and making decisions, loss of energy, and thoughts of death. These symptoms must be present nearly every day, represent a change from the individual's usual self, and cause clinically significant distress or impairment in social, occupational, or other areas of life. In addition, the symptoms cannot be attributable to other conditions, such as substance abuse or general medical conditions.

DSM-5 details changes in depressive disorders from the previous version of the *DSM*. Disruptive mood dysregulation disorder for children under eighteen years of age is newly included for diagnosing children who exhibit persistent irritability and frequent episodes of extreme behavioral dyscontrol. Premenstrual dysphoric disorder was moved from the section "Criteria Sets and Axes Provided for Further Study" in *DSM-IV*. Dysthymia is now categorized as a persistent depressive disorder. While bereavement (depressive symptoms lasting less than two months following the death of a loved one) was placed in the above exclusion criteria in *DSM-IV* (APA, 2000), it was removed from *DSM-5*. This change was made because MDD typically occurs in the context of a psychosocial stressor, which includes bereavement.

In addition to the *DSM* classification system, the International Classification of Diseases (ICD) is used as an official coding system for billing health management and diagnostically for monitoring the incidence and prevalence of disease and other health problems in the United States. *DSM-5* provides the current and forthcoming ICD codes in the text and appendix (APA, 2013). The implementation of the latest version of the ICD (ICD-10-CM) is scheduled for October 1, 2015 (Moran, 2014); providers continue to use the ICD-9-CM for billing and may use either *DSM-IV-TR* or *DSM-5* criteria for diagnosis and treatment until that date (Regier and Narrow, 2014). The latest news and information on ICD-10-CM is available via the websites of the American Psychiatric Association (*http://www.dsm5.org*) and Centers for Medicare and Medicaid Services (*http://www.cms.gov/Medicare/Coding/ICD10/index.html*).

PREVALENCE The lifetime prevalence of MDD among U.S. adults is estimated as 16.2% (Kessler et al., 2003). The same study reports that MDD affects 6.6% of adults in a given year, and 38% of these cases (2.0% of U.S. adults) are classified as severe and 12.9% as very severe (Kessler et al., 2003). A number of demographic factors reported to be associated with an increased prevalence of MDD during one's lifetime include being female, middle-aged, never or previously married, having a low income, being unemployed, or having a disability. Women are 63% more likely than men to experience depression during their lifetime. Non-Hispanic Blacks were found to be 38% less likely than non-Hispanic Whites to experience depression during their lifetime (Kessler et al., 2003).

A recent study also shows a similar twelve-month prevalence rate. According to the National Survey on Drug Use and Health (NSDUH), the twelve-month prevalence rate of major depressive episode in 2012 was 6.9%, or 16 million community-residing adults (Substance Abuse and Mental Health Services Administration [SAMHSA], 2013). Consistent with other data, the past year rate of major depressive episode was higher for women than men (8.4% versus 5.2%) and showed similar ethnic variations: American Indian or Alaska Native (10%), two or more racial groups

(7.7%), White (7.1%), Hispanic (7.0), Black (6.3%), Asian (3.2%). Among those adults who had a major depressive episode in the past year, 10.9 million individuals (68.0%) received treatment (e.g., medication, counseling) for depression within the year. The National Institute of Mental Health (NIMH) provides updates on mental health statistics regularly at *http://www.nimh.nih.gov/statistics/index.shtml*

COMORBIDITY Depression may coexist with other mental or physical disorders and this co-occurrence has an adverse impact on the course of the depression. Among those who reported experiencing MDD during their lifetime, 72.1% reported having other *DSM-IV* disorders: 59.2% reported having an anxiety disorder, 24.0% had a substance use disorder, and 30.0% reported impulse control disorders (Kessler et al., 2005). Other psychiatric disorders, such as panic disorder, obsessive-compulsive disorder, eating disorders, and borderline personality disorder frequently co-occur with MDD (APA, 2013).

Among people with physical health conditions, there is a greater prevalence of MDD than in the general population. Some medical conditions are known to directly cause mood symptoms (e.g., stroke, hypothyroidism) while others tend to act as ongoing stressors, making individuals vulnerable to depression. Common physical illnesses known to be associated with depression include stroke, hypertension, heart disease, diabetes, cancer, and osteoarthritis (APA, 2010).

RISK FACTORS It is commonly believed that the combination of genetic, biological, environmental, and temperamental factors largely determine vulnerability to depression. Major psychosocial stressors include bereavement, culture and ethnicity, older age, gender, pregnancy and postpartum, and family history. First-degree family members of individuals with MDD are two to four times more likely to develop MDD than individuals without a family history (APA, 2013). Adverse childhood experiences are potential risks for developing depression.

COURSE Although MDD can develop at any age, the likelihood of onset increases with puberty and seems to reach its peak in individuals in their twenties (APA, 2013). The course of MDD varies across individuals in terms of having or not having symptom free periods (remission) between depressive episodes. While most individuals with MDD experience recovery within one year of onset, the following factors are associated with lower recovery rates: having psychotic symptoms, prominent anxiety, personality disorders, and severe depressive symptoms. The risk of recurrence tends to become lower over time as the duration of remission increases. However, the risk of recurrence is higher for individuals with previous multiple episodes, severe symptoms, mild depressive symptoms during remission, and those who are young (APA, 2013).

ASSESSMENT A number of instruments are available to assess the presence and severity of depressive symptoms. They are often used for the purpose of screening, diagnosing, and monitoring treatment outcomes as well as for research. There are two formats of instruments: standardized rating scales or semi-structured interview format. Some of the standardized rating scales based on self-reports include the Center for Epidemiological Studies-Depression Scale (CES-D; Radloff, 1977), Beck Depression Inventory (BDI, Beck and Beck, 1972; BDI-II, Beck, Steer, and Brown, 1996), and the Patient Health Questionnaire-9 (PHQ-9, Kroenke and Spitzer, 2002). One of the most commonly used semi-structured interviews is the Structured Clinical Interview for *DSM-IV* Axis I Disorders (SCID), which inquires about current and past symptoms (see more information on *http://www.scid4.org*). *Another tool, the Composite International* Diagnostic Interview (CIDI), also assesses MDD as defined by *DSM-IV* and International Classification of Diseases (ICD-10). This diagnostic interview, developed by the World Health Organization (WHO) to be administered by non-clinicians (see Kessler and Üstün, 2004 for more information) has been used widely in epidemiological studies (Kessler et al., 2003). Another clinician-interview instrument includes the Hamilton Rating Scale for Depression (HAM-D, Hamilton, 1960). Most psychiatric rating scales for depression are available at *http://www.neurotransmitter.net/depressionscales.html*

TREATMENT The two main treatment modalities for depression are pharmacological treatment and psychosocial intervention. Selection of intervention is influenced by severity and chronicity of symptoms, any coexisting conditions and ongoing stressors, as well as preferences of individuals receiving services. Psychosocial interventions are often recommended as first-line treatments in mild cases. However, a combination of pharmacological and psychosocial intervention has been considered as the best practice for moderate to severe depression treatment (APA, 2010; de Maat, Dekker, Schoevers, and Jonghe, 2007).

Pharmacological Intervention. There are three major classes of antidepressants in the United States: tricyclic antidepressants (TCAs), monoamine oxidase inhibitors (MAOIs), and selective serotonin reuptake inhibitors (SSRIs). The antidepressants work on neurotransmitters, such as norepinephrine, serotonin, and dopamine (APA, 2010). TCAs, such as imipramine (Tofranil) and amitriptyline (Elavil), were the standard treatment for depression before the introduction of SSRIs. TCAs work by blocking reuptake of serotonin and norepinephrine in the brain. While many studies showed that TCAs are as effective as SSRIs in treatment of depression, in a meta-analysis TCAs were found to be more effective than SSRIs in treatment of inpatient adults with depression (Anderson, 2000). The same study reported less tolerability of TCAs compared to SSRIs due to negative side effects such as dry mouth, constipation, bladder problems, sexual problems, blurred vision, and drowsiness. TCAs are one of the common medications taken in self-poisoning and are highly lethal in medication overdoses (Kerr, McGuffie, and Wilkie, 2001). MAOIs are the oldest class of antidepressants and can be effective for some people. However, due to potential health risks caused from interaction of this drug with food and other drugs, people taking MAOIs need to be monitored closely by doctors (APA, 2010). The SSRIs are the most commonly used antidepressants, and they include fluoxetine (Prozac), citalopram (Celexa), sertraline (Zoloft), paroxetine (Paxil), and escitalopram (Lexapro). Other types of antidepressants are serotonin and norepinephrine reuptake inhibitors (SNRIs), such as venlafaxine (Effexor) and duloxetine (Cymbalta). Bupropion (Wellbutrin) is another antidepressant that is commonly used and it works on dopamine. SSRIs and SNRIs are popular because they do not cause as many side effects as older classes of antidepressants (Anderson, 2000). Some of the common side effects of SSRIs and SNRIs are headache, nausea, sleep disturbance, agitation, and sexual problems.

While medications have been largely considered as the first line of treatment for people with moderate to severe depression, recent studies have raised questions about the effectiveness of antidepressants, especially the SSRIs. A study reviewing all clinical trials submitted to the U.S. Food and Drug Administration (FDA), including unpublished studies, reported that the efficacy of the SSRIs depended on the severity of initial depression, and the difference between SSRIs and placebo was evident only for people in the very severely depressed group (Kirsch et al., 2008). Another meta-analytic study reported that the effect of the antidepressant did not significantly differ from placebo for mild or moderate symptoms of depression (Fournier et al., 2010). Generalizing findings from the study by Fournier and his colleagues to the efficacy of all SSRIs might be difficult due to the small number of studies reviewed (six studies) and the inclusion of only one SSRI (three studies with paroxetine) and one TCA (three studies with imipramine). Research and development of new antidepressants continues at a rapid pace and so it is vital that social workers keep up with the latest findings. More information on medication is available at *http://www.nimh.nih. gov/health/publications/mental-health-medications/ index.shtml*, and the latest information on antidepressants is available on the FDA website (*http://www.fda. gov/Drugs/*).

Psychosocial Interventions. Psychosocial interventions have been demonstrated to be effective in depression treatment. Overall, cognitive behavioral therapy (CBT) and interpersonal therapy (IPT) are considered as evidence-based interventions for MDD, and several interventions show promise, such as psychodynamic psychotherapy, problem-solving therapy, marital and family therapy, and group therapy.

Cognitive behavioral approaches emphasize the role of a person's thoughts on emotional and behavioral responses to life events (Beck, 1976; Ellis, 1994). Based on the seminal work of Aaron Beck (see resources and training information from the Beck Institute for Cognitive Behavior Therapy at *http:// www.beckinstitute.org*), cognitive behavior therapy (CBT) helps individuals with depression reframe negative views of self, environment, and the future in a positive and realistic way (APA, 2010). Studies have shown that CBT is particularly effective for treating mild or moderate depression. CBT has been extensively studied in controlled trials and the efficacy of CBT has been examined in many studies, including meta-analyses. When CBT is compared to no or minimal treatment, its effectiveness has been robust and fairly consistent (Blackburn and Moore, 1997; Dobson, 1989; Gaffan, Tsaousis, and Kemp-Wheeler, 1995; Gloaguen, Cottraux, Cucherat, and Blackburn, 1998). Evidence also shows that the effectiveness of CBT is comparable to medication in acute treatment of depressed outpatients in terms of rates of response and remission in individuals with moderate to severe MDD (DeRubeis et al., 2005; Hollon et al., 2005; Honyashiki et al., 2014; Jarrett et al., 1999). Unlike medication, it appears to have long-lasting effects: Some studies have shown that CBT decreases the risk of relapse even after the treatment is terminated

(Hollon et al., 2005) and continuing CBT in a maintenance phase further decreases this risk (Bockting et al., 2005; Paykel et al., 1999). However, the effectiveness of CBT has also been shown as comparable to other short-term psychotherapies such as IPT and brief dynamic psychotherapy (Jakobsen, Hansen, Simonsen, Simonsen, and Gluud, 2012; Jarrett and Rush, 1994). Several CBT manuals for treatment of depression have been published and the information is available at the following website: *https://hss.semel .ucla.edu/Resources/CBT.html*.

Interpersonal therapy (IPT) is based on the notion that life events influence the onset and expression of depression. The main goal of IPT is to help individuals better understand and cope with depression by making connections between current life events and the onset of symptoms. This is achieved, in part, by helping individuals to overcome interpersonal problems in an effort to improve life circumstances and relieve depression. Its focus is on current events and relationships rather than on past relationships or problems (Klerman, Weissman, Rounsaville, and Chevron, 1984; Weissman, Markowitz, and Klerman, 2000). In general, IPT is superior to treatment as usual and is an effective augmentation strategy for people receiving pharmacotherapy. A meta-analysis of thirteen studies of IPT conducted from 1974 to 2002 reported that, in nine of the studies, IPT was superior to placebo and more efficacious than CBT (de Mello, de Jesus Mari, Bacaltchuk, Verdeli, and Neugebauer, 2005). Another meta-analysis study reported that IPT is as effective as CBT (Jakobsen et al., 2012; Parker, 2007). Several IPT manuals for treatment of depression have been published and the information is available at the following website: *http://interpersonalpsychotherapy .org/about-ipt*.

Other Interventions. Along with pharmacological and psychosocial interventions for depression treatment, increased attention has been paid to other approaches, including complementary and alternative medicine, physical exercise, and brain stimulation therapies. Complementary treatment is used with conventional treatment, while an alternative treatment is used in place of a conventional treatment. Some of the widely used complementary and alternative treatments include St. John's wort, light therapy, acupuncture, omega-3 fatty acid, and folate. However, evidence is largely lacking in using those treatments alone for depression treatment (APA, 2010). Also, potential interaction between complementary/alternative treatments and prescription medication has been reported (APA, 2010). Many studies have reported the beneficial effect of physical exercise on depression (Mura, Sancassiani, Machado, and Carta, 2014; Singh, Clements, and Singh, 2001). While exercise seems to improve depressive symptoms compared with no treatment or control intervention, the effect in favor of exercise decreases when only methodologically robust trials are included (Rimer et al., 2012). Considering the lack of evidence using physical exercise as a sole treatment for depression, combined use of physical exercise with conventional interventions may be the approach to take in reducing depression symptoms (Mura, Sancassiani, Machado, and Cartal, 2014).

Brain stimulation therapies to treat depression involve activating the brain directly with electricity, magnets, or implants. Among these brain stimulation therapies, electroconvulsive therapy (ECT) has been used the longest and researched the most. ECT is usually considered as a treatment option for individuals with severe depression or those who are in life-threatening situations due to suicidality or severe malnutrition (APA, 2010). The efficacy of ECT in the treatment of depression has been shown via a high remission rate for people with severe MDD (Kellner et al., 2006) and also through reducing the relapse rate with follow-up treatment (Fink and Taylor, 2007). Other types of brain stimulation therapies have been introduced recently to treat severe depression, including vagus nerve stimulation (VNS) and repetitive transcranial magnetic stimulation (rTMS). A few studies have suggested that VNS show promise in treatment-resistant depression (Aaronson et al., 2013; George et al., 2005). However, these methods are still experimental in nature (George and Aston-Jones, 2010), and the effects on depression are not established.

SPECIAL CONSIDERATIONS FOR TREATMENT Special attention is required in treating depression, particularly concerning the issues of suicidality, depression during pregnancy and postpartum, and depression in older adults. Risk factors for completed suicide include being male, being single or living alone, and having prominent feelings of hopelessness. The comorbidity with borderline personality disorder significantly increases risk for future suicide attempts (APA, 2013). The Columbia-suicide severity rating scale (C-SSRS) has standardized questions to assess varying levels of suicidal ideations to suicidal behaviors, and it can be administered in both psychiatric and non-psychiatric settings by either clinicians or others with brief training. Different versions of the scales and training information are available at the following website: http://www.cssrs.columbia.edu/index.html

Postpartum depression affects 10% to 15% of women and it remains underdiagnosed and undertreated (Kessler et al., 2003). Risk factors for depression during pregnancy and postpartum include a history of anxiety, mood or eating disorders, a depression during a previous pregnancy, and increased life stressors (Josefsson et al., 2002; O'hara and Swain, 1996). While depression is less prevalent among older adults than among young age groups (Hasin, Goodwin, Stinson, and Grant, 2005), it is often missed or untreated, resulting in devastating consequences (Blazer, 2003). The presentation of symptoms, etiology, risk, and protective factors and potential outcomes of depression in older adults differs from symptoms found earlier in the lifespan, requiring knowledge and consideration of age in the assessment and treatment of older adults with depression (Fiske, Wetherell, and Gatz, 2009).

SERVICE UTILIZATION While advances have been made in treatment guidelines and increased outreach efforts, a majority of people with depression still remain untreated or undertreated (Kessler et al., 2003; Young, Klap, Sherbourne, and Wells, 2001). Approximately 51% who experienced MDD in the past year received treatment for MDD, although treatment was considered adequate in only 21% of the cases (Kessler et al., 2003). Members of ethnic and racial minority communities are far less likely than others to be treated (U.S. Department of Health and Human Services, 2001). Among adults who have experienced depression in the past twelve months, all ethnic and racial minority groups reported significantly lower mental health service use, compared with non-Latino Whites (59.8%): 31.3% of Asian Americans, 36.3% of Latinos, and 41.2% of African Americans (Alegria et al., 2008).

Reducing racial and ethnic disparities in access to, and quality of, mental health care remains a key challenge of the mental health system. To improve the early detection of symptoms, access to formal mental health services, and quality of mental health services, various innovative interventions have been suggested and implemented. Those programs include collaborative care models implemented for Hispanics (Ell et al., 2009; Ell et al., 2010) and collaborative treatment models implemented in primary care (Kwong, Chung, Cheal, Chou, and Chen, 2013; Yeung, Shyu, Fisher, Wu, Yang, and Fava, 2010). Recent meta-analysis of depression treatment for racial and ethnic minority older adults showed that collaborative or integrated care shows promise for African Americans and Latinos (Fuentes and Aranda, 2012). In addition, collaboration between mental health agencies and faith-based communities has been frequently recommended (Taylor, Ellison, Chatters, Levin, and Lincoln, 2000; Yamada, Lee, and Kim, 2011).

INTERNATIONAL PERSPECTIVES ON DEPRESSION

Depression is a significant public health issue across the world. Depression is a leading cause of disability worldwide, as 350 million people are estimated to have some form of depression (World Health Organization, 2012), and it is strongly believed to be related to conditions found in the society. A study that reviewed international epidemiological data for 18 countries on depression (Bromet et al., 2011) reported that more MDD have been reported in 10 high-income countries (15% of the population in a lifetime) compared to middle/low-income countries (11%). However, many similarities across different countries exist in several aspects of MDD. For example, women were two times more likely to have MDD and several sociodemographic factors were consistently associated with adverse outcomes: Difficulties in role transitions were associated with low education, high teen pregnancy, martial disruption, and unstable employment; reduced role functioning was found with low marital quality, low work performance, and low earnings. In addition, elevated risk of onset, persistence, and severity of a wide range of secondary disorders as well as increased risk of early mortality due to physical disorders and suicide were reported among people with MDD (Kessler and Bromet, 2013).

Despite some of these similarities, differences in working with affected individuals from different cultures may stem from the cultural explanation for the illness (for example, definition, cause) and the behaviors associated with it, such as coping and seeking help (APA, 2013). The DSM-5 includes cultural variations in its description and a Cultural Formulation Interview (CFI) that clinicians can use to better understand an individual's understanding of his or her own problem and solution for it (APA, 2013).

Bipolar Disorders

Bipolar disorder (BPD) is a serious mental illness and often results in high direct and indirect costs (Kleinman et al., 2003). The annual direct and indirect costs for treating bipolar disorder in 2009 were estimated to reach $151 billion in the United States alone (Dilsaver, 2011). Bipolar disorder is a leading cause of premature mortality due to suicide and associated medical conditions, such as diabetes mellitus and cardiovas-

cular disease (Kupfer, 2005; Osby, Brandt, Correia, Ekbom, and Sparen, 2001). Also, bipolar disorder causes widespread role impairment (Calabrese et al., 2003; Dean, Gerner, and Gerner, 2004). The individuals with BPD are more likely to be non-employed, and to have more social, cognitive, and work limitations, compared to individuals with depressive disorders (Shippee et al., 2011).

DIAGNOSIS According to the DSM-5 (APA, 2013), bipolar and related disorders include bipolar I disorder, bipolar II disorder, cyclothymic disorder, substance/medication-induced bipolar and related disorder, bipolar and related disorder due to another medical condition, other specified bipolar and related disorder, and unspecified bipolar and related disorder. The focus here is on issues related to bipolar I disorder and bipolar II disorder. Complete descriptions for other bipolar and related disorders, including their full diagnostic criteria, are available in DSM-5 (APA, 2013).

For an individual to be diagnosed with bipolar I disorder, he or she must meet the criteria for at least one manic episode. While hypomanic episodes or major depressive episodes (MDE) are common in bipolar disorder, they are not required for the diagnosis of bipolar I disorder. The central feature of a manic episode is a profound and persistent mood disturbance characterized by elation, irritability, or expansiveness and increased activity or energy that lasts at least one week. Three or more of the following seven symptoms are present during the episode: Grandiosity, diminished need for sleep, excessive talking or pressured speech, racing thoughts or flight of ideas, clear evidence of distractibility, increased level of goal-focused activity or psychomotor agitation, or sexually, excessive pleasurable activities, often with painful consequences. These symptoms are severe enough to cause impairment in social and work functioning, lead to hospitalization, or are presented as combined with psychotic features. The manic episode is assessed as part of the mental illness, and it must not be attributable to the effect of substances or other medical condition (APA, 2013).

Bipolar II disorder requires at least one episode of major depression disorder and at least one hypomanic episode during one's lifetime. If a person ever had a manic episode, this person must be diagnosed with bipolar I disorder. To meet the criteria for a hypomanic episode, the same symptoms must be present but with a shorter duration (at least four consecutive days instead of one week as required in a manic episode), and with less severe impairment in social or occupational functioning. The diagnostic criteria for a MDD are listed in the depression section of this article. Bipolar II disorder is no longer considered a condition milder than bipolar I disorder, mainly due to the extended amount of time people suffer from depression and serious impairment in social and occupational functioning (APA, 2013).

Bipolar disorder was considered to be a mood disorder in the *DSM-IV*. In the *DSM-5*, bipolar and related disorders are separated from mood disorders and placed between schizophrenia spectrum disorders and depressive disorders. This change reflects the observation that individuals with bipolar disorder often experience psychotic symptoms, and recent evidence from genetic and family studies shows shared vulnerabilities for these disorders (APA, 2013).

Although people may also present with symptoms of mania, more people present with symptoms of a major depressive episode when they initially seek treatment. Studies report that approximately 40% of individuals with bipolar disorder are initially misdiagnosed with unipolar depression (Ghaemi, Boiman, and Goodwin, 2000), which delays the initiation of specific bipolar treatment (Beesdo et al., 2009; Perlis et al., 2004). Therefore, inquiring about the history of manic or hypomanic episode is critical to assure a correct diagnosis and treatment planning (Bowden, 2001).

PREVALENCE Bipolar disorder affects approximately 9 million adults, or 4.4% of U.S. adults in their lifetime: 1.0% for bipolar I disorder, 1.1% for bipolar II disorder, and 2.4% for subthreshold bipolar disorder (Kessler, Merikangas, and Wang, 2007). The same study reports that bipolar disorder affects approximately 2.8% of U.S. adults, equivalent to more than 5 million U.S. adults in a given year: 0.6% for bipolar I disorder, 0.8% for bipolar II disorder, and 1.4% for subthreshold bipolar disorder. Bipolar disorder is inversely related to age and educational level and to the unemployed-disabled compared to the employed. Bipolar disorder is unrelated to sex, race/ethnicity, and family income. Sex-specific (male and female) prevalence estimates are 0.8% and 1.1% for bipolar I disorder, 0.9% and 1.3% for bipolar II disorder (Merikangas et al., 2007).

COMORBIDITY Bipolar disorder is associated with high rates of psychiatric, substance, and medical illnesses. Over 70% of persons with bipolar disorder met criteria for at least one other mental disorder in their lifetime (Merikangas et al., 2011). More specifically,

63.1% to 86.7% of respondents with lifetime bipolar disorder also met criteria for at least one lifetime comorbid anxiety disorder and 35.5% to 60.3% met criteria for at least one lifetime comorbid substance use disorder (Merinkangas et al., 2007). High rates of medical comorbidity have been reported, including hypertension, diabetes, pulmonary disease, hepatitis C, and other conditions, especially among veterans with bipolar disorder (Kilbourne et al., 2004). Comorbidity affects evaluation, course, and treatment of the affected individuals and also affects social and economic costs (Merikangas and Kalaydjian, 2007). A higher number of medical comorbidities was associated with a longer duration of lifetime depression and lifetime inpatient depression treatment, severe depression symptoms, and higher service utilization for depressive episode and increased suicidal behavior among individuals with bipolar disorder (Thompson, Kupfer, Fagiolini, Scott, and Frank, 2006).

RISK FACTORS It is commonly believed that the combination of genetic, biological, and environmental factors largely determine vulnerability to bipolar disorder. Marital disruption (separation, divorce, or widowed) is associated with higher rates of bipolar I disorder. On average, adult relatives of individuals with bipolar I and bipolar II disorder are ten times more likely to develop the illness as are individuals without a family history (APA, 2013).

COURSE The age of onset of bipolar disorder usually falls between 15 and 24 years (Bauer et al., 2010; Perlis et al., 2004): bipolar I disorder at 18.2 years and bipolar II disorder at 20.3 years (Merikangas et al., 2007). The effect of depressive episodes in individuals with bipolar disorder, in terms of duration of episodes and quality of life, is considerably worse than the effect of manic episodes (Calabrese, Hirschfeld, Frye, and Reed, 2004; Judd et al., 2002). The vast majority of people who have one manic episode tend to experience a recurrent mood episode. More than half of manic episodes occur immediately before a MDE. Individuals who have four or more mood episodes in any one year receive a "with rapid cycling" specifier (APA, 2013).

ASSESSMENT One of the widely used assessment tools for bipolar disorders is the Structured Clinical Interview for *DSM-IV* (SCID). However, the SCID has been found to have limitations for diagnosing bipolar disorder, especially bipolar II disorder (Benazzi and

Akiskal, 2009). The three main screening tools used for bipolar disorder are the Mood Disorder Questionnaire (MDQ; Hirschfeld et al., 2000), Hypomania Checklist (HCL-32; Angst et al., 2005), and Bipolar Spectrum Diagnostic Scale (BSDS; Phelps and Ghaemi, 2006). These tools have been employed in a number of recent cross-sectional studies to examine the level of undetected bipolar spectrum disorders. However, currently no single screening tool is reliable enough to be used alone for the purpose of diagnosis. Therefore, assessment by a mental health specialist or additional information on the history of past episodes is necessary to confirm the diagnosis.

TREATMENT With medication, psychotherapy, or combined treatment, most people with bipolar disorders can be effectively treated and resume productive lives.

Pharmacological Interventions. Bipolar disorder is treated with medication and treatment depends on the presenting phase of illness (for example, mania, hypomania, MDE, mixed state, or maintenance) and its severity. For acute manic episode, lithium, some anticonvulsants (e.g., valproate, carbamazepine), and several atypical antipsychotics (for example, aripiprazole, haloperidol, olanzapine, quetiapine, risperidone) are used either by themselves or as a combination (Grunze et al., 2009; Hirschfeld, 2005; Yatham et al., 2009). For depressive episode in bipolar I disorder, evidence shows that olanzapine-fluoxetine combination, quetiapine, and lamotrigine are most effective. While combined use of antidepressants and mood stabilizers has modest effects, use of antidepressants without a mood stabilizer is not recommended (Hirschfeld, 2005).

Psychosocial Interventions. Some psychosocial interventions have shown effectiveness when used with pharmacotherapy. Family-focused therapy (FFT) is a manualized psychosocial program, involving all available family members in weekly psychoeducation, communication enhancement training, and problem-solving skills training. Several studies have found FFT to be effective in helping a patient become stabilized and preventing relapses (Miklowitz et al., 2007; Miklowitz, George, Richards, Simoneau, and Suddath, 2003; Rea et al., 2003). Cognitive Behavioral Therapy (CBT) can help a person cope with bipolar symptoms and learn to recognize when a mood shift is about to occur. A systematic review and meta-analysis of randomized or quasi-randomized controlled trials re-

ported that CBT may be effective for relapse prevention in stable individuals with bipolar disorders (Beynon, Soares-Weiser, Woolacott, Duffy, and Geddes, 2008). One randomized, controlled study examined the utility of cognitive therapy in conjunction with pharmacotherapy and found significant beneficial effects of cognitive therapy in terms of fewer bipolar episodes, episode days, and number of hospital admissions over a 12-month period (Lam et al., 2003; Lam, Hayward, Watkins, Wright, and Sham, 2005). Interpersonal and social rhythm therapy (IPSRT), a variation of interpersonal therapy, focuses on addressing interpersonal problems and regulating daily routines during acute treatment in individuals with bipolar I. IPSRT combined with medications is as effective as other types of psychotherapy combined with medication in helping to extend the time to new episode and prevent a relapse of bipolar symptoms (Frank et al., 2005).

Special Considerations for Treatment. Researchers estimate the lifetime prevalence of at least one suicide attempt among individuals with bipolar disorder as between 25% and 60% and completed suicide as between 4% and 19%. One study found that the prevalence of suicide attempts was 36.3% in individuals diagnosed with bipolar I disorder and 32.4% in individuals with bipolar II disorder (Novick, Swartz, and Frank, 2010). The majority of suicides occur during the depressed or mixed-mood phase of the illness. Among the best-known risk factors for suicide are having a family history of suicide, the early onset of affective symptoms, young age, a history of prior suicide attempts, and comorbidity of anxiety and substance abuse disorders (Gonda et al., 2012).

SERVICE UTILIZATION There is often a 5- to 10-year interval between onset of a bipolar disorder and receipt of treatment (Baldessarini, Tondo, and Hennen, 2003). Forty-nine percent of those with these disorders are receiving treatment, and 38.8% of those receiving treatment receive minimally adequate treatment. Lifetime treatment of emotional problems by the time of the interview was reported by 80.1% of respondents with lifetime bipolar disorder. A history of treatment for bipolar I disorder and bipolar II disorder ranges from 89.2% to 95.0%. Psychiatrists were the most common providers for bipolar I (64.9%) and bipolar II disorder (62.2%) (Wang et al., 2005).

INTERNATIONAL PERSPECTIVES ON BIPOLAR DISORDER A World Mental Health Survey Initiative includes data from 11 countries in the Americas, Europe, Asia, the Middle East, and New Zealand and reports that prevalence rates of bipolar disorder vary considerably across studied countries: The highest prevalence rate is reported in the United States (4.4%), while India had the lowest rate (0.1%). Despite varied prevalence, some similarities exist in rates of comorbidity and underutilization of mental health services. About 75% of those with bipolar symptoms had at least one other disorder, with the majority having an anxiety disorder. Overall, less than half of those with bipolar symptoms received mental health services, but the rate of receiving services is as low as 25% in low-income countries (Merikangas et al., 2011).

According to a 2004 Global Burden of Disease study (World Health Organization, 2008), bipolar disorder was reported to be the seventh and eighth leading cause of years lived with a disability (YLD) for men and women, respectively. Similar to U.S. study results, the extent of disability and impairment is higher in bipolar disorder than in other mental disorders except for schizophrenia in Australia (Morgan, Mitchell, and Jablensky, 2005). Adults with bipolar disorder have a higher absence of working days compared to those with other mental disorders in the Netherlands (ten Have, Vollebergh, Bijl, and Nolen, 2002).

IMPLICATIONS FOR SOCIAL WORK PRACTICE For many decades, social workers have been involved in addressing issues of depression and bipolar disorder either as members of interdisciplinary teams or as independent providers in micro, mezzo, and macro levels of practice. The services typically provided by social workers include individual, group, and family therapy; case management; care coordination; and community education and advocacy. While many professionals are involved in the care of people with depression and bipolar disorder, social workers are in a unique position to care for the affected individuals, as these illnesses are influenced by the environment and may also exert influence on the environment. Social workers, as a profession, are uniquely well trained to identify environmental factors that may contribute to, trigger, or prolong the illness or relapse. These factors include unhealthy relationships; unsafe neighborhoods in inner-city areas; poverty; isolation and lack of social support in rural areas; discrimination based on race, gender, ability, etc.; and lack of availability of, or access to, community resources. When people have no means to escape such undesirable environments (due to fewer resources and less support), social workers can intervene to create more favorable environmental conditions by assessing needs and providing, or connect individuals to, resources, playing the role of case manager. At the same time, social workers can offer interventions that take into account environmental stress and empower people with depression to develop skills to systematically identify and solve their problems. In macro practice, social workers may be actively involved in efforts to change social policies and practices that may act as structural barriers to upward mobility for people with depression in poverty. Therefore the person-in-environment approach in social work is invaluable in understanding the impact of the environment on the development of depression and bipolar disorder and in providing effective treatment.

Social workers in the mental health field working directly with individuals with depression or bipolar disorder need to be aware of, and to be trained in, the latest developments in treatment as they become available, not only to benefit themselves, but also to translate the knowledge for clients and families with whom they work. Some of the emerging practice models and trends emphasize integrated health and mental health care. As integrated care becomes more of a norm, social workers need to be ready to provide services either imbedded in primary care setting or closely aligned with health professionals. Therefore, social workers need to acquire a knowledge of common physical health issues that people with mood disorders often face and skills to work collaboratively with medical providers who may or may not share the same values and beliefs in working with people with mood disorders. Another trend is using technology to provide mental health services. Telehealth uses technology to deliver mental health services to hard-to-reach populations such as home-bound older adults or people in remote locations. Social workers can make a significant impact on affected individuals as well as their family members. The majority of primary caregivers who provide direct support for those with mental illness have reported distress, as in the case of bipolar disorder (Perlick, Rosenbeck, et al., 2007). Therefore, social workers may provide necessary emotional and instrumental support as well as psychoeducation for the affected individuals and their families. Individuals suffering from recurrent episodes and their family members can benefit from learning ways to manage the illness and prevent relapse.

While social workers in mental health fields are more likely to be involved with individuals with depression or bipolar disorder or their families, social workers in other settings may also encounter individuals and their families affected by depression or bipolar disorders in settings such as schools, community centers, and agencies offering older adult services. Likewise, social workers in health-care settings may encounter people presenting physical complaints associated with depression or bipolar disorders. While their primary job responsibilities may not include the treatment of depression or bipolar disorder, social workers in non-mental health settings need to have an ability to recognize symptoms, community resources for referral, and the means to advocate access to services for the affected individuals and families.

Many studies have reported stigma associated with depression and bipolar disorder and its impact on various aspects of the lives of affected individuals, including treatment seeking behavior (Interian, Martinez, Guarnaccia, Vega, and Escobar, 2007; Sirey et al., 2001). Stigma affects not only individuals with depression or bipolar disorder, but also their family members (Perlick, Miklowitz, et al., 2007). Social workers need to continue working collaboratively with affected individuals and their families to reduce self (or internalized) stigma to improve their social functioning and quality of life. At the same time, social workers may engage in ongoing work to reduce negative attitude toward mental illness in the communities. In addition, all social workers must work to reduce disparities in access to treatment, quality of care, and treatment outcomes, and they need to advocate on behalf of ethnic minorities or other underserved populations in the practice.

REFERENCES

Aaronson, S. T., Carpenter, L. L., Conway, C. R., Reimherr, F. W., Lisanby, S. H., Schwartz, T. L., ... Bunker, M. (2013). Vagus nerve stimulation therapy randomized to different amounts of electrical charge for treatment-resistant depression: Acute and chronic effects. *Brain Stimulation*, 6(4), 631–640.

Alegria, M., Chatterji, P., Wells, K., Cao, Z., Chen, C., Takeuchi, D., ... Meng, X. L. (2008). Disparity in depression treatment among racial and ethnic minority populations in the United States. *Psychiatric Services*, 11(1), 264–1272. doi:10.1176/appi.ps.59.11.1264

American Psychiatric Association. (2000). *Diagnostic and statistical manual of mental disorders: DSM-IV-TR*. Washington, DC: Author.

American Psychiatric Association. (2010). *Practice guideline for the treatment of patients with major depressive disorder* (3rd ed.). Arlington, VA: Author. doi: 10.1176/appi.books.9780890423387.654001

American Psychiatric Association. (2013). *Diagnostic and statistical manual of mental disorders: DSM-5*. Arlington, VA: Author.

Anderson, I. M. (2000). Selective serotonin reuptake inhibitors versus tricyclic antidepressants: A meta-analysis of efficacy and tolerability. *Journal of Affective Disorders*, 58(1), 19–36. doi:10.1016/S0165-0327(99)00092-0

Angst, J., Adolfsson, R., Benazzi, F., Gamma, A., Hantouche, E., Meyer, T.D., ... Scott, J (2005). The HCL-32: Towards a self-assessment tool for hypomanic symptoms in outpatients. *Journal of Affective Disorders*, 88, 217–233.

Baldessarini, R. J., Tondo, L., & Hennen, J. (2003). Lithium treatment and suicide risk in major affective disorders: Update and new findings. *Journal of Clinical Psychiatry*, 64 (Suppl. 5), 44–52.

Bauer, M., Glenn, T., Rasgon, N., Marsh, W., Sagduyu, K., Munoz, R., ... Whybrow, P. C. (2010). Association between age of onset and mood in bipolar disorder: Comparison of subgroups identified by cluster analysis and clinical observation. *Journal of Psychiatric Research*, 44(16), 1170–1175. doi:10.1016/j.jpsychires.2010.04.009

Beck, A. T. (1976). *Cognitive therapy of the emotional disorders*. New York: Penguin.

Beck, A. T., & Beck, R. W. (1972). Screening depressed patients in family practice: A rapid technic. *Postgraduate Medicine*, 52(6), 81–85.

Beck, A. T., Steer, R. A., & Brown, G. K. (1996). *Manual for the Beck Depression Inventory-II*. San Antonio, TX: Psychological Corporation.

Beesdo, K., Höfler, M., Leibenluft, E., Lieb, R., Bauer, M., & Pfennig, A. (2009). Mood episodes and mood disorders: Patterns of incidence and conversion in the first three decades of life. *Bipolar Disorders*, 11(6), 637–649. doi: 10.1111/j.1399-5618.2009.00738.x

Benazzi, F., & Akiskal, H. S. (2009). The modified SCID Hypomania Module (SCID-Hba): A detailed systematic phenomenologic probing. *Journal of Affective Disorders*, 117(3), 131–136.

Beynon, S., Soares-Weiser, K., Woolacott, N., Duffy, S., & Geddes, J. R. (2008). Psychosocial interventions for the prevention of relapse in bipolar disorder: Systematic review of controlled trials. *British Journal of Psychiatry*, 192(1), 5–11. doi: 10.1192/bjp.bp.107.037887

Blackburn, I. M., & Moore, R. G. (1997). Controlled acute and follow-up trial of cognitive therapy and pharmacotherapy in out-patients with recurrent depression. *British Journal of Psychiatry*, 171(4), 328–334.

Blazer, D. G. (2003). Depression in late life: Review and commentary. *Journals of Gerontology Series A: Biological Sciences and Medical Sciences*, 58(3), M249–M265.

Bockting, C. L., Schene, A. H., Spinhoven, P., Koeter, M. W., Wouters, L. F., Huyser, J., & Kamphuis, J. H. (2005). Preventing relapse/recurrence in recurrent depression with cognitive therapy: A randomized controlled trial. *Journal of Consulting and Clinical Psychology*, 73(4), 647–657. doi:10.1037/0022-006X.73.4.647

Bowden, C. L. (2001). Strategies to reduce misdiagnosis of bipolar depression. *Psychiatric Services*, 52(1), 51–55. doi: 10.1176/appi.ps.52.1.51

Bromet, E., Andrade, L. H., Hwang, I., Sampson, N. A., Alonso, J., de Girolamo, G., ... Kessler, R. C. (2011). Cross-national epidemiology of *DSM-IV* major depressive episode. *BMC Medicine, 9*(1), 90.

Calabrese, J. R., Hirschfeld, R. M., Frye, M. A., & Reed, M. L. (2004). Impact of depressive symptoms compared with manic symptoms in bipolar disorder: Results of a U.S. community-based sample. *Journal of Clinical Psychiatry, 65*(11), 1499–1504.

Calabrese, J. R., Hirschfeld, R. M., Reed, M., Davies, M. A., Frye, M. A., Keck, P. E.,...Wagner, K. D. (2003). Impact of bipolar disorder on a U.S. community sample. *Journal of Clinical Psychiatry, 64*(4), 425–432.

de Maat, S. M., Dekker, J., Schoevers, R. A., & de Jonghe, F. (2007). Relative efficacy of psychotherapy and combined therapy in the treatment of depression: A meta-analysis. *European Psychiatry, 22*, 1–8.

de Mello, M. F., de Jesus Mari, J., Bacaltchuk, J., Verdeli, H., & Neugebauer, R. (2005). A systematic review of research findings on the efficacy of interpersonal therapy for depressive disorders. *European Archives of Psychiatry and Clinical Neuroscience, 255*(2), 75–82. doi:10.1007/s00406-004-0542-x

Dean, B. B., Gerner, D., & Gerner, R. H. (2004). A systematic review evaluating health-related quality of life, work impairment, and healthcare costs and utilization in bipolar disorder. *Current Medical Research and Opinion, 20*(2), 139–154. doi:10.1185/030079903125002801

DeRubeis, R. J., Hollon, S. D., Amsterdam, J. D., Shelton, R. C., Young, P. R., Salomon, R. M.,...Gallop, R. (2005). Cognitive therapy vs medications in the treatment of moderate to severe depression. *Archives of General Psychiatry, 62*(4), 409–416. doi:10.1001/archpsyc.62.4.409

Dilsaver, S. C. (2011). An estimate of the minimum economic burden of bipolar I and II disorders in the United States: 2009. *Journal of Affective Disorders, 129*(1), 79–83. doi:10.1016/j.jad.2010.08.030

Dobson, K. S. (1989). A meta-analysis of the efficacy of cognitive therapy for depression. *Journal of Consulting and Clinical Psychology, 57*(3), 414–419. doi:10.1037/0022-006X.57.3.414

Ell, K., Katon, W., Cabassa, L. J., Xie, B., Lee, P. J., Kapetanovic, S., & Guterman, J. (2009). Depression and diabetes among low-income Hispanics: design elements of a socio-culturally adapted collaborative care model randomized controlled trial. *International Journal of Psychiatry in Medicine, 39*(2), 113–132.

Ell, K., Katon, W., Xie, B., Lee, P. J., Kapetanovic, S., Guterman, J., & Chou, C. P. (2010). Collaborative care management of major depression among low-income, predominantly Hispanic subjects with diabetes: A randomized controlled trial. *Diabetes Care, 33*(4), 706–713.

Ellis, A. (1994). *Reason and emotion in psychotherapy: A comprehensive method of treating human disturbances: Revised and updated*. New York: Citadel.

Fink, M., & Taylor, M. A. (2007). Electroconvulsive therapy evidence and challenges. *Journal of the American Medical Association, 298*(3), 330–332. doi:10.1001/jama.298.3.330

Fiske, A., Wetherell, J. L., & Gatz, M. (2009). Depression in older adults. *Annual Review of Clinical Psychology, 5*, 363–389. doi: 10.1146/annurev.clinpsy.032408.153621

Fournier, J. C., DeRubeis, R. J., Hollon, S. D., Dimidjian, S., Amsterdam, J. D., Shelton, R. C., & Fawcett, J. (2010). Antidepressant drug effects and depression severity: A patient-level meta-analysis. *Journal of the American Medical Association, 303*(1), 47–53. doi:10.1001/jama.2009.1943

Frank, E., Kupfer, D. J., Thase, M. E., Mallinger, A. G., Swartz, H. A., Fagiolini, A. M.,... Monk, T. (2005). Two-year outcomes for interpersonal and social rhythm therapy in individuals with bipolar I disorder. *Archives of General Psychiatry, 62*(9), 996. doi:10.1001/archpsyc.62.9.996

Fuentes, D., & Aranda, M. P. (2012). Depression interventions among racial and ethnic minority older adults: A systematic review across 20 years. *American Journal of Geriatric Psychiatry, 20*(11), 915–931.

Gaffan, E. A., Tsaousis, J., & Kemp-Wheeler, S. M. (1995). Researcher allegiance and meta-analysis: The case of cognitive therapy for depression. *Journal of Consulting and Clinical Psychology, 63*(6), 966–980. doi:10.1037/0022-006X.63.6.966

George, M. S., & Aston-Jones, G. (2010). Noninvasive techniques for probing neurocircuitry and treating illness: Vagus nerve stimulation (VNS), transcranial magnetic stimulation (TMS) and transcranial direct current stimulation (tDCS). *Neuropsychopharmacology, 35*, 301–316. doi:10.1038/npp.2009.87

George, M. S., Rush, A. J., Marangell, L. B., Sackeim, H. A., Brannan, S. K., Davis, S. M.,...Goodnick, P. (2005). A one-year comparison of vagus nerve stimulation with treatment as usual for treatment-resistant depression. *Biological Psychiatry, 58*(5), 364–373.

Ghaemi, S. N., Boiman, E. E., & Goodwin, F. K. (2000). Diagnosing bipolar disorder and the effect of antidepressants: A naturalistic study. *Journal of Clinical Psychiatry, 61*(10), 804–808. doi:10.4088/JCP.v61n1013

Gloaguen, V., Cottraux, J., Cucherat, M., & Blackburn, I. M. (1998). A meta-analysis of the effects of cognitive therapy in depressed patients. *Journal of Affective Disorders, 49*(1), 59–72. doi: 10.1016/S0165-0327(97)00199-7

Gonda, X., Pompili, M., Serafini, G., Montebovi, F., Campi, S., Dome, P.,...Rihmer, Z. (2012). Suicidal behavior in bipolar disorder: Epidemiology, characteristics and major risk factors. *Journal of Affective Disorders, 143*(1), 16–26.

Greenberg, P. E., Stiglin, L. E., Finkelstein, S. N., & Berndt, E. R. (1993). The economic burden of depression in 1990. *Journal of Clinical Psychiatry, 54*, 405–418. doi:10.4088/JCP.v64n1211

Grunze, H., Vieta, E., Goodwin, G. M., Bowden, C., Licht, R. W., Möller, H. J., & Kaspar, S. (2009). The World Federation of Societies of Biological Psychiatry (WFSBP) guidelines for the biological treatment of bipolar disorders: Update 2009 on the treatment of acute mania. *World Journal of Biological Psychiatry, 10*(2), 85–116. doi:10.1080/15622970902823202

Hamilton, M. (1960). A rating scale for depression. *Journal of Neurology, Neurosurgery and Psychiatry, 23*, 56–61.

Hasin, D. S., Goodwin, R. D., Stinson, F. S., & Grant, B. F. (2005). Epidemiology of major depressive disorder: Results from the National Epidemiologic Survey on Alcoholism and Related Conditions. *Archives of General Psychiatry*, 62(10), 1097–1106.

Hirschfeld, R. M., Williams, J. B., Spitzer, R. L., Calabrese, J. R., Flynn, L., Keck, P. E.,...Zajecka, J. (2000). Development and validation of a screening instrument for bipolar spectrum disorder: The Mood Disorder Questionnaire. *American Journal of Psychiatry*, 157(11), 1873–1875. doi: 10.1176/appi.ajp.157.11.1873

Hirschfeld, R. M. A. (2005). *Guideline watch: Practice guideline for the treatment of patients with bipolar disorder*. Arlington, VA: American Psychiatric Association. Retrieved from http://www.psych.org/psych_pract/treatg/pg/prac_guide.cfm

Hollon, S. D., Jarrett, R. B., Nierenberg, A. A., Thase, M. E., Trivedi, M., & Rush, A. J. (2005). Psychotherapy and medication in the treatment of adult and geriatric depression: Which monotherapy or combined treatment? *Journal of Clinical Psychiatry*, 66, 455–468. doi:10.4088/JCP.v66n0408

Honyashiki, M., Furukawa, T. A., Noma, H., Tanaka, S., Chen, P., Ichikawa, K.,...Caldwell, D. M. (2014). Specificity of CBT for depression: A contribution from multiple treatments meta-analyses. *Cognitive Therapy and Research*, 38(3), 249–260. doi:10.1007/s10608-014-9599-7

Interian, A., Martinez, I. E., Guarnaccia, P. J, Vega, W. A., & Escobar, J. I. (2007). A qualitative analysis of the perception of stigma among Latinos receiving antidepressants. *Psychiatric Services*, 58(12), 1591–1594. doi:10.1176/appi.ps.58.12.1591

Jakobsen, J. C., Hansen, J. L., Simonsen, S., Simonsen, E., & Gluud, C. (2012). Effects of cognitive therapy versus interpersonal psychotherapy in patients with major depressive disorder: A systematic review of randomized clinical trials with meta-analyses and trial sequential analyses. *Psychological Medicine*, 42(07), 1343–1357. doi:10.1017/S0033291711002236

Jarrett, R. B., & Rush, A. J. (1994). Short-term psychotherapy of depressive disorders: Current status and future directions. *Psychiatry*, 57(2), 115–132

Jarrett, R. B., Schaffer, M., McIntire, D., Witt-Browder, A., Kraft, D., & Risser, R. C. (1999). Treatment of atypical depression with cognitive therapy or phenelzine: A double blind, placebo-controlled trial. *Archives of General Psychiatry*, 57(11), 1084–1085. doi: 10.1001/archpsyc.56.5.431

Josefsson, A., Angelsiöö, L., Berg, G., Ekström, C. M., Gunnervik, C., Nordin, C., & Sydsjö, G. (2002). Obstetric, somatic, and demographic risk factors for postpartum depressive symptoms. *Obstetrics and Gynecology*, 99(2), 223–228.

Kellner, C. H., Knapp, R. G., Petrides, G., Rummans, T. A., Husain, M. M., Rasmussen, K.,...Fink, M. (2006). Continuation electroconvulsive therapy vs pharmacotherapy for relapse prevention in major depression: A multisite study from the Consortium for Research in Electroconvulsive Therapy (CORE). *Archives of General Psychiatry*, 63(12), 1337–1344. doi: 10.1001/archpsyc.63.12.1337

Kerr, G. W., McGuffie, A. C., & Wilkie, S. (2001). Tricyclic antidepressant overdose: A review. *Emergency Medicine Journal*, 18, 236–241.

Kessler, R. C., & Bromet, E. J. (2013). The epidemiology of depression across cultures. *Annual Review of Public Health*, 34, 119–138. doi:10.1146/annurev-publhealth-031912-114409

Kessler, R. C., & Üstün, T. B. (2004). The world mental health (WMH) survey initiative version of the World Health Organization (WHO) composite international diagnostic interview (CIDI). *International Journal of Methods in Psychiatric Research*, 13(2), 93–121. doi:10.1002/mpr.168

Kessler, R. C., Berglund, P., Demler, O., Jin, R., Koretz, D., Merikangas, K. R.,...Wang, P. S. (2003). The epidemiology of major depressive disorder: Results from the National Comorbidity Survey Replication (NCS-R). *Journal of the American Medical Association*, 289(23), 3095–3105. doi: 10.1001/jama.289.23.3095

Kessler, R. C., Berglund, P. A., Demler, O., Jin, R., & Walters, E. E. (2005). Lifetime prevalence and age-of-onset distributions of *DSM-IV* disorders in the National Comorbidity Survey Replication (NCS-R). *Archives of General Psychiatry*, 62(6), 593–602. doi:10.1001/archpsyc.62.6.593

Kessler, R. C., Merikangas, K. R., & Wang, P. S. (2007). Prevalence, comorbidity, and service utilization for mood disorders in the United States at the beginning of the twenty-first century. *Annual Review of Clinical Psychology. 3*, 137–158. doi:10.1146/annurev.clinpsy.3.022806.091444

Kilbourne, A. M., Cornelius, J. R., Han, X., Pincus, H. A., Shad, M., Salloum, I.,...Haas. G. L. (2004). Burden of general medical conditions among individuals with bipolar disorder. *Bipolar Disorders*, 6(5), 368–373. doi:10.1111/j.1399-5618.2004.00138.x

Kirsch, I., Deacon, B. J., Huedo-Medina, T. B., Scoboria, A., Moore, T. J., & Johnson, B. T. (2008). Initial severity and antidepressant benefits: a meta-analysis of data submitted to the Food and Drug Administration. *PLoS Medicine*, 5(2), 260–268. doi:10.1371/journal.pmed.0050045

Kleinman, L., Lowin, A., Flood, E., Gandhi, G., Edgell, E., & Revicki, D. (2003). Costs of bipolar disorder. *PharmacoEconomics*, 21, 601–622. doi:10.2165/00019053-200321090-00001

Klerman, G. L., Weissman, M. M., Rounsaville, B. J., & Chevron, E. S. (1984). *Interpersonal psychotherapy of depression: A brief, focused, specific strategy*. New York: Basic Books.

Kroenke, K., and Spitzer, R. (2002). The PHQ-9: a new depression diagnostic and severity measure. *Psychiatric Annals*, 32(9), 509–515.

Kupfer, D. J. (2005). The increasing medical burden in bipolar disorder. *Journal of the American Medical Association*, 293(20), 2528–2530. doi:10.1001/jama.293.20.2528

Kwong, K., Chung, H., Cheal, K., Chou, J. C., & Chen, T. (2013). Depression care management for Chinese Americans in primary care: A feasibility pilot study. *Community Mental Health Journal*, 49(2), 157–165.

Lam, D. H., Hayward, P., Watkins, E. R., Wright, K., & Sham, P. (2005). Relapse prevention in patients with bipolar disorder: Cognitive therapy outcome after 2 years. *American Journal of Psychiatry*, 162(2), 324–329. doi:10.1176/appi.ajp.162.2.324

Lam, D. H., Watkins, E. R., Hayward, P., Bright, J., Wright, K., Kerr, N., . . . Sham, P. (2003). A randomized controlled study of cognitive therapy for relapse prevention for bipolar affective disorder: Outcome of the first year. *Archives of General Psychiatry, 60*(2), 145–152. doi:10.1001/archpsyc.60.2.145

Merikangas, K. R., & Kalaydjian, A. (2007). Magnitude and impact of comorbidity of mental disorders from epidemiologic surveys. *Current Opinion in Psychiatry, 20*(4), 353–358.

Merikangas, K. R., Akiskal, H. S., Angst, J., Greenberg, P. E., Hirschfeld, R., Petukhova, M., . . . Kessler, R. C. (2007). Lifetime and 12-month prevalence of bipolar spectrum disorder in the National Comorbidity Survey Replication. *Archives of General Psychiatry, 64*(5), 543. doi:10.1001/archpsyc.64.5.543

Merikangas, K. R., Jin, R., He, J. P., Kessler, R. C., Lee, S., Sampson, N. A., Zarkov, Z. (2011). Prevalence and correlates of bipolar spectrum disorder in the world mental health survey initiative. *Archives of General Psychiatry, 68*(3), 241–251.

Miklowitz, D. J., George, E. L., Richards, J. A., Simoneau, T. L., & Suddath, R. L. (2003). A randomized study of family-focused psychoeducation and pharmacotherapy in the outpatient management of bipolar disorder. *Archives of General Psychiatry, 60*(9), 904–912. doi:10.1001/archpsyc.60.9.904

Miklowitz, D. J., Otto, M. W., Frank, E., Reilly-Harrington, N. A., Wisniewski, S. R., Kogan, J. N., Sachs, G. S. (2007). Psychosocial treatments for bipolar depression: A 1-year randomized trial from the Systematic Treatment Enhancement Program. *Archives of General Psychiatry, 64*(4), 419–426. doi:10.1001/archpsyc.64.4.419

Moran, M. (2014, September 11). ICD-10 transition postponed to October 2015. *Psychiatric News.* Retrieved September 20, 2014 from http://psychnews.psychiatryonline.org

Morgan, V. A., Mitchell, P. B., & Jablensky, A. V. (2005). The epidemiology of bipolar disorder: Sociodemographic, disability and service utilization data from the Australian National Study of Low Prevalence (Psychotic) Disorders. *Bipolar Disorders, 7*(4), 326–337. doi:10.1111/j.1399-5618.2005.00229.x

Muñoz, R. F., Cuijpers, P., Smit, F., Barrera, A. Z., & Leykin, Y. (2010). Prevention of major depression. *Annual Review of Clinical Psychology, 6*, 181–212. doi:10.1146/annurev-clinpsy-033109-132040

Mura, G., Sancassiani, F., Machado, S., & Carta, M. G. (2014). Efficacy of exercise on depression: A systematic review. *International Journal of Psychosocial Rehabilitation, 18*(2), 23–36.

National Institute of Mental Health. (2010). *Mental health medications.* Rockville, MD: Author. Retrieved September 10, 2014 from http://www.nimh.nih.gov/health/publications/mental-health-medications/nimh-mental-health-medications.pdf

Novick, D. M., Swartz, H. A., & Frank, E. (2010). Suicide attempts in bipolar I and bipolar II disorder: A review and meta-analysis of the evidence. *Bipolar Disorders, 12*(1), 1–9. doi:10.1111/j.1399-5618.2009.00786.x

O'hara, M. W., & Swain, A. M. (1996). Rates and risk of postpartum depression: A meta-analysis. *International Review of Psychiatry, 8*(1), 37–54.

Osby, U., Brandt, L., Correia, N., Ekbom, A., & Sparen, P. (2001). Excess mortality in bipolar and unipolar disorder in Sweden. *Archives of General Psychiatry, 58*(9), 844–850. doi:10.1001/archpsyc.58.9.844

Parker, G. (2007). What is the place of psychological treatments in mood disorders? *International Journal of Neuropsychopharmacology, 10*(1), 137–145.

Paykel, E. S., Scott J., Teasdale, J. D., Johnson, A. L., Garland, A., Moore, R., . . . Pope, M. (1999). Prevention of relapse in residual depression by cognitive therapy: A controlled trial. *Archives of General Psychiatry, 56*, 829–835. doi:10.1001/archpsyc.56.9.829

Perlick, D. A., Miklowitz, D. J., Link, B. G., Struening, E., Kaczynski, R., Gonzalez, J., . . . Rosenheck, R. A. (2007). Perceived stigma and depression among caregivers of patients with bipolar disorder. *British Journal of Psychiatry, 190*(6), 535–536.

Perlick, D. A., Rosenheck, R. A., Miklowitz, D. J., Chessick, C., Wolff, N., Kaczynski, R., . . . Desai, R. (2007). Prevalence and correlates of burden among caregivers of patients with bipolar disorder enrolled in the Systematic Treatment Enhancement Program for Bipolar Disorder. *Bipolar Disorders, 9*(3), 262–273. doi:10.1111/j.1399-5618.2007.00365.x

Perlis, R. H., Miyahara, S., Marangell, L. B., Wisniewski, S. R., Ostacher, M., DelBello, M. P., . . . Nierenberg, A. A. (2004). Long-term implications of early onset in bipolar disorder: Data from the first 1000 participants in the systematic treatment enhancement program for bipolar disorder (STEP-BD). *Biological Psychiatry, 55*(9), 875–881. doi:10.1016/j.biopsych.2004.01.022

Phelps, J. R., & Ghaemi, S. N. (2006). Improving the diagnosis of bipolar disorder: Predictive value of screening tests. *Journal of Affective Disorders, 92*(2–3), 141–148.

Philip, S. W., Gregory, S., & Ronald, C. K. (2003). The economic burden of depression and the cost effectiveness of treatment. *International Journal of Methods in Psychiatric Research, 12*, 22–33. doi:10.1002/mpr.139

Radloff, L. (1977). The CES-D Scale: A self-report depression scale for research in the general population. *Applied Psychological Measurement, 1*(3), 385–401. doi:10.1177/014662167700100306

Rea, M. M., Tompson, M. C., Miklowitz, D. J., Goldstein, M. J., Hwang, S., & Mintz, J. (2003). Family-focused treatment versus individual treatment for bipolar disorder: Results of a randomized clinical trial. *Journal of Consulting and Clinical Psychology, 71*(3), 482–492. doi:10.1037/0022-006X.71.3.482

Regier, D. A., & Narrow, W. E. (2014). Understanding ICD-10-CM and DSM-5: A quick guide for psychiatrist and other mental health clinicians. Retrieved September 20, 2014 from http://www.dsm5.org/Documents/Understanding%20ICD%204-1-14.pdf

Rimer, J., Dwan, K., Lawlor, D. A., Greig, C. A., McMurdo, M., Morley, W., & Mead, G. E. (2012). Exercise for depression. *Cochrane Database Systematic Reviews, 7*, Art. No.: CD004366. doi:10.1002/14651858.CD004366.pub5

Shippee, N. D., Shah, N. D., Williams, M. D., Moriarty, J. P., Frye, M. A., & Ziegenfuss, J. Y. (2011). Differences in demographic composition and in work, social, and functional limitations among the populations with unipolar depression and bipolar disorder: Results from a nationally representative sample. *Health and Quality of Life Outcomes*, 9, 90–98. doi:10.1186/1477-7525-9-90

Singh, N. A., Clements, K. M., & Singh, M. A. F. (2001). The efficacy of exercise as a long-term antidepressant in elderly subjects: A randomized, controlled trial. *Journals of Gerontology Series A: Biological Sciences and Medical Sciences*, 56(8), M497–M504.

Sirey, J. A., Bruce, M. L., Alexopoulos, G. S., Perlick, D. A., Raue, P., Friedman, S. J., & Meyers, B. S. (2001). Perceived stigma as a predictor of treatment discontinuation in young and older outpatients with depression. *American Journal of Psychiatry*, 158(3), 479–481.

Substance Abuse and Mental Health Services Administration. (2013). *Results from the 2012 National Survey on Drug Use and Health: Mental health findings*. Rockville, MD: Author. Retrieved September 18, 2014 from http://www.samhsa.gov/data/NSDUH/2k12MH_FindingsandDetTables/2K12MHF/NSDUHmhfr2012.pdf

Taylor, R. J., Ellison, C. G., Chatters, L. M., Levin, J. S., & Lincoln, K. D. (2000). Mental health services in faith communities: the role of clergy in black churches. *Social Work*, 45(1), 73–87.

ten Have, M., Vollebergh, W., Bijl, R., & Nolen, W. A. (2002). Bipolar disorder in the general population in the Netherlands (prevalence, consequences and care utilisation): Results from the Netherlands Mental Health Survey and Incidence Study (NEMESIS). *Journal of Affective Disorders*, 68(2), 203–213. doi:10.1016/S0165-0327(00)00310-4

Thompson, W. K., Kupfer, D. J., Fagiolini, A., Scott, J. A., & Frank, E. (2006). Prevalence and clinical correlates of medical comorbidities in patients with bipolar I disorder: Analysis of acute-phase data from a randomized controlled trial. *Journal of Clinical Psychiatry*, 67(5), 783–788.

U.S. Department of Health and Human Services. (2001). *Mental health: Culture, race, and ethnicity—A supplement to mental health: A report of the surgeon general*. Rockville, MD: U.S. Department of Health and Human Services, Substance Abuse and Mental Health Services Administration, Center for Mental Health Services. Retrieved September 18, 2014 from http://www.ncbi.nlm.nih.gov/books/NBK44243/

Wang, P. S., Lane, M., Olfson, M., Pincus, H. A., Wells, K. B., & Kessler, R. C. (2005). Twelve-month use of mental health services in the United States: Results from the National Comorbidity Survey Replication. *Archives of General Psychiatry*, 62(6), 629–640. doi:10.1001/archpsyc.62.6.629

Weissman, M. M., Markowitz, J. C., & Klerman, G. L. (2000). *A comprehensive guide to interpersonal psychotherapy*. New York: Basic Books.

World Health Organization. (2012) *Depression*. Geneva, Switzerland: Author. Retrieved November 14, 2014 from http://www.who.int/mediacentre/factsheets/fs369/en/

World Health Organization. (2008). *The global burden of disease: 2004 update*. Geneva, Switzerland: Author. Retrieved September 18, 2014 from http://www.who.int/healthinfo/global_burden_disease/GBD_report_2004update_full.pdf

Yamada, A.-M, Lee, K. K., & Kim, M. A. (2011). Community mental health allies: Referral behavior among Asian American immigrant Christian clergy. *Community Mental Health Journal*, 48(1), 107–113. doi:10.1007/s10597-011-9386-9

Yatham, L. N., Kennedy, S. H., Schaffer, A., Parikh, S. V., Beaulieu, S., O'Donovan, C., . . . Kapczinski, F. (2009). Canadian Network for Mood and Anxiety Treatments (CANMAT) and International Society for Bipolar Disorders (ISBD) collaborative update of CANMAT guidelines for the management of patients with bipolar disorder: Update 2009. *Bipolar Disorders*, 11(3), 225–255. doi:10.1111/j.1399-5618.2009.00672.x

Yeung, A., Shyu, I., Fisher, L., Wu, S., Yang, H., & Fava, M. (2010). Culturally sensitive collaborative treatment for depressed Chinese Americans in primary care. *American Journal of Public Health*, 100(12), 2397–2402.

Young, A. S., Klap, R., Sherbourne, C. D., & Wells, K. B. (2001). The quality of care for depressive and anxiety disorders in the United States. *Archives of General Psychiatry*, 58(1), 55–61. doi:10.1001/archpsyc.58.1.55

FURTHER READING

Beck, A. T., & Dozois, D. J. (2011). Cognitive therapy: Current status and future directions. *Annual Review of Medicine*, 62, 397–409.

Bentley, K. J., Price, S. K., & Cummings, C. R. (2014). A psychiatric medication decision support guide for social work practice with pregnant and postpartum women. *Social Work*, 59(4), 303–313. doi:10.1093/sw/swu039

Choi, N. G., Hegel, M. T., Marti, C. N., Marinucci, M. L., Sirrianni, L., & Bruce, M. L. (2014). Telehealth problem-solving therapy for depressed low-income homebound older adults. *American Journal of Geriatric Psychiatry*, 22(3), 263–271.

Craighead, W. E., & Dunlop, B. W. (2014). Combination psychotherapy and antidepressant medication treatment for depression: For whom, when, and how. *Annual Review of Psychology*, 65, 267–300.

Drake, R. E., Frey, W., Bond, G. R., Goldman, H. H., Salkever, D., Miller, A., . . . Milfort, R. (2013). Assisting Social Security disability insurance beneficiaries with schizophrenia, bipolar disorder, or major depression in returning to work. *American Journal of Psychiatry*, 170(12), 1433–1441.

González, H. M., Tarraf, W., Whitfield, K. E., & Vega, W. A. (2010). The epidemiology of major depression and ethnicity in the United States. *Journal of Psychiatric Research*, 44(15), 1043–1051.

Gotlib, I. H., & Joormann, J. (2010). Cognition and depression: Current status and future directions. *Annual Review of Clinical Psychology*, 6, 285–312.

Kupfer, D. J., Frank, E., & Phillips, M. L. (2012). Major depressive disorder: New clinical, neurobiological, and treatment perspectives. *The Lancet*, 379(9820), 1045–1055.

National Institute of Mental Health science news at http://www.nimh.nih.gov/news/science-news/index.shtml

Reamer, F. G. (2013). Social work in a digital age: Ethical and risk management challenges. *Social Work*, 58(2), 163–172.

SAMHSA-HRSA Center for Integrated Health Solutions at http://www.integration.samhsa.gov/integrated-care-models

Singh, M. K., & Gotlib, I. H. (2014). The neuroscience of depression: Implications for assessment and intervention. *Behaviour Research and Therapy*, 62, 60–73. doi:10.1016/j.brat.2014.08.008

KAREN KYEUNGHAE LEE

MILITARY SOCIAL WORK

ABSTRACT: The history of military social work in the United States is rooted in the civilian professional social work community and is a microcosm of that sector. Military social work has a rich history of providing services to military men and women and their families during periods of peace, conflict, and national crises. They have been involved in humanitarian operations and have participated in multinational peace-keeping operations. Social work in the Army, Navy, and Air Force is tailored to the mission of their particular service. However, joint operations between the services are becoming more frequent. Military social workers adhere to the NASW code of ethics while providing service to an institution with its own unique culture, standards, and values.

KEY WORDS: armed forces; military social work

Characteristics

Social work practice in the 21st-century U.S. military continues the rich tradition of commitment to at-risk populations that began over 145 years ago during the Civil War. The U.S. Armed Forces have employed active-duty, uniformed, professional social workers for more than two-thirds of a century. Since World War II, military social work practice has evolved into a well-defined career option for social workers who serve in every branch of the military as commissioned officers and as civilian employees. Military social work began as social casework in mental health settings and now encompasses multiple fields of practice and intervention methods at all levels in the U.S. Department of Defense (DoD), including military family policy, child welfare, health care, substance abuse, mental health, hostage repatriation, combat stress, and humanitarian relief. The number of social workers employed at any given time by DoD varies according to the size of the military establishment. The influence of military social workers on DoD policy relating to the social welfare of the military community and on military missions involving a social welfare or mental health component has also expanded over time.

History of Military Social Work

Social Work services for uniformed personnel and their families were provided by the American Red Cross from World War I to the end of World War II. From 1942 to 1945 about 1,000 American Red Cross psychiatric social workers were assigned to named general and regional hospitals in the United States and overseas. (NASW, 1965). In 1942 six professionally qualified psychiatric social workers were assigned to the newly formed Mental Hygiene Consultation Service at Ft. Monmouth, New Jersey, in an enlisted status. In October 1943 the War Department published the Military Occupational Specialty 263 for Psychiatric Social Work Technicians (War, 1943). It was not until June 1945 that an Army social work branch was incorporated into the office of the surgeon general. The position of psychiatric social work consultant was created to head that branch.

Over the last decade, Reserve and National Guard personnel (Ready Reserve) have been more meaningfully involved with the active military than ever before. Increased participation of citizen soldiers in military missions has also resulted in a growing need for social work services to these military members and their families.

Military social work encompasses a full range of generalist and specialist settings and requires skills that range from individual therapy to policy practice. Military social workers practice in settings that include military combat units, mental health facilities, substance abuse treatment programs, hospitals, prisons and confinement facilities, community service agencies, research facilities, and commander's staffs in major military headquarters. Military social workers' functions include child and family welfare, medical social work, mental health, substance abuse treatment, research, program administration, policy formulation, and in humanitarian and peacekeeping missions. Under special conditions, other populations may become recipients of military assistance, including civilians who have been victims of war and victims of natural disasters.

Each of the services requires social workers to obtain a Master's Degree in Social Work from an institution accredited by the Council of Social Work Education. Social workers who qualify and become uniformed social workers will be commissioned as a social work officer.

Several factors inherent in military life contribute to the development of generalist skills by active-duty military social workers. A typical military career includes multiple and diverse professional assignments that are often dictated by organizational need rather than by personal choice. Therefore, military social workers must exercise both personal and professional flexibility and develop a broad range of generalist social work skills applicable to their changing professional assignments. Nearly all social work officers will serve in an isolated or overseas tour of duty at some point in their military career. The limited availability of resources in these assignments requires the individual practitioner to develop and provide a broad range of services.

All military services facilitate the development of macro skills by their social work officers. As a routine part of their career education, military social workers are provided training in military leadership, management, and administration. This education process begins with a basic officer orientation course and continues through senior service school. For a select few an opportunity will be given for them to obtain their doctorate degrees. They will be utilized in research and high-level leadership positions, upon completion of their education.

The Military Family Lifestyle

Regardless of their age, gender, or racial and ethnic mix, military personnel and their families have a different lifestyle from that of other groups of Americans. As Whitworth (1984) so aptly noted over 22 years ago, eight factors make military family life unique: (a) mobility, (b) separation, (c) periodic absence of parents, (d) adjustment of children, (e) overseas living, (f) high-stress and high-risk jobs, (g) conflicts between those of the military system, and (h) authoritarian management requirements. These eight unique factors remain accurate in today's military. Military families are likely to experience all of these factors—many of them repeatedly and some of them simultaneously—during their affiliation with the armed forces.

The attitude of today's military leaders toward families is significantly different than in previous years when the military viewed marriage and family life as unrelated to the military mission. Each of the services has family support policies, programs, and services designed to meet the unique needs of military families. In today's married and family-focused U.S. Armed Forces, health care and social service delivery systems are firmly in place to address the needs of service members and their families.

Army Social Work

Historically, social workers have embraced the Army's mission by providing support to soldiers and families through the entire deployment cycle (peace and war). Social workers have functioned as an integrated part of the military with social workers most recently deploying with U.S. forces to assist "Operation Iraq Freedom" (2003 to present) with the goal of implementing programs that reduce stress (including combat stress) and substance abuse.

Social workers provide a variety of services, including individual counseling, group counseling, and command consultation. They emphasize preventive health in primary care clinics, including screening for depression and other psychological or psychosocial issues.

Army social workers are deployed with the soldiers they serve and thus are in a position to provide "front line" intervention. They are supported by an equal complement of Reserve component social workers in the Combat Support Hospitals and Combat Stress Control units. There are close to 400 civil servant social workers plus contract staff who practice along with uniformed social workers (although not in areas of direct combat).

Social workers have also deployed with units involved in peacekeeping and as part of multinational forces observers. Specifically, they have been deployed to the Sinai Peninsula, Bosnia, and Kosovo. They were the sole mental health asset in Croatia and Somalia (personal conversation with chief of army social workers, Col. Yvonne Tucker-Harris, August 2007). Major changes in Army doctrine in the early 21st century have had an impact in social work practice. As a result of past experiences, there is a greater emphasis on educating military leaders on combat stress; how to prevent it, how to detect it, and the resources that are available, including Combat Operational Stress Control Teams. The Army's Training and Doctrine Command along with the Army's Medical Department Center and School share the responsibility for training in combat stress for our fighting force. There has also been a trend toward deployment with brigade combat teams, which seems to work extremely well in support of the soldiers in the theater of operation (Field Manual 8–51, 1994).

Although there has been a trend toward integration into behavioral health teams, social work maintains a separate department or service in most hospitals.

Social Work in the Navy

The Navy's social work program was provided by civilian social workers assigned to the Red Cross and large Navy relief offices, as well as by other volunteer agencies in the Navy. The first professional social worker was employed by the Navy Relief Society in 1945, the end of World War II (Raiha, 1999). Social work programs in the Navy include behavioral science support to Navy and Marine Corps commanders and personnel, medical and psychiatric social work at naval hospitals, research on the military family, family advocacy, and drug and alcohol prevention and rehabilitation.

In 1973, with the repatriation of American prisoners of war from Southeast Asia, the Navy developed a prevention-oriented social work program designed to provide outreach services to families of servicemen missing in action and to returning prisoners of war and their families. This program has since ended, but social workers have remained in naval hospitals to provide a variety of services. There are currently about 200 civilian social workers employed in naval hospitals.

In 1979 the Navy Family Support Program was established. In 2006, around 75 Fleet and Family Support Centers (FFSCs) operated throughout the world. These centers provide the on-site means by which the Family Support Program is implemented; they are multifunctional centers managed by Navy personnel (as opposed to medical personnel) that offer a variety of services, including deployment readiness services (for service members and families), Ombudsman programs are designed to support military families, personal financial services, support programs for new parents, transition assistance services for military members and families preparing to return to civilian life, family employment services, relocation assistance to help families during the frequent military moves, family advocacy services designed to prevent and intervene in child abuse and neglect and spouse abuse cases, sexual assault prevention and support services, life skills programs, and a variety of volunteer services. Approximately 400 civilian social workers are employed full time in these centers.

Active duty Navy social workers were first deployed in a wartime mission to Kuwait in 2007 to support the Navy's Warrior Transition Program designed to screen returning Sailors and Marines for potential combat stress and mental health issues and to help prepare them mentally and emotionally for return to the continental United States.

Social workers in today's Navy serve as staff officers at Navy headquarters, program managers for the Family Advocacy Program in the Bureau of Medicine and Surgery and the Rape/Sexual Assault Program at the Bureau of Naval Personnel, regional Family Advocacy Program managers in Navy and Marine Corps installations, directors and practitioners of hospital social work, and Family Advocacy Program managers, representatives, and practitioners in Family Service Centers.

Social Work in the Air Force

The position of social work consultant to the Air Force surgeon general and the commissioning of Air Force social work officers dates back to 1952. Since then, the role of active duty social workers has continued to expand in both peace-time and war-time missions.

The history of Air Force social work reflects a profession that has continuously risen to meet the needs of airmen and their families. The Children Have a Potential (CHAP) program is an early example of this kind of support. Established in 1961, the program was designed to promote military readiness by supporting families with disabilities. Air Force social workers provided counseling and referral, client advocacy and case management while ensuring access to medical care and appropriate educational resources for children with special needs. The program was later expanded to include adult family members of airmen, and became known as the Exceptional Family Member Program.

In 1996, the Air Force established the Integrated Delivery System (IDS), a working group representing the helping agencies of an Air Force base. Utilizing their community organization and networking skills, social workers immediately became key IDS participants in efforts to promote coordinated responses to the challenges of the Air Force community.

In 2006, the Air Force claimed the largest number of active duty social workers in the Department of Defense. With 190 officers serving across the world, social workers' presence within the Air Force Medical Services has risen to new heights. As part of the Air Force Biomedical Sciences Corps, which consists of 16 diverse allied health fields, social work officers have successfully competed for leadership roles ranging from Headquarters Air Force to commanding entire medical treatment facilities or their associated squadrons. Career-broadening opportunities have seen social work skills utilized in psychological operations, medical readiness, recruiting, family support, and health and wellness. In the aftermath of the terrorist attack on the World Trade Center and the Pentagon on

September 11, 2001, the role of the Air Force social worker dramatically changed. Social workers were increasingly called upon to support airmen and their families at home, with family support programs that addressed the impact of family separation, and abroad, in the midst of the front lines of the global war on terrorism.

Traumatic stress response teams incorporated the most current concepts in crisis management and were activated in the aftermath of terrorist bombings as well as natural disasters such as Hurricane Katrina. Social workers used specialized training in grief counseling and posttraumatic stress disorder to help airmen deal with the effects of these events. They also played prominent roles in postdeployment health risk appraisals, hoping to avert another Gulf War Syndrome, as well as assisting families in coming back together through reunion and reintegration programs. The Air Force continues to successfully deploy social workers in support of Operation Enduring Freedom (Afghanistan), Operation Iraqi Freedom, and in a variety of other locations in the Middle East. Air Force social workers now operate throughout the area of responsibility, traveling to forward operating bases where they support soldiers, sailors, and mariners, in the same way they have always supported airmen.

Challenges and Trends

Recent events related to war and terrorism have had a significant impact on our way of living our politics and on our sense of survival. The psychological and psychosocial implications of future conflicts are as yet unclear. What is clear however is that military social workers will have a major role in any future encounter with enemy forces, whether in support of our soldiers in direct combat, or in support of peacekeeping activities. Social workers of the different services will increasingly be in support of one another as they intervene in the problems of the military and the military family. It is also clear that the "citizen soldier," that is, members of the reserve components, will continue to be a vital part of our national defense and of the military social work community.

Acknowledgments

The authors thank the following individuals who made significant contributions to this article. Yvonne Tucker Harris, Social Work Consultant to the Army Surgeon General, Col. MSC, U.S. Army, Barry Adams LCDR, MSC, U.S Navy, Bureau of Medicine and Surgery, and Robert J. Campbell, Lt Col Social Work Consultant to the Air Force Surgeon General.

REFERENCES

Field Manual 8–51. (1994, September), Combat stress control in a theater of operations tactics, techniques, and procedures. Directorate of Combat Doctrine, Development, AMEDD Center and School.

National Association of Social Workers. (1965). *Mental health and psychiatric services.* New York: National Association of Social Workers.

Raiha, N. K. (1999). Medical social work in the U.S. Armed Forces. In *Social work practice in the military* (pp. xxviii, 358 p.). New York: Haworth Press.

War Department Letter. (1943, October 18). *Psychiatric social workers,* SSN 263. Washington, DC.

Whitworth, S. (1984). Testimony on military families. Hearings of the select Committee on Children, Youth and Families, U.S. House of Representatives, 98th Congress 2nd Session, Washington, DC: U.S. Government Printing Office.

FURTHER READING

Applewhite, L., Brintzenhofe-Szoc, K., Hamlin, E., & Timberlake, E. (1995, January). Clinical social work practice in the U.S. Army: An update. *Military Medicine, 160,* 288.

Bureau of Labor Statistics. (2004, September). Current population file.

Daley, J. (Ed.). (1999). *Social work practice in the military.* Binghamton, NY: The Hayworth Press.

Department of the Army Deputy Chief of Staff, Office of Army Demographics. (2004, September 15). Data from the Defense Manpower Data Center.

Garber, D. L., & McNelis, P. J. (1995). Military social work. In R. L. Edwards (Ed.), *Encyclopedia of social work* (19th ed., Vol. 2: pp. 1726–1736). Washington, DC: NASW Press.

Hamlin, E. R., Pehrson, K. L., & Gimmill, R. (1996). Social work service in Army medical treatment facilities: Are they reorganizing? *Military Medicine, 16*(1), 33–36.

Harris, J. J. (1993). Military social work as occupational practice. In P. A. Kurzman & S. H. Akabas (Eds.), *Work and well-being: The occupational social work advantage* (pp. 276–290). Washington, DC: NASW Press.

Harris, J. J. (1999). History of Army social work. In Daley (Ed.), *Social work practice in the military* (pp. 3–22). Binghamton, NY: The Hayworth Press.

Office of the Assistant Secretary of Defense. (1993). *Military family demographics: Profile of the military community.* Arlington, VA: Military Family Clearing House.

Pehrson, K. L. (2002). Retention and the social work officer. *Journal of the Army Medical Department,* July–September, 43–51.

Torgerson, F. G. (1956). A historical study of the beginnings of individualized social services in the United States Army. Unpublished doctoral dissertation, University of Minnesota.

JESSE J. HARRIS AND KYLE L. PEHRSON

MOTIVATIONAL INTERVIEWING

ABSTRACT: Motivational interviewing (MI) is a collaborative, goal-oriented conversation style designed to strengthen intrinsic motivation for and commitment to change. The spirit of MI includes four elements: partnership, acceptance, compassion, and evocation. MI is often employed as a therapeutic intervention, and it clinical effectiveness is well documented across more than 200 randomized controlled trials. Research has also documented wide variation in MI effectiveness across counselors, studies, and sites within studies.

KEY WORDS: intervention; motivation to change; motivational interviewing; substance abuse

Introduction

Motivational interviewing (MI) and other brief motivational interventions have gained considerable popularity as alternative or adjunctive approaches to more traditional psychotherapeutic approaches designed to produce behavior change among clients (Ryder, 1999; Walitzer, Dermen, & Connors, 1999; Yahne & Miller, 1999). As of 2013, there are more than 1,200 publications, including more than 200 randomized controlled trials, about MI (Miller & Rollnick, 2013). While initially used with addictive-behavior problems, such interventions have been implemented with success for a variety of behaviors ranging from diabetes self-management (Doherty, Hall, James, Roberts, & Simpson, 2000) to water disinfection practices (Thevos, Quick, & Yanduli, 2000) to treatment adherence among psychiatric patients (Swanson, Pantalon, & Cohen, 1999) to fruit and vegetable intake (Resnicow et al., 2001).

Empirical Support

The empirical literature has demonstrated the effectiveness of brief motivational interventions with substance-abusing populations (Burke, Arkowitz, & Mechola, 2003; DiClemente, Bellino, & Neavins, 1999; Miller, Andrews, Wilbourne, & Bennett, 1998; Vasilaki, Hosier, & Cox, 2006). In a meta-analysis of controlled clinical trials of the briefest form of motivational interventions, motivational interviewing (MI), for drinking problems, Vasilaki et al. (2006) concluded "that brief MI is an efficacious strategy for reducing alcohol consumption." In a broader meta-analysis, Burke et al. (2003) included studies targeting marijuana and other drug-use problems. These researchers concluded that motivational interviewing was "equivalent to other active treatments and supe-

rior to no treatment or placebo controls for problems involving alcohol [or] drugs" (p. 856). Moreover, these investigators documented an average within-treatment-group effect size of 0.82, with MI treatment assignment accounting for a remarkable 48% of the variance in outcomes among marijuana and other drug abusers. Moreover, MI effects were found to generalize beyond substance-use behaviors. Burke, Arkowitz, and Dunn (2002) found a treatment-group effect size of 0.90 for social impact outcomes for marijuana and other drug abusers. Thus, there is strong support for considering MI-interventions to be "empirically supported therapies" (ESTs), which are defined by Hall (2001) as "treatments that have been demonstrated to be superior in efficacy to a placebo or another treatment" (p. 503).

Principles

Miller and Rollnick (2013) characterize MI as "a person-centered counseling style for addressing the common problem of ambivalence about change" (p. 24). The underlying spirit of MI includes four key elements: partnership, acceptance, compassion, and evocation. Acceptance is critical for engaging clients and building a working therapeutic relationship, and it includes the four key aspects: absolute worth, accurate empathy, autonomy support, and affirmation. In contrast to traditional approaches, motivational interventions are intended, through support and persuasion, to increase the likelihood that people will make changes in their behavior by helping them to recognize that problems exist in their lives and to overcome ambivalence about change. This directive, client-centered counseling style has as an overarching goal of pinpointing and magnifying discrepancies between client goals and current behavior, and thus increasing ambivalence. Ambivalence is expressed through clients' change talk (pro-change arguments) and sustain talk (pro-status quo, anti-change arguments), and is considered a normal human process on the pathway to change. Change talk, which MI is designed to promote, is captured by the acronym DARN-CAT: when preparing to make changes, change talk is evidenced by statements expressing desire, ability, reasons, and need; when mobilizing for change, change talk is evidenced by statements expressing commitment, activation, and taking steps.

Interventions and Techniques

Core therapeutic skills in MI are represented by the acronym OARS: asking open-ended questions, affirming, reflecting, and summarizing. Providing information and advice may also be part of MI, but only with the client's permission. Therapeutic applications of MI typically involve four sequential processes: (a) engaging, in which both parties establish a helpful connection and a working relationship; (b) focusing, which involves clarifying direction and identifying the agenda; (c) evoking, which involves eliciting the client's own motivations for change and having the client voice the arguments for change; and (d) planning, in which commitment to change is supported and expanded, and a specific plan of action is formulated. In clinical practice, MI can be used in individual face-to-face consultation, or with couples, families, or groups. Moreover, there is empirical support for its effective delivery via telephone, televideo, computer, and print. Finally, MI has been adapted for use across a variety of cultures and special populations, and it can be implemented as a stand-alone treatment or a component of a larger, integrated-treatment package.

Effectiveness with Adolescents

A growing empirical literature supports the effectiveness of motivational interviewing (MI) with adolescent marijuana users and drinkers (Naar-King & Suarez, 2011). Published reports of randomized controlled trials (RCTs) of MI with adolescent marijuana users (for example, D'Amico, Miles, Stern, & Meredith, 2008; Martin, Copeland, & Swift, 2005; McCambridge & Strang, 2004, 2005; Stein et al., 2006; Walker, Roffman, Stephens, Berghuis, & Kim, 2006) and underage drinkers (for example, Borsari & Carey, 2000; Larimer et al., 2001; Marlatt et al., 1998; Monti et al., 1999; Roberts, Neal, Kivlahan, Baer, & Marlatt, 2000) support its effectiveness for reducing adolescent substance-use problems.

Thus, motivational interviewing, when used with late adolescent drinkers, meets Hall's (2001) criterion for an empirically supported therapy (that is, superior in efficacy to a placebo or another treatment). Across these clinical trials, treatment effects were independent of putative moderator variables including gender, parental history of alcoholism, history of conduct disorder, and stage of change. It should be noted, however, that each study involved predominantly non-Hispanic white youths (80%+), and included only older adolescents. To address these limitations, NIH, in the early 2010s, began supporting major clinical trials examining the efficacy of MI with younger and more diverse adolescent drinkers and drug users (for example, in 2012, NIDA grant R01 DA029779 [Co-PI's: E.F. Wagner & J. Lowe] examined the impact of MI on drinking and drug use among Native American 9th–12th graders).

Interest in MI has burgeoned since the 1990s, and many social workers and most addiction-treatment clinicians were, 20 years later, at least somewhat familiar with the approach. Certification in MI, both as a practitioner and a trainer, is available, and theoretical and empirical publications on the approach have been widely disseminated. MI may be particularly appealing to social workers because it is consistent with harm-reduction approaches to addictive behaviors. Harm reduction has been conceptualized as a peace movement, and it is aligned with the humanistic values around which social work is organized (Brocato & Wagner, 2003). MI specifically, and harm reduction approaches generally, may reduce the ethical conflicts confronted by social workers conducting more traditional and coercive interventions for substance-use problems. Moreover, MI is strongly consistent with strengths-based practice in social work; as such, MI has been identified as having important implications for social work research, practice, and education (Manthey, Knowles, Asher, & Wahab, 2011).

REFERENCES

Borsari, J. B., & Carey, K. B. (2000). Effects of a brief motivational intervention with college student drinkers. *Journal of Consulting and Clinical Psychology, 68*, 728–733.

Brocato, J., & Wagner, E. F. (2003). Harm reduction: A social work practice and social justice agenda. *Health and Social Work, 28*, 117–125.

Burke, B. L., Arkowitz, H., & Dunn, C. (2002). The efficacy of motivational interviewing. In W. R. Miller & S. Rollnick (Eds.), *Motivational interviewing: Preparing people for change* (2nd ed., pp. 217–250). New York: Guilford Press.

Burke, B. L., Arkowitz, H., & Mechola, M. (2003). The efficacy of motivational interviewing: A meta-analysis of controlled clinical trials. *Journal of Consulting & Clinical Psychology, 71*, 843–861.

D'Amico, E. J., Miles, J. N. V., Stern, S. A., & Meredith, L. S. (2008). Brief motivational interviewing for teens at risk of substance use consequences: A randomized pilot study in a primary care clinic. *Journal of Substance Abuse Treatment, 35*, 53–61.

DiClemente, C. C., Bellino, L. E., & Neavins, T. M. (1999). Motivation for change and alcoholism treatment. *Alcohol Research & Health, 23*, 86–92.

Doherty, Y., Hall, D., James, P. T., Roberts, S. H., & Simpson, J. (2000). Change counselling in diabetes: The development of a training programme for the diabetes team. *Patient Education & Counseling, 40*, 263–278.

Hall, G. C. N. (2001). Psychotherapy research with ethnic minorities: Empirical, ethical, and conceptual issues. *Journal of Consulting and Clinical Psychology, 69*, 502–510.

Larimer, M. E., Turner, A. P., Anderson, B. K., Fader, J. S., Kilmer, J. R., Palmer, R. S., & Cronce, J. M. (2001).

Evaluating a brief alcohol intervention with fraternities. *Journal of Studies on Alcohol*, 62, 370–380.

Marlatt, G. A., Baer, J. S., Kivlahan, D. R., Dimeff, L. A., Larimer, M. E., & Quigley, L., et al. (1998). Screening and brief intervention for high-risk college student drinkers: Results from a 2-year follow-up assessment. *Journal of Consulting & Clinical Psychology*, 66, 604–615.

Manthey, T. J., Knowles, B., Asher, D., & Wahab, S. (2011). Strengths-based practice and motivational interviewing. *Advances in Social Work*, 12, 126–151.

Martin, G., Copeland, J., & Swift, W. (2005). The adolescent cannabis check-up: Feasibility of a brief intervention for young cannabis users. *Journal of Substance Abuse Treatment*, 29, 207–213.

McCambridge, J., & Strang, J. (2004). The efficacy of a single-session motivational interviewing in reducing drug consumption and perceptions of drug-related risk and harm among young people: Results from a multi-site cluster randomized trial. *Addiction* 99, 39–52.

McCambridge, J., & Strang, J. (2005). Deterioration over time in effect of motivational interviewing in reducing drug consumption and related risk among young people. *Addiction*, 100, 470–478.

Miller, W. R., Andrews, N. R., Wilbourne, P., & Bennett, M. E. (1998). A wealth of alternatives: Effective treatments for alcohol problems. In W. R. Miller & N. Heather (Eds.), *Treating addictive behaviors* (2nd ed., pp. 203–216). New York: Plenum Press.

Miller, W. R., & Rollnick, S. (Eds.). (2013). *Motivational interviewing: Helping people change* (3rd ed.). New York: Guilford Press.

Monti, P. M., Colby, S. M., Barnett, N. P., Spirito, A., Rohsenow, D. J., Myers, M., et al. (1999). Brief intervention for harm reduction with alcohol-positive older adolescents in a hospital emergency department. *Journal of Consulting & Clinical Psychology*, 67, 989–994.

Naar-King, S., & Suarez, M. (2011). *Motivational interviewing with adolescents and young adults*. New York, US: Guilford Press.

Resnicow, K., Jackson, A., Wang, T., De, A. K., McCarty, F., & Dudley, W. N., et al. (2001). A motivational interviewing intervention to increase fruit and vegetable intake through black churches: Results of the eat for life trial. *American Journal of Public Health*, 91, 1686–1693.

Roberts, L. J., Neal, D. J., Kivlahan, D. R., Baer, J. S. & Marlatt, G. A. (2000). Individual drinking changes following a brief intervention among college students: Clinical significance in an indicated preventive context. *Journal of Consulting and Clinical Psychology*, 68, 500–505.

Ryder, D. (1999). Deciding to change: Enhancing client motivation to change behaviour. *Behaviour Change*, 16, 165–174.

Stein, L. A. R., Colby, S. M., Barnett, N. P., Monti, P. M., Golembeske, C., & Lebeau-Craven, R. (2006). Effects of motivational interviewing for incarcerated adolescents on driving under the influence after release. *American Journal of Addictions*, 15, 50–57.

Swanson, A. J., Pantalon, M. V., & Cohen, K. R. (1999). Motivational interviewing and treatment adherence among psychiatric and dually diagnosed patients. *Journal of Nervous & Mental Disease*, 187, 630–635.

Thevos, A. K., Quick, R. E., & Yanduli, V. (2000). Motivational interviewing enhances the adoption of water disinfection practices in Zambia. *Health Promotion International*, 15, 207–214.

Vasilaki, E. I., Hosier, S. G., & Cox, W. M. (2006). The efficacy of motivational interviewing as a brief intervention for excessive drinking: A meta-analytic review. *Alcohol and Alcoholism*, 41(3), 328–335.

Walitzer, K. S., Derman, K. H., & Connors, G. J. (1999). Strategies for preparing clients for treatment: A review. *Behavior Modification*, 23, 129–151.

Walker, D. D., Roffman, R. A., Stephens, R. S., Berghuis, J. A., & Kim, W. (2006). Motivational enhancement therapy for adolescent marijuana users: A preliminary randomized controlled trial. *Journal of Consulting and Clinical Psychology*, 74, 628–632.

Yahne, C. E., & Miller, W. R. (1999). Enhancing motivation for treatment and change. In B. S. McCrady & E. E. Epstein (Eds.), *Addictions: A comprehensive guidebook* (pp. 235–249). New York: Oxford University Press.

FURTHER READING

Motivational Interviewing: http://www.motivationalinterview.org/

Substance Abuse and Mental Health Services Administration: http://www.samhsa.gov/co-occurring/topics/training/motivational.aspx

Motivational Interviewing Network of Trainers (MINT): http://www.motivationalinterviewing.org/

ERIC F. WAGNER

MULTICULTURALISM

ABSTRACT: This article defines the concept of multiculturalism and explains, from a historical and contemporary perspective, its evolution and significance in social work. The relationship between multiculturalism and socioeconomic justice, oppression, populations at risk, health disparities, and discrimination is explained. The importance of preparatory training for social workers to meet the challenges of multiculturalism is highlighted and examples of cross-cultural training models are provided. Implications of multiculturalism for clinical practice and policy development are discussed.

KEY WORDS: cross-cultural practice; cultural competency; cultural diversity; multicultural social work; multiculturalism

Definitions, Assumptions, and Shifting Demographics

Several terms, including *multiculturalism*, *diversity*, *cultural diversity*, *cultural competency*, and *cross-cultural practice*, are often used in the literature to describe patterns of interaction and awareness of and sensitivity to "populations at risk." These populations are typically nonwhite and often considered oppressed, disenfranchised, and marginalized. Multiculturalism has been defined as an ideology that suggests that society should consist of, or at least recognize and include with equal status, diverse cultural groups (Sue, 2006). Multiculturalism is often considered as the opposite of monoculturalism, which implies a normative cultural unity and preexisting homogeneity. As monoculturalism assumes the rejection of differences and a belief in the superiority of dominant culture, multiculturalism represents acceptance, appreciation, utilization, and celebration of similarities and differences (Fong, 2005; Gutiérrez, Zuñiga, & Lum, 2004).

Multiculturalism as an ideal has been regarded both as the entitlement of cultural groups and as a form of civil rights grounded in human dignity and the equality of cultures. It is seen as a move toward interculturalism, the beneficial exchange where cultures learn about one another (Andersen & Collins, 2013). Cultural diversity is an essential component of multiculturalism, leading to a broader representation of perspectives, worldviews, lifestyles, language, and communication styles. Acknowledging diversity suggests that subordinate groups are not required to give up their identity or assimilate to dominate norms (Lum, 2004; Weaver, 2005). For dominant groups, this may mean that new ways of relating to those of different cultures need to be acquired.

Multiculturalism is even more essential as the U.S. population becomes increasingly diversified. According to the 1980 census, one in every five Americans was nonwhite, and in that year there were about 14 million foreign-born residents. A decade later, one in five Americans identified as nonwhite, and there were about 20 million foreign-born residents (Gould, 1996). On the basis of 2010 census data, white non-Latinos accounted for 63.7% of the population, while Latinos (who can be of any race) made up 16.3%, African Americans 13.6%, and Asian Americans 4.8% (Humes, Jones, & Ramirez, 2011). In 2010, 12.9%, or approximately 40 million of the U.S. population, were foreign-born (Grieco et al., 2012). In 2010, 36.3% of the U.S. population was identified as nonwhite minorities, and Asians were the largest and fastest-growing minority group.

As of 2013, there were five states—California, Texas, Hawaii, New Mexico, and California—and the District of Columbia in which the combined population of minorities exceeded the majority population (Humes et al., 2011). By 2050, non-Hispanic whites are predicted to make up just 50% of the population, with Latinos accounting for 24%, African Americans 15%, and Asian Americans 8% (Liao et al., 2004).

Simultaneously, the United States is in the midst of a dramatic shift in age distribution. By 2030 more than 20% of Americans will be 65 years or older (Council on Social Work Education [CSWE]/SAGE-SW, 2001). With this population shift, social workers are facing growing demands for formulating policy and providing services to enhance the physical, mental, and social well-being of people who have been historically marginalized. Practitioners must be prepared for multicultural social work practice and therefore to use modalities consistent with the life experiences and cultural values of diverse clients and client systems (Lum, 2004; Sue, 2006).

Background and Significance: Historical and Contemporary Perspectives

Although much of the literature suggests the need for Anglo-Americans to accept other cultures, the reality is that many of these other cultural groups were actually on U.S. soil long before Europeans arrived. A close look at history reveals a country in which the original settlers, Native Americans, were exploited. Many were killed and displaced by European Americans (Weaver, 2005). Africans were forcibly brought to the country, enslaved, and treated as property by Anglo-Americans (Davis & Proctor, 1989). In fact, much of the labor force used to build this country consisted of Africans, Chinese, Japanese, and Latinos (Schmitz, Stakeman, & Sisneros, 2001).

To examine the evolution of multiculturalism in social work practice, it is necessary to examine the origins of the social work profession. In its earliest conceptualization, the profession evolved from the need to address growing social problems related to industrialization, urbanization, and immigration at the end of the 19th century (Popple, 1995). The early Settlement House workers tried to be "neighbors" to the poor and employed a "pluralist" approach based on the belief in the equal value of some (especially white) immigrant cultures. By the early 1900s, staff members of the Charity Organization Societies were becoming professionally trained to provide direct services to mostly white immigrant children and families. At the time, it was believed that in America immigrants would be better off if they left their culture behind, assimilated, adapted, and became a part of the "melting pot" (Martinez-Brawley & Brawley, 1999).

By the 1930s and 1940s, a number of factors—including the Depression, the passage of the Social Security Act of 1935, World War II, and the Cold War—led to a sense of national pride in the United States and reinforced the belief that people of color should "abandon" their distinct identities and attempt to assimilate to the white norm (Logan, 2003; Van Soest, 1995). In the post–World War II era, social work saw a renewed focus on psychotherapeutic approaches, as a growing number of middle- and upper-income clients sought therapy from social workers. Practice methods and theories were considered culturally neutral and universally appropriate to all client groups regardless of demographic characteristics (Schiele, 2007).

However, the civil rights movement of the 1960s brought attention to growing racial and economic inequalities. This necessitated growing recognition of pluralistic perspectives and encouraged both the nation and the profession of social work to recognize and value diverse populations and cultural differences. For example, Norton (1978) used the term "the dual perspective" to emphasize that the worldview of persons of color and whites is different. During this period, the Council on Social Work Education (CSWE) developed accreditation standards of nondiscrimination in schools of social work in the United States and developed five ethnic minority task forces to address issues specifically pertinent to American Indians, Asian Americans, Chicanos, Puerto Ricans, and African Americans (Newsome, 2004).

By the mid-1970s, social work programs were required by the CSWE to address issues of difference, privilege, oppression, and discrimination at both the baccalaureate and graduate levels. In their attempts to focus on race, racism, and people of color, some schools began offering courses on institutional racism (Dumpson, 1970). Beginning in 1978, accredited schools of social work were required by CSWE to consider cultural diversity in admissions, faculty hiring, and curricula (McMahon & Allen-Meares, 1992).

From the mid-1970s to the mid-1980s, schools of social work also began to add gender and feminist practice theories to the curriculum, and CSWE established commissions on people of color and women (Spencer, Lewis, & Gutiérrez, 2000). From the mid-1980s to the mid-1990s, the concept of diversity was broadened again to include sexual orientation, and the CSWE Commission on Gay, Lesbian, Bisexual and Transgender (GLBT) Issues was established. Despite these proactive initiatives, a 1988 study of the impact of content on special populations in social work practice revealed a lack of clear understanding of the special needs of minority populations (Moore & Isherwood, 1988). Similarly, McMahon and Allen-Meares (1992) charged that the social work professional literature portrayed social work practice as focusing on individual interventions and "virtually ignores the societal context of the client" (p. 536).

In fact, CSWE (2008) expanded the definition and scope of diversity as curriculum content, listing 14 sources of oppression in CSWE's educational policy and the accreditation standards. These standards stipulated that social work education should prepare "social workers to practice without discrimination, with respect. And with knowledge and skills related to clients' age, class, color, culture, disability, ethnicity, family structure, gender, marital status, national origin, race, religion, sex, and sexual orientation" (p. 5). The trend to broaden the scope of multiculturalism in social work beyond ethnically sensitive practice is illustrated by the infusion of content on GLBT issues (Crisp, 2006; Sanders & Kroll, 2000), aging (Volland, & Berkman, 2004), disabilities (Gilson & DePoy, 2002), immigration (Chang-Muy & Congress, 2008), and social class (Shapiro, 2004) in the MSW curriculum. Some have called for the inclusion of religion and spirituality in education and practice as a diversity component and as part of a holistic spirituality assessment (Canda, Nakashima, & Furman 2004). Moreover, the expansion of many schools to focus on international social work practice has broadened the concept of multiculturalism to embrace aspects of globalization, immigration, and refugee issues (Healy, 2004). In fact, due to the growth of immigration in the United States, it is predicted that the U.S. foreign-born population will grow from 36 million in 2005 to 81 million in 2050 (Lum, 2011; Passel & Cohn, 2008).

Schiele (2007) expressed concern that expanding these definitions of diversity may serve to dilute the lesson of racism's persistence. According to Schiele, the "equality of oppressions" paradigm suggests that all groups are equally oppressed and may serve to even further minimize the content in social work education on people of color. Instead of increasing the number of oppressions, Schiele proposed a model of "differential vulnerability," which acknowledges that some groups are at greater risk than others.

There continues to be insufficient content on racism and people of color in the social work curriculum. Despite social work accreditation policies calling for the infusion of content related to minorities into the curriculum, Van Soest (1995) reported that the white European norm for social work practice is still dominant. Similarly, Lum (2004) conducted an extensive review of social work journals and found that only 9% of the articles addressed multicultural issues, and that people of color were largely absent in publications over a more than 30-year history. Clearly, incorporating multicultural perspectives and applying these concepts in various practice settings and with diverse populations continues to be a challenge.

Multicultural Training for Social Work Professionals

Building cultural competence is the primary goal for multicultural social work practice. Cultural competence is the integration and transformation of knowledge about individuals and groups of people into specific standards, policies, practices, and attitudes used in appropriate cultural settings to increase the quality of services (Lum, 2004; Weaver, 2005). This means learning new patterns of behavior and effectively applying them in appropriate settings and populations. The board of directors for the National Association of Social Workers (2001) approved 10 NASW Standards for Cultural Competence in Social Work Practice. These standards not only called for understanding and having knowledge of different cultures, but also for social workers to be aware of the impact of social policies and programs on diverse populations, and to advocate for clients when needed.

Almost all multicultural training to promote cultural competence begins by encouraging a social worker to become aware of one's own assumptions, values, and biases about human behaviors, which may facilitate or hinder one's ability to be an effective practitioner (Lum, Zuñiga, & Gutiérrez, 2004). Pinderhughes (1989) recommends that social workers be knowledgeable about culture, race, class, and ethnicity *and* their interrelationship with power or powerlessness. Through a process of developing cultural self-understandings, as well as an understanding of the client's cultural identity and perceptions of power, the practitioner is able to use this knowledge to enhance cross-cultural practice outcomes.

The next step is to understand the worldview of culturally different clients. Such understanding is followed by developing and applying appropriate intervention strategies with diverse client groups (Weaver, 2005). Martinez-Brawley and Brawley (1999) have extended the multiculturalism teaching debate even further and called for a contemporary "transcultural perspective" in which a social worker can have

"multi-consciousness" and cultural competence. In this state a social worker can be engaged with many cultural influences and enriched by the experience of interacting with other groups. These authors envision social workers going beyond cultural sensitivity and growing transculturally through interactions that provide an opportunity to gain in-depth knowledge about different cultures, disciplines, and cultural perspectives.

Another training approach, referred to as "critical multiculturalism," involves a profound exploration of oppression, differences, and prejudice (Schmitz et al., 2001). Such an examination of white privilege and understanding of internalized oppression often provokes resistance, fear, and denial. However, the educational process of critical self-awareness can lead to the destruction of stereotypes and improved understanding and appreciation of diversity.

Multicultural specialists have also adopted innovative strategies and training models via curriculum development and field education. Case examples that contain lived experiences and narratives of GLBT individuals demonstrate the need to incorporate the coming-out process within the study of the minority identity development (Schope, 2004). Other teachers have used experiential learning such as simulation exercises regarding aging and disability (Kane, 2003). Applying yet another training method, geriatric education rotational field placement models are used to teach students about diversity in the aging field (Netting, Hash, & Miller, 2002).

Ultimately, understanding organizational and institutional forces that enhance and negate cultural competence is critical in multicultural social work. It is based on the premise that an organization that values diversity is in a better position to provide culturally relevant services to its multicultural population. The Ackerman Institute for the Family created the Diversity and Social Work Training Program, in which Kaplan and Small (2005) identified elements critical to the program's success over 12 years. These include multicultural recruitment strategies, mentorships, partnerships with outside organizations, the provision of a long-term institutional commitment, biracial collaborations, and institutional change.

Recognizing the need to improve cultural competence in field education, Armour, Bain, and Rubio (2004) have called for field supervisors to stop "avoiding" racial issues. Their pilot study of diversity training for 11 field instructors illustrated successful adaptation of a transferable model of multicultural training, which seeks to increase comfort with diversity, attention to issues of power and control in field instructor–student relationships, and knowledge about oppressed groups. Their pretraining, posttraining, and six-month follow-up evaluation revealed significant decreases in field supervisors' avoidant behaviors with students over time.

Lee, Blythe, and Goforth (2009) explored an educational intervention to teach racism and social injustice while bringing a contemporary, global perspective by examining an educational case study of a multicultural human service agency in Mexico. Innovative teaching strategies using online discussion forums as a tool to help MSW students to talk about sensitive issues have been developed (Lee, Brown, & Bertera 2010).

Implications for Clinical Practice and Social Policy

The preceding literature review reveals two main streams of multicultural social work practice trends: (a) culture-specific interventions and (b) cross-cultural-universal approaches. In clinical social work, the standard used to diagnose normality and abnormality is derived from Anglo-American perspectives. As such, cross-cultural-universal approaches are culturally bound and may be inadequate in application to ethnically diverse groups. Multicultural specialists have called for culture-specific interventions that take into account issues of race, culture, gender, behavioral norms, and sexual orientation (Ewalt, Freeman, Fortune, Poole, & Witkin, 1999; Weaver, 2005).

A cross-cultural study by Wells, Klap, Koike, and Sherbourne (2001) demonstrates greater unmet needs for alcoholism and drug abuse treatment and mental health care among African Americans and Hispanics relative to whites. Similarly, such findings on racial disparities in mental health (Alegria Vallas & Pumariega, 2010) call for interventions targeted at specific cultural groups such as American Indians (Williams & Ellison, 1996), African Americans (McRoy, 2007), Latinos (Garcia & Zuñiga, 2007), and Asian Americans (Fong, 2007).

Disparities in outcomes for persons of color as compared to whites have led to more focused attention on the need for understanding how policies and practices differentially impact populations of color. For example, although there have been improvements in the overall health of Americans in the past several decades, compelling evidence demonstrates that members of racial and ethnic minority groups suffer increasing disparities in terms of incidence, prevalence, mortality, burden of diseases, and adverse health outcomes, when compared with white Americans (Williams & Mohammed, 2009).

Some populations, especially African Americans, are differentially impacted by poverty and racism, justifying greater attention to reducing their disparate outcomes (Schiele, 2007). Children of color are disproportionately represented among the population of children in the nation's foster care system, and African Americans are disproportionately represented in the child welfare, juvenile, and criminal justice systems (Green, Belanger, McRoy & Bullard, 2011; McRoy, 2004). Despite current affirmative action policies, racial minorities and students from lower socioeconomic statuses are underrepresented in higher educational systems (Moller, Stearns, Potochnick, & Southworth, 2011). The fact that such disparities continue to exist, despite the many successes of the Great Society and other programs, indicates that much work is still to be done in the area of social justice in American society. Lum (2011) suggests that culturally competent social work practice "should encompass the scope of human rights and social justice and economic justice" (p. 21). Unfortunately, the social work profession has yet to fulfill its social justice mission through more involvement in social activism on behalf of oppressed people (Davis & Bent-Goodley, 2004; Van Soest & Garcia, 2003).

Acknowledging the significance of multicultural practice, some practitioners continue to support universal, cross-cultural interventions. Particularly, macro practitioners argue that social programs need to be universally based and not targeted to specific populations and groups (Specht & Courtney, 1994). Dewees (2001) presents a postmodern approach to clinical practice that links the perspectives of cultural competence, diversity, and social constructionism and a generalist strengths-based orientation for work with families. Freeman and Couchonnal (2006) provide guidelines for using narrative approaches with culturally diverse clients in a range of practice settings in combination with task-centered, solution-focused family systems and crisis intervention models.

Multicultural practice has been applied to group work with GLBT clients (DeLois & Cohen, 2000) and cultural sensitivity training for transracial adoptive parents (Vonk, 2001). Also highlighted are intersections between cultural diversity and social problems such as family violence and substance abuse (Fong, McRoy, & Hendricks, 2006). Davis and Proctor (1989) have identified the significance of race, gender, and class in individual, family, and group treatment. Their use of empirical data and practice theories to examine the interrelationships between socioeconomic status and family problems, choice of treatment approach, group dynamics, and treatment outcomes provide social workers with much-needed concrete guidelines to consider when grappling with differences in the helping process of working with Muslim clients, GLBT individuals, older adults, and persons with disabilities (Lum, 2011).

With multiculturalism's focus on the interrelationships between race, class, gender, ethnicity, and age, the social work profession can produce the next generation of practitioners who are not only competent in working within communities of color but also cognizant of the differential impact of social policies on diverse client populations. The roles of advocate and translator of diverse client groups require a sophisticated understanding of diversity not only across groups but also within cultural groups. By the same token, social workers need to expand their knowledge and skill base to embrace and comprehend the impact of sexual orientation, religious background, immigration, and aging on human behavior and social problems.

Multicultural social work practice will enhance the effectiveness of social work intervention in all fields of practice on the individual and family intervention level. It also enhances social workers' ability to identify macro intervention strategies and to collaborate with policy makers on alleviating inequality, while reducing prejudice, poverty, oppression, and other forms of social injustice (Van Soest & Garcia, 2003). An understanding of multiculturalism leads social workers to examine how race and class may interact to perpetuate disproportional and disparate outcomes in all levels of practice. It will heighten their sensitivity to diversity both among and within different ethnic and racial groups and, therefore, result in more effective intervention outcomes. Training in "undoing racism" is beginning to be used by some agencies seeking to examine how unconscious or conscious racism can potentially differentially impact service delivery (People's Institute for Survival and Beyond, 2007). This awareness is just one aspect of the importance in multicultural practice.

Assessment

This examination of the evolution of social work's focus on multiculturalism reveals a pattern of shifting from assimilation perspectives in the early formative years of the profession to a focus on cultural pluralism and racism. Progressively, the profession endorsed an expansion of the multicultural concepts beyond racial groups to include gender issues, sexual orientation, social class, and abilities. Multiculturalism is closely related to important social work values such as self-determination, empowerment, advocacy, strengths

perspectives, and a client-centered approach. Social workers need to balance the importance of a client's cultural values in the process of assessment, intervention, and evaluation, advocating the use of universal and culture-specific strategies in the helping process. Continued racial disparities in health outcomes and access to care necessitate that social workers are sensitive to and aware of how group differences impact social problems at the individual and group level. Enhanced multicultural awareness moves members of the profession forward in intervention strategies at the individual, familial, group, and societal levels that take into account how culture, values, norms, and behaviors all interact in resolving social problems. Hence, multicultural social work continues to be an exciting and challenging field of practice in an ever-changing global age.

REFERENCES

Alegria, M., Vallas, M., & Pumariega, A. J. (2010). Racial and ethnic disparities in pediatric mental health. *Child and Adolescent Psychiatric Clinics of North America, 19*(4), 759–774.

Andersen, M. L., & Collins, P. H. (2013). *Race, class and gender: An anthology* (8th ed.). Belmont, CA: Wadsworth.

Armour, M. P., Bain, B., & Rubio, R. (2004). An evaluation study of diversity training for field instructors: A collaborative approach to enhancing cultural competence. *Journal of Social Work Education, 40*(1), 27–38.

Canda, E. R., Nakashima, M., & Furman, L. D. (2004). Ethical considerations about spirituality in social work: Insights from a national qualitative survey. *Families in Society, 85*(1), 27–35.

Chang-Muy, F., & Congress, E. P. (2008). *Social work with immigrants and refugees: Legal issues, clinical skills, and advocacy.* New York: Springer.

Council on Social Work Education. (2008). *Educational policy and accreditation standards.* Alexandria, VA: Author.

Council on Social Work Education/SAGE-SW. (2001). *Strengthening the impact of social work to improve the quality of life for older adults and their families: A blueprint for the new millennium.* New York: Author.

Crisp, C. (2006). The Gay Affirmative Practice Scale (GAP): A new measure for assessing cultural competence with gay and lesbian clients. *Social Work, 51*(2), 115–126.

Davis, K. E., & Bent-Goodley, T. B. (Eds.) (2004). *The color of social policy.* Alexandria, VA: Council on Social Work Education.

Davis, L. E., & Proctor, E. K. (1989). *Race, gender, and class: Guidelines for practice with individuals, families, and groups.* Englewood Cliffs, NJ: Prentice Hall.

DeLois, K., & Cohen, M. B. (2000). A queer idea: Using group work principles to strengthen learning in a sexual minorities seminar. *Social Work with Groups, 23*(3), 53–67.

Dewees, M. (2001). Building cultural competence for work with diverse families: Strategies from the privileged side.

Journal of Ethnic and Cultural Diversity in Social Work, 9(3–4), 33–51.

Dumpson, J. R. (1970). Special committee on minority groups. *Social Work Education Reporter,* 18, 30.

Ewalt, P. L., Freeman, E. M., Fortune, A. E., Poole, D. L., & Witkin, S. L. (1999). *Multicultural issues in social work: Practice and research.* Washington, DC: NASW Press.

Fong, R. (2005). The future of multicultural social work. *Advances in Social Work,* 6(1), 43–50.

Fong, R. (2007). Cultural competence with Asian Americans. In D. Lum (Ed.), *Culturally competent practice: A framework for understanding diverse groups and justice issues* (3rd ed., pp. 328–350). Belmont, CA: Thomson Brooks/Cole.

Fong, R., McRoy, R., & Hendricks, C. O. (2006). *Intersecting child welfare, substance abuse, and family violence: Culturally competent approaches.* Alexandria, VA: Council on Social Work Education.

Freeman, E. M., & Couchonnal, G. (2006). Narrative and culturally based approaches in practice with families. *Families in Society,* 87(2), 198–208.

Garcia, B., & Zuñiga, M. E. (2007). Cultural competence with Latino Americans. In D. Lum (Ed.), *Culturally competent practice: A framework for understanding diverse groups and justice issues* (3rd ed., pp. 299–327). Belmont, CA: Thomson Brooks/Cole.

Gilson, S. F., & DePoy, E. (2002). Theoretical approaches to disability content in social work education. *Journal of Social Work Education,* 38(1), 153–165.

Gould, K. H. (1996). The misconstruing of multiculturalism: The Stanford Debate and social work. In P. L. Ewalt, E. M. Freeman, S. Kirk, & D. L. Poole (Eds.), *Multicultural issues in social work* (pp. 29–42). Washington, DC: NASW Press.

Green, D., Belanger, K., McRoy, R., & Bullard, L. (2011). *Challenging racial disproportionality in child welfare: Research, policy, and practice.* Washington, DC: Child Welfare League of America.

Grieco, E. M., Acosta, Y. D., de la Cruz, G. P., Gambino, C., Gryn, T., Larsen, L. J., et al. (2012). *The Foreign-Born Population in the United States: 2010.* American Community Survey Reports, ACS-19, Washington, DC: U.S. Census Bureau.

Gutiérrez, L., Zuñiga, M., & Lum, D. (2004). *Education for multicultural social work practice: Critical viewpoints and future directions.* Alexandria, VA: Council on Social Work Education.

Healy, L. M. (2004). The international dimensions of multicultural social work. In L. Gutiérrez, M. Zuñiga, & D. Lum (Eds.), *Education for multicultural social work practice: Critical viewpoints and future directions* (pp. 307–318). Alexandria, VA: Council on Social Work Education.

Humes, K. R., Jones, N. A., & Ramirez, R. (2011). Overview of race and hispanic origin: 2010. *2010 Census Briefs,* C2010BR-02. Washington, DC: U.S. Census Bureau.

Kane, M. N. (2003). Teaching direct practice techniques for work with elders with Alzheimer's disease: A simulated group experience. *Educational Gerontology,* 29(9), 777–779.

Kaplan, L., & Small, S. (2005). Multiracial recruitment in the field of family therapy: An innovative training program for people of color. *Family Process,* 44(3), 249–265.

Lee, E. O., Blythe, B., & Goforth, K. (2009). Can you call it racism?: An educational case study and role-play approach. *Journal of Social Work Education,* 45(1), 123–130.

Lee, E. O., Brown, M., & Bertera, E. (2010). The use of an online diversity forum to facilitate social work students' dialogue on sensitive issues: A quasi-experimental design. *Journal of Teaching in Social Work,* 30(3), 272–285.

Liao, Y., Tucker, P., Okoro, C. A., Giles, W. H., Mokdad, A. H., & Harris, V. B. (2004). REACH 2010 surveillance for health status in minority communities—United States, 2001–2002. *Morbidity and Mortality Weekly Report,* 52(SS06), 1–36. Available at http://www.cdc.gov/MMWR/preview/mmwrhtml/ss5306a1.htm

Logan, S. (2003). Issues of multiculturalism: Multicultural practice, cultural diversity and competency. In R. Edwards (Ed.), *Encyclopedia of social work* (19th ed., 2003 Supplement, pp. 95–105). Washington, DC: NASW Press.

Lum, D. (2004). *Social work practice and people of color: A process-stage approach* (5th ed.). Belmont, CA: Brooks/Cole–Thomson Learning.

Lum, D. (2011). *Culturally competent practice: A framework for understanding diverse groups and justice issues* (4th ed.). Belmont, CA: Brooks/Cole.

Lum, D., Zuñiga, M., & Gutiérrez, L. (2004). Multicultural social work education: Themes and recommendations. In L. Gutiérrez, M. Zuñiga, & D. Lum (Eds.), *Education for multicultural social work practice: Critical viewpoints and future directions* (pp. 319–325). Alexandria, VA: Council on Social Work Education.

Martinez-Brawley, E. E., & Brawley, E. A. (1999). Diversity in a changing world: Cultural enrichment or social fragmentation? *Journal of Multicultural Social Work,* 7 (1–2), 19–35.

McMahon, A., & Allen-Meares, P. (1992). Is social work racist? A content analysis of recent literature. *Social Work,* 37(6), 533–539.

McRoy, R. (2004). The color of child welfare. In K. E. Davis & T. B. Bent-Goodley (Eds.), *The color of social policy* (pp. 36–63). Alexandria, VA: Council on Social Work Education.

McRoy, R. (2007). Cultural competence with African Americans. In D. Lum (Ed.), *Culturally competent practice: A framework for understanding diverse groups and justice issues* (3rd ed., pp. 276–298). Belmont, CA: Thomson Brooks/Cole.

Moller, S., Stearns, E., Potochnick, S. R., & Southworth, S. (2011). Student achievement and college selectivity: How changes in achievement during high school affect the selectivity of college attended. *Youth and Society,* 43(2), 656–680.

Moore, V. L., & Isherwood, J. T. (1988, March). Utilizing professional knowledge and values: Practice dilemmas for workers with oppressed populations. Paper presented at the Council on Social Work Education's Annual Program Meeting in Atlanta, Georgia.

National Association of Social Workers. (2001). NASW standards for cultural competence in social work practice. Washington, DC: Author. Available at http://www.naswdc.org/practice/standards/NAswculturalstandards.pdf

Netting, F. E., Hash, K., & Miller, J. (2002). Challenges in developing geriatric field education in social work. *Journal of Gerontological Social Work, 37*(1), 89–110.

Newsome, M., Jr. (2004). Analysis of past and present movements in cultural competence theory and practice knowledge in social work education. In L. Gutiérrez, M. Zuñiga, & D. Lum (Eds.), *Education for multicultural social work practice: Critical viewpoints and future directions* (pp. 3–18). Alexandria, VA: Council on Social Work Education.

Norton, D. (1978). *The dual perspective: Inclusion of ethnic minority content in the social work curriculum.* New York: Council on Social Work Education.

Passel, J. S., & Cohn, D. (2008). *U.S. population projections: 2005–2050.* Washington, DC: Pew Research Center.

People's Institute for Survival and Beyond. (2007). Undoing racism. Retrieved April 13, 2013, from http://www.pisab.org/our-principles

Pinderhughes, E. (1989). *Understanding race, ethnicity and power: The key to efficacy in clinical practice.* New York: Free Press.

Popple, P. (1995). Social work profession: History. In R. Edwards (Ed.), *Encyclopedia of social work* (19th ed., pp. 2282–2291). Washington, DC: NASW Press.

Sanders, G. L., & Kroll, I. T. (2000). Generating stories of resilience: Helping gay and lesbian youth and their families. *Journal of Marital and Family Therapy, 26*(4), 433–442.

Schiele, J. H. (2007). Implications of the equality-of-oppressions paradigm for curriculum content on people of color. *Journal of Social Work Education, 43*(1), 83–100.

Schope, R. D. (2004). Practitioners need to ask: Culturally competent practice requires knowing where the gay male client is in the coming out process. *Smith College Studies in Social Work, Special Issue: Pedagogy and Diversity, 74*(2), 257–270.

Schmitz, C. L., Stakeman, C., & Sisneros, J. (2001). Educating professionals for practice in a multicultural society: Understanding oppression and valuing diversity. *Families in Society, 82*(6), 612–622.

Shapiro, T. M. (2004). *The hidden cost of being African American: How wealth perpetrates inequality.* New York: Oxford University Press.

Specht, H., & Courtney, M. E. (1994). *Unfaithful angels: How social work has abandoned its mission.* New York: Free Press.

Spencer, M., Lewis, E., & Gutiérrez, L. (2000). Multicultural perspectives on direct practice in social work. In P. Allen-Meares & C. Garvin (Eds.), *The handbook of social work direct practice* (pp. 131–149). Thousand Oaks, CA: Sage Publications.

Sue, D. W. (2006). *Multicultural social work practice.* Hoboken, NJ: Wiley.

Van Soest, D. (1995). Multiculturalism and social work education: The non-debate about competing perspectives. *Journal of Social Work Education, 31*(1), 55–65.

Van Soest, D., & Garcia, B. (2003). *Diversity education for social justice: Mastering teaching skills.* Alexandria, VA: Council on Social Work Education.

Volland, P. J., & Berkman, B. (2004). Educating social workers to meet the challenge of an aging urban population: A promising model. *Academic Medicine, 79*(12), 1192–1197.

Vonk, M. E. (2001). Cultural competence for transracial adoptive parents. *Social Work, 46*(3), 246–255.

Weaver, H. N. (2005). *Explorations in cultural competence: Journeys to four directions.* Belmont, CA: Thomson Brooks/Cole.

Wells, K., Klap, R., Koike, A., & Sherbourne, C. (2001). Ethnic disparities in unmet need for alcoholism, drug abuse, and mental health care. *American Journal of Psychiatry, 158*(12), 2027–2032.

Williams, D. R., & Mohammed, S. A. (2009). Discrimination and racial disparities in health: Evidence and needed research. *Journal of Behavioral Medicine, 32*(1), 20–47.

Williams, E. E., & Ellison, F. (1996). Culturally informed social work practice with American Indian clients: Guideline for non-Indian social workers. *Social Work, 41*(2), 147–151.

FURTHER READING

Council on Social Work Education. (2008). *Educational Policy and Accreditation Standards.* Alexandria, VA: Author.

EUN-KYOUNG OTHELIA LEE AND RUTH MCROY

MULTIETHNIC AND MULTIRACIALISM

ABSTRACT: Although the year 2000 marked the first time U.S. citizens were allowed to report more than one race in the Census, multiraciality and multiethnicity are certainly not new in the United States or globally. The history of multiracial America is inextricably linked to its history of immigration, slavery, racism, and the very construction of single-race identities as master statuses during colonialism. Who is multiracial, as well as the idea that such an identity or population can or should exist, is highly complex and has shifted along with societal attitudes and laws governing race identity options and the sanctioning of multiracial families through marriage and adoption. The understanding in the early 21st century of this growing multiracial population is mired in this history, but also idealized as proof of a new and possibly "postrace" America. To examine multiraciality, this article begins by defining root concepts including race, ethnicity, nationality, and culture to then examine and define multiraciality. This article will include a brief historical discussion of multiraciality in the United States and will also explore demographic and health trends using such statistics as are available and examine identified risks, disparities, strengths, and resiliencies among this diverse population. Effective and ethical social-work practices with multiracial persons require expansion beyond the black–white dichotomy and monocentric paradigm of race to consider both strengths and vulnerabilities navigated by the increasing number of persons and families who identify as multiracial and multiethnic. Approaches to social work that promote multiracially attuned practices and engagement of the diverse resources for various communities of multiracial persons and families conclude this article.

KEY WORDS: cultural competence; culturally responsive/attuned; cultural identity; ethnicity; multiethnic; multiethnicity; multiracial; multiraciality; monoracialism; microaggression; race; racial identity; transracial adoption

Introduction

Mapping the history of multiracial America is complicated and constrained by several factors. First, no consistently formatted statistical record allowing all persons to check more than one race is available before the year 2000. Second, in both Census 2000 and Census 2010, statistics represent only self-reports about identity. Consequently, Census statistics indicate the number of persons who voluntarily identify as multiracial, but cannot be thought to represent the total number of persons who actually do have more than one racial–ethnic heritage. Despite long histories of race and ethnic mixing in the United States, most persons still only report a single-race identity on the U.S. Census form (U.S. Census, 2010). Finally, race identities are only more complicated by genetic research that traces present-day human beings back to a common biological, and thus genetic, history (Olsen, 2003) originating in Southwestern Africa (Wells, 2003). Genetic arguments of "we are all the same" have been critiqued (see, for example, Jorde, 2002) as based on improbable assumptions (for example, continuous random mating, constancy in population size, and open and malleable geographies). Still, understanding what is meant in claiming or reporting any racial or ethnic "identity" is often an inconsistent amalgamation of known or assumed heritages and personal choice in the context of contemporary social conventions, norms, and laws.

Discussing multiraciality requires a definition of race, ethnicity, culture, and nationality, terms that are often misused as synonyms. This section will briefly define these terms. Later sections will draw attention to how multiraciality highlights the problematic but pervasive assumption in society, research, and practice that these identity constructs are dependent on one another. I will also illuminate the ongoing tensions between genetic and biological understandings of racial and ethnic heritage and more self-chosen or socially imposed race and ethnic identities irrespective of heritage.

Race

Race is a socially and legally constructed concept that derives from the classification system used for plants and animals. It is important to note that the origins of human beings have been traced to a single region of Africa, suggesting that we are all descendants of a single racial–ethnic group of people (Wells, 2003). Despite that probability, our contemporary systems of meaning, manufactured and institutionalized across several centuries, have solidified a contemporary understanding of racial classifications as natural labels for identifying human (and genetic) differences. Across several iterations of race labels, colors were often used as early referents of race groups: black, brown, yellow, white, red. The common understanding of race in the United States is biological and is used as a method for identifying and explaining human differences (that is, abilities, traits, characteristics) through attaching a race category to a cluster of phenotypes (for example, skin tone, hair texture, body shape, facial features). This classification system is not a neutral system of meaning, however; it derived from America's history of colonialism, white supremacy, and slavery in an attempt to restrict legal, social, and economic privileges and rights of personhood solely to white Americans (Roediger, 2008). However, because race is a socially, not genetically, constructed concept, it is not a scientifically reliable way of distinguishing the genetic differences and traits that do exist between human beings (Brown & Armelagos, 2001; Zack, 1993). This is particularly true in societies like the United States that have evolved from myriad ethnic immigrants and indigenous populations living in close proximity. Yet in the United States, despite its history of racial mixing, because of the stigmas and privileges attached to membership in a specific race group, race remains a powerful influence on social hierarchies, personal identity development, and life outcomes. Legal and social privileges (such as housing, marriage, employment, education, freedom, and legal protection) have been restricted based on racial group membership. Consequently, disparities tied to racial group membership persist in the United States, including for multiracial Americans, in physical, social–emotional, and economic well-being across the life course (U.S. Department of Health and Human Services, 2010). Because of this history and the myriad flawed as well as racist assumptions attached to the social meaning and significance of race, race will not be considered in this paper as a proper noun to deliberately call the readers' attention to these issues. Race labels will not be capitalized in this article.

Ethnicity

Ethnicity is a social identity that is often assumed to correspond to a racial group, but to expand beyond more than the group's assumed external characteristics of physical appearance. It is a learned identity that is transmitted through one's family and social networks and is typically thought of as including cultural markers of language, food, values, religion, dress, and customs. Because of the constraints of race as a social construct, some social scientists use ethnicity as a more inclusive and less problematic label. Although all persons have ethnic heritages, not all persons identify with their ethnic heritage. The term "ethnic" is sometimes used only to identify racial minorities, erroneously constructing European heritage as a nonraced and nonethnic identity (Frankenberg, 1995) or as an "optional" identity for persons of European descent (Waters, 1990). Ethnic labels are capitalized in this article.

Culture

"Culture" refers to socially and relationally transmitted patterns of behavior and belief including language, food, values, religion, dress, customs, humor, aesthetic preference (art, what indicates beauty), and music. Culture also informs our understandings of class, gender, sexuality, and other social identities. Cultural identities are learned through one's family, peers, and community memberships. Given increasing multiculturalism in the United States, it is possible for persons to identify with cultural traditions that do not represent their own heritage, but that of the communities in which they live.

Nationality

"Nationality" refers to the nation or country in which a person holds citizenship (for example, American, Brazilian, and South African). It can also be used to represent a person's country of origin, but a place where she or he no longer lives. Nationality does not automatically indicate a specific race or ethnic heritage, particularly in multiracial and multiethnic coun-

tries like the United States. Therefore, a group of people can share a national identity as American, but not share an ethnic or racial identity or heritage.

Multiracial

The term "multiracial" has grown in popularity over other terms such as "biracial" as a more inclusive way of labeling persons who identify with more than one race category. Yet, given the concerns stated previously, some argue this term only reinforces and legitimizes the highly problematic elements of race rather than dismantling an inherently flawed system of meaning from our social consciousness (Spencer, 1997). After substantial debate and controversy, the U.S. Census 2000 chose a *check all that apply* approach, rather than use a pan-racial term *multiracial*, as an opportunity to obtain maximally accurate data on the demographic diversity among persons claiming more than one race. Census race reporting now allows for 57 racial combinations among the categories: Hispanic/Latino, black/African American, American Indian/Alaskan Native, Asian, Pacific Islander/Native Hawaiian, white, and other. This also permits statistical analyses of distinct groups of multiracial individuals and understanding of social shifts in self-identification as well as growth in birth rates. Again, such statistics must be understood as underestimates of the actual number of persons in the United States whose heritages include ancestors from more than one racial category. For example, it has been estimated that 75% to 90% of the African American/black population in the early 21st century also has white heritage (Davis, 1991; Winters & DeBose, 2003). Despite this history and contemporary growth in the number of persons who do claim multiracial identities, most persons in the United States do not claim more than one race identity on Census surveys. Some of the reasons for this will be discussed in later sections. According to the 2010 Census, the population reporting multiracial identities grew to 9 million people from 6.8 million reports in the 2000 Census (Jones & Bullock, 2013). Persons who identify multiracially may not have matching multicultural or multiethnic identifications. For example, someone of Japanese Mexican heritage who grew up in a predominantly white-populated town may identify as multiracial, but may not identify culturally or ethnically with being Japanese or Mexican.

Multiethnic

The term "multiethnic" refers to persons who identify with more than one ethnicity. Persons who are multiethnic may not identify as multiracial. For example, a person who identifies monoracially as white may identify multiethnically because her ethnic heritage includes Italian, Irish, and Norwegian. Similarly, someone whose father identifies as Puerto Rican and his mother as Mexican may not identify as multiracial, but rather as a Latino with multiethnic heritage. Because of the high rates of interethnic marriage within socially constructed pan-racial groups in the United States, most Americans could claim multiethnic identities (Waters, 1990; Zack, 1993).

SOCIAL AND LEGAL HISTORY OF MULTIRACIALITY AND MULTIETHNICITY IN THE UNITED STATES

Our nation's methods for categorizing race and ethnicity have reflected enduring obsessions and ambiguities around human "difference" and represent the use of law to institutionalize a social hierarchy into which persons are sorted according to race. This history has been characterized as a formal practice to "legalize racism" by erecting a system embedded in biological notions of genetic superiority of one race group (whites) over the genetic inferiority of all others (Haney López, 1996; Menchaca, 2008; Zack, 1993).

The U.S. Census has made many previous attempts to count the multiracial, multiethnic, and multinational heritages of its citizens. For example, identifying fractions of blackness through categories including "mulatto" and "quadroon" existed until the 1930s Census. After this time, choices then changed to white, Negro, Indian, and five Asian ethnic options (Hochschild & Powell, 2008). Ethnic groups that were allowed to select the racial category "white" have also changed drastically over time (Haney López, 1996). These facts illustrate that our national understanding of racial and ethnic diversity in the United States is in part linked to choices allowed by the U.S. government and the Census in which options they provide to citizens. But Census options also reflect the legal and social constructions of race embedded in a history of colonialism, slavery, and white supremacy. The nation's understanding of multiraciality is inextricably tied to this history. Below, several such historical markers significant to multiracial Americans are noted.

The Laws of Hypodescent and the "One-Drop Rule"

The first black–white multiracial individuals in the United States predated slavery and were the offspring of indentured European and African servants and farmers. Both socially occupied a class and social status of poor but free Americans, and their mixed-race children shared this status (Davis, 1991). However,

as the African slave trade took hold in the South, the numbers of black–white children were rapidly increasing. Yet this population increase was now primarily a result of the practice of rape by white slave-owners against their female slaves. In an effort to contain the slave population in the face of an ever-growing black–white multiracial population, laws were enacted to include black–white multiracial persons of any black heritage to the category black and, thus, to the social status "slave" (Zack, 1993). Simply stated, this one-drop rule indicated that a person with black heritage to any degree (that is, one drop of black blood) must identify solely as black. The one-drop rule not only provided legal clarity on designating multiracial individuals with white heritage as slaves, but also defined and thus protected whiteness and its privileges as restricted to those with racially "pure" white heritages. Thus whiteness was linked to purity and superiority, and membership within any other race group was linked to impurity and inferiority (Samuels, 2006). The one-drop rule is considered the strictest system of laws and methods for categorizing people in the world and was stricter than methods used by the Third Reich for identifying Jews (Zack).

Although laws of hypodescent do not formally exist in the early 21st century, the one-drop rule continues to inform social constructions of acceptable identity options for all persons of mixed race, but particularly for those of black heritage (Lee & Bean, 2010). Because the one-drop rule has been deeply internalized in U.S. culture, even persons who are of mixed race may still follow these norms and self-identify monoracially with their non-white heritage. The one-drop rule and its role in contributing to distinct stereotypes, forms of prejudice, and discrimination toward multiracial persons and families will be discussed further in the section on contemporary contexts for this population's identity and development.

Antimiscegenation Laws

Sexual segregation laws prohibiting interracial coupling, cohabitation, and marriage were common not only to the United States, but also in countries including Germany and South Africa. Although interracial coupling was not illegal in early colonial America, it was severely stigmatized and considered taboo. The persons involved received public whippings, and by the early 1700s interracial relationships were labeled as bestiality (Davis, 1991; Williamson, 1980). Analyses of 19th- and 20th-century legal rulings against interracial marriage indicate protecting the racial purity of whites as the leading justification to uphold antimiscegenation laws (Haney López, 1996). Conventional thought and even scientific theories of the time posited interracial coupling was unnatural and that disease, genetic frailty, infertility, and severe psychological maladies befell the offspring of such unions (Park, 1931). The original label used during slavery for black–white multiracial persons, "mulatto"—the root word referencing the mule, a sterile mixed-breed animal)—reflects these folk theories of race and multiraciality (Samuels, 2006).

In the 1660s, the states of Maryland and Virginia were the first to outlaw relationships between whites, blacks, and "Malays" (that is, persons of Asian descent) (Martyn, 1979). Between 1861 and 1890, Nevada, followed by five other Western states, passed laws specifically prohibiting intermarriage between Asians and whites (Sohoni, 2007). This was in direct response to the growing population in the West of male Chinese laborers, but these laws often also included (or were amended to include) growing numbers of Japanese, Asian Indian, Hindu, Filipino, and Korean immigrants (Martyn). Also governed were marriages for multiracial and multiethnic persons. States varied significantly in how multiraciality was interpreted within a single pan-racial/ethnic group. For example, in some Southwest states, light-skinned multiracial Mexicans who throughout various times in history have been allowed to racially classify as white (Haney López, 1996) were prohibited from marrying darker-skinned multiracial and multiethnic Mexicans racially classified as black, Indigenous/Indian, or Mestizo (Menchaca, 2008). Attitudes toward interracial marriage began to change, however, after World War II.

In 1948, Andrea Perez, a Mexican American woman, and Sylvester Davis, an African American man, sued the Los Angeles County Clerk (W. G. Sharp) after being denied a marriage certificate years earlier. After winning their case in the California Supreme Court, California became the first state to overturn its antimiscegenation laws by finding that such laws violate the constitution's 14th Amendment (*Perez vs. Sharp*, October 1, 1948). It took nearly 20 years for the U.S. Supreme Court to follow suit.

Loving v. Virginia and the Legalization of Interracial Marriage

Ironically, the U.S. Supreme Court case that ultimately found antimiscegenation laws unconstitutional in 1967 is named after an interracial couple whose last name is Loving. Mildred Jeter, a black woman, and Richard Loving, a white man, married in the District of Columbia in 1958 and then returned to their home state of Virginia. However, 8 years earlier, in 1959, the Lovings pled "guilty" to a grand jury indictment for interracial marriage in a Carolina County Court in Virginia. After suspending the sentence for 25 years on condition that they left the state of Virginia, the trial judge shared his biblical interpretation and personal opinion against interracial marriage: "Almighty God created the races white, black, yellow, malay and red, and he placed them on separate continents. And but for the interference with his arrangement there would be no cause for such marriages. The fact that he separated the races shows that he did not intend for the races to mix" (*Loving v. Virginia*, 388 U.S. 1, 1967, 395). Clearly this judge's understanding of the origins of human beings is in contrast with 21st-century genetic science regarding "the races" as not God-driven, but human fabrications that mask our shared origins and placement on a single contentment, not separate ones (Olsen, 2003; Wells, 2003).

Although antimiscegenation laws existed throughout the United States, with the exception of only seven Northern states, this Supreme Court decision made marriage discrimination based on race a violation of citizens' 14th-Amendment rights (*Loving v. Virginia*, 388 U.S. 1, 1967). Although this decision made antimiscegenation laws unconstitutional, this did not end the taboo and social stigma attached to interracial sex, partnering, or marriage. As recently as 2009, Keith Bardwell, a white justice of the peace in southeastern Louisiana, refused to marry Beth Humphrey, racially identified as white, and Terence McKay, racially identified as black. When interviewed by the Associated Press shortly after the news went public, Judge Bardwell explained, "I'm not a racist. I just don't believe in mixing the races that way" (Associated Press, 2009). Using the familiar concern about problems with mixed-race children, he justified his refusal by stating he did not want to take part in creating a situation that would cause their children pain and rejection from whites and blacks. Although this example may appear extreme, continued stereotypes that normalize social and emotional problems for multiracial families and their children, coupled with continued social patterns of racial and ethnic segregation, contribute to the reality that the vast majority of marriages, intimate partnering, and creations of family continue to be racially homogenous.

According to U.S. Census 2010, only 10% of heterosexual marriages are between persons who identify as different races (Lofquist, Lugaila, O'Connell, & Feliz, 2012). This number is only slightly higher among nonmarried couples, with 18% of unmarried opposite-sex couples and 21% of same-sex couples reporting as interracial (Lofquist et al.).

Census 2000 and the Multiracial Movement

What is now widely referred to as the "multiracial movement" initially represented a dispersed and loosely organized collection of white parents and, to a lesser extent, multiracial persons, primarily from the West Coast and Midwest in the early 1970s (Dalmage, 2000). Increasingly, these groups engaged in civil rights discourse to advocate inclusion for persons whose racial experience was ignored or pathologized by the dominant use of single-race categories. Kicking off the decade with the first edited volume on multiraciality by Maria P. P. Root (1992), later followed by a second (Root, 1996), and an explosion of multiracial births, the 1990s was quickly becoming known as the "biracial baby boom." As attention grew to what was becoming framed as a "new" U.S. population of multiracial persons, so too did the opposition to ideas of multiraciality as a legitimate population or identity (Dalmage, 2004; Spencer, 1997).

What is novel about Census 2000 is not that it records the presence of multiracial Americans. In fact, up until the 1930s racially mixed blacks were sometimes given the option to self-report in fractions of blackness (e.g., mulatto, quadroon). Other multiracial populations with black, Native American, and white heritage were recorded under their family names (for example, the Jackson Whites), which marked their distinct and known multiracial lineages (Samuels, 2006). Census 2000 is novel because it recognizes that persons can associate with more than one race label or category, including white, as opposed to having their own pan-racial/ethnic category (for example, multiracial, quadroon). It is also significant in that it makes data available to extend the conversation about mixed-race identity beyond the black–white paradigm, including populations of multiracial and multiethnic persons who do not have white heritage and desire public and official acknowledgment of their multiracial and multiethnic heritage.

Such proposed changes to the official enumeration of race and ethnicity to allow for more than one choice incited substantial controversy, some of which was expressed during the 1993 hearings by the U.S. House Subcommittee on Census Statistics. These hearings were preceded by several efforts among multiracial activist groups across the United States, but namely the Association for Multiethnic Americans. The association was founded in 1988 in California by a collection of smaller multiracial activists and groups across the West Coast (such as iPride) as well

as a large network in Chicago, the Biracial Family Network. The first president of the association, Carlos Fernandez, was a representative of iPride, and the vice present, Ramona Douglass, was from Biracial Family Network. Those arguing for a multiracial option on Census 2000 cited the need for recognition outside of the option "other," asserted the Bill of Rights from Root's first volume on multiraciality (1996), and called for identity options that do not "keep the races separate within me" (Root, 1996, p. 7).

Arguments against multiracial options or selecting more than one race were viewed as *statistical passing*, expressing fears that persons who earlier would never be considered white now had an option to select that race identity. Pan-racial organizations including the National Association for the Advancement of Colored People, the Urban League, and LaRaza voiced these concerns but also mistrust for how such data would be used to deplete the numbers of racial–ethnic minorities and, thus, undercut hard-won civil rights programs erected to alleviate racial disparities caused by institutionalized race discrimination (Fernández, 1996). The fact that conservative anti–affirmative action politicians including Newt Gingrich came out in support of a multiracial option only served as strong confirming evidence for these fears. There were also strong reactions against the idea of multiracial individuals as a legitimate population and identity. Books were written during this time that labeled mixed-race and multiracial persons who expressed multiracial identities as "race traitors" who were solely motivated by their desires to access white racial privileges and abandon stigmatized race identities and racial minority status and, by default, abandon the persons and communities attached to these identities. This position is clearly stated by the multiracial critic Jon Spencer, who asserted that although "some multiracialists begin down the road of racial bigotry by cock-a-doodling about their alleged specialness... they subtly assault the identity and self-esteem of Black Americans" (1997, p. 128). Over 15 years later, these contentious debates about the identities of multiracial people continue, particularly targeting the identities of black multiracial persons (Lee & Bean, 2010; Samuels, 2006). In fact, scholars have now labeled these dynamics as "monoracism," referring to the distinct racism and microaggressions faced by persons of mixed race (Johnston & Nadal, 2010). Dimensions of monoracism and multiracial microaggressions will be examined further in the sections that explore enduring elements of the normative developmental context navigated among contemporary multiracial populations.

Multiraciality and Adoption

Most children are adopted by parents who share their racial identity. Only 17% of adopted children under the age of 18 are reported as living with parents of a different race (Census, 2010). However, there is some indication that multiracial children may experience higher rates of placement with white parents both in the United States and globally (Miranda, 2004). The first wave of transracial placements of black children with white parents almost exclusively involved black–white multiracial children (Davis, 1991). Early research on transracial adoption reflects this reality, with this subpopulation of children dominating the "transracial adoptee" sample populations: 82% of Grow and Shapiro's (1974) sample, 73% of McRoy and Zurcher's (1983) transracial adoptee sample, 68% of Simon's (1996) sample, and 78% of the adoptee respondents in Vroegh's (1997) study. Even more recent transracial adoption scholarship indicates their sample populations are over 70% black–white biracial adoptees (see Patton, 2000; Simon & Roorda, 2000). Multiracial children have also been a dominant population in early waves of international adoptions. For example, mixed-race Korean children represented the largest wave of international adoptees from Korea who were offspring of Korean mothers and U.S. military men (Fruendlich & Leiberthal, 2000). Few scholars have directly addressed the issue of multiraciality in the study of adoption and identity outcomes (see, for exceptions, Samuels, 2009, 2010; Sweeney, 2013).

We face many challenges in accessing and collecting reliable data on multiraciality in the context of child welfare, foster care, and adoption. First, similar to U.S. Census data, reports on multiracial heritage are dependent upon self-reports. Such reports are limited to voluntary disclosures of biological parents' race (information that may be unobtainable when paternity is unknown) or to the disclosures of agency professionals who might or might not ask about a child's racial heritage or might assume a racial heritage and identity based on the child's physical appearance. It is also complicated by the fact that many adoptions occur outside of agencies and institutions and, thus, are not part of any federal administrative reporting systems. Our understanding of contemporary adoption and multiraciality is limited by these realities. However, Census 2010 data now collect far more complex household information on adopted children and race, and it also includes "more than one race" reporting options. This provides a first-time look at the under-18 adoptee population in ways that are not limited to agency reports of administrative

data, but remain underreport. In analyzing these data, further evidence emerges that multiracial children, particularly those with white heritage, may have distinct adoption outcomes. In an analysis conducted by Kreider and Raleigh (2011), the number of multiracial children under 18 living with white adoptive parents (19%) outnumbered black children (16%) with white adoptive parents. Although it is more difficult to discern unreported multiraciality, there were also notable findings for the racial reporting of identities for Latino transracial adoptees. Latino children (who, like anyone of Latino heritage, can record both ethnicity and race) comprise the second largest group of transracial adoptees in the United States (29%); Asian adoptees comprise the largest group, at 34%. Over half of Latino transracial adoptees were reported by their white adoptive parents as ethnically Latino, but racially as white, and fewer than 1% indicated the child's ethnicity as Latino but race as black. Research on multiraciality in adoption suggests that because adopters have a choice in the children they adopt, children with multiracial white heritage (or those who appear to have this heritage) may have higher rates of placement with white adopters (McRoy & Grape, 1999; Miranda, 2004). U.S. Census statistics are beginning to provide support for this, as well as insight for understanding how white heritage or light skin may contribute to the race disparities in placement outcomes that have existed within the child welfare system for decades (Davis, 1991; Smith, McRoy, Freundlich, & Kroll, 2008). Issues related to adoptive families and multiracial adoptees' development and outcomes will be discussed further in the sections on identity development and implications for social-work practice.

The Multiracial Population in the Early 21st Century

Between Census 2000 and Census 2010 the number of citizens claiming multiracial identities increased by 2.2 million (Jones & Bullock, 2013). These statistics indicate a larger percentage of growth among individuals claiming multiracial identities (32%) than among those claiming single-race identities (9%). Even with this growth, 97% of people in the United States continue to report only single-race identities, again highlighting the independence between one's biological heritage and one's self-chosen (or socially imposed) identity.

Within the population claiming two or more races, several shifts are emerging, most notably among multiracial persons with white heritage. The number of people claiming black–white identities grew by 134%

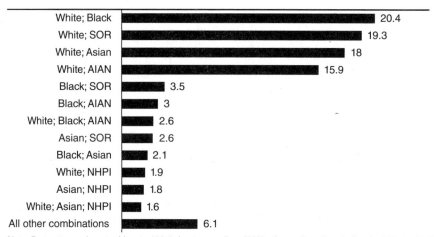

Note: Percentages do not add up to 100.0 due to rounding. AIAN refers to American Indian and Alaska Native; Black refers to Black or African American; NHPI refers to Native Hawaiian and Other Pacific Islander; and SOR refers to Some Other Race.

FIGURE 1 Two or More Races Population by Largest Combinations, 2010.
Source: Jones & Bullock, 2012, *2010 Two or More Race Population*, U.S Census Bureau, http://www.census.gov/prod/cen2010/briefs/c2010br-13.pdf

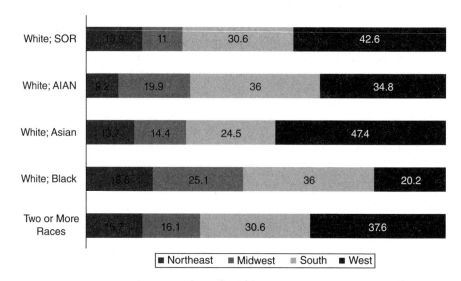

Note: Percentages may not add up to 100.0 due to rounding. AIAN refers to American Indian and Alaska Native; Black refers to Black and African American, and SOR refers to Some Other Race.

FIGURE 2 Regional Distribution of Multiracial Populations with Population Sizes of 1 Million or More.
Source: Jones & Bullock, 2012, *2010 Two or More Race Population*, U.S. Census Bureau, http://www.census.gov/prod/cen2010/briefs/c2010br-13.pdf

since the 2000 Census, making this racial combination the largest group of persons to identify multiracially (see Figure 1). This was followed by white–Asian multiracial persons (87% growth in reporting) and white–American Indian/Alaska Natives (an increase of 32%) (Jones & Bullock, 2013).

Those individuals claiming multiracial identities are not evenly dispersed across the United States. Not surprisingly, types of multiraciality reflect general patterns of racial and ethnic diversity across the United States (see Figure 2), with most persons who claim multiracial identities living in the West (37%).

Normative Context of Development for Multiracial and Multiethnic Persons and Families

As the literature on multiraciality and multiethnicity has developed, scholars have articulated distinct and shared experiences of racism, discrimination, and prejudice among this population and other racial–ethnic minority groups (Rockquemore & Brunsma, 2002). Like other groups of color in the United States, multiracial people can and do experience racism and discrimination, despite assumptions that indicate particularly those with white heritage may experience less racism (Nadal et al., 2010; Samuels, 2009). Earlier sections outlined historical discrimination specific to the formation of interracial marriages, multiracial families, and the creation of multiracial children. Multiracial persons in the early 21st century also report experiencing a distinct discrimination attached to their mixed-race heritage. This prejudice can come from family members who are not of mixed race or from nonmultiracial persons within their communities and close personal networks (Nadal et al., 2013; Rockquemore & Laszloffy, 2005; Root, 1998; Samuels, 2009).

In an attempt to distinguish racial biases against multiraciality, Johnston and Nadal (2010) developed a taxonomy to articulate dimensions of what they term *monoracism* and *multiracial microaggressions* (for a definition and more in-depth discussion of microaggressions, see Sue, 2010). Microaggressions are small but emotionally and psychologically toxic and taxing interactions that are often subtle and outside of others' awareness and thus hard to prove. Sometimes even the perpetrators may be unaware that they are microaggressing (for example, thinking one is complimenting her black–white biracial friend by telling her, "I don't even think of you as black!"). Drawing the offender's attention to his or her microaggressive behavior may pose more negative consequences for the victim, rather than offer a path to an apology or interpersonal resolution. Microaggressions are normative to the developmental and daily contexts of any person or family who exists outside of dominant mainstream norms (for example, persons who are racial/ethnic/cultural minorities, persons with disabilities, or persons who are sexual minorities). For multiracial persons, the primary driver of their microaggressions exists in society's idealization of monoraciality (that is, being or claiming one race identity) as normative and thus healthy for all, what Nadal et al. (2013) term "monoracism." Monoracist microaggressions can include (a) exclusion and isolation based on mixed-race status; (b) exoticization and objectification; (c) assumed racial identity; (d) denial or invalidation of multiracial identity and experience, and (e) pathologizing of multiracial identity and experience as psychologically unhealthy. Added to Nadal et al.'s (2013) analysis are scores of literature and research that examine both intrafamilial and extrafamilial monoracist microaggressions including *racial identity patrolling* by peers and others (Dalmage, 2000) to pressure or shame multiracial persons into claiming single race identities and allegiances, *racial litmus testing* (for example, evaluative judgments interrogating a person's identity in monoracial terms as not being "Asian enough" or as being "too white"), and general suspicions of *racial passing* (that is, that multiracial people claiming multiracial identities are "passing" as white or inherently wish to do so) (Bolatagici, 2004; Favor, 1999; McCubbin et al., 2010; Rancarati, Ravenna, Perez, & Navarro-Pertusa, 2009; Zack, 1993). Perhaps the single defining microaggression that nearly all multiracial or racially ambiguous persons report experiencing in daily life from acquaintances and even strangers in public is the question "What are you?" (Gaskins, 1999). Research is beginning to illuminate the ways in which experiences of monoracism contribute to negative psychological and socioemotional outcomes (Jackson, Wolven, & Aguilera, 2013). This will be discussed further in a later section.

There are also myriad "positive" stereotypes that shape the developmental context of multiracial persons. This includes the belief that multiracial people have "the best of both worlds," that they experience less racism, are natural bridge-builders across racial divisions, and are more attractive or exotic (Bolatagici, 2004; Gaskins, 1999; Streeter, 2003). Although these stereotypes can offer multiracial individuals more positive images of self, some arguably come at the cost of objectifying a physical attribute—race—that does not have any real causal or predictive function in driving personality, universal attractiveness, temperament, or other traits or interpersonal abilities. There are also social and developmental risks attached to some of these so-called positive stereotypes (for example, that they are more attractive and exotic or that they experience less racism and discrimination) that will be discussed in a later section.

Understanding Development in Multiracial Children and Youth

In terms of basic human development, there is no reason to consider multiracial children unique; all children, regardless of race or ethnicity, share basic developmental needs for healthy attachment, parental nurturing, and a family and community ecology that promotes their resilience and well-being

(Bronfenbrenner, 1986). Parental and familial support is consistently found to be a critical component of positive youth development across the life course, even into adulthood (Arnett, 2000). Among racial and ethnic minority children, the development of biculturalism (having cultural capital and competence in more than one culture) is understood as a protective factor, giving resilience in navigating racism and prejudice (LaFramboise, Coleman, & Gerton, 1993), and this has been found to be true for multiracial persons as well (Jackson, Wolven, & Aguilera, 2013). Factors such as moderate parental control, high engagement in family routines and rituals, parental emotional attunement and responsiveness, and parental support have all been positively linked to well-being among all youth (Bamaca, Umana-Taylor, Shin, & Alfaro, 2005; Lorenzo-Blanco, Bares, & Delva, 2013). The degree to which youth, particularly in adolescence, report positive relationships with a parent is also a strong protective factor against engaging in risky behaviors that compromise their positive life outcomes (Bronte-Tinkew, 2006).

Incipient research on outcomes among multiracial youth is mixed, but is beginning to outline areas of both concern and strength. When compared to monoracial and monoethnic youth, multiracial youth are sometimes found to be at higher risk for socioemotional and physical problems (Udry, Li, & Hendrickson-Smith, 2003). Similarly, multiracial youth often report lower levels of community cohesion and lower access to adult or peer co-ethnics (that is, other multiracial persons) in their daily social networks—protective factors that promote biculturalism and positive adjustment for youth of color. As mentioned previously, multiracial youth adopted by white parents may be at increased risk for experiencing childhood contexts that are not racially or ethnically diverse or affirming; Asian transracial adoptees are at the highest risk for such developmental/familial contexts in their multiracial families (Kreider & Raleigh, 2011). Multiracial children (both adopted and nonadopted) may not have access to essential social or familial supports in navigating their racialized environments and multiracial identities (Lorenzo-Blanco et al., 2013; Samuels, 2009). Unlike other groups of racial–ethnic minority children, this lack of access to co-ethnics includes lacking a shared experience of race with parents or extended family who are not multiracial themselves (Lorenzo-Blanco et al.). Some added risks for adopted multiracial children with white heritage may include erroneous beliefs about racial salience for multiracial children with white heritage, including that they will experience less racism, that they will fit in more easily within white families and communities, and that their adoptions will not be viewed as taking a child away from a racial–ethnic minority community (Samuels, 2009; Sweeney, 2013). Yet assumptions about the salience of race and racism for multiracial individuals with white heritage are also present among the biological parents of these multiracial children (see, for example, Lee & Bean, 2010; Rollings & Hunter, 2013). This raises questions about the types of critical support known to promote biculturalism and affirm healthy development among racial–ethnic minorities that may be fundamentally absent in the natural environments of many multiracial youth during childhood and even into adulthood (Samuels, 2009, 2010). It also suggests a need for attention in practice and parenting to take seriously the racial–ethnic and cultural identity development of this population as an essential, rather than optional, component of their healthy functioning and well-being.

In promoting resilience, family socialization has received consistent focus in promoting the healthy development of multiracial children. In a review of literature related to multiracial identity outcomes, several key influencing factors are emerging as critical to promoting positive outcomes and resilience in multiracial children and youth, including (a) parental awareness and sophistication of knowledge around issues of race; (b) family structure, and (c) openness in discussing race within the family (Allen, Garriott, Reyes, & Hsieh, 2013; Crawford & Allagia, 2008). It is also clear that how parents racially socialize their children (including the use of more indirect methods that allow for a stronger role for extrafamilial contribution) is directly tied to their own racial identity development and parents' own experiences with race, ethnicity, and culture in their families and communities of origin (Rockquemore & Laszloffy, 2005; Samuels, 2009, 2010).

Racial Labels and Identity Development

In the first theories on race identity development (see, for example, Cross, 1971; Helms, 1995) predictive stage-based models were popular for use in research and clinical practice. Persons of color were thought to be healthy if they were able to move away from early stages of internalizing negative stereotypes and seeking assimilation into whiteness as the privileged status or distancing themselves from their own minority group (Cross, 1971). Healthy developmental stages increasingly required the person to feel positive and secure in his or her minority group identity and label and have meaningful relationships with whites, but not to identify as white. Therefore, the healthy identity for a racial minority person inherently required nonidentification with whiteness racially or culturally. Similarly, theories of white racial identity development described a process of moving toward race consciousness and antiracist identities, developing an awareness of their unearned racial privileges without overidentification or exploitation of relationships with persons of color (Helms). Again, the healthy identity was to reject internalized stereotypes that privileged whites as the norm or ideal/superior racial group. In both cases, healthy identities were single-race identities with a matching cultural identity (that is, being Native American meant one was Native American racially, ethnically, and culturally).

Such models have been limited, particularly for understanding processes of multiracial identity development, as well as for adopted persons who may grow up in racial and cultural contexts that do not match their own heritages. Additionally, some multiracial persons may not only seek to have meaningful relationships with white people (that is, their parents, relatives, or peers), but also seek to identify in a range of ways with their own white heritage.

In the 1980s, biracial identity models copied these stage-based theories and proposed theories for healthy biracial identity that simply replaced a single identification outcome with a dual one. These models (see, for example, Poston, 1990) proposed increasing levels of acceptance of all of one's heritages, including white, and the use of a biracial label to indicate their multiraciality and healthy identity development. However, these models assumed a single option for healthy identity—ignoring potential diversity in how multiracial individuals might integrate their multiracial or multiethnic heritages in healthy ways over the life course. These models assumed dual but not multiple (more than two) racial–ethnic heritages and were fully silent about healthy identity processes for multiracial persons without white heritage.

During the explosion of multiracial literature and research from the 1990s into the 21st century, increasingly stage-based models were being rejected or expanded. Instead, identities are now thought to be healthy when they promote a child's resilience and well-being, regardless of the use of a specific label (Rockquemore & Laszloffy, 2005). In this way, healthy identity development becomes less about what one calls him- or herself (for example, using a multiracial or monoracial label), but rather how a person negotiates his or her multiraciality in daily life in ways that

promote social and emotional well-being. Today, multiracial children experience enduring monocentricity but increasing identity options and are beginning to assert their own identities and identity labels. Labels coined by younger cohorts of multiracial individuals to indicate their specific racial–ethnic heritages are emerging: blaxican (black Mexican), hapa (Asian white), latinegra (Latina black).

There is also a move away from understanding healthy identity as something that is fixed or limited to (or resolved by) adolescence. Instead, identity development is conceived as a lifelong process. Race identities can change and grow over the life course, and this can be especially true for persons of multiracial and multiethnic heritage who may not have had childhood access to certain racial or ethnic communities (Jackson, 2009; McCubbin et al., 2010; Samuels, 2009; Wijeyesinghe, 1992). Theories of intersectionality also enrich the understanding of racial identities by emphasizing the salience of myriad other social identities, such as sexuality, class, gender, and spirituality, that critically shape how one navigates, experiences, and expresses race identities (Samuels & Ross-Sheriff, 2007; Wijeyesinghe, 1992). Changes in identities no longer necessarily indicate unhealthy outcomes or "identity confusion/conflict," just as stability in one's identity does not necessarily indicate health or a positive feeling about that identity.

Identities are generally considered healthy when they are not grounded in denial, shame, or rejection of a particular heritage (Rockquemore & Laszloffy, 2005). However, this does not mean that multiracial persons always must use labels that publicly identify all of their racial, ethnic, cultural, or national backgrounds all of the time. There are several trends across research on multiple subpopulations of multiracial persons indicating active ingredients of healthy identity development that begin to point toward important elements of healthy identity processes: (a) parental/family openness and dialogues about race, racism, and discrimination; (b) color-conscious rather than colorblind race philosophy; (c) balancing an emphasis on sameness with difference in people; (d) effective strategies for actively combatting racial stigmas and stereotypes as an individual and family; (e) everyday environments that provide positive and natural access to relationships with co-ethnics including multiracial persons/families; (f) engaging multiculturalism in family culture; and (g) nurturing, validating, and affirming a child's self and identity (Allen et al., 2013; Childs, 2002; McCubbin et al., 2010; Rockquemore & Laszloffy, 2005; Rollins & Hunter, 2013; Samuels, 2009).

Need for More Research and Theory on Racial and Cultural Identity Processes Promoting Resilience

The empirical study of multiraciality has primarily been restricted to exploring identity outcomes and processes, as opposed to other elements of well-being and adjustment (for example, physical behavioral, psychological, or social/relational health). Overwhelmingly, this research has focused on the identities of black–white multiracial individuals in early adulthood (for exceptions see Allen et al., 2013; Jackson et al., 2013; Lee & Bean, 2010; McCubbin et al., 2010). To a lesser extent, racial and cultural socialization of multiracial children (both adopted and nonadopted) have also been explored. However, there is an overwhelming focus on how parents of multiracial youth racially classify their children (see, for example, Bratter & Heard, 2009; Brunsma, 2005; Holloway, Wright, Ellis, & East, 2009; Lee & Bean). We know very little, however, about processes of racial socialization as it occurs in families beyond racial label choice and even less about cultural socialization processes that support healthy development across the life course. There is a great need for research in this area to extend beyond understanding how multiracial persons label themselves and how parents and others racially socialize to a preferred label to instead understand processes and factors central to their healthy development and resilience across the life course. This includes not only the use and development of culturally relevant quantitative measures, but also the use of more ethnographic and naturalist observational methods of actual socialization processes in context (Ortiz & Samuels, n.d.). However, several factors are emerging within the extant research as important elements of socialization processes that promote positive adjustment and resilience among multiracial persons.

Studies involving multiracial youth and overall adjustment indicate "identity integration" as a protective factor in psychological adjustment and health (Jackson, Yoo, Guevarra, & Harrington, 2012). Youth exhibit identity integration when they report feeling supported and affirmed in their identification choices and experience low levels of conflict or distancing between their race identifications in their daily lives. Research has also identified elements of multiracial resilience, including developing an ability for racial–ethnic flexibility (Jackson et al., 2013; Vasquez, 2010) and the social capital to identify as an insider (that is, be bicultural) with more than one racial–ethnic community when they desire to do so (Shih & Sanchez, 2005). Research increasingly challenges the assumption that most multiracial persons experience dissatisfaction, sadness, or discomfort with their mixed-race identities or display weakened racial–ethnic identities. In fact, multiracially identified persons in some samples were found to have stronger ethnic identities (Bracey, Bamaca & Umana-Taylor, 2004) and were more socially well adjusted and felt more positive about themselves (Binning, Unzueta, Huo, & Molina, 2009) than their nonmultiracial peers.

Much more research is needed to understand meaningful differences in the developmental contexts of multiracial individuals and the role nonmultiracial parents can play in socializing their multiracial children by providing family and community contexts that affirm their positive development. There is also a need to understand cultural socialization rather than racial socialization and to engage samples of multiracial persons who do not have white heritage.

Health and Wellness

We know very little about the physical health of multiracial individuals. Often health statistics for persons of multiracial descent are combined within single pan-racial groups, thus masking any distinct health disparities for this population. However, as norms for reporting race in Census influence racial reporting among other federal and state institutions, such statistics are becoming available. For example, although mentioned previously as both a microaggression and a positive stereotype, it is concerning that multiracial persons may be exoticized and sexually objectified in ways that pose health and safety risks. Findings from the National Intimate Partner and Sexual Violence Survey indicated alarming outcomes for multiracial individuals nationally (Black et al., 2011). According to their 2010 report, multiracial persons experience the highest rates of intimate partner and sexual violence than any other racial–ethnic group in the United States. This was true for both males and females. One in every 3 multiracial women (33.5%) and nearly 1 in 3 multiracial men (31.6%) reported being raped at some point in their lives (Black et al.). In combining all forms of violence (rape, physical violence, and/or stalking by an intimate partner), 1 in 2 multiracial women and 4 in 10 multiracial men (39.3%) report being victims (Black et al.). Given the microaggressions and stereotypes of multiraciality discussed previously, specifically images and perceptions that portray both male and female multiracial persons as more attractive or exotic may negatively contribute to their disproportionate risk for sexual victimization.

Resilience and Community Building—The Multiracial Diaspora

Multiracial youth in the 21st century have access to a range of resources and communities not available to earlier generations of multiracial persons and families. The Internet provides unparalleled potential for connecting to other persons who share their identities. This is particularly important for persons and families who live in areas that are not racially diverse or areas where the diversity of the population does not reflect their own heritage or identities. There are also increasing numbers of national organizations, books, and other published resources led or authored by multiracial persons.

In an effort to reshape social understandings of "the multiracial experience" as diverse and examine the developmental contexts both shared and distinct among multiracial populations, MAVIN Foundation (*http://www.mavinfoundation.org*), a national organization, was founded by Matt Kelley. In 2007, MAVIN Foundation launched its Mixed Heritage Center (*http://www.mixedheritagecenter.org*), claiming status as the first comprehensive online resource of information and tools to support the multiracial community (including transracial adoptive multiracial families). MAVIN also published the edited text by Maria Root and MAVIN founder, Matt Kelley, *Multiracial Child Resource Book: Living Complex Identities* (Root & Kelley, 2003). In addition to the publication of this book, scholars, bloggers, and educators have continued to pursue opportunities to convey the diversity of experiences among the group "multiracial," to dispel social myths attached to multiraciality, and to complicate our social narratives about race mixing and multiracial families and persons in general (Root, 2003). There are unlimited resources both published and online that seek to provide an affirming community and set of resources to the multiracial diaspora. Examples of only a few of the many transracial adoption online resources and organizations include Adopted and Fostered Adults of the African Diaspora (AFAD), PACT, North American Council on Adoptable Children, and blogs by transracial adoptees and adoptive parents: *http://loveisntenough.com*, *http://johnraible.wordpress.com*, and *http://JaeRanKim.wordpress.com* Examples of multiracial web-based resources and organizations include *http://interracialfamily.org*, Association for Multiethnic Americans, *http://mixedmarrow.org* (an organization that seeks bone marrow donors for multiracial persons in need), Swirl Inc., and iPride.

Multiracially Attuned Social-Work Practices
There is a dearth of literature on empirically informed or theory-driven practices with multiracial persons and families across all academic fields, but particularly in social work. Much of the education, policy, and practice discourse around "cultural competence"

and culturally responsive or attuned practice models in our field, including the National Association of Social Workers' code of ethics, remain monocentric. In a review of social-work literature on multiracial persons and families, Jackson and Samuels (2011) ultimately propose to the profession a set of knowledge, skills, and increased awareness to promote more multiracially attuned and responsive practices for the social-work profession. Drawing from the National Association of Social Workers' code of ethics and an interdisciplinary body of scholarship, social-work professionals and scholars are challenged to build critical awareness of their own biases and internal assumptions that are informed by societal stereotypes and monocentricity. This includes not assuming that all problems faced by multiracial persons are caused by their mixed-race heritage or that it is normal for multiracial families and persons to have problems because of their multiracial status. Professionals are encouraged to integrate multiracial literature and research into their practice wisdom and to use relevant assessment tools and practice approaches for this highly diverse population (Jackson & Samuels). As discussed previously, there are unique and overlapping histories of multiraciality in the United States; these legacies shape contemporary microaggressions. Jackson and Samuels encourage researchers in the field to increase our awareness of how a child or family's immediate environment promotes or inhibits their well-being. This requires social workers to be attuned to the unique race dynamics within their own locals and to knowledge about both the available and the missing resources for multiracial families and persons in their communities and online.

Finally, theories and models of identity development now indicate a range of "healthy" identities for multiracial persons and show that identities can and do change across context, age, or development and even differ between siblings within families that share a biological heritage (Jackson & Samuels, 2011; Wijeyesinghe & Jackson, 2012). As practitioners evaluate so-called "normative" or healthy development in children, youth, and families, it is important that they use theories, interventions, and assessment tools to evaluate and promote healthy functioning that are culturally relevant and responsive to the lived experiences of their multiracial and multiethnic clientele.

REFERENCES
Allen, G. E. K., Garriott, P. O., Reyes, C. J., & Hsieh, C. (2013). Racial identity, phenotype, and self-esteem among biracial Polynesian/white individuals. *Family Relations*, 62, 82–91.

Arnett, J. J. (2000). Emerging adulthood: A theory of development from the late teens through the twenties. *American Psychologist*, 55, 469–480.

Associated Press. (2009, 15 October). Interracial couple denied marriage license by Louisiana Justice of the Peace. New York, NY: Associated Press.

Bamaca, M. Y., Umana-Taylor, A. J., Shin, N., & Alfaro, E. C. (2005). Latino adolescents' perception of parenting behaviors and self-esteem: Examining the role of neighborhood risk. *Family Relations*, 54, 621–632.

Binning, K. R., Unzueta, M. M., Huo, Y. J., & Molina, L. E. (2009). The interpretation of multiracial status and its relation to social engagement and psychological well-being. *Journal of Social Issues*, 65(1), 35–50.

Black, M. C., Basile, K. C., Breiding, M. J., Smith, S. G., Walters, M. L., Merrick, M. T., et al. (2011). *The National Intimate Partner and Sexual Violence Survey (NISVS): 2010 summary report*. Atlanta, GA: National Center for Injury Prevention and Control, Centers for Disease Control and Prevention.

Bolatagici, R. (2004). Claiming the (n)either/(n)or of "third space": (Re)presenting hybrid identity and the embodiment of mixed race. *Journal of Intercultural Studies*, 25(1), 75–85.

Bracey, J. R., Bamaca, M. Y., & Umana-Taylor, A. J. (2004). Examining ethnic identity and self-esteem among biracial and monoracial adolescents. *Journal of Youth and Adolescence*, 33, 123–131.

Bratter, J., & Heard, H. E. (2009). Mother's, father's, or both? Parental gender and parent–child interactions in the racial classification of adolescents. *Sociological Forum*, 24(3), 658–688.

Bronfenbrenner, U. (1986). Ecology of the family as a context for human development: Research perspectives. *Developmental Psychology*, 22, 723–742.

Bronte-Tinkew, J. J. (2006). The father–child relationship, parenting styles, and adolescent risk behaviors in intact families. *Journal of Family Issues*, 27, 850–881.

Brown, R., & Armelagos, G. J. (2001). Apportionment of racial diversity: A review. *Evolutionary Anthropology*, 10, 34–40.

Brunsma, D. L. (2005). Interracial families and the racial identification of mixed-race children: Evidence from the early childhood longitudinal study. *Social Forces*, 84(2), 1131–1157.

Childs, E. C. (2002). Families on the color-line: Patrolling borders and crossing boundaries. *Race & Society*, 5(2), 139–161.

Crawford, S. E., & Alaggia, R. (2008). The best of both worlds?: Family influences on mixed race youth identity development. *Qualitative Social Work*, 7(81).

Cross, W. E. (1971). The Negro to Black conversion experience: Towards a psychology of Black liberation. *Black World*, 20(9), 13–27.

Dalmage, H. (2000). *Tripping on the color line: Black–White multiracial families in a racially divided world*. New Brunswick, NJ: Rutgers University Press.

Dalmage, H. (2004). *The politics of multiracialism: Challenging racial thinking*. Albany: SUNY Press.

Davis, F. J. (1991). *Who is Black?* University Park, PA: Pennsylvania State University Press.

Favor, J. M. (1999). *Authentic Blackness*. Durham, NC: Duke University Press.

Fernandez, C. (1996). Government classification of multiracial/multiethnic people. In M. M. P. Root (Ed.), *The multiracial experience: Racial borders as the new frontier*. Thousand Oaks, CA: SAGE.

Frankenberg, R. (1995). Whiteness as an "unmarked" cultural category. In K. Rosenblum & T. Travis (Eds.), *The meaning of difference* (pp. 92–98). New York, NY: McGraw–Hill.

Freundlich, M., & Lieberthal, J. K. (2000). *The gathering of the first generation of adult Korean adoptees: Adoptees' perceptions of international adoption*. New York, NY: Evan B. Donaldson Institute.

Gaskins, P. F. (1999). *What are you? Voices of mixed-race young people*. New York, NY: Macmillan.

Grow, L. J., & Shapiro, D. (1974). *Black children, white parents*. Washington, DC: Child Welfare League of America.

Haney López, I. (1996). *White by law: The legal construction of race*. New York, NY: New York University Press.

Helms, J.E. (1995). An update of Helms's White and people of color racial identity models. In J. G. Ponterotto, J.M. Casas, L.A. Suzuki, & C. M. Alexander (Eds.), *Handbook of multicultural counseling* (pp. 181–191). Thousand Oaks, CA: SAGE.

Hochschild, J. L., & Powell, B. M. (2008). Racial reorganization and the United States Census 1850–1930: Mulattoes, half-breeds, mixed parentage, Hindoos, and the Mexican race. *Studies in American Political Development*, 22(1), 59–96.

Holloway, S. R., Wright, R., Ellis, M., & East, M. (2009). Place, scale, and the racial claims made for multiracial children in the 1990 US census. *Ethnic and Racial Studies*, 32(3), 522–547.

Jackson, K. F. (2009). Beyond race: Examining the facets of multiracial identity through a life-span developmental lens. *Journal of Ethnic and Cultural Diversity in Social Work*, 18, 309–326.

Jackson, K. F., & Samuels, G. M. (2011). Multiracial competence in social work: Recommendations for culturally attuned work with multiracial persons. *Social Work*, 56(3), 235–245.

Jackson, K. F., Wolven, T., & Aguilera, K. (2013). Mixed resilience: A study of multiethnic Mexican American stress and coping in Arizona. *Family Relations*, 62, 212–225.

Jackson, K. F., Yoo, H. C., Guevarra, R., Jr., & Harrington, B. A. (2012). Role of identity integration on the relationship between perceived discrimination and psychological adjustment of multiracial people. *Journal of Counseling Psychology*, 59(2), 240–250.

Johnston, M. P., & Nadal, K. L. (2010). Multiracial microaggressions: Exposing monoracism in everyday life and clinical practice. In D. W. Sue (Ed.), *Microaggressions and marginality: Manifestation, dynamics, and impact* (pp. 123–144). New York, NY: Wiley.

Jones, N. A., & Bullock, J. J. (2013). Understanding who reported multiple races in the U.S.: Results from Census 2000 and the 2010 Census. *Family Relations*, 62(1), 5–16.

Jorde, L. (2002). Book review. [Mapping human history: Discovering the past through our genes. By Steve Olson. Boston, MA: Houghton Mifflin, 2002.] *The American Journal of Human Genetics*, 71(6), 1484–1485.

Kreider, R. M., & Raleigh, E. (2011). *Contexts of racial socialization: Are transracial adoptive families more like multiracial or white monoracial families? SEHSD, working paper. Presented at the Annual Meeting of the Population Association of America.* Washington, DC. http://www.census.gov/population/www/socdemo/KreiderRaleighPAA2011.pdf

LaFramboise, T., Coleman, H. L. K., & Gerton, J. (1993). Psychological impact of biculturalism: Evidence and theory. *Psychological Bulletin*, 114, 395–412.

Lee, J., & Bean, F. D. (2010). *The diversity paradox: Immigration and the color line in 21st century America.* New York, NY: Russell Sage Foundation Press.

Lofquist, D., Lugaila, T., O'Connell, M., & Feliz, S. (2012). *Households and families 2010. Census 2010 Census brief.* Washington, DC: U.S. Census Bureau.

Lorenzo-Blanco, E. I., Bares, C. B., & Delva, J. (2013). Parenting, family processes, relationships, and parental support in multiracial and multiethnic families: An exploratory study of youth perceptions. *Family Relations*, 62, 125–139.

Loving. v. Virginia 388 U.S. 1 388 U.S. 1, Loving Et Ux. V. Virginia. (1967). Appeal from the Supreme Court of Appeals of Virginia, No. 395. Argued April 10, 1967. Decided June 12, 1967.

Martyn, B. (1979). *Racism in the United States: A history of the anti-miscegenation legislation and litigation.* PhD dissertation, Department of History, University of Southern California.

McCubbin, H., Ontai, K., Kehl, L., McCubbin, L., Strom, I., Hart, H., et al. (Eds.). (2010). *Multiethnicity and multiethnic families: Development, identity, and resilience.* Honolulu, HI: Leʻa.

McRoy, R. G., & Zurcher, L. A. (1983). *Transracial and inracial adoptees: The adolescent years.* Springfield, IL: Charles C. Thomas.

Menchaca, M. (2008). The anti-miscegenation history of the American southwest, 1837 to 1970: Transforming racial ideology into law. *Cultural Dynamics*, 20(3), 279–318.

Miranda, G. E. (2004, Spring/Summer). Reading between the lines: Black-white heritage and transracial adoption. *African American Research Perspectives*, 10(1), 174–187.

Nadal, K. L., Sriken, J., Davidoff, K. C., Wong, Y., & McLean, K. (2013). Microaggressions within families: Experiences of multiracial people. *Family Relations*, 62, 190–201.

Nadal, K. L., Wong, U. Y., Griffin, D., Sriken, J., Vargas, V., Wideman, M., et al. (2010). Microaggressions and the multiracial experience. *International Journal of Humanities and Social Sciences*, 1, 36–44.

Olsen, S. (2003). *Mapping human history: Genes, race, and our common ancestry.* Boston, MA: Mariner Books.

Ortiz, C., & Samuels, G. M. (n.d.). *Parental racial socialization: An argument for the inclusion of naturalistic observational methods.* Unpublished manuscript in progress.

Park, R. E. (1931). Mentality of racial hybrids. *American Journal of Sociology*, 36, 534–551.

Patton, S. (2000). *Birth Marks: Transracial adoption in contemporary America.* New York, NY: New York University Press.

Poston, W.S.C. (1990). The biracial identity development model: A needed addition. *Journal of Counseling and Development*, 69, 152–155.

Rancarati, A., Ravenna, M., Perez, J. A., & Navarro-Pertusa, E. (2009). Mixing against cultures vs mixing against nature: Ontologization of prohibited interethnic relationships. *International Journal of Psychology*, 44(1), 12–19.

Rockquemore, K. A., & Brunsma, D. L. (2002). *Beyond Black: Biracial identity in America.* Thousand Oaks, CA: SAGE.

Rockquemore, K. A., & Laszloffy, T. (2005). *Raising biracial children.* Lanham, MD: Altamira Press.

Roediger, D. R. (2008). *How race survived US history: From settlement and slavery to the Obama phenomenon.* New York, NY: Verso.

Rollins, A. and Hunter, A. G. (2013). Racial socialization of biracial youth: Maternal messages and approaches to address discrimination. *Family Relations*, 62, 140–153.

Root, M. P. P. (Ed.). (1992). *Racially mixed people in America.* Newbury Park, CA: SAGE.

Root, M. P. P. (1996). *The multiracial experience: Racial borders as the new frontier.* Thousand Oaks, CA: SAGE.

Root, M. P. P. (1998). Experiences and processes affecting racial identity development: Preliminary results from the biracial sibling project. *Cultural Diversity and Mental Health*, 4(3), 237–247.

Root, M. P. P. (2003). Bill of rights for racially mixed people. In M. P. P. Root & M. Kelley (Eds.), *Multiracial child resource book: Living complex identities* (pp. 32–33). Seattle, WA: MAVIN Foundation.

Root, M. P. P., & Kelley, M. (Eds.). (2003). *Multiracial child resource book: Living complex identities.* Seattle, WA: MAVIN Foundation.

Samuels, G. M. (2006). Beyond the rainbow: Multiraciality in the 21st century. In D. W. Engstrom & L. M. Piedra (Eds.), *Our diverse society: Race and ethnicity—Implications for 21st century American society.* Washington, DC: NASW Press.

Samuels, G. M. (2009). "Being raised by white people": Navigating racial difference among adopted multiracial adults. *Journal of Marriage and Family*, 71(1), 80–94.

Samuels, G. M. (2010). Building kinship and community: Relational processes of bicultural identity among adult multiracial adoptees. *Family Process*, 49(1), 26–42.

Samuels, G. M., & Ross-Sheriff, F. (2007). Identity, oppression, and power: Feminism and intersectionality theory. *Affilia: Journal of Women and Social Work*, 23, 5–9.

Shih, M., & Sanchez, D. T. (2005). Perspectives and research on the positive and negative implications of having multiple racial identities. *Psychological Bulletin*, *131*, 569–591.

Simon, R. J., & Roorda R. (2000). *In their own voices*. New York, NY: Columbia University Press.

Smith, S., McRoy, R., Freundlich, M., & Kroll, J. (2008). *Finding families for African American children: The role of race & law in adoption from foster care*. New York, NY: Evan B. Donaldson Institute.

Sohoni, D. (2007). Unsuitable suitors: Anti-miscegenation laws, naturalization laws, and the construction of Asian identities. *Law & Society Review*, *41*(3), 587–618.

Spencer, R. (1997). *The new colored people: The mixed-race movement in America*. New York, NY: New York University Press.

Streeter, C. A. (2003). The hazards of visibility: "Biracial" women, media images, and narratives of identity. In L. I. Winters & H. L. DeBose (Eds.), *New faces in a changing America: Multiracial identity in the 21st century* (pp. 194–221). Thousand Oaks, CA: SAGE.

Sue, D. W. (2010). *Microaggressions in everyday life: Race, gender, and sexual orientation*. Hoboken, NJ: Wiley.

Sweeney, K. A. (2013). Race-conscious adoption choices, multiraciality, and colorblind racial ideology. *Family Relations*, *62*(1), 42–57.

Udry, J. R., Li, R. M., & Hendrickson-Smith, J. (2003). Health and behavior risks of adolescents with mixed race identity. *American Journal of Public Health*, *93*, 1865–1870.

U.S. Department of Health and Human Services. (2011). *National Center for Health Statistics. Health, United States, 2010: With special feature on death and dying*. Hyattsville, MD: Author.

Vasquez, J. M. (2010). Blurred borders for some but not others: Racialization, "flexible ethnicity," gender, and third-generation Mexican American identity. *Sociological Perspectives*, *53*, 45–72.

Vroegh, K. S. (1997). Transracial adoptees: Developmental status after 17 years. *American Journal of Orthopsychiatry*, *67*(4), 568–575.

Waters, M. C. (1990). *Ethnic options: Choosing identities in America*. Berkeley, CA: University of California Press.

Wells, S. (2003). *The journey of man: A genetic odyssey*. Princeton, NJ: Princeton University Press.

Wijeyesinghe, C. (1992). *Towards an understanding of the racial identity of bi-racial people: The experience of racial self-identification of African-American/Euro-American adults and the factors affecting their choices of racial identity*. Electronic Doctoral Dissertations for UMass Amherst. Paper AAI9305915.

Wijeyesinghe, C., & Jackson, B. W. (2012). *New perspectives on racial identity development*. New York, NY: New York University Press.

Williamson, J. (1980). *New people: Miscegenation and mulattoes in the United States*. Baton Rouge, LA: Louisiana State University Press.

Winters, L. I., & DeBose, H. L. (Eds.). (2003). *New faces in a changing America: Multiracial identity in the 21st century*. Thousand Oaks, CA: Sage.

Zack, N. (1993). *Race and mixed race*. Philadelphia, PA: Temple University Press.

FURTHER READING

American Anthropological Association. (1998, 17 May). Statement on "race."

Anzaldua, G. (1987). *Borderlands, la frontera—The new mestiza*. San Francisco, CA: Aunt Lute Books.

Appiah, K. (1990). Race. In F. Lentricchia & T. McLaughlin (Eds.), *Critical terms for literary study* (pp. 274–287). Chicago, IL: University of Chicago Press.

Awkward, M. (1995). *Negotiating difference, race, gender, and politics of positionality*. Chicago, IL: University of Chicago Press.

Daniel, R. G. (2002). *More than Black? Multiracial identity and the new racial order*. Philadelphia, PA: Temple University Press.

Daniel, R. G. (2003). Multiracial identity in global perspective: The United States, Brazil, and South Africa. In L. I. Winters & H. L. DeBose (Eds.), *New faces in a changing America: Multiracial identity in the 21st century* (pp. 247–286). Thousand Oaks, CA: SAGE.

Graves, J. L., Jr. (2004). *The race myth: Why we pretend race exists in America*. New York, NY: Penguin Books.

Spencer, R. (1999). *Spurious issues: Race and multiracial identity politics in the United States*. Boulder, CO: Westview Press.

GINA MIRANDA SAMUELS

N

THE NASW CODE OF ETHICS

Abstract: Ethical standards in social work have matured significantly in recent years. As in most professions, social work's principal code of ethics has evolved from a brief, broadly worded document to a detailed, comprehensive guide to ethical practice. This article summarizes the diverse purposes and functions of professional codes of ethics and the historical trends and changes in social work's codes of ethics. The key components of the *NASW Code of Ethics*—the code's preamble, broad ethical principles, and more specific ethical standards—are described.

Key Words: Code of Ethics; ethical principles; ethical standards; NASW; National Association of Social Workers; social work ethics; social work values

One of the hallmarks of a profession is its willingness to establish ethical standards to guide practitioners' conduct (Greenwood, 1957; Hall, 1968; Lindeman, 1947). Ethical standards are created to address ethical issues in practice and to provide guidelines for determining what ethically acceptable or unacceptable behavior is.

Professions typically publicize their ethical standards in the forms of codes of ethics (Bayles, 1986; Banks & Gallagher, 2009; Kultgen, 1982; Reamer, 2006). According to Jamal and Bowie (1995), codes of ethics are designed to address three major issues. First, codes address problems of moral hazard, or instances when a profession's self-interest may conflict with the public's interest (for example, whether accountants should be obligated to disclose confidential information concerning serious financial crimes that their clients have committed, or whether dentists should be permitted to refuse to treat people who have a serious immune disease, such as HIV-AIDS). Second, codes address issues of professional courtesy—that is, rules that govern how professionals should behave to enhance and maintain a profession's integrity (for example, whether lawyers should be permitted to advertise and solicit clients, whether physicians should accept gifts and free trips from pharmaceutical company representatives, or whether psychotherapists should be permitted to engage in sexual relationships with former patients).

Finally, codes address issues that concern professionals' duty to serve the public interest (for example, the extent of nurses' or social workers' obligation to assist when faced with a public emergency or to provide low-income people with pro bono services).

Like other professions such as medicine, nursing, law, psychology, counseling, and engineering, social work has developed a comprehensive set of ethical standards. These standards have evolved over time, reflecting significant changes in the broader culture and in social work's mission, methods, and priorities. They address a wide range of issues, including, for example, social workers' handling of confidential information and electronic communications, dual relationships and boundary issues, conflicts of interest, informed consent, termination of services, administration, supervision, education and training, research, and political action.

Ethical standards in social work appear in various forms. The *NASW Code of Ethics* (NASW, 2008) is the most visible compilation of the profession's ethical standards. Ethical standards can also be found in codes of ethics developed by other social work organizations (for example, the National Association of Black Social Workers [NABSW] and the Clinical Social Work Association [CSWA]), regulations promulgated by state legislatures and licensing boards, and codes of conduct adopted by social service organizations and other employers. In addition, social work literature contains many discussions on ethical norms in the profession (Banks, 2012; Barsky, 2010; Dolgoff, Harrington, & Loewenberg, 2012; Reamer, 2006, 2013).

The Profession's Early Years

During the earliest years of social work's history, few formal ethical standards existed. The earliest known attempt to formulate a code was an experimental draft code of ethics printed in the 1920s and attributed to Mary Richmond (Pumphrey, 1959). Although several other social work organizations formulated draft codes during the profession's early years (for example, the American Association for Organizing Family Social Work and several chapters of the American Association of Social Workers [AASW]), it was not until 1947 that the AASW, the largest organization of social workers of that era, adopted a formal code (Johnson, 1955). In 1960 NASW adopted its first code of ethics, five years after the association was formed. Over time, the *NASW Code of Ethics* has been recognized as the most visible and influential code of ethics in the United States.

In 1960 the *NASW Code of Ethics* consisted of 14 proclamations concerning, for example, every social worker's duty to give precedence to professional responsibility over personal interests; to respect the privacy of clients; to give appropriate professional service in public emergencies; and to contribute knowledge, skills, and support to human welfare programs. First-person statements (that is, "I give precedence to my professional responsibility over my professional interests" and "I respect the privacy of the people I serve" [p. 1]) were preceded by a preamble that set forth social workers' responsibility to uphold humanitarian ideals, maintain and improve social work service, and develop the philosophy and skills of the profession. In 1967 a 15th principle pledging nondiscrimination was added to the proclamations.

Soon after the adoption of the code, however, NASW members began to express concern about its level of abstraction, its scope and usefulness for resolving ethical conflicts, and its provisions for handling ethics complaints about practitioners and agencies (McCann & Cutler, 1979). In 1977 NASW established a task force to revise the code and enhance its relevance to practice; the result was a new code adopted by NASW in 1979.

The 1979 code included six sections of brief, unannotated principles with a preamble setting forth the code's general purpose and stating that the code's principles provided standards for the enforcement of ethical practices among social workers. The code included major sections concerning social workers' general conduct and comportment and ethical responsibilities to clients, colleagues, employers, employing organizations, the social work profession, and society. The code's principles were both prescriptive ("The social worker should act to prevent the unauthorized and unqualified practice of social work" [principle V.M.3]) and proscriptive ("The social worker should not exploit relationships with clients for personal advantage" [principle II.F.2]). Several of the code's principles were concrete and specific ("The social worker should under no circumstances engage in sexual activities with clients" and "The social worker should respect confidences shared by colleagues in the course of their professional relationships and transactions" [principle III.J.2]), whereas others were more abstract, asserting ethical ideals ("The social worker should promote the general welfare of society" [principle VI.P] and "The social worker should uphold and advance the values, ethics, knowledge, and mission of the profession" [principle V.M]).

The 1979 code was revised twice (NASW 1990, 1993), eventually including 70 principles. In 1990 several principles related to solicitation of clients and fee splitting were modified following an inquiry into NASW policies by the U.S. Federal Trade Commission (FTC), begun in 1986, concerning possible restraint of trade. As a result of the FTC inquiry, principles in the code were revised to remove prohibitions concerning solicitation of clients from colleagues of one's agency and to modify wording related to accepting compensation for making a referral. NASW also entered into a consent agreement with the FTC concerning issues raised by the inquiry.

In 1993 the NASW Delegate Assembly voted to further amend the code of ethics to include five new principles, three related to the problem of social worker impairment and two related to the challenge of dual and multiple relationships. The first three principles addressed instances when social workers' own problems and impairment interfere with their professional functioning, and the latter two addressed the need to avoid social, business, and other nonprofessional relationships with clients because of the possibility of conflicts of interest (NASW, 1993).

The 1993 Delegate Assembly also passed a resolution to establish a task force to draft an entirely new code of ethics for submission to the 1996 Delegate Assembly. The task force was established in an effort to develop a new code of ethics that would be far more comprehensive in scope and relevant to contemporary practice. Since the adoption of the 1979 code, social workers had developed a keener grasp of a wide range of ethical issues facing practitioners, many of which were not addressed in the NASW code. The broader field of professional ethics (also called practical ethics), which had emerged in the early 1970s, had matured considerably, resulting in the identification and greater understanding of novel and challenging ethical issues not addressed in the 1979 code. Especially during the 1980s, scholarly analyses of ethical issues in the professions generally, and social work in particular, burgeoned. (For discussion of this development and the factors that accounted for it, see the article "Ethics and Values" elsewhere in this volume).

The Current NASW Code of Ethics

The Code of Ethics Revision Committee was appointed in 1994 and spent two years drafting a new code. The committee, which was chaired by this author and included a professional ethicist and social workers from a variety of practice and educational settings, carried out its work in three phases. The committee first reviewed literature on social work ethics and professional ethics generally to identify key concepts and issues that might be addressed in the new code. The committee also reviewed the 1979 code to identify content that should be retained or deleted and areas where content might be added. The committee then discussed possible ways of organizing the new code to enhance its relevance and use in practice.

During the second phase, which overlapped with phase one activities, the committee issued formal invitations to all NASW members and to members of various social work organizations to suggest issues that might be addressed in the new code. The committee then reviewed its list of relevant content areas drawn from the literature and from public comment and developed a number of rough drafts, the last of which was shared with a small group of ethics experts in social work and other professions for their comments.

In the third phase, the committee made a number of revisions based on the feedback it received from the experts who reviewed the document, published a copy of the draft code in the January 1996 issue of the *NASW News*, and invited NASW members to submit comments to be considered by the committee as it prepared the final draft for submission to the 1996 Delegate Assembly. In addition, during this last phase, members of the committee met with each of the NASW Delegate Assembly regional coalitions to discuss the code's development and receive delegates' comments and feedback. The code was then presented to and ratified by the Delegate Assembly in August 1996 and implemented in January 1997.

Several modest changes have been made to the current code since its ratification. In 1999 a clause was deleted from one standard (1.07[c]) because of concern about possible misinterpretation and risk to clients. The problematic clause stated that social workers are obligated to disclose confidential information without clients' permission when laws or regulations require disclosure. Some social workers were concerned that this statement might require members of the profession to disclose the identity of, and sensitive information about, undocumented immigrants, contrary to social workers' commitment to clients. In 2008, the NASW Delegate Assembly approved adding the phrase "gender identity or expression" to standards pertaining to cultural competence and social diversity; respect for colleagues; discrimination; and social and political action. This added language supplemented references in the code to insensitivity and discrimination related to individuals' race, ethnicity, national origin, color, sex, sexual orientation, age, marital status, political belief, religion, immigration status, and mental or physical disability.

The code, which contains the most comprehensive statement of ethical standards in social work, includes four major sections. The first section, "Preamble," summarizes social work's mission and core values. This is the first time in NASW's history that its code of ethics has contained a formally sanctioned mission statement and an explicit summary of the profession's core values. The mission statement emphasizes social work's historic and enduring commitment to enhancing human well-being and helping meet the basic needs of all people, with particular attention to the needs and empowerment of people who are vulnerable, oppressed, and living in poverty. The mission statement clearly reflects social work's unique concern about vulnerable populations and the profession's simultaneous focus on individual well-being and the environmental forces that create, contribute to, and address problems in living. The preamble also highlights social workers' determination to promote social justice and social change with and on behalf of clients.

The preamble also identifies six core values on which social work's mission is based: service, social justice, dignity and worth of the person, importance of human relationships, integrity, and competence. The Code of Ethics Revision Committee settled on these core values after systematically reviewing the literature on the subject.

The second section, "Purpose of the NASW Code of Ethics," provides an overview of the code's main functions and a brief guide for dealing with ethical issues or dilemmas in social work practice. This section alerts social workers to the code's various purposes:

- to set forth broad ethical principles that reflect the profession's core values and establish ethical standards to guide social work practice;
- to help social workers identify relevant considerations when professional obligations, conflicts, or ethical uncertainties arise;
- to familiarize practitioners new to the field with social work's mission, values, and ethical standards;
- to provide ethical standards to which the general public can hold the social work profession accountable, and
- to articulate standards that the profession itself (and other bodies that choose to adopt the code, such as licensing and regulatory boards, professional liability insurance providers, courts of law, agency boards of directors, and government agencies) can use to assess whether social workers have engaged in unethical conduct.

This section's brief guide for dealing with ethical issues highlights various resources social workers should consider when faced with difficult ethical decisions. Such resources include ethical theory and decision making, social work practice theory and research, laws, regulations, agency policies, and other relevant codes of ethics. Social workers are encouraged to obtain ethics consultation when appropriate, perhaps from an agency-based or social work organization's ethics committee, regulatory bodies (for example, a state licensing board), knowledgeable colleagues, supervisors, or legal counsel.

One of the key features of this section of the code is its explicit acknowledgement that instances sometimes arise in social work in which the code's values, principles, and standards conflict. The code does not provide a formula for resolving such conflicts and "does not specify which values, principles, and standards are most important and ought to outweigh others in instances when they conflict" (NASW, 2008, p. 3). The code states that "reasonable differences of opinion can and do exist among social workers with respect to the ways in which values, ethical principles, and ethical standards should be rank-ordered when they conflict. Ethical decision making in a given situation must apply the informed judgment of the individual social worker and should also consider how the issues would be judged in a peer review process where the ethical standards of the profession would be applied.… Social workers' decisions and actions should be consistent with the spirit as well as the letter of this "Code" (NASW, 2008, p. 3).

The code's third section, "Ethical Principles," presents six broad ethical principles that inform social work practice, one for each of the six core values cited in the preamble. The principles are presented at a fairly high level of abstraction to provide a conceptual base for the profession's more specific ethical standards. The code also includes a brief annotation for each of the principles. For example, the ethical principle associated with the value "importance of human relationships" states that "social workers recognize the central importance of human relationships" (p. 6). The annotation states that "social workers understand that relationships between and among people are an important vehicle for change. Social workers engage people as partners in the helping process. Social workers seek to strengthen relationships among people in a purposeful effort to promote, restore, maintain, and enhance the well-being of individuals, families, social groups, organizations, and communities" (p. 6).

The code's final section, "Ethical Standards," includes 155 specific ethical standards to guide social workers'

conduct and provide a basis for adjudication of ethics complaints filed against NASW members. The standards fall into six categories concerning social workers' ethical responsibilities to clients, to colleagues, in practice settings, as professionals, to the profession, and to society at large. The introduction to this section of the code states explicitly that some of the standards are enforceable guidelines for professional conduct and some are standards to which social workers should aspire. Furthermore, the code states, "the extent to which each standard is enforceable is a matter of professional judgment to be exercised by those responsible for reviewing alleged violations of ethical standards" (p. 7).

In general, the code's standards concern three kinds of issues (Reamer, 2003, 2009, 2013). The first includes what can be described as "mistakes" social workers might make that have ethical implications. Examples include leaving confidential documents displayed in public areas in such a way that they can be read by unauthorized persons or forgetting to include important details in a client's informed consent document. The second category includes issues associated with difficult ethical decisions—for example, whether to disclose confidential information to protect a third party from harm, barter with low-income clients who want to exchange goods for social work services, or terminate services to a noncompliant client. The final category includes issues pertaining to social worker misconduct, such as exploitation of clients, boundary violations, or fraudulent billing for services rendered.

Ethical Responsibilities to Clients

The first section of the code's ethical standards is the most detailed. It addresses a wide range of issues involved in the delivery of services to individuals, families, couples, and small groups of clients. In particular, this section focuses on social workers' commitment to clients, clients' right to self-determination, informed consent, professional competence, cultural competence and social diversity, conflicts of interest, privacy and confidentiality, client access to records, sexual relationships and physical contact with clients, sexual harassment, the use of derogatory language, payment for services, clients who lack decision-making capacity, interruption of services, and termination of services.

Unlike the 1960 and 1979 codes, the current *NASW Code of Ethics* acknowledges that although social workers' primary responsibility is to clients, instances can arise when "social workers responsibility to the larger society or specific legal obligations may on limited occasions supersede the loyalty owed clients" (standard 1.01, p. 7). Examples include when a social worker is required by law to report that a client has abused a child or has threatened to harm self or others. In a similar vein, the code also acknowledges that clients' right to self-determination, which social workers ordinarily respect, may be limited when clients' actions or potential actions pose a serious, foreseeable, and imminent risk to themselves or others.

Standards on informed consent were added to the current code specifying the elements that should be included when social workers obtain consent from clients or potential clients for the delivery of services; the use of electronic media such as computers, telephone, radio, and television, to provide services; audio- or videotaping of clients; third-party observation of clients who are receiving services; and release of information.

Another section added to the current code pertains to the subject of cultural competence and social diversity. In recent years social workers have enhanced their understanding of the relevance of cultural and social diversity in their work with clients, in communities, and in organizations. The code requires that social workers take reasonable steps to understand and be sensitive to clients' cultures and social diversity with respect to race, ethnicity, national origin, color, sex, sexual orientation, gender identity or expression, age, marital status, political belief, religion, and mental or physical disability.

Unlike earlier versions of the code of ethics, the current code pays substantial attention to the topics of conflicts of interest and problematic dual or multiple relationships, for example, involving social workers' social relationships with former clients or when social workers provide services to two or more persons who have a relationship with each other.

The current code substantially expands the profession's standards on privacy and confidentiality. Noteworthy are details concerning social workers' obligation to disclose confidential information to protect third parties from serious harm; confidentiality guidelines when working with families, couples, or groups; disclosure of confidential information to third-party payers; discussion of confidential information in public and semipublic areas; disclosure of confidential information during legal proceedings (privileged information); protection of clients' written and electronic records; the use of case material in teaching and training; and protection of the confidentiality of deceased clients. The code requires social workers to discuss confidentiality policies and guidelines as soon as possible in the social worker–client relationship and as needed throughout the course of the relationship.

The current code has also expanded standards related to social workers' sexual relationships with current and former clients, clients' relatives, and other individuals with whom clients maintain a close, personal relationship. Also included is a standard concerning appropriate and inappropriate physical contact with clients.

An unprecedented section of the code focuses on social workers' use of barter—that is, accepting goods or services from clients as payment for professional service. After considerable discussion, the Code of Ethics Revision Committee decided to stop short of banning bartering outright, recognizing that in some communities bartering is a widely accepted form of payment. However, the code advises social workers to avoid bartering because of the potential for conflicts of interest, exploitation, and inappropriate boundaries in social workers' relationships with clients.

The code also includes extensive guidelines concerning social workers' termination of services to clients. The code focuses primarily on termination of services when clients no longer need services, when clients have not paid an overdue balance, and when social workers leave an employment setting.

Ethical Responsibilities to Colleagues
This section of the code addresses issues concerning social workers' relationships with professional colleagues. These include respect for colleagues; proper treatment of confidential information shared by colleagues; interdisciplinary collaboration and disputes among colleagues; consultation with colleagues; referral for services; and sexual relationships with and sexual harassment of colleagues.

The current code particularly strengthens ethical standards pertaining to impaired, incompetent, and unethical colleagues. Social workers who have direct knowledge of a social work colleague's impairment (which may be caused by personal problems, psychosocial distress, substance abuse, or mental health difficulties, and which interferes with practice effectiveness), incompetence, or unethical conduct, are required to consult with that colleague when feasible; assist the colleague in taking remedial action; and if these measures do not address the problem satisfactorily, take action through appropriate channels established by employers, agencies, NASW, licensing bodies, and other professional organizations.

Ethical Responsibilities in Practice Settings
This section of the code addresses a wide range of issues pertaining to social work supervision; consultation; education and training; performance evaluation; client records; billing for services; client transfer; agency administration; continuing education and staff development; commitments to employers; and

labor–management disputes. Standards in this section state that social work supervisors, consultants, educators, and trainers should avoid engaging in any dual or multiple relationships when there is a risk of exploitation or potential harm. Another standard requires that social workers who function as educators or field instructors for students should take reasonable steps to ensure that clients are routinely informed when services are being provided by students.

Several standards pertain to client records. The current code enhances documentation standards to which social workers are held. In particular, the code requires that records include sufficient, accurate, and timely documentation to facilitate the delivery of services and ensure continuity of services provided to clients in the future. Documentation should avoid gratuitous detail and include only information that is directly relevant to the delivery of services. The code also spells out expectations concerning protection of clients' privacy, record storage and retention, and accurate billing for services.

The code urges social workers to be particularly careful when an individual who is receiving services from another agency or colleague contacts a social worker for services. Several standards are designed to protect clients from exploitation and to avoid conflicts of interest. The code requires social workers to discuss with potential clients the nature of their current relationship with other service providers and the implications, including possible benefits and risks, of entering into a relationship with a new service provider. If a new client has been served by another agency or colleague, social workers should discuss with the client whether consultation with the previous service provider is in the client's best interest.

The code greatly expands coverage of ethical standards related to agency administration. Key issues involve social work administrators' obligation to advocate for resources to meet clients' needs; provide adequate staff supervision; allocate resources fairly; ensure a working environment consistent with code standards; and arrange for appropriate continuing education and staff development.

The code also includes a number of ethical standards for social work employees, for example, related to unethical personnel practices and misappropriation of agency funds. Especially important are standards concerning social workers' obligation to address employing organizations' policies, procedures, regulation, or administrative orders that interfere with the ethical practice of social work.

A novel feature of the code is the acknowledgement of ethical issues social workers sometimes face

as a result of labor–management disputes. Although the code does not prescribe how social workers should handle dilemmas related to going on strike, it does permit social workers to engage in organized labor-related actions to improve services to clients and working conditions.

Ethical Responsibilities as Professionals

This section of the code focuses on issues primarily related to social workers' professional integrity. In addition to emphasizing social workers' obligation to be proficient, the code exhorts social workers to routinely review and critique the professional literature; participate in continuing education; and base their work on recognized knowledge, including empirically based knowledge, relevant to social work practice and ethics.

Several standards address social workers' values and personal conduct. The code states that social workers should not practice, condone, facilitate, or collaborate with any form of discrimination and should not permit their private conduct to interfere with their ability to fulfill their professional responsibilities. The code further obligates social workers to make clear distinctions between statements and actions engaged in as a private individual and those engaged in as a social worker.

A prominent theme in the code concerns social workers' obligation to be honest in their relationships with all parties, including accurately representing their professional qualifications, credentials, education, competence, and affiliations. Also, social workers are obligated to take responsibility and credit, including authorship credit, only for work they have actually performed and to which they have contributed. In addition, the code requires that social workers not engage in uninvited solicitation of potential clients who, because of their circumstances, are vulnerable to undue influence, manipulation, or coercion.

One of the most important standards in the code concerns social workers' personal impairment. The code mandates that social workers must not allow their personal problems, psychosocial distress, legal problems, substance abuse, or mental health difficulties to interfere with their professional judgment and performance or jeopardize others for whom they have a professional responsibility. In instances where social workers find that their personal difficulties interfere with their professional judgment and performance, they are obligated to seek professional help, make adjustments in their workload, terminate their practice, or take other steps necessary to protect clients and others.

Ethical Responsibilities to the Profession

Social workers' ethical responsibilities are not limited to clients, colleagues, and the public at large; they also include the social work profession itself. Standards in this section of the code focus on the profession's integrity and social work evaluation and research. The principal theme concerning the profession's integrity pertains to social workers' obligation to maintain and promote high standards of practice by engaging in appropriate study and research, teaching, publication, presentations at professional conferences, consultation, service to the community and professional organizations, and legislative testimony.

The code also includes a substantial series of standards concerning evaluation and research. The standards emphasize social workers' obligation to monitor and evaluate policies, implementation of programs, and practice interventions. In addition, the code requires social workers to critically examine and keep current with emerging knowledge and to use evaluation and research evidence in their professional practice.

The code requires social workers involved in evaluation and research to follow widely accepted guidelines concerning the protection of evaluation and research participants. Standards focus specifically on the role of informed consent procedures in evaluation and research; the need to ensure that evaluation and research participants have access to appropriate supportive services; the confidentiality and anonymity of information obtained during the course of evaluation and research; the obligation to report results accurately; and the handling of potential or real conflicts of interest and dual relationships involving evaluation and research participants.

Ethical Responsibilities to Society at Large

The social work profession has always been committed to social justice. This commitment is clearly reflected in the code's preamble and in the final section of the code's standards. The standards explicitly highlight social workers' obligation to engage in activities that promote social justice and the general welfare of society, including local, national, and international efforts. These activities may include facilitating public discussion of social policy issues; providing professional services in public emergencies; engaging in social and political action (for example, lobbying and legislative advocacy) to address basic human needs; promoting conditions that encourage respect for the diversity of cultures and socieeties; and acting to prevent and eliminate domination, exploitation, and discrimination against any person, group, or class of people.

Conclusion

Ethical standards in social work, particularly as reflected in the NASW Code of Ethics, have changed dramatically during the profession's history. Along with all other professions, and largely as a result of the emergence of the professional ethics field beginning in the 1970s, social work's ethical standards have matured considerably. The current NASW Code of Ethics reflects social workers' increased understanding of ethical issues in the profession and the need for comprehensive ethical standards.

By themselves, ethical standards in social work cannot guarantee ethical behavior. Ethical standards can certainly guide practitioners who encounter ethical challenges and establish norms by which social workers' actions can be judged. However, in the final analysis, ethical standards in general, and codes of ethics in particular, are only one tool in social workers' ethical arsenal. In addition to specific ethical standards, social workers must draw on ethical theory, concepts, and decision-making guidelines; social work theory and practice principles; and relevant laws, regulations, and agency policies. Most of all, social workers must consider ethical standards within the context of their own values and ethics. As the NASW Code of Ethics states, ethical principles and standards "must be applied by individuals of good character who discern moral questions and, in good faith, seek to make reliable ethical judgments" (p. 4).

REFERENCES

Banks, S. (2012). Ethics and values in social work. Basingstoke, Hampshire, England: Palgave Macmillan.

Banks, S., & Gallagher, A. (2009). Ethics in professional life. Basingstoke, Hampshire, England: Palgave Macmillan.

Barsky, A. (2010). Ethics and values in social work. New York: Oxford University Press.

Bayles, M. (1986). Professional power and self-regulation. Business and Professional Ethics Journal, 5, 26–46.

Dolgoff, R., Harrington, D., & Loewenberg, F. (2012). Ethical decisions for social work practice (9th ed.). Belmont, CA: Brooks/Cole.

Greenwood, E. (1957). Attributes of a profession. Social Work, 2, 44–55.

Hall, R. H. (1968). Professionalization and bureaucratization. American Sociological Review, 33, 92–104.

Jamal, K., & Bowie, N. (1995). Theoretical considerations for a meaningful code of ethics. Journal of Business Ethics, 14, 703–714.

Johnson, A. (1955). Educating professional social workers for ethical practice. Social Service Review, 29, 125–136.

Kultgen, J. (1982). The ideological use of professional codes. Business and Professional Ethics Journal, 1, 53–69.

Lindeman, E. (1947). *Social work matures in a confused world*. Albany, NY: State Conference on Social Workers.

McCann, C. W., & Cutler, J. P. (1979). Ethics and the alleged unethical. *Social Work, 24*, 5–8.

National Association of Social Workers. (1960). *NASW code of ethics*. Washington, DC: Author.

National Association of Social Workers. (1979). *NASW code of ethics*. Silver Spring, MD: Author.

National Association of Social Workers. (1990). *NASW code of ethics*. Washington, DC: Author.

National Association of Social Workers. (1993). *NASW code of ethics*. Washington, DC: Author.

National Association of Social Workers. (1996). *NASW code of ethics*. Washington, DC: Author.

National Association of Social Workers. (2008). *NASW code of ethics*. Washington, DC: Author.

Pumphrey, M. W. (1959). *The teaching of values and ethics in social work education*. New York: Council on Social Work Education.

Reamer, F. G. (2003). *Social work malpractice and liability: Strategies for prevention* (2nd ed.). New York: Columbia University Press.

Reamer, F. G. (2006). *Ethical standards in social work: A review of the NASW code of ethics* (2nd ed.). Washington, DC: NASW Press.

Reamer, F. G. (2009). *The social work ethics casebook: Cases and commentary*. Washington, DC: NASW Press.

Reamer, F. G. (2013). *Social work values and ethics* (4th ed.). New York: Columbia University Press.

FREDERIC G. REAMER

OPPRESSION

ABSTRACT: If social workers are to avoid unintended collusion with pervasive oppressive systems and if they are to be successful in promoting social and economic justice, a firm grasp of the nature of oppression with its dynamics of power and its systemic character is required. The concept of oppression is presented here, followed by discussion of its dynamics and common elements and the need for social workers to engage in anti-oppressive practice in order to expose and oppose oppressive relationships and systemic power arrangements.

KEY WORDS: discrimination; power; diversity; racism; privilege; anti-oppressive social work practice

The social work profession has a historic mandate to oppose oppression—a commitment usually stated in terms of challenging social injustice and promoting social and economic justice—that is expressed in the *National Association of Social Workers' Code of Ethics* (NASW, 2008), the *International Declaration of Ethical Principles of Social Work of the International Federation of Social Workers* (IFSW, 2012), and the *Educational Policy and Accreditation Standards of the Council on Social Work Education* (CSWE, 2008).

Oppression Defined

Oppression is a multidimensional social phenomenon, a dynamic and relational group-based concept that is not accidental—though usually unintentional—and which, once integrated into societal institutions and individual consciousness, comes to permeate almost all relations and, depending on the circumstances, involves all individuals in the role of both oppressor and oppressed at one time or another (Gil, 1998; Mullaly, 2002). There are multiple definitions of oppression, all of which have an underlying theme related to the use and misuse of power in human relationships. Oppression is commonly understood as the domination of a powerful group—politically, economically, socially, culturally—over subordinate groups. Another common definition is that oppression is an institutionalized, unequal power relationship—prejudice plus power (Rothenberg, 1988).

Bulhan (1985) defined oppression more specifically as a situation in which one segment of the population acts to prevent another segment from attaining access to resources or acts to inhibit or devalue them to dominate them. Lipman-Blumen (1984, 1994) focused on the institutional nature of oppression as the act of molding, immobilizing, or reducing opportunities, which thereby restrains, restricts, or prevents social, psychological, or economic movement of an individual or group. Pinderhughes (1973) defined oppression as a relatively constant pattern of prejudice and discrimination between a privileged, favored individual and one who is exploited and deprived of privilege due to membership in a devalued group.

Young (2000) suggested that oppression is not based on any one group membership and, as a means of distinguishing among various experiences, identified "five faces" of oppression—exploitation, marginalization, powerlessness, cultural imperialism, and violence—emphasizing that the presence of any of these five experiences or faces constitutes oppression, and that most people experience some combination of these. Frye's (1995) definition focused on the lived experience of oppression as "living...one's life...confined and shaped by forces and barriers which are not accidental or occasional and hence avoidable, but are systematically related to each other in such a way as to catch one between and among them and restrict or penalize motion in any direction" (p. 39).

Dynamics and Common Elements of Oppression

Elements that are common to all oppressions regardless of the target population (Pharr, 1988) serve to both rationalize and maintain oppressive systems. First, oppression always bestows power and advantage on certain people who are regarded as the norm and denies power and advantage to others based on their status as "other" or different. The defined norm (for example, White, male, heterosexual) is the standard of *rightness* against which all "others" are judged; the "other" (that is, not White, not male, not heterosexual) is not only different from the norm, but is also believed and perceived to be inferior and deviant, which then justifies conferring advantage on those who fit the norm and disadvantaging the "other."

A second common element is that all types of oppression are held in place by ideology and violence or the threat of violence. The ideology on which racial oppression is based is that of superiority based on race (that is, white supremacy). Likewise, the ideology on which sexual oppression is based is that of superiority based on gender (that is, male), and the basis for homosexual oppression is an ideology of superiority based on sexual orientation (that is, heterosexuality). Violence, which is used to enforce and maintain all oppressions, comes in many forms and may be physical and direct (for example, lynching, rape, battering, gay bashing) or personal and psychological (for example, name-calling based on dominant ideology and negative stereotypes). Violence may be indirect or institutionalized. For example, it may be associated with high poverty rates, the predominance of men of color in the criminal justice system and on death row, and the reality of police brutality.

A third common element of all oppression is that it is institutionalized. This means that racism, sexism, and heterosexism are built into the norms, traditions, laws, and policies of a society, so that even those who have nonracist, nonsexist, and nonheterosexist beliefs are compelled to act in accordance with institutional interests, that is, "business as usual." Institutionalized racism, for example, ensures white entitlement and benefits regardless of the intentions of individuals in those institutions.

A fourth common element of oppression is the invisibility endured by groups who are oppressed. By keeping the oppression structurally invisible, individuals and groups are socially defined in a way that inhibits recognition of the group's heterogeneity by the dominant group. In addition, the internalization of external sociopolitical judgments that devalue aspects of one's identity inevitably leads to individuals undervaluing and ignoring substantive parts of their own origins and history.

The issue of multiple identities further complicates the dynamics of oppression. Individual conditions of oppression often involve a convergence between aspects of one's experience where one is a target of oppression (for example, as a low-income, disabled female, a Latina, an African American, a gay woman) with other aspects of one's experience as privileged (for example, a middle- or high-income gay person, a disabled Euro American male) (Rose, 2002). Understanding the presence of power, privilege, advantage, or constraints introduced through oppression in one's life draws attention to experiences and realities that may have been denied or minimized and lays the foundation for connecting with others different from oneself.

Implications for Social Work and Future Trends

In well-established oppressive relationships, their structures are invisible to both the subordinate party and the more powerful party. The sources of oppression are embedded within the psychological makeup of all parties, thereby obscuring the realities of the relationships. Thus, the greatest challenge for social work professionals is to uncover, make visible, expose, and oppose oppressive relationships and systemic power arrangements that give privilege and advantage to one group over another. Adopting oppression as the major explanation for social problems and an anti-oppressive social work practice as a way of dealing with problems helps to avoid blaming the victims of social problems, links the personal with the political, and addresses the systemic nature of oppression and thus avoids technical or minor social reform solutions (Mullaly, 2001).

REFERENCES

Council on Social Work Education. (2008). *Educational policy and accreditation standards*. Alexandria, VA: Author.

Frye, M. (1995). Oppression. In M. L. Andersen & P. H. Collins (Eds.), *Race, class, and gender: An anthology* (2nd ed., pp. 37–41). Belmont, CA: Wadsworth.

Gil, D. (1998). *Confronting injustice and oppression: Concepts and strategies for social workers*. New York: Columbia University Press.

International Federation of Social Workers. (2012). *International declaration of ethical principles of social work*. Oslo, Norway: Author.

Lipman-Blumen, J. (1984). *Gender roles and power*. Englewood Cliffs, NJ: Prentice Hall.

Lipman-Blumen, J. (1994). The existential bases of power relationships: The gender role case. In H. L. Radtke & H. J. Stam (Eds.), *Power/gender: Social relations in theory and practice* (pp. 108–135). Thousand Oaks, CA: Sage.

Mullaly, R. (2001). Confronting the politics of despair: Towards the reconstruction of progressive social work in a global economy and postmodern age. *Social Work Education, 20*(3), 303–320.

Mullaly, R. (2002). *Challenging oppression: A critical social work approach*. Don Mills, Ontario: Oxford University Press.

National Association of Social Workers. (2008). *Code of ethics*. Washington, DC: Author.

Pharr, S. (1988). *Homophobia: A weapon of sexism*. Inverness, CA: Chardon Press.

Pinderhughes, C. A. (1973). Racism and psychotherapy. In C. Willie, B. Kramer, & B. Brown (Eds.), *Racism and mental health* (pp. 61–121). Pittsburgh: University of Pittsburgh Press.

Rose, S. (2002, March). Social work at a crossroads: A reflection paper. Presented at the Social Work at the Crossroads

Conference, California State University, Fresno, Department of Social Work Education.

Rothenberg, P. (1988). *Racism and sexism: An integrated study.* New York: St. Martin's Press.

Young, I. M. (2000). Five faces of oppression. In M. Adams, W. J. Blumenfeld, R. Castenada, H. W. Hackman, M. L. Peters, & X. Zuniga (Eds.), *Readings for diversity and social justice* (pp. 35–49). New York: Routledge.

Further Reading

Adams, M., Blumenfeld, W. J., Castenada, R., Hackman, H. W., Peters, M. L., & Zuniga, X. (Eds.), *Readings for diversity and social justice.* New York: Routledge.

Bulhan, H. A. (1985). *Frantz Fanon and the psychology of oppression.* New York: Plenum Press.

Garcia, B., & Van Soest, D. (2006). *Social work practice for social justice: Cultural competence in action, a guide for students.* Alexandria, VA: Council on Social Work Education.

Van Soest, D., & Garcia, B. (2008). *Diversity education for social justice: Mastering teaching skills* (2nd ed.). Alexandria, VA: Council on Social Work Education.

Dorothy Van Soest

ORGANIZATIONAL CHANGE IN HUMAN SERVICE ORGANIZATIONS

Abstract: This is an overview of the field of organizational change as it applies to human service organizations (HSOs). It offers definitions, conceptual models, and perspectives for looking at organizational change, and notes common reasons that organizational change efforts fail. The overview takes the perspective of an agency executive or manager who has the responsibility for initiating and implementing a planned organizational change initiative. It offers a comprehensive, evidence-based model for tactics to use and steps to take, from assessing change readiness and change capacity to institutionalizing and evaluating change outcomes within the organization. Common change methods are reviewed, including those particularly relevant to HSOs, such as implementation science; the use of consultants; and change efforts, which can be initiated by lower-level employees. A research agenda, with particular attention to change tactics, is offered.

Key Words: organizational change; organization development; organizational performance; implementation science; evidence-based practice; leadership; continuous quality improvement; process consultation; action research; planned change; employee attitude surveys; change leadership

Introduction

For the foreseeable future, leaders of human service organizations (HSOs) will need to become increasingly adept at managing and leading change in their organizations. However, the vast literature on organizational change, ranging from scholarly articles to books in the popular management press, which are typically based on only authors' experiences as consultants or on profiles of allegedly successful change leaders, to an academic literature that often focuses on only a limited number of possible variables or on individual case studies, has notable limitations in guiding practice. Defining and measuring success are particularly complex and challenging, and perhaps for that reason success is rarely documented adequately. A particularly rich literature is growing in the area of implementation science; but this literature often focuses only on implementation of evidence-based practices, with less consideration of other types of organizational change.

After a brief review of theories of organizational change, the literature on organizational change in HSOs and some perspectives for viewing organizational change will be reviewed. A conceptual model will be presented, including detailed attention to phases and tactics. Some common organizational change methods, the use of consultants, and change by lower-level staff will be addressed, ending with some implications for research and practice.

Key Theories of Organizational Change

At the broadest level, several theories commonly used to frame discussions of organizational change (Fernandez & Rainey, 2006; Schmid, 2010) are highlighted here, suggesting how they shape views of organizational change.

- *Life cycle theories* suggest that managers should anticipate normal stages of growth (such as needs for a new organization to create formal administrative systems), and that when an organization becomes "mature," it will still need to continue to adapt and change.
- *Evolution theories* suggest that organizations will have to adapt to environmental challenges to survive.
- *Institutional theory* suggests that an organization will follow the trends in its field, such as in the human services, incorporating evidence-based practices, or developing advanced accountability systems.
- *Stakeholder theories* focus on how the organization adapts to satisfy key stakeholders, including funding organizations and community groups.
- *Rational adaptation* approaches suggest that managers can use their human agency to respond to external and internal forces for change.

The focus here is on planned change employing rational adaptation approaches, which see managers as change agents who can assess their environments and other conditions and then purposefully drive change within their organizations, as distinct from organizational change that *happens* to organizations such as when funding is cut or environmental conditions seem to dictate what change must occur. This latter dynamic, change that comes without intention from the organization, can, however, be followed by purposeful, planned organizational change to deal with such negative changes affecting an organization.

Schmid (2010, p. 456) defines organizational change as "the process that occurs in an HSO as a result of external constraints imposed on it or as a result of internal pressures that cause alterations and modifications in the organization's core activity, goals, strategies, structures, and service programs." More specifically, planned organizational change involves leadership and the mobilizing of staff to move the organization to a desired future state using change processes that involve both human and technical aspects of the organization.

Because substantive organizational change often confronts indifference or resistance and leads to discomfort or stress on the part of employees, it is not surprising that many change efforts fail. Many initiatives fail because they are introduced in an authoritarian way. Kotter (1996) found several commonalities in failed change efforts, including allowing too much complacency, undercommunicating the change vision, permitting obstacles such as existing systems to block the new vision, declaring victory too soon, and neglecting to anchor changes firmly in the corporate culture. The change model described below addresses these factors and others that contribute to failed efforts.

Organizational Change in Human Service Organizations

In HSOs, seminal writing on organizational change began over 30 years ago (Resnick & Patti, 1980), and has been addressed sporadically in the human services literature. In recent years, it has received increasing attention.

Austin (2004) and others described over 20 cases of change in public human service agencies, with many based on the expectations of the Federal welfare reform legislation of 1996. Implementing evidence-based practices (Austin, 2008), knowledge management processes (Austin, Claassen, Vu, & Mizrahi, 2008), and implementation science (for example, Proctor et al., 2009) are other examples.

There have been some attempts to develop comprehensive models of organizational change in the

human services. Glisson (2012) has provided evidence of the usefulness of the ARC (availability, responsiveness, and continuity) organizational intervention model, which involves the use of trained change agents to help change culture, climate, and performance in human service programs. This model notes the critical importance of the organizational context, specifically, social, strategic, and technical factors that impact prospects for improving program operations and outcomes. Models from Proehl (2001) and Lewis, Packard, and Lewis (2012, ch. 11) suggest steps to be taken in the change process, while acknowledging that tactics and principles are applied at different points based on the uniqueness of a situation. The Sanctuary Model (Esaki et al., 2013) is another model of organizational change in HSOs, and includes training, skill development through technical assistance and consultation, and the use of tools such as fidelity checklists and manuals.

Ultimately, in spite of the importance of organizational change in the human services, research to support theory and practice models has been "fragmented, inconclusive, and sometimes even contradictory" (Jaskyte, 2003, p. 26). Glisson (2012) eloquently summarized the limitations in this literature, from poor specification of intervention strategies to inadequate outcome measures. With the exception of the research on ARC by Glisson and colleagues (for example, Glisson et al., 2010) and implementation science, much published research involves case studies only, often with weak theory; quantitative studies generally do not build on or connect with relevant earlier research or models.

Perspectives on Organizational Change

There are multiple perspectives from which to view organizational change. At the broadest level, organizational change may be planned or unplanned. The focus here will be on planned change, as defined above.

Organizations and staffs change in small ways, such as developing new procedures, perhaps without even considering that change is occurring. Beyond daily changes, there are three levels of increasing intensity of change. Anderson and Ackerman-Anderson (2010) have described these levels of organizational change. *Developmental change* involves adjustments to existing operations or improving a skill, method, or process that does not currently meet the organization's standard. This level of change is the least threatening to employees and the easiest to manage. Examples include simple problem solving, routine training, and improving communications. *Transitional change* involves implementing something new and abandoning old ways of functioning. This move through a transitional period to a new future state requires patience and time. Examples include basic reorganizations, new technology systems, and implementing a new program. The most extreme form of change is *transformational change*, which requires major shifts in vision, strategy, structure, or systems. This might evolve out of necessity, for example, as a result of major policy changes such as managed care or a shift to outcomes measurement or performance-based contracting required by funding organizations. The new state after such change involves a new culture, new beliefs, and awareness of new possibilities.

While minor changes can happen on an almost regular basis, *punctuated equilibrium theory* (Gersick, 1991) suggests that sometimes an organization in a state of equilibrium is forced to deal with "revolutionary" forces, such as, in HSOs, welfare reform and evidence-based practice. For such larger-scale changes, the use of the process discussed below should enhance the prospects of the organization reaching its desired new state. Consultants may also be brought into any change process as appropriate.

Organizational change can be described based on the distinctions between change *content* and change *process*. Change *content*, according to Anderson and Ackerman-Anderson (2010), looks at "what in the organization needs to change, such as structure, systems, business processes, technology, products, or services" (p. 52). Change *process* includes, according to Armenakis and Bedeian (1999), the phases of change and what is referred to as change tactics. Similarly, Anderson and Ackerman-Anderson see the change process as the way in which the content changes will be planned, designed, and implemented, including the human dynamics of change, such as individual mindsets and organizational culture.

Organizational change can also be viewed in terms of its context (Armenakis & Bedeian, 1999). Change context includes both external and internal factors. External contextual factors include environmental changes such as new governmental policies, decreases in funding, and expectations for greater accountability to funding organizations. Developments such as welfare reform, evidence-based practice, performance-based contracting, and managed care have precipitated needs for organizational change, requiring that HSOs adapt to these new expectations and make changes to organizational systems.

Internal contextual factors such as management capacity and program capacity (Sowa, Selden, & Sandfort, 2004) can suggest needs for change and can affect the way an organization responds to change. These need to be addressed when assessing, planning, and implementing change and are discussed in more detail in the Assessment section.

Change content includes the goals and targets for change: a desired future state and the aspects of the organization that need to be changed, such as changing organizational structures. Change process includes the tactics and methods used by change leaders, including methods such as Total Quality Management and organization development (OD).

A Conceptual Model of Planned Organizational Change

Within these perspectives, planned change can be seen as a series of steps, including setting a change goal, assessing organizational conditions, choosing a strategy, implementing the change process using change tactics and specific change technologies (methods), and assessing outcomes of the change process.

While this can be seen as a phase model suggesting sequential activities, it is in fact dynamic: steps may be repeated or modified based on experiences during the process. A change process typically starts with identifying a change need or opportunity and framing it as a goal. An assessment process may have begun before goal setting, but in any case, an assessment of the organization's current state is a necessary step. This would typically be followed by strategy selection and decisions about tactics and methods. After completion of the change process, outcomes would be assessed with reference to original change goals.

A non-linear aspect of this model can be seen by the notion that an executive should be routinely assessing the organization's current state (external and internal contexts) and looking for opportunities for improvement. Assessment thus includes looking at current conditions in terms of what needs to be addressed, and what internal factors need to be considered in developing a change goal and plan.

The Change Goal

A planned change initiative typically begins by identifying a need or opportunity, often through an organization's executive assessing the organization's external and internal conditions. External conditions include changing priorities or demands from the organization's funders or other stakeholders, threats such as decreases in funding, and new opportunities for the organization based on identified community needs. Internal conditions could include program quality or the need to adopt more evidence-based models, the need for enhanced cultural competence, management process issues such as an inadequate performance measurement system, or significant morale issues with staff.

After some amount of assessment, the organization's leaders (typically upper management staff) identify the *content* of the change needed. This may range from addressing funding cuts to creating a new service delivery system. Changing organizational culture (Glisson, 2007) or implementing an evidence-based practice (Austin & Claassen, 2008) are common change goals.

Any change initiative should be driven by and be consistent with the organization's current and planned strategy. If the agency does not have a current strategic plan, then a strategic planning process may be the first change activity. At a deeper level, if the absence of a strategic plan is reflective of inadequate management capacity overall, then a first change activity may involve building management capacity, through management consultation, training, and/or leadership development.

In the absence of an urgently needed change, an agency executive may simply have a desire to improve the organization's functioning or outcomes in some way, and may thus need to do a full assessment of organizational functioning to identify specific areas for improvement. Assessment in this sense, which typically precedes the identification of a change goal, is addressed in the next section.

In either case, once a change goal has been identified, doing an assessment of organizational conditions can help to both identify leverage points and targets for change and also identify additional change opportunities.

Assessment

Doing an assessment as part of organizational change involves two layers: process and content. Assessment regarding the process of change looks at factors including the organization's readiness and capacity for change and possible sources of resistance. Assessment regarding content includes identification of problems, issues, or conditions in the organization that may benefit from organizational change.

ASSESSING THE PROCESS ASPECTS OF CHANGE   Early work on assessing the process of change focused on *resistance* to change. While resistance has received considerable attention, the concept has recently been reexamined (Ford & Ford, 2009). It is now seen in a broader context, which includes *readiness* (Bouckenooghe, 2010). Readiness can be simply defined as "the extent to which an individual or individuals are

cognitively and emotionally inclined to accept, embrace, and adopt a particular plan to purposefully alter the status quo" (Holt, Armenakis, Feild, & Harris, 2007, p. 239).

Assessments of readiness typically consider factors such as staff beliefs in the need for the change, staff feeling capable of implementing a proposed change, the proposed change being seen as beneficial to staff and appropriate for and beneficial to the organization, leader commitment to the proposed change (that is, management support), and a supportive organizational climate (for example, cohesion, trust, support, communication, low stress).

Several instruments to assess readiness for change have been developed (for example, Bouckenooghe, Devos, & Van den Broeck, 2009). Cinite, Duxbury, and Higgins (2009) have developed a measure of readiness for public sector organizations.

More recently, the concept *capacity for change*, defined as "a combination of managerial and organizational capabilities that allows an enterprise to adapt more quickly and effectively than its competition to changing situations" (Judge & Douglas, 2009, pp. 635–636), has received attention. A change capacity scale developed by Judge and Douglas includes these dimensions:

- Trustworthy leaders
- Trusting followers
- Capable champions
- Involved mid-management
- Innovative culture
- Accountable culture
- Systems thinking
- Systems communication

Readiness and change capacity should also look at the styles and philosophies of the change leaders, such as participative or directive styles of leadership. According to Burke (2011, p. 248), a change leader should have a tolerance for ambiguity, accept not being able to control everything, understand how feelings affect behavior, and be open to shared decision making. Battilana, Gilmartin, Sengul, Pache, and Alexander (2010) noted the importance of competencies including person-oriented behaviors such as interpersonal skills and emotional intelligence, and task-oriented behaviors including a focus on goals and outcomes of the change process. Gilley, McMillan, and Gilley (2009) identified coaching, motivating, communicating, and team building as characteristics of leadership effectiveness in organizational change.

Some research has examined individual employee factors that are relevant in organizational change implementation, including commitment to change (Jaros, 2010; Parish, Cadwaller, & Busch, 2008), tolerance for ambiguity, cynicism, and beliefs about change (Walker, Armenakis, & Bernerth, 2007); self-competence, self-confidence, and self-efficacy (Austin & Claassen, 2008); and feelings of empowerment (Lamm & Gordon, 2010).

Beyond the individual level, organizational culture and climate are seen as essential factors when planning organizational change (Austin & Claassen, 2008), particularly in terms of assessing possible reactions to the change.

The change agents can use this assessment to identify strengths that can be used to support the process, and, perhaps more importantly, to identify aspects of readiness and change capacity that should be increased before beginning the process. Increasing readiness and capacity can, in fact, be seen as a preliminary change goal and activity.

Assessing Content: What Needs to be Changed

If there is a clearly defined goal, such as implementing an evidence-based practice, the only assessment needed may be regarding the process of change discussed above. However, if an administrator does not have a clearly focused change goal but thinks that change is needed because of factors such as poor service quality or low morale, a full assessment may be needed to identify factors contributing to organizational problems: the *content* of change.

Assessing at the content level involves examining the current functioning of the organization: how well it is doing with respect to factors such as leadership, management processes and systems, program quality, mission and strategy, organizational structure, the transformation processes (for example, service delivery), and employee perspectives (for example, satisfaction, organizational climate), considering how each of these affect desired outputs or outcomes. Also important are organizational system dynamics and alignment or fit across these factors. Diagnostic models (for example, Burke, 2011) provide conceptual frameworks for assessing these and other factors. Assessments of management capacity (the effectiveness of management processes) and program capacity (effectiveness of programs) (Sowa et al., 2004) are increasingly being used in the nonprofit arena.

Strategies

Based on the change goals and assessment of conditions outside and within the organization, broad change strategies are selected. A change strategy may be defined as "the general design or plan of action," contrasted with tactics, "the concrete and specific actions that flow from the strategy" (Lauer cited in Connor, Lake, & Stackman, 2003, p. 122).

One classic conceptualization of change strategies suggests that organizational change can be based on rational and analytical methods, attention to individual and interpersonal processes, or the use of power (Burke, 2011, pp. 183–186). Empirical-rational strategies assume that "people are rational and that they will follow their rational self-interest once it is made apparent to them" (p. 183). In this approach, research findings and analytical techniques are used by change leaders to show what needs to be done and what change processes should be used. Normative-reeducative strategies assume that "people conform and are committed to sociocultural norms" (pp. 184–185). This strategy is reflected in the use of extensive employee participation in the change process through techniques such as group problem solving. Power-coercive strategies suggest using power, for example, by applying "political and economic sanctions for noncompliance with the proposed change" (p. 186). The literature on organizational change seems to tend toward a use of a normative-reeducative strategy, sometimes augmented by the use of analytical techniques such as Total Quality Management. The tactics discussed next are generally most compatible with a normative-reeducative strategy.

Organizational Change Steps and Tactics

Much has been written about change tactics, often in a "how to" format, suggesting specifically what change leaders should do in working with people in the organization to make the change happen. However, much of this literature is not based on strong evidence, suggesting promising opportunities to assess evidence on the use of commonly proposed change tactics. A preliminary study of the use of the tactics below (Packard, 2010) found statistically significant differences in their use between successful and unsuccessful change processes.

The model of organizational change presented here is appropriate for transitional and transformational change as described above. A leader may initiate an organizational change process to meet a particular need or goal, such as moving the organization from a process-oriented to an outcomes-oriented culture, implementing an evidence-based practice, or addressing significant funding cuts. This model includes eight steps. Within each step, specific tactics are used to implement the process.

Although the steps below are presented in a linear fashion, they may at times overlap or be addressed in a different sequence, based on specific organizational conditions. Throughout the process, change leaders should be alert to human factors, including staff resistance and their need to be informed of activities. Involving staff in the process should have a significant effect on creating staff commitment, as well as leading to better ideas and outcomes.

1. Assess the present

A change initiative typically starts with a change leader such as the executive and her or his management team, and perhaps other staff, who need to develop a clear understanding of the problem, the need for change (the current state), and the desired outcome (the future state). This may involve gathering and assessing available data to focus the change.

Next, the change leader or team can assess the scope of the change and determine the type of change needed. Transitional or transformational change would suggest the use of this change management process.

Change leaders should also determine the extent to which important preconditions for change are present. In a HSO, a core level of management competence, clearly articulated humanistic values, and a participative management philosophy would be desirable preconditions. Substantive change will be less likely with ineffective or authoritarian management, an excessively bureaucratic or political culture, or heavily conflicted management-staff relations. If these conditions exist, then they should be the first targets for change and will require outside consultation.

Other aspects of organizational readiness to consider are likely levels of support and enthusiasm for the change and the capabilities of staff (their skills and abilities).

The leader should also engage in some self-assessment. Burke (2011) has suggested that a change leader should begin a major organizational change initiative with self-examination, focusing on her or his self-awareness, motives, and values, and use insights from this assessment when deciding on change tactics.

2. Create a sense of urgency

The change leader will need to clearly and persuasively communicate the need, desirability, and urgency for the change. Staff may be comfortable and happy with the status quo and feel overworked enough as it is, and therefore may be disinclined to take on a significant change in the way they or their programs operate. A change formula (Beckhard & Pritchard, 1992, p. 75) suggests that change can occur when (a) there is dissatisfaction with the current state, (b) staff has a clear vision of an ideal future state of the organization, (c) there is a clear and feasible process for reaching the desired state, and (d) these factors considered together outweigh the perceived costs of

changing. From an employee's point of view, costs of change can include changes in employees' sense of competence, power or status, workplace relationships, rewards, and identity or roles. Therefore, the change leader can create conditions for change by creating dissatisfaction with the status quo, providing a clear and compelling vision for the new state, and establishing and using an effective and efficient process that minimizes the "costs" to participants.

The change leader can use data to show that if a change is not made, the organization and staff will suffer undesirable consequences, such as loss of clients, loss of funding, a decrease in service quality or productivity, or a serious morale problem. Problems can range from new directives from funders, funding cutbacks, or expectations for improved services to low staff morale, burnout, or inadequate management systems. As much as possible, existing data should be used to demonstrate the urgency for change.

3. Communicate the change vision

In addition to fully articulating the problem needing attention, the vision for success—outcomes for the change—need to be clearly communicated. There needs to be a clear and specific plan for how the change initiative will be implemented, including a basic strategy, who will be involved, and planned activities and persons accountable for them. The plan should also describe how any additional data will be collected and analyzed, and the use of task forces and other change processes. The timeframe for the project and available resources (especially staff time and any necessary financial support) should be noted.

4. Develop and maintain support

Throughout the process, change leaders will need to continuously show support for the process and anticipate and address resistance. Top management, such as the organization's executive, and in some cases the agency's board, should formally show support for the process. A senior executive may take the role of "championing" the cause for change on a regular basis through frequent communication with employees.

Other key individuals and organizations inside and outside the organization (for example, community partner organizations) should be solicited for their support.

The assessments described above to examine change capacity, readiness, and resistance factors can be used to develop plans to enhance change capacity through training, build trust between leaders and followers, create a culture of accountability, enhance readiness through involving staff, and provide managerial and supervisory support.

Adequate resources in terms of staff time and any necessary financial and technological support should be made available. There should be widespread participation of staff in the change process, but staff should not overtaxed.

Resistance will need to be thoughtfully addressed. As Proehl (2001) summarized, people resist for three possible reasons: not knowing about the change, not being able to change, or not being willing to change. Those who do not know about the change can be influenced by change leaders communicating the who, what, when, why, and how of the change, and by getting them involved in the process. Those who feel unable to change can be educated regarding the new knowledge and skills that will be needed during and after the change. This might involve training in problem-solving methods, new management skills, team building, or conflict management. A small number of staff may be unwilling to change. Their concerns should be recognized and addressed through feedback and coaching, showing how they may benefit. Rewards and performance management may be used as needed.

5. Develop an action system

Change leaders should clearly and fully communicate with employees how the change process will be implemented, including basic change activities and people and groups to be involved. Building a broad-based action system with designated responsibility for implementing and overseeing the change initiative serves several functions. If many staff members are involved, then multiple talents can be brought to bear to address the challenges and tasks ahead. Spreading the workload can help ensure that the additional demands of change do not significantly disrupt ongoing work. Additionally, getting staff members involved can increase their sense of ownership of the results.

A large-scale change initiative can be guided and overseen by a "change coalition" (Kotter, 1996) such as an organizational change steering committee that has representatives from all key stakeholder groups in the organization, including different levels of the hierarchy (from executives to line staff), different program and administrative areas, and labor organization representation if appropriate. Most members of the organization must consider this group to be legitimate.

Specific roles should be delineated. An executive can serve as a *sponsor*, who demonstrates organizational commitment to the process and ensures that necessary resources (especially including staff time) are allocated. The key staff person responsible for day-to-day operation of the initiative, perhaps the HR manager, can serve as a *champion* who not only oversees implementation, but also provides ongoing

energy and focus for staff. There will probably be multiple change agents who are responsible for implementation at the unit or team level. They may be task force or problem-solving group chairs, facilitators, or external consultants.

Many other staff should be involved as task force or committee members or involved in data collection and analysis and the design and implementation of new systems or processes. Employees from various management and staff levels should be invited to participate based on their relevant knowledge and skills. People with credibility in the organization, formal or informal power, and particular interest in the problem should be especially considered. People who are directly affected by the problem are particularly important for inclusion.

Finally, organizational systems need to be set up to ensure effective functioning of the process. This includes structural arrangements, such as the reporting relationships of the various committees and task forces, and communication processes to ensure that all staff members are aware of what is happening. Newsletters, email bulletins, all-staff meetings, and reports at regular unit meetings should all be used on an ongoing basis. Communication systems for all the involved groups to coordinate with each other and several mechanisms for communicating progress on the initiative should be developed. Kotter (1996) has said that when it comes to organizational change, "you cannot overcommunicate." Messages about the need for change and what is being done need to be ongoing and frequent.

It is important to address the "human factor." In addition to designing structures, processes, and communication systems, provisions should be made for team building and conflict resolution. Consultants or staff, such as the change champion or human resources staff with relevant training, can fill these roles. Widespread staff participation can be a powerful force in creating staff buy in and commitment while also improving the quality of the change results through the expertise that staff bring to the process.

6. Implement the plan for change

Strategies and processes to implement the change should begin by providing necessary information and training to give staff the capacities to complete assigned change activities. Several of these are more fully detailed in the "Change Methods" section below.

Problem-solving groups, going by various names such as task forces or action teams, are always needed in planned organizational change. Change efforts should usually include the analysis of existing organizational performance data to identify where quality, efficiency, and effectiveness improvements need to be made. Additional data may be gathered as needed. Employee attitude surveys (Burke, 2011) are a very useful way to develop a deeper understanding of employee concerns and needs, and perhaps to assess the current culture and climate of the organization. Survey results can provide guidance for issues to address and strategies for ensuring staff commitment to the process.

For organization-wide change, Business Process Reengineering can be used to identify workflow and coordination improvement opportunities and eliminate processes that do not add value. Organization redesign, if necessary, should include not only traditional restructuring, but also changes in decision-making and communication processes across organizational functions. Workshops using trained facilitators for team building, role clarification, conflict management, and other concerns can often augment the change effort.

An action planning and monitoring system including tasks, persons responsible, and timelines should be used to track progress. Project activities should be revised as appropriate based on new information or changing conditions. Monitoring systems should also be able to identify staff concerns, so that these can be addressed. Progress on the change process should be regularly and fully communicated to all staff. Kotter (1996) and others have emphasized the need for quick successes, to show staff progress that will build credibility for the process, reward those involved, and build momentum.

7. Institutionalize the change

Implementation of new systems should be monitored, with further adjustments made as needed. If goals are not met, then conditions can be reassessed and new plans made and implemented. Changes need to be institutionalized. For example, when a new system is designed, procedures will need to be written and a staff training program developed. Staff will need to be retrained, and training for new staff should reflect the new system. Job descriptions and performance appraisal systems may need to be modified to support the new systems. If culture change was a goal, this, too, will need to be monitored, perhaps using follow-up staff surveys.

Staff should be made aware of the results of the change process. Changes and successes should be celebrated in ways consistent with the organization's culture. Special events can be held when major milestones are met, and smaller successes can be rewarded and celebrated in staff meetings and other arenas. Ideally an outcome of the process would be the creation of organizational systems and an organizational culture committed to ongoing change and development.

8. Evaluate the change

Any changes made should be evaluated to ensure success, using whatever data and evaluation methods are appropriate, such as pre-post data on factors identified for change and improvement. The outcomes of an organizational change effort can be evaluated in terms of both process and content. Evaluation of the change process typically assesses the extent of implementation of the change process as designed (for example, the extent to which the change process plan was followed). If a specific change model, such as ARC, was used, then the change process can be evaluated in terms of model fidelity: the extent to which the model was implemented according to defined standards. Evaluating the content of an organizational change examines its impact in terms of some important aspect of performance such as improved outcomes for consumers, client, and/or stakeholder satisfaction, improved efficiency or cost savings, a better service delivery model, a more appropriate culture and climate, lower turnover, new staff knowledge and skills, increased organizational learning capacity enhanced management capacity, or improved employee quality of working life.

Another important evaluation element is assessing the extent to which the results are institutionalized through formal changes in policies, procedures, staffing structures, or other changes in organizational operations.

Use of Consultants

The process just outlined is a complex one, and may be more manageable with the use of consultants. Such consultants could be internal to the organization, with skilled staff providing guidance on the process and perhaps serving as a coach to executives. In situations in which an administrator or the organization does not have the knowledge or skills to respond to a particular need for change, external consultants can help by providing expertise in specific organizational change methods.

TYPES OF CONSULTATION Yankey and Willen (2006) described two broad types of consultation. The *expert model* involves a content expert, such as a specialist in program evaluation, who applies specific expertise to address a goal the organization identifies. Organizational change typically involves the other type, a *process model*, in which the consultant is in more of a facilitator role, using expertise in change management processes but not giving expert advice on what an organization should do to solve its problem, except by suggesting change technologies to use.

Consultants and clients should thoughtfully consider the needs of the situation and arrange for the best approach. The expert model can be used, for example, if a program has identified a specialized need such as training on work with incest victims or automating an information system. The organization can then solicit consultants with the needed expertise. For complicated situations ranging from poor morale to funding crises, process skills will likely be needed because there will be no easy "right" answer. Ideally, a consultant would have both process skills and expertise in selected areas. For example, in a funding crisis, process skills would be needed to help the client organization sort things out, identify issues, and consider actions; and expertise skills in areas such as strategic planning, budgeting, cost analysis, and fund development would be valuable as well.

SELECTING AND USING CONSULTANTS Yankey and Willen (2006) provide useful guidelines for selecting and using consultants and guidelines for making the consultation useful. They have suggested (2006, p. 414) that consultant interviews should cover not only consultant expertise and previous work, but a consultant's compatibility with the organization's beliefs and values regarding organizational change, ethics, and appreciation for confidentiality.

There should be clarity regarding the consultation goals, reflected in both the request for proposals, if one is used, and in the contract with the consultant chosen. A contract should outline responsible parties and their roles, the problem and goal, individuals and/or units or programs to be involved, consultant "deliverables" (for example, a report, recommendations, services provided), ground rules, fees, and a schedule.

A few commonly used consultation methods to enhance organizational performance will be mentioned here. These are used more frequently in for-profit businesses, which usually have greater resources available for consultation.

Some Common Organizational Change Methods

ORGANIZATION DEVELOPMENT The most fully developed organizational change method is *organization development* (OD): a comprehensive and broad-based set of intervention options including action research, survey feedback, process consultation, and team building. It can be defined as "a system wide application and transfer of behavioral science knowledge to the planned development, improvement, and reinforcement of the strategies, structures, and processes that lead to organization effectiveness" (Cummings & Worley, 2009, pp. 1–2).

An OD initiative often includes the formation of a steering committee with broad representation of different components of the workforce to guide the goal setting, data collection, intervention planning, implementation, and evaluation of the process. Employee involvement in planning and decision making is an important principle of OD. Ultimately, OD is intended to improve organizational functioning and to help achieve the strategic goals of the organization. Change methods, such as those mentioned below, can be used as part of an OD initiative. Many of these can be used individually to address specific problems in a work unit, division, or even the whole organization.

Common OD interventions include team building, problem-solving sessions, training programs to enhance organizational skills, and survey feedback (using employee surveys, which provide diagnostic data about the organization and its current norms and processes through surveys of staff). Process consultation (Schein, 1999), in which the consultant meets individually with a manager to discuss issues and alternatives, much as a counselor does, is another common OD method.

The key to defining an intervention as OD is not the specific strategy used but the roles of the consultant and staff that might be affected by a change. This assumes that the organization and its members must have some control over the change process. Also, regardless of specific consultation activities, an effective OD consultant will follow clear procedures that include problem identification, contracting, assessment, planning, intervention, and evaluation.

In many situations, the assessment process leads not to training or group process interventions, but to changes in organizational systems. If members of an organization are actively involved in the process, then they are likely to be as actively involved in supporting the implementation of solutions.

ACTION RESEARCH *Action research* is a core technology of OD. An OD process typically begins when an agency executive identifies a need for change, such as inadequate program performance, significant employee morale issues, or the need for a new organizational culture. An OD consultant guides the organization through the action research process: data collection to identify problems, issues, or visions; data feedback to staff; analysis of data and action planning; implementation of action plans; additional data collection to assess results; and continuation of the cycle. Common data collection methods are employee attitude surveys, reviews of administrative data such as program performance data, and interviews or focus groups with staff and outside stakeholders.

Problem solving groups are often formed after survey results are fed back to employees to address problems identified by the survey. If team building workshops are being used, they begin with data collection, usually interviews by the consultant, followed by off-site sessions to address issued identified during data collection.

APPRECIATIVE INQUIRY A recent approach to organizational change that offers an option for traditional action research is *appreciative inquiry*. It uses a strengths-based mindset, which looks at what is going well and envisioning even more positive possibilities. It involves "the discovery of what gives 'life' to a living system when it is most effective, alive, and constructively capable in ecological, economic, and human terms" (Cooperrider, Whitney, & Stavros, 2003, p. 3). This innovative approach emphasizes asking positive questions to reveal the positive elements of an organization to help achieve its ideal future.

BUSINESS PROCESS REENGINEERING *Business Process Reengineering* (BPR), sometimes referred to as simply reengineering, reached fad status in the business and government sectors in the 1990s. It has been defined as "a fundamental rethinking and radical redesign of business processes to achieve dramatic improvements in critical contemporary measures of performance such as cost, quality, capital, service, and speed" (Hammer & Champy, 1993, as cited in Grobman, 2008, p. 297).

Reengineering typically involves a thorough examination of the whole organization, focusing on structures and processes. The current organization is assessed, and a new, ideal organization is proposed that eliminates all processes that do not add value for clients or organizational outcomes. Reengineering is sometimes seen as a euphemism for downsizing, and a common result of reengineering is the elimination of management layers and positions. When positions are eliminated, an organization should do everything possible to retain employees in other still-needed positions.

TOTAL QUALITY MANAGEMENT OR CONTINUOUS QUALITY IMPROVEMENT *Total Quality Management* (TQM), more commonly known recently as *Con-* *tinuous Quality Improvement* (CQI), is an organization-wide philosophy and process of continuous improvements in quality by focusing on the control of variation to satisfy customer requirements, including top management support and employee participation and teamwork (Grobman, 2008, pp. 295–296). As contrasted with reengineering, TQM focuses on the line worker level rather than the larger administrative systems and structures. TQM uses structured problem-solving methods such as workflow or process analysis and cause and effect diagrams to analyze work processes, eliminate unnecessary steps, and improve quality.

MANAGEMENT ANALYSIS *Management analysis* is a generic term for expert analysis and audits of management structures, goals and objectives, and processes including organization charts, staff utilization, coordination mechanisms, roles and responsibilities, and work methods to improve efficiency and reduce costs. Recommendations include reorganization, consolidation, downsizing/rightsizing, and, in government settings, sometimes privatization. This is a clear example of Yankey and Willen's "expert" model, although some management analysts attempt to include employees in an analysis of findings and preparation of recommendations to have "buy-in."

LEARNING ORGANIZATIONS AND ORGANIZATIONAL LEARNING *Organizational learning* can be seen as organizational change to the extent that it involves having the organization create a new culture, which is focused on ongoing learning for organizational improvement. In the simplest terms, according to Peter Senge, who popularized the term, learning organizations "are organizations where people continually expand their capacity to create the results they truly desire, where new and expansive patterns of thinking are nurtured, where collective aspiration is set free, and where people are continually learning how to learn together" (2006, p. 3). A related term is organizational learning. According to Gill (2010), "An organization is learning when people are continuously creating, organizing, storing, retrieving, interpreting, and applying information. This information becomes knowledge (and hopefully, wisdom) about improving the work environment; improving performance; improving operational . . . processes; and achieving long-range goals" (p. 6).

CAPACITY BUILDING In the nonprofit arena, *capacity building* can be seen broadly as a change method that can address specifics ranging from improving board of directors functioning to fundraising and management development. Defined as "actions that improve nonprofit effectiveness" (Blumenthal, 2003), capacity building is primarily focused on the *content* of change as defined above, such as strategic planning or fund development.

IMPLEMENTATION SCIENCE As noted above, the implementation of evidence-based practices can be seen as a specific method for organizational change in HSOs, now typically defined as *implementation science*, or *implementation research* (Proctor et al., 2009). After program interventions have been tested for efficacy and effectiveness and have been determined to be evidence-based, thoughtful attention needs to be paid to how they are implemented in organizational settings. While specific implementation models are still evolving, the implementation process typically four stages (Aarons, Hurlburt, & Horwitz, 2011).

At the *exploration* stage, leaders in the organization note a need for change which may come from, for example, a funding organization which requires the use of an evidence-based practice. Assessment of organizational capacity and readiness for the change begins at this stage and needs continuing attention through implementation. At the *adoption decision/ preparation* phase, the organization's leaders decide to implement an EBP, giving particular attention to the allocation of necessary resources and creating a culture and climate in which staff will "take ownership of the process" (p. 11). The *active implementation* phase typically involves allocation of implementation roles for involved staff and intervention developers who offer expertise regarding the practice to be implemented, including ensuring fidelity to the model. After the practice has been implemented, continued use of it needs to be assured through *sustainment* of the practice, including ongoing fidelity to the model and institutionalizing it in the organization's policies, practices, and culture. These stages align well with the stages of generic organizational change described above, but will continue to be informed by the growing body of research on the specifics of implementation science.

STAFF-INITIATED ORGANIZATIONAL CHANGE One final method of organizational change, very different from the others, warrants attention. Often, employees at the line staff level see a need or opportunity for change before administrators do. Change strategies which are initiated by lower-level employees, sometimes referred to as *staff-initiated organizational change*

(SIOC), have been rarely discussed in the professional literature since their appearance in some publications more than twenty five years ago (Holloway, 1987). A recent exception is a book by Cohen and Hyde (2014a) which uses the term "change from below" to offer conceptual frameworks and cases to describe this change method. The model which follows is based primarily on these two sources.

This process as initiated by line workers involves five steps. First, a great deal of attention is given to assessment, including the identification of a problem and selection of a change goal. Data collection, through methods including interviews and focus groups with staff and clients, surveys, and review of agency documents, can be used to refine the problem statement and the change goal. Assessment also includes identifying key actors within the organization, with particular attention to those in decision-making roles. According to Cohen and Hyde (2014b, p. 39), these actors can be classified into three groups. Critical actors are decision makers who have the power to implement the change goal. Their support will be essential. Facilitating actors may have formal or informal power in the organization, and can be helpful in influencing the decision makers. Allies are staff who can support the change effort in other ways.

Cohen and Hyde (2014b) describe the use of a classic organization development technique, the force field analysis (Brager & Holloway, 1993), as a way to provide detailed assessment of these actors and other forces: driving forces which can support or facilitate the change, and restraining forces which will make the change difficult. Unless restraining forces outweigh driving forces so extensively that the change seems impossible, change agents then determine ways to enhance and use the driving forces and minimize or modify the restraining forces. These change agents can be seen as an action system: individuals who have a commonality of interests and concerns regarding the problem and change goal. The potential influence of staff as change agents is assessed, as are the organizational context, risks and benefits to change agents, and attention to the interests and concerns of the organizational decision makers involved.

Based on the force field analysis and analysis of other data gathered, an overall change strategy is chosen. A collaborative strategy is appropriate where there is high agreement among all actors on the change goal. A campaign strategy may be used when the decision makers may not see the need for the change, and a conflict strategy may be needed if the decision makers oppose the change. Cohen and Hyde recommend using the "principle of least contest" (Cohen and Hyde,

2014b, p. 47), which suggests using the least conflictual strategy that can achieve the change goal. After a strategy is chosen, specific tactics can be developed. These can range from persuasion and presenting data on the problem and proposed solutions to decision makers (collaborative) to negotiation or threats (campaign), or demands and actions such as protests and strikes (conflict).

The next stage in Holloway's model, preinitiation, involves change agents assessing and developing their influence and credibility (social capital) and inducing or augmenting stress so that the problem will be addressed. Workers who have been supportive of the organization and in the past have taken initiative to support agency strategies will have built up social capital which should result in upper administration paying more attention to their ideas.

At the initiation stage, the change goal is introduced, with consideration of how it will be seen as conforming to the interests of key decision makers. Representatives meet with decision makers and introduce the change goal and proposal. If the change goal is approved, then the implementation stage includes gaining support and commitment of staff involved and managing resistance, ensuring that implementation expectations are understood.

Finally, institutionalization involves making any necessary adjustments to the plan and then developing standardized procedures for the proposal and linking it with other organizational elements (for example, the policies and procedures manual and agency information systems).

This summary may make the process seem too easy; and, in fact, Holloway also acknowledged the risks faced by lower-level employees proposing potentially controversial ideas.

IMPLICATIONS FOR RESEARCH AND PRACTICE Notable progress has been made in extracting new knowledge and practice principles from case studies (for example, Austin, 2004); but with rare exceptions such as the ARC model (Glisson, 2012), research which can show relationships among preconditions such as change capacity, change interventions, and specific aspects of organizational performance is limited, offering opportunities for further research. There is a rich and growing body of research regarding the implementation of evidence-based programs. However, there is not equivalent research on organizational change initiatives which have goals beyond the implementation of an evidence-based model, such as organizational restructuring, cutback management, and quality improve-

ment. The research agenda suggested here could assess the implementation and effects of such broader change initiatives. Armenakis and Bedeian (1999) asserted that "research reporting what processes have been used to implement changes should be extended to include how well and when specific tactics and strategies for change have been successful" (p. 312).

Future research should go beyond individual case studies of successful change and use both qualitative methods, such as observation and interviewing, and quantitative methods, such as surveys of participants in change processes and analysis of documents and organizational outcomes data. Such broad-based survey research should provide even stronger evidence than does the more common approach of gathering data from only a few managers or allegedly successful cases.

Such research could examine relationships among different combinations of important variables including contextual factors such as organizational size or structure, change capacity, leadership style, organizational culture, change methods, and change tactics as they impact change process outcomes. Ultimately, the implementation of change processes should be correlated with organizational outcomes, such as improved client conditions and organizational efficiency and effectiveness.

Existing research and practice principles do offer some guidance to practitioners such as agency managers who need to implement change in their organization. To the extent that administrators and other staff as change leaders can use existing research, and more refined research such as that suggested here, to guide their use of change tactics, organizational change may be more impactful, resulting in improvements in organizational functioning and client outcomes.

REFERENCES

Aarons, G., Hurlburt, M., & Horwitz, S. (2011). Advancing a conceptual model of evidence-based practice implementation in public service sectors. *Administration and Policy in Mental Health and Mental Health Services Research, 38*(1), 4–23.

Anderson, D., & Ackerman-Anderson, L. (2010). *Beyond change management* (2nd ed.). San Francisco, CA: Pfeiffer.

Armenakis, A., & Bedeian, A. (1999). Organizational change: A review of theory and research in the 1990s. *Journal of Management, 25*(3), 293–315.

Austin, M. J. (Ed.). (2004). *Changing welfare services: Case studies of local welfare reform programs.* New York, NY: The Haworth Press.

Austin, M. J. (2008). "Introduction." *Journal of Evidence-Based Social Work, 5*(1–2), 1–5.

Austin, M. J., & Claassen, J. (2008). Impact of organizational change on organizational culture: Implications for introducing evidence-based practice. *Journal of Evidence-Based Social Work, 5*(1/2), 321–359.

Austin, M. J., Claassen, J., Vu, C. M., & Mizrahi, P. (2008). Knowledge management: Implications for human service organizations. *Journal of Evidence-Based Social Work, 5*(1–2), 361–389.

Battilana, J., Gilmartin, M., Sengul, M., Pache, A., & Alexander, J. (2010). Leadership competencies for implementing planned organizational change. *Leadership Quarterly, 21*, 422–438.

Beckhard, R., & Pritchard, W. (1992). *Changing the essence.* San Francisco, CA: Jossey-Bass.

Blumenthal, B. (2003). *Investing in capacity building: A guide to high-impact approaches.* New York, NY: The Foundation Center. Retrieved from http://www.foundationcenter.org/getstarted/onlinebooks/blumenthal/text.html

Bouckenooghe, D. (2010). Positioning change recipients' attitudes toward change in the organizational change literature. *The Journal of Applied Behavioral Science, 46*(4), 500–531.

Bouckenooghe, D., Devos, G., & Van den Broeck, H. (2009). Organizational change questionnaire–climate of change, processes, and readiness: Development of a new instrument. *Journal of Psychology: Interdisciplinary and Applied, 143*(6), 559–599.

Brager, G., & Holloway, S. (1993). Assessing the prospects for organizational change: The use of force field analysis. *Administration in Social Work, 16*(3/4), 15–28.

Burke, W. (2011). *Organization change: Theory and practice* (3rd ed.). Thousand Oaks, CA: Sage.

Cinite, I., Duxbury, L. E., & Higgins, C. (2009). Measurement of perceived organizational readiness for change in the public sector. *British Journal of Management, 20*(2), 265–277.

Cohen, M., & Hyde, C. (2014a). *Empowering workers & clients for organizational change.* Chicago, IL: Lyceum Books.

Cohen, M., & Hyde, C. (2014b). Organizational assessment for change. In M. Cohen, & C. Hyde. *Empowering workers and clients for organizational change* (pp. 34–51). Chicago, IL: Lyceum Books.

Connor, P., Lake, L., & Stackman, R. (2003). *Managing organizational change* (3rd ed.) Westport, CT: Praeger.

Cooperrider, D., Whitney, D., & Stavros, J. (Eds.). (2003). *Appreciative inquiry handbook: The first in a series of AI workbooks for leaders of change.* San Francisco, CA: Berrett-Koehler.

Cummings, T., & Worley, C. (2009). *Organization development and change* (9th ed.). Mason, OH: South-Western Cengage Learning.

Esaki, N., Benamati, J., Yanosy, S., Middleton, J., Hopson, L., Hummer, V., et al. (2013). The sanctuary model: Theoretical framework. *Families in Society, 94*(2), 87–95.

Fernandez, S., & Rainey, H. (2006). Managing successful organizational change in the public sector: An agenda for research and practice. *Public Administration Review 66*(2): 1–25. Retrieved from http://www.aspanet.org/scriptcontent/custom/staticcontent/t2pdownloads/FernandezRainey.pdf

Ford, J., & Ford, L. (2009). Resistance to change: A reexamination and extension. In Woodman, R., Pasmore, W., & Shani, A. (Eds.). *Research in organizational change and development* (Vol. 17, pp. 211–239). Burlington: Emerald Group Publishing Limited.

Gersick, C. (1991). Revolutionary change theories: A multilevel exploration of the punctuated equilibrium paradigm. *Academy of Management Review, 16*, 10–36.

Gill, S. (2010). *Developing a learning culture in nonprofit organizations.* Thousand Oaks, CA: Sage.

Gilley, A., McMillan, H., & Gilley, J. (2009). Organizational change and characteristics of leadership effectiveness. *Journal of Leadership & Organizational Studies, 16*(1), 38–47.

Glisson, C. (2007). Assessing and changing organizational culture and climate for effective services. *Research on Social Work Practice, 17*(6), 736–747.

Glisson, C. A. (2012). Interventions with organizations. In Glisson, C., Dulmus, C., & Sowers, K. (Eds.). *Social work practice with groups, organizations, and communities* (pp. 159–190). Hoboken, NJ: Wiley.

Glisson, C., Schoenwald, S. K., Hemmelgarn, A., Green, P., Dukes, D., Armstrong, K. S., & Chapman, J. (2010). Randomized trial of MST and ARC in a two-level evidence-based treatment implementation strategy. *Journal of Consulting and Clinical Psychology, 78*(4), 537–550.

Grobman, G. (2008). *The nonprofit handbook* (5th ed.). Harrisburg, PA: White Hat Communications.

Holloway, S. (1987). Staff-initiated organizational change. In A. Minahan (Ed.), *Encyclopedia of social work* (18th ed., pp. 729–736). Washington, DC: NASW Press.

Holt, D., Armenakis, A., Feild, H., & Harris, S. (2007). Readiness for organizational change: The systematic development of a scale. *Journal of Applied Behavioral Science, 43*(2), 232–255.

Jaros, S. (2010). Commitment to organizational change: A critical review. *Journal of Change Management, 10*(1), 79–108.

Jaskyte, K. (2003). Assessing changes in employees' perceptions of leadership behavior, job design, and organizational arrangements and their job satisfaction and commitment. *Administration in Social Work, 27*(4). 25–39.

Judge, W., & Douglas, T. (2009). Organizational change capacity: The systematic development of a scale. *Journal of Organizational Change Management, 22*(6), 635–649.

Kotter, J. (1996). *Leading change.* Boston, MA: Harvard Business School Press.

Lamm, E., & Gordon, J. (2010). Empowerment, predisposition to resist change, and support for organizational change. *Journal of Leadership & Organizational Studies. 17*(4), 426–437.

Lewis, J., Packard, T., & Lewis, M. (2012). *Management of human service programs* (5th ed., Ch. 11). Belmont, CA: Thompson/Brooks Cole.

Packard, T. (2010, November). Organizational change in human services organizations: comparing successful and unsuccessful interventions. *Association for Research on Nonprofit Organizations and Voluntary Action Annual Conference*, Alexandria, VA.

Parish, J., Cadwaller, S., & Busch, P. (2008). Want to, need to, ought to: employee commitment to organizational change. *Journal of Organizational Change Management, 21*(1), 32–52.

Proctor, E., Landsverk, J., Aarons, G., Chambers, D., Glisson, C., & Mittman, B. (2009). Implementation research in mental health services: An emerging science with conceptual, methodological, and training challenges. *Administration and Policy in Mental Health and Mental Health Services Research, 36*(1), 24–34.

Proehl, R. (2001). *Organizational change in the human services.* Thousand Oaks, CA: Sage.

Resnick, H., & Patti, R. (1980). *Change from within.* Philadelphia, PA: Temple University Press.

Schein, E. (1999). *Process Consultation.* Reading, MA: Addison-Wesley.

Schmid, H. (2010). Organizational change in human service organizations: Theories, boundaries, strategies, and implementation. In Y. Hasenfeld (Ed.), *Human services as complex organizations* (2d ed., pp. 455–479). Thousand Oaks, CA: Sage.

Senge, P. (2006). *The fifth discipline* (rev. ed.). New York, NY: Doubleday Currency.

Sowa, J., Selden, S., & Sandfort, J. (2004). No longer unmeasurable? A multidimensional integrated model of nonprofit organizational effectiveness. *Nonprofit and Voluntary Sector Quarterly, 33*(4), 711–728.

Walker, H., Armenakis, A., & Bernerth, J. (2007). Factors influencing organizational change efforts: An integrative investigation of change content, context, process and individual differences. *Journal of Organizational Change Management, 20*(6), 761–773.

Yankey, J., & Willen, C. (2006). Consulting with nonprofit organizations: Roles, processes, and effectiveness. In R. Edwards & J. Yankey (Eds.), *Effectively managing nonprofit organizations* (pp. 407–428). Washington, DC: NASW Press.

FURTHER READING

Administration for Children and Families, Child Welfare Information Gateway. *Continuous Quality Improvement.* Retrieved from https://www.childwelfare.gov/management/reform/soc/communicate/initiative/soctoolkits/cqi.cfm#phase=pre-planning

Barbee, A. P., Christensen, D., Antle, B., Wandersman, A., & Cahn, K. (2011). Successful adoption and implementation of a comprehensive casework practice model in a public child welfare agency: Application of the getting to outcomes (GTO) model. *Children and Youth Services Review, 33*(5), 622–633.

By, R. (2007). Ready or not.... *Journal of Change Management, 7*(1), 3–11.

Curran, C., & Bonilla, M. (2010). Taking OD to the bank: Practical tools for nonprofit managers and consultants. *Journal for Non Profit Management, 14*, 1–7.

Eadie, D. (2006). Building the capacity to lead innovation. In R. Edwards & J. Yankey (Eds.), *Effectively managing nonprofit organizations* (pp. 29–46). Washington, DC: NASW Press.

Judge, W. (2011). *Building organizational capacity for change.* New York, NY: Business Expert Press.

Organization Development Network http://www.odnetwork.org/

Packard, T. (2013). Organizational change: A conceptual framework to advance the evidence base. *Journal of Human Behavior and the Social Environment, 23*(1), 75–90.

Palmer, I., Dunford, R., & Akin, G. (2009). *Managing organizational change: A multiple perspectives approach* (2nd ed.). Boston, MA: McGraw-Hill.

Proctor, E., Powell, B., & McMillen, J. (2013). Implementation strategies: Recommendations for specifying and reporting. *Implementation Science, 8*(1), 139.

Whelan-Berry, K., & Somerville, K. (2010). Linking change drivers and the organizational change process: A review and synthesis. *Journal of Change Management, 10*(2), 175–193.

Young, M. (2009). A meta model of change. *Journal of Organizational Change Management, 22*(5), 524–548.

THOMAS PACKARD

OUTCOME MEASURES IN HUMAN SERVICES

ABSTRACT: Throughout history, measuring outcomes has been a goal and priority in the human services. This entry chronicles the history of outcomes measurement in the human services in the United States and discuss present-day outcome measurement activities as well as trends and some of the key areas for outcomes measurement in several human service domains.

KEY WORDS: outcome measures; outcomes measurement; performance measurement; human services

Broadly defined, outcome measures are "outputs" (Hatry, 2011) or "results of a program['s or policy's] activity compared to its intended purpose" (Mullen, 2004, p. 84; Government Performance and Results Act, 1993), or indicators of functioning for individuals, organizations, systems, or communities. During the last three decades the development of outcome measures, and outcome measurement activities, has exponentially increased (Magnabosco & Manderscheid, 2011; Mullen & Magnabosco, 1997) in every human services area. This growth has largely been due to increased demands for accountability by funders, managers, and consumers; competition for survival; and a myriad of research and evaluation efforts. Consequently, outcomes measurement has simultaneously been broadened and deepened, with an amalgam of definitions, measures, and defined purposes that have become important and/or essential to improving human lives.

Outcome measures can be field-(for example, health, mental health, addictions, education, child welfare), discipline-(for example, psychology, social work, medicine), or sector-(for example, private, public, nonprofit) specific. The development, selection, use, monitoring, and reporting of outcome measures is a complex, values-based, culturally and historically based process that often spans across, and integrates, bodies of knowledge, lessons learned, and goals. Examples of outcome measures are increased access to services or total number of participants served; number of evidence-based practices, strategies, and policies implemented; and abstinence from alcohol or drug use (CSAP & DCCC, 2006). Outcome measures are generated to answer a variety of questions, such as "To what extent can documented outcomes be attributed to the intervention?" (Patton & Gornick, 2011).

Outcome measures are distinct from performance measures. They have similar, yet different meanings and are frequently (and sometimes inappropriately) referred to interchangeably. Performance measures "cover not only the measurement of service outcomes, but also the measurement of the amount of physical output produced by an organization, such as the number of sessions held with clients" (Hatry, 2011, p. 18). Performance measures are often used in the private sector, no matter the industry, while outcome measures are most often used in the public and nonprofit sectors. Government has typically used both types of measures. While the distinction between the two types of measures is blurring more these days, for purposes of this article the focus will be on outcome measures.

Lists and descriptions of outcome measures can be found in almost any type of informational medium—from more traditional sources such as books, magazines, and published articles and reports, to more contemporary sources such as Web sites, blogs, and professional discussions on social media engines such as LinkedIn. Some professional journals (such as the *Journal of Outcome Measurement* and *Journal of Patient Related Outcome Measures*) specifically target the topic of outcomes measurement. However, any professional journal that reports on human service issues may contain articles or essays that focus primarily or partially on outcome measurement.

Outcome Measures and Outcomes Measurement: History and Trends

The evolution of societies has largely been predicated on quests to determine the value or measurement—of progress, accomplishments, power, wealth, relationships, and quality of life. Such quests have been laden with age-old controversies embodying questions such as, *How do we know what we know?*

Can any concept, perception, behavior, or effect truly be measured? And how do we "best" establish the validity of quantitative and qualitative approaches to outcomes measurement and hence prioritize use of the "best" or most fitting outcome measures? While the scope of this article does not allow for chronicling a complete history associated with outcomes measurement, several important points in time and trends that have helped to shape outcomes measurement in the human services in the United States will be described.

OUTCOMES MEASUREMENT IN THE 19TH CENTURY

The origins of present-day outcomes measurement can be traced to the mid-1800s after the Civil War when "America underwent a spectacular expansion of productive facilities and output that was without parallel in the history of the world" (Trattner, 1989, p. 76). While this "expansion" created new industrial jobs and urbanization, it "displaced" much of the "craftsmanship" that was America's initial hearth of success. The "hardship and destitution" that ensued, as well as cycles of poverty that were already established, forged a "new era of philanthropy" (Trattner). Here, the "organized charity movement...formed the basis of [the] science of social therapeutics," (Trattner, p. 87) which sought to make relief (that is, charity, aid) a "matter of the head as well as the heart" (p. 87).

In addition to this epiphany in decision making, the advent of modern-day "organized" public health was also under way during this time. State boards of health were established. More laws (building on the Elizabethan Poor Law of 1692), reforms, and movements (for example, child welfare, settlement house, Poorhouse) emerged that developed and supported more systematic procedures to prevent and treat disease, filth, neighborhood decay, and delinquent behaviors. Analyses and reports of various sorts were being created to document basic statistics, and descriptive measures, of community needs and progress in health, mental health, crime, child welfare, public health, poverty, and other dimensions of society.

OUTCOMES MEASUREMENT IN THE 20TH CENTURY

By the early 1900s assessments of society had become more the norm. Simultaneous to this development was the "quest for professionalization" of social workers and others devoted to the betterment, treatment, and assessment of society's needs (Trattner, 1989). This set the stage for emerging organizations, and prominent individuals, to develop workplace and philanthropic guidelines, standards, and measures regarding assessment, workflow, and outputs within newly organized disciplinary frameworks.

By the mid-20th century, the United States' welfare state had solidified, and a foundation for a "science" of outcomes measurement had gelled in both the public and private sectors. However, outcomes measurement was very mechanistic, basic in statistical nature, and disparate (that is, uncoordinated, not comparable) at best. (This trend continues today. For example, "statistical and qualitative data collected on public mental health systems in the 19th and 20th centuries [has been] difficult to organize into comparable measures between organizations, programs and government agencies" (Magnabosco, 2001, p. 11).) The theories and practices of "scientific management" that were associated with Frederick W. Taylor's "assembly-line" approach to management, production, and measurement (for example, "minimiz[ing] complexity [to] maximize efficiency" and quality) promulgated the service and manufacturing industries (Walton, 1986).

The 1970s ushered in new approaches to management, economics, outcomes measurement, and production as the legislation and programs from the 1960s Great Society (that is, set of legislative reforms and programs geared to address America's poverty, racial injustice, education, transportation, and other human service issues) led to widespread bureaucracy (Wilson, 1989); decentralization; advances in theories and models of organizations (Morgan, 1986); recognition that "managing by objectives" (Drucker, 1954) had limitations for reaching and measuring goals; minimal or no requirements for measuring outcomes of many government-sponsored human service programs; and more "comprehensive" (Magnabosco, 2001) planning strategies to deal with social welfare issues.

New perspectives on implementation, and its role in the social policy process, also came to light during this time. Before the 1970s it was "assumed that policy decisions were automatically carried through the policy system as intended and with the desired outcomes" (Magnabosco, 2001, p. 27; Younis & Davidson, 1990). Consequently, "implementation" was "established as the missing link in policy-making" (Hargrove, 1976; Magnabosco, p. 28; Sabatier & Mazmanian, 1981) with four main supporting models or theoretical approaches [that is, top-down or "forward mapping" (Elmore, 1982; Sabatier & Mazmanian), bottom-up or "backward mapping" (Elmore), adaptive (Berman, 1980), and evolutionary (Majone & Wildavsky, 1979)]. This expanded perspective on implementation had important implications for outcomes measurement. Stakeholders in both the private and public sector began to forge a less linear and hierarchical way of perceiving the intra- and interworkings of organizations, planning of goals and objectives, and measuring outcomes. Hence, organizations had evolved to be perceived as "complex" (Perrow, 1986) entities, with both intended and unintended outcomes. As a result, measuring outcomes was recast from solely a "top-down" approach, to one that also encompassed "bottom-up" or "street-level" (that is, direct line worker and consumer or client; Lipsky, 1980) influences.

The 1980s were laden with "deregulatory and decentralization philosophies and strategies" that included "budget cuts"; "block grant policy" (that is, "in 1981, the Omnibus Reconciliation Act changed federal-local categorical grant relationships to federal-state-local arrangements...where 77 categorical grants were reorganized into 7 block grants" (Magnabosco, 2001; pp. 29–30)); and "vague reporting and outcomes measurement requirements for human services" (Magnabosco). Despite being "left to do more with less" (Talbott, 1980), biases toward quantitative methods, and fears associated with potential consequences of organizational or program assessment, an abundance of outcome measurement and evaluation studies ensued in various human sectors. Even so, many "human service programs [failed] to demonstrate their efficacy" (Martin & Kettner, 1996, p. 2) during this time.

In the 1990s, rising health care costs; a growing emphasis on total quality management principles and consumer satisfaction; the implementation of managed health care principles and programs; and legislative initiatives, like the 1993 Government Performance and Results Act (GPRA; Mullen & Magnabosco, 1997) signaled the need for a renewed focus on results-based human services. GPRA (and its subsequent modifications like PART) "specifie[d] that beginning with fiscal year 1998, all federal departments must begin reporting on effectiveness, [outcomes and] performance measures" (Gore, 1993; Martin & Kettner, 1996, p. 12).

This renewed focus included a commitment to "reinventing government" (Osbourne & Gaebler, 1992) that was geared to reform how government worked; anchor measures of progress and success on meaningful, useful, and scorecard metrics (such as the Balanced Scorecard and process developed by Kaplan and Norton (1996)); and promote the participation of the public (Kettle & Milward, 1996) in how human services—and government activities—were conducted. This focus coincided with similarly spirited and suggested reforms in specific human services. For example, the Institute of Medicine (IOM) was fostering support for health care system reform that was largely based on a shift from system- or physician-driven care to "patient (consumer)-driven" or "patient (consumer)-

centered" care, which included input from patients (consumers) in the development, selection, and recommended use of process (for example, how health care is provided) and outcome measures (Committee on Quality of Health Care in America, Institute of Medicine, 2001).

OUTCOMES MEASUREMENT IN THE 21ST CENTURY

Like the 20th century, outcomes measurement in the 21st century has been impacted, and directed, by various reforms, domestic and global factors, and greater focus on competitive accountability. At the time of this writing, "our nation has once again just completed a thorough examination of how our health, mental health, and child and family services and systems are to be delivered and managed. Having just recently witnessed the passing of national health care reform, mental health parity, and new procedures to overhaul state child and welfare accountability systems, citizens in the United States are living in an unprecedented time of systemic change within our human services. Such historic change, once again, directs much attention to human service outcomes and measurements" (Magnabosco & Manderscheid, 2011, p. 1).

New Contexts for Outcomes Measurement. A few new contexts for the delivery of human services, such as prevention, recovery, and strengths-based care (Magnabosco & Manderscheid, 2011), have come into their own and, in turn, are providing new roots for outcomes measurement. Here, Campbell (2011) defines recovery as "having hope for the future: living a self-determined life, maintaining self-efficacy, and achieving meaningful roles in society" (p. 233). Recovery is also considered to be comprised of "10 fundamental components of recovery...self-direction, individualism, person centeredness, empowerment, holism, nonlinearity, strengths-based, peer support, respect, responsibility, and hope" (Campbell, p. 233; Onken, Craig, Ridway, Ralph, & Cook, 2007). Strengths-based approaches to care focus on "elevating and magnifying" one's positive attributes instead of targeting problem areas (Magnabosco & Manderscheid; Seligman, 2002; Seligman & Csikszentmihalyi, 2000). Such contexts seem to be complementing, and not supplanting, some well-established frameworks associated with outcomes measurement, such as quality improvement or quality management (Shortell et al., 1995), and evidence-based practice (Thyer, 2011).

Trends in Outcomes Measurement. In addition to new contexts, several other trends in outcomes meas-

urement are emerging, with seemingly minimal risk of fading. In 2011, two experts who have devoted their careers to the development of outcome measures and outcomes measurement systems, and evaluating human services in the United States and abroad summarized some of these trends.

Core Outcomes Measurement Questions. Harry Hatry (2011) raises several questions in response to today's "expansion in interest, requirements and need for outcomes measurement" by funders, government agencies, service providers, policy makers, researchers, advocates, and consumers. Such questions include the following: "Are outcome data that are being collected sufficiently valid and comprehensive? Do the data cover enough of the outcomes dimensions important to [human service organizations] and others, and especially the clients they serve? How is outcomes and performance measurement information being used? To what extent are the data being used to improve services and programs, and thus improve outcomes for the clients of [human services organizations]?" (pp. 21–22).

Hatry (2011) notes that "key issues related to answering these questions" include the examination of the "need to intertwine and balance outcomes measurement and program evaluations" (p. 22), "address disparities" (p. 23), "improve strategies that integrate outcomes across programs and agencies" (p. 25), "improve quality and comparability of outcome measurement data, [and assess] the increasing use of outcome information to motivate service providers [and] use of outcome information to improve services" (p. 28).

Core Outcomes Measurement Issues. Likewise, Brian Yates (2011) describes four issues that have become increasingly important to outcomes measurement, especially for "measuring outcomes quantitatively across [human service organizations]." His first premise is that "twentieth century standard methods for quantifying outcomes still apply in the 21st century, but new approaches are emerging to measure and compare outcomes quantitatively" (p. 48). Here, Yates explains that typical "modeling approach[es]" (for example, statistical tests of the null hypothesis and significance testing) for measuring quantitative outcomes serve their purposes but do not take "into account the entire service process." He discusses "one type of cognitive social learning model, the Resource/Activity/Process/Outcome Analysis (RAPOA) model" (Yates, 2002, p. 49) that does just that. RAPOA is innovative in that it also includes "costs and benefits," thereby providing comprehensive and "useful" information about client changes that can be used in decision making and evaluation by funders, providers, and other stakeholders.

Second, Yates (2011) states that "issues concerning the reliability and validity of quantitative outcomes are no longer based only on science" (p. 51). He points out that many "believe" that the "essential framework for quantitative measurement and research can [and should] be modified...[to take] into account... [the]...context of specific cultures, interest groups and other value sets" (p.51; see also Siegert & Brisolara, 2002) in which they have been "created." He goes on to say that this would help to create "fairer" contexts for standardization, and comparability, between outcome measures.

The last two issues that Yates highlights are interrelated: He describes how "the process of selecting and quantifying outcomes for funders and other stakeholders (including clients) is not standardized" (p. 53), and that "attitudes about quantifying outcomes [in human service organizations] will continue to vary among stakeholders" (Yates, 2011, p. 54). His best suggestions for dealing with these two facts is for stakeholders to integrate perspectives on how to measure outcomes (for example, combine outcome measures into composites, value interdisciplinary approaches), increase comfort levels with numeric representations of outcomes, and become more "consumer oriented" (Yates, 2002).

Newly Valued Approaches to Outcomes Evaluation. A few other current trends in outcomes measurement are worth noting because they also are becoming mainstays in the development, use, and analysis of outcomes. While quantitative outcomes—and quantitative methods to evaluate outcomes—have been more traditionally valued and used, "qualitative evaluation of outcomes" has been "increasing in value" and "making an important contribution by identifying and validating especially effective, evidence-based practices" (Patton & Gornick, 2011, p. 31). Over the past decade the "science and art" (Magnabosco, 1997) of "qualitative outcomes evaluation" (or "large-scale, multi-site, comparative case study projects" that use qualitative data from "open-ended interviews, focus groups, observations and documents like client case files and organization reports") has developed due to the "increased importance of comparative analysis in...outcomes measurement" (Patton & Gornick, p. 31). Interestingly enough, this type of evaluation has been made more "manageable" by new developments in technology—software programs that organize large amounts of qualitative data into units that can be used to analyze themes and numeric counts.

Outcomes Measurement and Leadership. Finally, like other times in our history, meeting the challenges associated with outcomes measurement in the human services requires "attention to...the impact that leadership [at all levels] has on implementing organizational change and achieving positive human services outcomes" (Packard & Beinecke, 2011, p. 90). Leadership has been shown to "make a difference in the ability of [human service organizations] to achieve their goals" (Packard & Beinecke, p. 98). Hence, "implementing an outcomes measurement culture in [human service organizations]" (Kelly, 2011; Packard & Beinecke, p. 192) is extremely important to the future of those served in any sector, and to any type of human services organization (including those that are consumer driven or consumer run).

Outcome Measures and Outcome Measurement Activities: Present Day

Like outcome measures, *outcome measurement activities* encompass many forms and are engaged in varying degrees, depending on whether they are mandated or voluntary, and carried out in human service organizations that have the commitment, capacity, and availability of human capital and financial resources. Such activities include the following:

> *Outcomes measurement* is "a systematic way to assess the extent to which a program [policy or set of other factor(s)] has achieved its intended results"; it differs from *evaluation* in that it will explore what [a] program provides, what its intended impacts are, and whether it achieves them. It will not prove that [the] changes [that] have taken place are a result [or are caused by] the program, policy, or other factors (Compassion Capital Fund National Resource Center, n.d.). Relatedly, *performance measurement* is defined as the "regular collection and reporting of information about the efficiency, quality, and effectiveness of human service programs" (Martin & Kettner, 1996, p. 3; Urban Institute, 1980). Performance measurement is also considered "only one of many...approaches to program accountability...[others include] process accountability, fiscal accountability, legal accountability, [and] service delivery accountability" (Martin & Kettner, p. 3; Rossi & Freeman, 1993).

Outcomes management is the "use of outcome information by organization managers to help them manage better, such as better allocated resources and better formulated and justified budgets" (Hatry, 2011, p. 18). Here, "*cost and outcome analysis* has become an increasingly popular complement to traditional evaluation findings in informing human services policy [and programming] decisions" (Kilburn, 2011, p. 283). Three typical types of cost and outcome analysis approaches—cost analysis, cost-effectiveness analysis, and cost-benefit analysis—require different types of outcomes data (Kilburn, p. 283).

Outcomes research (regardless of quantitative, qualitative, or mixed-method approach) seeks to provide evidence about which interventions work best for which types of patients, or clients, and under what circumstances. *Outcomes evaluation* similarly uses designs to determine the results and impacts of intervention[s] (Patton & Gornick, 2011). *Outcome surveys*, such as *self-report patient (consumer or client) surveys*, have been increasingly used to measure the "extent to which a patient is satisfied with the health [or other] care he or she received" by "health plans, provider groups, individual physicians, [and] a variety of settings" (Cherepanov & Hays, 2011, p. 138).

The passage of the 2010 Affordable Care Act (health reform) established the Patient-Centered Outcomes Research Institute to shift greater attention to *comparative effectiveness research* in certain human service areas (for example, health, mental health, addictions, child services, complementary and alternative medicine). Comparative effectiveness research (CER) can be defined as the "generation and synthesis of evidence that compares the benefits and harms of alternative methods to prevent, diagnose, treat, and monitor a clinical condition or to improve the delivery of care. The purpose of CER is to assist consumers, clinicians, purchasers, and policymakers to make informed decisions that will improve health care at both the individual and population levels" (Coulter & Khorsan, 2011, p. 173; Sox & Greenfield, 2009, p. 203).

Quantitative (meta-analysis) and qualitative (research synthesis) systematic reviews that assess human service outcomes have mainly been conducted using research studies as their unit of analysis; that is, their focus has been the analysis of results from studies, not so much the actual use of particular outcome measures and their credibility. Nonetheless, information about the validity and reliability of outcome measures is often provided in *descriptions* of instruments, toolkits, and outcome research study reports or publications. Certain *professional forums*, such as the Cochrane Collaboration (for health topics), The

Campbell Collaboration (for social welfare topics), and the Agency for Healthcare Research and Quality (ARHQ)—as well as individual researchers (for example, Littell & Corcoran, 2009)—also publish reviews of measures, evidence-based practices, protocols of assessment tools, and use of some outcomes. Thyer (2011) predicts that in the near future, the "emerging *Cochrane Handbook of Systematic Reviews of Diagnostic Test Accuracy* will likely prove to be a definitive resource for use in deciding what measures to adopt or exclude" (p. 69).

Expert panel meetings and other consensus-building forums have been convened to discuss the development, selection, use, research, and dissemination of outcome (and performance) measures. A variety of entities, and efforts, have been part of such activities, including the following:

- *national* (for example, ARHQ, Institute of Medicine, National Forum on Quality, National Committee for Quality Assurance, National Council for Community Behavioral Health, Child Welfare League of America, Joint Commission for Accreditation of Healthcare Organizations), *professional* (for example, the National Association of Social Workers, American Medical Association, American Pediatrics Association, American Psychological Association, American Psychiatric Association, and American Psychiatric Nurse Association), and *consumer-based organizations* (for example, the National Alliance on Mental Illness);

- federal (for example, the Department of Health and Human Services Substance Abuse Mental Health Services Administration, Administration for Children and Families, Health Resources and Services Administration, Center for Substance Abuse Treatment; Office of the Assistant Secretary for Planning and Evaluation; Centers for Medicare and Medicaid Services; and Department of Veterans Affairs), state, and local *government agencies*;

- national, state, and local *initiatives and task forces* (for example, Healthy People 2020, National Research Council Panel on Performance Measures and Data for Public Health Performance Partnership Grants, Task Force for Good Practices for the Assessment of Patient-Reported Outcomes in Children and Adolescents, and Task Force on Developing Obesity Outcomes and Learning Standards);

- *researchers*, providers, consumers, advocates, policymakers and payors in the United States and internationally.

Many of these endeavors share foundational philosophies and information, have occurred simultaneously, and/or been maintained for their own purposes, without synchronization. Regardless of this fact, one result of consensus building is that outcomes measurement *within* certain human service arenas has begun to centralize and/or produce agreed-upon domains of measurement. For example, in *health*, HEDIS measures are the accepted "gold standard" for performance, outcomes and quality (National Committee for Quality Assurance [NCQA], 2013); the short and long versions of the SF-36, and Consumer Assessment of Healthcare Providers and Systems (CAHPS) surveys are also widely used to measure patient-reported outcome (PRO) and health-related quality of life (HRQoL) outcomes (Cherepanov & Hays, 2011).

In *mental health and substance use*, National Outcome Measures (NOMs) outcome domains are being used for adults and children served by federal grants (CSAP & DCCC, 2006; Kelly, 2011); the Mental Health Statistics Improvement Pilot (MHSIP) Report Card (Campbell, 2011) is used by public and private sector organizations to measure satisfaction and quality of life outcomes.

In *child welfare*, child welfare agencies (and other organizations that serve children and families) utilize the three main outcome measurement domains designated by the U.S. Children's Bureau of the Administration for Children and Families—safety, permanency, and family and child well-being (McGowan & Walsh, 2011).

And, in *gerontology*, researchers and practitioners are working on developing and refining outcomes measurement to align with the National Institutes of Health's priority areas—maintaining health and functioning, improving quality of life in chronic conditions, enhancing the end-of-life experiences, and reducing health disparities (Berkman & Kaplan, 2011).

While these examples are representative of how outcomes measurement *within* the human services is deepening, benefits that consensus building can bring for measurement across the field of human services have not yet been realized.

Summary

Today, outcome measures are as various and plentiful (Corcoran & Hozack, 2011) as the populations, organizations, communities, and purposes they delineate.

Outcome measures permeate planning, decision making, financing, contracting, research and evaluation, organizational change endeavors, advocacy, and legislation. Outcome measures can be developed, and exist, for all levels of analysis: individual (person-centered), organizational, and system (including population and community). While outcome measures are often discussed in and of themselves, their meaning and interpretation should take into account their underlying values, and cultural and historical bases, and the larger frameworks from which they are cast (for example, academic discipline, sector, theoretical underpinnings, and/or human service area).

Many outcomes measurement activities, and historical events, have helped to evolve the development, evaluation, and use of outcome measures. Even so, outcomes measurement in the human services remains "fractured" (Mullen & Magnabosco, 1997). Fortunately, it is now commonly recognized that integrating outcome measurement efforts across fields and disciplines is important, and that furthering the science that supports achieving positive human service outcomes can be beneficial to stakeholders and human service recipients (Magnabosco & Manderscheid, 2011). As such, the future of outcomes measurement in the human services largely depends on exercising carefully crafted plans to further this recognition in ways that effectively, efficiently, and collaboratively improve human lives.

REFERENCES

Berkman, B., & Kaplan, D. B. (2011). Outcomes measurement and gerontology: What the United States needs as it grows older. In J. L. Magnabosco & R. W. Manderscheid (Eds.), *Outcomes measurement in the human services: Cross cutting issues and methods in the era of health reform* (pp. 147–162). Washington, DC: NASW Press.

Berman, P. (1980). Thinking about programmed and adaptive implementation. In H. Ingram & D. Mann (Eds.), *Why policies succeed or fail* (pp. 205–230). Beverly Hills, CA: Sage.

Campbell, J. (2011). Outcomes measurement and the mental health consumer movement: Research, recovery, and recognition in the human services. In J. L. Magnabosco & R. W. Manderscheid (Eds.), *Outcomes measurement in the human services; Cross cutting issues and methods in the era of health reform* (pp. 233–250). Washington, DC: NASW Press.

Center for Substance Abuse Prevention Data Coordination and Consolidation Center. (2006). *Overview of the national outcome measures for the CSAP substance abuse prevention and treatment block grant and discretionary grants.* Washington, DC: Author.

Cherepanov, D., & Hays, R. D. (2011). Health and quality-of-life outcomes: The role of patient-reported measures. In J. L. Magnabosco & R. W. Manderscheid (Eds.), *Outcomes measurement in the human services: Cross cutting issues and methods in the era of health reform* (pp. 129–146). Washington, DC: NASW Press.

Committee on Quality of Health Care in America, Institute of Medicine. (2001). *Crossing the quality chasm.* Washington, DC: The Institute of Medicine.

Compassion Capital Fund National Resource Center. (n.d.). *Intermediary development series: Measuring outcomes*. Rockville, MD: Department of Health & Human Services, Administration of Children & Families.

Corcoran, K., & Hozack, N. (2011). Rapid assessment instrument as outcomes measures: Past and current use. In J. L. Magnabosco & R. W. Manderscheid (Eds.), *Outcomes measurement in the human services: Cross cutting issues and methods in the era of health reform* (pp. 223–232). Washington, DC: NASW Press.

Coulter, I. D., & Khorsan, R. (2011). Complementary alternative and integrative medicine: Current challenges for outcomes measurement. In J. L. Magnabosco & R. W. Manderscheid (Eds.), *Outcomes measurement in the human services: Cross cutting issues and methods in the era of health reform* (pp. 163–178). Washington, DC: NASW Press.

Drucker, P. F. (1954). *The practice of management*. New York, NY: Harper Collins.

Elmore, R. F. (1982). Backward mapping: Implementation research and policy decisions. In Aaron Wildavsky (Ed.), *Studying implementation: Methodological and administrative issues*. Chatham, NJ: Chatham House.

Gore, A. (1993). *Creating a government that works better and costs less: Report of the national performance review*. Washington, DC: Government Printing Office.

Government Performance and Results Acts, 1993, Pub. L. No. 103-162. #1115, 107 State. 285. (1993).

Hargrove, E. C. (1976). *The missing link: The study of the implementation of social policy*. Washington, DC: The Urban Institute.

Hatry, H. (2011). *Outcomes measurement in the human services: Lessons learned from the private and public sectors*. In J. L. Magnabosco & R. W, Manderscheid (Eds.), *Outcomes measurement in the human services: Cross cutting issues and methods in the era of health reform* (pp. 17–30). Washington, DC: NASW Press.

Kaplan, R. S., & Norton, D. P. (1996). *Translating strategy into action: The balance scorecard*. Boston, MA: Harvard Business School Press.

Kelly, T. A. (2011). New directions for outcome-oriented mental health system transformation. In J. L. Magnabosco & R. W. Manderscheid (Eds.), *Outcomes measurement in the human services: Cross cutting issues and methods in the era of health reform* (pp. 191–206). Washington, DC: NASW Press.

Kettle, D. F., & Milward, H. B. (Eds.). (1996). *The state of public management*. Baltimore, MD: The Johns Hopkins University Press.

Kilburn, M. R. (2011). Cost and outcomes analysis of child well-being. In J. L. Magnabosco & R. W. Manderscheid (Eds.), *Outcomes measurement in the human services: Cross cutting issues and methods in the era of health reform* (pp. 283–296). Washington, DC: NASW Press.

Lipsky, M. (1980). *Street-level bureaucracy: Dilemmas of the individual in public services*. New York, NY: Russell Sage Foundation.

Littell, J. H., & Corcoran, J. (2009). Systematic reviews and evidence-based practice. In A. R. Roberts (Ed.), *Social worker's desk reference* (2nd ed., pp. 1152–1156). New York, NY: Oxford University Press.

Magnabosco, J. L. (1997). Book review: Evaluation and quality improvement in the human services. In A. G. Peter & M. G. Richard. *Research on social work practice* (Vol. 7, No. 2, pp. 278–280). Newbury Park, CA: Sage Periodicals Press.

Magnabosco, J. L. (2001). *An evaluation of state public mental health systems performance for adult persons with serious mental illness: Effects of state political culture and state mental health planning and implementation characteristics on state public mental health system comprehensiveness*. Ann Arbor, MI: UMI Dissertation Services, Bell & Howell Information and Learning Company.

Magnabosco, J. L., & Manderscheid, R. W. (Eds.). (2011). Conclusion. In *Outcomes measurement in the human services: Cross cutting issues and methods in the era of health reform* (pp. 1–16, 375–378). Washington, DC: NASW Press.

Majone, G., & Wildavsky, A. B. (1979). Implementation as evolution. In J. L. Pressman & A. B. Wildavsky (Eds.), *Implementation* (pp. 163–180). Berkeley: University of California Press.

Martin, L. L., & Kettner, P. M. (1996). *Measuring performance of human service programs*. Thousand Oaks, CA: Sage.

McGowan, B. G., & Walsh, E. M. (2011). Research-to-practice examples: Implementation of child and family services reviews: Progress and challenges. In J. L. Magnabosco & R. W. Manderscheid (Eds.), *Outcomes measurement in the human services: Cross cutting issues and methods in the era of health reform* (pp. 297–314). Washington, DC: NASW Press.

Morgan, G. (1986). *Images of organization*. Newbury Park, CA: Sage.

Mullen, E. J. (2004). Outcomes measurement: A social work framework for health and mental health policy and practice. In A. Metteri, T. Krogan, A. Pohjohn, & P. L. Rauhala (Eds.), *Social work approaches in health and mental health from around the globe* (pp. 77–94). Binghamton, NY: Haworth Press.

Mullen, E. J., & Magnabosco, J. L. (Eds.). (1997). *Outcomes measurement in the human services: Cross cutting issues and methods in the era of health reform*. Washington, DC: NASW Press.

National Committee for Quality Assurance (NCQA). (2013). *HEDIS 2013*. Washington, DC: Author.

Onken, S., Craig, C., Ridgway, P., Ralph, R., & Cook, J. (2007). An analysis of the definitions and elements of recovery: A review of the literature. *Psychiatric Rehabilitation Journal, 31*, 9–22.

Osbourne, D., & Gaebler, T. (1992). *Reinventing government: How the entrepreneurial spirit is transforming the public sector*. Menlo Park, CA: Addison-Wesley.

Packard, T., & Beinecke, R. H. (2011). Leadership in the human services: Models for outcomes-driven organizational cultures. In J. L. Magnabosco & R. W. Manderscheid (Eds.), *Outcomes measurement in the human services: Cross cutting issues and methods in the era of health reform* (pp. 89–112). Washington, DC: NASW Press.

Patton, M. Q., & Gornick, J. K. (2011). Qualitative approaches to outcomes evaluation. In J. L. Magnabosco & R. W. Manderscheid (Eds.), *Outcomes measurement in the human services: Cross cutting issues and methods in the era of health reform* (pp. 31–46). Washington, DC: NASW Press.

Perrow, C. (1986) *Complex organizations: A critical essay*. San Francisco, CA: McGraw-Hill.

Rossi, P., & Freeman, H. (1993). *Evaluation: A systematic approach*. Newbury Park, CA: Sage.

Sabatier, P. A., & Mazmanian, D. A. (1981). The implementation of public policy: A framework for analysis. In D. A. Mazmanian & P. A. Sabatier (Eds.), *Effective policy implementation* (pp. 3–38). Lexington, MA: Lexington Books.

Seligman, M. (2002). Positive psychology, positive prevention, and positive therapy. In C. R. Snyder & S. J. Lopez (Eds.), *The handbook of positive psychology* (pp. 3–12). New York, NY: Oxford University Press.

Seligman, M., & Csikszentmihalyi, M. (2000). Positive psychology: An introduction. *American Psychologist, 55,* 5–14.

Shortell, S. M., O'Brien, J. L., Carman, J. M., Foster, R. W., Hughes, E. F. X., Boerstler, H., & O'Connor, E. J. (1995). Assessing the impact of continuous quality improvement/total quality management: Concept versus implementation. *Health Services Research, 30*(2), 377–401.

Siegert, D., & Brisola, S. (2002). Feminist evaluation. *New Directions for Evaluation, 96,* 123–152.

Sox, H., & Greenfield, S. (2009). Comparative effectiveness research: A report from the Institute of Medicine. *Annals of Internal Medicine, 151,* 203–205.

Talbott, J. A. (1980). Toward a public policy on the chronic mentally ill patient. *American Journal of Orthopsychiatry, 50*(1), 43–53.

Thyer, B. A. (2011). Outcomes measurement in the human services: The role of evidence-based practice. In J. L. Magnabosco & R. W. Manderscheid (Eds.), *Outcomes measurement in the human services: Cross cutting issues and methods in the era of health reform* (pp. 59–72). Washington, DC: NASW Press.

Trattner, W. I. (1989). *From poor law to welfare state: A history of social welfare in America*. New York, NY: The Free Press.

Urban Institute. (1980). *Performance measurement*. Washington, DC: Author.

Walton, M. (1986). *The Deming management method*. New York, NY: Perigee Books.

Wilson, J. A. (1989). *Bureaucracy*. New York, NY: Basic Books.

Yates, B. T. (2002). Roles for psychological procedures, and psychological processes, in cost-offset research: Cost/procedures/process/outcome analysis. In N. A. Cummings, W. T. O'Donohue, & K. E. Ferguson (Eds.), *The impact of medical cost offset on practice and research: Making it work for you* (pp. 91–123). Reno, NV: Context Press.

Yates, B. T. (2011). Quantitative approaches to outcomes measurement. In J. L. Magnabosco & R. W. Manderscheid (Eds.), *Outcomes measurement in the human services: Cross cutting issues and methods in the era of health reform* (pp. 47–58). Washington, DC: NASW Press.

Younis, T., & Davidson, I. (1990). The study of implementation. In T. Younis (Ed.), *Implementation in public policy* (pp. 3–14). Aldershot, U.S.A.: Dartmouth.

JENNIFER L. MAGNABOSCO

P

PERSON-IN-ENVIRONMENT

ABSTRACT: The person-in-environment perspective in social work is a practice-guiding principle that highlights the importance of understanding an individual and individual behavior in light of the environmental contexts in which that person lives and acts. The perspective has historical roots in the profession, starting with early debates over the proper attention to be given to individual or environmental change. Theoretical approaches that have attempted to capture the meaning of person-in-environment are presented, as are promising, conceptual developments.

KEY WORDS: person-in-environment perspective; person-in-situation (person-in-context); ecosystem framework; ecological theory; general systems theory

The person-in-environment perspective in social work is a practice-guiding principle that highlights the importance of understanding an individual and his or her behavior in light of the various environmental contexts in which that person lives and acts (CSWE, 2004). These contexts include (but are not limited to) social, economic, political, communal, historical, religious, physical, cultural, and familial environments. This definition incorporates the notion that there is a reciprocity to the person–environment relationship, such that the individual can impact the various elements of the environment, just as the environment can exert a conducive or inhibiting influence on the individual. The definition also includes the notion that an understanding of the person in his or her total context creates opportunities for assessment and interventions that are directed at individual functioning, at environmental conditions, or both. It is important to note that this definition is not coextensive with the various theoretical or operational formulations that have attempted to give more substance to the person-in-environment perspective. For example, this perspective is not the same as the various ecosystem models with which it is commonly identified, and which it predates in the literature and in practice.

The person-in-environment perspective has been linked to definitions of social work practice since the concept's earliest articulation in the first working definition of practice (Bartlett, 2003, reprinted from Bartlett, 1958). The preambles to both the current *Educational Policy and Accreditation Standards of the Council on Social Work Education* and the most recent *National Association of Social Work Code of Ethics* identify attention to the individual in environmental context as a crucial element in defining social work practice, as does the definition of practice promulgated by the International Federation of Social Workers (CSWE, 2004; IFSW, 2006; NASW, 1996).

Historical Background

The notion that both person and his/her environment are central considerations in social work practice has strong historical roots. Although emphasis assigned to either personal change or environmental change has varied over time, neither the "person" nor the "environment" half of this equation was ever completely eclipsed within the practice and academic communities.

This early history is best exemplified by the public debate between Jane Addams and the founders of the settlement movement, on the one hand, and Mary Richmond and other leaders in the Charity Organization Society, on the other (Germain & Hartman 1980; Peterson, 1979). Addams underscored the importance of the social, cultural, and policy environment in the lives of individuals and families, and embraced social-environmental change as a way of improving the lives of people in poverty and social distress (Austin, 2001; Germain & Hartman 1980). By contrast, Richmond adopted a medical model defined by a process of diagnosis and treatment that was focused on identifying and correcting individual deficits (Germain & Hartman 1980; Peterson, 1979). A careful reading of the historical literature, however, suggests that while the debate between proponents of these two positions was often lively, in practice both Richmond and Addams intervened with individuals, families, and larger systems (Germain & Hartman 1980).

The medical model favored by Richmond provided fertile ground for implanting the emerging theory and practice of psychotherapy into social casework during the post–World War I period. Many in mainstream social work at this time eschewed emphasis on promoting environmental or system change, adopting instead a concern for psychodynamic factors thought to determine human functioning. However, even with this trend toward more psychological approaches to case work, there were countervailing voices continuing to insist on the importance of the social, economic, political, and cultural environments in explaining social problems and in defining strategies to improve the lives of individuals and families. Ada Sheffield, for example, expanded on the concept of a client's "total situation," in which individuals and their immediate environments were interrelated (Sheffield, 1931). Bertha Reynolds and Harry Laurie also advocated for the importance of social and economic aspects of the environment as cause and potential solution for social problems (Germain & Hartman 1980; Schriver, 1987a, 1987b).

While the professional practice community was experiencing the tension between proponents of psychological approaches and those advocating the importance of environmental strategies, leaders in the profession were also preoccupied with a quest to define social work's scope and purpose. An early attempt was the Milford Conference and the 1929 final conference report. The report specifically mentioned adjustments in the environment and use of community resources as a proper concern of social work (Brieland, 1977; Holosko, 2003). Following the formation of the National Association of Social Workers (NASW) in 1955, a study group, headed by Harriet Bartlett, was commissioned to develop a working definition of social work practice. The group report identified three generic methods as proper to social work practice: (a) changing the individual in relation to the social environment, (b) changing the social environment in relation to the individual, or (c) both in relation to their interaction (Bartlett, 2003). Although the original working definition had its share of critics, including Gordon's (1962) reexamination of the definition and Wakefield's (2003) reconsideration of both Gordon's critique and the working definition itself, the notion that the person-in-environment was the proper domain of social work practice remained intact.

Theoretical Conceptualizations

As early as the 1950s, a few social work scholars had begun to look for ways to better conceptualize the so-called person–environment perspective. By the 1970s this quest had become a major preoccupation in disciplinary discourse. Over the next several decades, two major, interrelated frameworks were advanced specifically for the purpose of giving theoretical substance to the person–environment perspective: (a) general systems theory and (b) ecological theory and life model.

General Systems Theory

Hearn (1958, 1969) is usually credited with introducing general systems theory into the social work literature (Drover & Shragge 1977). Other early contributors to the application of general systems theory to social work include Pincus and Minihan (1973), Meyer (1976), Goldstein (1973), Gordon (1969), and Lathrope (1969). General system theory, based largely on the work of theoretical biologist Bertalanffy (1950, 1969), became ascendant in the social work literature in the 1960s and 1970s, and remained the prevailing paradigm until the introduction of ecological systems theory (or ecosystems theory) in the late 1970s and 1980s.

Bertalanffy was concerned with what he saw as the increasingly mechanistic and atomized view projected by contemporary science, in which parts and processes of a given phenomenon were identified and studied as isolated entities. He argued that an element is best understood in relation to its constituent parts (subsystems) and in relation to larger or more complex elements of which it is a constituent part. He defined "system" as "sets of elements standing in interrelation" (1969, p. 38). Bertalanffy identified two kinds of systems: "closed systems," that is, "systems that are considered to be isolated from their environment" (1969, p. 39) and "open systems," characteristic of living organisms, which are in constant interaction with their environments. Other concepts he emphasized included "subsystems," the constituent elements of a larger system in a hierarchical order, and "feedback," or the flow of information in an open system that allows regulation (change) and stability (homeostasis) in relation to other systems.

The concept of a hierarchy of systems, in which a system was comprised of a set of subsystems and in turn constituted a subsystem of a larger entity/system, was crucial to the application of systems theory in social work. Persons and other systems were understood to be influenced by contiguous systems and by larger systems of which they were a part. System theory reinforced the notion that the focus of social work practice should be on neither person nor environment, but rather on *transactions* between person (a system) and systems in the environment (Gordon, 1969; Lathrope, 1969; Pincus & Minihan, 1973).

Because of system theory emphasis on linkages between systems of differing sizes and complexity, early theorists were convinced that systems theory would aid in unifying social work practice, including the dual focus on person and environment (Gordon, 1969; Hearn, 1969; Pincus & Minihan, 1973). However, not everyone was enthusiastic about system theory's potential. Drover and Shragge (1977), for example, argued that systems theory did not account for values and ideology. Leighninger (1977, 1978) shared the concern for values, particularly with regard to what he viewed as an implicit acceptance of the status quo (emphasis on achieving homeostasis) and consequent inadequacy of the theory to deal with larger social change or conflict. Others suggested that the level of abstraction of the model was somewhat distant from the human phenomena the model was said to describe (Drover & Shragge, 1977; Germain, 1978a). Still others argued that the systems theory focus on *transactions* took attention away from the "person," and, therefore, was inconsistent with social work's commitment to the centrality of the individual (Mishne, 1982).

The general system paradigm was the major influence in social work theorizing for approximately two decades. At the time it provided a useful challenge to psychodynamic theory as the reigning conceptual model for practice, and brought renewed attention to larger elements in the social environment (Leighninger, 1977). Although largely replaced by ecological (ecosystem) theory, general system theory concepts are still operative in a number of family therapy models, particularly in "structural family therapy" developed by Minuchin (1974).

Ecosystems Theory and the Life Model

Ecosystems theory in social work draws on general systems theory and the science of ecology, the study of living organisms within their environments. The ecological or ecosystem perspective is usually associated with the work of Germain and Gitterman (Germain, 1973, 1977, 1978a, 1978b, 1981; Germain & Gitterman, 1996; Gitterman & Germain, 1981) and Meyer (1983).

Although general systems theory provided useful tools for organizing assessments and planning interventions with various systems (macro and micro) relevant to a particular case, many came to view systems theory as too mechanistic and too abstract to deal effectively with the phenomena of people's daily lives (Germain, 1978a; Peterson, 1979). The discipline of ecology, based as it is on living organisms in relationship to other systems with which they interact in an environment, appeared to offer a more concrete and lifelike metaphor for conceptualizing the traditional person-in-environment perspective.

The core principle of the ecosystem perspective is that each individual (family, group) is in an interdependent and constant relationship with the larger environment and with other elements that make up his or her environment (Germain & Gitterman, 1996). This means that an individual cannot be understood adequately without reference to the environmental context the individual inhabits (Brower, 1988). The perspective emphasizes that the environment can exert a facilitative or an inhibiting effect on well-being of individuals, just as individuals can impact the environment in ways that promote or damage the ability of the environment to facilitate life (Germain, 1981). To a greater extent than general systems theory, ecosystems theory stressed the mutuality of person–environment relationships (Germain, 1973, 1981). Similarly, while general systems theory helped practitioners think systematically about influences external to the individual, the ecosystem framework and the life model of practice based on this framework went further by insisting on the absolute necessity of considering the whole human context in any practice situation.

The most comprehensive critique of the ecosystem framework was leveled by Wakefield (1996a, 1996b). Two of his arguments are pertinent to this discussion. First, he challenged the notion that social work needs one all-encompassing conceptualization like the ecosystem framework to give coherence to disparate forms of practice, including interventions with differing emphasis on person and environment. He further argued that the ecosystem perspective "loses the specialness of the person" with its identification of person as one system among many others and a focus on transactions rather than persons (1996b, pp. 198–199). Gitterman (1996) responded to Wakefield by arguing that an overarching conceptualization like the ecosystem framework helps us to understand that no one domain-specific theory or model accounts for all of social reality. He further argued that the ecosystem model, rather than dismissing the importance of the person, captures the uniqueness of each person in his or her singular context. Other critiques of the ecosystem perspective have generally accepted the framework, but have suggested that typical conceptualizations of the ecosystem framework lacked attention to identified aspects of person or cultural–social–physical environment (Besthorn & Canda, 2002; Devore, 1983; Epple, 2004; Saleeby, 1992, 2004). Despite its critics, the ecosystem framework continues to have a great deal of currency as a conceptualization of person-in-environment, so much so that the ecosystem framework is sometimes treated (erroneously) as synonymous with the person-in-environment perspective. The perspective continues to be identified in theoretical and research literature as a guiding framework (Rogge & Cox, 2001).

Recent Conceptual Developments

A series of new theoretical approaches have emerged in the literature since the early 1990s, providing alternate formulations for the person–environment relationship. These perspectives offer a fresh look at the relationship between individuals and their contexts, with the possibility of new avenues for intervention and research.

Nonlinear, Dynamical Systems Theory

Several theorists have begun to extend systems theory by applying nonlinear, dynamical systems theories to complex clinical problems. Proponents argue that human behavior is frequently more complex and apparently unpredictable than can be explained by simple, linear cause and effect relationships (Warren, Franklin, & Streeter, 1998; Warren & Knox, 2000). Dynamical systems theories attempt to account for change in systems over time, including feedback loops that may recursively alter the process of change in unexpected ways (Warren et al., 1998). Warren and Knox (2000) have successfully applied mathematical formulae based on dynamical systems theory to the behavior of adolescent sex offenders. These authors suggest that the model may be useful for other types of compulsive behavior.

Risk and Resilience Theory as an Ecosystem Approach

Linking ecological theory with concepts drawn from epidemiology and public health, theorists posit that there are risk factors and protective factors inherent in the environment and in the person (Fraser, Richman, & Galinsky, 1999, 2004). Risk factors increase the likelihood of harm or the continuation of a harmful situation; protective factors support positive outcomes even in situations of risk (Fraser, Richman, & Galinsky, 1999, 2004). What makes this framework useful for social workers and researchers is the conceptual and operational support it provides for multilevel assessment, intervention, and evaluation. There is a growing body of social work literature, including empirical studies, supporting this perspective, particularly (though not exclusively) in child welfare (Corcoran & Nichols-Casebolt, 2004; Early & Vonk, 2001; Fraser, 1996, 2004; Fraser, Richman, & Galinsky, 1999; Greene & Cohen, 2005; Little, Axford, & Morpeth, 2004; Unger, 2001). A more recent, intriguing development in risk-resilience theory is the suggestion that the fields of genetics and social epidemiology may have something to offer social workers through promising work on gene–environment interactions (McCutcheon, 2006).

Person and Environment in Social Constructivist Theory

Since the 1990s, the social work literature has seen increasing interest in the implications of social constructionist theories. Those who adopt some form of constructivist perspective agree that the impact of the environment on individuals is not direct, but rather is mediated by various meaning-making processes through which people make sense of their environmental realities (Allen, 1993; Carpenter, 1996; Gergen, 1999; Kondrat, 2002; Laird, 1993). Social constructionism serves as the basis for newer forms of therapy with individuals and families, including solution-focused and narrative therapies (Berg & De Jong, 1996; Franklin, 1996; Gergen, 1999). Consistent with a belief that knowledge and reality are humanly constructed, constructivist researchers adopt qualitative, interpretivist approaches to inquiry (Schwandt, 1994). More than earlier person-in-environment conceptualizations, constructivism advances the notion of the human beings as active agents in constituting their own social environments. However, social constructionist theorizing has tended to focus on the construction of micro (interpersonal) realities, and has not consistently accounted for the macro environment, except to suggest that larger social structures do impact individual realities (Kondrat, 1999, 2002; Laird, 1993). In an effort to include larger systems more securely in constructivist thinking, Kondrat (1999, 2002) proposed a macro-constructivist conceptualization of person-in-environment, based on Giddens' Structuration Theory (1979, 1984, 1987). This formulation suggests that larger social structures and institutions, even society itself, are all social constructions, constituted and maintained by the social actions and interactions of people over time. She suggests that the individual is in the environment not so much the way a smaller box is within a larger box (the historical metaphor) as Germain (1978a) proposed, but rather the way players are in the football game or dancers in the ballet. The game and the dance do not exist without the players/dancers. This conceptualization is said to offer a more dynamic link between individuals and their environments, both micro and macro (Kondrat, 2002).

Operationalizing Person-in-Environment

A number of attempts have been made to operationalize the terms "environment" and "person" to provide practitioners with a consistent tool to guide assessment and intervention across practice situations. By and large, these efforts have been atheoretical; that is to say, have formulated operational terms directly from the person–environment practice principle, without reference to given theories. The "genogram" and "eco-map" are familiar examples (Hartman, 1978; Walton & Smith, 1999). The most comprehensive attempt to operationalize person-in-environment was the PIE classification system developed by Karls and Wandrei (1992, 1994) (Karls, Lowery, Mattaini, & Wandrei, 1997; Williams, Karls, & Wandrei, 1989). The PIE classification system is described as an instrument for coding common problems of adult clients. It is a four-factor system (a) person's problems in social functioning, (b) problems in the environment affecting a person's functioning, (c) mental health problems (using the DSM), and (d) health problems (Karls & Wandrei, 1994). A number of studies and case applications were described in the book that presented the system. This system held the initial promise of doing for social work what the DSM does for psychiatry—that is, provide a common nomenclature to guide assessment and intervention. Critics, however, suggested that the system was too focused on aggregating discrete problems, that it may have limited cultural applicability particularly in more collectivist cultures, and that it was too reliant on the medical model (Karls et al., 1997). The strong problem focus may also be incompatible with more recent emphases on client strengths, not captured in the PIE formula. For whatever reason, the PIE system has not been further developed in the literature in any systematic way.

Conclusion

Wakefield's (1996a, 1996b) provocative question as to whether the profession's historical quest for one all-encompassing theory to capture the disparate forms of social work practice may have been answered by recent history. Currently, there are a number of alternate and coexisting conceptualizations for the relationship between person and environment that are bridging interdisciplinary boundaries in unexpected and promising ways. For better or worse, the search for one discipline-unifying conceptualization may not have been realized. Nevertheless, to date, the principle that social work practice is characterized by a person-in-environment perspective seems to have stood the test of time.

REFERENCES

Allen, J. A. (1993). The constructivist paradigm: Values and ethics. *Journal of Teaching in Social Work*, 8, 31–54.

Austin, D. (2001). Guest editor's foreword. *Research on Social Work Practice*, 11(2), 147–151.

Bartlett, H. M. (2003). Working definition of social work practice. *Research on Social Work Practice*, 13(3), 267–270.

(Reprinted from Bartlett, H. (1958). Working definition of social work practice. *Social Work*, 3(2), 5–8.)

Berg, I. K., & De Jong, P. (1996). Solution-building conversations: Co-constructing a sense of competence with clients. *Families in Society*, 77(6), 376–391.

Bertalanffy, L. V. (1950). The theory of open systems in physics and biology. *Science*, 111, 23–29.

Bertalanffy, L. V. (1969). *General system theory*. New York: George Braziller.

Besthorn, F. H., & Canda, E. R. (2002). Revisioning environment: Deep ecology for education and teaching in social work. *Journal of Teaching in Social Work*, 22(1), 79–101.

Brieland, D. (1977). Historical overview. *Social Work*, 22(5), 341–346.

Brower, A. M. (1988). Can the ecological model guide social work practice? *Social Service Review*, 62(3), 411–429.

Carpenter, D. (1996). Constructivism and social work treatment. In F. J. Turner (Ed.), *Social work treatment: Interlocking theoretical approaches* (4th ed., pp. 146–167). New York: Free Press.

Corcoran, J., & Nichols-Casebolt, A. (2004). Risk and resilience ecological framework for assessment and goal formation. *Child and Adolescent Social Work Journal*, 21(3), 211–235.

Council on Social Work Education. (2004). Educational policy and accreditation Standards, Retrieved on December 9, 2006, from http://www.cswe.org

Devore, W. (1983). Ethnic reality: The life model and work with black families. *Social Casework*, 64(9), 525–531.

Drover, G., & Shragge, E. (1977). General systems theory and social work education: A critique. *Canadian Journal of Social Work Education*, 3(2), 28–39.

Early, T. J., & Vonk, M. E. (2001). Effectiveness of school social work from a risk and resilience perspective. *Children and Schools*, 23(1), 9–31.

Epple, D. M. (2004). Encounter with soul. *Clinical Social Work Journal*, 31(2), 173–188.

Franklin, C., & Nurius, P. S. (1996). Constructivist therapy: New directions in social work practice. *Families in Society*, 77(6), 323–325.

Fraser, M. W. (1996). Aggressive behavior in childhood and early adolescence: An ecological-developmental perspective. *Social Work*, 41(4), 347–361.

Fraser, M. W. (2004). The ecology of childhood: A multisystems perspective. In M. W. Fraser (Ed.), *Risk and resilience in childhood* (2nd ed., pp. 1–12). Washington, DC: National Association of Social Workers.

Fraser, M. W., Richman, J. M., & Galinsky, M. J. (1999). Risk, protection and resilience: Toward a conceptual framework for social work practice. *Social Work Research*, 23(3), 131–143.

Gergen, K. J. (1999). *An invitation to social construction*. Thousand Oaks, CA: Sage.

Germain, C. B. (1973). An ecological perspective in casework practice. *Social Casework*, 54, 323–330.

Germain, C. B. (1977). An ecological perspective on social work practice in health care. *Social Work in Health Care*, 3(1), 67–76.

Germain, C. B. (1978a). General-systems theory and ego psychology: An ecological perspective. *Social Service Review, 52*(4), 535–550.

Germain, C. B. (1981). The ecological approach to people-environment transactions. *Social Casework, 62*(6), 323–331.

Germain, C. B. (1987). Human development in contemporary environments. *Social Service Review, 61*(4), 565–580.

Germain, C. B., & Gitterman, A. (1996). *The life model of social work practice* (2nd ed.). New York: Columbia University.

Germain, C. B., & Hartman, A. (1980). People and ideas in the history of social work. *Social Casework, 61*(1), 323–331.

Giddens, A. (1979). *Central problems in social theory: Action, structure and contradiction in social analysis.* Berkeley and Los Angeles, CA: University of California Press.

Giddens, A. (1984). *The constitution of society.* Oxford: Polity Press.

Giddens, A. (1987). *Social theory and modern sociology.* Stanford: Stanford University Press.

Gitterman, A. (1996). Ecological perspective: Response to Professor Jerry Wakefield. *Social Service Review, 70*(3), 472–476.

Goldstein, H. (1973). *Social work practice: A unitary approach.* Columbia, SC: University of South Carolina.

Gordon, W. (1962). A critique of the working definition. *Social Work, 7*(4), 3–13.

Gordon, W. (1969). Basic constructs for an integrative and generative conception of social work. In G. Hearn (Ed.), *General Systems Approach: Contributions toward a holistic conception of social work* (pp. 5–11). New York: Council on Social Work Education.

Greene, R. R., & Cohen, H. L. (2005). Social work with older adults and their families: Changing practice paradigms. *Families in Society, 86*(3), 367–374.

Hartman, A. (1978). Diagrammatic assessment of family relationships. *Social Casework, 59*(8), 465–476.

Hearn, G. (1958). *Theory building in social casework.* Toronto, Ontario: University of Toronto.

Hearn, G. (Ed.). (1969). *General systems approach: Contributions toward a holistic conception of social work.* New York: Council on Social Work Education.

Holosko, M. J. (2003). Guest editor's foreword. *Research on Social Work Practice, 13*(3), 265–266.

International Federation of Social Workers. (2006). Definition of social work. Retrieved December 3, 2006, from http://www.ifsw.org/en/p38000208.html

Karls, J. M., Lowery, C. T., Mattaini, M. A., & Wandrei, K. E. (1997). The use of PIE (person-in-environment) system in social work education. *Journal of Social Work Education, 33*(1), 49–58.

Karls, J. M., & Wandrei, K. E. (1992). PIE: A new language for social work. *Social Work, 37*(1), 80–85.

Karls, J. M., & Wandrei, K. E. (Eds.). (1994). *Person-in-environment system.* Washington, DC: NASW.

Kondrat, M. E. (1999). Who is the self in self-aware: Professional self-awareness from a critical theory perspective. *Social Service Review, 73*(4), 451–477.

Kondrat, M. E. (2002). Toward an actor-centered social work: Re-visioning person-in-environment through a critical theory lens. *Social Work, 47*(4), 435–448.

Laird, J. (1993). Family-centered practice: Cultural and constructionist reflections. *Journal of Teaching in Social Work, 8,* 77–109.

Lathrope, D. (1969). The general systems approach in social work practice. In G. Hearn (Ed.), *General systems approach: Contributions toward a holistic conception of social work* (pp. 45–62). New York: Council on Social Work Education.

Leighninger, R. (1977). Systems theory and social work. *Journal of Education for Social Work, 13*(3), 44–49.

Leighninger, R. (1978). Systems theory. *Journal of Sociology and Social Welfare, 5*(4), 446–480.

Little, M., Axford, N., & Morpeth, L. (2004). Research review: Risk and protection in the context of children in need. *Child and Family Social Work, 9*(1), 105–117.

McCutcheon, V. V. (2006). Toward an integration of social and biological research. *Social Service Review, 80*(1), 159–178.

Meyer, C. (1976). *Social work practice* (2nd ed.). (1970). New York: Free Press.

Meyer, C. (1983). *Clinical social work in the eco system perspective.* New York: Columbia University Press.

Minuchin, S. (1974). *Families and family therapy.* Cambridge: Harvard University.

Mishne, J. M. (1982). The missing system in social work's application of systems theory. *Social Casework, 63*(9), 547–553.

National Association of Social Workers. (1996). Code of ethics. Retrieved December 3, 2006, from http://www.socialworkers.org/pubs/code/code.asp

Peterson, K. J. (1979). Assessment in the life model: A historical perspective. *Social Casework, 60*(10), 586–596.

Pincus, A., & Minihan, A. (1973). *Social work practice: Model and method.* Itasca: Peacock.

Rogge, M. E., & Cox, M. E. (2001). The person-in-environment perspective in social work journals: A computer-assisted content analysis. *Journal of Social Services Research, 28*(2), 47–68.

Saleeby, D. (1992). Biology's challenge to social work: Embodying the person-in-environment perspective. *Social Work, 37*(2), 112–118.

Saleeby, D. (2004). 'The power of place': Another look at the environment. *Families in Society, 85*(1), 7–16.

Schriver, J. M. (1987a). Harry Lurie's critique: Person and environment in early casework practice. *Social Service Review, 61*(6). 514–532.

Schriver, J. M. (1987b). Harry Lurie's assessment and prescription: An early view of social workers' roles and responsibilities regarding political action. *Journal of Sociology and Social Welfare, 14*(2), 111–127.

Schwandt, T. A. (1994). Constructivist, interpretivist approaches to human inquiry. In N. K. Denzin & Y. S. Lincoln (Eds.), *Handbook of qualitative inquiry* (pp. 118–137). Thousand Oaks, CA: Sage.

Sheffield, A. (1931). The situation as the unit of case study. *Social Forces, 9,* 465–474.

Unger, M. (2001). The social construction of resilience among problem youth in out-of-home placement: A study of health-enhancing deviance. *Child and Youth Care Forum, 30*(3), 137–154.

Wakefield, J. C. (1996a). Does social work need the eco-systems perspective? Part 1. Is the perspective clinically useful? *Social Service Review, 70*(1), 1–32.

Wakefield, J. C. (1996b). Does social work need the eco-systems perspective? Part 2. Is the perspective clinically useful? *Social Service Review, 70*(2), 183–213.

Wakefield, J. C. (2003). Gordon versus the working definition: Lessons from a classic critique. *Research on Social Work Practice, 13*(3), 284–298.

Walton, E., & Smith, C. (1999). The genogram: A tool for assessment and intervention in child welfare. *Journal of Family Social Work, 3*(3), 3–20.

Warren, K., Franklin, C., & Streeter, C. L. (1998). New directions in systems theory: Chaos and complexity. *Social Work, 43*(4), 357–373.

Warren, K., & Knox, K. (2000). Offense cycles, thresholds and bifurcations: Applying dynamical systems theory to the behaviors of adolescent sex offenders. *Journal of Social Service Research, 27*(1), 1–27.

Williams, J. B. W., Karls, J., and Wandrei, K. (1989). The person-in-environment (PIE) system for describing problems of social functioning. *Hospital and Community Psychiatry, 40*, 1125–1126.

FURTHER READING

Berger, P., & Luckmann, T. (1966). *The social construction of reality.* Garden City, NY: Doubleday.

Buffum, W. E. (1988). Measuring person-environment fit in nursing homes. *Journal of Social Service Research, 11*(2/3), 35–54.

Coulton, C. J., Holland, T. P., & Fitch, V. (1984). Person-environment congruence and psychiatric patient outcome in community care homes. *Administration in Mental Health, 12*(2), 71–88.

Dean, R. G. (1993). Teaching a constructivist approach to clinical practice. *Journal of Teaching in Social Work, 8*, 55–75.

Kemp, S. P. (2001). Environment through a gendered lens: From person-in-environment to woman-in-environment. *AFFILIA, 16*(1), 7–30.

Lutz, W. A. (1956). *Concepts and principles underlying social casework practice.* New York: National Association of Social Workers.

Minahan, A. (1977). Introduction to special issue. *Social Work, 22*(5), 339.

Minahan, A. (1981). Purpose and objectives of social work revisited. *Social Work, 26*(1), 5–6.

Monkman, M. M. (1991). Outcome objectives in social work practice: Person and environment. *Social Work, 36*(3), 253–258.

MARY E. KONDRAT

POVERTY

ABSTRACT: Poverty has been a subject of concern since the beginnings of social work. This is a review of three key research areas. First, the extent and dynamics of poverty are examined, including the measurement of poverty, patterns of cross-sectional and comparative poverty rates, the longitudinal dynamics of poverty, and poverty as a life-course risk. Second, reasons for poverty are discussed. These are divided into individual versus structural level explanations. The concept of structural vulnerability is offered as a way of bridging key individual and structural determinants in order to better understand the existence of poverty. Third, strategies and solutions to poverty are briefly reviewed.

KEY WORDS: causes of poverty; human capital; labor market; life course; poverty dynamics; poverty measures; poverty rates; residential segregation; social welfare state; solutions to poverty; structural vulnerability

Context

The subject of poverty has been of central importance to the profession of social work. In fact it could be argued that addressing poverty lies at the heart of what the profession stands for. As Simon notes, the original twin missions of social work were "those of relieving the misery of the most desperate among us and of building a more just and humane social order" (1994, p. 23). This mission rings true today as well. The National Association of Social Work's *Code of Ethics* begins by stating, "the primary mission of the social work profession is to enhance human well-being and help meet the basic human needs of all people, with particular emphasis to the needs and empowerment of people who are vulnerable, oppressed, and living in poverty" (1996, p. 1). Likewise, the Council on Social Work Education's curriculum policy statement declares that the purpose of the social work profession is to "enhance human well-being and alleviate poverty, oppression, and other forms of social injustice" (2003, p. 4).

Social work has placed a heavy emphasis on alleviating poverty for at least two reasons. First, poverty has been viewed as undermining the concept of a just society. In an affluent nation such as the United States, it appears patently unfair that not only are many left out of such prosperity, but that they also live in debilitating economic conditions. Second, social workers have long understood that poverty underlies many of the problems and issues that they confront on a daily basis. Whether the discussion revolves around racial or gender inequalities, family stress, health disparities, child welfare, economic development, or a host of other topics that social workers routinely confront, research indicates that poverty is intricately connected to each of these subjects. The alleviation of poverty is therefore perceived to be essential in striving toward the enhancement of human well-being and helping to "meet the basic human needs of all people" (NASW, 1996, p. 1). As a result, the profession has historically engaged in research, practice, organizing, and advocacy on the local, state, and federal levels with respect to poverty alleviation.

This article addresses the scope and nature of poverty, with a particular emphasis upon poverty in the United States. Three fundamental questions are addressed. First, what are the parameters and dynamics of poverty? Second, how can the existence of poverty be best understood? And third, what can be done to alleviate the conditions of poverty?

The Extent, Prevalence, and Dynamics of Poverty

Poverty has been conceptualized and measured in a number of different ways. Over 200 years ago, Smith, in his landmark treatise, *Wealth of Nations* (1776), defined poverty as a lack of those necessities that "the custom of the country renders it indecent for creditable people, even of the lowest order, to be without." This type of definition is what is known as an absolute approach. A minimum threshold for living conditions is determined, and individuals falling below that threshold are considered poor. An example of this approach is the manner in which the official poverty line is drawn in the United States. The U.S. poverty line is calculated by estimating the income needed for different sizes of households to obtain what is considered a minimally adequate basket of goods and services for the year. For example, in 2011 a family of four was considered in poverty if its total income fell below $23,021 (U.S. Census Bureau, 2012). The often used standard of defining poverty as living on less than a dollar or two a day in developing countries is another example of an absolute measure of poverty.

Alternatively, poverty can be constructed in a relative rather than absolute sense. A frequently used relative measure is one that defines the poor as being in households whose incomes fall below 50% of the population's median household income. This measure is often found within a European context, as well as in comparative analyses across industrialized countries.

A third type of measure attempts to incorporate more than just low income by factoring in additional aspects of deprivation such as illiteracy, high mortality rates, and chronic unemployment. The focus here is on the concept of social exclusion or "the inability to participate in the activities of normal living" (Glennerster, 2002, 89). This type of measure has been used by the United Nations in its construction of a human poverty index for both the developing and developed nations (United Nations Development Programme, 2012), and has been discussed most notably in the work of Sen (1992).

Beyond the various approaches to measuring poverty, the dimension of time is fundamental in understanding the extent and dynamics of poverty. Poverty can be understood from a cross-sectional, longitudinal, or life-course perspective.

CROSS-SECTIONAL RATES In 1959 the U.S. poverty rate stood at 22.4% (U.S. Census Bureau, 2012). During the 1960s the rate fell sharply, such that by 1973 it had reached a low of 11.1%. Since 1973, the overall rate of poverty has fluctuated between 11% and 15% (Hoynes, Page, & Stevens, 2006; Meyer & Wallace, 2009). It has tended to rise during periods of economic recession (early 1980s, early 1990s, middle to later 2000s), and has fallen during periods of economic expansion (middle to later 1980s, middle to later 1990s).

The poverty rate in 2011 stood at 15.0%, which represented 46.2 million individuals, or about one out of every seven Americans (U.S. Census Bureau, 2012). The percentage of the population falling into poverty or near poverty (125% of the poverty line) was 19.8% (or 60.9 million Americans), whereas 6.6% of the population (or 20.4 million Americans) experienced extreme poverty (falling below 50% of the poverty line). Of those who fell into poverty in 2011, 44% were living below 50% of the poverty line (U.S. Census Bureau, 2012). Consequently, a significant proportion of the poor in America are also experiencing extreme poverty.

In addition, Census Bureau data indicate that certain characteristics put individuals at a greater risk of experiencing cross-sectional poverty. These include having less education, being young, non-Whites, living in single-parent families, residing in economically depressed inner cities or rural areas, or having a disability (U.S. Census Bureau, 2012). In combination, these characteristics can substantially raise the risk of poverty. For example, families with Black children under the age of 5 residing in a female-headed household had an overall poverty rate of 57.8% (U.S. Census Bureau, 2012).

Cross-sectional poverty rates have also been analyzed from a comparative perspective. The Luxembourg Income Study (LIS) has gathered income and demographic information on households in ~30 industrialized nations from 1967 to the present. Variables have been standardized across the various national data sets, allowing researchers to conduct cross-national analyses regarding poverty and income inequality. This body of research shows that U.S. poverty rates (and income inequality) tend to be the highest in the developed world. Whether one looks at relative or absolute poverty among working-age adults, children, or the elderly, the story is much the same (Smeeding, 2005a). For example, in a study of international poverty rates among children, the United States ranked second highest among 26 industrialized countries with a poverty rate of 21.9% (poverty was measured as falling below one half of the country's median income). The only country with a higher rate of poverty among children was Mexico at 27.7%. In contrast, the poverty rate for children in Denmark stood at 2.4% (UNICEF, 2005). For American children in married couple families, single-parent families, or cohabiting families, the story is much the same—a far greater percentage of American children are at risk of poverty compared with their counterparts in nearly all other developed countries (Weinshenker & Heuveline, 2006).

LONGITUDINAL DYNAMICS Since the 1970s, researchers have increasingly sought to uncover the longitudinal dynamics of poverty. The focus has been on understanding the extent of turnover in the poverty population from year to year and determining the length of poverty spells. These studies have relied on several nationally representative panel data sets, including the Panel Study of Income Dynamics (PSID), the National Longitudinal Survey of Youth (NLSY), and the Survey of Income and Program Participation (SIPP). Results from these longitudinal analyses have shed considerable light on understanding the patterns of U.S. poverty. Several broad conclusions can be drawn from this body of work.

First, most spells of poverty in the United States are fairly short. The typical pattern is that households are impoverished for one or two years and then manage to get out of poverty (Bane & Ellwood, 1986; Blank, 1997; Cellini, McKernan, & Ratcliffe, 2008; Duncan, 1984; Walker, 1994). They may stay there for a period of time, only to experience an additional

fall into poverty at some point (Stevens, 1999). Since their economic distance above the poverty line is often not that far, a detrimental economic event such as the loss of a job, the breakup of a family, or a medical problem can easily throw a family back below the poverty line (Duncan et al., 1995; Iceland, 2012; McKernan & Ratcliffe, 2005).

Analysts that have looked at monthly levels of poverty have found even greater fluctuation in poverty spell dynamics. For example, Iceland (2003) examined the monthly fluctuations in and out of poverty from 1996 to 1999 and found that 34% of Americans experienced poverty for at least two months during this time period, while half of all poverty spells were over within four months, and four-fifths were completed at the end of one year.

On the other hand, this body of work has also shown that there is a small number of households that do indeed experience chronic poverty for years at a time. Typically they have characteristics that put them at a severe disadvantage vis-a-vis the labor market (for example, individuals with serious work disabilities, female headed families with large numbers of children, racial minorities living in economically depressed inner city areas). Their prospects for escaping poverty for any significant period of time are greatly diminished (Devine & Wright, 1993; Wilson, 2009).

Finally, research into the dynamics of poverty shows that many households who encounter poverty will re-experience poverty at some point in their future. Using annual estimates of poverty from the PSID data, Stevens (1994) calculated that of all persons who had managed to get themselves above the poverty line, over half would return to poverty within 5 years.

The picture of poverty drawn from this body of research is thus characterized by fluidity. Individuals and households tend to weave their way in and out of poverty, depending upon the occurrence or non-occurrence of particular detrimental events (for example, job loss, family disruption, ill health). Similar findings have been found with respect to the longitudinal patterns of welfare use (Bane & Ellwood, 1994; Blank, 1997; Duncan, 1984; Rank, 1985, 1994a).

LIFE-COURSE RISK A third approach for assessing the scope of poverty has been to analyze poverty as a life-course event. Rowntree's (1901) description of 11,560 working-class families in the English city of York was pioneering in developing this approach. Likewise, Hunter (1904) in his book *Poverty* sought to locate impoverishment within the context of the life course.

Recently, the work of Rank and Hirschl has attempted to gauge the extent of poverty across the American life course. Their results indicate that between the ages of 20 and 75, nearly 60% of Americans will experience at least one year of impoverishment, while 68% of Americans will encounter poverty or near poverty (125% below the official poverty line). The odds of encountering poverty across adulthood are significantly increased for African Americans and those with lower levels of education—91% of Blacks will encounter poverty between the ages of 20 and 75 versus 53% for Whites, while 75% of those with less than 12 years of education will experience at least a year of poverty compared with 48% for those with 12 or more years of education (Rank, 2004; Rank & Hirschl, 1999a). In addition, the life course risk of experiencing poverty has increased for those in their 20s, 30s, and 40s from the 1970s through the 1990s (Sandoval, Rank, & Hirschl, 2009).

Consistent with earlier studies of poverty dynamics, individuals experiencing poverty often do so for only one or two consecutive years. However, once an individual experiences poverty, they are quite likely to encounter poverty again (Rank & Hirschl, 2001a, 2001b).

Rank and Hirschl's analyses (1999b) also indicate that poverty is quite prevalent during childhood. Between the time of birth and age 17, 34% of American children will have spent at least one year below the poverty line, while 40% will have experienced poverty or near poverty (125% of the poverty line). In addition, 40% of the elderly will encounter at least one year of poverty between the ages 60 and 90, while 48% will encounter poverty at the 125% level (Rank & Williams, 2010).

The likelihood of using a social safety net program is also exceedingly high. Consequently, 65% of all Americans between the ages 20 and 65 will at some point reside in a household that receives a means-tested welfare program (including food stamps, Medicaid, Supplemental Security Income, Aid to Families with Dependent Children (AFDC), or other cash assistance). Furthermore, 40% of the American population will use a welfare program in five or more years (although spaced out at different points across the life course). As with the life-course patterns of poverty, the typical pattern of welfare use is that of short spells. Consequently, only 15.9% of Americans will reside in a household that receives a welfare program in five or more consecutive years (Rank, 2004; Rank & Hirschl, 2002).

One program that has a particularly wide reach is the Food Stamp Program (also known as the Supplemental Nutrition Assistance Program or SNAP). For example, approximately half (49.2%) of all U.S. children between the ages 1 and 20 will at some point reside in a household that receives food stamps (Rank & Hirschl, 2009). For the majority of Americans, it would appear that the question is not if they will encounter poverty, but rather, when, which entails a fundamental shift in the perception and meaning of poverty (Rank, 2004).

The Causes of Poverty

A second major area of research has examined the factors and causes underlying poverty. Much of the debate in the literature has centered upon the extent to which poverty can be understood as a result of individual versus structural failings. As O'Connor (2001) notes in her history of 20th-century poverty research, the thrust of this research has shifted from an examination of industrial capitalism as a fundamental cause of poverty at the turn of the century, to a highly technical analysis of the demographic and behavioral characteristics of the poor and welfare recipients being modeled as the causes for poverty by the end of the 20th century.

One reason for this shift has been the growing importance of survey research within the social sciences. Such an approach lends itself more readily to an empirical analysis of individual characteristics, rather than the structural conditions underlying poverty. For example, race and gender are often treated as individual demographic attributes to be controlled for within multivariate models, rather than as structural dimensions of social and economic stratification in their own right (O'Connor, 2001). As is argued below, focusing upon particular individual factors helps to explain who loses out in the competition to find economic opportunities, while the more structural dynamics in society help to explain why there are not enough viable economic opportunities in the first place.

INDIVIDUAL FACTORS The notion of poverty resulting from individual deficits goes back hundreds of years. Survey research confirms that a majority of Americans continue to believe that this is a very important reason for the existence of poverty (Feagin, 1975; Gans, 1995; Gilens, 1999; Kluegel & Smith, 1986; Smith & Stone, 1989). In particular, the argument has been that the poor lack the correct attitudes, motivation, or morals to get ahead (Sawhill, 2003;

Schwartz, 2000). A variation on this argument has been that generous welfare programs have created work and marriage disincentives, leading to counterproductive behaviors such as out-of-wedlock teenage childbearing and avoidance of work, which in turn creates government dependency that further traps individuals and families into a cycle of poverty (Mead, 1986; Murray, 1984; Olasky, 1992).

Researchers examining the attitudes of the poor have found little evidence for the position that the poor have a different set of attitudes which have contributed to their poverty (Duncan, 1984; Edwards, Plotnick, & Klawitter, 2001; Rank, 1994a, 1994b; Seccombe, 1999). Contrary to popular opinion, the poor tend to amplify and reiterate mainstream American values such as the importance of hard work, personal responsibility, and a dislike of the welfare system. Although poverty is accompanied by increasing levels of stress and frustration, the vast majority of the poor express a similar set of core attitudes and motivations as middle-class Americans (Lichter & Crowley, 2002). Furthermore, the impact of social welfare programs on altering individual behavior and thereby fostering dependency has been shown to be minimal (Blank, 1997; Hays, 2003; Moffitt, 1992; Rank, 1989). In short, there is little empirical support for the argument that the counterproductive attitudes of the poor or the generosity of the U.S. welfare system creates or exacerbates poverty.

On the other hand, evidence overwhelmingly confirms the importance of human capital in affecting earnings (and consequently the risk of poverty). Human capital refers to the skills, education, and credentials that individuals bring with them into the labor market (Becker, 1964). The importance of human capital has been studied extensively within the labor economics and social stratification literatures. Individuals acquiring greater human capital tend to be in greater demand in the market place. As a result, they are able to pursue more lucrative careers resulting in higher paying and more stable jobs. Those lacking in human capital are unable to compete as effectively in the labor market, and therefore must often settle for unstable, low-wage work.

The effect of human capital upon the risk of poverty has been shown to be substantial (Karoly, 2001; Schiller, 2008). In particular, greater levels of education, skills, and training are strongly associated with higher levels of earnings (U.S. Census Bureau, 2012). Conversely, those lacking in marketable job skills and education are at a much greater risk of experiencing poverty.

Additional research has demonstrated that levels of human capital are highly dependent upon levels of parental human capital and economic resources. Children of parents with greater income, wealth, education, and so on, are more likely to acquire greater human capital than children coming from lower-income backgrounds. These differences, in turn, affect children's future life chances and outcomes, including the risk of poverty. Recent research has demonstrated a strong association between parents and their children with respect to levels of education, occupational status, income, and wealth (Bowles, Gintis, & Groves, 2005; d'Addio, 2007; Ermisch, Jantti, & Smeeding, 2012; Levine & Mazumder, 2007).

Beyond human capital, several other individual and family characteristics have been shown to be important in increasing or decreasing the risk of poverty. These include family structure, number of children, work disabilities, and age (Blank, 1997; Iceland, 2012). Each of these factors can be conceptualized as impacting individuals' ability to take advantage of labor market opportunities. Specifically, poverty rates tend to be higher for single-parent families, households with large numbers of children, those with work disabilities, and younger adults (U.S. Census Bureau, 2012).

STRUCTURAL FACTORS Various structural factors have been shown to be critical in understanding the existence of poverty in the United States and elsewhere. Perhaps the most important of these has been an emphasis on the failure of the economy to provide enough viable economic opportunities and jobs for all. Several pioneering studies of poverty conducted at the end of the 19th and beginning of the 20th century focused heavily on the importance of labor market failings to explain poverty. The work of Booth (1892–1897), Rowntree (1901), Hull House (1895), Hunter (1904), and DuBois (1899) all emphasized the importance of inadequate wages, lack of jobs, and unstable working conditions as primary causes of poverty.

Recent research has also demonstrated a mismatch between the number of decent paying jobs that can adequately support a family versus the number of individuals in search of such jobs (Harvey, 2000; Quigley, 2003). For example, Bartik (2001) used several different approaches and assumptions to estimate the number of jobs that would be needed to significantly address the issue of poverty in the United States. He concluded that even in the booming U.S. economy of the late 1990s, between five and nine million more jobs were needed in order to meet the needs of the poor and disadvantaged. During the economic downturn beginning in 2008, this mismatch between the number of jobs needed versus those seeking such jobs was significantly greater.

In addition to the imbalance between numbers of jobs versus those in need of jobs, during the past 25 years, the American economy has been producing an increasing percentage of low-paying jobs, jobs that are part-time, and jobs that are lacking in benefits (Fligstein & Shin, 2004; Kalleberg, 2011; Hacker, 2006). Studies analyzing the percentage of the U.S. workforce falling into the low-wage sector have shown that far more American workers fall into this category than do their counterparts in other developed countries. For example, Smeeding et al. (2001) found that 25% of all U.S. full-time workers could be classified as employed in low-wage work (defined as earning less than 65% of the national median earnings for full-time jobs). This was by far the highest of the countries analyzed (the overall average was 12.9%). The result is that more Americans are working at jobs that simply do not support a family at an adequate income level.

A second structural factor affecting a society's overall rate of poverty is the effectiveness of the social welfare state in pulling individuals and families out of economic destitution. Countries with a more comprehensive welfare state (such as the Scandinavian and Benelux countries) are able to cut poverty much more than countries with a weak safety net (such as the United States or Australia). Research has repeatedly demonstrated the significant impact that a social welfare state exerts on poverty reduction (Alesina & Glaeser, 2004; Brady, 2009; Ritakallio, 2002; Smeeding, 2005a).

A third set of structural factors examined has been the impact of racial and gender discrimination. Substantial research has shown that economic, social, and political discrimination remains prevalent in American society (Feagin, 2010; Massey, 2007) and impacts the life chances of racial minorities and women in various ways, resulting in higher rates of poverty among these groups. For example, Oliver and Shapiro (2006), Shapiro (2004), and Johnson (2006) have demonstrated the legacy of discrimination through historical racial differences in wealth and asset inequalities.

Considerable work has also examined the role of residential segregation in combination with other patterns of discrimination, as a further structural cause of poverty, particularly for African American and Latino populations. This body of work has demonstrated that residential segregation on the basis of race is widespread, leading to deteriorating economic

and social conditions within neighborhoods (Massey & Denton, 1993). Residential segregation restricts the opportunities available to urban Black and Latino families through social isolation and increasing levels of deprivation. These, in turn, ensure high levels of poverty and widespread social disorganization (Charles, 2003, 2006; Jargowsky, 1997; Yinger, 1995). Wilson (1987, 1996, 2008, 2009) and Anderson (1990, 1999) have also emphasized the importance of collapsed economic opportunities combined with patterns of social isolation and residential segregation resulting in high rates of urban poverty among minorities.

THE ROLE OF STRUCTURAL VULNERABILITY The concept of structural vulnerability (Rank, 1994, 2004; Rank, Yoon, & Hirschl, 2003) bridges the earlier discussed importance of human capital with the broader significance of structural forces. This framework recognizes that human capital and other labor market attributes are associated with who loses the economic game (and hence will be more likely to experience poverty), but that the structural elements in society ensure that there will be losers in the first place.

Consequently, it is argued that a certain percentage of the American population will experience economic vulnerability as a result of the structural failings mentioned earlier. Individuals experiencing such economic deprivation are likely to have characteristics putting them at a disadvantage in terms of competing in the economy (less education, fewer skills, single-parent families, illness or incapacitation, minorities residing in inner cities, and so on). These characteristics help to explain who in particular is at a greater risk of poverty. However, given the overall structural failings, a significant percentage of the American population will experience economic vulnerability regardless of what their individual characteristics are.

The critical mistake that social scientists have often made is equating the question of who loses out at the game, with the question of why the game produces losers in the first place. They are, in fact, distinct and separate questions. While deficiencies in human capital and other marketable characteristics help to explain who in the population is at a heightened risk of encountering poverty, the fact that poverty exists in the first place results not simply from these characteristics, but rather from the lack of decent opportunities and supports in society (for example, jobs that pay a living wage, access to health care, affordable child care, low cost housing). By focusing solely on personal characteristics, such as education, individuals can be shuffled up or down in terms of their being more likely to land a job with good earnings, but someone still loses out if there are not enough decent paying jobs to go around. In short, the structural vulnerability perspective argues that we are playing a large-scale version of a musical chairs game with many more players than available chairs.

Poverty Alleviation

The social policies of the United States have largely emphasized altering the incentives and disincentives for those playing the game through welfare reform, or in a very limited way, upgrading their skills and ability to compete in the game through job training programs, while at the same time leaving the structure of the game untouched. While ensuring that individuals have good quality human capital and skills are certainly important, in and of themselves, they are insufficient for reducing overall poverty.

When the overall poverty rates in the United States do in fact go up or down, they do so primarily as a result of structural impacts that increase or decrease the number of viable opportunities. In particular, the performance of the economy has been historically important. Why? Because when the economy expands, more opportunities are available for the competing pool of labor and their families. The reverse occurs when the economy slows down and contracts. Consequently, during the 1930s, early 1980s, and later 2000s when the economy was doing badly, poverty rates went up, while during periods of economic prosperity such as the 1960s or the middle to late 1990s, the overall rates of poverty declined (Hoynes et al. 2006; U.S. Census Bureau, 2012).

Similarly, changes in various social supports and the social safety net available to families make a difference in terms of how well such households are able to avoid poverty or near poverty. When such supports were increased through the War on Poverty initiatives in the 1960s, poverty rates declined. Likewise, when Social Security benefits were expanded during the 1960s and 1970s, the elderly poverty rate declined precipitously (Katz & Stern, 2006). Conversely, when social supports have been weakened and eroded, as in the case of children's programs since the mid-1970s, their rates of poverty have gone up (Seccombe, 2000).

Consequently, social policies with the potential to effectively reduce the extent of poverty are largely those that increase and enhance the overall pool of opportunities as well as improving the living conditions and capacities of those seeking such opportunities. As Rank (2004) discusses, these policies can take several different forms. Of foremost importance is ensuring the existence of decent paying jobs that can support a family above the poverty line (Kenworthy, 2004; Quigley, 2003; Schiller, 2008). This includes job creation strategies, as well as raising and indexing the minimum wage up to a living wage and continuing support for the Earned Income Tax Credit (EITC).

A second fundamental poverty alleviation strategy is to increase the affordability and access to several key social and public goods, including a quality education, health care, available housing, and child care. These social goods are vital in building and maintaining healthy and productive citizens, yet are often in short supply for low-income U.S. households in the United States (Esping-Andersen, 2007). In addition, ensuring that a strong and effective safety net is in place when economic setbacks occur is essential (Zuberi, 2006).

A third strategy targets the lingering patterns of discrimination found in both the housing market and occupational structure for racial minorities and women. Vigilant enforcement of fair housing laws and antidiscrimination policies in the work place are essential for breaking down decades of discriminatory practices (Blau, Brinton, & Grusky, 2006; Stainback & Tomaskovic-Devey, 2012; Yinger, 1995). In addition, stronger enforcement of child support laws would help millions of women at risk of poverty who are heading families with children (Cancian & Meyer, 2006), as well as other family supportive employment policies (Waldfogel, 2009).

A final poverty reduction strategy is the development and implementation of asset-building policies for lower-income households and communities (Schreiner & Sherraden, 2007; Shapiro & Wolff, 2001). These include individually based policies such as Individual Development Accounts, as well as community revitalization and reinvestment policies that have been implemented across the United States.

Taken as a whole, these policies have the potential to dramatically reduce the extent of poverty and economic vulnerability that currently exists in the United States. Social work practice and advocacy should strive toward the development and implementation of such poverty alleviation strategies. By doing so, the profession of social work will be proactively engaging in its primary mission to enhance "human well-being and help meet the basic human needs of all people, with particular emphasis to the needs and empowerment of people who are vulnerable, oppressed, and living in poverty" (NASW, 1996, 1).

REFERENCES

Alesina, A., & Glaeser, E. L. (2004). *Fighting poverty in the US and Europe: A world of difference*. New York: Oxford University Press.

Anderson, E. (1990). *Streetwise: Race, class and change in an urban community*. Chicago: University of Chicago Press.

Anderson, E. (1999). *Code of the street: Decency, violence, and the moral life of the inner city*. New York: W. W. Norton.

Bane, M. J., & Ellwood, D. T. (1986). Slipping into and out of poverty: The dynamics of spells. *Journal of Human Resources, 21*, 1–23.

Bane, M. J., & Ellwood, D. T. (1994). *Welfare realities: From rhetoric to reform*. Cambridge, MA: Harvard University Press.

Bartik, T. J. (2001). *Jobs for the poor: Can labor demand policies help?* New York: Russell Sage Foundation.

Becker, G. S. (1964). *Human capital*. New York: Columbia University Press.

Blank, R. M. (1997). *It takes a nation: A new agenda for fighting poverty*. Princeton, NJ: Princeton University Press.

Blau, F. D., Brinton, M. C., & Grusky, D. B. (2006). *The declining significance of gender?* New York: Russell Sage Foundation.

Booth, C. (1892–1897). *Life and labour of the people of London, first series: Poverty*. London: Macmillan.

Bowles, S., Gintis, H., & Groves, M. O. (2005). *Unequal chances: Family background and economic success*. New York: Russell Sage Foundation.

Brady, D. (2009). *Rich democracies, poor people: How politics explain poverty*. New York: Oxford University Press.

Cancian, M., & Meyer, D. R. (2006). Child support and the economy. In R. M. Blank, S. H. Danziger, & R. F. Schoeni (Eds.), *Working and poor: How economic and policy changes are affecting low-wage workers* (pp. 338–365). New York: Russell Sage Foundation.

Cellini, S. R., McKernan, S. M., & Ratcliffe, C. (2008). The dynamics of poverty in the United States: A review of data, methods, and findings. *Journal of Policy Analysis and Management, 27*, 577–605.

Charles, C. Z. (2003). The dynamics of racial residential segregation. *Annual Review of Sociology, 29*, 167–207.

Charles, C. Z. (2006). *Won't you be my neighbor? Race, class, and residence in Los Angeles*. New York: Russell Sage Foundation.

Council on Social Work Education. (2003). *Handbook of accreditation standards and procedures*. Alexandria, VA: Commission on Accreditation.

d'Addio, A. C. (2007). Intergenerational transmission of disadvantage: Mobility or immobility across generations? A review of the evidence for OECD countries. *OECD Social, Employment and Migration Working Papers*, No. 52. Paris: OECD publications service.

Devine, J. A., & Wright, J. D. (1993). *The greatest of evils: Urban poverty and the American underclass*. New York: Aldine de Gruyter.

DuBois, W. E. B. (1899). *The Philadelphia Negro*. Philadelphia: University of Pennsylvania Press.

Duncan, G. J. (1984). *Years of poverty, years of plenty: The changing economic fortunes of American workers and families*. Ann Arbor, MI: Institute for Social Research.

Duncan, G. J., Gustafsson, B., Hauser, R., Schmaus, G., Jenkins, S., Messinger, H., et al. (1995). Poverty and social-assistance dynamics in the United States, Canada, and Europe. In K. McFate, R. Lawson, & W. J. Wilson (Eds.), *Poverty, inequality and the future of social policy: Western states in the new world order* (pp. 67–108). New York: Russell Sage Foundation.

Edwards, M. E., Plotnick, R., & Klawitter, M. (2001). Do attitudes and personality characteristics affect socioeconomic outcomes? The case of welfare use by young women. *Social Science Quarterly, 82*, 827–843.

Ermisch, J., Jantti, M., & Smeeding, T. (2012). *From parents to children: The intergenerational transmission of advantage*. New York: Russell Sage Foundation.

Esping-Andersen, G. (2007). Equal opportunities and the welfare state. *Contexts, 6*, 23–27.

Feagin, J. R. (1975). *Subordinating the poor: Welfare and American beliefs*. Englewood Cliffs, NJ: Prentice-Hall.

Feagin, J. R. (2010). *Racist America: Roots, current realities, and future reparations*. New York: Routledge.

Fligstein, N., & Shin, T. J. (2004). The shareholder value society: A review of the changes in working conditions and inequality in the United States, 1976 to 2000. In K. M. Neckerman (Ed.), *Social inequality* (pp. 401–432). New York: Russell Sage Foundation.

Gans, H. J. (1995). *The war against the poor: The underclass and antipoverty policy*. New York: Basic Books.

Gilens, M. (1999). *Why Americans hate welfare: Race, media, and the politics of antipoverty policy*. Chicago: University of Chicago Press.

Glennerster, H. (2002). United States poverty studies and poverty measurement: The past twenty-five years. *Social Service Review, 76*, 83–107.

Hacker, J. S. (2006). *The great risk shift*. New York: Oxford University Press.

Harvey, P. (2000). Combating joblessness: An analysis of the principal strategies that have influenced the development of American employment and social welfare law during the 20th century. *Berkeley Journal of Employment and Labor Law, 21*, 677–758.

Hays, S. (2003). *Flat broke with children: Women in the age of welfare reform*. New York: Oxford University Press.

Hoynes, H. W., Page, M. E., & Stevens, A. H. (2006). Poverty in America: Trends and explanations. *Journal of Economic Perspectives, 20*, 47–68.

Hull House. (1895). *Hull House maps and papers*. New York: Thomas Y. Crowell.

Hunter, R. (1904). *Poverty: Social conscience in the progressive era*. New York: Macmillan.

Iceland, J. (2003). Dynamics of economic well-being: Poverty 1996–1999. Current Population Reports, Series P70–91. Washington, DC: U.S. Government Printing Office.

Iceland, J. (2012). *Poverty in America: A handbook*. Berkeley, CA: University of California Press.

Jargowsky, P. A. (1997). *Poverty and place: Ghettos, barrios, and the American city.* New York: Russell Sage Foundation.

Johnson, H. B. (2006). *The American Dream and the power of wealth: Choosing schools and inheriting inequality in the land of opportunity.* New York: Routledge.

Kalleberg, A. L. (2011). *Good jobs, bad jobs: The rise of polarized and precarious employment systems in the United States, 1970s to 2000s.* New York: Russell Sage Foundation.

Karoly, L. A. (2001). Investing in the future: Reducing poverty through human capital investments. In S. H. Danziger & R. H. Haveman (Eds.), *Understanding poverty* (pp. 314–356). Cambridge, MA: Harvard University Press.

Katz, M. B., & Stern, M. J. (2006). *One nation divisible: What America was and what it is becoming.* New York: Russell Sage Foundation.

Kenworthy, L. (2004). *Egalitarian capitalism: Jobs, incomes, and growth in affluent countries.* New York: Russell Sage Foundation.

Kluegel, J. R., & Smith, E. R. (1986). *Beliefs about inequality: Americans' views of what is and what ought to be.* New York: Aldine de Gruyter.

Levine, D. I., & Mazumder, B. (2007). The growing importance of family: Evidence from brothers' earnings. *Industrial Relations, 46,* 7–21.

Lichter, D. T., & Crowley, M. L. (2002). Poverty in America: Beyond welfare reform. *Population Bulletin, 57,* 1–36.

McKernan, S. M., & Ratcliffe, C. (2005). Events that trigger poverty entries and exits. *Social Science Quarterly, 86,* 1146–1169.

Massey, D. S. (2007). *Categorically unequal: The American stratification system.* New York: Russell Sage Foundation.

Massey, D. S., & Denton, N. A. (1993). *American apartheid: Segregation and the making of the underclass.* Cambridge, MA: Harvard University Press.

Mead, L. (1986). *Beyond entitlement: The social obligations of citizenship.* New York: Free Press.

Moffitt, R. (1992). Incentive effects of the U.S. welfare system: A review. *Journal of Economic Literature, 30,* 1–61.

Murray, C. (1984). *Losing ground: American social policy, 1950–1980.* New York: Basic Books.

National Association of Social Workers. (1996). *Code of ethics.* Washington, DC: NASW Press.

O'Connor, A. (2001). *Poverty Knowledge: Social science, social policy, and the poor in twentieth-century U.S. history.* Princeton, NJ: Princeton University Press.

Olasky, M. (1992). *The tragedy of American compassion.* Washington, DC: Regnery Publishing.

Oliver, M. L., & Shapiro, T. M. (2006). *Black wealth/white wealth: A new perspective on racial inequality.* New York: Routledge.

Quigley, W. P. (2003). *Ending poverty as we know it: Guaranteeing a right to a job at a living wage.* Philadelphia: Temple University Press.

Rank, M. R. (1985). Exiting from welfare: A life-table analysis. *Social Service Review, 59,* 358–376.

Rank, M. R. (1989). Fertility among women on welfare: Incidence and determinants. *American Sociological Review, 54,* 296–304.

Rank, M. R. (1994a). *Living on the edge: The realities of welfare in America.* New York: Columbia University Press.

Rank, M. R. (1994b). A view from the inside out: Recipients' perceptions of welfare. *Journal of Sociology and Social Welfare, 21,* 27–47.

Rank, M. R. (2004). *One nation, underprivileged: Why American poverty affects us all.* New York: Oxford University Press.

Rank, M. R., & Hirschl, T. A. (1999a). The likelihood of poverty across the American adult lifespan. *Social Work, 44,* 201–216.

Rank, M. R., & Hirschl, T. A. (1999b). The economic risk of childhood in America: Estimating the probability of poverty across the formative years. *Journal of Marriage and the Family, 61,* 1058–1067.

Rank, M. R., & Hirschl, T. A. (1999c). Estimating the proportion of Americans ever experiencing poverty during their elderly years. *Journal of Gerontology: Social Sciences, 54B,* S184–S193.

Rank, M. R., & Hirschl, T. A. (2001a). Rags or riches? Estimating the probabilities of poverty and affluence across the adult American life span. *Social Science Quarterly, 82,* 680–686.

Rank, M. R., & Hirschl, T. A. (2001b). The occurrence of poverty across the life cycle: Evidence from the PSID. *Journal of Policy Analysis and Management, 20,* 737–755.

Rank, M. R., & Hirschl, T. A. (2002). Welfare use as a life course event: Toward a new understanding of the U.S. safety net. *Social Work, 47,* 237–248.

Rank, M. R., & Hirschl, T. A. (2009). Estimating the risk of food stamp use and impoverishment during childhood. *Archives of Pediatrics and Adolescent Medicine, 163,* 994–999.

Rank, M. R., & Williams, J. H. (2010). A life course approach to understanding poverty among older American adults. *Families in Society, 91,* 337–341.

Rank, M. R., Yoon, H. S., & Hirschl, T. A. (2003). American poverty as a structural failing: Evidence and arguments. *Journal of Sociology and Social Welfare, 30,* 3–29.

Ritakallio, V. M. (2002). Trends of poverty and income inequality in cross-national comparison. *European Journal of Social Security, 4,* 151–177.

Rowntree, B. S. (1901). *Poverty: A study of town life.* London: Thomas Nelson and Sons.

Sandoval, D. A., Rank, M. R., & Hirschl, T. A. (2009). The increasing risk of poverty across the American life course. *Demography, 46,* 717–737.

Sawhill, I. (2003). The behavioral aspects of poverty. *The Public Interest, 153,* 79–93.

Schiller, B. R. (2008). *The economics of poverty and discrimination.* Englewood Cliffs, NJ: Prentice Hall.

Schreiner, M., & Sherraden, M. (2007). *Can the poor save?: Saving and asset building in individual development accounts.* New Brunswick, NJ: Transaction.

Schwartz, J. (2000). *Fighting poverty with virtue: Moral reform and America's urban poor, 1825–2000.* Bloomington, IN: Indiana University Press.

Seccombe, K. (1999). *So you think I drive a Cadillac? Welfare recipients' perspectives on the system and its reform.* Needham Heights, MA: Allyn & Bacon.

Seccombe, K. (2000). Families in poverty in the 1990s: Trends, causes, consequences, and lessons learned. *Journal of Marriage and the Family, 62,* 1094–1113.

Sen, A. (1992). *Inequality reexamined.* New York: Russell Sage Foundation.

Shapiro, T. M. (2004). *The hidden cost of being African American: How wealth perpetuates inequality.* New York: Oxford University Press.

Shapiro, T. M., & Wolff, E. N. (2001). *Assets for the poor: The benefits of spreading asset ownership.* New York: Russell Sage Foundation.

Simon, B. L. (1994). *The empowerment tradition in American social work: A history.* New York: Columbia University Press.

Smeeding, T. A. (2005a). Public policy, economic inequality, and poverty: The United States in comparative perspective. *Social Science Quarterly, 86,* 955–983.

Smeeding, T. A. (2005b). Poor people in rich nations: The United States in comparative perspective. Luxembourg Income Study Working Paper, No. 419. Syracuse, NY: Maxwell School of Citizenship and Public Affairs.

Smeeding, T. A., Rainwater, L., & Burtless, G. (2001). U.S. poverty in a cross-national context. In S. H. Danziger & R. H. Havemen (Eds.), *Understanding poverty* (pp. 162–189). Cambridge, MA: Harvard University Press.

Smith, A. (1776). *An inquiry into the nature and causes of wealth of nations.* London: W. Strahan and T. Cadell.

Smith, K. B., & Stone, L. H. (1989). Rags, riches, and bootstraps: Beliefs about the causes of wealth and poverty. *Sociological Quarterly, 30,* 93–107.

Stainback, K., & Tomaskovic-Devey, D. (2012). *Documenting desegregation: Racial and gender segregation in private-sector employment since the Civil Rights Act.* New York: Russell Sage Foundation.

Stevens, A. H. (1994). The dynamics of poverty spells: Updating Bane and Ellwood. *American Economic Review, 84,* 34–37.

Stevens, A. H. (1999). Climbing out of poverty, falling back in: Measuring the persistence of poverty over multiple spells. *The Journal of Human Resources, 34,* 557–588.

UNICEF. (2005). Child poverty in rich countries. Innocenti Report Card, No. 6.

United Nations Development Programme. (2012). *Human development report 2012.* New York: Oxford University Press.

U.S. Census Bureau. (2012). Income, poverty, and health insurance coverage in the United States: 2011. Current Population Reports, Series P60—243. Washington, DC: U.S. Government Printing Office.

Waldfogel, J. (2009). The role of family policies in antipoverty policy. In M. Cancian & S. Danziger (Eds.), *Changing poverty, changing policies* (pp. 242–265). New York: Russell Sage Foundation.

Walker, R. (1994). *Poverty dynamics: Issues and examples.* Aldershot, UK: Avebury.

Weinshenker, M., & Heuveline, P. (2006). The international child poverty gap: Does demography matter? Luxembourg Income Study Working Paper, No. 441. Syracuse, NY: Maxwell School of Citizenship and Public Affairs.

Wilson, W. J. (1987). *The truly disadvantaged: The inner city, the underclass, and public policy.* Chicago: University of Chicago Press.

Wilson, W. J. (1996). *When work disappears: The world of the new urban poor.* New York: Knopf.

Wilson, W. J. (2008). The political and economic forces shaping concentrated poverty. *Political Science Quarterly, 123,* 555–571.

Wilson, W. J. (2009). *More than just race: Being black and poor in the inner city.* New York: W. W. Norton.

Yinger, J. (1995). *Closed doors, opportunities lost: The continuing costs of housing discrimination.* New York: Russell Sage Foundation.

Zuberi, D. (2006). *Differences that matter: Social policy and the working poor in the United States and Canada.* Ithaca, NY: Cornell University Press.

MARK R. RANK

PRACTICE INTERVENTIONS AND RESEARCH

ABSTRACT: Social work is distinguishable from other disciplines by its emphasis on producing change that affects clients and their environment. This emphasis has influenced the nature of social work practice research, which calls for attention to the development, design, and implementation of change strategies through the use of the science of intervention research. This overview provides a definition of intervention research, highlights its culturally congruent elements, and addresses its implications for social work evidence-based practice and practice guidelines.

KEY WORDS: social work; practice; intervention

Introduction

The social work profession has long been preoccupied with the extent to which its research is able to inform and guide practice and policy (Briar & Miller, 1971; Fortune & Reid, 2003; Rosen, Proctor, & Staudt, 1999). Although there has been an increase in the production of intervention research, and improvement in its theoretical and methodological scientific sophistication, intervention research remains scarce (Fraser, 2004).

What Is Intervention Research?

Intervention research is conducted to understand, design, and test the feasibility, efficacy, and effectiveness of intervention strategies, with the goal of improving practice and policy (Rubin, 2000; Shilling, 1997; Thyer, 2000). Thomas and Rothman's (1994) science of intervention research paradigm, which has extensively guided social work intervention studies, defines intervention research as an intrusion into the environment of an individual, couple, family, or other target unit that is intended to bring about beneficial changes for the individual or others involved. By providing a systematic model of intervention planning, design, and implementation, this paradigm promotes the involvement of the client, community, and agency contexts in all stages of the research.

The paradigm encompasses three phases: (a) knowledge development, (b) knowledge utilization, and (c) design and implementation (Thomas & Rothman 1994). The knowledge development stage focuses on the use of social and behavioral sciences to generate practical information related to the problem(s) that the intervention attempts to address. This step is conducted through (a) a literature review, (b) qualitative and quantitative data collection where the researcher defines the problem of concern, (c) identifying risk and protective risk factors, (d) specifying conceptual frameworks and theories that inform the design and delivery of the intervention components, and (e) identifying existing empirical research. In the knowledge development stage, it is critical to use practice experience to inform the intervention content and study implementation. The knowledge utilization stage, which employs data generated in the knowledge development stage, aims to inform and pilot the intervention content and delivery strategies. This stage allows the researcher to make decisions about the feasibility and acceptability of the study, effect size, and the type of control group to be used in the efficacy trial. The purpose of the design and implementation stage encompasses the methodologies used to test the design and effectiveness of the intervention. Controlled field testing employs a systematic evaluation of the intervention and randomized controlled designs. Finally, if the trial proves effective, dissemination can take place. Thus, this research paradigm encourages innovation and facilitates the systematic development of efficacious intervention models.

Fraser (2004) has identified recent social work intervention research advances: First, more culturally and contextually relevant theoretical models are available. Second, new methods for dealing with randomization, attrition, and selection biases now exist, along with culturally congruent measures. Although randomized controlled clinical trials are viewed by many researchers as the "Gold Standard," alternatives (for example, interrupted time-series designs, regression discontinuity

designs) have been encouraged and used in intervention science. Third, analytical approaches, such as mixture modeling, propensity score matching, and approaches for dealing with missing data, have grown in sophistication. To strengthen the integrity and effectiveness of the research, use of manualized treatment protocols and quality assurance and quality control measures to assure fidelity of the study's implementation have increased.

Culturally Congruent Intervention

Over the past decade, a strong emphasis has been placed on the importance of the design of culturally congruent social work interventions to meet the needs of the profession's diverse client population. Thomas and Rothman's (1994) development intervention model allows researchers to incorporate values, practice wisdom, and agency context as well as worldviews of the clients, agency, and community into the early stages of the design, and later, into implementation of the studies (Galinsky, Turnbull, Meglin, & Wilner, 1993; Zayas, 2003). Culturally congruent intervention research must (a) include consumers, stakeholders, and the community in the early stages of the research so as to assure that the intervention fits well with real-world settings and encompasses the client's and the community's worldviews and their belief systems (Coulton, 2005); (b) employ culturally congruent recruitment and retention strategies (Witte et al., 2004); (c) be guided by conceptual theoretical frameworks and measurements that are culturally relevant to the population (El-Bassel et al., 2001); (d) employ culturally competent researchers (El-Bassel et al., 2001; Witte et al., 2004); and (e) involve a community advisory board in every stage of the research (Sormanti, Pereira, El-Bassel, Witte, & Gilbert, 2001; Witte et al., 2004).

How Intervention Research in Social Work Affects Evidence-Based Practice

Social work intervention research plays a fundamental role in the development and progress of evidence-based practice (EBP) and practice guidelines that make up essential core elements of social work practice (Gambrill, 1994; Proctor, 2004; Reid, 2002; Rosen, 2003). Social workers are expected to understand and use research evidence in defining client problems and in selecting interventions that lead to best outcomes (Proctor, 2003). Rooted in intervention studies, practice guidelines advise social workers how to apply EBP in their practice (Proctor, 2003). Unfortunately, the social work profession has limited access to evidence-based interventions to guide the use of EBP (Howard & Jenson 2003; Mullen & Bacon, 2003; Proctor & Rosen, 2003) and inform practice guidelines (Fortune & Reid 2003; Fraser, 2004; Gambrill, 1994; Proctor & Rosen, 2003). Each year, less than a dozen published studies focus on intervention research that practitioners may be able to replicate (Fraser, 2004). To advance the social work profession and to continue to promote EBP and practice guidelines, intervention research should remain in the forefront of the profession's mission.

Conclusion

Intervention research remains extremely valued in the social work profession because it provides empirically based solutions, advances the profession's ability to help clients by providing the best social work practices, improves and enhances clients' social conditions, leads to efficacious service delivery systems and social policies that change clients' lives (Shilling, 1997; Thomas & Rothman, 1994), and informs EBP and practice guidelines (Proctor & Rosen, 2003).

References

Briar, S., & Miller, H. (1971). *Problems and issues in social casework.* New York: Columbia University Press.

Coulton, C. (2005). The place of community in social work practice: Conceptual and methodological developments. *Social Work Research, 29*(2), 73–87.

El-Bassel, N., Witte, S., Gilbert, L., Sormanti, M., Moreno, C., Pereira, L., et al. (2001). HIV prevention for intimate couples: A relationship-based model. *Families, Systems and Health, 19*(4), 379–395.

Fortune, A. E., & Reid, W. (2003). Empirical foundations for practice guidelines in current social work. In A. Rosen & E. K. Proctor (Eds.), *Developing practice guidelines for social work intervention* (pp. 59–79). New York: Columbia University Press.

Fraser, M. W. (2004). Intervention research in social work: Recent advances and continuing challenges. *Research on Social Work Practice, 14*(3), 210–222.

Galinsky, M. J., Turnbull, J. E., Meglin, D. E., & Wilner, M. E. (1993). Confronting the reality of collaborative practice research: Issues of practice design, measurement, and team development. *Social Work, 38*, 440–449.

Gambrill, E. (1994). Social work research: Priorities and obstacles. *Research on Social Work Practice, 4*(3), 359–388.

Howard, M. O., & Jenson, J. M. (2003). Clinical guidelines and evidence-based practice in medicine, psychology, and allied professions. In A. Rosen & E. K. Proctor (Eds.), *Developing practice guidelines for social work intervention* (pp. 83–107). New York: Columbia University Press.

Mullen, E. J., & Bacon, W. F. (2003). Practitioner adoption and implementation of practice guidelines and issues of quality control. In A. Rosen & E. K. Proctor (Eds.),

Developing practice guidelines for social work intervention (pp. 223–235). New York: Columbia University Press.

Proctor, E. K. (2003). Research to inform the development of social work interventions. *Social Work Research, 27*(1), 3–6.

Proctor, E. K. (2004). The search for social work treatments of choice: What interventions work better than others? *Social Work Research, 28*(2), 67–69.

Proctor, E. K., & Rosen, A. (2003). The structure and function of social work practice guidelines. In A. Rosen & E. K. Proctor (Eds.), *Developing practice guidelines for social work intervention* (pp. 108–127). New York: Columbia University Press.

Reid, W. (2002). Knowledge for direct social work practice: An analysis of trends. *The Social Service Review, 76*(1), 6–35.

Rosen, A. (2003). Evidence-based social work practice: Challenges and promise. *Social Work Research, 27*(4), 197.

Rosen, A., Proctor, E. K., & Staudt, M. M. (1999). Social work research and the quest for effective practice. *Social Work Research, 23*(1), 4–14.

Rubin, A. (2000). Social work research at the turn of the millenium: Progress and challenges. *Research on Social Work Practice, 10*, 9–14.

Shilling, R. F. (1997). Developing intervention research programs in social work. *Social Work Research, 21*(3), 173–180.

Sormanti, M., Pereira, L., El-Bassel, N., Witte, S., & Gilbert, L. (2001). The role of community consultants in designing an HIV prevention intervention. *AIDS Education and Prevention, 13*(4), 311–328.

Thomas, E. J., & Rothman, J. (1994). An integrative perspective on intervention research. In J. R. E. Thomas (Ed.), *Intervention research: Design and development for human service* (pp. 3–20). Binghamptom, NY: Haworth Press.

Thyer, B. A. (2000). A decade of research on social work practice. *Research on Social Work Practice, 10*, 5–8.

Witte, S., El-Bassel, N., Gilbert, L., Wu, E., Chang, M., & Steingless, P. (2004). Recruitment of minority women and their main sexual partners in an HIV/STI prevention trial. *Journal of Women's Health, 13*(10), 1137–1147.

Zayas, L. H. (2003). Service-delivery factors in the development of practice guidelines. In A. Rosen & E. K. Proctor (Eds.), *Developing practice guidelines for social work intervention* (pp. 193–220). New York: Columbia University Press.

Nabila El-Bassel

PRIMARY HEALTH CARE

Abstract: The passage of the Affordable Care Act (ACA) has injected new life into primary health care by establishing the primary care medical home (PCMH) as a cornerstone of health-care reform legislation. In addition to the PCMH, the ACA has a number of primary-care components that can open opportunities for social workers. Concerns remain for payment reform in the implementation of the PCMH. The implementation of the ACA is still a work in progress, with anticipated modifications and changes as issues arise.

KEY WORDS: Affordable Care Act; behavioral health; primary health; primary health care; neighborhood health centers

Definition of Primary Health Care

The Institute of Medicine (IOM) definition of primary health care (IOM, 1978) included the importance of primary care as multidimensional with its five attributes of accessibility, comprehensiveness, coordination, continuity, and accountability. In 1996, the IOM Committee on the Future of Primary Care reaffirmed the 1978 components in a new definition of primary health care: "Primary care is the provision of *integrated, accessible health care* services by clinicians who are *accountable* for addressing a large *majority of personal health care needs*, developing a *sustained partnership* with *patients*, and practicing in the *context of family and community*" (Donaldson, Yordy, Lohr, & Vanselow, 1996). This definition identifies three additional perspectives to the 1978 definition: (a) patient and family, (b) community, and (c) integrated delivery system. The definition acknowledges the context of family and community in understanding the patient's living conditions and cultural background and the need to function within the broader health-care delivery system.

In both the 1978 and the 1996 reports, the committee affirmed a team approach with a variety of medical and allied medical professionals, including social workers as part of the team. Disease prevention and health promotion are the major themes in the delivery of primary health care given its focus on life stages, health-care access, and the inclusion of family and community.

The 2008 article on primary health care for the *Encyclopedia of Social Work* (Ashery, 2008) found consensus that primary health care was a fragmented system that had not lived up to its promises and was threatened by new forms of health-care delivery and a decline in primary-care physicians. The spectrum of primary health-care activities as defined by the IOM were mainly performed in clinics such as the Federally Qualified Health Centers (FQHCs) or by some health maintenance organizations such as Kaiser Permanente.

Affordable Care Act

Much is anticipated to change in the area of primary health care with the passage of the Affordable Care Act (ACA) in 2010 (Public Law 111–148). Also referred to as the Patient Protection and Affordable Care Act or Health Care Reform, the ACA represents the most significant legislative change in the U.S. health-care system since the passage of Medicare and Medicaid in 1965. When fully implemented in 2019, it will provide access to coverage for an estimated 32 million nonelderly Americans who are now uninsured by expanding Medicaid eligibility. Since 2014 it has prohibited the exclusion of coverage for people with preexisting conditions and prohibit annual or lifetime caps on coverage (Substance Abuse and Mental Health Services Administration, 2010). However, approximately 26 to 27 million nonelderly are still uninsured, with about a third of these being unauthorized immigrants who are not covered by the law (Congressional Budget Office, 2012). These individuals will most likely seek health care through the FQHCs and other clinics.

It should be noted that the ACA is still a work in progress, with some proposed rules and guidelines pending. In addition, as components are implemented and more research studies are completed, modifications may be made to accommodate unanticipated barriers and issues and to incorporate best practices.

This article will highlight key components of the ACA that are specific to primary health care. The key components are interrelated and may work in tandem. They are the primary care medical home (PCMH), the essential health benefits (EHBs), the accountable care organizations (ACOs), and workforce development.

Primary Care Medical Home

The ACA has established as its cornerstone the concept of the PCMH encompassing the five functions and attributes of the IOM definition of primary health care and adding three additional functions: health information technology, workforce development, and fundamental payment reform (Agency for Healthcare Research and Quality, n.d.). The vision of the PCMH is the provision of comprehensive care emphasizing prevention and wellness services, patient management, doctor/patient partnerships, and links to community resources. An emphasis of the PCMH is on managing patient populations with chronic diseases such as diabetes and congestive heart failure rather than just individual patients (Substance Abuse and Mental Health Services Administration, 2010). The services of the PCMH can be provided on the same premises or through linkages and a referral network.

This means that chronic disease management care coordinators are embedded within the practice to help manage high-risk patients. The reduction of both hospital admissions and visits to the emergency department has been shown to be the greatest cost savings in the PCMH model, mainly because of its emphasis on patient populations and patient-care coordinators. It is not clear how the care coordinators will be funded. There is anticipation that documentation of dollars saved by decreases in hospital emergencies and emergency department visits will pay for the care coordinators through some type of cost savings and bonuses that will be shared through the insurance companies and various governmental agencies (Longworth, 2011).

Common concerns among primary-care practices that have initiated the transition to the PCMH are promoting physician buy-in; changing office culture, care coordination, staffing, and space allocations; and leveraging electronic medical records. Other concerns are obstacles in terms of payment reform (Green, Wendland, Carver, Rinker, & Mun, 2012). Additional studies also warn that the PCMH will need adequate capital funding from a combination of federal, state, local, insurance industry, and health systems participation (Nutting et al., 2009).

A primary model for the PCMH are the FQHCs (also referred to as the Community Health Centers). They have been performing across the spectrum of primary health care for over 45 years to patients, regardless of their ability to pay. In the early 21st century there are nearly 9,000 service delivery sites that provide care to more than 21 million patients. The ACA established the Community Health Center Fund, which provides $11 billion over a 5-year period for the operation, preventive, and primary-care service expansion and the establishment of new health center sites. Health centers are also facilitating the enrollment of their service populations into affordable health insurance coverage (Bureau of Primary Health Care, 2013).

To ensure quality, standards have been developed by the National Committee for Quality Assurance (NCQA) to assess the ways in which practices function as medical homes. The PCMH practices earning NCQA recognition may qualify for additional bonuses or payments. The NCQA standards for the PCMH include elements in six standard categories with three different qualifying levels that a PCMH can meet. These standards include "must pass" elements to achieve recognition at any level such as care management, access during office hours, and referral tracking and follow-up (NCQA, 2011).

Essential Health Benefits
Tying into the concept of the PCMH are the EHB categories. Small-group and individual insurance policies that are sold within a state, including those offered through an exchange, must cover EHBs in each of 10 categories beginning in 2014. The EHB requirements do not apply to fully insured large-group plans or any grandfathered plans. Among the 10 general categories of covered benefits, many include primary-care services such as preventive and wellness services, chronic disease management, pediatric services including oral and vision care, behavioral health, and ambulatory patient services (Kaiser Family Foundation, 2012; United Health Care, 2013).

It should be noted that behavioral health (mental health) and substance-use disorder services are part of the EHBs and will have parity protections, which means that this coverage must be generally comparable to coverage for medical and surgical care. In addition, most health plans must now cover preventive services such as depression screening for adults and behavioral assessments for children at no cost. Since 2014, plans have been restricted from denying coverage or charging more because of preexisting mental illness (White House, 2013).

Accountable Care Organizations
The focus of the ACOs is on delivering comprehensive care coordinated across the entire continuum of health care—primary care, specialists, hospitals, home health, etc.—with a strong focus on prevention and care management of individuals with chronic disease. The foundation of the ACO is the PCMH. A driving force for the formation of the ACOs is the spiraling cost of chronic disease management within the Medicare and Medicaid populations. Although the emphasis is on the Medicare population, ACOs are also for private insurers (Gold, 2011). Four types of organizations are envisioned to be designed as ACOs: integrated health systems, multispecialty provider groups, physician–hospital organizations, and independent provider associations. Other models may emerge (Marcoux, Larrat, & Vogenberg, 2012). The ACO must meet a number of criteria, particularly in terms of standards of care. When an ACO succeeds in both delivering high-quality care and spending health-care dollars more wisely, it will share in the savings it achieves for the Medicare program. The ACO shares risk, but also shares financial incentives for meeting patient outcomes (Centers for Medicare and Medicaid Services, 2013). Although many ACOs are currently being formed, Correia questions whether the financial incentive to form an ACO is strong enough, given the administrative burden, implementation costs, and financial risks that the ACO must assume. (Correia, 2011).

Additional Forms of Health-Care Delivery

Two additional forms of health-care delivery related to primary care and deserving attention are urgent care and concierge care. They are not part of the ACA; however, they are fast-growing forms of health care with potential links to primary care. This growth reflects the fact that they are filling the needs of both patients and providers.

The broadest definition of urgent care as defined by the Urgent Care Association of America (UCAOA) is health care provided on a walk-in, no-appointment basis for acute illness or injury that is not life or limb threatening and is beyond either the scope or the availability of the typical primary-care practice or retail clinic. Approximately 9,000 facilities in the United States meet this definition, with a growth rate of 300 per year (UCAOA, 2011). These centers are state or county regulated, and in addition, the UCAOA has a certified Urgent Care Designation to help the public identify standards of an urgent-care center. Many of these centers are for-profit and will take various insurance plans, but may not take Medicaid. Some hospitals are also establishing urgent-care centers.

The urgent-care centers offer quick services for patients who cannot get a "sick call" appointment with their primary-care provider or who may not even have a primary-care provider. Urgent-care centers have met the needs of after-hours and weekend visits and have demonstrated savings from the avoidance of emergency room encounters (Patwardhan, Davis, Murphy, & Ryan, 2012).

The UCAOA claims that the urgent-care centers can play a role in linking the PCMH and primary-care physicians. With PCMH requirements for enhanced access and expanded office hours, urgent-care centers can handle this need and unscheduled visits. The UCAOA notes that urgent-care centers have rarely been included in solution development at the legislative level. The UCAOA wants the roles of the urgent-care center explored, piloted, and incorporated into the delivery system and planning at state, federal, and local levels (UCAOA, 2011). Some physicians worry that an overreliance on urgent-care centers can complicate efforts to improve health through better coordination of care (Galewitz, 2012).

Concierge medicine is also referred to as boutique medicine or retainer medicine. Concierge medicine enables physicians to reduce their case load and spend more time with their patients. It is an arrangement in which primary-care physicians contract with patients who are willing to pay a flat annual fee, either for all primary services or for services beyond those covered by conventional insurance. Fees may vary from less than $1,000 to $20,000 and involve "luxury primary care including extended office visits, 24 hour accessibility, streamlined specialty referrals and other perquisites. Practice size is limited to a manageable number with more time for the patient" (Huddle & Centor, 2011). Physicians may still take insurance with the annual fee covering additional services not covered by insurance. A concierge practice could be a PCMH, especially because many people willing to pay a flat annual fee may have chronic illnesses that will require the coordination of services and prevention of further illness. Whereas some physicians contend that this type of practice is ethical, others disagree, claiming it is unethical, and still others have a live-and-let-live attitude. Some fear that the primary-care shortage will worsen if physicians leave primary care for a concierge practice. There is concern regarding a two-tiered system that separates the wealthy from others, although some physicians have included individuals with an inability to pay under their concierge practice. There is a lack of documentation regarding higher quality care for concierge practices (Annals of Internal Medicine, 2012). There is no indication that the growth of concierge medicine will slow with the passage of the ACA. According to the American Academy of Private Physicians, the professional association for concierge physicians, there has been a 30% growth in concierge doctors since 2012. Concierge doctors are making money. Corporate interests, venture capitalists, and private equity firms are getting involved. Some are considering how to build a new model for primary care (Leonard, 2012).

Workforce

PRIMARY-CARE WORKFORCE Estimates indicate the United States will need 52,000 additional primary-care physicians by 2025 to meet demands that are growing as a result of three trends: population growth, population aging, and insurance expansion (Robert Wood Johnson Foundation, 2012; Sanders, 2013).

The ACA includes financial incentives to improve and strengthen the primary-care physician workforce including increases in Medicare and Medicaid payments, special modifications for federal student loans for medical students specializing in primary care, and scholarship and loan repayment programs for primary-care physicians in exchange for 2 years of service in a community-based area of high need (Teitelbaum, 2011).

Primary-care providers such as physician assistants and nurse practitioners currently make up one fourth of the primary-care workforce. Although their numbers may be adequate, the manner in which they are deployed may be insufficient because rural and low-income urban areas often lack a primary-care workforce (Hill, 2012). Money is also available through the ACA Prevention and Public Health Fund for training physician assistants in primary care, supporting nursing students to attend school full-time, and establishing nurse practitioner–led clinics that provide comprehensive primary-care services to populations living in medically underserved communities (Health and Human Services, 2010). The Primary Care Extension Program is another provision of the ACA based on the model of the Agricultural Extension Service. These programs are required to (a) assist primary-care clinicians in implementing a PCMH; (b) develop and support primary-care learning communities; (c) participate in a national network of Primary Care Extension Program hubs to develop a process to share best practices; and (d) develop a plan for financial sustainability after the initial 6-year period of funding under this section is completed (American College of Physicians, 2011).

In addition, the ACA included a total of $1.5 billion in new, dedicated funding for the National Health Service Corps (NHSC) over 5 years to Fiscal Year 2015, in addition to discretionary funding appropriated annually. The NHSC was established over 40 years ago and has a school loan repayment program for primary-care medical, dental, and behavioral- and mental-health clinicians in exchange for providing health care at NHSC-approved sites, which are mainly in areas identified as experiencing a health profession shortage. The NHSC includes social workers.

SOCIAL-WORK WORKFORCE The ACA specifically recognizes social workers by their inclusion as part of the health professional workforce. The law has a number of provisions to help build the workforce, as well as provisions that will enable students to reduce their educational debt. The law authorizes millions of dollars to specifically help develop the social-work workforce through grant funding to institutions that train social workers. It also expands the geriatric career awards available to clinical social workers and psychologists. In addition, the law authorizes grants to schools of social work and graduate psychology for professional training in child and adolescent mental health (Malamud, 2010).

ROLES FOR SOCIAL WORK IN PRIMARY HEALTH CARE Social work in primary health care through the ACA includes both micro/clinical and macro roles in terms of advocacy, policy, management, and direct

work with the community: (a) working with other stakeholders in setting up state health insurance exchanges and developing essential health benefits packages; (b) care coordination for mental and substance-abuse services (Collins, 2011); (c) integration of physical and mental-health needs; (d) direct clinical delivery of mental-health and substance-abuse services; (e) case management services for nonmedical resources; (f) motivational interviewing for patients with understanding of social, economic, and cultural barriers to health; (g) consultation on the individual, family, and community levels; and (h) advocacy to insure that appropriate local and national policies are developed (Allen, 2012). Although social workers are already engaged in many of these activities, the ACA will expand the demand with the creation of the PCMH and the expansion of the Medicaid population. Also, with the Mental Health Parity and Addiction Equity Act of 2008, the PCMH will likely provide comprehensive care that addresses physical and mental-health needs, integrating both in prevention and treatment and further expanding the social-work role (Allen). In addition, Golden (2011) points out that the ACA also creates promising models for improving care in which social workers should be playing key roles such as community-care transition, independence at home, and interdisciplinary community health teams. Although social workers could make a number of contributions under the ACA, their roles have not been made explicit because there has been no funding for new social-work positions. It is hoped that Congress will acknowledge the need to strengthen the profession and recognize social work's contribution by passing the Social Work Reinvestment Initiative related to social-work recruitment, training, retention, and research (National Association of Social Workers, n.d.).

REFERENCES

Affordable Care Act (Public Law 111–148). (2010). Retrieved from http://www.healthcare.gov/law

Agency for Healthcare Research and Quality Patient Center Medical Home Resource Center. (n.d.). Retrieved February 15, 2013, from http://pcmh.ahrq.gov/portal/server.pt/community/pcmh__home/1483/pcmh_tools___resources_foundations_v2

Allen, H. (2012). Health care reform and the future of medical social work. *Health and Social Work, 37*(3), 183–186.

American College of Physicians. (2011). Primary care extension programs. Retrieved February 1, 2013, from http://www.acponline.org/advocacy/where_we_stand/assets/iii5-primary-care-extension.pdf

Annals of Internal Medicine. (2012). Can the practice of retainer medicine improve primary care. Comments and responses. *Annals of Internal Medicine, 156*(5), 399–401.

Ashery, R. S. (2008). Social work and primary health care. In *Encyclopedia of Social Work*. New York, NY: Oxford University Press and National Association of Social Workers.

Bureau of Primary Health Care, Health Resources, and Services Administration. (2013). *The affordable care act and health centers*. Retrieved October 20, 2013, from http://bphc.hrsa.gov/about/healthcenterfactsheet.pdf

Centers for Medicare and Medicaid Services. (2013). Retrieved February 10, 2013, from http://innovation.cms.gov/initiatives/aco/index.html

Collins, S. (2011, April). The medical home model: What is it and how do social workers fit in? *Practice Perspectives, 10*. Washington DC: The National Association of Social Workers.

Congressional Budget Office (2012, March 13). *Updated estimates for the insurance coverage provisions of the Affordable Care Act*. Retrieved February 21, 2013, from http://www.cbo.gov/publication/43080

Correia, E. W. (2011, August). Accountable care organizations: The proposed regulations and the prospects for success. *American Journal of Managed Care, 17*(8), 560–568.

Donaldson, M. S., Yordy, K. D., Lohr, K. N., & Vanselow, N. A. (Eds.). (1996). *Primary care: America's health in a new era* (pp. 27–51). Washington, DC: National Academy Press.

Galewitz, P. (2012, September 17). *Urgent care centers are booming, which worries some doctors*. Retrieved January 4, 2013, from http://www.kaiserhealthnews.org/Stories/2012/September/18/urgent-care-centers.aspx?p=1

Gold, J. (2011, October 21). *FAQ on ACOs: Accountable care organizations, explained*. Retrieved January 31, 2013, from http://www.kaiserhealthnews.org/stories/2011/january/13/aco-accountable-care-organization-faq.aspx

Golden, R. L. (2011). Viewpoint: coordination, integration and collaboration: A clear path for social work in health care reform. *Health and Social Work, 36*(3), 227–228.

Green, E. P., Wendland, J., Carver, M. C., Rinker, C. H., & Mun, S. K. (2012). Lessons learned from implementing the Patient Centered Medical Home. *International Journal of Telemedicine and Applications, 2012*, Article ID 103685. Retrieved from http://www.hindawi.com/journals/ijta/2012/103685/

Health and Human Services. (2010, June 16). *News release: Sebelius announces new $250 million investment to strengthen primary health care workforce*. Retrieved December 4, 2012, from http://www.hhs.gov/news/press/2010pres/06/20100616a.html

Hill, I. (2012). Will there be enough providers to meet the need? Provider capacity and the ACA: Cross-cutting issues. *ACA Implementation—Monitoring and Tracking, November*. Retrieved from http://www.urban.org/UploadedPDF/412699-Will-There-Be-Enough-Providers-to-Meet-the-Need.pdf

Huddle, T. S., & Centor, R. M. (2011). Retainer medicine: An ethically legitimate form of practice that can improve primary care. *Annals of Internal Medicine, 155*, 633–635.

Institute of Medicine (IOM). (1978). Primary care in medicine: A definition. In *A manpower policy for primary health care: report of a study* (Chapter 2). Washington, DC: National Academy Press.

Kaiser Family Foundation. (2012, December 7). *Quick take, essential health benefits: What have states decided for their benchmarks?* Retrieved January 17, 2013, from http://kff.org/health-reform/fact-sheet/quick-take-essential-health-benefits-what-have-states-decided-for-their-benchmark/

Leonard, D. (2012, November 29). *Is concierge medicine the future of health care? Business Week*. Retrieved February 10, 2013, from http://www.businessweek.com/articles/2012-11-29/is-concierge-medicine-the-future-of-health-care

Longworth, D. L. (2011). Medical ground rounds. Accountable care organizations, the patient-centered medical home and health care reform: what does it all mean? *Cleveland Clinic Journal of Medicine, 78*(9), 571–582.

Malamud, M. (2010). Law recognizes social workers as leading providers of health care in the U.S. *NASW News, 55*(5). Retrieved February 28, 2013, from https://www.socialworkers.org/pubs/news/2010/05/health-care-reform2.asp?back=yes

Marcoux, R. M., Larrat, E. P., & Vogenberg, F. R. (2012). Accountable Care Organizations—An improvement over HMOs? *Pharmacy and Therapeutics, 37*(1), 629–630.

National Association of Social Workers. (n.d.). *Social work reinvestment initiative*. Retrieved February 19, 2013, from http://www.socialworkreinvestment.org

National Committee for Quality Assurance (NCQA). (2011). *Patient Centered Medical Home 201: Health care that revolves around you*. Retrieved from http://www.ncqa.org/portals/0/programs/recognition/2011PCMHbrochure_web.pdf

National Health Service Corps (NHSC). (n.d.). Retrieved October 20, 2013, from http://www.acponline.org/advocacy/state_health_policy/hottopics/nhsc_grants.pdf

Nutting, P. A, Miller, W. L., Crabtree, B. F., Jaen, C. R., Stewart, E. E., & Strange, K. C. (2009). Initial lessons from the First National Demonstration Project on practice transformation to a patient-centered medical home. *Annals of Family Medicine, 7*(3), 254–260.

Patwardhan, A., Davis, J., Murphy, P., & Ryan S. F. (2012). After-hours access of convenient care clinics and cost savings associated with avoidance of higher-cost sites of care. *Journal of Primary Care and Community Health, 3*(4), 243–245.

Robert Wood Johnson Foundation. (2012, November 20). *Study: More primary care physicians needed by 2025*. Retrieved December 29, 2012, from http://www.rwjf.org/en/blogs/human-capital-blog/2012/11/study_more_primary.html

Sanders, B. (2013). *Primary care access: 30 million new patients and 11 months to go: Who will provide their primary care? Hearing before the subcommittee on primary health and aging, January 29, 2013*. U.S. Senate Committee on Health, Education, Labor & Pensions.

Substance Abuse and Mental Health Services Administration. (2010, May–June). Health reform: Overview of the Affordable Care Act. *SAMHSA News, 18*(10). Retrieved February

13, 2013, from http://www.samhsa.gov/samhsanewsletter/
volume_18_Number_3/AffordableHealthCareAct.aspx

Teitelbaum, J. (2011). *Primary care physician workforce*. Retrieved
December 29, 2012, from http://healthreformgps.org/
resources/primary-care-physician-workforce/

United Health Care. (2013). *Essential health benefits overview*.
Retrieved February 16, 2013, from http://www.uhc.com/
live/uhc_com/Assets/Documents/EssentialHealthBenefits_
overview.pdf

Urgent Care Association of America (UCAOA). (2011).
The case for urgent care (White Paper, September 1, 2011).
Retrieved January 5, 2013, from http://www.ucaoa.org/
docs/WhitePaperTheCaseforUrgentCare.pdf

White House. (2013, August 21). *The Affordable Care Act and
expanding mental health coverage*. Retrieved October 19,
2013, from http://www.whitehouse.gov/blog/2013/08/
21affordable-care-act-and-expanding-mental-health-
coverage

REBECCA S. ASHERY

PSYCHOSOCIAL FRAMEWORK

ABSTRACT: The psychosocial framework is a distinctive practice model that originated early in the profession's history. Its goals are to restore, maintain, and enhance the personal and social functioning of individuals. Drawing on psychological and social theories, it has evolved considerably from its Freudian and ego psychological underpinnings. It has incorporated new knowledge on gender and diversity. Assessment, the client–worker relationship, respect for diversity, and an appreciation of client strengths are fundamental to the psychosocial approach. It uses both individual and environmental interventions and can be applied to a broad range of client populations. There is empirical evidence for the utility of psychosocial intervention but more research on the psychosocial framework is needed.

KEY WORDS: psychosocial framework; practice approach; person–situation perspective; diagnostic model; clinical social work

Although a psychosocial or person–situation perspective is at the core of all social work practice, the psychosocial framework has been a distinctive practice model that had its origins in the early history of the profession. It has evolved considerably over time in response to new theoretical and practice developments and greater understanding of the needs of diverse and vulnerable populations. It continues to be used widely by social work practitioners, particularly those who consider themselves to be clinical social workers.

The goals of the psychosocial framework are to restore, maintain, and enhance the personal and social functioning of individuals through mobilizing strengths, supporting coping capacities, building self-esteem, modifying dysfunctional patterns of thinking, feeling, and relating to others, linking people to necessary resources, and alleviating environmental stress. It draws on diverse theories of human behavior and the social environment. Although it has been mainly used with individuals, it can also be utilized in work with families and groups (Northen, 1969; Woods & Hollis, 1990).

History

The psychosocial framework had its earliest origins in the beginning of social casework and the writings of Richmond (1917). Viewing environmental conditions as crucial in affecting individuals, Richmond nevertheless saw each person as unique in the way he or she dealt with these social factors. The "diagnostic school" or "differential" approach emerged in the 1920s, taking its name from the fact that it emphasized diagnosis as the foundation of all intervention. It developed further during the period of the "psychiatric deluge" after World War I when Freud's views began to gain acceptance in certain segments of the social work profession. At the end of the 1930s and throughout the post-World War II period, ego psychological concepts also were incorporated into the diagnostic model (Goldstein, 1984, 1995). They helped to bridge the psychological and social spheres and were used to help correct some of the excesses of the Freudian emphasis.

In 1940, Hamilton published the widely used text, *Theory and practice of social casework*, which puts forth the principles of the evolving diagnostic approach. Hamilton began to use the term "psychosocial." Diagnostic social workers such as Austin (1948), Garrett (1958), Hollis (1949), among others, tried to define the goals and techniques of social casework as differentiated from psychotherapy during the 1940s and 1950s.

In the early 1960s, Florence Hollis wrote *Casework: A psychosocial therapy* (1964), which became a text that was widely used by several generations of social workers in the United States and other countries. Hollis' thinking evolved over the years as seen in later editions of the book (Hollis, 1972; Hollis & Woods, 1981; Woods & Hollis, 1990), the most recent of which was published after her death in 1987.

More recently, the psychosocial framework is no longer associated mainly with Hollis' writings. Others have made important contributions to updating the model with newer theoretical and practice developments and have tried to carry forth the psychosocial tradition in their writings (Applegate & Bonovitz, 1995; Berzoff, Flanagan, & Hertz, 1996; Brandell & Perlman, 1997; Elson, 1986; Goldstein, 1984, 1995, 2001; Mishne, 1993; Strean, 1979). Nevertheless, Hollis' writings constitute the most systematic statement of the psychosocial framework.

Theoretical Underpinnings and Related Theory

The person–situation perspective is central to the psychosocial approach, which draws on many developmental and environmental theories that help to understand the person, the situation, and the interactions between them. It focuses on the psychological and social factors that limit successful or optimal coping and cause various forms of suffering and maladaptation.

To understand the personality in depth and the coping capacities that people bring to their life transactions, the psychosocial framework employs contemporary psychodynamic theories, including Freudian psychoanalysis, ego psychology, attachment and object relations theory, self psychology, relational theory, and intersubjectivity (Berzoff, Flanagan, & Hertz, 1996; Brandell & Perlman, 1997; Goldstein, 2001). It places importance on integrating knowledge with respect to emotional disorders and serious forms of psychopathology. It embodies new perspectives on female development, the adult life cycle, the impact of trauma, gay and lesbian development, and cultural, ethnic, and racial diversity. It incorporates the findings of observational studies of infants and small children that enlarge and to some extent modify our understanding of developmental processes. Cognitive theory and new knowledge about the influence of biological factors on personality and psychopathology add an important dimension to our understanding of human functioning. Communications, family, and small group theories shed light on the nature of interpersonal interactions. Role theory provides an important link between social and environmental influences and personality development. Crisis theory adds an important dimension to showing how stressful circumstances disrupt an individual's usual means of coping. Knowledge regarding the impact of organizational structure and processes, the service delivery system, the community, and the society are also essential to understanding person–environmental transactions (Woods & Hollis, 1990).

Major Components

Diagnosis or assessment of the client's current and past functioning and life circumstances is fundamental to the psychosocial framework. Because each individual presents with a unique constellation of biological predispositions, needs, coping capacities, interpersonal relationships, stressors, cultural background, and environmental resources, correct assessment of the client's total person–situation functioning must be individualized and related to developing and implementing an appropriate interventive plan. Although time constraints may require that the assessment process be abbreviated and focused, accurate understanding is just as important in crisis and short-term intervention as in ongoing work.

Understanding and empathizing with the client's perception of his or her needs and difficulties is essential to the assessment process. The use of clinical or medical diagnoses may provide important information about symptom constellations and discrete disorders that have a certain etiology and course but should be augmented by a fuller psychosocial assessment. Thus concluding that a client has a learning disability, medical problem, emotional disorder, and the like has important implications but is not sufficient for the purposes of assessment and the planning of intervention. The focus and nature of intervention follows from the assessment and the client should be involved in establishing the treatment plan.

The client–worker relationship is a crucial element in the psychosocial framework. The worker shows human concern for clients and conveys certain key attitudes and values. These include acceptance of the client's worth, empathy, genuineness, a nonjudgmental attitude toward the client, appreciation of the client's individuality or uniqueness, respect for the client's right to self-determination, and adherence to confidentiality (Woods & Hollis, 1990). The worker may use the relationship with the client to help bring about change in keeping with the assessment of the client's needs and interventive goals. Sometimes the worker functions as a role model or provides corrective experiences for the client. The worker, however, must guard against imposing his or her own values on the client, using the client to meet the worker's needs, or encouraging too much dependence on the worker.

An important interventive principle, particularly in the engagement phase, is being where the client is. It is advisable for the worker to show respect for the client's diversity and recognize the factors that are influencing the client's participation in the helping relationship. These involve the client's motivation and expectations, previous experiences in getting help, values, gender, religion, sexual orientation, class, ethnicity, race, ego functioning, current life situation, and the characteristics of the service delivery setting itself.

Both participants influence the client–worker relationship. Sometimes, however, the client's or worker's past relationships influence and distort the real relationship between client and worker. These latter responses are termed transference and counter-transference reactions and may become disruptive (Woods & Hollis, 1990). In these instances, they need to be managed effectively. When ending the relationship because the work is complete or prematurely disrupted, the worker must consider the meaning the relationship has to the client and help the client deal with the feelings involved.

The psychosocial approach tries to mobilize client strengths. In codifying and refining the psychosocial framework, Hollis (1964, 1972) and Hollis and Woods (1981) described and studied individual techniques that can be used flexibly in the interventive process. These included sustainment, direct influence, exploration-description-ventilation, person-in-situation reflection, pattern-dynamic reflection, and developmental reflection. Hollis classified environmental intervention according to the type of resource employed, the type of communication used, and the type of role assumed. The latter consisted of provider, locator, creator of a resource, interpreter, mediator, and aggressive intervener. Although the psychosocial framework did not generate the use of cognitive-behavioral and other types of evidence-based practice techniques, many of these interventions can be incorporated into the psychosocial approach.

Because of shared theoretical assumptions about human behavior and basic practice principles, the psychosocial approach and the crisis intervention model are consistent with one another (Golan, 1978) and other forms of dynamically oriented short-term treatment (Reid & Epstein, 1972). The crisis and brief treatment models require somewhat different skills than do more extended forms of treatment because the constraints of time dictate faster assessments and more active and focused interventions. An important issue today is the degree to which briefer forms of intervention are used because they are indicated or as a blanket approach irrespective of client need in order to save money.

Diverse and Special Populations

With its early roots in Freudian theory and ego psychology, the psychosocial approach came under attack in the 1960s for viewing difference as pathology or deviance, and for not being attuned to the needs, problems, and strengths of diverse, oppressed, and vulnerable populations (Wasserman, 1974). Since that time, the psychosocial framework has expanded to encompass new perspectives on women's development and roles and the unique experiences, characteristics, strengths, and coping strategies of African

Americans, Latinos, Asians, and other people of color, and of other oppressed groups such as gays and lesbians (Goldstein, 1995). It has attempted to incorporate many of the principles that have been suggested by more sensitive, affirmative, and empowering interventive models (Collins, 1986; Drescher, 1998; Falco, 1991; Goldstein, 2003; Gutierrez, 1990; Hirayama & Cetingok 1988; Jordan, 1990; Phillips & Gonzalez-Ramos, 1989; Robinson, 1989; Ryan, 1985). Likewise, changes in society and in the clients needing help have focused greater attention on the application of the psychosocial approach to special populations. Psychosocial intervention has been utilized with every conceivable type of client populations and client problem, including victims and perpetrators of rape and other forms of violent assault, child abuse, domestic violence, substance abuse the homeless and chronically mentally ill, adult survivors of sexual abuse, and persons with AIDS (Turner, 1983, 1995).

Issues in Research

Historically, the psychosocial approach derived considerable strength from the extensive experiences of practitioners, that is, from "practice wisdom." In the late 1960s and throughout the 1970s, critics of the psychosocial framework drew attention to its lack of an empirical base and to the disappointing results of research on casework effectiveness (Mullen, Dumpson, & Associates, 1972). It later came to light that the studies in question were seriously flawed as the interventive goals, processes, and treatment outcomes were not well selected, defined, operationalized, and measured (Perlman, 1972). More rigorous research methodology was advocated (Bloom, 1983, pp. 560–582; Blythe & Briar, 1985, pp. 483–488; Fischer & Hudson, 1983, pp. 673–693; Levy, 1983, pp. 583–602; Reid, 1983, pp. 650–672).

In the years since these early studies, the evidence on treatment outcomes for psychosocial intervention reflects more positive results (Rubin, 1985, pp. 469–476; Thomlison, 1984, pp. 51–56). Greater sophistication in research methodology and design and more willingness on the part of theorists to subject their ideas to investigation have led to more systematic study of the theories that inform the psychosocial model. For example, there is significant research on child and adult development and the ways in which people cope with stress, crisis, and various types of life demands and events. Tools for assessing adaptive and maladaptive personality functioning also have evolved. In contrast to these developments, intervention research has lagged considerably but there have been significant research studies that address psychotherapy process and outcome based on psychosocial principles (Fonagy, 2006; Lambert & Hill, 1994; Weston, Novotny, & Thompson-Brenner, 2006).

An important thrust of process-oriented studies has addressed the common factors that are associated with positive outcomes across different therapeutic models. Lambert and Bergin (1994, p. 163) list 33 such features. Perhaps the two most important foci in these studies have been on the therapeutic alliance and therapist characteristics such as accurate empathy, positive regard, nonpossessive warmth, and congruence or genuineness (Howard & Orlinsky, 1986).

There is a good deal of evidence for the effectiveness of psychosocial interventions and psychotherapy based on psychodynamic principles that are not often integrated into courses on evidence-based practice (Fonagy, 2006; Rubin, 1985; Thomlison, 1984). Nevertheless, isolating the specific factors that are associated with effectiveness has been more difficult. The task of operationally defining psychosocial variables, interventions, and outcomes remains a challenging task and there is a dearth of evidence for psychosocial interventions in comparison to cognitive-behavioral approaches. Thus, research on psychosocial intervention still is at an early stage.

Outcome evaluation, while important, is not the only type of research methodology that can be used to study practice. Although systematic studies of the effectiveness of intervention with specific target problems and populations are needed, qualitative and other diverse research strategies are equally necessary (Reamer, 1992). Further, those involved in clinical practice should play a greater role in the formulation, design, and implementation of such studies either by acquiring practice research expertise themselves or through collaboration with researchers interested in and challenged by the problems inherent in conducting clinical studies.

Challenges and Dilemmas

Although the strength of the psychosocial framework approach has been its openness to new knowledge over the years and its willingness to discard ideas that are not useful, it is now more difficult to delimit its knowledge base precisely and to present a fully integrated view of its theoretical underpinnings. Ironically, it may be more accurate today to describe the psychosocial framework as a perspective that guides practice rather than as discrete practice model. Nevertheless, it does rely on a core of theoretical concepts and practice principles.

The continuing popularity of the psychosocial framework among social work practitioners shows

that it has stood the test of time (Mackey, Urek, & Charkoudian, 1987). There has been lingering criticism, however, that the psychosocial framework is too pathology oriented, psychotherapeutic in nature, and appropriate to the treatment of the "worried well" rather than work with clients presenting with difficult problems in living (Specht & Courtney, 1994). No doubt, some of this criticism stems from the fact that many private practitioners utilize the psychosocial framework. This criticism ignores its broadened application and considerable evolution. Although the psychosocial model includes psychotherapy, it has a broader scope and interventive repertoire (Strean, 1978; Turner, 1978). It may be short-term or long-term in nature and involve discharge planning, case management, and linkage to community and social resources, the support of functioning, or modification of longstanding personality or interpersonal difficulties. Moreover, the view that the goals of psychotherapy itself are only self-understanding or self-actualization rather than helping clients cope more effectively with their life circumstances represents a gross misunderstanding of the treatment process (Goldstein, 1996). Likewise, even those in private practice work with clients who present with complex problems and sometimes tragic life situations. The psychosocial model originated in and has been used extensively in agency-based practice since its inception. Social work practitioners have applied its principles and techniques in work with a broad range of clients and client problems. Nevertheless, it is important for there to be a continuing effort to apply the psychosocial framework to the problems of diverse, oppressed, economically disadvantaged, and special populations in today's agency practice arena and to study its effectiveness in work with these and other populations.

REFERENCES

Applegate, J. S., & Bonovitz, J. M. (1995). *The facilitating partnership*. Northvale, NJ: Jason Aronson.

Austin, L. (1948). Trends in differential treatment in social casework. *Social Casework*, 29, 203–211.

Berzoff, J. L., Flanagan, M., & Hertz, P. (Eds.). (1996). *Inside out and outside in*. Northvale, NJ: Jason Aronson.

Bloom, M. (1983). Empirically based clinical research. In A. Rosenblatt & D. Waldfogel (Eds.), *Handbook of clinical social work* (pp. 560–582). San Francisco: Jossey-Bass.

Blythe, B. J., & Briar, S. (1985). Developing empirically based models of practice. *Social Work*, 30, 483–488.

Brandell, J. R., & Perlman, F. T. (Eds.). (1997). *Theory and practice in clinical social work*. New York: Free Press.

Collins, B. G. (1986). Defining feminist social work. *Social Work*, 31, 214–220.

Drescher, J. (1998). *Psychoanalytic therapy and the gay man.* Hillsdale, NJ: The Analytic Press.

Elson, M. (1986). *Self psychology in clinical social work.* New York: W. W. Norton.

Falco, K. L. (1991). *Psychotherapy with lesbian clients: Theory into practice.* New York: Brunner/Mazel.

Fischer, J., & Hudson, W. (1983). Measurement of client problems for improved practice. In A. Rosenblatt & D. Waldfogel (Eds.), *Handbook of clinical social work* (pp. 673–693). San Francisco: Jossey-Bass.

Fonagy, P. (2006). *Evidence-based psychotherapies. In Psychodynamic diagnostic manual* (pp. 765–818). Silver Spring, MD: Alliance of Psychoanalytic Organizations.

Garrett, A. (1958). *Modern casework: The contributions of ego psychology.* In H. J. Parad (Ed.), Ego psychology and dynamic casework (pp. 38–52). New York: Family Service Association of America.

Golan, N. (1978). *Treatment in crisis situations.* New York: Free Press.

Goldstein, E. G. (1984). *Ego psychology and social work practice.* New York: Free Press.

Goldstein, E. G. (1995). *Ego psychology and social work practice* (2nd ed.). New York: Free Press.

Goldstein, E. G. (1996). What is clinical social work? Looking back to move ahead. *Clinical Social Work Journal, 24,* 89–104.

Goldstein, E. G. (2001). *Object relations theory and self psychology in social work practice.* New York: Free Press.

Goldstein, E. G., & Horowitz, L. (2003). *Lesbian identity and contemporary psychotherapy: A framework for clinical practice.* Hillsdale, NJ: The Analytic Press.

Gutierrez, L. M. (1990). Working with women of color: An empowerment perspective. *Social Work, 35,* 149–154.

Hamilton, G. (1940). *Theory and practice of social casework.* New York: Columbia University Press.

Hirayama, H., & Cetingok, M. (1988). Empowerment: A social work approach for Asian immigrants. *Social Casework: The Journal of Contemporary Social Work, 69,* 41–47.

Hollis, F. (1949). The techniques of casework. *Journal of Social Casework, 30,* 235–244.

Hollis, F. (1964). *Casework: A psychosocial therapy.* New York: Random House.

Hollis, F. (1972). *Casework: A psychosocial therapy* (2nd ed.). New York: Random House.

Hollis, F., & Woods, M. E. (1981). *Casework: A psychosocial therapy* (3rd ed.). New York: Random House.

Howard, K. I., & Orlinsky, D. E. (1986). Process and outcome. In S. L. Garfield & A. E. Bergin (Eds.), *Handbook of psychotherapy and behavior change* (3rd ed., pp. 311–381). New York: Wiley.

Jordan, J. V. (1990). *Relational development through empathy: Therapeutic applications. In Empathy revisited, Work in progress* (No. 40, pp. 11–14). Wellesley, MA: Wellesley College, Stone Center.

Lambert, M. J., & Bergin, A. (1994). Psychodynamic approaches. In A. Bergin & S. L. Garfield (Eds.), *Handbook of psychotherapy and behavioral change* (4th ed., pp. 467–508). New York: Wiley.

Lambert, M. J., & Hill, C. E. (1994). Assessing psychotherapy outcomes and process. In A. Bergin & S. L. Garfield (Eds.), *Handbook of psychotherapy and behavioral change* (4th ed., pp. 72–113). New York: Wiley.

Levy, R. L. (1983). Overview of single-case experiments. In A. Rosenblatt & D. Waldfogel (Eds.), *Handbook of clinical social work* (pp. 583–602). San Francisco: Jossey-Bass.

Mackey, R. A., Urek, M. B., & Charkoudian, S. (1987). The relationship of theory to clinical practice. *Clinical Social Work Journal, 15,* 368–383.

Mishne, J. M. (1993). *The evolution and application of clinical theory.* New York: Free Press.

Mullen, E. J., & Dumpson, J. R., & Associates (Eds.). (1972). *Evaluation of social intervention.* San Francisco: Jossey-Bass.

Northen, H. (1969). *Social work with groups.* New York: Columbia University Press.

Perlman, H. H. (1972). Once more with feeling. In E. J. Mullen, J. R. Dumpson, & Associates (Eds.), *Evaluation of social intervention* (pp. 191–209). San Francisco: Jossey-Bass.

Phillips, L. J., & Gonzalez-Ramos, G. (1989). Clinical social work practice with minority families. In S. M. Ehrenkranz, E. G. Goldstein, L. Goodman, & J. Seinfeld (Eds.), *Clinical social work with maltreated children and their families: An introduction to practice* (pp. 128–148). New York: New York University Press.

Reamer, F. J. (1992). The place of empiricism in social work. *Journal of Social Work Education, 28,* 260–269.

Reid, W. J. (1983). Developing intervention methods through experimental designs. In A. Rosenblatt and D. Waldfogel (Eds.), *Handbook of clinical social work* (pp. 650–672). San Francisco: Jossey-Bass.

Reid, W. J., & Epstein, L. (1972). *Task-centered casework.* New York: Columbia University Press.

Richmond, M. L. (1917). *Social diagnosis.* New York: Russell Sage Foundation.

Robinson, J. B. (1989). Clinical treatment of black families: Issues and strategies. *Social Work, 34,* 323–329.

Rubin, A. (1985). Practice effectiveness: More grounds for optimism. *Social Work, 30,* 469–476.

Ryan, A. S. (1985). Cultural factors in casework with Chinese Americans. *Social Casework: The Journal of Contemporary Social Work, 66,* 333–340.

Specht, H., & Courtney, M. (1994). *Unfaithful Angels.* New York: Free Press.

Strean, H. S. (1978). *Clinical social work.* New York: Free Press.

Strean, H. S. (1979). *Psychosocial theory and social work practice.* New York: Free Press.

Thomlison, R. J. (1984). Something works: Evidence from practice effectiveness studies. *Social Work, 29,* 51–56.

Turner, F. J. (1978). *Psychosocial therapy: A social work perspective.* New York: Free Press.

Turner, F. J. (Ed.). (1983). *Differential diagnosis and treatment in social work practice* (3rd ed.). New York: Free Press.

Turner, F. J. (Ed.). (1995). *Differential diagnosis and treatment in social work practice* (4th ed.). New York: Free Press.

Wasserman, S. L. (1974). Ego psychology. In F. J. Turner (Ed.), *Social work treatment* (pp. 42–83). New York: Free Press.

Weston, D., Novotny, C. M., & Thompson-Brenner, H. (2006). *The empirical status of empirically supported psycho-therapies: Assumptions, findings, and reporting in controlled clinical trials. In Psychodynamic Diagnostic Manual* (pp. 631–663). Silver Spring, MD: Alliance of Psychoanalytic Organizations.

Woods, M. E., & Hollis, F. (1990). *Casework: A psychosocial therapy.* New York: McGraw Hill.

EDA G. GOLDSTEIN

QUALITATIVE RESEARCH

ABSTRACT: The term *qualitative methods* is relatively new. There is no single definition, although they share features in common, that is, flexibility, holism, naturalism, and insider perspectives. Epistemological debates continue among qualitative researchers, and the diverse methodological approaches often reflect the influence of constructivist critiques. The basic approaches—ethnography, grounded theory, case studies, narrative, phenomenological, and action research—are described along with the fundamentals of data collection and analysis, the role of theory, standards for rigor, ethical issues, and social work values. Rapid growth in the popularity of these methods ensures that they will play a key role in the profession's knowledge development in the future.

KEY WORDS: qualitative methods; epistemology; constructivism; postpositivism; ethnography; grounded theory; rigor

The term *qualitative methods* is relatively new to the research lexicon compared with the venerable age of some of its constituent approaches, such as ethnography. Historically rooted in 19th-century anthropological studies of non-Western cultures, these methods have become increasingly complex and diverse as they have been embraced by researchers in sociology, psychology, nursing, medicine, and social work (Creswell, 2007; Marshall & Rossman 2006; Miles & Huberman 1994; Morse, 1994; Padgett, 2008).

Distinguishing Features of Qualitative Methods

There is no single definition for "qualitative methods." The distinction between them and quantitative research, that is, "a mile wide and an inch deep" versus "a mile deep and an inch wide," is often invoked to increase understanding of their special features (Padgett, 2008).

Other contrasts include the following:
- Insider rather than outsider
- Person-centered rather than variable-centered
- Holistic rather than particularistic
- Depth rather than breadth

Qualitative methods are *inductive* rather than *hypothetico-deductive*. They favor *naturalistic* observation and interviewing. As such, they imply a degree of *closeness* and an *absence of controlled conditions* that stand in contrast to the distance and control of experimental studies.

Qualitative studies seek to convey the complex worlds of respondents in a holistic, on-the-ground manner. Furthermore, they assume a *dynamic reality*, a state of flux that can only be captured via intensive engagement with respondents. Unlike the pre-coded standardized questionnaire, the qualitative researcher must be a sensitive instrument of observation, capable of flexibility, and on-the-spot decision-making about following promising leads.

Paradigmatic and Epistemological Underpinnings

A primary source of epistemological difference among qualitative researchers is between *postpositivism* and *pragmatism* on the one hand and *constructivism* and *interpretivism* on the other (Denzin & Lincoln 2005; Padgett, 2008; Patton, 2002). Coming into full flower by the 1990s, epistemological debates centered on fundamental questions about the nature of reality (a single "objective" reality versus subjectively derived multiple realities) and the relationship between the researcher and study participants (detachment versus immersion). Although the salience of these differences tends to be felt more deeply on the constructivist side and within the halls of academia, most qualitative researchers accept the premise of multiple interpretations and reject the notion of "pure" objectivity and neutrality.

Much of the vocal opposition to positivism has come from scholars in the field of education such as Yvonna Lincoln, Egon Guba, Harry Wolcott, and John Creswell. Along with sociologist Norman Denzin, these individuals pioneered the development of interpretivist and social constructivist approaches as stand-alone alternatives. Similar disagreements over epistemological stance can be found in anthropology, sociology, psychology, nursing, and social work.

The rapid growth in the popularity of qualitative methods in recent years has done little to increase consensus about these issues. Philosophical pragmatism is often cited as a foundation for avoiding such debates entirely and focusing instead on matching method to subject matter to optimize "what works." In practice, much of the qualitative research taking place in social work and elsewhere implicitly adopts a pragmatic stance in that epistemological allegiances are not given priority.

Primary Approaches to Qualitative Research

The following sections provide brief descriptions of six of the primary types of qualitative methods, described in rough chronological order (beginning with the earliest).

ETHNOGRAPHY Ethnography has its roots in the study of non-Western people and cultures (Bernard, 2000). Though rarely explicated as a set of skills imparted in a classroom, ethnography is defined by its commitment to prolonged engagement using a holistic perspective. Data collection is done by observation (with varying amounts of participation) and through interviews conducted with selected informants. Pioneered by anthropologists and adapted by the "Chicago School" of sociology to studies of urban life, ethnography has endured as the primary means of understanding a social group or culture and its requisite beliefs and values (Emerson, 2001). Despite its pedigree as the first qualitative method, ethnography does not preclude use of quantitative techniques, for example, measuring caloric intake or quantifying social networks.

Ethnography and its parent discipline of anthropology underwent a profound identity crisis by the late 1970s in which previous canons of objectivity and the invisibility of the researcher were questioned. The methodological self-consciousness that resulted has produced new approaches such as "auto-ethnography" in which the authors' role in the inquiry becomes the focus of interest. Adopted by researchers in other disciplines (including social work), ethnography has retained its value as a method for naturalistic research using its hallmark technique of participant observation.

GROUNDED THEORY The most commonly used of all qualitative methods, grounded theory (GT) has its roots in the Chicago School of sociology and its parentage in the collaboration of Barney Glaser and Anselm Strauss dating back to the 1960s (Charmaz, 2006; Glaser & Strauss, 1967; Strauss & Corbin 1990). GT has emerged as the most systematized and

documented of qualitative methods. Glaser and Strauss developed GT as a means of generating theory relying upon an iterative process of data collection and analysis, using inductive thinking and *constant comparative analysis*. Data analysis in GT involves coding, comparison, and thematic interpretation of data to reveal conceptual frameworks and "mid-range" theories of human social behavior and interaction. GT's attractions include its flexibility and transparency of method. Distinct from *content analysis* (which involves identifying and usually counting occurrences of specified phenomena within texts), GT is designed to yield conceptually rich understanding.

NARRATIVE TECHNIQUES Narrative techniques share a focus on the form and content of speech, whether monologic or dialogic. Rooted in philosophy, literary criticism, linguistics, and psychotherapy, narrative analyses assume that much can be learned from the ways that individuals tell stories and converse with one another. Pioneers of these methods include William Labov, Elliott Mishler, Gordon Gee, and Catherine Reissman. Two basic variants of narrative techniques include analysis of interviews about life experiences (with an emphasis upon natural story-telling) and analyses of conversation and discourse. The former approach shares some features in common with narrative therapy in which story-making is part of the therapeutic encounter. The latter reflect a sociolinguistic focus upon the ways that social status (gender, social class, race, age, ethnicity, and so on) is revealed during speech events (Reissman, 1993).

PHENOMENOLOGICAL ANALYSIS Phenomenological analysis (PA) owes much to the philosophers Edmund Husserl and Alfred Schutz and to the developmental work of Duquesne University psychologist Amedeo Giorgi. As a qualitative method, PA seeks to grasp holistically the "lived experience" and the life worlds of study participants who share a particular experience in common. Its technique of repeated interviews and reflective immersion in the data requires the researcher to "bracket" his or her own personal experiences and feelings in order to fully capture the experience of others, for example, being a cancer survivor, a crime victim, or a first-time parent (Giorgi, 1985).

CASE STUDY ANALYSIS The intensive study of a bounded entity, that is, a single case or group of cases, has long been recognized as an important form of inquiry in the social and natural sciences. Case study analyses in research are different from their use in clinical training (where cases, or vignettes, are presented for pedagogic reasons). A "case" may be an individual, an agency, a village, an innovation, or an important event—its selection as the focus of study is an indication of its capacity to inform and expand understanding on a deeper level. To achieve maximum depth, case studies involve multiple forms of data (which may also be quantitative). Multiple case studies, which usually entail *within-case* and *across-case analyses*, are appropriate when the phenomenon encompasses more than one entity and comparisons are needed (Stake, 1995).

ACTION AND COMMUNITY-BASED APPROACHES These approaches, rooted in 1960s liberation movements, are united by their commitment to research as a vehicle for social change and community empowerment. Although not necessarily qualitative, these approaches tend to emphasize community immersion and involvement, which, in turn, favor in-depth interviewing and rapport-building. Action researchers often engage in partnerships with community members to ensure that local needs are being served and that the research findings are beneficial to the community (Israel, Eng, Schulz, & Parker 2005).

Qualitative Designs: Methods of Data Collection and Analysis

Qualitative studies may be longitudinal or cross-sectional, single-site or multi-site, and single-group or group-comparative. Some general principles characterizing the vast majority of qualitative designs include the following: flexibility, multiple sources of data (when applicable), multiple interviews with each participant (when possible), iterative phases of data collection and analysis, and careful documentation of all activities during the study (Padgett, 2008).

The three primary means of data collection in qualitative research are interviews, observation, and analysis of documents. A qualitative interview is *minimally structured* and intended to yield lengthy and rich accounts from study participants, which are audio-recorded and transcribed verbatim. Observational data produce field notes, which are also analyzed as texts. Some researchers use photography and video recording, although these bring greater ethical concerns regarding confidentiality. Existing documents might include case records, personal diaries, minutes from meetings, and so on. Although the specifics of data analysis depend upon the type of method, all share in common immersion in the data, inductive thinking, and a search for deeper meaning (Padgett, 2008).

Sampling in qualitative research is typically *purposive* and designed to maximize the retrieval of rich, meaningful data. Sample sizes can range from a single case to fewer than 10 (as in PA) to 25 or more (as in GT). The ultimate size of a study's sample depends upon the quality of the data and when *saturation* (redundancy) is achieved. A design emphasis on *multiple interviews with each participant* is an important factor in addressing concerns about small samples and shallow, insufficient data. For these reasons, qualitative studies are not expected to be generalizable in the traditional scientific sense, but their findings should have credibility and wider applicability (Padgett, 2008).

Use of qualitative data analysis (QDA) computer software has become increasingly common, with programs such as NVIVO and ATLAS/ti providing tools for data management and retrieval with the following caveat: QDA software does not perform the most important functions of qualitative analysis, that is, conceptualization, categorization, and comparison.

The Role of Theory in Qualitative Research

While a strength of qualitative studies lies in their avoidance of strict allegiance to any given theory (or theories), this does not preclude drawing upon theories to inform the study. Often easier to incorporate when broken down into conceptual building blocks, theories contribute *sensitizing concepts* that may (or may not) be found relevant during analysis (Charmaz, 2006) Though not designed to test theories deductively, qualitative studies offer fertile ground for their application (Padgett, 2008).

Standards for Quality and Rigor

Qualitative research adheres to different standards than quantitative research, though there is little consensus on what those standards should be. Under the general heading of "trustworthiness," qualitative studies are judged by their ability to convey deeper understanding of a phenomenon through use of systematic application of the methods of choice. A successful qualitative study is informative and thought-provoking; it also "rings true" in the sense of reflecting the insider perspective obtained from immersion and analyses based upon the participants' own words (Charmaz, 2006; Padgett, 2008).

A number of strategies for rigor have been put forth, including *data triangulation* (use of more than one source of data), *peer debriefing* to minimize investigator bias, *keeping an audit trail*, or documentation of data and analytic decisions, *negative case analysis* to avoid premature and untested conclusions, *member checking* to seek participant input, and *prolonged engagement*.

The deployment of one or more of these strategies enhances study rigor and credibility.

Ethical Issues

In addition to seeking voluntary informed consent and protecting confidentiality, qualitative researchers must address concerns specific to their methods, that is, the sensitivity of personal revelations and fears of identity disclosure. The sharing of personal and sometimes painful information is not uncommon in qualitative studies, but such emotions almost always resolve without harm. Nevertheless, qualitative researchers anticipate this and build into the study referral mechanisms for outside counseling if warranted. Unintended disclosure of a study participant's identity is another risk, given the detailed description found in a qualitative report, but changing unimportant details helps mitigate against this. The inherent flexibility of qualitative inquiry ensures that ethical issues require attention at all times. In addition, social work researchers must make allowances for mandated reporting of child abuse and imminent threats of harm.

Social Work Values in Qualitative Research

Qualitative methods attract researchers with a predisposition toward being socially responsible (and socially active), in part because there is no expectation that they be "value-neutral" as there is in quantitative methods. In addition to action- and community-based research, feminist studies, critical race theory, and queer theories (among others) are explicitly devoted to addressing inequality and injustice.

The researcher's choice of topic consonant with social advocacy is one manifestation of this ethos, for example, studying the health problems of poor children as opposed to those of middle-class children, but the conduct of qualitative research is also considered a means to this end. Two primary ways that this occurs are (a) the emphasis on egalitarian partnership of researcher and researched; and, (b) an emphasis on participants voicing their responses freely and in their own words.

Trends

Growing recognition that qualitative methods "go where quantitative methods cannot go" has led to a boom in their popularity in recent years. The National Institutes of Health, a major source of funding and prestige in the United States, has issued helpful guidelines for qualitative researchers and has funded an increasing number of studies on drug abuse, AIDS, mental illness, and immigrant health. This trend toward widespread acceptance has also spawned increased interest in *mixed methods* studies using both quantitative and qualitative methods (Padgett, 2004). Although mixed methods studies carry a risk of short-changing the qualitative portion of the study, their attraction is likely to continue into the future. It is also noteworthy that the heterogeneity of qualitative methods has contributed to "internal mixing" (for example, case studies combined with GT analyses in the same study) and to new combinations (for example, the *constructivist grounded theory* of Kathy Charmaz).

Qualitative methods have also gained greater prominence as research, practice and policy have "gone global," for example, AIDs, violence against women, the aftermath of wars and natural disasters, drug trafficking. Qualitative methods have a number of advantages in this regard, including their multidisciplinary foundation, attention to cultural sensitivity, flexible designs, and ability to adapt to local conditions of other cultures. Increased interest in community-based approaches, rapid assessment, and culturally-appropriate partnerships is evidence of the growing awareness of the globalization of many social problems and their potential solutions.

Within social work, qualitative research had tremendous relevance, given the complexity of human problems and its ethos of egalitarianism. This is especially visible among the membership of the Society for Social Work and Research (SSWR), an organization that has grown rapidly since the mid-1990s, in part because of its inclusion of qualitative methods content within its annual conference program.

REFERENCES

Bernard, H. R. (Ed.). (2000). *Handbook of methods in cultural anthropology*. Walnut Creek, CA: Altamira Press.

Charmaz, K. (2006). *Constructing grounded theory*. Thousand Oaks, CA: Sage.

Creswell, J. W. (2007). *Qualitative inquiry and research design*. Thousand Oaks, CA: Sage.

Denzin, N. K., & Lincoln, Y. S. (Eds.). (2005). *Handbook of qualitative research*. Thousand Oaks, CA: Sage.

Emerson, R. M. (2001). *Contemporary field research*. Prospect Heights, IL: Waveland Press.

Giorgi, A. (1985). *Phenomenology and psychological research*. Pittsburgh, PA: Duquesne University Press.

Glaser, B. G. & Strauss, A. L. (1967). *The discovery of grounded theory*. Chicago: Aldine.

Israel, B. A., Eng, E., Schulz, A. J., & Parker, E. A. (Eds.). (2005). *Methods in community-based participatory research for health*. San Francisco: Jossey-Bass.

Marshall, C., & Rossman, G. B. (2006). *Designing qualitative research*. Thousand Oaks: Sage.

Miles, M., & Huberman, A. (1994). *Qualitative data analysis*. Thousand Oaks, CA: Sage.

Morse, J. M. (Ed.). (1994). *Critical issues in qualitative research methods*. Thousand Oaks, CA: Sage.

Padgett, D. K. (2008). *Qualitative methods in social work research*. Thousand Oaks, CA: Sage.

Padgett, D. K. (Ed.). (2004). *The qualitative research experience*. Pacific Grove, CA: Brooks/Cole Publishers.

Patton, M. (2002). *Qualitative research and evaluation methods*. Thousand Oaks, CA: Sage.

Reissman, C. (1993). *Narrative analysis*. Newbury Park, CA: Sage.

Stake, R. (1995). *The art of case study research*. Thousand Oaks, CA: Sage.

Strauss A., & Corbin, J. (1990). *The basics of qualitative research*. Newbury Park, CA: Sage.

FURTHER READING

http://www.nsf.gov/pubs/2004/nsf04219/start.htm (Proceedings from workshop on qualitative methods at the National Science Foundation)

http://obssr.od.nih.gov/Documents/ConferencesAnd_Workshops/Qualitative.PDF (Document produced by the National Institutes of Health in 1999)

http://www.uofaweb.ualberta.ca/iiqm/Conferences.cfm (Comprehensive site from the University of Alberta's International Institute for Qualitative Methodology)

http://www.ualberta.ca/~ijqm/ (*International Journal of Qualitative Methods*)

http://www.nova.edu/sss/QR/web.html (includes the journal *The Qualitative Report* and other resources)

http://www.c4qi.org/ (International Center for Qualitative Inquiry and annual conference headed by Professor Norman Denzin)

http://www.qualitativeresearch.uga.edu/QualPage/ (Resources provided through Professors Judith Norris and Judith Preissle)

http://www.quarc.de (German–English site with links to other resources)

http://www.lsoft.com/scripts/wl.exe?SL1=QUALRS-L&H=LISTSERV.UGA.EDU (multi-disciplinary resources and listserv from the University of Georgia)

http://qualitative-research.net (German–English site with on-line journal)

http://sophia.smith.edu/~jdrisko/qualres.htm (Professor James Drisko's compendium of resources)

http://www.nova.edu/ssss/QR/QR1-4/wark.html (listing of qualitative journals)

http:///www.scolari.com (information and downloadable software demos for Atlas.ti, NVIVO, The Ethnograph, etc.)

http://www.researchtalk.com (training and workshops on Long Island, NY)

http://caqdas.soc.surrey.ac.uk/ (support for computer-assisted qualitative data analysis)

http://onlineqda.hud.ac.uk/Introduction/index.php (assistance in qualitative data analysis using computer software)

DEBORAH PADGETT

R

RIGHTS-BASED FRAMEWORK AND SOCIAL WORK

ABSTRACT: The early 21st century has seen a surge in efforts to incorporate rights-based approaches in programming. The rise has been spearheaded by growing awareness that human rights may be the most effective way to reduce or eradicate poverty and injustice while advancing human dignity and welfare. The profession of social work has played a major role in issues of welfare and human rights. In fact, at the core of social work is the "intrinsic" value of every person and the mandate to promote social justice while upholding human dignity. Also reflected in the profession's code of ethics are the profession's ethical responsibilities to the broader society (NASW, 1999). This review looks at the basic underpinnings of the rights-based discourse as it relates to programming and assessment. An historical overview is presented. Approaches to rights-based programming along with tools supporting the approach are highlighted. Areas of intersection between social work and rights-based programming are also identified.

KEY WORDS: duty bearer; human rights; indicators; principles of human rights; right holder; rights-based assessment; rights-based programming

Introduction to the Rights-Based Perspective

The rights-based perspective is a conceptual and organizational framework for ensuring that human rights principles are reflected in program and policy initiatives at both local and national levels (OHCHR, 2012; UNICEF, 1998; 2004). It is also seen as both a process and approach underscoring steps and strategies that need to be undertaken to ensure that the rights of vulnerable individuals and groups are respected, promoted, protected, and fulfilled. The perspective is based upon the values, standards, and principles reflected in the United Nations Charter, the Universal Declaration of Human Rights, and subsequent legally binding human rights conventions and treaties (Nyamu-Musembi & Cornwall, 2004; OHCHR, 2008/9). The rights-based perspective reflects the recognition of human rights as essential for people to live in freedom and dignity (Gil, 1998; OHCHR, 2012; 2008/9).

The framework facilitates translation of needs into rights and acknowledges the human person as an active subject of rights and as a claim-holder. It further identifies the duties and obligations of those against whom a claim can be brought to ensure that rights and entitlements are realized. In a sense, it defines the relationship between the right holder and duty bearer and outlines mechanisms by which duty bearers can be held accountable (see Figure 1). Rights holders are identified as those who are entitled to claim rights and entitlements. These may include vulnerable groups such as women, children, youth, older adults, persons with disabilities, racial minorities, and gays, lesbians, transgender, and queer people. Duty bearers are those who have a responsibility to protect, respect, and fulfill claimed rights. The primary duty bearer is said to be the state and non-state actors (OHCHR, 2012). The framework also enables enhancement of stakeholder capacities to meet their respective obligation: as a right holder or as a duty bearer.

The rights-based perspective is increasingly being adopted as an organizing framework by actors in diverse fields, including public health and development. The perspective has also been articulated and adopted in policies by bilateral and international development agencies including the United Nations. The value of the rights-based perspective lies in the transformative potential of human rights to highlight and alleviate injustice, inequality, and poverty, as well as other forms of vulnerabilities. Through utilization of the human rights principles of universality, indivisibility, interdependence, equality, and non-discrimination, the framework helps identify individuals and groups that are marginalized or excluded, or that are at risk for marginalization or exclusion, and guides implementation of remediation strategies.

Moreover, the framework facilitates the creation of an enabling environment, one that strengthens the capabilities of vulnerable individuals and groups and enables them to demand and exercise their rights. Indeed, the rights-based perspective is about empowering vulnerable individuals and groups to make decisions about their lives; it recognizes that success in tackling vulnerability requires an environment that allows vulnerable individuals and groups to have a stake and a voice and that makes channels available for meaningful participation in issues that affect their welfare.

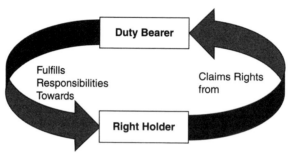

FIGURE 1 *The Reciprocal Relationship between the Right Holder and Duty Bearer*

Historical Overview

The rights-based perspective is enshrined in the discourse of human rights. It has a long tradition entrenched in the history of human societies, which, for thousands of years, have established moral and legal codes to regulate the relationship between the individual and the community (Roosevelt, 1948; Theis, 2004). Examples of these include the Vedas, the Torah, the Bible, and the Qur'an.

Human rights constitute a modern set of individual and collective rights that have been formally established and promoted through international and domestic law since the Universal Declaration of Human Rights in 1948 (UN, 1948). Given that the Declaration was not legally binding, state actors and their allies have put in place a series of international treaties that are legally binding for state parties. While some of these have focused on collective rights, such as the International Covenant on Civil and Political Rights (ICCPR) and the International Covenant on Economic, Social, and Cultural Rights (ICECSR), others have emphasized rights of individuals and groups in need of special protection, for example, the Convention on the Elimination of All Forms of Discrimination against Women (CEDAW) and the Convention of the Rights of the Child (CRC). These conventions have expanded both the scope and depth of rights that should be protected (UNICEF, 1998; UNIFEM, 2005; UNDP, 2005; WHO, 2005).

The rights-based perspective came into the global discourse during the 1990s. A number of factors facilitated the convergence between human rights and social welfare. Primary among these was the 1993 Vienna Conference on Human Rights whose main focus was strengthening commitment to human rights. The Conference examined the link between human rights and development and affirmed the indivisibility of human rights and development. This culminated in the United Nations' reform of 1997, which proposed the integration of human rights into all United Nations systems and activities (Annan, 2005).

Since 2000, several organizations, including international financial institutions such as the World Bank, international non-governmental organizations such as CARE and Save the Children, as well as bilateral donor agencies such as the Norwegian Agency for Development Cooperation (NORAD) and the United Kingdom's Department for International Development (DFID) started to incorporate rights-based approaches in their programs (DFID, 2005; 2000; Piron & O'Neil, 2005; Piron & Watkins, 2004; Save the Children, 2004; Theis, 2004). Rights and development gained further impetus in the 2000s when the United Nations Development Program (UNDP) made considerable effort in connecting human rights and development. The UNDP, in its 2000 Human Development Report, presented a compelling argument for an integrated approach to development drawing upon the principles of international human rights and strategies of human development to advance dignity and welfare. The profession of social work has also endorsed the framework both in its preamble and ethical standards; specifically ethical standard no. 6, which highlights the profession's ethical responsibility to the broader society (NASW, 1999).

Other factors associated with the popularity of this framework include globalization and growing awareness that human rights and development offer greater hope to reduce or eradicate poverty and injustice (Gil, 1998; Moser & Norton, 2001; Nyamu-Musembi, 2002; OHCHR, 2004, 2002; UNDP, 2005, 2003a, b). The emphasis on human rights as an essential component of development effort also has been taken up in the Millennium Declaration of 2000, which has been adopted by world leaders. Alongside development goals on poverty, water, and education, commitments have been made to promote and respect human rights. In fact, in recent years, there has been a call for policies,

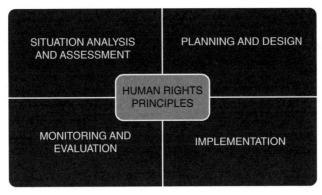

FIGURE 2 *Incorporation of Human Rights Principles in Programming*

programs of development cooperation, and technical assistance to further the realization of human rights as laid down in the Universal Declaration of Human Rights and other international human rights instruments. Although other fields are slowly embracing rights-based programming, the approach is stronger in the field development, a field in which the approach has been extensively utilized.

Strategies and Approaches to Rights-Based Assessment and Programming

Rights-based programing is generally understood as a set of program activities that is normatively based on international human rights standards whose ultimate goal is to promote and protect human rights through realization of program goals and objectives (UNICEF, 1998, 2004; OHCHR, 2012). Rights-based programming is premised on the assumption that attainment of welfare goals cannot be divorced from fulfillment of human rights (see Figure 2 for a conceptual model). Emphasis is on the centrality of the human person in programming; it stresses active participation of vulnerable individuals and groups throughout the process. In this way, the framework represents a shift in programming from one that is engrained in needs or deficiencies to one that perceives the recipient of services as an agent endowed with rights.

Various approaches exist with respect to rights-based strategies in programming. These are dictated by the nature of the program as well as context. However, common elements are generally reflected in rights-based approaches. This section reviews these elements.

It is important to acknowledge that a rights-based approach has many elements that are shared with other mechanisms utilized by human service agencies. Human service agencies, for example, underscore stakeholder participation, a key element in the rights-based framework. Moreover, the concept of accountability, which is

an important component of any good program, holds a central position in rights-based programming. In short, most interventions and techniques employed to promote welfare, for example, food, shelter, health, and education, reflect human rights ideals to some extent.

The rights-based approach to programming is nevertheless unique. It starts with creation of an enabling environment: one that attempts to improves access to resources and services by facilitating respect protection and fulfillment of human rights. The approach supports those who have the obligation to respect, protect and fulfill rights by helping them develop capacities to perform their duties adequately. It also empowers the right holders to develop capabilities to claim entitlements and participate meaningfully in political, economic, and social exchange. To this end, a rights-based programming demands participation of diverse segments of the population, especially vulnerable individuals and groups, in the programming process—from initial planning and design to implementation, monitoring, and evaluation. The participatory requirement stems from the idea that people are not passive recipients of services or commodities, but rather actors or agents with the capacity to influence outcomes in their favor (Nyamu-Musembi, 2002; Veneklasen, Miller, Cark, & Reilly, 2004; OHCHR, 2004). This perspective also focuses on increasing program impact and strengthens sustainability by addressing the root causes of vulnerability (Theis, 2004).

Rights-based programming follows four main stages: assessment, planning and design, implementation of operational commitments, and monitoring and evaluation (these are reviewed below).

ASSESSMENT This stage involves a situation or context analysis with the goal of understanding stakeholder capacities and vulnerabilities as well as causes and effects. The aim is to identify the human rights claims of rights holders and corresponding obligations of duty bearers. The assessment also provides data on the immediate, underlying, and structural causes impinging on attainment of human rights.

Coping mechanisms as well as current responses to the problem or issue of focus are examined. The main objective of the assessment is to guide implementation of strategies to help strengthen the capacity of rights holders to claim their rights and of duty bearers to fulfill their obligations.

Planning and Design This stage outlines action based on data from the assessment stage. It establishes goals and objectives with respect to program commitments. Attention is devoted to ensuring that programming is informed by human rights standards and meets the recommendations of international human rights bodies. Identification of resources for planned commitments is also important at this stage. Plans for monitoring and evaluation may be adopted at this stage.

Implementation of Operational Commitments This stage involves putting the plan into action. It may build on existing programs and, where possible, may link new responses to existing initiatives. The goal is to ensure that human rights are reflected in operational commitments while addressing program mandates. This may require advocacy to help create an enabling environment. Primary activities may include putting in place planned commitments and establishing mechanisms to support service delivery systems.

Impact Monitoring and Evaluation Activities to be undertaken at this stage may include measurement of:
- Impact
- Outputs
- Efficiency and effectiveness

In addition, evaluation and monitoring activities could focus on:
- Strengthening accountability
- Facilitating organizational learning
- Strengthening collaborations and team building
- Supporting advocacy efforts
- Influencing organizational culture

Key activities at this stage may include establishing a participatory monitoring and evaluation processes (such as the inclusion of vulnerable individuals and groups) as well as identifying tools to guide monitoring and evaluation. Attention may be on the selection of metrics and data collection mechanisms. Focus may

be on outcomes with greater potential for impact and sustainability.

Human rights principles guide program decisions at all stages. These include: universality and inalienability; indivisibility; interdependence and interrelatedness; nondiscrimination and equality; participation and inclusion; and accountability and the rule of law (an overview of each principle is presented in the ensuing subsection).

Utilization of human rights principles in programming guarantees that human rights are incorporated at every stage of the program. It is also recognition that participation of marginalized, disadvantaged, and excluded individuals and groups is both a means and a goal. Indeed, inclusive participation enhances representation of multiple stakeholders groups, and empowers and ensures that programs reflect stakeholder interests, among many other things.

Principles of Human Rights-Based Perspective Human rights principles establish conditions to enable the realization of human rights through social welfare programs. These principles are often divided into two groups: ones that are directly related to human rights (these include universality, indivisibility, equality and nondiscrimination, and accountability), and those that are associated with the notion of good governance (these consist of participation along with accountability and rule of law).

Universality and inalienability. The principle of the universality of human rights means all human are born free and have equal dignity and rights simply by virtue of their humanity. The concept of universality transcends time, space, and culture. It, in fact, distinguishes human rights from other rights such as citizenship or contractual rights (OHCHR, 2012, 2008/9). The principle of inalienability suggests that rights are entitlements that cannot be taken away or voluntarily given up. These principles identify all human as subjects of rights and demand that programs attend to issues of exclusion and injustices—all which impinge on these principles. A major component of this is raising awareness among both the right holders and the duty bearers (Goonesekere & De Silva-de Alwis, 2005).

Indivisibility. The principle of indivisibility suggests a holistic span for a rights-based approach. It recognizes the interdependence of rights and acknowledges that all rights are equally important and essential for realization of a life of respect and dignity (OHCHR, 2012). With respect to programming, while all rights—

civic, political, economic, social, and cultural—are to be treated with the same importance, the context or problem might dictate that certain rights take precedence. However, the principle of non-retrogression, which demands that the prioritization of some rights must not deliberately affect attainment of other rights, may be utilized as guide (Boesen & Martin, 2004; OHCHR, 2012; UNICEF, 2005).

Inter-dependence and Inter-relatedness. The principle of inter-dependence or inter-relatedness acknowledges that rights are intricately connected. Non-attainment of one may affect realization of others (UN Philippines, 2002; UNICEF, 2005). For example, the failure to realize the right to health may affect the right to work. The attribute of interdependence/relatedness is especially useful at the assessment stage in that it allows identification of the root causes of a problem and guides formulation of remedial strategies (UNICEF, 2005).

Equality and nondiscrimination. The principle of equality and nondiscrimination requires that access to available goods and services that are necessary to fulfillment of basic human needs is enjoyed by all (UNICEF, 2005). This principle prohibits discrimination in any field that is regulated and protected by public authorities. Within the rights-based framework, the principle of equality and nondiscrimination denotes that program efforts should target excluded groups who, for instance, have limited access to social services. A rights-based assessment may help identify prevailing discriminatory patterns, social stigmas, and other forms of inequality experienced by marginalized groups. This may be especially important during emergency situations because emergencies often exacerbate existing vulnerabilities.

Participation and inclusion. The principle of participation is recognized as a right in itself; it is an entitlement guaranteed by international law and thus an imperative in the rights framework (UNICEF, 2005). It demands free, active, and meaningful participation of all in civil, economic, social, and political exchange. The principle also implies that all people are entitled to participate in society to the maximum of their potential. This, in turn, necessitates taking steps to facilitate participation through provision of an enabling environment. Within the rights-based framework, the principle highlights the importance of involving the locals at all stages of programming. In effect, attention is devoted to both the processes of achieving goals as well as the goals themselves.

Accountability and rule of law. This principle lies at the core of human rights principle and requires that human rights be protected by law. The principle demands that states and other duty bearers that assist governments in fulfilling their obligations, for example, donors, aid organizations, NGOs, and development practitioners, are answerable for the observance of human rights (UNICEF, 2005). The principle entails that aggrieved rights holders have access to fair and just judicial processes. This observation is notable and suggests that rights-based programming may need to take into account the state of the judicial system, in a given context, along with its capacity to claimed rights. Consideration should also be given to religious and cultural practices that may affect the welfare and rights of vulnerable individuals and groups.

Accountability directly relates to rule of law. It is derived from the fact that rights imply duties, which in turn demand accountability (UNICEF, 2005). This is, in fact, one of the key aspects of the rights-based approach; it moves the discourse from the realm of needs to that of obligation. In relation to the rights-based framework, accountability requires transparency and clearly articulated mechanisms for seeking redress for decisions and actions that affect rights negatively. Moreover, while it is up to duty bearers to determine the appropriate mechanisms of accountability, all mechanisms must be accessible, transparent, and effective (OHCHR, 2002).

Tools Supporting the Implementation of Rights-Based Programming

The rights-based framework is relatively new; hence, few tools exist to guide operational decisions (OHCHR, 2002; Piron & O'Neil, 2005; Piron & Watkins, 2004; Save the Children, 2004; UNDG, 2004; UNDP, 2005, 2003a, b; WHO, 2005). Many of the tools currently in place are in the fields of development and humanitarian aid. Most of these have been put in place by major international organizations such as the United Nations and its systems, international financial institutions such as the World Bank, as well as governmental organizations such as the Norwegian Agency for Development Cooperation (NORAD) and the United Kingdom's Department for International Development (DFID). This section provides a brief overview of resources to guide implementation of rights-based programs.

Examples of these include a compilation on approaches to poverty reduction put together by the World Bank in collaboration with the United Nations (OHCHR 2002); a checklist on rights-based programming developed by UNDP and OHCHR for program staff (UNDP, 2003a); a manual outlining government-to-government assistance with respect to human rights obligations created by the Victorian Equal Opportunity and Human Rights Commission (2008), Human Rights Council of Australia; and a handbook on human rights assessment developed by NORAD (2001).

Effort has also been devoted to development of performance indicators. A performance indicator is defined as a measure that is used to demonstrate change in a situation, or progress in, or results of, an intervention, activity, or program (Green, 2001; UNDP Oslo Governance Centre, 2006; Theis, 2003; UN Philippines, 2002; UNAIDS, 2005a, b). Performance indicators, typically, fall into five broad categories as follows:

- Impact. These measure the quality and quantity of long-term results generated by program outputs (for example, measurable change in quality of life, reduced incidence of diseases, increased income for women, or reduced mortality).
- Outcome. This captures the intermediate results generated by program outputs. They often correspond to any change in people's behavior as a result of program actions and activities.
- Output. This identifies the quantity, quality, and timeliness of goods or services resulting from an intervention, activity, or program.
- Process. This measures the flow of program activities and the way these are carried out (for example, it attempts to capture what happens from entry into a program to exit).
- Input. This reflects the quantity, quality, and timeliness of resources provided for an intervention, activity, or program and may include human, financial and material, technological, and information assistance.

Within the context of programming, indicators provide useful information on the degree to which rights have been realized. They help identify the capacity of state institutions with respect to their human rights obligations as well as the capacities of individuals/groups to claim their rights. Indicators also provide information on the context as well as socioeconomic and political processes that are related to realization or failure to attain human rights. In addition to this, they facilitate the process of monitoring and evaluation. Headways have been made in development of indicators with respect to rights-based approaches (see, e.g., Carr Center for Human Rights Policy, 2006; UNDP Oslo Governance Centre, 2006). Despite this effort, development of indicators to guide programming remains a challenge. Primary resources currently in place include:

UNITED NATIONS PUBLICATIONS:

Indicators for human rights based approaches to development in UNDP Programming: A Users' Guide (2006). http://gaportal.org/sites/default/files/HRBA%20indicators%20guide.pdf

A Human Rights Based Approach to Development Programming in UNDP – Adding the Missing Link (2004). http://www.undp.org/content/dam/aplaws/publication/en/publications/democratic-governance/dg-publications-for-website/a-human-rights-based-approach-to-development-programming-in-undp/HR_Pub_Missinglink.pdf

United Nations Office of the High Commissioner for Human Rights (2002). *OHCHR Principles and Guidelines for a Human Rights Approach to Poverty Reduction Strategies*, Geneva: United Nations Office of the High Commissioner for Human Rights. http://www.ohchr.org/EN/Issues/Poverty/DimensionOfPoverty/Pages/Guidelines.aspx

The Human Rights Based Approach to Development Cooperation: Towards a Common Understanding Among UN Agencies, Inter-Agency Workshop on a Human Rights Based Approach in the context of UN Reform (2003). http://www.unescobkk.org/fileadmin/user_upload/appeal/human_rights/UN_Common_understanding_RBA.pdf

OTHER PUBLICATIONS:

Ball, P.B. with Cifuentes, R., Dueck, J., Gregory, R., Salcedo, D., and Saldarriaga, C. (1994). *A Definition of Database Design Standards for Human Rights Agencies*, Washington, DC: American Association for the Advancement of Science.

Norwegian Agency for Development Cooperation (2001). *Handbook in Human Rights Assessment: State Obligations Awareness and Empowerment*, Oslo: NORAD. https://www.norad.no/globalassets/import-2162015-80434-am/www.norad.no-ny/filarkiv/vedlegg-til-publikasjoner/handbook-in-human-rights-assessment.pdf

Filmer-Wilson, E. (2006). *An Introduction to the Use of Human Rights Indicators for Development Programming. Netherlands Human Rights Quarterly*, 24(1), 155-162.

Social Work and Rights-Based Programming

Social workers are concerned with social problems, their causes, solutions, and impact on society. In fact, at the core of social work is the "intrinsic" value of *every* person, and the mandate to promote social justice while upholding human dignity (IFSW, 2012; 1988; NASW, 1999). Also reflected in the profession's values are principles of human rights (CSWE, 2008). Furthermore, the Code of Ethics of the National Association of Social Work espouses the rights-based framework both in its preamble and ethical standards, such as ethical standard #6, which highlights the profession's ethical responsibilities to the broader society (IFSW, 2012; NASW, 1999).

This section highlights the relationship between the profession of social work and rights-based programming with a specific focus on practice implications in the areas of advocacy, policy, and research.

PRACTICE IMPLICATION

Advocacy. A rights-based perspective adds legitimacy/value to social work's agenda of social justice by drawing attention to the structure of accountability that defines the relationship between the right holder and duty bearer. Increased focus on accountability may hold the key to improved program effectiveness and transparency as well as achievement of sustainable results. Human rights are reflected in social work's ideals—promotion of a just world, securing freedom for all, and promotion of welfare and dignity of all people everywhere. Using right-based principles, social workers could work toward reducing inequality and promoting human rights. Attention could focus on identification of structure barriers that hinder attainment of human rights. Another area of focus could be creating awareness of the welfare responsibilities of the right holder along with the corresponding obligations of the duty bearer. Alongside this, advocacy effort could encourage national authorities and civil society to engage in policy dialogue with the ultimate goal of promoting, protecting, and fulfilling claimed rights. Advocacy, in this area, has potential to bring new energy and strengthen social work's commitment to the human rights agenda.

Programming. Application of rights-based programming requires knowledge of the role of human rights in programs especially as they relate to vulnerable individuals/groups. This is important for social work in that vulnerable groups are at the center of the social work profession. Social work's mandate of promoting the welfare of vulnerable individuals/groups is also underscored by the Council of Social Work Education (CSWE) which states that "service, social justice, dignity and worth of the person ..." are among the core values of social work (CSWE, 2008). These values frame the profession's commitment to respect for all people and the quest for economic and social justice. Rights-based programming ensures these commitments are accomplished through realization of program goals and objectives.

A value added by the application of a human rights-based approach is the focus on the most marginalized and excluded; groups whose human rights, in many spheres e.g., the social, economic, political, civil and/or cultural, are often denied or left unfulfilled (UNAIDS, 2005a, b). Utilization of rights-based programming has potential to lead more focused strategies/interventions. Rights-based programming has potential to bring about social transformation through empowerment of right holders and enhancement of the capacity of duty bearers to meet their obligations.

Research. The profession of social work is deeply entrenched in scientific inquiry. This can be traced throughout the profession's history. In fact, scientific inquiry and the centrality of the human person in social work practice are among the core values emphasized by the Council of Social Work Education (CSWE) through its Educational Policy and Accreditation Standards (EPAs Policy 1.1). Assessment and program monitoring demanded by rights-based programming help in understanding legal frameworks as well as factors that create and perpetuate discrimination and social exclusion and hinder people from realizing their potential. Social work has a unique role to play in this regard. An area of focus may be the development of indicators to guide assessment and program monitoring. Characteristics of these indicators may include the following:

- Accessible
- Measurable
- Robust & statistically validated
- Reliable
- Sufficiently comparable across cultures
- Amenable to adaptation
- Relevant
- Sensitive to context
- Multi-dimensional
- Timely

Conclusion

This article set out to provide an overview of the rights-based approaches in programming with respect to social work. Specifically, we reviewed the basic underpinnings of the rights-based discourse as it relates to programming and assessment. An historical overview of the rights-based framework along with approaches to rights-based programming was presented. We also highlighted areas of intersection between social work and rights-based programming. Furthermore, tools supporting the approach were identified. As observed, the popularity of rights-based approaches is rooted in the growing popularity of social justice and rising awareness that human rights may be the most effective way to reduce/eradicate poverty, inequality, and injustice. The profession of social work has played and continues to play a major role in issues of welfare and human rights. In fact, at the core of social work is the "intrinsic" value of *every* person and the mandate to promote social justice while upholding human dignity.

REFERENCES

Annan, K. (2005). In larger freedom: Decision time at the UN. *Foreign Affairs.* May/June 2005. http://www.foreignaffairs

.com/articles/60799/kofi-annan/in-larger-freedom-decision-time-at-the-un

Boesen, J. & Martin, T. (2004). Applying a rights-based approach: An inspirational guide for civil society. Retrieved from http://www.humanrights.dk/files/pdf/Publikationer/applying%20a%20rights%20based%20approach.pdf

Carr Center for Human Rights Policy. (2006). Measurement of human rights: A guide to tackle challenges. Retrieved from http://www.hks.harvard.edu/cchrp/mhr/publications/index.php#FullReports

CSWE. (2008). Educational Policy and Accreditation Standards. http://www.cswe.org/File.aspx?id=13780

Department for International Development. (2005). Developing a human rights-based approach to addressing maternal mortality: Desk review. Retrieved from http://www.hurilink.org/tools/Developing_aHRBA_to_Maternal_Mortality-DFID.pdf

Department for International Development. (2000). Realising human rights for poor people. Strategy paper. Retrieved from http://www2.ohchr.org/english/issues/development/docs/human_rights_tsp.pdf

Gil, G. D. (1998). Confronting Injustice and Oppression: Concepts and Strategies for Social Workers. New York: Columbia University Press.

Green, M. (2001). What we talk about when we talk about indicators: current approaches to human rights measurement. Human Rights Quarterly, 23(4), 1062–1097.

Goonesekere, S., & De Silva-de Alwis, R. (2005). Women's and children's rights: In a human rights-based approach to development. Retrieved from http://www.unifem.org/cedaw30/attachments/resources/WomensAndChildrensRightsInAHumanRightsBasedApproach.pdf

International Federation of Social Workers. (1988). Human rights and social work: A manual for schools of social work and the social work profession. Retrieved from http://cdn.ifsw.org/assets/ifsw_24626-7.pdf

International Federation of Social Workers. (2012). Statement of ethical principles. Retrieved from http://ifsw.org/policies/statement-of-ethical-principles/

Moser, C. & Norton, A. (2001). To claim our rights: Livelihood security, human rights and sustainable development. Overseas Development Institute. Retrieved from http://www.odi.org.uk/pppg/publications/books/tcor.pdf

National Association of Social Workers. (1999). Code of ethics. Washington, DC: Author.

NORAD. (2001). Handbook in human rights assessment: State obligations, awareness and empowerment. Retrieved from http://www.norad.no/en/tools-and-publications/publications/publication?key=109343

Nyamu-Musembi, C. (2002). Towards an actor-oriented perspective on human rights. IDS working paper 169, Institute of Development Studies, October 2002. Retrieved from http://www.drc-citizenship.org/system/assets/1052734370/original/1052734370-nyamu-musembi.2002-towards.pdf

Nyamu-Musembi, C., & Cornwall, A. (2004). What is the "rights-based approach" all about? Perspectives from the international development agencies. IDS working paper 234, Institute of Development Studies. Retrieved from http://www.gsdrc.org/go/display/document/legacyid/1317

Office of the United Nations High Commissioner for Human Rights. (2012). Principles and guidelines for a human rights approach to poverty reduction strategies. Asia and the Pacific, Retrieved from http://www.ohchr.org/Documents/Publications/PovertyStrategiesen.pdf

OHCHR. (2008/2009). Annual Report. Retrieved from http://www.ohchr.org/EN/PUBLICATIONSRESOURCES/Pages/AnnualReportAppeal.aspx

OHCHR. (2002). OHCHR Principles and Guidelines for a Human Rights Approach to Poverty Reduction Strategies. Retrieved from http://www.ohchr.org/EN/Issues/Poverty/DimensionOfPoverty/Pages/Guidelines.aspx

OHCHR. (2004). Human rights and poverty reduction: A conceptual framework (New York and Geneva, United Nations. Retrieved from http://www2.ohchr.org/english/issues/poverty/docs/povertyE.pdf

Piron, L. & O'Neil, T. (2005). Integrating human rights into development: A synthesis of donor approaches and experiences, Overseas Development Institute. Retrieved from http://www.odi.org.uk/sites/odi.org.uk/files/odi-assets/publications-opinion-files/4403.pdf

Piron, L. & Watkins, F. (2004). DFID Human rights review: A review of how DFID has integrated human rights into its work. Overseas Development Institute. Retrieved from http://www.odi.org.uk/sites/odi.org.uk/files/odi-assets/publications-opinion-files/2289.pdf

Roosevelt, E. (1948). Speech upon adoption of UDHR. Retrieved from http://www.americanrhetoric.com/speeches/eleanorrooseveltdeclarationhumanrights.htm

Save the Children UK (East and Central Africa). (2004). Child rights programming: A resource for planning. Retrieved from http://images.savethechildren.it/f/download/Policies/ch/child-rights-handbook.pdf

The Victorian Equal Opportunity & Human Rights Commission. (2008). From principle to practice: Implementing the human rights-bases approach in community organizations. Retrieved, 2013, from http://www.humanrightscommission.vic.gov.au/index.php/our-resources-and-publications/toolkits/item/303-from-principle-to-practice-implementing-the-human-rights-based-approach-in-community-organisations-sept-2008

Theis, J. (2004). Promoting rights-based approaches: Experiences and ideas from Asia and the Pacific. Retrieved from www.crin.org/docs/resources/publications/hrbap/promoting.pdf

Theis, J. Save the Children (2003). Rights-based approach to monitoring human rights Child Rights Information Network. Retrieved 2012, from http://www.crin.org/docs/resources/publications/hrbap/RBA_monitoring_evaluation.pdf

UNAIDS. (2005a). HIV-related stigma, discrimination and human rights violations: Case studies of successful programmes. UNAIDS best practice collection. Retrieved from http://data.unaids.org/publications/irc-pub06/jc999-humrightsviol_en.pdf

UNAIDS. (2005b). Monitoring the declaration of commitment on HIV/AIDS: Guidelines on construction of core indicators. Retrieved from http://data.unaids.org/publications/irc-pub06/jc1126-constrcoreindic-ungass_en.pdf

UNDG. (2004). Guidelines for UN country teams preparing for a CCA and UNDAF. Retrieved from http://www.undp.org/documents/4874-CCA---UNDAF_Guidelines-1.doc

UNDP. (2005). Programming for justice: Access for all. A practitioner's guide to a human rights-based approach to access to justice. Retrieved from http://www.hrea.org/index.php?base_id=104&language_id=1&erc_doc_id=3746&category_id=587&category_type=2&group=

UNDP. (2003a). Poverty reduction and human rights: A practice note. Retrieved from http://www.undp.org/content/dam/aplaws/publication/en/publications/poverty-reduction/poverty-website/poverty-reduction-and-human-rights/povertyreduction-humanrights0603_1_.pdf

UNDP. (2003b). Human rights-based reviews of UNDP programmes: Working guidelines. Retrieved from http://hdr.undp.org/en/media/HRBA_Guidelines.pdf

UNDP Oslo Governance Centre. (2006). How to use indicators for assessing human rights standards in development programmes? Retrieved from http://www.eldis.org/go/topics&id=43106&type=Document#.UgPJQqzAFOQ

UNICEF. (2005). Women's and children's rights in a human rights based approach to development. Retrieved, 2012, from http://www.unifem.org/cedaw30/attachments/resources/WomensAndChildrensRightsInAHumanRightsBasedApproach.pdf

UNICEF. (2004). A human rights-based approach to programming. Retrieved 2012, from http://www.unicef.org/sowc04/files/AnnexB.pdf

UNICEF. (1998). A human rights approach to UNICEF programming for children and women: what it is, and some changes it will bring (CF/EXD/1998-04, April 21, 1998). Retrieved from http://www.unhcr.org/refworld/pdfid/3f82adbb1.pdf

UNIFEM. (2005). Women's human rights. Retrieved from http://www.unifem.org/gender_issues/human_rights/

United Nations. (1948). Universal declaration of human rights. Retrieved from http://www.un.org/en/documents/udhr/index.shtml

VeneKlasen, L. Miller, Cark & Reilly. (2004). Rights-based approaches and beyond: challenges of linking rights and participation. IDS working paper 235, Institute of Development Studies. Retrieved from http://www.ids.ac.uk/files/Wp235.pdf

WHO. (2005). Human rights, health and poverty reduction strategies, Health and Human Rights Publication Series, No. 5. Retrieved from http://www.who.int/hhr/news/HHR_PRS_19_12_05.pdf

FURTHER READING

OHCHR. (2006). Frequently asked questions on a human rights-based approach to development cooperation. UN, New York and Geneva. Retrieved from http://www.ohchr.org/Documents/Publications/FAQen.pdf

United Nations Philippines. (2002). What is a rights-based approach to development? In *Rights-based approach to development programming: Training manual* (pp. 11–18). Retrieved 2012, from http://www.un.org.ph/publications/RBAManual.pdf

SUGGESTED LINKS

CARE International. Principles into practice: Learning from innovative rights-based programmes, http://www.handicap-international.fr/bibliographie-handicap/3ApprocheDroit/OutilProgMEO/CarePrinp.pdf

Child Rights Information Network (CRIN). http://www.crin.org/hrbap/

Interaction. Resources links on human rights based approach to development. http://www.interaction.org/

International Human Rights Network http://www.ihrnetwork.org/

OHCHR. International human rights instruments. http://www2.ohchr.org/english/law/

OHCHR. Lessons learned project, on a human rights-based approach to development in the Asia–Pacific region. http://hrbaportal.org/wp-content/files/RBA-in-AP-region3.pdf

OHCHR. Resource database on human rights approaches to development for practitioners in rights information network (CRIN), "Rights based programming" resource page, http://www.crin.org/hrbap/

Overseas Development Institute. Rights in action, http://www.odi.org.uk/rights/index.html

Stamford Inter-Agency Workshop. Statement of common understanding of a human rights-based approach to development cooperation, http://www.hrea.org/index.php?base_id=104&language_id=1&erc_doc_id=3107&category_id=44&category_type=3&group=

United Nations Development Group. (2004). Guidelines for UN country teams preparing a CCA and UNDAF. http://www.globalgovernancewatch.org/resources/common-country-assessment-and-united-nations-development-assistance-framework--guidelines-for-un-country-teams-on-preparing-a-cca-and-undaf

UNDP. Human Rights Strengthening (HURIST) joint programme between UNDP and OHCHR, http://www.undp.org/governance/programmes/hurist.htm

UNDP. Poverty reduction and human rights: A practice note. http://www.undp.org/content/dam/aplaws/publication/en/publications/poverty-reduction/poverty-website/poverty-reduction-and-human-rights/povertyreduction-humanrights0603_1_.pdf

UNICEF. Rights and results, http://www.unicef.org/rightsresults/index_23693.html

UNIFEM. Pathway to Gender Equality: CEDAW, Beijing and the MDGs, http://www.unifem.org/attachments/products/385_PathwayToGenderEquality_screen.pdf

MARGARET LOMBE

S

SCHOOL SOCIAL WORK

ABSTRACT: In 2006, school social work celebrated 100 years as a vibrant profession. This overview details the genesis and development of this particular specialization to the early 21st century, exploring the history of the profession, including policy and legislation that has either resulted from or affected schools on a national level. Additionally, the article explains the knowledge base of school social work, examines the regulation and standards for both practice and practitioners, and considers future trends for the field.

KEY WORDS: children and adolescents; education; schools; service delivery; public education

As practitioners and scholars alike continue to seek solutions and interventions for ever-changing social problems, school social work will continue to be defined by research and new knowledge developments in social work and related fields.

School social workers started as and remain an integral link among school, home, and community. Those who choose this particular field of social work provide direct services, as well as specialized services such as mental-health intervention, crisis management and intervention, and facilitating community involvement in the schools. Working as an interdisciplinary team member, school social workers not only continue to provide services to school children and their families, but also continue to evaluate their roles, services, and consequently modify them to meet organizational, contextual, and contemporary needs.

School social work as a discipline continues to develop in relation to social issues, needs of the school systems, continuing education, and evolving research, perhaps more so than other school-based disciplines. Statistics indicate a recent upswing in the number of school social workers or social-work services in schools. As a result, the Bureau of Labor Statistics (2012) estimates that employment of child, family, and school social workers will have increased by 20% between 2010 and 2020.

In the 21st century, practitioners will face evolving definitions of personhood and family, disparities in terms of quality education and health care, and job opportunities that will affect how children learn and function, not only in a school environment but also in their communities. Through it all, school social work will continue to change, thrive, and provide evidence-based solutions for children and families. Before discussing more fully the current trends and issues that are impacting, or have the potential to impact, school social-work practice, it is vital to revisit and examine its historical evolution.

History

Social work in schools began between 1906 and 1907 (Allen-Meares, 2006), with initial development outside the school system, as private agencies and civic organizations took on the work (Costin, 1969). It was not until 1913 that the first Board of Education initiated and financed a formal visiting teacher program, placing visiting teachers in special departments of the school under the administration and direction of the superintendent of schools.

EARLY INFLUENCES As the school social-work movement gained momentum, the early 20th century proved to be a fruitful period in its development. Several important influences included the following:

1. *The passage of compulsory school attendance laws:* Concern regarding the illiteracy of youth brought attention to a child's right to receive a minimum education and the states' responsibility for providing it. This attention led to support for the enactment of compulsory attendance statutes, and by 1918 each state had passed its own version. The lack of effective enforcement led to the idea that school attendance officers were needed, and Abbott and Breckinridge (1917) held that this responsibility should be assigned to the school social worker.

2. *Knowledge of individual differences:* As the scope of compulsory education laws expanded, states were required to provide an educational experience for a variety of children. At the same time, new knowledge about individual differences among children began to emerge. Previous to this, there had been no real concern about whether children had different learning needs; those who presented a challenge were simply not enrolled.

EXPANSION During the 1920s the number and the influence of school social workers increased, largely as a result of a series of demonstrations held over 3 years, organized and funded by the Commonwealth Fund of New York (Oppenheimer, 1925), which provided financial support to the National Committee of Visiting Teachers and increased experimentation in the field of school social work.

The 1920s were also the beginning of a therapeutic role for school social workers in public schools. According to Costin (1978), the increasing recognition of individual differences among children and interest on the part of the mental hygienists in understanding behavior problems led to an effort on the part of visiting teachers to develop techniques for the prevention of social maladjustment.

SHIFTING GOALS The development of social-work service was greatly hindered during the Depression, with services either abolished or reduced in volume (Areson, 1923). As the Depression worsened, the social-work activity that did take place centered on ensuring that people's basic needs were met. During this time, visiting teachers began viewing their role in a different way, with their early responsibilities as attendance officers being replaced by the burgeoning role of social caseworker.

EMPHASIS ON SOCIAL CASEWORK By 1940, the shift to social caseworker was complete. No longer were social change and neighborhood conditions seen as the sole points of intervention. Instead, the profession was beginning to build its clinical base, with the personality needs of the individual child taking primary attention.

CHANGING GOALS AND METHODS Public schools came under attack in many different ways during the 1960s. There were those who argued that public education was not sufficient. Several studies documented adverse school policies and claimed that inequality in educational opportunity existed as a result of racial segregation. There was considerable discussion about the need for change, including change in the practices of both social workers and guidance counselors.

During this time, group work, which had previously been introduced to the school system, was becoming a prominent method. In a research progress report, Robert Vinter and Rosemary Sarri described the effective use of group work in dealing with such school problems as high-school dropouts, undera-chievement, and academic failure (Vinter & Sarri, 1965).

CHANGING DEMOGRAPHICS AND INCREASED RECOGNITION IN EDUCATIONAL LEGISLATION During the 1970s the number of school social workers increased, and at the same time more emphasis was being placed on family, community, teaming with workers in other school-related disciplines, and the education of handicapped pupils.

Congress passed The Education for All Handicapped Children Act (1975), which had "impacted social work services in schools profoundly," as "[s]ocial workers were named specifically as one of the related services required to help individuals with disabilities benefit from special education" (Atkins-Burnett, 2010, p. 177). This would be the first time, but not the last, that the importance of school social workers was recognized and codified.

Educational legislation continues to play a major role in the definition and function of school social workers and in shaping and expanding the services they provide. In the 1980s school social workers were included as "qualified personnel" in Part H of the Education of the Handicapped Act Amendments of 1986, the Early Intervention for Handicapped Infants and Toddlers, and the Elementary and Secondary School Improvement Amendments of 1988.

The 1990s brought with them many more changes. National organizations grew and offered added support to the specialty. Codified standards for school social workers were edited and tailored for relevance, and states themselves began to take an active role in what it means to be a school social worker.

In 1994 school social workers were once again included in a major piece of legislation—the American Education Act, which included eight national goals, of which the major objectives were research promotion, consensus building, and systemic change, to ensure equality of educational opportunities for all students.

Additionally, two key pieces of legislation have influenced the job and roles of school social workers. In 1990, the Individuals with Disabilities Education Act was authorized. Amended several times, the Individuals with Disabilities Education Act further refined services, eligibility, parent involvement, assessment and testing, and learning opportunities for students with disabilities or special needs (IDEA, 1991).

In 2002, President George W. Bush signed into law a comprehensive and controversial piece of federal legislation titled the No Child Left Behind Act

(2002). Reauthorized in 2006, the act was conceived as a way to hold school systems and students accountable for learning and includes standards for those with special needs. The most recent No Child Left Behind legislation, enacted by the Obama administration in 2011, was the Elementary and Secondary Education Act Flexibility. The Elementary and Secondary Education Act Flexibility legislation allowed states to request waivers of specific provisions of No Child Left Behind to avoid unintentional barriers to state and local educational reforms (U.S. Department of Education, 2012).

Knowledge Base of School Social Work

As school social work evolved, so too did different practice models. A practice model may be defined as "a coherent set of directives which state how a given kind of treatment is to be carried out. . . . It usually states what a practitioner is expected to do or what practitioners customarily do under given conditions" (Reid & Epstein, 1972, pp. 7–8).

Alderson (1972) offered four models of school social-work practice: the traditional clinical model, the school change model, the community school model, and the social interaction model.

TRADITIONAL CLINICAL MODEL The best known and most widely used model is the traditional clinical model, which focuses on individual students with social and emotional problems that interfere with their potential to learn. The model's primary base is psychoanalytic and ego psychology. The model's major assumption is that the individual child or the family is experiencing difficult times or dysfunction. As a result, the school social worker's role is that of a direct caseworker—providing services to the child or the family and not focusing on the school itself. School personnel are only involved as a source of information about the child's behavior.

SCHOOL CHANGE MODEL In contrast, the school change model's target is, in fact, the school and changing any institutional policies, conditions, and practices that were seen as causing student dysfunction or malperformance. The school itself is considered the client, and school personnel are involved in discussion, identification, and change.

COMMUNITY SCHOOL MODEL The community school model focuses primarily on communities with limited social and economic resources. The social

worker's role is to educate these communities about the school's offerings, organize support for the school's programs, and explain to school officials the dynamics and societal factors affecting the community. This model assumes that school personnel require ongoing and up-to-date information about social problems and their effects on school children to have a complete understanding.

SOCIAL INTERACTION The social interaction model emphasizes reciprocal influences of the acts of individuals and groups. The target of intervention is the type and the quality of exchanges between parties (the child, groups of children, families, the school, and the community). The school social worker takes on the role of mediator and facilitator, with the goal of seeking common ground and common solutions.

COSTIN'S MODEL Another important model grew out of a demonstration project of a multiuniversity consortium for planned change in pupil personnel services. An amalgamation of several methods, Lela B. Costin's school–community–pupil relations model (Costin, 1973) emphasized the complexity of the interactions among students, the school, and the community. Especially relevant in today's schools, its primary goal serves to bring about change in the interaction of this triad and, thus, to modify to some extent harmful institutional practices and policies of the school. In a national survey of school social work, authors found that school social workers largely provided mental-health services to at-risk children and their families. In addition, most of the services provided were tier-three services (Kelly et al., 2010).

Demographics and Standards

STATE-BY-STATE REGULATION AND REQUIREMENTS Since the early 1970s, the number of state associations of school social workers has risen. These organizations play an important part in heightening this field's visibility and regulate the profession. Information on specific state associations for school social workers may be found at http://www.sswaa.org/display common.cfm?an=1&subarticlenbr=67 (School Social Work Association of America, 2012a).

NATIONWIDE NUMBER OF SOCIAL WORKERS In 2010, there were approximately 650,000 social workers employed in the United States. Estimates suggest that 290,000 of these social workers were child, family, and school social workers. This number includes child protective services, many other government jobs, and school social workers (*http://careerplanning.about .com/od/occupations/p/social_worker.htm*).

EDUCATIONAL REQUIREMENTS In most states a Master's of Social Work is required. However, some states allow certification at the entry level with a bachelor's degree (School Social Work Association of America, 2012b).

STANDARDS FOR SOCIAL-WORK SERVICES IN SCHOOLS In 1976, the National Association of Social Workers (NASW) developed the first standards for school social-work services, which were grouped into three areas: attainment of competence, organization and administration, and professional practice. The NASW continues to provide guidelines, standards, and a *Code of Ethics* (NASW, 2008) for the social-work community, as well as specific standards for school social workers (NASW, 2012). Over the years, the NASW standards have been revised to contextualize this field of practice within new knowledge, new policies, and laws.

RESOURCES FOR SCHOOL SOCIAL WORKERS In addition to its specific standards for school social work, the NASW offers specialized certification as a Certified School Social Work Specialist, as well as a dedicated specialty practice section.

In 1994, spearheaded by the school social-work leadership, the School Social Work Association of America was formed, independent of the NASW (School Social Work Association of America, 2012c). In addition, a new national organization has recently been developed, the American Council for School Social Work, which offers school-based social-work practitioners resources for educators and parents, recommended reading (through journals, articles, and books), and practice evaluation tools. Several regional councils also support school social work.

In addition, important journals supported by major organizations such as *Children and Schools* (NASW) and the *School Social Work Journal* (Lyceum Books) provide research, theoretical practice, and policy information.

Trends and Directions

NEW STRUCTURES, NEW PARTNERS As we look into the future of school social work, concerns about the quality and cost of education, student learning outcomes, accountability, increased demand to serve more diverse student populations, and increased social problems among children and families will challenge the profession to think creatively and differently about their services and how to organize them for greater effectiveness and efficiency. Frey et al. (2012) proposed a national model for social work that considers social justice, an ecological perspective, ethical and legal policies, and a data-driven approach for the advancement of school social-work practice. What does this mean for school social-work services?

Although many school social workers are employed by local school districts, trends indicate that some school systems are implementing new organizational structures and creating new partnerships. Some districts are contracting with external mental-health service providers or other agencies in what they believe to be a cost-efficient way to serve their students. Schools have also formed relevant partnerships, termed *school-linked* or *integrated services*, with organizations such as health providers, which provide their services through the school system (Franklin, 2004).

Among its most pressing issues, this field of practice will be facing a myriad of changes and issues, including the following:

1. Increased global competition and educational excellence. School social workers will need to empirically demonstrate their contributions to the national focus on performance measures and standardized tests and warn the school system about misuse and problems facing vulnerable pupils. Specifically, as education reform has become a top political priority (The White House, 2009), there have been growing pressures for school social workers to tie interventions to specific learning outcomes (such as test scores, grades, and attendance).

2. Social, economic, and educational policy and its impact on education. School social workers must be knowledgeable of those policies, advocate for those that are just, and lobby for the elimination of those that are problematic. For example, the topics of violence and bullying have become substantial in the media. Although these topics are of great relevance, rates of school violence have declined steadily since the 1990s (Pitner, Astor & Benbenishty, 2014). Social workers should be knowledgeable about the literature associated with these important issues and should keep school administrators informed when political pressures call for radically changing a system that may already be working.

3. Technological advances. The gap between those who are technologically literate and those who

are not will have an effect on poverty and unemployment rates. Working with other relevant school personnel, school social workers must also make others aware of these inequities.

4. Growing diversity and new immigrant populations. Multicultural competency, including knowledge about new immigrants, will challenge our public schools and consequently the profession. In response, school social workers will need to increase their knowledge to remain effective assessors, advisors, and advocates for these students.

5. The focus on evidence-based interventions and outcomes, particularly within the context of the three-tier model (Response to Intervention and Positive Behavioral Intervention and Supports; Thompson, 2013). Practitioners will need to keep abreast of and incorporate evidence-based interventions, new problem-solving approaches, and innovative partnerships to address the needs of all students.

Conclusion

The American public-education system is subject to numerous criticisms and challenges. Yet it has proven to be resilient and essential to the core values of our democracy. As adaptations or new innovations develop, the profession of social work must not only respond, but also be proactive in shaping the future. School social workers provide crucial social services in one of the most accessible settings, playing an integral role in prevention, intervention, and positive change for school-age children and their families.

REFERENCES

Abbott, E., & Breckinridge, S. (1917). *Truancy and nonattendance in the Chicago schools: A study of the social aspects of the compulsory education and child labor legislation of Illinois.* Chicago, IL: University of Chicago Press.

Alderson, J. J. (1972). Models of school social work practice. In R. Sarri & F. Maple (Eds.), *The school in the community* (pp. 151–160). Washington, DC: NASW.

Allen-Meares, P. (2006). One hundred years: A historical analysis of social work services in schools. *School Social Work Journal, Special Issue,* 24–43.

Areson, C. W. (1923). Status of children's work in the United States. *Proceedings of the national conference of social work* (p. 398). Chicago, IL: University of Chicago Press.

Atkins-Burnett, S. (2010). Children with disabilities. In P. Allen-Meares (Ed.), *Social work services in schools* (6th ed.). Needham Heights, MA: Allyn & Bacon.

Bureau of Labor Statistics. (2012). Social workers: *Occupational outlook handbook.* Retrieved March, 2013, from http://www.bls.gov/ooh/Community-and-Social-Service/Social-workers.htm#tab-6

Costin, L. B. (1969). An analysis of the tasks in school social work. *Social Service Review, 43,* 274–285.

Costin, L. B. (1973). School social work practice: A new model. *Social Work, 20,* 135–139.

Costin, L. B. (1978). Social work services in schools: Historical perspectives and current directions. Continuing education series #8 (pp. 1–34). Washington, DC: NASW.

Education for All Handicapped Children Act. Federal Register. Pub. L. No. 94–142 41:46977. (1975).

Franklin, C. (2004). The delivery of school social work services. In P. Allen-Meares (Ed.), *Social work services in the school* (4th ed., pp. 295–326). Boston, MA: Allyn & Bacon.

Frey, A. J., Alvarez, M. E., Sabatino, C. A., Lindsey, B. C., Dupper, D. R., Raines, J. C., et al. (2012). The Development of a National School Social Work Practice Model. *Children & Schools, 34*(3), 131–134.

Individuals With Disabilities Education Act. Congressional Information Service Annual Legislative Histories for U.S. Public Laws. Pub. L. No. 101–476. (1991).

Kelly, M. S., Frey, A. J., Alvarez, M., Berzin, S. C., Shaffer, G., & O'Brien, K. (2010). School social work practice and response to intervention. *Children & Schools, 32*(4), 201–209.

National Association of Social Workers (NASW). (2008). *NASW code of ethics.* Retrieved May 2, 2013, from http://www.socialworkers.org/pubs/code/code.asp

National Association of Social Workers (NASW). (2012). *Standards for school social work services.* Washington, DC: Author. Retrieved May 2, 2013, frm http://www.socialworkers.org/practice/standards/naswschoolsocialwork-standards.pdf

No Child Left Behind Act of 2001. Pub.L. No. 107–110 (2002).

Oppenheimer, J. (1925). *The visiting teacher movement, with special reference to administrative relationships* (2nd ed., p. 5). New York, NY: Joint Committee on Methods of Preventing Delinquency.

Pitner, R., Astor, R. A., & Benbenishty, R. 2014. Violence in schools. In P. Allen-Meares (Ed.), *Social Work Services in Schools* (7th ed.). Boston, MA: Pearson.

Reid, W., & Epstein, L. (1972). *Task-centered casework.* New York, NY: Columbia University Press.

School Social Work Association of America. (2012a). *State associations.* Retrieved May 1, 2013, from http://www.sswaa.org/displaycommon.cfm?an=1&subarticlenbr=67

School Social Work Association of America. (2012b). *School social work as a career.* Retrieved May 1, 2013, from http://sswaa.affiniscape.com/displaycommon.cfm?an=1&subarticlenbr=99

School Social Work Association of America. (2012c). *SSWAA history.* Retrieved May 1, 2013, from http://www.sswaa.org/displaycommon.cfm?an=1&subarticlenbr=60

Thompson, A. M. (2013). Improving classroom conflict management through positive behavior supports. In C. Franklin, M. B. Harris, & P. Allen-Meares (Eds.), *The school services sourcebook: A guide for school-based professionals* (2nd ed.). New York, NY: Oxford University Press.

U.S. Department of Education. (2012). *Bringing flexibility and focus to education law*. Retrieved from http://www .whitehouse.gov/sites/default/files/fact_sheet_bringing_ flexibility_and_focus_to_education_law_0.pdf

Vinter, R., & Sarri, R. (1965). Malperformance in the public school: A group work approach. *Social Work, 10*, 38–48.

The White House. (2009). Fact sheet: The race to the top. Retrieved March, 2013, from http://www.whitehouse.gov/ the-press-office/fact-sheet-race-top

PAULA ALLEN-MEARES

SOCIAL JUSTICE

ABSTRACT: This is an examination of the concept of social justice and its significance as a core value of social work. Diverse conceptualizations of social justice and their historical and philosophical underpinnings are examined. The influence of John Rawls' perspectives on social justice is addressed as are alternative conceptualizations, such as the capabilities perspective. The roots of social justice are traced through social work history, from the Settlement House Movement to the Rank and Film Movement, Civil Rights Movement, and contemporary struggles in the context of globalization. Challenges for social justice-oriented practice in the 21st century are addressed. The discussion concludes with concrete example of ways in which social workers are translating principles of social justice into concrete practices.

KEY WORDS: social justice; distributive justice; John Rawls; capabilities perspective; Settlement House Movement; participatory democracy; globalization

Social justice is one of the core values guiding social work, a hallmark of its uniqueness among the helping professions. It is a concept deeply rooted in social work history. The *Social Work Dictionary* defines social justice as:

> ...an ideal condition in which all members of a society have the same rights, protections, opportunities, obligations, and social benefits. Implicit in this concept is the notion that historical inequalities should be acknowledged and remedied through specific measures. A key social work value, social justice entails advocacy to confront discrimination, oppression, and institutional inequities. (Barker, 2003, p. 405).

The concept of social justice draws attention to institutional arrangements and systemic inequities that further the interests of some groups at the expense of others in the distribution of material goods, social benefits, rights, protections, and opportunities (Delaney, 2005; Dewees, 2006). Social justice can be thought of as a perspective through which social workers recognize and address the connection between personal struggles and structural arrangements of society (Fisher & Karger 1997). It can also be conceived as a goal for an equitable, sustainable society.

The *NASW Code of Ethics* mandates social workers to work toward social justice with all people but particularly with those marginalized from full participation in society because of discrimination, poverty, or other forms of social, political, and economic inequality. It emphasizes that social workers need to develop an understanding of oppression and cultural and ethnic diversity. It highlights a fundamental principle of social justice: the promotion of participatory processes to enable all people to engage in decision making that affects their lives (NASW, 1999). However, as indicated by Banerjee (2005), while the *NASW Code of Ethics* refers to a practice informed by social justice, it does not provide a clear definition of the term.

Meanings of Social Justice

The meanings of social justice are far reaching and ambiguous; translation into concrete practice is fraught with challenges. Social justice is a contextually bound and historically driven concept, and as such it has been a subject of ongoing debate in social work (Banerjee, 2005; Caputo, 2002; McGrath Morris, 2002; Miller, 1999; Pelton, 2001; Reisch, 2002; Saleebey, 1990; Scanlon & Longres, 2001; Van Soest, 1995; Van Soest & Garcia, 2003). Political theorists, philosophers, and social workers alike have explored what it means to be in "right relationship" between and among persons, communities, states, and nations. As McCormick (2003) notes, "There is not even agreement about whether liberty, equality, solidarity or the common good is the primary cornerstone on which the edifice of justice is to be constructed" (p. 8).

Understandings of social justice in U.S. social work are largely derived from Western philosophy and political theory and Judeo-Christian religious tradition. Conceptions of justice are abstract ideals that overlap with beliefs about what is right, good, desirable, and moral. Notions of social justice generally embrace values such as the equal worth of all citizens, their equal right to meet their basic needs, the need to spread opportunity and life chances as widely as possible, and finally, the requirement that we reduce and, where possible, eliminate unjustified inequalities. As Caputo (2002) remarks, the concept of social justice invoked by social work has largely been one steeped in liberalism, which may serve to maintain the status quo. However, Caputo also contends that social justice remains relevant as a value and goal of social work.

Some students of social justice consider its meaning in terms of the *tensions* between individual liberty and common social good, arguing that social justice is promoted to the degree that we can promote collective good without infringing upon basic individual freedoms. Some argue that social justice reflects a concept of *fairness* in the assignment of fundamental rights and duties, economic opportunities, and social conditions (Miller, 1976, p. 22, as cited in Reisch, 1998). Others frame the concept in terms of three components – legal justice, which is concerned with what people owe society; commutative justice, which addresses what people owe each other; and distributive justice, or what society owes the person (Reichert, 2003, p. 12; U.S. Catholic Bishops, 1986; Van Soest, 1995, p. 1811). From a distributive perspective, the one most often referenced by social workers, social justice entails not only approaches to societal choices regarding the distribution of goods and resources, but also consideration of the structuring of societal institutions to guarantee human rights and dignity and ensure opportunities for free and meaningful social participation.

Discussions of social justice in the context of social work generally address the differing philosophical approaches used to inform societal decisions about the distribution or allocation of resources. These discussions refer to three dominant theories of resource distribution: Utilitarian, libertarian, and egalitarian.

Utilitarian theories emphasize actions that bring about the greatest good and least harm for the greatest number. From this perspective, individual rights can be infringed upon if so doing helps meet the interests and needs of the majority (McCormick, 2003; Van Soest, 1994). Libertarian theories reject obligations for equal and equitable distribution of resources, contending instead that each individual is entitled to any and all resources that he or she has legally acquired (Nozick, 1974). They emphasize individual autonomy and the fundamental right to choose; they seek to protect individual freedom from encroachment by others. Proponents support minimal state responsibility for protecting the security of individuals pursuing their own separate interests (McCormick, 2003). Egalitarian theories contend that every member of society should be guaranteed the same rights, opportunities, and access to goods and resources. From this theoretical perspective the *redistribution* of societal resources should be to the advantage of the most vulnerable members of society. Thus, redistribution is a moral imperative to ensure that unmet needs are redressed (e.g., Rawls, 1971). However, as Reichert (2003) notes, the idea of social justice, expressed variously in these theories, remains elusive, especially in terms of concrete applicability to practice.

A number of social workers concerned about questions of social justice have turned to the work of the political philosopher John Rawls (1971), whose theory of justice is grounded in the egalitarian approach addressed above. Drawing from liberal thought, Rawls critiqued utilitarian and libertarian conceptualizations of social justice for their justification of personal hardships in lieu of a greater common good (Swenson, 1998). Rawls' theory asks, what would be the characteristics of a just society in which basic human needs are met, unnecessary stress is reduced, the competence of each person is maximized, and threats to well-being are minimized? For Rawls, distributive justice denotes "the value of each person getting a fair share of the benefits and burdens resulting from social cooperation," both in terms of material goods and services and also in terms of nonmaterial social goods, such as opportunity and power (Wakefield, 1988, p. 193). In *Justice as Fairness: A Restatement*, Rawls (2001) provides two basic principles of social justice, modified from his earlier work:

a. Each person has the same indefeasible claim to a fully adequate scheme of equal basic liberties, which scheme is compatible with the same scheme of liberties for all; and

b. Social and economic inequalities are to satisfy two conditions: first, they are to be attached to offices and positions open to all under conditions of fair equality of opportunity; and second, they are to be to the greatest benefit of the least-advantaged members of society (the difference principle). (pp. 42–43)

Jerome Wakefield (1988) argues that Rawls' notion of distributive justice is the organizing value of social work. He proposes that a Rawlsian perspective helps social work integrate its micro and macro practice divide and that it contains "the power to make sense of the social work profession and its disparate activities" (p. 194). Michael Reisch (1998) draws on Rawls' principle of "redress," that is, to compensate for inequalities and to shift the balance of contingencies in the direction of equality, in articulating the relationship between social work and social justice. He argues that a social justice framework for social work and social welfare policy would "hold the most vulnerable populations harmless in the distribution of societal resources, particularly when those resources are finite. Unequal distribution of resources would be justified only if it served to advance the least advantaged groups in the community" (Reisch, 1998, p. 20). Banerjee (2005), following a thorough review of the literature, claims that social work scholars and practitioners most often refer to Rawls' theory of social justice primarily because of its emphasis on egalitarianism, attention to distributive principles, and potential to bridge micro and macro levels of practice.

The concept of distributive justice is central to a number of discussions of social justice and social work. For example, according to Dorothy Van Soest and Betty Garcia (2003, p. 44), "Our conception of social justice is premised on the concept of distributive justice, which emphasizes society's accountability to the individual. What principles guide the distribution of goods and resources?" Van Soest and Garcia address five perspectives on distributive justice that help us grasp the complexity of the concept. Three of these perspectives, addressed previously—utilitarian, libertarian, and egalitarian—are prescriptive in nature, speaking of what social justice should be. A fourth, the racial contract perspective, offers a description of the current state of society and the unequal system of privilege and racism therein. The racial contract perspective argues that the notion of the "social contract" as the basis of Western democratic society is a myth. The contract did not extend beyond white society. Thus white privilege is a constitutive part of the "social contract" and must be dismantled in the struggle for social justice. A fifth view, the human rights perspective, makes human rights central to the discussion of social justice (p. 45). From this perspective, social justice encompasses meeting basic human needs, equitable distribution of resources, and recognition of the inalienable rights of all persons, without discrimination.

Stanley Witkin (1998), Jim Ife (1997, 2001), and Elizabeth Reichert (2003) have argued for the possibilities of the Universal Declaration of Human Rights as a conceptual frame for social work practice. Reichert contends that a human rights approach encompasses "a more comprehensive and defined set of guidelines for social work practice than social justice" (2003, p. 13). As Catherine MacDonald claims (2006, p. 176), "Social work practice can be seen as promoting a universalist view of social justice balanced by and expressed through a relativist view of human needs, varying from person to person, context to context." She suggests that a human rights-based practice has a moral and political clarity that can provide social

work with legitimacy for action, something lacking in more ambiguous constructions of social justice.

The work of Iris Marion Young (1990, 2001) on processual justice has also influenced social work thought and practice (Caputo, 2002). Processual justice "refers to the decision-making processes that lead to decisions about the distribution [of social goods and resources] and to the relationships between dominant and subordinate groups, such as racial majorities and people of color, that affect decisions about distribution" (Longres & Scanlon 2001, p. 448). In sum, Young argues that distributive issues are important, but that "the scope of justice extends beyond them to include the political as such, that is, all aspects of institutional organization insofar as they are potentially subject to collective decision" (1990, p. 8). In contrast to Rawls, Young's view of social justice is grounded in an explicit critique of capitalism and its inherently unjust social and economic relations. Her approach calls for participatory processes in decision making regarding issues of social allocation and distribution, rather than focusing solely on outcomes.

Patricia McGrath Morris (2002) calls social workers' attention to another approach to social justice— the capabilities perspective. This perspective addresses the limitations of the Rawlsian perspective, the foundation for which is grounded on fairness in the distribution of liberties and social primary goods. The capabilities perspective builds on the work of economist Amartya Sen; it focuses "on the fair distribution of capabilities—the resources and power to exercise self-determination—to achieve well being" (p. 368). It goes beyond the importance of securing social primary goods and sees these as an essential part of a process toward achieving social justice but not the ultimate goal: "Capability is based on what a person wants to achieve and what power she or he has to convert primary goods to reach her or his desired goals" (p. 368). Whereas the Rawlsian perspective of social justice defines societal principles, the capabilities perspective begins at the individual level and imagines what a person is capable of doing and of becoming (Nussbaum, 2002). Martha Nussbaum (2002, 2004) has generated a list of capabilities, such as bodily health, affiliation, and play, that can be changed and expanded in congruence with social and cultural context. Thus, the list is suggestive and meant to facilitate discussion and decision making by providing "a focus for quality of life assessment and for political planning." (Nussbaum, 2002, p. 131). In addition, Nussbaum (2004) presents a cogent argument for the structural inadequacies of Rawlsian-influenced perspectives when applied to a global context. She argues that solutions to problems of global justice cannot be addressed through an approach that denies the fundamental inequalities of nations and views them as equals in terms of power and resources. Instead, she advocates for a perspective that resurrects "the richer ideas of human fellowship that we find in Grotius and other exponents of the natural law tradition" (p. 4). Nussbaum views the capabilities perspective as emergent and calls for it to be further informed by the perspectives of those whose lived experiences makes them experts in the day-to-day struggles to achieve a modicum of justice in what Reisch (2002, p. 343) refers to as a "socially unjust world."

McGrath Morris (2002) advocates for the capabilities perspective because it expands on a distributive justice perspective commonly referred to in social work and includes and emphasizes the importance of other social work values such as self-determination, well-being, and human dignity. She highlights the compatibility of the capabilities framework with the underlying principles set forth in social work's dominant theoretical approaches that focus on strengths, person-in-environment, and empowerment. Banerjee (2005) also notes the need to rethink social work's emphasis on Rawls' view of social justice and to more thoroughly critique its application to social work practice. He contends that drawing on other justice theorists such as Nussbaum guides practice toward advocacy, especially "when society and life's circumstances outside of one's control do not permit some people, especially people of color and particularly women, to develop their capabilities" (p. 53).

Historical Perspective

In claiming the roots of social justice in social work history, the early settlement house movement has generally served as a starting point. Through the movement, social workers were developing a critical consciousness about dramatically changing social, economic, and political conditions and their differential impacts in the lives of poor and vulnerable groups, particularly immigrants. Settlement house workers located their work in contrast to the "charity" approach to social work gaining prominence in the late 19th century. They began to make the connections between individual misery and societal arrangements and to address both the logic and the impacts of structural inequalities. Citing the National Conference on Charities and Corrections in 1909, McGrath Morris (2002) evokes the fervor of the time when social workers were challenged to "dare to repeat

the creed of the Hebrew prophet – justice, justice shalt thou pursue ... We have had the age of chivalry, the age of generosity, and the age of mercy, and now we need the age of justice" (Wise, 1909, p. 29 as cited in McGrath Morris, 2002, p. 365).

As Eleanor Stebner (1997) notes, the concept of the "social" was acquiring new power at the turn of the 20th century. Settlement houses were experiments in social democracy; their residents were advocates of social reform, and often, followers of the social gospel. When Jane Addams made the decision to cast her lot with the poor she embraced a concept of social justice. In her presidential address to the 1910 National Conference on Charities and Corrections, Addams spoke directly of the limits of charity and the challenges of social justice (Addams, 1960, pp. 85–87). However, as Sharon Berlin (2005, p. 490) notes, Addams' efforts were also "constrained by her own ideological blind spots," which kept her from finding common cause with early-20th-century African American women reformers whose activism against racism and segregation was also shaped by a strong spiritual commitment (Carlton-LaNey, 1999).

Other noted Hull-House residents, such as Florence Kelly, engaged in trenchant critiques of industrial capitalism and its relationship to the lived experience of the urban poor. Their work in documenting exploitative labor practices, unsafe housing conditions, and the vulnerability of women and children, made explicit links between personal struggles and public issues. While invoking the language of social reform and social democracy, they modeled a philosophy and practice of social justice that called for them to see the world from the vantage point of the less powerful; to invite participation of those affected in the understanding and resolution of social problems; to construct new forms of social life grounded in belonging, respect, and participation; and to hold to a vision of a just world.

"Groups were the primary modus operandi from which the settlement house agenda was to be achieved," and were, therefore, a vehicle of social justice (Jacobson & Rugeley, 2007). Group work theory and practice were firmly embedded in democratic principles that embodied humanitarian concerns, social responsibility, human relationships, and social justice (Andrews, 2001; Lee, 1986, 1992; Schwartz, 1986). Addams envisioned the group as a means for learning about democracy as people engaged in democratic group processes. She emphasized the need to exchange "the music of isolated voices [for] the volume and strength of the chorus" (as cited in Schwartz, 1986, p. 12). Throughout social work's history, organizing efforts to combat social injustice were forged through the development of groups. For example, in the midst of the Great Depression of the 1930s, the Rank and File Movement arose from within service organizations, provoked by unfair labor conditions, oppressive bureaucratic structures, and an economic system that favored corporate interests over human need. Bertha Capen Reynolds, a leader of the movement, helped form unions, and she illustrated through her work "a justice-oriented social work practice" (Reisch, 2002, p. 348). Reynolds' principles of practice emphasized belonging, mutuality, power sharing, and "forming and joining coalitions with clients, community groups, and like-minded colleagues from all disciplines" (Reynolds, 1963, pp. 173–175). She recognized groups as arenas and relations through which social justice principles and aims can play out on the broader landscape.

As the emphasis on group work within social work waxed and waned through the 1940s and 1950s so did the profession's attention to issues of social justice. One of the most damaging impacts to the profession's concern for social justice and participatory democracy came by way of McCarthyism: "By the 1940s, particularly after the War, many activities engaged in by social workers, especially the practice and ideology of group workers, came under attack by anti-Communists" (Andrews, 2001, p. 52). As cited in Andrews' historical analysis of group work, Harold Lewis believed that group work was a significant casualty of the post-WWII period:

> This was a serious loss, since this method was the most democratic in the profession. The core concept of group work and the goal of its major proponents was participatory democracy.... What survived was the method's narrower function, therapeutic aid. (Lewis, 1992, pp. 41–42, as cited in Andrews, 2001, pp. 52–53)

The powerful social and political movements of the 1960s pressed the social work profession to further examine its commitment to social justice. The civil rights movement, poor people's and welfare rights movements, women's movement, and anti-war movement demanded public and professional attention to deeply embedded social and economic inequalities and to the workings of structural as well as physical forms of violence. In 1973 NASW published an edited volume titled *Social Work Practice and Social Justice* that grappled with stark examples of racism and inequality as manifest in correctional, health, education, and welfare systems; the complicity of social work and social workers in perpetuating systemic injustices;

and the responsibility of the profession to advocate for justice-oriented social change. The contributors critiqued the dominance of individual pathology approaches to theory and practice, which tended to bracket attention to social structures. They argued that social work had failed to live up to its professed values of human dignity, worth, and self-determination by ignoring social structures, failing to identify basic social problems and participate in their resolutions, and claiming a stance of professional neutrality regarding issues that are fundamentally political. Bess Dana (1973) challenged social workers to advocate for health care as a right. She argued that social justice honors knowledge that illuminates human possibility, values respect for others, and demonstrates a willingness to give up power and prestige. She called for a practice of social justice based on partnership, collaborative action, promotion of rights, pursuit of new knowledge, and advocacy. The contributors advocated for the right to a minimum standard of living for all and for the right to involvement in the issues that affect one's life.

As Bernard Ross concluded (1973, p. 152), "Social justice is concerned not just with the equitable distribution of goods and services but with the right and power of persons and groups to obtain their fair share. Thus social workers necessarily accept as a goal the redistribution of goods, services, and power." However, despite the evocation of a language of rights and calls for a rights-based practice, general knowledge of human rights and specific attention to human-rights based practice have not played a dominant role in social work in the United States. Questions of power, on the other hand, have become central to emergent theoretical directions of late 20th century social work, where empowerment perspectives, envisioned as a route toward social-justice-oriented practice, have gained prominence.

Social Work and Social Justice in a Global Context

Each year the United Nations completes a Human Development Report documenting global disparities that highlight life expectancies, access to material and social goods, and inequalities based on gender, race, age, and other markers of difference. The report points to the growing divide between those with an abundance of resources and those with little or no access to basic necessities. These issues raise questions of social justice. As Nussbaum (2004) indicates, "Any theory of justice that proposes political principles defining basic human entitlements ought to be able to confront these inequalities and the challenge they pose, in a world in which the power of the global market and of multinational corporations has considerably eroded the power and autonomy of nations" (pp. 3–4). The global economy and its penetration into every aspect of human existence link people through what Polack (2004) refers to as "a complex web of economic relationships" (p. 281). Therefore, social workers need to locate and understand many domestic social justice issues within a larger global context.

Lynne Healy (2001) argues for the need to pay simultaneous attention to global interdependence and social exclusion, or the forces of social and economic marginalization that deny whole populations the right to participate in opportunities available in society. Karen Lyons (1999) argues that attention to social justice on a global scale requires critical thinking and action to address poverty, migration, disasters, and their global impacts (1999, p. 14). Polack (2004) notes that the NASW Code of Ethics puts forth a global mandate for the promotion of social justice. In making explicit that the ethical responsibilities of social workers extend beyond national boundaries, NASW challenges social workers to broaden and deepen their knowledge base. Polack argues that, in order to address the structures of privilege and inequality in the global economy, social workers need a critical understanding of colonialism and its legacies; the global structuring of debt; the logic and function of structural adjustment programs; and shifting forms of labor and movements of labor forces.

Echoing Polack's concerns, Caputo (2002) argues that a commitment to social justice and the "ethics of care" are critical counter forces for social change in the context of the ascendancy of neoliberalism and the infiltration of market principles in all aspects of social life. These conceptualizations of justice speak of broad societal responsibilities that cannot be readily confined to the concerns and obligations of particular states or nations. If social workers limit their focus to the situation of social justice within a given state, they miss fundamental inequalities among states and the transnational policies and practices that maintain and justify them. As Lyons (1999) notes, citizenship as it is conceptualized and practiced at the national level is inherently exclusionary when we consider the differences in power and access to resources among states.

Social workers in both the United States and abroad have reported on the insidious impacts of marketization, managerialism, and fragmentation of social welfare systems and social work practices in the era of neoliberal globalization (Clarke, Gewirtz, & McLaughlin 2000; Harris, 2005; Jones; 2005). Healy (2005, p. 220) warns of the trend toward "reprivatization of public concerns, such as poverty" and the implications for a justice-oriented practice of social work. In this new environment of marketization and managerialism, Healy (2001) expresses concern that increasing demands by funding agencies and service managers for cost-effectiveness and evidence of service outputs may constrain practice grounded in the profession's core values. Similarly, Dominelli (1996) has expressed concern over the "commodification of social work" that moves the focus of practice away from concern about people and relationships toward a "product that is being purchased from a contractor" (pp. 163–164). Rossiter (2005) challenges social workers to think specifically about the clinical, legal, and ethical implications of social work within the neoliberal global order. She asks: "Can we picture our current students working for a private child protection service owned by an American multinational?" (p. 190). If social workers take principles of social justice seriously then they have to develop an international or transnational perspective of the obligations of both citizenship and the profession. These are fundamental challenges for social work in the 21st century.

Linking Social Justice and Social Work Practice

The meaningful incorporation of social justice principles into social work practice calls for an ongoing examination of the questions of difference, power, and oppression (Saleebey, 2006). As Beth Glover Reed and colleagues (Reed, Newman, Suarez, & Lewis, 1997, p. 46) argue, "recognizing and building on people's differences is important and necessary, but not sufficient for a practice that has social justice as a primary goal." For social justice-oriented practice, "both *difference* and *dominance* dimensions must be recognized and addressed. Developing and using individual and collective critical consciousness are primary tools for understanding differences, recognizing injustice, and beginning to envision a more just society" (Reed et al., 1997, p. 46). Translating the value of social justice into practice requires that social workers align themselves with those who have experienced the world from positions of oppression and challenge the practices and conditions that reproduce inequality. Social work becomes a transformative process in which both social conditions and participants, including the social worker, are changed in the pursuit of a just world (Adams, Domenelli, & Payne, 2005; Witkin, 1998).

Social workers are translating the principle of social justice into concrete practices. For example, Lynn

Parker (2003) argues that a social justice perspective informed by feminism calls attention to questions of power, privilege, and oppression in all aspects of social work, including clinical practice. Lorraine Gutiérrez and Edith Lewis (1999) have drawn from the experiences of women of color to promote social justice through an empowerment-based model of practice (Gutiérrez & Lewis, 1999). Janet Finn and Maxine Jacobson (2007) have put forth the "just practice framework," as a guide to social justice-oriented practice. The framework brings together five interrelated concepts—meaning, context, power, history, and possibility—as a basis for critical inquiry and action. Advocacy practice provides another direction for social justice-oriented social work. Richard Hoefer (2006, p. 8) defines advocacy practice as "that part of social work practice where the social worker takes action in a systematic and purposeful way to defend, represent, or otherwise advance the cause of one or more clients at the individual, group, organizational, or community level in order to promote social justice."

Charles Waldegrave and colleagues at the Family Centre in Wellington, New Zealand, have developed a model for "Just Therapy," which makes social justice the heart of direct practice (Waldegrave, 2000). The approach is characterized by three main concepts: belonging, sacredness, and liberation. Waldegrave describes the emergence of Just Therapy in a "reflective environment" in which diverse stakeholders came together and critically examined the ways in which helping systems and demands of help seeking have served to reproduce inequalities and experiences of marginalization. Waldegrave describes Just Therapy as a demystifying approach that involves a wide range of practitioners in addressing the deep social pain experienced by people who have been systematically marginalized.

Elizabeth Mulroy (2004) presents a framework for thinking about organizational and community practice in an increasingly complex context of "shifting resources and constraints." It highlights social justice as a core principle of macro-level practice and the need to "understand how the forces of oppression operate across a metropolitan landscape in order to devise strategies capable of bringing about lasting change" (p. 81). Mulroy emphasizes the need for environmental surveillance in order to stay alert to a rapidly changing social environment where organizational survival is predicated on mobilizing power through inter-organizational collaboration, gaining legitimacy by reaching out to the community and maintaining relationships, and sustaining vertical and horizontal linkages to economic resources.

Using a social justice lens helps organizations to reframe issues generally viewed as individual in origin to include broader social, political, economic, and cultural understandings. These open up possibilities for new solutions. The examples cited here are but a few of social workers' efforts to translate the principles of social justice to a practice level. Efforts along these lines continue to grow stronger as social, economic, and political disparities increase. They signal that a commitment to social justice remains an imperative of the profession and a core value guiding social work into the 21st century.

REFERENCES

Adams, R., Domenelli, L., & Payne, M. (Eds.). (2005). *Social work futures: Crossing boundaries and transforming practice.* New York: Palgrave/MacMillan.

Addams, J. (1960). *A centennial reader.* New York: MacMillan.

Andrews, J. (2001). Group work's place in social work: A historical analysis. *Journal of Sociology and Social Welfare,* 28(4), 45–65.

Banerjee, M. (2005). Apply Rawlsian social justice to welfare reform: An unexpected finding for social work. *Journal of Sociology and Social Welfare,* 32(2), 35–57.

Barker, R. (2003). *The social work dictionary* (5th ed.). Washington, DC: NASW Press.

Berlin, S. (2005). The value of acceptance in social work direct practice: A historical and contemporary view. *Social Service Review,* 79(3), 482–510.

Caputo, R. (2002). Social justice, the ethics of care, and market economies. *Families in Society,* 83(4), 355–364.

Carlton-LaNey, I. (1999). African American social work pioneers' response to need. *Social Work,* 44(4), 311–321.

Clarke, J., Gewirtz, S., & McLaughlin, E. (2000). *New managerialism, new welfare?* London: Sage.

Dana, B. (1973). Health, social work, and social justice. In B. Ross & C. Shireman (Eds.), *Social work practice and social justice* (pp. 111–128). Washington, DC: NASW.

Delaney, R. (2005). Social justice. In Francis J. Turner (Ed.), *Encyclopedia of Canadian social work.* Waterloo, Ontario: Wilfred Laurier University Press.

Dewees, M. (2006). *Contemporary social work practice.* Boston: McGraw-Hill.

Dominelli, L. (1996). Deprofessionalizing social work: Anti-oppressive practice, competencies and post-modernism. *British Journal of Social Work,* 26, 153–157.

Finn, J., & Jacobson, M. (2007). *Just practice: A social justice approach to social work* (2nd ed.). Peosta, IA: Eddie Bowers Publishing, Inc.

Fisher, R., & Karger, H. (1997). *Social work and community in a private world.* New York: Longman.

Gutiérrez, L., & Lewis, E. (1999). *Empowering women of color.* New York: Columbia University Press.

Harris, J. (2005). Globalisation, neo-liberal managerialism and UK social work. In I. Ferguson, M. Lavalette, & E. Whitmore (Eds.), *Globalisation, global justice and social work* (pp. 81–93). New York: Routledge.

Healy, K. (2005). Under reconstruction: Renewing critical social work practices. In S. Hick, J. Fook, & R. Pozzuto (Eds.), *Social work: A critical turn* (pp. 219–229). Toronto: Thompson Educational Publishing, Inc.

Healy, L. (2001). *International social work: Professional action in an interdependent world*. New York: Oxford University Press.

Hoefer, R. (2006). *Advocacy practice for social justice*. Chicago: Lyceum Press.

Ife, J. (1997). *Rethinking social work: Towards critical practice*. Melbourne: Longman.

Ife, J. (2001). *Human rights and social work: Towards rights-based practice*. Cambridge, UK: Cambridge University Press.

Jacobson, M., & Rugeley, C. (2007). Community-based participatory research: Group work for social justice and community change. *Social Work with Groups, 30*(4), 21–39.

Jones, C. (2005). The neo-liberal assault: Voices from the front line of British state social work. In I. Ferguson, M. Lavalette, & E. Whitmore (Eds.), *Globalisation, global justice and social work* (pp. 97–109). New York: Routledge.

Lee, J. A. B. (1986). Seeing it whole: Social work with groups within an integrative perspective. *Social Work with Groups, 8*(4), 39–49.

Lee, J. A. B. (1992). Jane Addams in Boston: Intersecting time and space. In J. Garland (Ed.), *Group work reaching out: People, places and power* (pp. 7–21). New York: Haworth Press.

Lewis, H. (1992). Some thoughts on my forty years in social work education. *Journal of Progressive Human Services, 3*(1), 39–51.

Longres, J., & Scanlon, E. (2001). Social justice and the research curriculum. *Journal of Social Work Education, 37*(3), 447–463.

McCormick, P. (2003). Whose justice? An examination of nine models of justice. *Social Thought, 22*(2/3), 7–25.

McDonald, C. (2006). *Challenging social work: The institutional context of practice*. New York: Palgrave.

McGrath Morris, P. (2002). The capabilities perspective: A framework for social justice. *Families in Society, 83*(4), 365–373.

Miller, D. (1976). *Social justice*. Oxford: Clarendon Press.

Miller, D. (1999). *Principles of social justice*. Cambridge, MA: Harvard University Press.

Mulroy, E. (2004). Theoretical perspectives on the social environment to guide management and community practice: An organization-in-environment approach. *Administration in Social Work, 28*(1), 77–96.

National Association of Social Workers. (1999). *Code of ethics of the national association of social workers*. Washington, DC: Author.

Nozick, R. (1974). *Anarchy, state, and utopia*. New York: Basic Books.

Nussbaum, M. (2002). Capabilities and social justice. *International Studies Review, 4*(2), 123–135.

Nussbaum, M. (2004). Beyond the social contract: Capabilities and global justice. *Oxford Development Studies, 32*(1), 3–18.

Parker, L. (2003). A social justice model for clinical social work practice. *Affilia, 18*(3), 272–288.

Polack, R. (2004). Social justice and the global economy: New challenges for social work in the 21st century. *Social Work, 49*(2), 281–290.

Rawls, J. (1971/1995). *A theory of justice* (1st & 2nd eds.). Cambridge, MA: Harvard University Press.

Rawls, J. (2001). *Justice as fairness: A restatement*. Cambridge, MA: Belknap Press of Harvard University Press.

Reed, B. G., Newman, P., Suarez, Z., & Lewis, E. (1997). Interpersonal practice beyond diversity and toward social justice: The importance of critical consciousness. In C. Garvin & B. Seabury (Eds.), *Interpersonal practice in social work: Promoting competence and social justice* (2nd ed., pp. 44–78). Boston: Allyn and Bacon.

Reichert, E. (2003). *Social work and human rights: A foundation for policy and practice*. New York: Columbia University Press.

Reisch, M. (1998). *Economic globalization and the future of the welfare state. Welfare reform and social justice visiting scholars program*. Ann Arbor: The University of Michigan School of Social Work.

Reisch, M. (2002). Defining social justice in a socially unjust world. *Families in Society, 83*(4), 343–354.

Reynolds, B. (1963). *An uncharted journey*. Washington, DC: NASW Press.

Ross, B. (1973). Professional dilemmas. In B. Ross & C. Shireman (Eds.), *Social work practice and social justice* (pp. 147–152). Washington, DC: NASW Press.

Rossiter, A. (2005). Where in the world are we? Notes on the need for a social work response to global power. In S. Hick, J. Fook, & R. Pozzuto (Eds.), *Social work: A critical turn* (pp. 189–202). Toronto: Thompson Educational Publishing, Inc.

Saleebey, D. (1990). Philosophical disputes in social work: Social justice denied. *Journal of Sociology and Social Welfare, 17*(2), 29–40.

Saleebey, D. (Ed.). (2006). *The strengths perspective in social work practice* (4th ed.). Boston: Pearson Education, Inc.

Schwartz, W. (1986). The group work tradition and social work practice. *Social Work with Groups, 8*(4), 7–27.

Stebner, E. (1997). *The women of hull house: Study in spirituality, vocation, and friendship*. Albany: State University of New York Press.

Swenson, C. (1998). Clinical social work's contribution to a social justice perspective. *Social Work, 43*(6), 527–537.

United States Catholic Bishops. (1986). *Economic justice for all: Pastoral letter on Catholic social teaching and the U.S. economy*. Washington, DC: National Conference of Catholic Bishops.

Van Soest, D. (1994). Strange bedfellows. A call for reordering national priorities from three social justice perspectives. *Social Work, 39*(6), 710–717.

Van Soest, D., & Garcia, B. (2003). *Diversity education for social justice: Mastering teaching skills*. Alexandria, VA: Council on Social Work Education.

Wakefield, J. (1988). Psychotherapy, distributive justice and social work: Part I – Distributive justice as a conceptual framework for social work. *Social Service Review, 62*(2), 187–210.

Waldegrave, C. (2000). Just therapy with families and communities. In G. Burford & J. Hudson (Eds.), *Family group conferencing: New directions in community-centered child and family practice* (pp. 153–163). New York: Aldine de Gruyter.

Wise, S. (1909). The conference sermon. Charity versus justice. *Proceedings of the National Conference of Charities and Corrections, 36*, 20–29.

Witkin, S. (1998). Human rights and social work. *Social Work, 43*(3), 197–201.

Young, I. M. (1990). *Justice and the politics of difference.* Princeton, NJ: Princeton University Press.

Young, I. M. (2001). Equality for whom? Social groups and judgments of injustice. *The Journal of Political Philosophy, 9*(1), 1–18.

FURTHER READING

Council on Social Work Education. (1994). *Handbook of accreditation standards and procedures.* Alexandria, VA: Author.

Dominelli, L. (2002). *Anti-oppressive social work theory and practice.* London: Macmillan.

Ferguson, I., Lavalette, M., & Whitmore, E. (2005). *Globalisation, global justice and social work.* New York: Routledge.

Harvey, D. (1989). *The condition of postmodernity: An enquiry into the origins of cultural change.* Oxford, UK: Basil Blackwell, Ltd.

Reisch, M. (2005). American exceptionalism and critical social work: A retrospective and prospective analysis. In I. Ferguson, M. Lavalette, & E. Whitmore (Eds.), *Globalisation, global justice and social work* (pp. 157–172). New York: Routledge.

Reisch, M., & Andrews, J. (2001). *The road not taken: a history of radical social work in the United States.* New York: Brunner/Routledge.

Ross, B., & Shireman, C. (Eds.). (1973). *Social work practice and social justice.* Washington, DC: NASW Press.

JANET L. FINN AND MAXINE JACOBSON

SOCIAL POLICY: OVERVIEW

ABSTRACT: Social policy is how a society responds to social problems. Any government enactment that affects the well-being of people, including laws, regulations, executive orders, and court decisions, is a social policy. In the United States, with its federal tradition of shared government, social policies are made by governments at many levels—local, state, and national. A broad view of social policy recognizes that corporations and both nonprofit and for-profit social-service agencies also develop policies that affect

customers and those they serve and therefore have social implications. Social policies affect society and human behavior, and their importance for social-work practice has long been understood by the social-work profession. Modern social welfare policies, which respond to basic human needs such as health care, housing food, and employment, have evolved since their introduction during the New Deal of the 1930s as responses to the Great Depression. In the aftermath of the recent "Great Recession" that began in 2006, the nation has once again experienced the kinds of social problems that led to the creation of innovative social welfare policies in the 1930s. How policy makers respond to human needs depends on who has the power to make policy and how they conceptualize human needs and the most effective ways to respond to them. In the early 21st century, the idea that the state should guarantee the welfare and well-being of its citizens through progressive welfare state policies and services has few adherents among policy makers. The complex social problems resulting from the recession—the highest unemployment since the Great Depression of the 1930s, escalating budget deficits at all levels of government, an unprecedented housing crisis exemplified by massive foreclosures, increasing social and economic inequality, a nation polarized by corrosive political conflict and incivility—create a context in which social policies are debated vociferously. Social workers, long committed to the ideal of social justice for all, are obligated to understand how policies affect their practice as well as the lives of those they serve and to advocate for policies that will improve social well-being as the United States recovers.

KEY WORDS: globalization; social policy; welfare

DEFINITIONS Social policies are created and function in dynamic social, economic, and cultural contexts. Conflicting ideas and interests exist over what kinds of policies are needed to address social problems and human needs.

The concept of *social welfare* refers broadly to what is needed to provide people with resources and opportunities to lead satisfying and productive lives (Midgley & Livermore, 2009). A broad array of economic and social policies affects social welfare, ranging from tax policy to educational policy. More narrowly, some social welfare policies focus on policies and programs that provide income assistance and social services to people in need. Conservatives have generally supported "residual" time-limited social welfare policies and services, whereas liberals have argued for "universal" or "institutional" social welfare policies that provide assistance to citizens as communal rights. Institutional social welfare polices adopted by European "welfare states" never received much political support in the United States, where residual programs providing limited assistance to those seen as having genuine needs were favored (Patterson, 2000). Poverty, unemployment, dependent children, family instability, inadequate health care, and the needs of the elderly have been targets of social welfare policies. Because social policy responds to social problems, how those problems are defined and legitimized is important. Social workers, with their intimate knowledge of human needs, can provide critical information to policy makers if they can influence the policy-making process.

Socially constructed family and gender norms influence social policy and the lives of beneficiaries. Current debates about the meaning of "family" and "marriage" exemplify how social policies, such as the Defense of Marriage Act of 1996, may enforce specific norms while delegitimizing behavior deemed inappropriate by those who hold power. The federal government and states have clashed over the meaning of marriage and whether state recognition of same-sex marriage violates federal policy. Such contentious debates are often resolved in the courts. Traditions of public debate and discourse encourage interest groups to lobby for policies that will advantage their members. Some social policy experts feel corporate and business sectors have become so powerful that they dominate policy making, making government less responsive to social needs (Stiglitz, 2012).

Sometimes policies enacted to benefit special interests produce disastrous social results. For example, opening public lands to oil, timber, and mineral corporations has harmed people and environments if appropriate safeguards are not in place (Gore, 2007). Foreign policy also has a social impact. During the Cold War in the second half of the 20th century, social policy enforced gendered family norms with a male breadwinner, supporting a workforce that would enable the United States to compete for international economic hegemony. In the early 21st century, in the wake of the terrorist attacks on the United States on September 11, 2001, and our involvement in wars in Iraq and Afghanistan, resources that could have been used to develop or expand social welfare programs such as accessible health care for all Americans have been allocated to national defense and military spending. Escalating national debt after the "Great Recession" and the demands of the competi-tive, globalized marketplace have adversely affected the industrial U.S. workforce as U.S. corporations downsized or disappeared. The American middle class has seen its well-being threatened by loss of income and reduced job opportunities, decreasing opportunities for upward social mobility. The obstacles facing the poor for social advancement are numerous.

Given the range and relative importance of policy choices, social welfare policies must compete with economic, political, and defense needs for attention and resources. At least since the presidency of the conservative Republican Ronald Reagan, government policies and programs directed at public social welfare provision have been attacked as ineffectual and inappropriate interferences in the marketplace. Social policies that transferred and redistributed income from the wealthy to the poor, such as programs assisting poor women with families, were harshly criticized. Efforts have been made to privatize social services and the Social Security system, our most universal social welfare program. In the early 21st century, our political parties debate how our nation can promote economic growth and social well-being, emphasizing the need for job growth, while the longstanding issues of poverty and social and economic inequality receive less attention.

Philosophical Underpinnings of U.S. Social Policy

The notion of citizenship carries specific rights and obligations. Individualism, personal liberty, and the rights of persons to pursue activities freely and without excessive governmental intrusion are hallmarks of U.S. political philosophy and they inform policy making. Political and social conservatives generally support market-oriented, limited government and private activities to promote social well-being or social welfare, whereas liberals, recognizing that social conditions often limit people's ability to access opportunities to become self-sufficient, have supported the use of government authority to achieve social welfare goals (Ginsberg, 2002). The conservative "Tea Party" of the early 21st century and its supporters proclaim government itself to be regressive and non-responsive to human needs. The radical left and progressive critics generally reject both conservative and liberal social policy perspectives because they believe that social inequality and social problems can be resolved most effectively by active social planning and government redistribution of wealth. The dominant philosophy of government in the United States in the early 21st century holds that the market, broadly defined, should be allowed to function with as little interference as possible by governments to provide opportunities for all. The Republican Party has long held that government should do less regulation of business, for example, to give entrepreneurs freedom to take risks that might create new jobs. To attack massive federal debts, they encourage cutbacks of government programs and services, including social welfare programs, while reducing taxes on "job creators." Democrats argue that the best way to attack national debt is to create a more progressive tax system that will increase taxes on the wealthiest Americans to help fund critical government social programs, while offering tax incentives and other supports for businesses.

Social Policy Development

During the Progressive Era, Jane Addams and other reformers argued that government had obligations to protect poor women and children, who were seen as victims of industrialization. Despite opposition from business and from organized labor, "maternalist" reform achieved some success. Many states enacted mothers' pensions that provided limited cash support to women and children in dire economic need (Gordon, 1994), as well as categorical assistance programs targeted at specific groups—the elderly and the blind. These programs were administered locally, with few consistent standards used to determine eligibility or payment levels, allowing local prejudices and biases about who were "worthy" recipients (Abramovitz, 1996).

Skocpol (1998) has argued that social policy analysis must recognize how political and institutional forces influence policy choices and the administration of services and benefits as evidenced by mothers' pensions and contemporary social welfare programs. Progressive-Era workers' compensation laws provided income support to injured workers and were supported by conservative businessmen who realized that it was better for the state to aid injured workers than to subject business to the uncertainties of injured workers' negligence lawsuits and unpredictable jury verdicts (Herrick, 2009).

Modern social welfare policy began with the New Deal enacted in the 1930s during the administration of the liberal Democrat Franklin D. Roosevelt in response to the Great Depression and unprecedented unemployment and social unrest. Policy makers understood that private charities, voluntary organizations, and local and state governments were unable to provide enough economic assistance to address the needs of millions of people who were unemployed. Nearly one-third of private social-service

agencies ceased operations between 1919 and 1932 (Trattner, 1998). The federal government assumed unprecedented authority to intervene in the economy, resulting in controversy and opposition from conservatives who felt New Deal policy innovations were unwarranted intrusions by government into the lives of Americans. The most sweeping New Deal social welfare legislation, the Social Security Act of 1935, created new social insurance and public-assistance programs. Social insurance included unemployment insurance and the Social Security pension program and Old Age, Survivors, and Disability Insurance financed by payroll taxes on employees and employers. Public assistance (or welfare) was limited to the most needy and was administered by local governments, which often denied benefits to persons of color.

Progressive and radical critics, including some social workers, felt that the liberal reforms of the New Deal did not go far enough in addressing social inequality and the needs of working Americans and they argued for national planning and an institutional welfare state to distribute national wealth and end poverty (Reynolds, 1951; Selmi, 2005).

American social welfare grew incrementally, subject to political pressures and changing priorities, and never adopted the progressive vision. Although the Social Security pension program expanded over the years to include agricultural workers and others not originally covered, many of whom were people of color living in the South, it was influenced by contemporary gender and racial norms. Although it has provided a measure of economic security for retired workers who earned high incomes for many years, it disadvantaged women workers, who were unable to work outside the home for extended periods because of home and family responsibilities, resulting in smaller contributions to Social Security and reduced pensions (Abramovitz, 1996).

Social welfare policy and programs were expanded in the liberal President Johnson's Great Society "War on Poverty" of the 1960s. Medicare and Medicaid provided health insurance for retired workers and medical assistance for the poor. Although the Social Security pension system has been successful in reducing poverty among elderly workers and has widespread public support, its public assistance or welfare programs have been controversial. Aid to Families with Dependent Children (AFDC), a New Deal program that was expanded in 1962, offered residual "means-tested" cash assistance to the poor, financed by the federal government and the states and administered locally. Between 1960 and 1967, welfare rolls doubled, encouraging critics to argue that welfare was being abused by "cheats" and "unworthy" recipients, many of whom were people of color. A work incentive program, WIN, which required work from AFDC recipients, began a long retreat from support for dependent women and families. Conservative pundits and writers, generously funded by "think tanks" such as the Heritage Foundation, itself funded by the billionaire Richard Mellon Scaife, went on the offensive against liberal welfare policies. Public opinion was galvanized against social welfare programs using media to spread stigmatizing gender and racial stereotypes of welfare recipients as indolent and irresponsible. Single African American mothers receiving AFDC assistance were denigrated and called "welfare queens" by President Reagan (Chappell, 2010). In 1995, President Clinton, a Democrat, campaigned to "end welfare as we know it" and collaborated with the conservative Republican legislators who took control of Congress in 1994 to pass the Personal Responsibility and Work Opportunity Reconciliation Act of 1996, abolishing the AFDC and ending the federal entitlement to public assistance that had existed since the New Deal. In its place, the new Temporary Assistance to Needy Families (TANF) program gave states "block grants" to establish welfare assistance programs consistent with changing social priorities. New rules required work from recipients and limited cash assistance to five years. The 1998 Workforce Investment Act required welfare recipients to seek work before receiving social services, which was criticized by social workers as ignoring the needs of women and children who needed long-term assistance and supportive services. By 2005, the number of persons receiving public assistance was half what it had been in the 1990s. Although it is certain that many single mothers and others left the welfare rolls, whether they have achieved economic and social self-sufficiency is debatable. Securing employment with employers who provide low wages and few, if any, benefits, such as health insurance, does not provide a decent standard of living or good job security. There is clear evidence of large increases in the numbers of individuals receiving Medicaid and Food Stamps since 1996, supporting the argument that former welfare recipients have joined the ranks of the working poor, struggling to obtain decent housing, medical care, and food for their families (Shipley, 2004). Policy makers face ongoing dilemmas as they attempt to promote work, decrease dependency, and alleviate need among the most vulnerable members of American society (Grogger & Karoly, 2005) as poverty and social inequality increase to levels not seen since the Depression of the 1930s.

Research shows that for the poor to become self-sufficient, they need support that will provide for their basic needs so they can engage in learning and hence acquire skills to obtain good jobs (Andersson, Holzer, & Lane, 2005; Austin, 2004). In the early 21st century, although many training and temporary assistance programs are offered by social workers and others working in government, nonprofit, and for-profit agencies that can assist those transitioning from welfare to work by matching them to supportive programs, including medical assistance, housing, and child care, increasing homelessness and scarce job opportunities reduce the chances of finding full-time employment. A "pluralist" model of social welfare provision that integrates government programs with nonprofit and for-profit agencies and community resources has evolved in an attempt to meet complex human needs. Funded from many sources, including federal and local governments, foundations, philanthropy, and private donations, social services attempt to meet specific needs, such as job retraining and employment assistance, child care, homelessness, and hunger. Despite many innovative services and programs aimed at poverty alleviation, its seeming intractability while the wealthiest Americans prosper remains a national dilemma.

Suggestions to privatize Social Security, our most large-scale and institutional social welfare program, were proposed during the Bush administration. Proponents argued that individual retirement accounts, under individual control, would reduce federal entitlement liabilities (Herrick & Midgley, 2002). President George W. Bush favored state and charitable programs rather than federally run programs as the most effective way of dealing with certain social problems. He proposed federal funding for faith-based community services, based on the premise that local service providers can deliver the most humane and cost-effective human services, and he used his executive authority to fund an array of nonprofit faith-based social services (Smith, 2007).

Social Policy Context

Since 2006 and the beginning of the Great Recession, the federal government has attempted to combat the recession's economic and social impact. Both President George W. Bush, a conservative Republican, and his successor, President Barack H. Obama, a moderate Democrat, used federal funds to shore up the shaky economy in an attempt to stave off a major economic depression. In 2009, the American Reinvestment and Recovery Act allocated $787 billion to shore up the states. The largest amount, $87.1 billion, went to states to assist Medicare funding. Money also was allocated to other social programs, including the Supplemental Nutrition Assistance Program, TANF, U.S. Department of Housing and Urban Development housing assistance, energy bill assistance, public schools in low-income areas, and child care, which primarily benefitted low-income persons (Smeeding, Thompson, Levanon, & Burak, 2011). These efforts and others, although controversial, seem to have kept the nation from falling into a major depression, although the economy remained unsteady. Millions of workers lost jobs as companies downsized or disappeared as demand weakened. In 2008, 3.1 million jobs were lost, followed by another 4.7 million in 2009 (Goodman & Mance, 2011). Rising unemployment challenged local and state governments and social-service agencies to respond to increasing needs for unemployment compensation, job retraining, and services to assist those who were economically and socially at risk. Social workers, long accustomed to the challenges of providing services in times of crisis, worked creatively and doggedly to respond to emerging challenges. By 2013, unemployment was slowly falling but sectors of the labor market, including older workers and new college graduates, continued to face dismal job prospects. The middle class faces an unknown economic future as the job market changes and retirees' pensions are threatened by erratic swings in the stock market. Social policies to address the unemployment crisis are issues in local, state, and federal politics. Many corporations and public employers demand pension and benefit cutbacks, arguing that such draconian measures are necessary to maintain economic viability. Retirees and public employees such as social workers and teachers face job loss and reduced retirement income, increasing their economic and social insecurity. Entitlement programs such as Social Security are targets for those bent on reducing the scope of government and are often characterized as failed "nanny state" experiments by conservative critics.

Escalating needs in areas of traditional concern to social workers present social policy challenges. Twenty-one percent of America's children lived in poverty in 2011, a higher rate than that of nearly all prosperous nations (Stanford University Center for the Study of Poverty and Inequality, 2012). A 2012 Indiana University white paper, "At Risk" (Seefeldt, Abner, Bolinger, Xu, & Graham, 2012), found many states losing revenues, resulting in cutbacks of "safety net" programs that have traditionally supported economically and socially vulnerable citizens. Age, ethnicity, and family composition contribute to poverty. Racial disparity among poor Americans is evident,

with 1 in 4 Hispanics and African Americans living in poverty compared to 1 in 10 Whites. In 2013, 46 million Americans lived in poverty, the largest number in 53 years of published poverty rates. Not since the Great Depression have so many families and children become homeless. In 2010, 1 in 45 children were homeless (Bassuk, Murphy, Coupe, Kenney, & Beach, 2010). Social security, food stamps, and other programs provide a safety net for millions of Americans, keeping them out of poverty.

President Obama's Affordable Care Act, "Obamcare," while controversial, promises affordable and accessible health care to millions of Americans, a goal long supported by social work.

Increasing Inequality

During the late 20th century as conservative, neoliberal market–oriented assumptions came to dominate approaches to social welfare provision, exemplified by President Clinton's welfare reforms, the issue of social inequality was ignored by many social scientists who focused on postmodernist themes of identity, gender, and culture in social policy analyses. In the early 21st century, inequality has been rediscovered by social scientists determined to understand the social structural issues that impede America's progress.

Nobel laureate economist Joseph Stiglitz notes that the income of the top 1% amounts to nearly 25% of the total national income. The top 1% also controls 40% of the total wealth (Stiglitz, 2012). Rates of economic and social mobility are lower than the rates of many of our national competitors. Forty-two percent of men raised in families in the bottom quintile of incomes remain there as adults. About 62 percent of male and female Americans raised in the top quintile stay in the top two fifths throughout their lives (Alterman, 2012). Growing inequality preceded the Great Recession and has persisted in its aftermath. Much of this may be explained by the responsiveness of our political and government systems to powerful interests that deploy massive financial resources to influence policy making, such as efforts to make the tax system favorable to corporate interests. The U.S. Supreme Court's ruling in the *Citizens United* decision has opened the door for unlimited amounts of money to be used in political campaigns, thereby allowing wealthy interests to disproportionately influence candidate selection as well as social policy agendas. The Great Recession brought considerable economic insecurity to the middle class. A 2012 study by the Federal Reserve showed the middle class lost nearly 40% of its wealth between 2007 and 2010, whereas the wealthiest Americans gained assets (Bricker, Kennick, Moore, & Sabelhaus, 2012). Effective social policy must acknowledge increasing inequality as a barrier to the creation of a more just and equitable society. Class divisions are becoming increasingly problematic given our long-held belief in America as an egalitarian society.

The Future of U.S. Social Policy

Debates among conservatives and liberals about the viability of Social Security, our most basic and universal social welfare program, reflect how economic uncertainty impacts social policy. The conservative belief that the free market, unfettered by constrictive social welfare policies, can best respond to human needs by offering short-term assistance when necessary and, more important, opportunities to acquire the skills necessary to succeed in the globalized marketplace, is widely held. Social problems exacerbated by the Great Recession demonstrate that bold new approaches are needed to deal with complex problems such as unemployment and homelessness. Liberals generally favor government-financed economic stimuli to bolster the economy, whereas conservatives favor cuts in spending to reduce deficits.

Liberal policy makers support education and training programs to promote job readiness for the unemployed, but these programs do not produce immediate results, leaving laid-off workers with few resources, particularly when unemployment benefits expire. As the labor market changes, residual social policy responses do not address increasing structural inequality in the United States (Stiglitz, 2012). Low-income jobs, often taken by single women with children, once supported by welfare, contribute to the wage gender gap (Gatta & Deprez, 2008; Kuttner, 2002). The income gap between the rich and the rest of Americans is growing. Chief executive officers of major corporations earn hundreds of times more than their workers (Anderson, Cavanagh, Collins, Pizzigati, & Lapham, 2007). Furthermore, the share of total national income earned by an increasingly smaller percentage of persons is growing. Tax policies have provided some relief to the working poor through the earned income tax credit but the middle class and the wealthy have benefited far more under the tax code as income has been redistributed upward, increasing class inequality.

Globalization has exacerbated social inequalities worldwide (Chomsky, 2000). The United Nations University, World Institute for Development Economics Research (2005), found that in 2000 1% of the world's population owned 40% of global assets and that half of the world's adults owned only 1% of its wealth. Some argue for progressive policies that alter social structures to reduce social, racial, and gender inequalities by giving people more power and control over government decision making (Bates, 2000; Chomsky, 2000). Others support pushback from the rush toward globalization, pointing out that although it has produced immense wealth for some nations and individuals, millions of others in the United States and worldwide have been left behind and their needs cannot be ignored (Bates, 2000). It seems clear in the early 21st century that social welfare policies face an uncertain future as the nation struggles to shore up a recession economy. Social workers' roles will change as programs and services dependent on public and private support cope with funding reductions and changing missions. Demands on private charities and local and state governments will increase as long as the safety net is threatened by calls for austere measures to reduce the national debt and state budget shortfalls.

Roles of Social Workers

The National Association of Social Workers (NASW) encourages social workers to get involved in policy making. Many opportunities to do so are available through state NASW chapters.

Social workers have been elected to local, state, and federal offices, including the U.S. House of Representatives and the Senate. The NASW, both nationally and through its state chapters, engages in lobbying to influence social policy development. Social-work educators, students, and practitioners advocate for social policies to assist women, children, AIDS victims, prisoners reentering society, victims of abuse, the homeless, military veterans, immigrants, and others in need. Social workers have the knowledge, skills, and values to be strong advocates for the poor (Marsh, 2005; Schneider, 2000), continuing the tradition of social action begun long ago by social-work pioneers Jane Addams, Bertha Reynolds, and Whitney Young. Social workers are challenged to continue advocacy to attack social injustice and social inequality (Rowntree & Pomeroy, 2010). The NASW-sponsored Social Work Policy Institute offers timely information on policy innovations and social-work research that can be easily accessed at http://www.socialworkpolicy.org/. As the nation recovers from the Great Recession, social work can play a vital role in the evolution of the new economy, which is increasingly international, high tech, and green. Social workers in Congress, working with the NASW, established the Congressional Social Work Caucus in 2010, which works for the creation of a strong safety net of services and programs to assist the diverse needs of Americans. Social workers, working through the broad membership of the NASW, utilize the practice experiences of social workers across the nation to issue policy recommendations through Social Work Speaks (2012) and Hoffler & Clark (2012).

REFERENCES

Abramovitz, M. (1996). *Regulating the lives of women: Social welfare policy from colonial times to the present* (rev. ed.). Boston: South End Press.

Alterman, E. (2012, June 11). All the media money can buy. *The Nation,* 9.

Anderson, S., Cavanagh, J., Collins, C., Pizzigati, S., & Lapham, M. (2007). *Executive excess 2007: The staggering social cost of U.S. business leadership.* Washington, DC/ Boston, MA: Institute for Policy Studies/United for a Fair Economy.

Andersson, F., Holzer, H., & Lane, J. (2005). *Moving up or moving on: Who advances in the low wage labor market.* New York, NY: Russell Sage Foundation.

Austin, M. (2004). *Changing welfare services: Case studies in local welfare reform programs.* Binghamton, NY: Haworth Press.

Bassuk, E., Murphy, C., Coupe, N., Kennesy, R., and Beach, C. (2010). *America's youngest outcasts 2010.* Needham, MA: National Center on Family Homelessness. Retrieved from http://www.homelesschildrenamerica.org/media/ NCFH_AmericaOutcast2010_web.pdf

Bates, J. (2000). *Globalization, poverty and inequality.* Washington, DC: Progressive Policy Institute.

Bricker, J., Kennickell, A., Moore, K., and J. Sabelhaus (2012, June). Changes in U.S. family finances from 2009 to 2010: Evidence from the survey of consumer finances. *Federal Reserve Bulletin,* 98(2), 1–80. Retrieved from http://www.federalreserve.gov/pubs/Bulletin/2012/PDF/ scf12.pdf

Chappell, M. (2010). *The war on welfare: Family, poverty, and politics in modern America.* Philadelphia, PA: University of Pennsylvania Press.

Chomsky, N. (2000). *Profit over people: Neoliberalism and global order.* New York, NY: Seven Stories Press.

Gatta, M., & Deprez, L. (2008). Introduction to the special issue. *Journal of Sociology and Social Welfare,* 35(3), 9–19.

Ginsberg, L. (2002). *Conservative social welfare policy: A description and analysis.* Chicago, IL: Nelson–Hall.

Goodman, C., & Mance, S. (2011). Employment loss and the 2007–9 recession: An overview. *Monthly Labor Review.* Retrieved April 3, 2012, from http://www.bls.gov/opub/ mlr/2011/04/art1full.pdf

Gordon, L. (1994). *Pitied but not entitled: Single mothers and the history of welfare.* New York, NY: The Free Press.

Gore, A. (2007). *The assault on reason.* New York, NY: Penguin.

Grogger, J., & Karoly, L. (2005). *Welfare reform: Effects of a decade of change.* Cambridge, MA: Harvard University Press.

Herrick, J. (2009). Social policy and the Progressive Era. In J. Midgley & M. M. Livermore (Eds.), *The handbook of social policy* (pp. 114–132). Thousand Oaks, CA: Sage.

Herrick, J., & Midgley, J. (2002). The United States. In J. Dixon & R. Scheurell (Eds.), *The state of social welfare: The twentieth century in cross-national review* (pp. 187–216). Westport, CT: Praeger.

Hoffler, E., & Clark, E. (Eds.) (2012). *Social work matters: The power of linking policy and practice.* Washington, DC: NASW Press.

Kuttner, R. (Ed.). (2002). *Making work pay: America after welfare.* New York, NY: New Press.

Marsh, J. (2005). Social justice: Social work's organizing value. *Social Work,* 50(4), 293–294.

Midgley, J., & Livermore, M. (Eds.). (2009). *The handbook of social policy* (2nd ed.) Thousand Oaks, CA: Sage.

Patterson, J. (2000). *America's struggle against poverty in the twentieth century.* Cambridge, MA: Harvard University Press.

Reynolds, B. (1951). *Social work and social living: Explorations in philosophy and practice.* New York, NY: Citadel.

Rowntree, M., & Pomeroy, E. (2010). Bridging the gaps among social justice, research, and practice. *Social Work,* 55(4), 293–295.

Schneider, R. (2000). *Social work advocacy.* New York, NY: Wadsworth.

Seefeldt, K., Abner, G., Bolinger, J., Xu, l., & Graham, J. (2012). *At risk: America's poor during and after the Great Recession.* Bloomington: Indiana University School of Public and Environmental Affairs. Retrieved from http:// www.indiana.edu/-spea/pubs/white_paper_at_risk.pdf

Selmi, P. (2005). Mary van Kleeck. In J. Herrick & P. Stuart (Eds.), *Encyclopedia of social welfare history* (pp. 413–415). Thousand Oaks, CA: Sage.

Shipley, D. (2004). *The working poor, invisible in America.* New York, NY: Knopf.

Skocpol, T. (1998). The limits of the New Deal system and the roots of contemporary welfare dilemmas. In M. Weir, A. Orloff, & T. Skocpol (Eds.), *The politics of social policy in the United States* (pp. 293–312). Princeton, NJ: Princeton University Press.

Smeeding, T., Thompson, J., Levavon, E., & Burak, E. (2011). Poverty and income inequality in the early stages of the great recession. In D. Grusky, B. Western, & C. Wimer (Eds.), *The great recession* (pp. 82–126). New York, NY: Sage Foundation.

Smith, S. (2007). Social services and social policy. *Society,* 44(3), 54–59.

Social Work Speaks (9th ed.). (2012). *NASW policy statements, 2012–2014.* Washington, DC: NASW Press.

Stanford University Center for the Study of Poverty and Inequality. (2012). *20 facts about US inequality that everyone should know.* Retrieved from http://www.stanford.edu/ group/scspi/cgi-bin/facts.php

Stiglitz, J. (2012). *The price of inequality.* New York, NY: Norton.

Trattner, W. (1998). *From poor law to the welfare state: A history of social welfare in America* (6th ed.). New York, NY: Free Press.

United Nations University, World Institute for Development Economics Research. (2005). *World economic income inequality database*. Retrieved from http://www.wider.unu.edu

FURTHER READING
Association for Policy Analysis and Management: http://www.appam.org/

Center for Law and Social Policy: http://www.clasp.org/

Center for Social Policy, Poverty and Homelessness Research at the John W. McCormack Graduate School of Policy Studies, University of Massachusetts, Boston: http://www.mccormack.umb.edu/csp/index.jsp/

Gilons, M. (1994). "Race coding" and white opposition to welfare. *American Political Science Review*, 90, 593–604.

National Association of Social Workers: http://www.social-workers.org

Progressive Policy Institute: http://www.ppionline.org/

Weiner Center for Social Policy, John F. Kennedy School of Government, Harvard University, Research on social problems and social policy: http://www.ksg.harvard.edu/socpol/

Urban Institute: http://www.urban.org/

U.S. GOVERNMENT SITES:
American Public Welfare Association: http://www.apha.org/

Census Bureau, http://www.census.gov/

Center for Budget and Policy Priorities: http://www.cbpp.org/

Common Cause: http://www.commoncause.org/

Democratic National Committee: http://www.democrats.org

Electronic Policy Network: http://cpn.org/

Federal Statistics: http://www.fedstats.gov/

General Accounting Office: http://www.gao.org/

League of Women Voters: http://www.lwv.org/

National Mental Health Association: http://nmha.org/

Republican National Committee: http://www.republicans.org/

Social Policy: http://www.socialpolicy.org/

Social Security Administration: http://www.ssa.gov/

U.S. House of Representatives: http://www.house.gov/

U.S. Senate: http://www.senate.gov/

White House: http:www.whitehouse.gov/

Republican National Committee: http://republicans.org

JOHN M. HERRICK

SOCIAL WORK MALPRACTICE, LIABILITY, AND RISK MANAGEMENT

ABSTRACT: Social workers have become increasingly aware of malpractice and liability risks. Disgruntled clients, former clients, and others may file formal ethics complaints and lawsuits against practitioners. Complaints often allege that social workers departed from widely embraced ethical and social work practice standards. This article provides an overview of the concept of risk management and common risks in social work practice pertaining to clients' rights, confidentiality and privacy, informed consent, conflicts of interest, boundaries and dual relationships, digital and electronic technology, documentation, and termination of services, among others. It describes procedures used to process ethics complaints, licensing-board complaints, and lawsuits. In addition, the author outlines practical strategies, including an ethics audit, designed to protect clients, third parties, and social workers.

KEY WORDS: ethics; lawsuit; liability; malpractice; negligence; risk management

Social workers are trained to provide competent services that meet widely accepted professional standards. A practitioner's principal goal is to assist people who struggle with mental and physical illness, addiction, relationships, aging, disabilities, poverty, family violence, and other challenges.

On occasion, disgruntled clients and other parties believe they have been harmed by social workers' conduct. Examples include clients who claim that a social worker did not provide competent care, breached confidentiality, terminated services without the client's consent, or engaged in an unethical dual relationship.

Many clients who are distressed about their social worker's conduct suffer in silence or address their concerns with the social worker informally. Others, however, decide to take formal action in the form of a lawsuit or ethics complaint. It is important for social workers to identify potential risks that can harm clients and lead to lawsuits and ethics complaints, learn about practical risk-management protocols, and implement strategies to minimize risks.

The Concept of Risk Management
Social workers expose themselves to risk when they practice in a manner that is inconsistent with prevailing professional standards (Barsky, 2009; Houston-Vega, Nuehring, & Daguio, 1997; Reamer, 2003). Risk management is generally defined as the identification, analysis, assessment, control, avoidance, minimization, or elimination of unacceptable risks and hazards (Coleman, 2011; Hopkin, 2010). Historically, risk management and assessment have been associated with financial investments, financial audits, and project management (for example, bridge, building, airport, or highway construction) in industry and commerce.

More recently, risk management has been applied to human-service professions.

Social work risks can arise as a result of practitioners' inadvertent mistakes, deliberate decisions, or misconduct (Reamer, 2003).

Mistakes Some lawsuits and ethics complaints arise out of social workers' mistakes and oversights. Examples include social workers who inadvertently disclose confidential information about a client on their personal Facebook site, fail to protect the confidentiality of clients' electronic records and communications (for example, email), or neglect to document an important clinical consultation. Social workers who are named in such complaints typically are competent and ethical practitioners who have had an uncharacteristic lapse in judgment. This may occur when a social worker is overwhelmed with personal and work-related tasks and simply fails to pay attention to important details.

Decisions Other ethics complaints and lawsuits arise from social workers' deliberate decisions—for example, when social workers disclose confidential information without clients' consent to law enforcement officials in order to protect a third party from harm, hire a former client to work in one's agency, accept a client's gift, or terminate services to a client who has a large unpaid bill. In these instances, social workers are fully aware that they must make a professional judgment, examine the relevant facts and professionals standards, and make a decision. Clients or other parties who are distressed by the social worker's decision may file a formal complaint.

Misconduct In addition, some ethics complaints and lawsuits are the result of practitioners' ethical misconduct. Examples include a social worker who becomes sexually involved with a client, bills insurance companies for services that the social worker did not render, or falsifies documents. In some instances, social workers who engage in serious misconduct expose themselves to the risk of criminal prosecution (for example, following sexual assault of a client, insurance fraud, or embezzlement of client funds) in addition to ethics complaints and civil suits.

Social workers can be held accountable for negligence and ethical violations in several ways. In addition to filing lawsuits, parties can file ethics complaints with the National Association of Social Workers (NASW) or with state licensing and regulatory boards.

In some instances, social workers are also subjected to review by other professional organizations to which they belong, such as the American Board of Examiners in Clinical Social Work and the Clinical Social Work Association. In exceptional circumstances, criminal charges may be filed against social workers.

Ethics Complaints Many social work membership associations throughout the world provide mechanisms for filing ethics complaints. In the United States, ethics complaints filed against NASW members are processed using a peer-review model that includes NASW members and, initially, the National Ethics Committee (NASW, 2012). If a request for professional review is accepted by the National Ethics Committee, a NASW Chapter Ethics Committee (or the National Ethics Committee in special circumstances, for example, if there is a conflict of interest at the state level) conducts a hearing during which the complainant (the person filing the complaint), the respondent (the person against whom the complaint is filed), and witnesses have an opportunity to testify. After hearing all parties and discussing the testimony, the committee presents a report to elected chapter officers that summarizes its findings and presents its recommendations. Recommendations may include sanctions (such as expulsion from NASW, suspension of NASW membership, notification of findings to a state licensing board and the respondent's malpractice insurer, or a letter of censure) or various forms of corrective action (such as mandated supervision, consultation, continuing education, restitution, notification of the respondent's supervisor or employer, or correction of a client case record). In some cases, the sanction may be publicized through local and national NASW publications.

NASW also offers mediation in some instances in an effort to avoid formal adjudication and adversarial proceedings, particularly involving matters that do not include allegations of extreme misconduct. If complainants and respondents agree to mediate the dispute, NASW will facilitate the mediation.

Licensing Board Complaints

In some nations, legislative bodies empower social work licensing boards and regulatory bodies to process ethics complaints filed against social workers. Ordinarily, these boards appoint a panel of colleagues to review the complaint and, when warranted, conduct a formal investigation and hearing; some boards include public members in addition to professional colleagues. In some jurisdictions, licensing boards have authority over social workers exclusively; in other jurisdictions licensing boards are interdisciplinary and have authority over several human-service professions, such as social work, mental health counseling, and marriage and family therapy.

In some jurisdictions, formal hearings are conducted by the licensing board itself. In other jurisdictions, formal hearings are conducted by administrative-law judges. Typically, cases are brought against social workers by prosecuting attorneys representing the licensing body. Social workers are usually represented by legal counsel.

Licensing boards typically have authority to impose sanctions and various forms of corrective actions. Sanctions may include suspension or revocation of a license, a term of probation, or a letter of reprimand, or all of those. Corrective action may include mandated supervision, consultation, continuing education, restitution, and notification of the respondent's supervisor or employer. Licensing boards may publicize findings on their formal websites or in prominent newspapers and professional publications.

Negligence Claims and Civil Lawsuits

Negligence claims or lawsuits filed against social workers typically allege that social workers engaged in malpractice in that the practitioners failed to adhere to specific standards of care. The standard of care is based on what ordinary, reasonable, and prudent practitioners with the same or similar training would have done under the same or similar circumstances (Johnson, 2011; Madden, 2003; Reamer, 2003; Woody, 1997).

Departures from the profession's standards of care may result from a social worker's acts of commission or acts of omission (Johnson, 2011). Acts of commission can occur as a result of misfeasance, malfeasance, or nonfeasance. Misfeasance is the commission of a proper act in a wrongful or injurious manner or the improper performance of an act that might have been performed lawfully. Examples include a social worker who discloses confidential information to a third party without the client's consent or inadvertently records inaccurate information about the client in an important case note or report.

Malfeasance is the commission of a wrongful or unlawful act. A social worker who has an intimate relationship with a client and exploits the client financially for personal benefit, or who deliberately falsifies client records, may be liable for malfeasance.

Nonfeasance, or an act of omission, occurs when a social worker fails to perform certain duties that ought to have been performed. For example, a social worker who fails to obtain a client's informed consent before releasing sensitive confidential information, take proper steps to prevent a client's suicide, or report suspected abuse or neglect of a child or older adult may be liable for nonfeasance.

Lawsuits and liability claims that allege malpractice are civil suits, in contrast to criminal proceedings. Ordinarily, civil suits are based on tort or contract law, with plaintiffs (the parties bringing the lawsuit) seeking some sort of compensation for injuries they claim to have incurred as a result of the defendant practitioner's negligence. These injuries may be economic (for example, the former client of a clinical social worker claims that she is unable to work because of emotional distress caused by her sexual relationship with her social worker), physical (for example, a client claims that a social worker mistreated him physically during a confrontation in a residential program), or emotional (for example, a client claims he became depressed when he received incompetent care from a practitioner).

As in criminal trials, defendants in civil lawsuits are presumed to be innocent until proved otherwise. In ordinary civil suits, defendants will be found liable for their actions based on the legal standard of preponderance of the evidence, as opposed to the stricter standard of proof beyond a reasonable doubt used in criminal trials. In some civil cases—for example, those involving contract disputes between a residential treatment facility for adolescents and the client's family—the court may expect clear and convincing evidence, a standard of proof that is greater than preponderance of the evidence but less than proof beyond a reasonable doubt.

In general, malpractice occurs when evidence exists that (a) at the time of the alleged malpractice a legal duty existed between the social worker and the client; (b) the social worker was derelict in that duty or breached the duty, either by commission (misfeasance or malfeasance) or omission (nonfeasance); (c) the client suffered some harm or injury; and (d) the harm or injury was directly and proximately caused by the social worker's dereliction or breach of duty.

In some cases, prevailing standards of care are relatively easy to establish, through citations of the profession's literature, expert testimony, statutory or regulatory language, or relevant code of ethics standards. Examples include standards concerning sexual relationships with current clients, disclosing confidential information to protect children or older adults who may have been abused or neglected, fraudulent billing, or falsified clinical records. In other cases, however, social workers disagree about standards of care (Austin, Moline, & Williams, 1990; Haas & Malouf, 2005). This may occur in cases involving controversial treatment methods or ambiguous clinical or administrative circumstances (Reamer, 2006a, 2006b). For example, social workers and others involved in the care of an elderly client may disagree about her right to live in her unsanitary home and risks associated with her hoarding behaviors and other mental health issues. Some social workers may believe that clients who have not been declared legally incompetent have the right to assume risk, even if doing so may endanger them. This, they argue, is consistent with social work's longstanding commitment to clients' right to self-determination. Other social workers might argue that professionals have a fundamental duty to protect clients from likely harm, and this may require overriding clients' wishes. That is, in the context of true ethical dilemmas, thoughtful, reasonable, and principled colleagues may disagree.

Key Risks in Social Work

Based on the best available data concerning patterns of ethics complaints and litigation involving social workers, risk-management efforts should focus on a number of areas (Reamer, 2001, 2006b; Strom-Gottfried, 2000, 2003). These include:

CLIENT RIGHTS Especially since the 1960s, social workers have developed a keen understanding of a wide range of clients' rights, many of which were established by legislation or court ruling. These include rights related to confidentiality and privacy, nondiscrimination, release of information, informed consent, access to services, use of the least restrictive alternative, refusal of treatment, options for alternative services, access to records, termination of services, and grievance procedures.

CONFIDENTIALITY, PRIVILEGED COMMUNICATION, AND PRIVACY Client confidentiality is one of the hallmarks of social work practice. Social workers must understand the nature of clients' confidentiality rights and exceptions to them (Bernstein & Hartsell, 2004). More specifically, social workers should have sound policies and procedures in place related to:

- Solicitation of private information from clients
- Disclosure of confidential information to protect clients from self-harm and to protect third parties from harm inflicted by clients
- Release of confidential information pertaining to alcohol and substance abuse assessment or treatment

- Disclosure of information about deceased clients
- Release of information to clients' guardians or conservators
- Sharing of confidential information among clients' family members
- Disclosure of confidential information to media representatives, law enforcement officials, child and elder protective-service agencies, other social service organizations, and collection agencies
- Protection of confidential written and electronic records, information transmitted to other parties through the use of computers, electronic mail, fax machines, telephones, and other electronic technology (such as social networking sites)
- Transfer or disposal of clients' records
- Protection of client confidentiality in the event of a social worker's retirement, death, disability, or employment termination
- Precautions to prevent social workers' discussion of confidential information in public or semipublic areas such as agency hallways, waiting rooms, elevators, and restaurants
- Disclosure of confidential information to third-party payers
- Disclosure of confidential information to consultants
- Disclosure of confidential information for teaching or training purposes, and
- Protection of confidential and privileged information during legal proceedings (such as termination-of-parental-rights proceedings, criminal trials, workers' compensation proceedings, divorce and child-custody proceedings, probate, guardianship, and conservatorship proceedings; and negligence lawsuits).

It is especially important for social workers to understand how to respond to subpoenas of confidential information. Many social workers misunderstand what a subpoena requires of them. Some believe that a subpoena requires them to appear in court and disclose the information requested; otherwise, they will be found in contempt of court and incarcerated or fined. In fact, however, a subpoena is merely an order to respond to the request for information (information that may be presented in the form of verbal testimony or in case records).

If clients have not given their social workers permission to disclose the information requested, social workers should do their best to convince the court that the information should not be disclosed. Social workers can argue that the information was shared in confidence and that disclosure in court without the client's permission would cause considerable harm. If possible, social workers should suggest alternative ways or sources through which the court can obtain the information being sought.

A court could formally order social workers to reveal subpoenaed information despite practitioners' or lawyers' attempts to avoid or limit disclosure. This may occur even in jurisdictions that recognize, by statute or regulation, that the clients of social workers have the right of privileged communication, that is, that social workers are permitted to disclose confidential information only when clients grant them permission to do so. Should a court issue such an order, the social worker must make a difficult decision about the extent to which the disclosure of confidential information is justifiable, that is, the extent to which the information is essential to prevent basic harm to the parties involved. In addition to considering how this decision may affect the client and people involved in the client's life, the social worker can legitimately consider as well how his decision may affect her own career.

To protect clients and minimize risk, social workers should discuss with clients and other interested parties (such as minor clients' parents and guardians) the nature of confidentiality and limitations of clients' right to confidentiality (Bernstein & Hartsell, 2004; Dickson, 1998; Polowy & Gorenberg, 1997). Depending on the setting, these topics can include the importance of confidentiality in the social worker-client relationship (a brief statement of why the social worker treats the subject of confidentiality so seriously):

- Laws, ethical standards, and regulations pertaining to confidentiality (relevant laws and regulations; ethical standards in social work)
- Measures the social worker will take to protect clients' confidentiality (storing records in a secure location, limiting colleagues' and outside parties' access to records)
- Circumstances in which the social worker would be obligated to disclose confidential information (for example, to comply with mandatory reporting laws related to child and elder abuse or neglect, to comply with a court order, or to protect a third party from harm or the client from self-injury)
- Procedures that will be used to obtain clients' informed consent for the release of confidential information and any exceptions to this (a summary of the purpose and importance of and the steps involved in informed consent)
- The procedures for sharing information with colleagues for consultation, supervision, and coordination of services (a summary of the roles of consultation and supervision, and coordination of services, and why confidential information might be shared)
- Access that third-party payers (insurers or healthcare officials) or employers will have to clients' records (social workers' policy for sharing information with managed-care organizations, insurance companies, insurance-company representatives, utilization-review personnel, supervisors, and regulatory agencies)
- Disclosure of confidential information by telephone, computer, fax machine, email, and the Internet
- Access to agency facilities and clients by outside parties (for example, people who come to the agency to attend meetings or participate in a tour), and
- Audiotaping and videotaping of clients.

Social workers should be aware that different ethnic and cultural groups view the concepts of privacy and confidentiality differently; some people are more likely than others to place a high premium on privacy and confidentiality and to insist on strong protections regarding disclosure (Cortese, 1999; Marsiglia & Kulis, 2009).

INFORMED CONSENT Informed consent is required in a variety of circumstances when working with clients, including release of confidential information, program admission, service delivery and treatment, videotaping, and audiotaping (Berg, Appelbaum, Parker, & Lidz, 2001). Although various courts, state legislatures, and agencies have somewhat different interpretations and applications of informed-consent standards, there is considerable agreement about the key elements that social workers and agencies should incorporate into consent procedures: clients should be given specific details about the purposes of the consent, a verbal explanation, information about their rights to refuse consent and withdraw consent, information about alternative treatment options, and an opportunity to ask questions about the consent process. Social workers who serve clients who struggle with mental illness and cognitive impairment (such as dementia) need to be assured that clients are competent to provide informed consent. Social workers should be aware that different ethnic and cultural groups view the concept of informed consent differently; some people are more likely to defer to professional authority while others may be more insistent on client's involvement in treatment and other services-related decisions (Cortese, 1999).

SERVICE DELIVERY Social workers must provide services to clients and represent themselves as competent only within the boundaries of their education, training, license, certification, consultation received, supervised experience, or other relevant professional experience. They should provide services in substantive areas and use practice approaches and techniques that are new to them only after engaging in appropriate study, training, consultation, and supervision from people who are competent in those practice approaches, interventions, and techniques. Social workers who use practice approaches and interventions for which there are no generally recognized standards should obtain appropriate education, training, consultation, and supervision. This is particularly important when social workers use novel and controversial intervention approaches.

USE OF DIGITAL AND ELECTRONIC TECHNOLOGY The proliferation and widespread use of digital and electronic technology has created novel and unprecedented risks for social workers. The popularity of Facebook, Twitter, email, mobile and smartphones, videoconferencing, and telephone and web-based therapies has triggered a wide range of challenging ethical and risk-management issues—especially related to boundaries and confidentiality—that did not exist when many contemporary practitioners concluded their formal education (Lamendola, 2010; Menon & Miller-Cribbs, 2002; Reamer, 2013; Zur, 2012). Practitioners who use Facebook must decide whether to accept clients' requests for friend status. Similarly, practitioners must decide whether they are willing to exchange email and text messages with clients and, if so, under what circumstances; share their personal mobile telephone numbers with clients; or offer clinical services by means of videoconferencing or other cybertherapy options, such as those that allow clients to represent themselves using graphical avatars rather than real-life images.

These novel electronic media have forced social workers to think in entirely new and challenging ways about the nature of professional ethics. Self-disclosure issues are no longer limited to practitioners' in-office sharing of information with clients about aspects of their personal lives. Practitioners' strategies for setting limits with regard to clients' access to them are no longer limited to office and landline telephone availability. Widespread use of email, text messaging, and cell phones has greatly expanded practitioners' availability, thus requiring them to think differently about boundary management.

Considerable controversy surrounds social workers' use of online interventions, social media, and electronic communications. Some practitioners are enthusiastic supporters of these technologies as therapeutic tools. Others are harsh critics or skeptics, arguing that heavy reliance on online interventions and social media compromises the quality of social work services and could endanger clients who are clinically vulnerable and who would be better served by in-person care.

To manage risk, social workers who consider engaging with clients electronically would do well to develop comprehensive policies and guidelines that address relevant ethical issues. For example, discussing these issues with clients at the beginning of the working relationship can help avoid boundary confusion and misunderstanding. Kolmes (2010) offers a useful template that addresses policies concerning practitioners' use of diverse social-media sites and services. Social workers are quickly discovering that a social-media policy reflecting current ethical standards can simultaneously protect clients and practitioners. Ideally, a comprehensive social-media ethics policy should address the most common forms of electronic communication used by clients and social workers.

BOUNDARY ISSUES, DUAL RELATIONSHIPS, AND CONFLICTS OF INTEREST Social workers should establish clear policies, practices, and procedures to ensure proper boundaries in their in-person and electronic relationships with current and former clients; relationships with clients' relatives or acquaintances; relationships with supervisees, trainees, students, and colleagues; physical contact with clients; friendships with current and former clients; encounters with clients in public settings; attending clients' social, religious, or lifecycle events; gifts to and from clients; performing favors for clients; the delivery of services in clients' homes; financial conflicts of interest; delivery of services to two or more people who have a relationship with one another (such as family members); bartering with clients for goods and services; managing relationships in small or rural communities; and self-disclosure to clients (Celenza, 2007; Gabriel, 2005; Jayaratne, Croxton, & Mattison 1997; Reamer, 2012). Some dual and multiple relationships are difficult to avoid, for example, in rural areas where social workers' and clients' paths are likely to cross in different settings.

Some dual and multiple relationships involve boundary crossings. A boundary crossing occurs when a social worker is involved in a dual relationship with a client in a manner that is not coercive, manipulative, deceptive, or exploitative (Gutheil & Simon, 2002; Zur, 2007). Boundary crossings are not inherently unethical; they often involve boundary bending as opposed to boundary breaking. Other dual and multiple relationships involve boundary violations. Boundary violations occur when a social worker engages in a dual relationship with a client that is coercive, manipulative, deceptive, or exploitative (Gutheil & Gabbard, 1993).

Dual relationships in social work fall into five conceptual categories: intimate relationships, pursuit of personal benefit, professionals' response to their own emotional and dependency needs, altruistic gestures, and responses to unanticipated circumstances (Reamer, 2012; Syme, 2003). Intimate relationships entail a sexual relationship or physical contact, although they may entail other intimate gestures, such as gift giving, friendship, and affectionate communications (Celenza, 2007; Zur, 2007). Examples of pursuit of personal benefit are social workers who market personal-care or other therapeutic products to clients or barter for goods and services. Boundary issues related to social workers' own emotional and dependency needs sometimes take the form of practitioners who are much too available to clients because of their own social isolation or loneliness. Social workers' altruistic instincts can also be problematic at times, for example, when practitioners give clients their home or mobile telephone numbers, give clients gifts, or write clients affectionate notes. Finally, it is not unusual for social workers to encounter challenging boundary issues entirely unexpectedly, such as when a client moves into a social worker's neighborhood and their children are in the same school class, a client is hired at a firm at which the practitioner's spouse is employed, or the social worker, who is a recovering alcoholic, and a client encounter each other at a local Alcoholics Anonymous meeting.

Documentation Careful documentation and comprehensive records are necessary to assess clients' circumstances; plan and deliver services appropriately; facilitate supervision; provide proper accountability to clients, other service providers, funding agencies, insurers, utilization review staff, regulatory agencies, and the courts; evaluate services provided; and ensure continuity in the delivery of future services (Kagle & Kopels, 2008; Reamer, 2005; Sidell, 2011; Wiger, 2005).

Thorough documentation also helps to ensure quality care if a client's primary social worker becomes unavailable because of illness, incapacitation, vacation, retirement, or employment termination. In addition, thorough documentation can help social workers who are named in ethics complaints or lawsuits (for example, when evidence is needed to demonstrate that a social worker obtained a client's informed consent before releasing confidential information, assessed for suicide risk properly, consulted with knowledgeable experts about a client's clinical issues or a potential conflict of interest, consulted ethics codes in order to make a difficult ethical decision, or referred a client to other service providers when services were terminated).

In typical clinical settings, documentation should ordinarily include:

- A complete social history, assessment, and treatment plan that states the client's problems, reason(s) for requesting services, objectives and relevant timetable, intervention strategy, planned number and duration of contacts, methods for assessment and evaluation of progress, termination plan, and reasons for termination
- Informed consent procedures and signed consent forms for release of information and treatment
- Notes on all contacts made with third parties (such as family members, acquaintances, and other professionals), whether in person or by telephone, including a brief description of the contacts and any important events surrounding them
- Notes on any consultation with other professionals, including the date the client was referred to another professional for service
- A brief description of the social worker's reasoning for all decisions made and interventions provided during the course of services
- Information summarizing any critical incidents (for example, suicide attempts, threats made by the client toward third parties, child abuse, family crises) and the social worker's response
- Any instructions, recommendations, and advice provided to the client, including referral to and suggestions to seek consultation from specialists (including physicians)
- A description of all contacts with clients, including the type of contact (for example, in person or via telephone or in individual, family, couples, or group counseling), and dates and times of the contacts
- Notation of failed or canceled appointments
- Summaries of previous or current psychological, psychiatric, or medical evaluations relevant to the social worker's intervention

- Information about fees, charges, and payment
- Reasons for termination and final assessment, and
- Copies of all relevant documents, such as signed consent forms, correspondence, fee agreements, and court documents (Reamer, 2001).

When documenting, social workers should be sure to include sufficient detail, avoid excessive detail, avoid ambiguous entries or inappropriate use of jargon that is not easily understood, acknowledge documentation errors, write legibly using proper spelling and grammar, document in a timely fashion, and not alter records.

DEFAMATION OF CHARACTER Social workers should ensure that their written and oral communications about clients, their family members, and others are not defamatory. Libel is the written form of defamation of character; slander is the oral form (McNamara, 2007). Defamation occurs when a social worker says or writes something about a client or another party that is untrue, the social worker knew or should have known that the statement was untrue, and the communication caused some injury to the client or third party (for example, a client on parole was terminated from a drug treatment program and arrested because of noncompliant behavior, or an elderly client's adult child's reputation was damaged because of a social worker's allegations that the adult child abused the elder). The best way to prevent defamation is to limit oral and written communications to known and verifiable facts.

RECORD STORAGE AND RETENTION Social workers should maintain and store records securely for the number of years required by law or relevant contracts. Practitioners should make special provisions for proper access to their records in the event of their disability, incapacitation, retirement, termination of practice, or death (Sidell, 2011; Wiger, 2005). This may include entering into agreements with colleagues who would be willing to assume responsibility for social workers' records if the social workers are unavailable for any reason.

SUPERVISION In principle, social workers can be named in ethics complaints and lawsuits alleging ethical breaches or negligence by those under their supervision (Thomas, 2010). Social work supervisors should ensure that they meet with supervisees regularly, address appropriate issues, and document the supervision provided. Social work supervisors should avoid any dual relationship with supervisees (for example,

close friendships and intimate relationships) that would compromise their objectivity and constitute a conflict of interest.

Supervisors (including those who supervise staff and social work students) should be concerned about several specific issues, including supervisors' failure to:
- Provide information necessary for supervisees to obtain clients' consent
- Identify and respond to supervisees' errors in all phases of client contact, such as the inappropriate disclosure of confidential information
- Protect third parties
- Detect or stop a negligent treatment plan or treatment carried out longer than necessary
- Determine that a specialist is needed for treatment of a particular client
- Meet regularly with the supervisee
- Review and approve the supervisee's records, decisions, and actions
- Provide adequate coverage in the supervisee's absence (Kadushin & Harkness 2002; Reamer 1989; Taibbi 2012)

CONSULTATION Social workers should be clear about when consultation with colleagues is appropriate and necessary, and the procedures they should use to locate competent consultants. Social workers who encounter ethical dilemmas may find it helpful to seek out ethics consultation in order to manage risk. In recent years, a number of professions—including social work—have developed a cadre of ethics consultants. Ethics consultation—first provided in hospitals—began in the late 1960s and early 1970s (Aulisio, Arnold & Youngner, 2003; Hester, 2007). Over the years, ethics consultation has assumed various forms and tasks that can be usefully incorporated into many social work settings. Ethics consultation is typically available to practitioners who encounter challenging, case-specific dilemmas, for example, related to disclosure of confidential information, conflicts of interest, dual relationships and boundary issues, client consent to treatment, and termination of services to noncompliant clients.

Ideally, ethics consultants have obtained formal education in ethical theory, practical ethics, and professional ethics to supplement their substantive expertise in their profession. Ethics consultants are trained to identify, analyze, and help resolve difficult ethical issues. Ethics consultants in social work can assume various roles, depending on their employment setting and responsibilities. These roles include those of professional colleague, educator, mediator, and advocate.

As a professional colleague, the ethics consultant's mission is to provide a social worker with a thoughtful reaction to ethical issues or dilemmas. This consultation may be relatively informal and may consist of little more than a focused discussion of complex issues that the consultant examines from a variety of angles.

An ethics consultant can also be an effective educator, especially regarding risk management. Many ethics consultants provide in-service training to agency staff about ethical issues they encounter. Through lectures, case illustrations, and group discussions, the ethics consultant can enhance staffers' ability to recognize and address ethical issues in practice. The consultant may acquaint staff with common ethical challenges and prevailing views on ethically appropriate responses. The consultant can also present staff with an overview of various models of ethical decision-making that can be used in practice.

As a mediator, the ethics consultant may help resolve differences of opinion among parties who have a vested interest in a particular case's outcome. An ethics consultant can also serve as an effective advocate, particularly in instances in which a client or social worker believes his or her rights have been violated.

CLIENT REFERRAL Social workers have a responsibility to refer clients to colleagues when those social workers do not have the expertise or time to assist clients in need. Practitioners should know when to refer clients to other professionals and how to locate competent colleagues. Social workers should be especially careful to avoid conflicts of interest when referring clients, for example, referring a clients to a colleague with whom the social worker has an intimate relationship, particularly when such a referral may not be in the client's best interest.

FRAUD Social workers should have strict procedures in place to prevent fraud related to, for example, documentation in case records, billing for clinical services provided to clients, and employment applications. One common risk pertains to insurance fraud. Social workers must be careful to avoid embellishing clients' clinical symptoms to be eligible for reimbursement (Kirk & Kutchins, 1988). Also, social workers should avoid having other professionals (for example, a psychiatrist) "sign off" on insurance forms, to obtain reimbursement, when the signers did not have direct contact with the client.

TERMINATION OF SERVICES Social workers expose themselves to risk when they terminate services improperly—for example, when a social worker leaves a home-care or mental-health agency suddenly without adequately referring a vulnerable client to another practitioner—or terminate clinical services to a very vulnerable client who has missed appointments or who has not paid an outstanding bill. Practitioners should develop thorough and comprehensive termination protocols to prevent client abandonment.

Abandonment is a legal concept that refers to instances in which a professional is not available to a client when needed (Pozgar, 2010). Once social workers begin to provide service to a client, they incur a legal responsibility to continue that service or to properly refer a client to another competent service provider. Of course, social workers are not obligated to serve every individual who requests assistance. A particular social worker might not have room to accept a new referral or may lack the special expertise that a particular client's case may require.

Nonetheless, once social workers begin service, they cannot terminate it abruptly. Rather, social workers are obligated to conform to the profession's standard of care regarding termination of service and referral to other providers in the event the client is still in need.

Some social workers have failed to terminate services when termination is in the client's best interest. For example, unscrupulous independent private practitioners—clearly a minority of private practitioners—have been known to encourage clients to remain in treatment longer than necessary in order to generate income. In the process, clients may be inconvenienced, they may be misled about the nature of their problems, and third-party payers, primarily insurance companies, may be spending money unnecessarily (which may lead to an increase in premiums for other policy holders). A similar phenomenon occurs when social workers in residential programs seek to extend residents' stay beyond what is clinically warranted in order to fill the program's coffers.

A more common problem occurs when clients' services are terminated prematurely, that is, before termination is clinically warranted. This may occur for several reasons. Clients may request termination of service, perhaps because of the expense or inconvenience involved. In these cases, termination of service may be against the advice of the social worker involved in the client's care. For example, clients in residential and nonresidential substance-abuse treatment programs may decide that they do not want to continue receiving services. They may leave residential programs against professional advice or may decide not to return for outpatient services.

In other instances, services may be terminated at the social worker's request or initiative, for instance, when a social worker believes that a client is not making sufficient progress to warrant further treatment or is not able to pay for services. In some cases, program administrators in a residential program may want to terminate a client whose insurance benefits have run out or in order to make a bed available for a client who will generate a higher reimbursement rate because of his particular insurance coverage. In a number of cases, social workers terminate services when they find clients to be uncooperative or too difficult to handle. Social workers may also terminate services prematurely because of poor clinical judgment; that is, social workers may believe that clients have made more (or less) progress than they have in fact made.

Premature termination of services can result in ethics complaints and lawsuits alleging that, as a result, clients were harmed or injured, or injured some third party because of their continuing disability. Family members of a client who commits suicide following premature termination from a psychiatric hospital may allege that the premature termination was the direct cause of the suicide. Family members who are physically injured by a client who was discharged prematurely from a substance-abuse treatment program may claim that their injuries are the direct result of poor clinical judgment.

On occasion, services must be terminated earlier than a social worker or client would prefer for reasons that are quite legitimate. This may occur because a client in fact does not make reasonable progress or is uncooperative, or because the social worker moves out of town or finds that she does not have the particular skills or expertise needed to be helpful to the client.

Adequate follow-through should include providing clients as much advance warning as possible, along with the names of several other professionals they might approach for help. Social workers should also follow up with clients who have been terminated to increase the likelihood that they receive whatever services they may need.

Social workers can also face ethics complaints or lawsuits if they do not provide clients with adequate instructions for times when the social workers are not available as a result of vacations, illness, or emergencies. Social workers should provide clients with clear and detailed information, verbally and in writing, about what they ought to do in these situations, such as whom to call, where to seek help, and so on.

Social workers who expect to be unavailable for a period of time—perhaps because of vacation or medical care—should be especially careful to arrange for competent coverage. The colleagues who are to provide the coverage should be given sufficient information about the clients to enable them to provide adequate care should the need arise. Social workers should obtain clients' consent to the release of this information about their cases and should disclose the least amount of information necessary to meet the clients' needs.

Practitioner Impairment, Misconduct, and Incompetence A significant percentage of ethics complaints and negligence claims are filed against social workers who meet the definition of impaired professional (impairment that may be due to factors such as substance abuse, mental illness, extraordinary personal stress, or legal difficulties). Social workers should understand the nature of professional impairment and possible causes, be alert to warning signs, and have procedures in place to prevent, identify, and respond appropriately to impairment in their own lives or colleagues' lives (Coombs, 2000; Reamer, 1992).

In addition, social workers occasionally encounter colleagues who have engaged in ethical misconduct or are incompetent. Examples include social workers who learn that a colleague is sexually involved with a client, exploiting an elder client financially, falsifying travel expense vouchers or client records, or providing services outside his or her areas of expertise (Strom-Gottfried, 2000, 2003).

In some instances, social workers can address these situations satisfactorily by approaching their colleague, raising their concerns, and helping the colleague devise an earnest, constructive, and comprehensive plan to stop the unethical behavior, minimize harm to affected parties, seek appropriate supervision and consultation, and develop any necessary competencies. When these measures fail or are not feasible—perhaps because of the seriousness of the ethical misconduct, impairment, or incompetence—social workers must consider "blowing the whistle" on their colleague. Whistleblowing entails taking action through appropriate channels—such as notifying administrators, supervisors, professional organizations, and licensing and regulatory bodies—in an effort to address the problem (Miceli, Near, & Dworkin, 2008). Before deciding to blow the whistle, social workers should carefully consider the severity of the harm and misconduct involved, the quality of the evidence of wrongdoing (one should avoid blowing the whistle without clear and convincing evidence), the effect of the decision on colleagues and one's agency, the whistle-blower's motives (that is, whether the whistle-blowing is motivated primarily by a wish for revenge), and the viability of alternative, intermediate courses of action (whether other, less drastic means might address the problem). Social work administrators need to formulate and enforce agency policies and procedures that support and protect staffers who disclose impairment, misconduct, and incompetence conscientiously and in good faith.

Management Practices Periodically, social work administrators should assess the appropriateness or adequacy of the agency's risk-management guidelines and ethical standards, ethical decision-making protocols (for example, staffers' use of supervision and agency-based ethics committees), staff training on risk management, government licenses, the agency's papers of incorporation and bylaws, the state licenses and current registrations of all professional staff, protocols for emergency action, insurance policies, staff-evaluation procedures, and financial-management practices (Chase, 2008; Kurzman, 1995).

Implementing a Comprehensive Risk Management Strategy: Conducting an Ethics Audit

One of the most effective ways to prevent ethics complaints and ethics-related lawsuits is to conduct an ethics audit (Reamer 2006a, 2001). An ethics audit provides social workers with a practical framework for examining and critiquing the ways in which they address a wide range of ethical issues (Kirkpatrick, Reamer, & Sykulski, 2006; McAuliffe, 2005). More specifically, an ethics audit provides social workers with an opportunity to:

- Identify pertinent ethical issues in their practice settings that are unique to the client population, treatment approach, setting, program design, and staffing pattern
- Review and assess the adequacy of their current ethics-related policies, practices, and procedures
- Design a practical strategy to modify current practices, as needed, to prevent lawsuits and ethics complaints, and
- Monitor the implementation of this quality-assurance strategy

Conducting an ethics audit involves several key steps:

1. In agency settings, a staff member should assume the role of chair of the ethics-audit committee. Appointment to the committee should be based on demonstrated interest in the agency's ethics-related policies, practices, and procedures. Ideally, the chair would have formal education or training related to professional ethics. Social workers in private or independent practice may want to consult with knowledgeable colleagues in a peer supervision group.

2. Using the list of major ethical-risk areas as a guide (client rights, privacy and confidentiality, informed consent, service delivery, boundary issues and conflicts of interest, documentation, defamation of character, client records, electronic communications and relationships, supervision, staff development and training, consultation, client referral, fraud, termination of services, practitioner impairment), the committee should identify specific ethics-related issues on which to focus. In some settings, the committee may decide to conduct a comprehensive ethics audit, one that addresses all the topics. In other agencies, the committee may focus on specific ethical issues that are especially important in those settings.

3. The ethics-audit committee should decide what kind of data it will need to conduct the audit. Sources of data include interviews conducted with agency staff and documents that address specific issues contained in the audit. For example, staff may examine the agency's clients' rights and informed consent forms or social-media policies. In addition, staff may interview or administer questionnaires to "key informants" in the agency about such matters as the extent and content of ethics-related training that they have received or provided, specific ethical issues that need attention, and ways to address compelling ethical issues. Committee members may want to consult a lawyer about legal issues (for example, the implications of confidentiality regulations and laws or key court rulings) and agency documents (for example, the appropriateness of the agency's informed-consent and release-of-information forms). Also, committee members should review all relevant regulations and laws and ethics codes in relation to confidentiality, privileged communication, informed consent, client records, electronic communications and relationships, termination of services, supervision, licensing, personnel issues, and professional misconduct.

4. Once the committee has gathered and reviewed the data, it should assess the risk level associated with each topic. The assessment for each topic has two parts, policies and procedures. The ethics

audit assesses the adequacy of various ethics-related policies and procedures. Policies (for example, official ones concerning confidentiality, informed consent, dual relationships, electronic communications and social media, and termination of services) may be codified in formal agency documents or memoranda. Procedures entail social workers' handling of ethical issues in their relationships with clients and colleagues (for example, concrete steps that staff members take to address ethical issues involving confidentiality or collegial impairment, routine explanations provided to clients concerning agency policies about informed consent and confidentiality, ethics consultation obtained, informed-consent forms completed, documentation placed in case records in ethically complex cases, and supervision and training provided on ethics-related topics). The committee should assign each topic addressed in the audit to one of four risk categories: (a) no risk—current practices are acceptable and do not require modification, (b) minimal risk—current practices are reasonably adequate, but minor modifications would be useful, (c) moderate risk—current practices are problematic, and modifications are necessary to minimize risk, (d) and high risk—current practices are seriously flawed, and significant modifications are necessary to minimize risk.

5. Once the ethics audit is complete, social workers need to take assertive steps to make constructive use of the findings. Social workers should develop a plan for each risk area that warrants attention, beginning with high-risk areas that jeopardize clients and expose social workers and their agencies to serious risk of lawsuits and ethics complaints. Areas that fall into the categories of moderate risk and minimum risk should receive attention as soon as possible.

6. Social workers also need to establish priorities among the areas of concern, based on the degree of risk involved and resources available.

7. Spell out specific measures that need to be taken to address the problem areas identified. Examples include reviewing all current informed-consent forms and creating updated versions; writing new, comprehensive confidentiality policies; creating a client rights statement; inaugurating training of staff responsible for supervision; developing a social-media policy; strengthening staff training on documentation and on boundary issues; and preparing detailed procedures for staff to follow when terminating services to clients. Identify all

the resources needed to address the risk areas, such as agency personnel, publications, staff-development time, a committee or task force (which may need to be appointed), legal consultants, and ethics consultants.

8. Identify which staff member or members will be responsible for the various tasks, and establish a timetable for completion of each. Have a lawyer review and approve policies and procedures to ensure compliance with relevant laws, regulations, and court opinions.

9. Identify a mechanism for following up on each task to ensure its completion and for monitoring its implementation.

10. Document the complete process involved in conducting the ethics audit. This documentation may be helpful in the event of a lawsuit alleging ethics-related negligence (in that it provides evidence of the agency's or practitioner's conscientious effort to address specific ethical issues).

Since the turn of the 21st century, social workers have learned a great deal about the risk of lawsuits and ethics complaints filed against practitioners and agencies. To minimize these risks, and especially to protect clients, social workers need to understand the nature of professional malpractice and negligence. They also need to be familiar with major risk areas and practical steps they can take to prevent complaints.

REFERENCES

Aulisio, M., Arnold, R., & Youngner, S. (2003). *Ethics consultation: From theory to practice.* Baltimore, MD: Johns Hopkins University Press.

Austin, K., Moline, M., & Williams, G. (1990). *Confronting malpractice: Legal and ethical dilemmas in psychotherapy.* Newbury Park, CA: Sage.

Barsky, A. E. (2009). *Ethics and values in social work: An integrated approach for a comprehensive curriculum.* New York: Oxford University Press.

Berg, J., Appelbaum, P., Parker, L., & Lidz, C. (2001). *Informed consent: Legal theory and clinical practice* (2nd ed.). New York: Oxford University Press.

Bernstein, B., & Hartsell, T. (2004). *The portable lawyer for mental health professionals* (2nd ed.). Hoboken, NJ: John Wiley.

Celenza, A. (2007). *Sexual boundary violations: Therapeutic, supervisory, and academic contexts.* Lanham, MD.: Aronson.

Chase, Y. (2008). Professional liability and malpractice. In T. Mizrahi and L. Davis (Eds.-in-Chief), *Encyclopedia of social work* (20th ed., vol. 3, pp. 425–429). Washington, DC: and New York: NASW Press and Oxford University Press.

Coleman, T. S. (2011). *A practical guide to risk management.* Charlottesville, VA: CFA Institute.

Coombs, R. (2000). *Drug-impaired professionals.* Cambridge, MA: Harvard University Press.

Cortese, A. (1999). Ethical issues in a subculturally diverse society. In T. Johnson (Ed.), *Handbook on ethical issues in aging* (pp. 24–58). Westport, CT: Greenwood Press.

Dickson, D. (1998). *Confidentiality and privacy in social work.* New York: Free Press.

Gabriel, L. (2005). *Speaking the unspeakable: The ethics of dual relationships in counseling and psychotherapy.* New York: Routledge.

Gutheil, T., & Gabbard, G. (1993). The concept of boundaries in clinical practice: Theoretical and risk-management dimensions. *American Journal of Psychiatry, 150,* 188–196.

Gutheil, T., & Simon, R. (2002). Non-sexual boundary crossings and boundary violations: The ethical dimension. *Psychiatric Clinics of North America, 25,* 585–592.

Haas, L., & Malouf, J. (2005). *Keeping up the good work: A practitioner's guide to mental health ethics* (4th ed.). Sarasota, FL: Professional Resources Press.

Hester, D. M. (Ed.). (2007). *Ethics by committee: A textbook on consultation, organization, and education for hospital ethics committees.* Lanham, MD: Rowman & Littlefield.

Hopkin, P. (2010). *Fundamentals of risk management: Understanding, evaluating, and implementing effective risk management.* London: Kogan Page.

Houston, V., Nuehring, E., & Daguio, E. (1997). *Prudent practice: A guide for managing malpractice risk.* Washington, DC: NASW Press.

Jayaratne, S., Croxton, T., & Mattison, D. (1997). Social work professional standards: An exploratory study. *Social Work, 42,* 187–199.

Johnson, V. (2011). *Legal malpractice in a nutshell.* St. Paul, MN: Thomson Reuters.

Kadushin, A., & Harkness, D. (2002). *Supervision in social work* (4th ed). New York: Columbia University Press.

Kagle, J., & Kopels, S. (2008). *Social work records* (3d ed.). Long Grove, IL: Waveland Press.

Kirk, S., & Kutchins, H. (1988). Deliberate misdiagnosis in mental health practice. *Social Service Review, 62,* 225–237.

Kirkpatrick, W., Reamer, F., & Sykulski, M. (2006). Social work ethics audits in health care settings: A case study. *Health and Social Work, 31,* 225–228.

Kolmes, K. (2010). Developing my private practice social media policy. *The Independent Practitioner, 30,* 140–142.

Kurzman, P. (1995). Professional liability and malpractice. In R. L. Edwards (Ed.-in-Chief), *Encyclopedia of social work* (19th ed., vol. 3, pp. 1921–1927). Washington, DC: NASW Press.

Lamendola, W. (2010). Social work and social presence in an online world. *Journal of Technology in the Human Services, 28,* 108–119.

Madden, R.G. (2003). *Essential law for social workers.* New York: Columbia University Press.

Marsiglia, F., & Kulis, S. (2009). *Diversity, oppression, and change: Culturally grounded social work.* Chicago: Lyceum.

McAuliffe, D. (2005). Putting ethics on the organisational agenda: The social work ethics audit on trial. *Australian Social Work, 58,* 357–369.

McNamara, L. (2007). *Reputation and defamation.* New York: Oxford University Press.

Menon, G. M., & Miller-Cribbs, J. (2002). Online social work practice: Issues and guidelines for the profession. *Advances in Social Work, 3,* 104–116.

Miceli, M., Near, J. & Dworkin, T. (2008). *Whistle-blowing in organizations.* New York: Routledge.

National Association of Social Workers (2012). *NASW procedures for professional review* (5th ed.). Washington, DC: Author.

Polowy, C., & Gorenberg, C. (1997). *Office of General Counsel law notes: Client confidentiality and privileged communications.* Washington, DC: National Association of Social Workers.

Pozgar, G. (2010). *Legal and ethical issues for health professionals* (2nd ed.). Sudbury, MA: Jones and Bartlett.

Reamer, F. (2012). *Boundary issues and dual relationships in the human services.* New York: Columbia University Press.

Reamer, F. (2005). Documentation in social work: Evolving ethical and risk-management standards. *Social Work, 50,* 325–334.

Reamer, F. (2006b). *Ethical standards in social work: Review and commentary* (2nd ed.). Washington, DC: NASW Press.

Reamer, F. (1989). Liability issues in social work supervision. *Social Work, 34,* 445–448.

Reamer, F. (2013). Social work in a digital age: Ethical and risk-management challenges. *Social Work, 58,* 163–172.

Reamer, F. (2003). *Social work malpractice and liability: Strategies for prevention* (2nd ed.). New York: Columbia University Press.

Reamer, F. (2006a). *Social work values and ethics.* (3rd ed.). New York: Columbia University Press.

Reamer, F. (1992). The impaired social worker. *Social Work, 37,* 165–170.

Reamer, F. (2001). *The social work ethics audit: A risk management tool.* Washington, DC: NASW Press.

Sidell, N. L. (2011). *Social work documentation: A guide to strengthening your case recording.* Washington, DC: NASW Press.

Strom-Gottfried, K. (2000). Ensuring ethical practice: An examination of NASW Code violations. *Social Work, 45,* 251–261.

Strom-Gottfried, K. (2003). Understanding adjudication: Origins, targets, and outcomes of ethics complaints. *Social Work, 48,* 85–94.

Syme, G. (2003). *Dual relationships in counselling and psychotherapy.* London: Sage.

Taibbi, R. (2012). *Clinical social work supervision: Practice and process.* Upper Saddle River, NJ: Pearson.

Thomas, J. (2010). *Ethics of supervision and consultation: Practical guidance for mental health professionals.* Washington, DC: American Psychological Association.

Wiger, D. (2005). *The clinical documentation sourcebook: The complete paperwork resource for your mental health practice.* Hoboken, NJ: Wiley.

Woody, R. (1997). *Legally safe mental health practice*. Madison, CT: Psychosocial Press.

Zur, O. (2007). *Boundaries in psychotherapy: Ethical and clinical explorations*. Washington, DC: American Psychological Association.

Zur, O. (2012). TelePsychology or TeleMentalHealth in the digital age: The future is here. *California Psychologist, 45*, 13–15.

FREDERIC G. REAMER

SOCIAL WORK PRACTICE: HISTORY AND EVOLUTION

ABSTRACT: Social work is a profession that began its life as a call to help the poor, the destitute, and the disenfranchised of a rapidly changing social order. It continues today in pursuing that quest, perhaps with some occasional deviations of direction from the original spirit.

Social work practice is the primary means of achieving the profession's ends. It is impossible to overstate the centrality or the importance of social work practice to the profession of social work. Much of what is important about the history of the profession is the history of social work practice.

We must consider both social work practice per se (the knowledge base, practice theories, and techniques) and the context for social work practice. The context of practice includes the agency setting, the policy framework, and the large social system in which practice takes place.

Social work practice is created within a political, social, cultural, and economic matrix that shapes the assumptions of practice, the problems that practice must deal with and the preferred outcomes of practice. Over time, the base forces that create practice and create the context for practice, change. Midgley (1981) correctly notes that practice created in one social order is often inappropriate for work in another social order. Since the social order changes over time, practice created at one point in time may no longer be appropriate in the future.

KEY WORDS: social work history; social work practice; social work profession; social work organizations

The Profession Develops

Social work, in the United States, is largely a product of the same industrial revolution that created the welfare state and industrial society. As Garvin and Cox (2001) note, industrialization led to the factory system, with its need for large numbers of concentrated workers, and subsequently created mass immigration, urbanization, and a host of consequent problems. Social work was a response to many urban problems such as mass poverty, disease, illiteracy, starvation, and mental health challenges.

Both the Charities Organization Society and the Settlement House Movement were responses to these problems. Both movements were imported from Great Britain and supplemented the efforts of religious groups and other associations, as well local and state governments in dealing with the problems of urbanization and industrialization. The Charities Organization Society and the Settlement Houses were important forces in shaping the development of American social work practice and the professionalization of social work.

The Charities Organization Society (COS) represented the cause of scientific charity, which sought to introduce more rational methods to charity and philanthropy (Trattner, 2004). The direct services component consisted of paid investigators, who worked for the COS, and "Friendly Visitors," who were volunteers that visited the clients. There were also Councils of Social Agencies, which coordinated the efforts of social services agencies. It can be argued that the paid investigators were probably the precursors of caseworkers while the Councils of Social Agencies gave rise to social planning in community practice. The United Way Movement, which credits its founding to the Denver COS, was another product of this group. Richmond's (1917) very important contribution was *Social Diagnosis*, which presented her observations on the nature of social casework. Perhaps the final contribution made to social work practice by the COS was the mark it made on social work education through its role in creation of the New York School of Philanthropy. As Austin (1986) notes, the scholar practitioner model, where faculty come from a social work practice (as opposed to a traditional academic model), is our prevailing mode of preparing social workers today.

The Settlement House Movement aimed at the inner city and created houses as community centers in urban area. This was a completely different approach from that used by the COS. The settlement house workers used social group work to help socialize new immigrants to the city. They offered adult education for their urban neighbors and provided help and advice. They worked on community problems together with the other residents of poor urban neighborhoods. The Settlement House Movement is often most thought of for its social action efforts (Trattner, 2004). Working in conjunction with organized labor and other community activists, the settlement house workers were instrumental in the creation of the juvenile court, mother's pensions, child labor laws, and workplace protections. This is often seen as the touchstone of social work's involvement in social action and policy practice. Jane Addams was well known in this regard. Because many of the settlement house workers were social scientists who worked in conjunction with university-based academic social scientists, they began important research into urban problems.

Between these two movements lies the foundation of much of the practice we see today, accounting for casework, social group work, community development, social planning, and social action. The beginning of research supporting social policy is also here.

The development of fields of practice began to occur with the emergence of psychiatric social work and medical social work (Dolgoff & Feldstein, 1980; Lubove, 1969). These new specialties allowed the creation of practice methodology refined for certain populations and many other practices specialties emerged.

All of this occurred during the process of professionalization described by Lubove (1969). This included the creation of professional organizations, a code of ethics, professional agencies, and the creation of professional schools and a knowledge base.

In 1915 Abraham Flexner questioned whether social work was actually a profession because of what he saw as the lack of a scientific knowledge base. This created an underlying theme in the profession that has occasionally led to unfortunate results (Austin, 1983; Eherenreich, 1985). Social workers, in response to this criticism, worked to find a knowledge base that would satisfy Flexner's critique. This quest continues to this day.

As the profession developed and changed, so did society. As America became more conservative, social action activities decreased. This was especially true during the first three decades of the 20th century. Eherenreich (1985) observes that the rediscovery of poverty and the changing national mood toward social programs created a crisis for the profession. It did not, on balance, lead to much in the way of changes in social work practice.

Freud and psychoanalysis became very influential in social work from the early part of the 20th century until the sixties. This period, often called the Psychoanalytical Deluge, saw social workers eagerly adopting psychoanalysis as a means to solve several of the profession's needs. While social work created its own variants that brought more social factors into the mix (ego psychology and psychosocial treatment), psychodynamic treatment became fashionable. Psycho-

analysis was popular with psychiatrists, which facilitated the creation of strong bonds with the medical profession and the emerging mental health movement (see Eherenreich, 1985). Although, it is not completely clear whether the profession as a whole endorsed Freud or just its leadership (see Alexander, 1972). The impact of psychoanalysis cannot be discounted. The individually centered nature of psychodynamic theory also served to push the profession further from social action. Although one can debate whether psychoanalysis was the cause or consequence of a disengagement from social action and the poor, it is clear that this extraordinarily individualistic practice method closed off many avenues of engagement. Casework was the dominant practice method, a trend that can be seen throughout the history of the professional, and this was, perhaps, its most individualistic form.

The Milford Conference (1923–1929) came to an agreement on the importance of casework to the profession (Eherenreich, 1985). The Lane Report in 1939 argued that community organizers deserved equal status to caseworkers and social group workers (Dolgoff & Feldstein, 1980).

There were dissenting voices in direct practice however. A group of social workers formed the Functionalist School, providing a challenge to psychoanalysis. Functionalist theory, based on the work of Otto Rank, advocated an agency-based view of practice, which was different from the psychodynamically based diagnostic school. The Functional-Diagnostic Debate continued, with the more psychodynamically based diagnostic school maintaining the upper hand.

There were also social workers who bucked both the more conservative national mood and the conservative orientation of the social work profession and engaged in social action. Perhaps the best known were Bertha Capen Reynolds and Mary Van Kleek who led a group called the Rank and File Movement during the Depression years. They advocated more progressive politics and a movement away from casework (Eherenreich, 1985). The response of the profession was less than positive and the conservative mood that characterized social work reflected a conservative political mood.

Until the end of the 1950s, social work was a far more unified profession. Disagreements had been worked out and the profession presented a singular face to the world. That was about to change as the nation and the profession encountered the 1960s.

The Profession Changes in the Sixties
The sixties changed the social policy, and the forces changing the context of practice changed the nature

of professional social work practice and ultimately the profession. The politically and culturally conservative fifties gave way to a new national mood and a series of social movements that changed the political agenda for a nation. Poverty was part of the national debate in a way that it had not been since the Depression. This time, the results were different for social work and social work practice.

There were major changes in social work practice during the 1960s. Those changes continued at least for the next four decades and will likely continue into the future. The most momentous change was the erosion of the psychodynamic influence in social casework. There are many possible explanations for this situation, but it is important to note this as a major change in the profession's view of practices. This does not mean that social workers no longer do psychodynamic practice, nor does it mean that social work schools no longer teach psychodynamic practice theory. The hold that Freudian and neo-Freudian approach had on social casework was, however, broken.

In the macro area, politically oriented community action reemerged. Certainly the War on Poverty and the Ford Foundation's Gray Areas project helped this to occur. Involvement in social planning was facilitated by the Model Cities Program and the regional planning agencies such as the Appalachian Regional Commission. Rothman's (1969) influential approach to community organization theory helped define and organize the field. This was less than 10 years before Lurie, writing in the Boehm Report, had questioned the lack of integration in the field.

It is fair to say that the 1960s began a pattern of fundamental change in the profession and within social work practice. This change continues even today.

The Changing Face of Social Work Practice
In the three decades that followed the 1960s there were a great many changes in the way that social work practice was described, conducted, and taught. This reflected an adaptation to changes in the context of practice, as well as the efforts of social workers to move beyond the older agreement.

Micro practice has taken advantage of models and approaches from the social sciences and from other helping groups. While some practitioners still use psychodynamic approaches, social workers also use behavioral and phenomenological approaches. Theories such as task-centered treatment, cognitive behavioral approaches, reality therapy, and so forth provide options for the social work micro practitioner. New approaches that look at social networks and other sets of relationships are also used and will continue to become more important as our knowledge of social networks evolves (Christakis & Fowler, 2009). Turner (1996) and Payne (2005) describe a vast variety of clinical approaches that move beyond the single theory approach of the profession prior to 1960.

Macro practice has matured since the 1960s and will continue to develop as time goes forth. Community practice has developed new approaches that encompass a wide variety of strategies and techniques. Political organizing, locality development, and social planning have matured and developed. Administration (frequently referred to as Social Administration) once had an unclear place in social work practice, but is now clearly established as a method of social work practice. This began with a series of reports and projects in the 1970s and evolved into eventual recognition of the approach. Recognition of policy practice as a practice field is also established in most of the profession. This brings in policy analysis and policy change (advocacy, lobbying, and so forth) together in a single social work role. These are developments that would have been unthinkable in the past but, in many ways, the profession still lags behind other fields in the training of practitioners for macro practice.

Going beyond the macro–micro divisions, the growth of generalist practice theory is noteworthy. Generalist social work means using an essentially constant set of approaches at multiple levels. Generalist practice has developed a robust set of theories and approaches to inform this perspective.

Ecological systems theory and the Life Model, the Strengths Perspective and Empowerment practice, as well as Feminist Social Work Practice Theory, provide explanations at multiple levels that can encompass several types of techniques. These are, in many ways, recognition of the limitations of earlier approaches.

Evidence-based practice (O'Hare, 2005) is a likely paradigm shift in social work, judging from the impact of evidence-based approaches on medicine, public health, and nursing. The use of research findings to guide practice is an attractive theory and one that promises further improvement in the quality of practice.

Also important are the developments in technology-based practice, including e-therapy, telemedicine, electronic advocacy, and other techniques that use high technology. These have grown in importance as the technology evolves, the online environment become more important and experience and research push the development of practice toward further refinement.

What Is Next?

The world is now in midst of a new economic and social transition, one that began in the 1970s and continues today. This transition will create an information economy that will be as different from our industrial economy as it was from the agricultural society that preceded it. It is already changing the nature of society in many profound ways and changing the environment of practice. Friedman (2005) identifies major changes in the political economy of the near future, including global competition, outsourcing, more technology, and so forth. This will have major impacts on policies, agencies, and clients. Also important will be the destruction of the physical environment and the rise of globalization as drivers of social policy decision-making. The profession will have to adapt, much in the way that social workers in the 1800s adapted.

The History of Social Work Practice Considered

There are a number of lessons that can be gleaned from this discussion of social work practice. It is undeniable that direct services/casework is the primary practice orientation in social work. The orientation of social work practice often conflicts with its concerns for social justice and systems change. When Specht and Courtney (1994) called social workers "Unfaithful Angels," there was significant evidence to back up that charge. Social work has evolved into a conservative profession that has a hard time resolving the conflict between its social justice values and its choice of primary practice methodologies. It often seems that whatever the problem is, casework or psychotherapy is often our primary answer. That does not mean that it is the correct answer.

Social work practice will face a number of challenges in the future. The change in political economy, coupled with other developments in culture, the environment and social organization, will create the need for new practice methods and make others less viable. The development of new knowledge will also create new practice theories and techniques. Social workers must resist the temptation to hold on to the past when the future is at our door.

REFERENCES

Alexander, L. B. (1972). Social work's Freudian deluge: Myth or reality? *Social Service Review, 46,* 517–538.

Austin, D. M. (1983). The Flexner Myth and the History of Social Work. *Social Service Review, 57,* 357–377.

Austin, D. M. (1986). A *History of social work education* (Monograph No. 1). Austin: University of Texas School of Social Work.

Christakis, N. A., & Fowler, J. H. (2009). *Connected: The surprising power of our social networks and how they shape our lives.* New York, NY: Little, Brown, and Company.

Dolgoff, R., & Feldstein, D. (1980). *Understanding social welfare.* New York: Harper & Row.

Eherenreich, P. (1985). *Altruistic imagination: A history of social work and social policy in the United States.* Ithaca, NY: Cornell.

Flexner, A. (1915). Is social work a profession? In *National Conference of Charities and Corrections, Proceedings of the National Conference of Charities and Corrections at the 42nd Annual Session,* Baltimore, Maryland, May 12–19. Chicago: Hildmann, pp. 581, 584–588, 590.

Friedman, T. L. (2005). *The world is flat: A brief history of the twenty-first century.* New York: Farrar, Straus and Giroux.

Garvin, C., & Cox, F. (2001). A history of community organization since the Civil War with special reference to oppressed communities. In J. Rothman, J. Erlich, & J. Tropman (Eds.), *Strategies of community intervention* (pp. 65–100). Itasca, MN: Peacock.

Lubove, R. (1969). *Professional altruist: The emergence of social work as a career 1880–1930.* New York: Macmillian.

Midgley, J. (1981). *Professional imperialism: Social work in the third world.* London: Heinemann.

O'Hare, T. (2005). *Evidence-based practices for social workers: An interdisciplinary approach.* Chicago: Lyceum Books.

Payne, M. (2005). *Modern social work theory* (3rd ed.). Chicago: Lyceum Books.

Richmond, M. (1917). *Social diagnosis.* New York: Russell Sage Foundation.

Rothman, J. (1969). Three models of community organization practice. In *Social work practice 1968* (pp. 16–47). New York: Columbia University Press.

Specht, H., & Courtney, M. (1994). *Unfaithful angels: How social work has abandoned its mission.* New York: Free Press.

Trattner, W. J. (2004). *From poor law to welfare state: A history of social welfare in America* (6th ed.). New York: The Free Press.

Turner, F. J. (Ed.). (1996). *Social work treatment: Interlocking theoretical approaches* (4th ed.). New York: The Free Press.

JOHN MCNUTT

SOCIAL WORK PROFESSION: HISTORY

ABSTRACT: The social work profession originated in volunteer efforts to address the "social question," the paradox of increasing poverty in an increasingly productive and prosperous economy, in Europe and North America during the late nineteenth century.

By 1900, working for social betterment had become an occupation and social work achieved professional status by 1930. By 1920, social workers could be found in hospitals and public schools, as well as in child welfare agencies, family agencies, and settlement hoses. During the next decade, social work focused on the problems of children and families. As a result of efforts to conceptualize social work method, expand social work education programs, and develop a stable funding base for voluntary social service programs, social work achieved professional status by the 1930s. The Great Depression and World War II refocused professional concerns, as the crises wrought by these events demanded the attention of social workers. After the war, mental health concerns became important as programs for veterans and the general public emphasized the provision of inpatient and outpatient mental health services. In the 1960s, social workers again confronted the problem of poverty. Since then, the number of social workers has grown even as the profession's influence on social welfare policy has waned.

KEY WORDS: social work; profession; professionalization; personal service; social services

Originating in volunteer efforts for social betterment in the late 19th century in Europe and North America, social work became an occupation in the early 20th century and achieved professional status by the 1920s. The 1930 Census classified social work as a profession for the first time. Social work began as one of several attempts to address the "social question," the paradox of increasing poverty in an increasingly productive and prosperous economy. Social workers initially focused on poverty, but were increasingly concerned with the problems of children and families in the 1920s. By the 1930s, the new occupation had achieved professional status as a personal service profession, as a result of the growth of professional organizations, educational programs, and publications (Walker, 1933). But current events refocused professional concerns on poverty, as the crises of the Great Depression and World War II demanded the attention of social workers. After the war, mental health concerns became important as programs for veterans and the general public emphasized the provision of inpatient and outpatient mental health services. In the 1960s, social workers again confronted the problem of poverty and continued to grow as a profession, so that by the 21st century social work was licensed in all 50 states. Since then, the number of social workers has grown

even as the profession's influence on social welfare policy has waned.

The Emergence of the Social Question

During the late 19th century, industrialization created an urban society in a globalizing economy. Steam power fueled an expansion of industrial production and revolutionized transportation, resulting in expedited communication and the worldwide movement of capital, manufactured goods, and people. Cities in the industrializing societies of Europe and North America grew larger and social problems seemed to reach a critical level, as industrial economies produced new problems—unemployment, neglected and abandoned children, chronic disability, and poverty in the midst of unprecedented wealth. While the United States remained a predominantly rural society, big cities seemed to portend the future, and many reacted with horror to the apparent misery of the urban poor—and to their potential for disruption (Bremner, 1956; Rodgers, 1998).

In the United States, interest in the social question, as concern with urban problems and the consequences of industrialization came to be known, had both religious and rationalistic roots. The sentimental reformism that had informed antislavery efforts before the Civil War turned to the problems of the poor, particularly children. In charity organization, child saving, and the settlements, religious people campaigned for reform in assistance to the poor. Protestant ministers professed a Social Gospel, proclaiming that Christians had a duty to campaign for social reform. Roman Catholic reformers heeded Pope Leo XIII's encyclical Rerum Novarum (1891), which called for justice in the relations between capital and labor. Jews in Germany and the United States embraced a reform movement that emphasized social justice. But the development of big business and its increasing reliance on technology and new models of formal organization also suggested directions for reform: modern charity work would be scientific and would borrow organizational structures from the emerging corporate world.

Boards of Charity, composed of prominent citizens who served without pay, attempted to rationalize state residential institutions created before the Civil War. Rational administration meant careful budgeting, civil service rules, and the collection of data on the performance of state institutions. Board members visited and inspected state institutions—mental hospitals, prisons, orphanages, and schools for persons with a variety of disabilities—and made recommendations for more efficient management. Beginning with Massachusetts in 1862, most states established boards of charities during the last third of the 19th century. Most boards had an advisory function, while others (usually called Boards of Control) had administrative oversight over state institutions.

In the nation's large cities, child-saving movements sought to improve the lives of orphans and poor children. Protestant minister Charles Loring Brace founded the New York Children's Aid Society (CAS) in 1853. Over the next half century, the CAS initiated a variety of child saving measures, notably the orphan trains, which placed poor New York children with Christian farm families in the Midwest. The orphan train movement stimulated the development of Jewish and Catholic orphanages and the child-saving movement soon outgrew its origins. Orphanage care of children increased during the late 19th century as states attempted to end the practice of placing children in poorhouses. By the turn of the century, reformers contemplated a mixed system of care for dependent children, involving both public and private institutions, community placement as well as institutional care, and preventive legislation, including laws regulating or prohibiting child labor and requiring school attendance.

In the 1880s, two new institutions were created that would be formative in creating a new occupation to provide assistance to the poor. Most large American cities, beginning with Buffalo in 1877, established charity organization societies (COS), modeled on the London Charity Organisation Society. Charity organization emphasized a controlled form of love extended to the poor. An organization of voluntary charities rather than a provider of direct material assistance, the COS organized a city's voluntary relief associations on a rational basis. District agents, paid COS employees, interviewed applicants for relief, determined appropriate assistance, and arranged for friendly visits by volunteers. The visitors provided good advice and an example of caring, while the district agents curbed potential abuse. During the 1880s, most COS work was done by volunteers called "friendly visitors." By the 1890s, however, paid employees supplanted volunteers (Lubove, 1965). COS also became increasingly active in environmental work. In 1898, the New York COS established the Summer School of Applied Philanthropy, which later became the New York School of Philanthropy (1904). The school was renamed the New York School of Social Work in 1919 and became part of Columbia University in 1940, becoming the Columbia University School of Social Work in 1963.

Settlement houses, also based on an English model, were established in large cities in the United States during the 1880s. Jane Addams and Ellen Gates Starr founded Chicago's Hull-House, the most famous settlement in the United States, in 1889 after a visit to London's Toynbee Hall, the first settlement house. Settlement workers were middle-class and affluent volunteers who "settled" in the immigrant districts of large cities. The settlements provided a vital service, Addams believed, both for the volunteer residents, who needed a purpose in life, and for the society at large, by building needed bridges between the classes in an increasingly stratified and fragmented society (Addams, 1893).

Members of the existing state boards of charities began to meet in 1874 as a section of the American Social Science Association. In 1879, the group formed its own organization, the Conference of Boards of Public Charities, which became the National Conference of Charities and Correction in 1880 and the National Conference of Social Work in 1917. Although the conference was initially an annual gathering of the members of state boards, child savers, COS workers, and settlement house residents, many others interested in the social question, became active in the organization. For much of the 20th century, the National Conference was the major meeting place for social workers (Bruno, 1957).

Social Work as an Occupation

By the first decade of the 20th century, a separate occupational status for charity workers had emerged. Schools of charity or philanthropy in five cities provided training to members of the new occupation. COS visitors, child care workers, and settlement house residents were joined by social workers in new settings—big city general hospitals, public schools, psychiatric clinics, and juvenile courts. Although the methods to be used by the new occupation were hardly defined, the emerging methods and techniques were applied to new populations in these new settings. The decade also saw the beginnings of investment in the new occupation, with the founding of the Russell Sage Foundation in 1907. For its first 40 years, the foundation supported the development of a profession of social work.

Career COS administrator Mary Richmond joined the new Russell Sage Foundation in 1908 as director of its Charity Organization Department. During the next 20 years, she and fellow staff member Francis McLean transformed charity organization. They worked on two fronts—the organizational and the conceptual. McLean worked with COS to form a new national organization of city charity organizations, the National Association of Societies for Organizing Charity, in 1911. Richmond worked to develop the conceptual base for social case work, which would become the primary method for social work practice with individuals and families. The foundation published Richmond's *Social Diagnosis* (1917), which quickly became an authoritative text in 1919. The National Association of Societies for Organizing Charity changed its name to the American Association for Organizing Family Social Work and in 1930 to the Family Welfare Association of America.

In addition to its efforts in charity organization, the Russell Sage Foundation supported the developing field of child welfare. A Child Welfare Department, headed by Hastings Hart, consulted with states on legislation and services for children. Campaigns for the codification of state laws on children, the Children's Code, energized child savers on the state level, as states codified the laws on children, adding or strengthening provisions regulating child labor, requiring school attendance, establishing juvenile courts, and providing payments for children in single parent households. In 1909, President Theodore Roosevelt called the first White House Conference on Dependent Children. The conference called for the creation of a Children's Bureau in the federal government "to investigate and report . . . upon all matters pertaining to the welfare of children." Congress established the Children's Bureau in 1912. Eight years later, in 1920, child welfare agency executives founded the Child Welfare League of America.

World War I, the United States' first European war, resulted in an expansion of the social work profession both in numbers and in scope. The Red Cross's Home Service provided linkage between soldiers and other service personnel and their families. Mary Richmond trained Red Cross home service workers, who provided social case work services to rural and small town families for the first time. Other war-related charities also expanded, as did the Army Medical Corps. Faced with a variety of psychological and neurological problems, the army used social workers, many of whom were Red Cross personnel detailed to army units in the field. Smith College established its School for Social Work in 1918 as a wartime measure. Graduates provided services to soldiers and veterans suffering from shell shock and other psychiatric disabilities. The war also resulted in an increase in social planning. Social worker Mary van Kleeck temporarily left the Russell Sage Foundation to help set up the Women in Industry Service in the U.S. Department of Labor.

From Occupation to Profession

Social work education programs expanded during the years 1913–1919 and even more rapidly during the next decade, as a result of changes in charity organization and the expansion of hospital social work, school social work, and child welfare. Educator Abraham Flexner's conclusion in a paper read at the National Conference of Charities and Correction in 1915 that social work was not a profession because it lacked original jurisdiction and an educationally transmissible technique stimulated the development of social work theory. During the 15 years following the delivery of the paper, professional education flourished. Schools of social work were established in the South and the West as well as in the Northeast and Midwest. Professional organizations and national federations of agencies were established and engaged in explorations of social work practice theory.

Perhaps the most important development of the 1920s was the expansion of federated fundraising. Before World War I, most social work agencies had survived by soliciting subscriptions and contributions from wealthy donors. Such financing was often unreliable, and fluctuations in agency budgets were not unusual. During World War I, a united "War Chest" raised money for war-related charities in many American cities. After the war, these war chests were converted to Community Chests, local agencies that raised money for the community's social work agencies, usually through an annual campaign that solicited funds from middle-class and working people as well as the wealthy. With its annual campaign targeted on a broad base of potential donors, incremental budgeting, and generally successful fund drives, the community chest provided voluntary agencies with financial stability during the 1920s. Although some social workers objected to the "stereotyped social work" that resulted from the budgeting process, most cities had adopted the Community Chest idea by the end of the decade.

Public social services had expanded enough by 1923 that a prominent social welfare administrator could write about a transformation "from charities and correction to public welfare" (Kelso, 1923). Most professional social work, however, was practiced in voluntary agencies. Social workers did practice in some correctional agencies, particularly in juvenile corrections and in law enforcement, during the 1920s. State hospitals and outpatient programs employed social workers as well. The Commonwealth Fund supported child guidance clinics, new children's mental health clinics staffed by social workers and other professionals, and school social work demonstration projects. The federal Sheppard-Towner Act of 1921 established a program of grants to the states to support maternal and child health programs administered by social workers in the Children's Bureau. State children's code campaigns resulted in the creation of statewide child welfare and public assistance programs in many states during the decade.

By the end of the decade, voluntary social work had a stable financial base, social workers had created a number of professional organizations, and public social services had expanded. In his 1929 presidential address to the National Conference of Social Work, social work educator Porter R. Lee could say that social work "once a cause" had become "a function of a well-ordered society." The project of professionalization now seemed complete, although Lee worried about how to maintain zeal in an increasingly routinized profession. The 1930 Census, which classified social work as a profession for the first time, enumerated over 30,000 social workers in the United States, but only 5,600 of them were members of the American Association of Social Workers, the largest professional organization of social workers (Walker, 1933).

The Great Depression: A Crisis for the New Profession

The worldwide economic contraction that began in 1929 resulted in economic and social crises as the demand for products slackened, workers lost their jobs, and political unrest toppled established governments around the world. In Europe, a fascist takeover of the German government led to the emigration of many, including leading social workers like Maida Solomon, to the United States and elsewhere. Ultimately, the worldwide depression of the 1930s resulted in World War II, which began in 1939 with the German invasion of Poland.

In the United States, voluntary and state-supported social welfare services contracted in response to reductions in funding. Community Chest donations declined in the early years of the Great Depression, and over one-third of the nation's voluntary social service agencies closed. Other agencies contracted with local governments to provide relief to the swelling ranks of the unemployed. The slowing economy resulted in declining tax receipts for property and sales taxes, making it difficult for state and local governments to meet increasing demands for unemployment relief. Cities that had resisted the Community Chest movement, notably Boston, Chicago, and New York, turned to federated fundraising to broaden the pool of potential donors. The federal government began to support state and local relief efforts, first with loans to the states beginning in 1932 during the Hoover administration and then with grants for unemployment relief during the Roosevelt administration.

Herbert Hoover, who served as President in the early years of the Depression (1929–1933), increased the federal budget but wanted states and the voluntary sector to take the lead in relief. In contrast, the Roosevelt administration, while it enlisted state governments, favored a strong federal role. President Franklin D. Roosevelt took office in 1933, promising a "New Deal" for the American people—a more vigorous federal government and renewed experimentation in recovery efforts. Roosevelt's Federal Emergency Relief administrator, Harry Hopkins, a social worker with a background in the administration of both public and voluntary agencies, required that states receiving federal grants for unemployment relief establish public agencies to administer the relief program, ending the practice of contracting with voluntary agencies (Trattner, 1999). In response, the general director of the Family Welfare Association of America charted a new course for private social work. Public agencies should provide relief to the unemployed while voluntary family agencies should concentrate on casework services for "disorganized families" (Swift, 1934).

The Social Security Act (1935) established a federal old age insurance program and state programs, supervised and partially funded by the federal government, of unemployment insurance, public assistance, and social services. States pressed new employees, most of them without social work experience, into service in the rapidly expanding state welfare systems. States established training programs and many state universities introduced undergraduate social work education programs. The established schools of social work, concentrated in urban areas and often in private universities, increasingly emphasized graduate education. Two social work education organizations, the American Association of Schools of Social Work (AASSW) and the National Association of Schools of Social Administration (NASSA), representing the two movements in social work education, attempted to represent education for the new profession.

While NASSA supported undergraduate education, the AASSW emphasized graduate education; in 1939, AASSW restricted membership to graduate programs. During the next few years, the master of social work (MSW) became the standard professional degree. To some in social work education, it appeared that two social work professions were emerging, a graduate profession based on the MSW degree and a baccalaureate profession based on the acquisition of a baccalaureate degree. While many MSWs continued to work in the voluntary social service sector, opportunities for public employment increased during the 1930s, as states implemented the services titles of the Social Security Act.

Social workers developed new conceptualizations of social work practice methods during the 1930s. Different branches of psychoanalytic casework, influenced by psychiatrists Otto Rank and Sigmund Freud, contested for dominance in social case work. Group workers and community organizers attempted to conceptualize their methods by sponsoring special sessions at the National Conference of Social Work in 1935 and 1939. The 1935 group work sessions resulted in the creation of a new group work organization, the Association for the Study of Group Work, and the 1939 session on community organization eventually led to another new organization, the Association for the Study of Community Organization.

Maturation

The United States entered World War II in December 1941 after an attack on Pearl Harbor in Hawaii by the Japanese Navy. By then the war was already being fought worldwide and some refugees from Hitler's Europe found sanctuary in the United States. Some, like Werner Boehm, had not been social workers in Europe but would become leaders in social work practice and education after the war. The growth of army camps and war-related industries ended the Depression and disrupted community life even before the United States entered the war. Congress passed the Lanham Act (1940) to provide assistance for war-impacted communities. Veteran social workers like Bertha Reynolds, who worked for the Personal Service Department of the National Maritime Union, devoted themselves to war work even as she challenged the direction of the profession. New social workers were recruited to war-related social work services.

Wars bring about psychological crises for service members whether they are called shell shock (World War I), battlefield neurosis (World War II), or post-traumatic stress disorder (Vietnam and Afghanistan/Iraq wars). During World War II, the Army Medical Corps deployed psychiatric social workers to treat service men and women suffering from war-related psychological trauma. In 1944, Congress enacted the Servicemen's Readjustment Act, or G.I. Bill, which provided health care, home and business loans, and postsecondary education grants for veterans of World War II. The Act, which some hailed as "completing the New Deal," created the postwar middle class by making home ownership and college education

available to veterans. The G.I. Bill also resulted in an expansion of the Veterans Administration (VA) hospital system. Social work became an important part of the VA health care system, which planners hoped would model an efficient public health system for the nation.

Congress enacted new social legislation after World War II. The National Mental Health Act (1946) created the National Institute of Mental Health (NIMH). Opportunities for social workers in health and mental health expanded as a result of the Hill-Burton Hospital Construction Act of 1946, the creation of NIMH, and the expansion of the VA Hospital System. The United States signed the charter of the United Nations in 1945, creating an international body that provided an arena for international exchange. Social workers in the United States were eager to share their expertise with development programs in war-ravaged Europe and Asia and later with developing nations in an era of decolonization. Unfortunately, the models were sometimes based on what was effective in the United States, with little effort to adapt practices to local conditions (Midgley, 2006). Social work in the late 1940s was a fragmented profession. Practitioners working in different fields of practice emphasized the special skills and knowledge needed by specialists, so that graduate education emphasized specialized rather than generic content. Separate education organizations accredited undergraduate and graduate programs. Many believed that the social work profession needed to speak with one voice. A movement for generic casework practice, initiated at the University of Chicago by Charlotte Towle, appeared to have promise for unifying social work practice. Social work practice organizations and social work education organizations amalgamated. In 1947, NASSA and AASSW formed the National Council on Social Work Education to explore professional unification. A study of social work education was commissioned, conducted by adult educator Ernest W. Hollis and social work educator Alice Taylor. The Hollis–Taylor Report, as the study was known, appeared in (1951); the following year, NASSA and AASSW merged to form the Council on Social Work Education (CSWE). CSWE moved quickly to require graduate status and university affiliation for institutional membership—social work would be a graduate profession.

Social work practitioner organizations presented a more confusing picture. The American Association of Social Workers (AASW), organized in 1921, attempted to represent all social workers, but specialized practitioner organizations existed for medical social workers (organized in 1918), school social workers (1919), psychiatric social workers (1926), group workers (1936), community organizers (1946), and researchers (1949). Several interorganizational committees met during the early 1950s to develop an agreement for a single social work practitioner organization. Although the early committees included the AASSW as a nonvoting member, consolidation of the education and practitioner organizations was not pursued. In 1955, the seven practitioner and researcher organizations joined to form the National Association of Social Workers (NASW), which had 22,000 members after the merger.

In 1958, an NASW Commission on Social Work Practice issued a Working Definition of Social Work Practice to provide a generic definition of social work practice (Bartlett, 1958). CSWE commissioned a comprehensive study of the social work curriculum, directed by Werner Boehm. Published in 1959, the 13-volume *Curriculum Study* included volumes on undergraduate education; specialized practice methods—administration, community organization, group work, and casework; fields of practice—corrections, public social services, and rehabilitation; and curriculum areas—human growth and behavior, research, social welfare policy and services, and values and ethics (Boehm, 1959). The intent of both efforts was to unify social work by providing a common set of concepts and educational experiences.

The Profession Broadens

In 1955, the Mental Health Study Act (PL 84–182) created the Joint Commission on Mental Illness and Health. The commission issued *Action for Mental Health* (1961), a report that called for renewed investment in mental health. The new liberal Kennedy administration in 1961 proposed an expansion in community mental health, based on the report and California's experience with community mental health centers. The Community Mental Health Centers Act (PL 88–164), enacted by Congress in 1963, provided grants-in-aid, administered by NIMH, to the states for local Community Mental Health Centers that would serve mentally ill persons outside of state facilities. By the end of the decade, social workers provided the majority of mental health care in the United States.

The Kennedy administration initiated other projects, notably in public welfare and delinquency prevention. After Kennedy delivered a special message on public welfare, Congress enacted the (1963) Public Welfare Amendments to the Social Security Act (PL 87–543), which provided federal funds for state social service programs and for training social workers

to work in state public welfare programs. The act increased opportunities for public welfare personnel to enter MSW programs and resulted in expanded opportunities in public welfare programs for professional social workers. Two years later, a federal task force projected an increased need for social work personnel and called for additional investment in social work education, including the development of undergraduate education for social work (U. S. Task Force on Social Work Education and Manpower, 1965).

President Kennedy's Committee on Juvenile Delinquency provided demonstration grants for antidelinquency programs. The example of the President's Committee led the new Johnson administration to propose a War on Poverty in 1964. A vigorous antipoverty program would be directed by quasi-public entities. Some social workers were involved in the design of the program, while others looked askance at its nonprofessional, some thought antiprofessional, approach to solving the problem of poverty. Voluntary social service agencies found new opportunities for contracting to provide services to the poor, from community organization to family counseling. Under President Johnson, a federal health insurance program for the elderly, Medicare, and a state-administered health assistance program for the poor, Medicaid, were passed by Congress as Titles XVIII and XIX of the Social Security Act, along with the Older Americans Act (PL 89–73) in 1965.

The effect of the expansion of government social welfare services during the Great Depression and after World War II was to shift the most important source of funding and practice for social work from the voluntary, nonprofit sector to the public sector, and to emphasize health and mental health programs. Other sectors, such as corrections and child welfare, medicalized their approaches, as talk of treatment for offenders and dependent children began to dominate professional discourse in these areas.

The increasing complexity of the emerging welfare state resulted in an increasing emphasis on policy, planning, and administration in social work curricula and in practice. Many programs in the Kennedy–Johnson era, from the antidelinquency programs of the Kennedy years to the community action, older Americans, and Model Cities programs of the Johnson administration, relied on increasingly complex federal relationships with state and local governments managed by community planners, many with social work credentials. If the decade was contentious, the social work profession seemed vibrant during the 1960s. In 1966, the membership of NASW reached nearly 46,000, doubling its membership in its first decade.

Social Work in a Conservative Era

In 1969, NASW, which had previously required the MSW for full membership, opened full membership to individuals with a baccalaureate degree from programs approved by CSWE. In doing so, NASW endorsed the conclusion of the Task Force on Social Work Education and Manpower that baccalaureate social workers were needed to fill the many social work positions created by the expansion of social welfare programs in the 1960s. CSWE subsequently developed standards and accreditation procedures for undergraduate social work programs. It seemed that the goal of NASSA for recognition of the undergraduate degree had been achieved. However, some believed that recognition of the BSW had "deprofessionalized" social work.

Federal spending for social welfare increased during the 1970s, but employment for social workers stagnated as a result of several related trends (Patterson, 2000). Congress and the Nixon administration favored "hard" services, such as material provisions, over such "soft" services as counseling. Hard services could be provided by anyone, many believed, resulting in reduced demand for MSWs and even BSWs. State public welfare departments separated social services from public assistance payments, reversing the logic of the 1963 Public Welfare Amendments. State and local public social service agencies reclassified jobs to require a BSW rather than an MSW—and sometimes any or no baccalaureate degree rather than a BSW. Often justified as cost-saving measures, these changes, which were particularly important in public child welfare services, limited employment opportunities for professional social workers even as they reduced the quality of services for clients. By the late 1970s, many social services were provided by private or quasi-public agencies or by private practitioners under contract to public authorities rather than by public agency employees.

These trends were exacerbated during the 1980s as the Reagan administration used the block grant mechanism to "return power to the states" while reducing federal commitments for social service spending. Many conservatives around Reagan were suspicious of social workers, whom they viewed as misguided philanthropists, harming poor people even as they attempted to assist them. In response, social work practitioner organizations lobbied for legal regulation. Licensing by the state, accomplished in varying degrees in all of the states by the 1990s, would assure the public of quality social services while increasing the demand for licensed social workers, advocates believed. Licensing also facilitated the growth of private practice,

as in many states it provided standards for independent practice. In 1988, the Director of NIMH appointed a Task Force on Social Work Research to study the status of research and research training in social work. The *Task Force Report*, published in 1991, recommended the creation of an Institute for the Advancement of Social Work (IASWR) and increased attention to social work research by NIMH, CSWE, and NASW (Task Force on Social Work Research, 1991).

Despite a new democratic administration in Washington, the trends of the 1980s continued during the Clinton administration—growth in government contracting with nonprofit and for profit organizations, increasing reliance on third-party payments, and privatization of social services. In spite of the creation of IASWR in 1993 and of a new national organization for social work researchers, the Society for Social Work and Research (SSWR) in 1994, social work was largely ignored when Congress enacted the Personal Responsibility and Work Opportunity Reconciliation Act of 1996 (PL 104–193), which eliminated a 40-year-old public assistance program for poor families, Aid to Families with Dependent Children (AFDC), replacing it with a block grant program Temporary Assistance to Needy Families (TANF), which imposed work requirements and time limits for the receipt of public assistance.

As the 21st century began, new organizations of practitioners, educators, and researchers had arisen to complement CSWE and NASW, creating a situation reminiscent of the 1940s. Research, increasingly emphasized by social work educators, did not seem to influence social work practice, signaling a potentially dangerous division between academics and practitioners. NASW held a Social Work Summit in 2002, which brought 43 different social work organizations together to discuss coalitions and collaborative undertakings, and a Social Work Congress in 2005 to identify common goals for the next 10 years.

Challenges and Trends

Although the social work profession seemed fragmented, a number of organizations of practitioners and educators were able to work together on interorganizational projects to promote social work research and focus the profession's political advocacy activities. The number of social work education programs at the BSW and MSW levels grew during the last decade of the 20th century and continue in the early 21st century. By 2012, there were over 500 social work education programs in the United States, including 479 baccalaureate programs, 218 masters programs, and 78 doctoral programs (Council on Social Work Education, 2012; Group for the Advancement of Doctoral Education, 2012). Over 800,000 people in the United States identified themselves as social workers. However, many of those employed as social workers were not professionally educated. Of over 400,000 licensed social workers, less than half belong to NASW. The Bureau of Labor Statistics predicted that the number of social work positions would increase more rapidly than the average for all occupations, particularly as the population aged. By the early 21st century, social workers were uncertain about the profession's mission and its relationship to the welfare state. Fragmentation, together with privatization, deprofessionalization, and competition with other professions in a shrinking human service arena, provided challenges for the profession.

References

Addams, J. (1893). *Philanthropy and social progress.* New York: T. Y. Crowell.

Bartlett, H. M. (1958). Toward clarification and improvement of social work practice. *Social Work, 3*(2), 3–9.

Boehm, W. W. (Ed.). (1959). *The curriculum study* (Vols. 1–13). New York: Council on Social Work Education.

Council on Social Work Education. (2007). *Statistics on social work education in the United States: 2004.* Alexandria, VA: CSWE.

Council on Social Work Education. (2012). Accreditation. Available at http://www.cswe.org/Accreditation.aspx

Group for the Advancement of Doctoral Education. (2012). Membership Directory. Available at http://www.gadephd.org/mbruniv.asp

Hollis, E. V., & Taylor, A. L. (1951). *Social work education in the United States: The report of a study made for the National Council on Social Work Education.* New York: Columbia University Press.

Joint Commission on Mental Illness and Health. (1961). *Action for mental health: Final report.* New York: Basic Books.

Kelso, R. W. (1923). The transition from charities and correction to public welfare. *Annals of the American Academy of Political and Social Science, 105,* 21–25.

Lee, P. R. (1929). Social work: Cause and function. *National Conference of Social Work, Proceedings, 56,* 3–20.

Midgley, J. (2006). International social welfare. In J. M. Herrick & P. H. Stuart (Eds.), *Encyclopedia of Social Welfare History in North America* (pp. 198–203). Thousand Oaks, CA: Sage Publications.

Richmond, M. E. (1917). *Social diagnosis.* New York: Russell Sage Foundation.

Swift, Linton B. (1934). *New alignments between public and private agencies in a community family welfare and relief program.* New York: Family Welfare Association of America.

Task Force on Social Work Research. (1991). *Building social work knowledge for effective services and policies: A plan for research development.* Austin, TX: Task Force on Social Work Research.

Trattner, W. I. (1999). *From poor law to welfare state* (6th ed.). New York: Free Press.

U.S. Task Force on Social Work Education and Manpower. (1965). *Closing the gap in social work manpower: Report of the departmental task force on social work education and manpower.* Washington, DC: U.S. Government Printing Office.

Further Reading

Huff, D. (n.d.). The social work history station. Retrieved November 18, 2097, from http://www.boisiestate.edu/socialwork/dhuff/central/core.htm

Leiby, J. (1978). *A history of social welfare and social work in the United States.* New York: Columbia University Press.

Leighninger, L. (1988). *Social work: Search for identity.* Westport, CT: Greenwood Press.

Lubove, R. (1965). *The professional altruist: The emergence of social work as a career, 1880–1930.* Cambridge, MA: Harvard University Press.

Maas, H. S. (1951). *Adventure in mental health: Psychiatric social work with the armed forces during World War II.* New York: Columbia University Press.

National Conference on Social Welfare. (1874–1982). Proceedings. Retrieved November 18, 2007, from http://www.quod.lib.umich.edu/n/ncosw/ (Also called: Conference of Boards of Public Charities, 1874; Conference of Charities, 1875–1879; Conference of Charities and Correction, 1880–1881; National Conference of Charities and Correction, 1882–1916; National Conference of Social Work, 1917–1956; National Conference on Social Welfare, 1957–1982.).

National Institutes of Health. (2005). NIH history. Retrieved November 18, 2007, from http://www.nih.gov/about/history.htm

Odum, H. W. (1933). Public welfare activities. In *Recent social trends in the United States: Report of the president's research committee on social trends* (Vol. 2, pp. 1224–1273). New York: McGraw-Hill.

Reynolds, B. C. (1971). *Social work and social living: Explorations in philosophy and practice.* NASW classics series. Washington, DC: National Association of Social Workers (originally published 1951).

Social Security Administration. (2007). Social security online: Social security history. Retrieved November 18, 2007, from http://www.ssa.gov/history/history.html

Trattner, W. I. (1999). *From poor law to welfare state: A history of social welfare in America* (6th ed.). New York: The Free Press.

Walker, S. H. (1933). Privately supported social work. In *Recent social trends in the United States: Report of the president's research committee on social trends* (Vol. 2, pp. 1168–1223). New York: McGraw-Hill.

Wenocur, S., & Reisch, M. (1989). *From charity to enterprise: The development of American social work in a market economy.* Urbana: University of Illinois Press.

PAUL H. STUART

SOLUTION-FOCUSED BRIEF THERAPY

ABSTRACT: Building on a strengths perspective and using a time-limited approach, solution-focused brief therapy is a treatment model in social work practice that holds a person accountable for solutions rather than responsible for problems. Solution-focused brief therapy deliberately utilizes the language and symbols of "solution and strengths" in treatment and postulates that positive and long-lasting change can occur in a relatively brief period of time by focusing on the solution-building process instead of focusing on the problems. Currently, this practice model has been adopted in diverse social work practice settings with different client populations, which could be partly accounted for by the fact that the assumptions and practice orientation of solution-focused brief therapy are consistent with social work values as well as the strengths-based and empowerment-based practice in social work treatment.

KEY WORDS: brief treatment; empowerment-based; social work treatment; solution-focused; strengths-based

History

The development of solution-focused brief therapy was originally inspired by the work of the husband and wife team Steve de Shazer and Insoo Kim Berg, along with their associates at the Brief Family Therapy Center in Milwaukee. The Brief Therapy Center was first established by de Shazer and Berg in 1978 and formally became the home of solution-focused brief therapy in 1982. With the passing of de Shazer in September 2005 and then Berg in January 2007, the stewardship of the Brief Therapy Center was transferred to the Solution-Focused Brief Therapy Association (SFBTA). De Shazer was instrumental in the development of SFBTA because he was the one who first invited the solution-focused community to meet in 2001. This group, including de Shazer, Berg, and 27 colleagues, founded the SFBTA in the fall of 2002. The European Brief Therapy Association (EBTA), which was established earlier in 1993, shares similar aims to promote the development and dissemination of solution-focused brief therapy. Both the SFBTA and the EBTA hold annual conferences, support research efforts, and further the development and promotion of solution-focused brief therapy in practice.

When de Shazer and Berg first conceptualized the approach, solution-focused brief therapy was atheoretical, and the focus was on finding "what works in therapy." Wary of the potentially limiting effects of assumptions or presumptions of theory-based practice approaches pertaining to clients, problems, and diagnoses, these pioneers of solution-focused brief therapy took a new and different approach in exploring the treatment process by asking one simple question: "What works in treatment?" They were interested in listening to what clients have to share, noticing what actually happens in session that helps positive improvement, and distancing themselves as much as possible from presumptions about what works as proposed by diverse treatment approaches. The original team regularly met and observed therapy sessions using a one-way mirror. While observing the therapeutic dialogues and process, the team behind the mirror diligently attempted to identify, discover, and converse about what brought beneficial positive changes in clients and families. In other words, the early development of solution-focused brief therapy was antithetical to the modernist epistemology of understanding human behavior and change based on a presumed understanding of the observed phenomena. Instead of taking a positivistic, hierarchical, or expert stance, the understanding is accomplished by a bottom-up and grounded approach, which strives for a contextual and local understanding of what works in therapy (Berg, 1994; Lee, 2011).

De Shazer, the co-founder of solution-focused brief therapy, was trained in brief therapy at the Mental Research Institute (MRI) in Palo Alto, CA. Consequently, the brief therapy tradition at MRI does have some legacy on the development of solution-focused brief therapy. Brief therapy, as based on MRI, is influenced by a systems perspective (Bateson, 1979), social constructivism (for example, see Berg & Luckmann, 1966; Neimeyer & Mahoney, 1993; Rosen & Kuehlwein, 1996), and the work of the psychiatrist Milton Erickson, who was an expert in observing and utilizing what clients brought to the session in order to solve their presenting problems. Erickson's work exemplified the belief that individuals have the strengths and resources to solve their problems (Erickson, 1985a; Erickson, 1985b). To note, a major difference between MRI and solution-focused brief therapy is that while the brief therapy approaches that were developed at MRI focus on disrupting the problem-maintaining pattern, solution-focused brief therapy emphasizes the solution-building process. Such a shift in treatment focus is influenced by a strong emphasis on the role of language in creating and sustaining reality as embraced by solution-focused brief therapy (de Shazer, 1994).

Practice Assumptions of Solution-Focused Brief Therapy

Insoo Kim Berg, Steve de Shazer, and the solution-focused community emphasized that solution-focused brief therapy is not simply a set of therapeutic techniques but instead represents a way of thinking (de Shazer, 1985). Mastering the techniques without embracing underlying assumptions and beliefs of solution-focused brief therapy toward clients and change is not helpful in the treatment process. While the original development of solution-focused brief therapy was atheoretical, the practice of solution-focused brief therapy is consistent with the views posed by a systems perspective, social constructivism, and the work of the psychiatrist Milton Erickson. The practice assumptions of solution-focused brief therapy are:

Focus on solutions, strengths, and health. Solution-focused brief therapy focuses on what clients can do versus what clients cannot do. Instead of focusing and exploring clients' problems and deficiencies, the focus is on the successes and accomplishments when clients are able to satisfactorily address their problems of living. The focus is on how to notice, identify, expand, and use these successes them more often (Berg & Kelly, 2000; de Shazer, 1985). The emphasis on solutions and successes is neither a consequence of "naive" beliefs regarding strengths in clients nor simplistic "positive thinking." It is a deliberate therapeutic choice, which is supported by repeated clinical observations that clients discover solutions more quickly when the focus is on what they can do, what strengths they have, and what they have accomplished (de Jong & Berg, 2013). Theoretically speaking, the focus on solutions and successes to facilitate positive changes in clients is supported by a systems perspective (Bateson, 1979) and the role of language in creating reality (de Shazer, 1994).

Systems perspective. One major proposition of a systems perspective is that change is constant in any system (Bateson, 1979). Because change is constant and there is movement in any system, every problem pattern includes an exception to the pattern (de Shazer, 1985). For example, no matter how conflicted a relationship is, there must be times that the dyads (that is, a couple or two people) are not fighting or bickering. The time when the dyad is doing something else to handle its differences constitutes an exception to the problem pattern, which also contains potential solution to the problem of fighting. Underlying such a view is a belief in the inherent strengths and potentials of clients to engage in behavior that is outside the problem pattern (De Jong & Berg, 2013). In other words, despite the multi-deficiencies and problems that clients may perceive that they have, there are times when clients handle their life situations in a more satisfying way or in a different manner. These exceptions provide the clues for solutions (de Shazer, 1985, 1988) and represent the client's "unnoticed" strengths and resources. The task for the solution-focused practitioner is to assist clients in noticing, amplifying, sustaining, and reinforcing these exceptions, regardless of how small or infrequent the exceptions may be (Berg & Kelly, 2000, Lee, Sebold, & Uken, 2003). Once clients are engaged in non-problem behavior, they are on their way to a solution-building process (Berg & Steiner, 2003).

Another major assumption of a systems perspective is the inter-relatedness of all parts of a system, which presumes that everything is connected. Change in one part of a system leads to change in other parts of the system (Bateson, 1972; Becvar & Becvar, 2012; Keeney & Thomas, 1986). As such, a systems perspective does not assume a one-to-one linear relationship between problem and solution. The focus is on circular relationships rather than linear relationships among different parts of a system. The complex inter-relatedness of different parts of systems also renders the effort to establish a causal understanding of problems essentially futile. It is almost impossible to precisely ascertain exactly why any problem occurs in the first place and the trajectory of development. As such, solutions to a problem can happen in multiple pathways and do not necessarily have to be directly related to the presenting problem (de Shazer, 1985). In other words, insight into the problem's origin is not necessary to initiate a process of change in clients. Without minimizing the importance of a person's experience and perception of the history of the problem, solution-focused brief therapy views what is going on in the present as more important than what caused the problem at the very beginning.

The choice of not drilling into the history and patterns of problem but focusing on what clients do well is further influenced by the power of language in shaping clients' experience of their reality (de Shazer, 1994; Lee et al., 2003).

Language and reality. There is a conscious effort in solution-focused brief therapy to stay focused on solution dialogues and to de-emphasize problem dialogues. Such a conscious effort grows out of a concern about the role of language in creating or sustaining reality. Solution-focused brief therapy views language as the medium through which personal meaning and understanding are expressed and socially constructed in conversation (de Shazer, 1991, 1994). Furthermore, the meaning of things is contingent on the contexts and the language within which issues are described, categorized, and constructed by clients (Wittgenstein, 1958). Wittgenstein (1958) suggested that the way an individual experiences the reality is framed and limited by the language available to him or her to describe it. As such, these meanings are inherently unstable and shifting (Wittgenstein, 1958). Consequently, a major therapeutic task for social work professionals is to consider how we can use language in treatment that will facilitate the description and construction of a "beneficial" reality that will open space for individuals to find solutions to their presenting problems.

Recognizing the power of language in creating and sustaining realities, the "conversation of change" is the preferred language of solution-focused brief therapy. The "conversation of change" uses language with the following characteristics (Lee, et al, 2003):

- Language that implies the person wants to change
- Language that implies that the person is capable
- Language that implies change has occurred or is occurring
- Language that implies the changes are meaningful
- Language that encourages the person to explore possibilities for change
- Language that suggests that the person can be creative and playful about life
- Language that conveys recognition of the persons' evolution of their personal story
- Language that does not encourage negative, blaming, or self-defeating descriptions

This "conversation of change" uses presuppositional language that assumes a possibility of change and thereby induces hopefulness in clients (Lee et al., 2003; Walter & Peller, 1992).

Accountability for Solutions

Practitioners of solution-focused brief therapy choose to hold the client responsible for solutions instead of problems in the treatment process in order to ethically and effectively facilitate positive changes in clients (de Shazer, 1985). The advantage of such a focus is that the practitioner and the client can direct therapeutic efforts toward supporting the client's responsibility

for building solutions and avoiding the potential negativity cycle that might be perpetrated by the language of blaming (Lee et al., 2003). However, holding clients to be accountable for solutions is neither simple nor easy. Clients usually seek treatment because they do not know or even feel that there are solutions to their presenting problems. Change requires hard work and a solution-building process requires discipline and effort (Berg & Kelly, 2000; De Jong and Berg, 2013). In solution-focused treatment, the "solution" is established in the form of a goal that is to be self-determined and attained by the client (Lee, Uken, & Sebold, 2007). Characteristics of useful goals are:

- personally meaningful and important to the clients;
- small enough to be achieved;
- concrete, specific, and behavioral so that indicators of success can be established and observed;
- positively stated so that the goal represents the presence rather than the absence of something;
- realistic and achievable within the context of the client's life; and
- perceived as involving hard work (Berg & Miller, 1992; Lee et al., 2007).

A Present and Future Orientation

People can take helpful actions to impact the present and the future, but obviously we cannot change what has already happened in the past. Solution-focused brief therapy believes that problems belong to the past while solutions exist in the present and future. Solution-focused brief therapy assumes that the meanings of a problem are artifacts of the context (de Shazer, 1991). Because one can never know exactly why a problem exists and because problem perceptions are not external objective "realities," insight into the problem's origin is not necessary to initiate a process of change in clients. Without minimizing the importance of the client's experience and perception of the history of the problem, a solution-focused practitioner listens attentively to clients' sharing of their stories and experiences. However, the practitioner does not reinforce this line of conversation and instead looks for opportunities to shift to a "conversation of change" that assists clients in "staying at the surface of their problems" (de Shazer, 1991). "Staying at the surface of problems" should not be equated with being superficial in the treatment process. The treatment process avoids going "deep" into the problem; rather, it aims to assist clients to do something attainable and observable in their present, immediate life context (de Shazer, 1994). Solution-focused brief therapy acknowledges that we cannot change the past but assumes that we can do something helpful in the present.

Solution-focused brief therapy also assumes that "the future exists in our anticipation of how it will be" (Cade & O'Hanlon, 1993, p. 109). In other words, how we construct a picture of a desirable future will influence how events will unfold in life. Consequently, the solution-focused practitioner asks questions that will help clients to describe a future that does not contain the problem. The more specific and clearer the vision of a desirable future, the more likely it will happen because the client will have a goal to aspire to and steps to follow. Consequently, the task of therapy is to help clients envision a desirable future and identify the first small step that they can take to attain a future without the problem (Berg, 1994, De Jong & Berg, 2013). Such descriptions also inspire hope and enhance motivation in clients to engage in beneficial behaviors that will lead to positive changes in their lives.

CLIENTS DEFINE THEIR GOALS: THE CLIENT AS ASSESSOR

Solution-focused brief therapy views goals as individually constructed by clients in a collaborative process during treatment. Aligned with social constructivism (Berg & Luckmann, 1966; Neimeyer & Mahoney, 1993; Rosen & Kuehlwein, 1996), solution-focused brief therapy believes that solutions to problems are not objective "realities" but rather individually constructed. Clients are the most legitimate "knower" of their life experiences and should be the center of the change process. Externally imposed therapeutic goals, as promoted by therapy approaches or society, may be inappropriate or irrelevant to the needs of clients. In addition, clients generally are willing to work harder if they define the goal of therapy and perceived the goal as personally meaningful (Lee et al., 2007). Consequently, a distinctive characteristic of solution-oriented assessment is its focus on the client as the assessor (Lee et al., 2003). Contrary to most medical models of assessment, which view professionals as possessing expert diagnostic knowledge and clients as the objects for assessment, solution-focused assessment emphasizes the client as the assessor who constantly self-evaluates what the problem is, what may be feasible solutions to the problem, what the desirable future is, what the goals of treatment are, what strengths and resources the client has, what may be helpful in the process of change, how committed or motivated the client is to make change a reality, and how quickly the client wants to proceed with the change, etc (Lee et al., 2003). Solution-focused practitioners are experts on the "conversation of change" and keep the dialogues going in search of a description of an alternative and beneficial reality (de Shazer, 1994).

Collaborative therapeutic relationship. This view of clients as the assessor fundamentally shifts the relationship between the client and the social work practitioner, so that it is no longer a hierarchal relationship but rather a collaborative one, with the client as the assessor and the social work practitioner as an expert of the conversation of change. Clients no longer simply provide "data" for professionals to use in determining a diagnosis and a treatment plan. The role of the solution-focused practitioner is to provide a therapeutic context for clients to construct and develop a personally meaningful goal. The practitioner enters into their perspective, adopts their frame of mind, listens to and understands their goals, and looks for strengths instead of weaknesses or diagnoses (Lee, 2011). Instead of being hierarchical, the solution-focused practitioner-client relationship is an egalitarian and collaborative relationship in which both the client and social work professional work together to facilitate positive changes (de Jong & Berg, 2013). This collaborative relationship inherently enhances the process of engagement and client's ownership of the treatment process.

Utilization. Milton Erickson was an expert in utilizing clients' symptoms to help resolve their presenting problems. He firmly believed that individuals have the strengths and resources to solve their problems and that the main therapeutic task is to uncover and activate these resources in clients (Haley, 1973). Influenced by Erickson's work, solution-focused practitioners utilize whatever resources clients bring with them, whether these are skills, knowledge, beliefs, motivations, behaviors, symptoms, social networks, circumstances, and personal idiosyncrasies, to uncover the solution (de Shazer, 1985; O'Hanlon & Wilk, 1987). Such a practice orientation is based on several beliefs: (1) there is the presence of exception in every problem situation (de Shazer, 1985); (2) instead of attempting to teach clients something new or foreign based on the practitioner's presumed notions of what is best for the client, it is usually more efficient to focus on what clients are doing when they engage in non-problem behaviors; (3) utilizing and building on exceptions is a more efficient and effective way for clients to develop solutions that are relevant to and viable in their unique life circumstances as opposed to suggestions from professionals; (4) people are usually more invested in solutions that they discover or identify by themselves. As such, the task for the solution-focused practitioner is to elicit, trigger, reinforce, expand, and consolidate the exceptions that the client generates. Solution-focused practitioners stay away from teaching clients skills or intervening in their lives in ways that may fit our "model" of what is good, but may not be appropriate or viable in their lives (Lee, et al., 2003; Lee, 2011).

Tipping the first domino: A small change. "A journey of a thousand miles begins with one step" (Laozi, *Dao Te Ching*, Chapter 100). Solution-focused brief therapy fully embraces the wisdom of beginning the change effort with the first, small step. There are many benefits of focusing on the first small step: (1) small changes are more feasible, doable, attainable, and manageable than big changes; (2) small steps provide indicators of improvement; (3) people are usually more encouraged and committed to the change process when they experience successes; and (4) small successes provide feedback for more successes in the process of change. Change requires both the vision of a "big" picture and a pragmatic plan for the first small step.

The emphasis on the first small step is also influenced by systems perspective. Introducing any change in a system may disturb a person's equilibrium in unpredictable ways as a result of reiterating feedback. Repetitive attempts at the same unsuccessful solution are precisely what create problems in the first place (Watzlawick, Weakland, & Fisch, 1974). Consequently, solution-focused brief therapy believes that the best responses to clients' problems involve minimal, but personally meaningful, intervention by the solution-focused practitioner into their lives (Lee et al., 2003). Clients should determine what constitutes acceptable solutions. The most important thing is for practitioners to help clients identify the first small behavioral step toward desirable change.

The Solution-Focused Treatment Manual adopted by SFBTA succinctly describes the basic tenants of solution-focused brief therapy. It can be found at: *http://www.sfbta.org/researchDownloads.html* (Trepper, McCollum, De Jong, Korman, Gingerich, & Franklin, 2010).

Solution-Focused Interventions

Solution-focused interventions engage the client in a "conversation of change" that is conducive to the solution-building process. In this conversation, the solution-focused practitioner invites the client to be the "expert of change." Collaboratively, the solution-focused practitioner and the client co-construct a desirable future that does not contain the problem. The practitioner listens intensely and explores the meaning of the client's perception of his or her situation. Practitioners utilize solution-oriented questions, including exception questions, outcome questions, coping questions, scaling questions, and relationship questions to assist clients in constructing a reality that does not contain the problem. De Shazer, Berg, and their colleagues develop these questioning techniques to fully utilize the resources and potential of clients (for example, Berg & Kelly, 2000; de Jong & Berg, 2013; de Shazer, 1985). Questions are perceived as better ways to create open space for clients to think about and self-evaluate their situation and solutions.

First session. In terms of the treatment process, clients are first oriented to a solution-focused frame in which the focus of therapy is to assist clients in finding solutions to their problems with as few sessions as needed. The clients are immediately encouraged to give a clear and explicit statement of their presenting complaint. Without focusing on the history of the problems, the solution-focused practitioner uses solution-building questions to begin assisting clients in identifying solutions for their problems. Specific interventions include:

- *Pre-session change.* Early in treatment, the solution-focused practitioner helps clients to notice positive changes in their natural environment before they receive any treatment. "What changes have you noticed that have happened or started to happen since you called to make the appointment for this session?" (Trepper et al., 2010). Pre-session change assumes that change is ongoing and is initiated by the clients and not the professionals.

- *Exception questions* inquire about times when the problem is either absent, less intense, or dealt with in a manner that is acceptable to the client (de Shazer, 1985). The solution-focused practitioner presupposes that change is happening in the client's problem situation. Such an effort shakes the rigid frames constructed by many clients with respect to the pervasiveness and permanency of their complaints. Examples of exception questions include: When was the last time that you didn't have this problem? When was the last time that you expected that you'd have the problem but it did not happen? When was the last time that you thought you would lose your temper but you didn't? What was different about these times?

- *Miracle questions* allow clients to separate themselves from their problem-saturated context and construct a future vision of life without the presenting complaint or with acceptable improvements in the problem. Miracle questions foster a sense of hopefulness and offer an opportunity for clients to develop a beneficial direction for improving their lives. The focus is on identifying small, observable, and concrete behaviors that are indicators of small changes, which can make a difference in the client's situation (de Shazer, 1985). A widely used format of miracle question is: *Suppose that after our meeting today, you go home, do your things, and go to bed. While you are sleeping, a miracle happens and the problem that brought you here is suddenly solved, like magic. The problem is gone. Because you were sleeping, you don't know that a miracle happened, but when you wake up tomorrow morning, you will be different. How will you know that a miracle has happened? What will be the first small sign that tells you that the problem is resolved?* (Berg & Miller, 1992). Variations of the miracle question include the dream question (Greene, Lee, Mentzer, Pinnell, & Niles, 1998) and the nightmare question (Reuss, 1997).

- *Coping questions* help clients to notice times when they are coping with their problems and what they are doing when they are successfully coping. Asking coping questions indirectly reframes the meaning frames of clients who have assumed that they are entirely helpless and thus they have no control over the problem situation (Berg, 1994; Berg & Steiner, 2003). Examples of coping questions include: *How have you been able to keep going despite all the difficulties you've encountered? How are you able to get up despite being so depressed?* A newly developed question is the "lemon question" that embraces personal pride and dignity in assisting clients to look for personal strengths in coping with difficult situation: *Suppose you came to see, with a new clarity, that _____ [a normalized statement of the difficult life predicament in which the clients find themselves], what would you be most proud of as your response to that situation?* (Taylor, 2012).

- *Scaling questions* ask clients to rank their situation or goal on a 1-to-10 scale (de Jong & Berg, 2013). Usually, 1 represents the worst scenario that could possibly be and 10 is the most desirable outcome. Scaling questions provide a simple tool for clients to quantify and evaluate their situation and progress so that they can establish a clear indicator of progress for themselves. Some examples of commonly used scaling questions are: *On a 1-to-10 scale, with 1 being the worst the problem could possibly be and 10 as the most desirable outcome, where would you put yourself on the scale? On a 1-to-10 scale with 1 being you don't believe you can do anything to change the situation and 10 meaning you are absolutely determined to do something to change the problem, how would you put yourself on the scale? What would your wife say using the same scale?*

- *Relationship questions* ask clients to imagine how significant others in their environment might react to their problem or situation and changes they make (Berg, 1994; de Jong & Berg, 2013). Relationship questions recognize the interactional aspect of many problems. These questions not only contextualize problem definition but also the client's desired goals and changes. In addition, relationship questions help establish multiple indicators of change as grounded in clients' real life context. Examples of relationship questions include: *Who would be the first to notice changes in you? What would your friends notice that is different about you if you are more comfortable with the new college environment? How would your mother rate your motivation to do something different and helpful on a 1-to-10 scale?*

Taking a break. Solution-focused practitioners are encouraged to take a break near the end of the session prior to wrapping up the session. The break serves several important functions: (1) the practitioner can consult with his or her team or supervisor about the session and solicit ideas and feedback for complimenting and providing solution-focused interventions to the client; (2) the practitioner can use the time to organize his or her thoughts and develop with compliments and ideas for possible interventions (Berg, 1994; Trepper et al., 2010); and (3) the break prepares the client or family to focus and receive the feedback from the solution-focused practitioner.

The end-of-session message usually consists of three components: a compliment, a bridging statement, and tasks. The compliment helps the client or family to clearly notice, register, and anchor what they have done well, what might be helpful in the change process, and what things that they should be proud of, and so on. Authentic compliments serve to motivate and direct clients for positive changes. A bridging statement serves to connect the compliment with the solution-focused tasks and experiments. An example of an end-of-session message is:

> Apparently, you are determined to be a better mom for your children despite your kids being in foster care right now. Some parents might choose to distance themselves from their children because of the pain of not being able to be with them and you are determined not to let that pain take control over you (compliment). Since you are such a keen observer (bridging statement), between now and next time we meet I would like you to observe what happens in your daily life and in particular your interaction with the child welfare people that you want to continue to have happen more often so that you have a better chance to reunite with your children in the near future (observation task).

Solution-focused tasks and experiments. Solution-focused brief therapy routinely uses task assignments and experiments to assist clients in noticing solutions in their natural life context (de Shazer & Molnar, 1984; Molnar & de Shazer, 1987). Some common solution-focused tasks and experiments are:

- If clients can identify exception behaviors to the problem, then clients are asked to "do more of what works."
- For clients who focus on the perceived stability of their problematic pattern and fail to identify any exceptions, an observation task is given: "Between now and next time we meet, we (I) want you to observe, so that you can tell us (me) next time, what happens in your (life, marriage, family, or relationship) that you want to continue to have happen" (Molnar & de Shazer, 1987). Another observation task directs clients to notice what they do when they overcome the temptation or urge to engage in the problem behavior.
- Other tasks that assist clients in interrupting their problem patterns and developing new solutions include: Do something different ("Between now and next time we meet, do something different and tell me what happened") and the prediction task, which asks the client to predict his or her behavior by tossing a coin ("If it is heads, do what you normally do; if it is tails, pretend that the miracle day has happened") (Berg, 1994).

Second session and after. The focus of second session and afterwards is on facilitating clients to notice and expand changes that have happened or were observed between sessions. A typical question is the "What's better?" question: So, what is better, even a little bit, since last time we meet? (Berg, 1994; Trepper

et al., 2010). Noticing change is a small but important step for clients to realize their desired future. The solution-focused practitioner continues to use solution-focused questions and interventions to elicit, amplify, and consolidate positive goal efforts that are demonstrated by the client. An important skill is to encourage clients to describe their small change effort in great detail so that the "ordinary" becomes "extraordinary" (Lee et al., 2003). Another important therapeutic task in the second session is to help clients notice the connection between their behaviors, feelings, thoughts, and their desired solutions. Examples of these questions include: How are you able to go out together for a walk four out of seven days last week? How did both of you do that? How did you feel when you decided to stop arguing instead of exploding despite your anger? What's in you mind when you chose not to talk back and argue with your parents?

It is not uncommon for clients become distracted by problems, for things to not get better, or for clients to have not acted on the solution-focused tasks, and so on. From a solution-focused perspective, there is no good or bad response, because clients' responses are just feedback to the practitioners to continue co-construct a beneficial reality with the clients (Lee et al., 2003). In other words, there is no failure because responses are just feedback (de Shazer, 1985). Oftentimes, clients might have overlooked the small change or been distracted by problems. The trick is for the solution-focused practitioners to remain persistent and patient. It is helpful to ask the client to restate in a different way his or her goal and the things that he or she has noticed. The task is to help the client to look for small changes that can be further amplified and expanded. Other times, the client might need to reevaluate his or her goals based on experimentation. People might need to experiment using trial and error to determine what is important and helpful to them. When clients do not improve or have done nothing by the second session, it is likely that the stated goals or tasks are not important, not appropriate, or not relevant to the extent that the clients are committed to do something different. It is important for the practitioner to offer choices as much as possible and to continue helping the clients to self-assess what might be beneficial for them. Solution-focused practitioners should not view clients as resistant or unmotivated. Instead, they should look for ways that clients are cooperating (Lee et al., 2003).

The solution-building process is allows the clients to notice a difference that can make a difference in their livesin their natural environment. The solution-focused practitioner cautiously refrains from providing or suggesting solutions. The solution-focused practitioner is responsible for creating a therapeutic dialogical context in which clients experience a solution-building process that is initiated from within and grounded in clients' cultural strengths as well as thier personal construction of the solution reality (Lee, 2003). It is for clients to discover what works for them in their unique life context.

Termination. The goals of termination in solution-focused brief therapy are to (1) review goals and discuss progress; (2) facilitate clients to own and take full credit for their improvement and positive changes; (3) assist clients in developing connections between their actions and positive change efforts; and (4) assist clients in establishing indicators of relapse and follow-up measures. Oftentimes, the solution-focused practitioners use scaling questions to help clients evaluate differences in their presenting problem between now and before: *Suppose when we first started meeting, your problem was at a 1 and where you wanted to be is at a 10. Where would you say you are at today on a scale of 1-to-10?* In addition, scaling questions are used to evaluate the clients' confidence in their ability to maintain change: *On a scale of 1-to-10, with a 10 meaning that you have every confidence that you will keep up with your progress and a 1 meaning that you have no confidence at all to maintain the change, where would you put yourself today? What would it take for you to move from a 5 to a 6?*

In addition to complimenting clients for the positive change efforts, one major solution-focused intervention at termination is to use questions that assist clients to make connections between their actions and positive changes as well as to take ownership of the change. *Looking back, what have you done to help you in making these changes? How do you decide that you are determined to make the change despite not being easy? When did you decide to do that? Where do you think it comes from for you, the commitment?*

Change will be more long lasting when clients are able to consolidate their changes into alternative, beneficial "self-descriptions" such as an honest man, a caring parent, or a loving husband. These descriptions encapsulate the overall change so that clients develop "the language of success" in place of the "language of problem" in describing the self (Lee et al., 2003). *How would you describe yourself as a husband now as compared to when we first met a few months ago?*

In addition to consolidating change efforts, it is important to help clients prepare for the ups and downs in life. Solution-focused practitioners use scaling and relationship questions to assist clients establish earliest indicator(s) of relapse and develop contingency plans: *What will need to happen in order for you to slide back again? What you will need to do to prevent that happening again? What would be the earliest sign to you that you are starting to go backward? When you notice that you are sliding back, what can you do differently to pull yourself up?*

Solution-focused brief therapy takes a developmental perspective in viewing change. In other words, there are always ups and downs in life, and clients might need to seek help again in the future for different problems of living, which is normal and not an indicator of failure. The important thing is for clients to learn something new and useful each time that they can use in addressing future problems.

In sum, solution-focused brief therapy advocates for an open process of self-evaluations and choice-making through a "conversation of change." There is no longer an objective problem or reality that exists independently outside the client. Treatment is essentially an ongoing and open process in which the client and the social work practitioner actively engage in co-constructing an inherently unstable reality that is different from the problem reality and contains the desirable future as defined by the client. The practitioner listens for and absorbs clients' descriptions, words, and meanings, and then formulates responses by building on clients' frames of reference and connecting to clients' words and meanings. This cyclical and ongoing process of listening, connecting, and responding allows solution-focused practitioners and clients to co-construct new, alternative, and beneficial solutions or desired futures as determined by the clients (Trepper, 2010). Assessment and treatment are no longer alienated procedures operated on the client by an expert. Instead, treatment focuses on co-constructing a "conversation of change" that deliberately utilizes the language of change, strengths, and resources to help clients developing useful goals, recognizing exceptions, amplifying change efforts, and consolidating the new behaviors in their life. It becomes an open process in which the clients continuously make evaluations and choices. Ownership, options, and choices become an integral part of the treatment process (Lee et al., 2003).

Clinical Applications of Solution-Focused Brief Therapy

Solution-focused brief therapy has gained prominence in social work practice despite its relatively short history as compared to other established practice approaches in social work treatment. One plausible reason is that solution-focused brief therapy has its roots in social work because social work professionals actively participate in its development and dissemination. The late Insoo Kim Berg and Steve de Shazer, the founders of solution-focused brief therapy, were social work professionals. Peter de Jong, Michelle Weiner-Davis, and Eve Lipchik, who all belonged to the original group at BFTC, were social work professionals. Cynthia Franklin, Johnny Kim, and Michael Kelly applied solution-focused brief therapy to family practice and school social work (Franklin & Jordan, 1998; Kelly, Kim, & Franklin, 2008). Mo Yee Lee, Adriana Uken, and John Sebold are social work professionals who use solution-focused brief therapy to work with domestic violence offenders (Lee et al., 2003). Wally Gingerich, who conducted the first systematic narrative review of solution-focused brief therapy outcome studies, is a social work professional (Gingerich & Esiengart, 2000). This list is certainly not exhaustive as there are many other social work professionals actively applying solution-focused brief therapy with their client populations in creative and beneficial ways. Because the founders of solution-focused brief therapy were social work professionals, it is not surprising that the practice and value orientation of solution-focused brief therapy are consistent with the social work overarching framework of person-in-environment as well as the social work values of respecting clients' dignity and self-determination (Karls, 2009; NASW, 1999). The practice of solution-focused brief therapy—being systems-based, collaborative, strengths-based, respectful, pragmatic, and focused—facilitates the adoption of this model by social work professionals in their work (Lee, 2011).

The increasing adoption of solution-focused brief therapy by social work professionals is plausibly related to its focus on clients' strengths and resources, which is consistent with the empowerment-based and strengths-based approaches in human services; approaches that have gained increased prominence since the late 1990s (Rees, 1998; Saleebey, 2009). In addition, solution-focused brief therapy provides a specific set of treatment skills and techniques that help to operationalize strengths-based and empowerment-based practice in daily social work practice. In other words, solution-focused brief therapy translates the concept of strengths and empowerment to every day practice of using the "language of empowerment" (Rappaport, 1985; Rees, 1998) and the "lexicons of strengths" (Saleebey, 2008) in social work treatment. Finally, while the development of solution-focused brief therapy is entirely independent of the development of managed care, its emphasis on being brief, efficient, and effective clearly aligns with the mandate of managed care, which is on cost-effectiveness and cost-containment.

To date, solution-focused brief therapy has been adopted in a variety of social work practice settings (Nelson & Thomas, 2007). Examples of these settings or practices include but are not limited to the followings:

- Child welfare, for example, the Sign of Safety (Berg & Kelly, 2000; Turner, 2007)
- Family practice (Berg, 1994; Franklin & Jordan, 1998)
- Child and adolescent practice (for example, Berg, & Steiner, 2003; Selekman, 1993, 1997).
- Students from single-parent families and their parents (Lee & Grover-Ely, 2013)
- Schools (for example, Franklin & Gerlach, 2007; Kelly, Kim, & Franklin, 2008; Metcalf, 2008)
- Substance use (for example, Berg & Reuss, 1998; Smock & Trepper et al., 2008)
- Mental health (Knekt & Lindfors, et al., 2008a; Knekt & Lindfors, et al., 2008b; Macdonald, 2007)
- Domestic violence (Lee, 2007; Lee et al., 2003; Lee et al., 2012; Uken, Lee, & Sebold, 2013)
- Health (O'Connell & Palmer, 2003)
- Suicide prevention (Fiske, 2008; Hendon, 2008)
- Restorative justice (Walker & Hayashi, 2009)
- Administration and management (Lueger & Korn, 2006)
- Culturally competent practice (Lee, 2003; Kim, 2013)
- Coaching (for example, Berg & Szabo, 2005; Szabo & Meier, 2009)
- Supervision (Triantafillou, 1997; Wheeler, 2007)

Relevant Research and Challenges

SFBT is gaining increased recognition as an evidence-based model. Solution-focused brief therapy is currently listed in the Office of Juvenile Justice and Delinquent Prevention Model Program Guide (*http://www.ojjdp.gov/mpg/mpgProgramDetails.aspx?ID = 712*) and is included in SAMHSA's National Registry of Evidence-based Programs and Practices. In addition, Franklin and her associates published the book *Solution-focused brief therapy: A handbook of evidence based practice* (Franklin, Trepper, Gingerich, & McCullum, 2012). These are important milestones for solution-focused brief therapy, in part because the history of solution-focused brief therapy is relatively recent compared to other established treatment approaches such as cognitive-behavioral approaches. In addition, solution-focused brief therapy was developed by social work professionals in practice and not by academics at universities or research institutes. Nonetheless, the founders of solution-focused brief therapy, Insoo Kim Berg and Steve de Shazer, had a clear vision and support for advancing research in solution-focused brief therapy (de Shazer & Berg, 1997). At the EBTA conference at Brugge, Belgium, in 1997, Berg facilitated a one-day post-conference meeting of people who were interested in solution-focused brief therapy research. This was probably the first "Research Day" to discuss research development in solution-focused brief therapy. The Solution-Focused Brief Therapy Association (SFBTA), which is the professional organization promoting solution-focused brief therapy in North America, continues its vision for promoting research of solution-focused brief therapy. The Research Committee of SBFTA is charged with the mission to promote, strengthen, and disseminate research pertaining to solution-focused brief therapy. This committee organizes a Research Day as part of the pre-conference activities. Since 2010, SFBTA has also funded the SFBTA Research Award, under the auspice of the Research Committee, to continue promote and support research in SFBT.

Outcome research. Over the years, numerous intervention studies have been conducted for solution-focused brief therapy in diverse practice settings. Gingerich and Eisengart (2000) conducted the first systematic narrative review of solution-focused brief therapy outcome study. They conducted a systematic review of 15 outcome studies on solution-focused brief therapy. More recently, Johnny Kim has conducted a meta-analysis that consisted of outcome studies that were conducted between 1988 and 2005 (Kim, 2008). This review included 22 studies that used a control or comparison group in their study design. In addition, the meta-analysis focused on external behavioral outcomes, internal behavioral outcomes, and family or relationship problem outcomes. In addition, Corcoran and Pillai (2009) reviewed 10 studies that used SFT in treatment. The analysis of these studies found about 50% of the studies can be viewed as showing improvement over alternative conditions or no-treatment control.

While there is increasing empirical evidence of the effectiveness of solution-focused brief therapy, the rigor of these studies is limited by numerous issues in research design. These limitations, however, are not unusual in intervention studies conducted in real life practice settings. The identified problems include small and non-representative samples, lack of randomized controlled procedures, lack of specific manualized protocol, problems with treatment fidelity, measurement

problems, and so on (Gingerich & Eisengart, 2000; Kim, 2008; Lee et al., 2007). To further develop and strengthen evidence for the efficacy of solution-focused brief therapy, future studies should consider a more rigorous research design that (1) uses larger and more representative samples; (2) includes control or comparison groups using randomized assignment procedures; (3) uses standardized measures that are sensitive enough to measure treatment changes; (4) uses observation-based rating systems in data collection when possible and appropriate, (5) further refines and develops the treatment manual for training purposes and fidelity analyses, (6) increases the rigor of the fidelity procedures by using observation-based approaches with a refined, specific, and rigorous fidelity measurement protocol; (7) carefully monitors the data collection process to reduce problems in measurement attrition; and (8) includes research sites that serve ethnically and racially diverse populations (Lee, 2011).

Process research. A unique development in solution-focused brief therapy research is its incorporation of microanalysis as a major research effort. Microanalysis is the close examination of moment-by-moment, utterance-by-utterance communicative actions in conversations, with an emphasis on how these sequences function in the interaction (Bavelas, McGee, Phillips, & Routledge, 2000). Microanalysis views communication as constructive and directive (Bavelas, Coates, & Johnson, 2000). Consequently, microanalysis as a research method allows us to closely examine the co-constructive process in treatment, which is a hallmark of solution-focused brief therapy. A group of researchers led by Janet Bevalas that includes Peter de Jong, Harry Korman, Sara Smock, Adam Froerer, Christine Tomori, and Sara Healing are using microanalysis to study therapeutic communication as a mechanism of change in solution-focused brief therapy. Their work includes the following types of research: (1) process research (for example, microanalysis of communication within therapy sessions) that assesses congruence between theory and practice and reveals similarities and differences in therapeutic approaches (De Jong & Bavelas, 2009; Froerer & Smock, 2009; Tomori & Bavelas, 2007), and the communication process such as formulation and grounding sequences in treatment (Bavelas, 2011); (2) basic experiments in a laboratory setting that provide evidence supporting fundamental assumptions such as co-construction in the treatment process (for example, Bavelas et al., 2000; 2002); and (3) experiments on therapeutic techniques, which test key techniques such as the miracle question in the laboratory using non-therapeutic tasks and populations (Healing & Bavelas, 2009). Such research program illuminates important mechanisms of change and other process issues involved in the solution-focused treatment process. In addition, microanalysis in itself introduces novel research methodologies in understanding the therapeutic processes that may be relevant to other types of social work treatment approaches.

The Future

Each social work treatment approach makes different assumptions about how problems of living should be approached as well as how change happens. Recognizing the power of therapeutic dialogues and the potentially harmful effects of a pathology-based and deficits-based perspective in sustaining the problem and disempowering clients, solution-focused brief therapy deliberately adopts the language and symbols of "solution and strengths" and fully embraces clients' voices and resources in the search for effective solutions. While doing so, it is important to evaluate the effectiveness of solution-focused brief therapy and carefully examine the associated mechanisms and processes that contribute to its effectiveness so that treatment is based on an informed position in addition to ethical choices or theoretical preferences (Lee, 2007).

Another challenge in the development of solution-focused brief therapy is the dilemma between fidelity adherence versus open flow. Solution-focused brief therapy emphasizes itself as a way of thinking and not just a set of techniques (de Shazer, 1985). The treatment process is a co-constructive process between the solution-focused practitioner and the client. Consequently, there are questions about how much the professional body, that is, SFBTA, can and should ensure strict fidelity to an "established" treatment protocol. If this is not feasible or desirable, how can we develop some structure (such as a national network of basic solution-focused brief therapy training), establish defining parameters, or the minimum amount of SF to ensure the adherence to the model (personal communication with Gallagher & Nelson, 2012).

Despite these challenges, helping professionals around the globe are practicing solution-focused brief therapy in a variety of settings with diverse client groups in beneficial ways.

REFERENCES

Bateson, G. (1972). *Steps to an ecology of mind*. New York: Ballantine Books.

Bateson, G. (1979). *Mind and nature: A necessary unity*. New York: Dutton.

Bavelas, J. (2011). From the lab to the therapy room. Microanalysis, co-construction, and solution-focused therapy. In C. Franklin, T. Trepper, W. J. Gingerich, & E. McCollum (Eds.), *Solution-focused Brief Therapy: From Practice to Evidence-Informed Practice* (pp. 144–162). Oxford: Oxford University Press.

Bavelas, J. B., Coates, L., & Johnson, T. (2000). Listeners as co-narrators. *Journal of Personality and Social Psychology, 79*, 941–952.

Bavelas, J. B., Coates, L., & Johnson, T. (2002). Listener responses as a collaborative process: The role of gaze. *Journal of Communication, 52*, 566–580.

Bavelas, J. B., McGee, D., Phillips, B., & Routledge, R. (2000). Microanalysis of communication in psychotherapy. *Human Systems, 11*, 47–66.

Becvar, D. S., & Becvar, R. J. (2012). *Family Therapy, A systematic integration* (8th ed.): Boston, MA: Allyn and Bacon.

Berg, I. K. (1994). *Family-based services: A solution-focused approach*. New York: W. W. Norton.

Berg, I. K., & Kelly, S. (2000). *Building solutions in child protective services*. New York: W. W. Norton.

Berg, I. K. & Miller, S. (1992). *Working with the problem drinker: A solution-focused approach*. New York: W. W. Norton & Co.

Berg, I. K. & Reuss, N. (1998). *Solutions step by step: A substance abuse treatment manual*. NY: W. W. Norton.

Berg, I. K., & Steiner, T. (2003). *Children's solution work*. New York: W. W. Norton.

Berg, I. K., & Szabo, P. (2005). *Brief coaching for lasting solutions*. New York: W. W. Norton.

Berg, P. L., & Luckmann, T. (1966). *The social construction of reality: A treatise in the sociology of knowledge*. New York: Doubleday.

Cade, B., & O'Hanlon, W. (1993). *A brief guide to brief therapy*. New York: W. W. Norton.

Corcoran, J., & Pillai, V. (2009). A Review of the Research on Solution-Focused Therapy. *British Journal Of Social Work, 39*(2), 234–242.

De Jong, P., Bavelas, J. (2009). *The role of formulations in co-constructing meanings in cognitive-behavioral therapy, motivational interviewing, and solution-focused brief therapy*. Presentation at 2009 Conference on Solution-Focused Practices, Solution-Focused Brief Therapy Association, November 4–9, Albany, New York.

De Jong, P., & Berg, I. K. (2013). *Interviewing for solutions*. (4th Ed.). Belmont, CA: Brooks/Cole.

de Shazer, S. (1985). *Keys to solutions in brief therapy*. New York: W. W. Norton.

de Shazer, S. (1988). *Clues: Investigating solutions in brief therapy*. New York: W. W. Norton.

de Shazer, S. (1991). *Putting difference to work*. New York: W. W. Norton.

de Shazer, S. (1994). *Words were originally magic*. New York: W. W. Norton.

de Shazer, S., & Berg, I. K. (1997). What works? Remarks on research aspects of solution focused brief therapy. *Journal of Family Therapy, 19*, 121–124.

de Shazer, S., & Molnar, A. (1984). Four useful interventions in brief family therapy. *Journal of Marital and Family Therapy, 10*, 297–304.

Erickson, M. (1985a). *Conversations with Milton H. Erickson, Volume I: Changing Individuals*, edited by Jay Haley. New York: W. W. Norton.

Erickson, M. (1985b). *Conversations with Milton H. Erickson, Volume I: Changing couples*, edited by Jay Haley. New York: W. W. Norton.

Fiske, H. (2008). *Hope in action: Solution-focused conversations about suicide*. New York: Routledge.

Franklin, C., & Gerlach, B. (2007). Clinical applications of solution-focused brief therapy in public schools. In T. S. Nelson & F.N. Thomas (Eds.), *Handbook of solution-focused brief therapy: Clinical applications* (pp. 168–169). Philadelphia: Haworth Press.

Franklin, C., & Jordan, C. (1998). *Family practice: Brief systems methods for social work*. Pacific Cove, CA: Brooks/Cole.

Franklin, C., Trepper, T. S., Gingerich, W. J., McCullum, E. E. (Eds.). (2012), *Solution-focused brief therapy: A handbook of evidence-based practice*. New York: Oxford University Press.

Froerer, A., & Smock, S. (2009). *Microanalysis of solution-focused formulations*. Presentation at 2009 Conference on Solution-Focused Practices, Solution-Focused Brief Therapy Association, November 4–9, Albany, New York.

Gallagher, D. & Nelson, T. (2012) Personal communication at Celebrating Solutions: 2012 SRBTA Conference, November 14–18, Minneapolis, MN.

Gingerich, W., & Eisengart, S. (2000). Solution-focused brief therapy: A review of outcome research. *Family Process*, 39, 477–496.

Greene, G. J., Lee, M. Y., Mentzer, R., Pinnell, S., Niles, D. (1998). Miracles, dreams, and empowerment: A brief practice note. *Families in Society*, 79, 395–399.

Haley, J. (1973). *Uncommon therapy: The psychiatric techniques of Milton H. Erickson, M. D.* New York: W. W. Norton.

Healing, S., & Bavelas, J. (2009). *An Experimental Study of Mechanisms of Change: Effects of Questioning on Attributions and Performance*. Unpublished manuscript.

Hendon, J. (2008). *Preventing suicide: The solution focused approach*. Hoboken, NJ: John Wiley.

Karls, J. M. (2009). Person-in-environment system. In A. R. Roberts (Eds.), *Social workers' desk reference*, 2nd ed. (pp. 371–375). New York: Oxford University Press.

Keeney, B. P., & Thomas, F. N. (1986). Cybernetic foundations of family therapy. In Piercy, F. P., Sprenkle, D. H. (Eds.)., *Family therapy sourcebook* (pp. 262–287). New York: Guilford Press.

Kelly, M. S., Kim, J. S., & Franklin, C. (2008). *Solution-focused brief therapy in schools: A 360-degree view of the research and practice principles*. New York: Oxford University Press.

Kim, J. S. (2008). Examining the effectiveness of solution-focused brief therapy: A meta-analysis. *Research on Social Work Practice*, 18, 107–116.

Kim, J. S. (2013). *Solution-focused brief therapy: A multicultural approach to working with minority clients*. Thousand Oaks, CA: Sage.

Knekt, P., Lindfors, O., et al. (2008a). "Randomized trial on the effectiveness of long-term and short-term psychodynamic psychotherapy and solution-focused brief therapy on psychiatric symptoms during a 3-year follow-up." *Psychological Medicine*, 38, 689–703.

Knekt, P., O. Lindfors, et al. (2008b). "Effectiveness of short-term and long-term psychotherapy on work ability and functional capacity: A randomized clinical trail on depressive and anxiety disorders." *Journal of Affective Disorders*, 107, 95–106.

Lee, M. Y. (2007). Discovering strengths and competencies in female domestic violence survivors: An application of Roberts' continuum of the duration and severity of woman battering. *Brief Treatment and Crisis Intervention*, 7, 102–114.

Lee, M. Y. (2003). A solution-focused approach to cross-cultural clinical social work practice: Utilizing cultural strengths. *Families in Society*, 84, 385–395.

Lee., M. Y. (2011). Solution-focused theory. In Turner, F. J. (Eds.). *Social work treatment*, 5th Ed, *(pp. 460–476)*. New York: Oxford University Press.

Lee, M. Y. & Ely, C. (2013). Effective intervening with students from single-parent families and their parents. In Franklin, C., Harris, M., & Allen-Meares, P. (Eds), *The School Services Sourcebook: A guide for School-Based professionals*, 2nd Ed. (chapter 51) New York: Oxford University Press.

Lee, M. Y., Sebold, J., Uken, A. (2003). *Solution-focused treatment with domestic violence offenders: Accountability for change*. New York: Oxford University Press.

Lee., M. Y., Uken. A., Sebold, J. (2007). Role of Self-Determined Goals in Predicting Recidivism in Domestic Violence Offenders. *Research on Social Work Practice*, 17, 30–41.

Lee, M. Y., Uken, A., & Sebold, J. (2012). Solution-focused model with court mandated, domestic violence offenders. In C. Franklin, T. Trepper, W. J. Gingerich, & E. McCollum (Eds.), *Solution-focused Brief Therapy: From Practice to Evidence-Informed Practice* (chapter 11, pp. 165–182). New York: Oxford University Press.

Lueger, G., & Korn, H-P. (Eds.) (2006). *Solution focused management*. München, Mering: Rainer Hampp Verlag.

Macdonald, A. J. (2007). Applying solution-focused brief therapy to mental health practice. In T. S. Nelson & F. N. Thomas (Eds.), *Handbook of solution-focused brief therapy: Clinical applications* (pp. 267–294). Philadelphia: Haworth Press.

Metcalf, L. (2008). *A field guide to counseling toward solutions*. San Francisco: Jossey-Bass.

Molnar, A. & de Shazer, S. (1987). Solution focused therapy: Toward the identification of therapeutic tasks. *Journal of Marital and Family Therapy*, 13(4), 349–358.

National Association of Social Workers 1999. *The NASW Code of Ethics*. Washington, DC: NASW.

Neimeyer, R. A., & Mahoney, M. J. (1993). *Constructivism in psychotherapy*. Washington, DC: American Psychological Association.

Nelson, T. S. & Thomas, F. N. (Eds.) (2007), *Handbook of solution-focused brief therapy: Clinical applications*. Philadelphia, PTH: Haworth Press.

O'Connell, B., & Palmer, S. (2003). *Solution focused therapy: A handbook for health care professionals*. London: Sage.

O'Hanlon, W., & Wilk, J. (1987). *Shifting contexts: The generation of effective psychotherapy.* New York: Guilford Press.

Rappaport, J. (1985). The power of empowerment language. *Social Policy, Fall, 16,* 15–21.

Rees, S. (1998). Empowerment of youth. In L. M. Gutierrez, R. J. Parsons, & E. O. Cox (Eds.), *Empowerment in social work practice: A sourcebook* (pp. 130–145). Pacific Grove, CA: Brooks/Cole.

Reuss, N. H. (1997). The nightmare question: Problem-talk in solution-focused brief therapy with alcoholics and their families. *Journal of Family Psychotherapy, 8(4),* 71–76.

Rosen, H., & Kuehlwein, K. T. (Eds.) (1996). *Constructing realities: Meaning-making perspectives for psychosolution-focused practitioners.* San Francisco: Jossey-Bass Publishers.

Saleebey, D. (2009). *Strengths perspective in social work practice,* 5th ed. Boston, MA: Allyn & Bacon.

Selekman, M. (1993). *Pathways to change: Brief therapy solutions with difficult adolescents.* New York: Guilford Press.

Selekman, M. (1997). *Solution-focused brief therapy with children.* New York: Guilford Press.

Smock, S. A., Trepper, T. S., et al. (2008). "Solution-focused group therapy for level 1 substance abusers." *Journal of Marital & Family Therapy, 34,* 107–120.

Szabo, P. & Meier, D. (2009). *Coaching plain & simple: Solution-focused brief coaching essentials.* New York: W. W. Norton.

Taylor, L. (2012). The lemon question: Pride as a useful resource in solution-focused interviewing. Presented at Celebrating Solutions: 2012 SRBTA Conference, November 14–18. Minneapolis, MN.

Tomori, C., & Bavelas, J. B. (2007). Using microanalysis of communication to compare solution-focused and client-centered therapies. *Journal of Family Psychotherapy, 18,* 25–43.

Trepper, T. S., McCollum, E. E., De Jong, P., Korman, H., Gingerich, W., & Franklin, C. (2010). *Solution focused therapy treatment manual for working with individuals.* SFBTA: Research Committee of the Solution Focused Brief Therapy Association. Retrieved from http://www.sfbta.org/researchDownloads.html

Triantafillou, N. (1997). A solution-focused approach to mental health supervision. *Journal of Systemic Therapies, 16,* 305–328.

Turner, A. (2007). Thinking and practicing beyond the therapy room: solution-focused brief therapy, trauma, and child protection. In T. S. Nelson & F.N. Thomas (Eds.), *Handbook of solution-focused brief therapy: Clinical applications* (pp. 295–314). Philadelphia: Haworth Press.

Uken, A., Lee, M. Y., & Sebold, J. (2013). The Plumas poject: Solution-focused treatment of domestic violence offenders. In P. DeJong & I. K. Berg, *Interviewing for solutions,* 4th Ed. (pp. 333–345). Belmont, CA: Brooks/Cole.

Walter, J., & Peller, J. (1992). *Becoming solution-focused in brief therapy.* New York: Brunner/Mazel.

Walker, L. & Hayashi, L. (June 2009). Pono Kaulike: Reducing violence with restorative justice and solution-focused approaches. *Federal Probation Journal, 73*(1), 23–27.

Watzlawick, P., Weakland, J. H., & Fisch, R. (1974). *Change: Principles of problem formulation and problem resolution.* New York: W. W. Norton.

Wheeler, J. (2007). Solution-focused supervision. In T. S. Nelson & F.N. Thomas (Eds.), *Handbook of solution-focused brief therapy: Clinical applications* (pp. 343–370). Philadelphia: Haworth Press.

Wittgenstein, L. (1958). *Philosophical investigation,* Translated by G. E. M. Anscombe. New York: Macmillan.

FURTHER READING

European Brief Therapy Association: http://blog.ebta.nu/

Solution-focused Brief Therapy Association: http://www.sfbta.org/

Solution-Focused Brief Therapy Evaluation List: http://www.solutionsdoc.co.uk/sft.html

MO YEE LEE

SPIRITUALITY IN SOCIAL WORK

ABSTRACT: This overview addresses the topic of spirituality in the social work profession, with an emphasis on the American context. Toward that end, the history of the relationship between the profession and spirituality is traced from the profession's origins, through secularization, to the present reemergence of spirituality as a legitimate subject in social work discourse. The diverse ways in which spirituality and religion are conceptualized are reviewed along with rationales that are advanced to support the inclusion of spirituality in social work. The topics of spiritual assessment and intervention are discussed and guidelines for using spiritual interventions in practice settings are presented with a brief review of the research on spiritual interventions from an evidenced-based perspective. Some of the organizations that help support and nurture spirituality in social work are delineated. The article concludes with a summary of prescriptions for advancing spirituality to the next stage in its professional development.

KEY WORDS: religion; secularization; spirituality; spiritual assessment; spiritual interventions

This entry focuses on social work in the United States and, to a lesser extent, social work internationally. However, it also draws on content from medicine, psychology, and other academic disciplines. As illustrated in the following section, the trend toward incorporating spirituality in the social work profession is part of a larger movement that encompasses all of these disciplines. This movement stems from changes in philosophical systems of belief—in essence, societal meta-narratives—that transcend these disciplines. The result is a broad trans-disciplinary movement that affirms the importance of spirituality.

Accordingly, the emergence of spirituality in the social work profession reflects broader historical currents that have affected many academic disciplines. These larger philosophical shifts have shaped how the social work profession has understood spirituality over the course of its history. In turn, this history serves to frame and illuminate the profession's present understanding of spirituality.

History of Spirituality in Social Work

The social work profession grew out of organized religion. Until at least the late 19th century, most social welfare was conducted in a religious setting or was animated by a spiritual impulse. For instance, around 370 AD, the Eastern Orthodox Church established the first major hospital, which was set among houses for the poor, buildings for people with diseases, homes for the elderly, and a special hospital for people with leprosy (Hanawalt & Lindberg, 1994; Koenig, King & Carson, 2012). If the history of welfare work in recorded human history was proportionally chronicled in a 100-page book, only the last 2½ pages would be devoted to the emergence of the social work profession in its present secular form (Marty, 1980). Thus, it is possible to understand the history of the relationship between the profession and spirituality in terms of three eras, which can be summarized under the rubrics of origination, secularization, and reemergence.

ORIGINATION The philosophical basis for social welfare is primarily found in religious teachings. Philosophically, the notion of justice requires the existence of a transcendent moral standard (Smith, 1996). If the norms of a given culture are used to assess the culture, then it is not logically possible to posit that something is unjust. The existing culture cannot provide a frame of reference that allows it to critique itself. Without the ability to, in a certain sense, rise above the status quo, it is impossible to recognize injustice.

To posit that a situation is unjust requires a moral framework that stands apart from the culture. In turn, this framework provides individuals with the ability to assess the present culture in relationship to this framework. It provides an independent position from which to posit what a just society looks like. An independent moral framework provides a lens through which to evaluate a given culture, to determine whether or not a status (poverty) or action (slavery) is just or unjust.

Religious traditions provide such a framework (Stark, 2003). Religions affirm moral standards—formal or informal notions about what is right, just, and fair. In turn, they provide an external framework for assessing a given culture. To the extent that the status quo does not conform to the standard, action is implicitly called for to set things right. Put differently, religions provide a framework for envisioning the world as it should be. It provides a vision of a just society (for example, a society free of poverty or slavery).

Buddhism, Christianity, Hinduism, Islam, and Judaism all provide adherents with a distinctive moral framework for determining just and unjust situations. Although different religions affirm different notions of justice, there is wide agreement across faith traditions that poverty and suffering represent deviations from what ought to be. Consequently, religions typically affirm the moral importance of efforts to address such concerns. In Islam, for instance, one of the five pillars of the faith is the zakat, in which a percentage of one's accumulated wealth and assets—usually 2.5% each year—is given to charity to address economic inequalities and to provide for the general welfare (Crabtree, Husain & Spalek, 2008).

Since the philosophical basis for social welfare is derived from religion, it is unsurprising that the earliest forms of organized social work were developed by spiritually motivated individuals in religious settings (Popple & Leighninger, 2011). Catholics, Jews, Muslims, and other religious believers have been providing assistance to disenfranchised people for centuries. As societies changed, new methods of service delivery were continually developed and implemented which, during a certain epoch, led to the creation of the social work profession.

In the United States, the roots of organized social work can be largely traced to the work of evangelical Christians in the second half of the 19th century (Magnuson, 1977; Smith, 1957). As industrialization spawned new problems, such as widespread urban poverty, new and more systematic approaches were needed to address these emerging issues. Accordingly, evangelical Christians, who were prominent societal actors during this era, led the way in developing new methods to deal with these problems. Included among these were innovations such as charity organization societies (COS), settlement houses, and organizational innovations such as foster care.

The first COS in the United States emerged in Philadelphia before the Civil War. By 1851, the city had been divided into sections that were assigned to

5,000 poverty relief workers, representing most of the 160 church-sponsored and 40 other charitable societies in Philadelphia. Through this systematic approach, assistance could be provided to virtually every family struggling with poverty in the city. In 1850, Phoebe Palmer founded what may be the first settlement house in the nation, the Five Points Mission in urban New York City. Emphasizing environmental factors in poverty, the Five Points Mission and House of Industry provided food, clothing, shelter, and employment. In 1853, Charles Loring Brace founded the Children's Aid Society in New York City, as an alternative to sending orphaned children to institutions which were often overcrowded, impersonal, and ineffective in meeting the developmental needs of children. Through this Society, essentially the first foster care agency in the nation, children were placed with families in the Midwest.

These three movements—the COS, settlement houses, and a broader movement that emphasized the development of institutions to deal with social problems—are widely considered to have provided the foundation for the social work profession as it presently exists in the United States. All of these movements expanded rapidly in the late 19th century, aided by efforts by Catholics and others who shared the same basic concern to alleviate human suffering. In turn, this growth led to the emergence of a distinct professional discourse. All three of these foundational pillars, however, grew out of the Christian church. In this sense, the church gave birth to the present day social work profession (Popple & Leighninger, 2011).

SECULARIZATION Despite the religious origination of social work, the profession experienced a rapid secularization process. Beginning in the late 19th century and continuing throughout the majority of the 20th century, religious and spiritual content was progressively eliminated from the profession's discourse. By the middle of the 20th century, the profession had been largely secularized.

The relatively rapid transformation of the profession was part of a larger trend stemming from the acceptance of modernism among cultural elites. Although many factors contributed to the development of modernism, the Enlightenment, which originated in 18th-century continental Europe, is widely considered to be the driving force behind modernism. A central tenet of the modernist meta-narrative is the privileging of human rationality over other ways of knowing (Gellner, 1992). Enlightenment thinkers rejected transcendent perspectives, such as Christianity, in favor of the notion of objective human reason. The application of rigorous, unbiased human logic was posited to lead to richer and more productive forms of human existence.

As modernist notions of reality were increasingly accepted across academic disciplines, secular values came to dominate academic discourse (Smith, 2003). In each discipline, the process of secularization was somewhat different. For instance, in social work, the desire to be viewed by other, more prestigious, academic disciplines as a genuine profession helped accentuate the rejection of religious perspectives in favor of secular perspectives (Holloway & Moss, 2010). Nevertheless, while the route toward secularization differed, the secular narrative affirmed by modernism was adopted across academic disciplines.

The affirmation of the secular narrative was apparent throughout the helping professions. Although neglect of religion was common, in many cases leading figures expressed direct animosity toward religion. Included among these were such influential individuals as Sigmund Freud and Albert Ellis.

Freud, the father of psychoanalysis, is perhaps the most influential person in the history of modern therapy. In *The Future of an Illusion*, Freud (1927/1964) posited that religion represents a form of "obsessional neurosis" or psychopathology. Ellis is widely viewed as founder of the modern cognitive behavior therapy (CBT) movement. In *The Case Against Religion*, Ellis (1980) argued that religion is a form of "emotional illness" that creates and maintains "neuroses and psychoses." In short, devout spirituality was framed as a form of mental illness that helping professionals should actively attempt to discourage.

These trends were also evident in social work. In a seminal study, Cnaan and colleagues (1999) examined 35,000 abstracts listed in Social Work Abstracts, 1,500 papers presented at five Annual Program Meetings (APMs) of the Council on Social Work Education (CSWE), 50 social welfare course outlines posted at two APMs, 20 widely used social work textbooks on social policy and social welfare history, and all editions of the *Social Work Yearbook* and the *Encyclopedia of Social Work*. In every content area, analysis revealed that religion received little or no mention. The efforts of spiritually animated individuals to assist people in need were either ignored or delegitimized.

To be clear, Christian organizations such as Catholic Charities and the Salvation Army continued to provide services to the poor and disenfranchised during this era. Similarly, some social work programs existed in Catholic, evangelical Christian, and Jewish universities. Through more informal mechanisms, American Indians, Muslims, and other religious groups continued to offer assistance to people in need. At best, however, these actors operated at the margins of the profession. The professional mainstream showed little interest in religion or spirituality for the better part of the last century.

REEMERGENCE The late 20th century was characterized by a renewed interest in spirituality in the social work profession that has carried on into the present. This interest was not confined to social work, but transcends the social sciences. As was the case with secularization, broad philosophical influences provided the foundation for this shift. More specifically, the advent of postmodernism created philosophical space for spirituality in academic discourse.

Beginning in the mid-20th century, postmodernism has increasingly challenged modernism as the intellectual dominant worldview among cultural elites in Western societies. Postmodernists posit that the events of the past century have undermined confidence in the notion of objective human reason (Lyotard, 1979/1984). The human reason that Enlightenment thinkers hypothesized would lead to the development of a secular, certain, universally applicable knowledge that would enhance humanity has not produced the promised results. Rather, it produced value-informed narratives that reflected the interests of those with power. Instead of the salutary benefits posited by Enlightenment thinkers, the application of secular human reason led to the creation of destructive meta-narratives such as Marxism, National Socialism or Nazism, and the French Revolution's reign of terror (Gellner, 1992). Accordingly, the Enlightenment project is no longer intellectually creditable from the vantage points of postmodernists.

Although the fundamental principles of postmodernism are still in the process of being negotiated, a number of suppositions serve to demarcate post-modernism as a distinct worldview. Among these is the de-centering of human rationality in favor of a plurality of ways of knowing. Rather than a single, objective material reality, multiple realities exist, incorporating both material and spiritual dimensions. Human relationships and subjectivity are emphasized.

The acceptance of the postmodern worldview has legitimized the topic of spirituality in academic discourse. In social work, interest in spirituality has increased dramatically since the 1980s (Canda & Furman, 2010). A number of social work programs provide specialized courses in spirituality and religion and an even greater number incorporate content on spirituality into their curricula. A few programs offer certificates and/or focused training in spirituality. CSWE's APM has a specialized track dedicated to spirituality and another dedicated to one specific religion: Islam and Muslims. More recently, CSWE convened a Religion and Spirituality Work Group in 2011 to promote ethical and effective practice in the area of spirituality and religion. Numerous books and articles on spirituality have appeared in the literature and prominent mainstream social work journals have devoted special issues to the topic.

Indeed, perhaps the best indicator of the reemergence of spirituality as a legitimate topic in academic discourse is the amount of content devoted to this subject in the peer-reviewed literature. Figure 1 depicts the results of a key word search (spirit* or religi*) of peer reviewed journals in Social Services Abstracts. As can be seen, the number of publications addressing spirituality and religion has increased exponentially over the last few decades. Beginning from a total of 13 articles in the 1950s, this increased to 48 in the 1960s, to 140 in the 1970s, to 337 in the 1980s, to 922 in the 1990s, and 2,937 articles in 2000s. As these

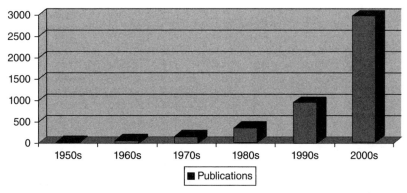

FIGURE 1 Number of peer-reviewed journal publications on spirituality and/or religion in Social Services Abstracts by decade.

data indicate, interest in spirituality has grown exponentially over the course of the past two decades.

In spite of these developments, spirituality remains controversial in some circles of the profession. Echoing Freud and Ellis, some individuals have continued to argue in favor of excluding spiritual perspectives, especially those of underrepresented groups such as evangelical Christians. The notion of spiritual diversity has been a particular source of contention. Some are willing to accept the inclusion of spiritual perspectives into professional discourse, but only those perspectives that are consistent with the values of the dominant secular narrative. In response, others have argued that the profession should expand its understanding of diversity in the area of spirituality—in the same way it has done with race, gender, ethnicity, and sexual orientation in the past—so the profession reflects the demographics of the increasingly multicultural society it is called to serve. These various tensions also animate conceptualizations of spirituality and religion, as well as understandings of the relationship between these two constructs.

Definitions

Traditionally, spirituality has been understood as a dimension within religion. In other words, religion was viewed as the broader, more encompassing concept. Spirituality referred to a subset of individuals who were deeply committed to the precepts of their religious tradition. New, more postmodern forms of spirituality, such as the syncretistic spirituality movement or the New Age movement, are viewed as representing new religions.

In keeping with this understanding, international human rights protocols typically mention religion. For example, the United Nations' (1948/1998) Universal Declaration of Human Rights repeatedly mentions religion as a human right that should be protected. Conversely, spirituality is not mentioned. Rather, it is implicitly incorporated into the wider concept of religion.

Reflecting the ascendance of postmodernism, this ordering is frequently reversed in recent scholarship on spirituality and religion. Religion is understood to be one venue in which spirituality is expressed. In other words, spirituality is viewed as the broader, more encompassing concept. Postmodern forms of spirituality are often viewed as being distinct from religion.

Although no consensus has emerged regarding the relationship between spirituality and religion, fairly wide agreement exists that they are overlapping but distinct constructs (Derezotes, 2006). Each construct is also widely understood to be multi-dimensional. In other words, both spirituality and religion are complex entities comprised of different, intertwined components.

Generally speaking, spirituality is defined as an individually oriented construct, while religion is defined as a socially oriented construct. More specifically, spirituality tends to be conceptualized in more individualistic, subjective, and experiential terms. In addition, spirituality is frequently posited to incorporate reference to God, the transcendent, or the divine. Conversely, religion tends to be conceptualized in communal, organizational, or structural terms. In addition, religion is often understood to be related to, or mediates, spirituality.

Beyond this very general framework, little agreement exists. A wide variety of definitions has appeared in the social work literature. Spirituality, in particular, has been conceptualized diversely. For example, spirituality has been defined as an individual's relationship with someone/something beyond the individual, the human search for meaning and purpose, and as a dimension of human personality/development. As implicitly reflected in these definitions, some scholars conceptualize spirituality as a unique aspect of human experience that is experienced by some individuals. Others define it as a universal dimension of human experience that is experienced by everyone (Crisp, 2010).

The lack of agreement, however, has not hindered the emergence of spirituality as a legitimate topic in the profession. Indeed, in many ways it has helped to advance the profession's still somewhat tentative embrace of the concept. Regardless of the philosophical influences that animate various definitions, the respective scholars using these various definitions believe in their validity. In turn, arguments are marshaled in favor of including spirituality—variously understood—as an important aspect of social work's professional conversation.

Rationales for Including Spirituality in Social Work Practice

At least five different rationales are commonly advanced to support the inclusion of spirituality in social work. These rationales are related to ethical standards, client self-determination, spiritual strengths, worldview knowledge, and policy requirements. Different authors articulate these rationales in different ways. Regardless of their specific formulation, these concepts are widely cited to support the importance of incorporating spirituality as a legitimate issue in social work practice.

It should be noted that these five rationales are highly intertwined and tend to overlap one another. For instance, respect for client self-determination is an important ethical standard or principle. As such, these rationales serve to reinforce one another in providing a philosophical foundation for recognizing spirituality in social work.

ETHICAL STANDARDS Professional ethics represent one reason why social workers should attend to spirituality. The National Association of Social Workers (NASW) *Code of Ethics* (2008) notes, "professional ethics are at the core of social work." Ethics are at the center of the profession. Social work can be seen as emanating from, or driven by, professional ethics.

Professional ethics codes have many purposes. A primary goal, however, is to provide standards that guide professional conduct. As the NASW *Code of Ethics* states, the *Code* sets forth certain values, principles, and standards to guide social workers' conduct. It enumerates specific ethical standards that should inform and direct social work conduct.

The NASW *Code of Ethics* refers to religion in numerous locations, either directly or indirectly. Spirituality is not explicitly mentioned. In this sense, the NASW *Code of Ethics* implicitly reflects the traditional understanding of religion being a broader, more encompassing construct than spirituality.

In the area of cultural competence and social diversity, the *Code* instructs social workers to obtain education about and to seek to understand the nature of diversity and oppression regarding religion (1.05c). When communicating with clients and colleagues, social workers should avoid unwarranted negative criticism, such as demeaning religious comments (2.01b). In a related standard, social workers are enjoined not to practice, condone, facilitate, or collaborate with any form of religious discrimination (4.02). In addition to these more micro-oriented standards, the *Code* also mentions religion in a macro context. For example, in the area of social and political action, social workers are called to prevent and eliminate religious discrimination.

As these ethical standards imply, social workers have an ethical responsibility to address spirituality. This includes both their work with individual clients and their efforts to promote a more equitable and just society. Fidelity to these ethical standards requires social workers to, for instance, fight against religious discrimination.

It is important to note that the ethical standards articulated in the NASW *Code of Ethics* are not unique to social work in the United States. The International Federation of Social Workers' (2004) Statement of Ethical Principles also mentions spirituality. More specifically, social workers are called to uphold and defend each person's spiritual integrity and well-being (4.1). In the area of social justice, social workers have a responsibility to challenge discrimination that stems from people's spiritual beliefs (4.2.1). The Statement also emphasizes the importance of advocating for the human rights articulated in international protocols, such as the United Nation's (1948/1998) Universal Declaration of Human Rights.

The Universal Declaration mentions religion in a number of places. For example, it prohibits religious discrimination (Art. 2, 16). Perhaps more importantly, however, the Declaration also lists religious freedom as a basic human right and then maps the terrain of this right. Article 18 stipulates that everyone has the right to change one's religion, and the right to manifest one's religion in teaching, practice, worship, and observance. This includes the right to manifest one's belief in private or public space, either alone or in community with others.

It is also worth noting that social work is not unique in terms of its ethical stipulations regarding spirituality. Many professional ethics codes in the helping professions mention spirituality or religion in a similar manner (Miller, 2003). This professional agreement serves to underscore the ethical importance of attending to spirituality in professional practice. To be congruent with the vision of practice depicted in professional ethics codes, social workers must address spirituality in their practice of social work.

CLIENT SELF-DETERMINATION A second rationale for addressing spirituality is related to client autonomy. Self-determination is an important social work value. For instance, the NASW *Code of Ethics* calls social workers to respect and promote clients' right to self-determination (1.02).

The salience of client preference is underscored by the evidence-based practice movement, which emphasizes the importance of incorporating clients' preferences into the therapeutic dialogue. Effective therapy is predicated on the creation of a non-coercive atmosphere in which clients' desires are respected. Tailoring therapy to incorporate clients' desires leads to better outcomes.

Spirituality is a salient life dimension for many people. According to Gallup data, approximately 90% of the general population in the United States believes in God or a universal spirit (Newport, 2012).

Forty-one percent are very religious and 28% are moderately religious. Although substantial variation exists among nations, at the global level, interest in spirituality and religion is increasing (Grim & Finke, 2010).

Many of these individuals want their spiritual values to be taken into account during service provision. To be clear, not everyone for whom spirituality is important wants to have their spiritual values integrated into service provision. Many, however, do. It is also important to note that spirituality tends to be even more salient among traditionally disenfranchised populations. For example, African Americans, Latinos, women, people who are poor, and the elderly tend to report disproportionately higher levels of spirituality (Newport, 2012). For instance, approximately 93% of older African Americans report that prayer is "very important" in dealing with stressful situations (Taylor, Chatters & Jackson, 2007). While social work is committed to assisting all people, it has a special ethical commitment to attend to the needs of people who are vulnerable, oppressed, and living in poverty (NASW Code of Ethics, 2008).

In short, numerous clients want to have their spiritual beliefs and practices incorporated into counseling and other forms of service provision. Social workers have an ethical obligation to respect clients' desires in this area. Integrating clients' spiritual values into service provision demonstrates respect for client self-determination, which, in turn, fosters better clinical outcomes.

SPIRITUAL STRENGTHS A third rationale for addressing spirituality pertains to clients' spiritual assets. Identifying and operationalizing assets, resources, and strengths is a central component of social work practice. Determining "what works" in clients' lives typically plays a foundational role in ameliorating problems, facilitating effective coping, and promoting health and wellness.

In addition to being a key component of practice, the importance of strengths is also highlighted in the NASW Code of Ethics. Social workers are called to recognize the strengths that exist in all cultures (1.05a). Once identified, these assets can be marshaled to help clients overcome the challenges they face.

Spirituality is often an important strength in clients' lives. A relatively large and expanding body of research exists on this topic. The modernist hypothesis advanced by individuals such as Freud (1964 /1927) and Ellis (1980)—that spirituality is linked to mental illness—is no longer tenable. In aggregate,

higher levels of spirituality are associated with higher levels of mental and physical health (Koenig et al., 2012). The breadth of the research is extensive. Literally thousands of studies indicate that spirituality is related to a wide variety of positive health outcomes.

For example, spirituality is positively associated with quality of life (typically when facing major life-challenges), psychological well-being (for example, happiness, joy, life satisfaction), meaning and purpose, internal sense of control, social support, self-esteem, hope, optimism, and less loneliness. It is also related to positive character traits, such as altruism, forgiveness, and volunteering, as well as social capital, which are commonly understood as social networks that facilitate cooperative and mutually supportive relationships. In terms of personality traits, spirituality is associated with agreeableness, conscientiousness, cooperativeness, in tandem with less risk taking, irresponsibility, hostility, and anger.

Spirituality is inversely related to anxiety, substance abuse, delinquency, crime, and marital instability (for example, spirituality predicts less divorce and separation, spousal abuse, infidelity, and greater commitment to the marriage and martial satisfaction). It is also associated with less depression and faster recovery from depression, lower levels of suicidal ideation, attempts, and completions.

In addition to better mental health outcomes, increased spirituality also predicts better physical health (Koenig et al., 2012). For instance, spirituality predicts less likelihood of Alzheimer's disease and dementia, cancer, heart disease, hypertension, and cerebrovascular disease (stroke). It predicts higher levels of immune functioning, self-rated health, and longevity.

To be clear, the relationship between spirituality and wellness is not universal (Koenig et al., 2012). Some studies report no or an inverse association between spirituality and health. Nevertheless, the state of the present research is such that it is no longer a question about whether or not spirituality is positively linked to health and wellness. Rather, the relationship between spirituality and wellness is so well established that research now tends to focus on understanding the mechanisms that explain the relationship.

One mechanism that tends to activate a spiritual response is major life challenges (Pargament, 2007). The salience of spirituality frequently becomes more significant during times of stress or difficulty, which may help explain why spirituality tends to play a more pronounced role in the lives of traditionally disenfranchised populations. For instance, people often turn to spirituality when coping with general medical illness, chronic pain, cancer, vision problems, HIV/AIDS, caregiving burden, psychiatric illness, bereavement, and end-of-life issues. Individuals wrestling with such problems tend to report that spirituality enhances their ability to cope and adapt.

Social workers often encounter individuals when they are facing major life challenges. To help clients deal with these challenges, they have an ethical obligation to identify all assets that may be relevant to this task. In many cases, spiritual assets can be marshaled to assist clients in ameliorating problems.

WORLDVIEW KNOWLEDGE A fourth rationale is to understand clients' worldviews. Successful practice is largely predicated upon understanding clients' value systems. This is particularly important when working with those from different cultures, who are often hesitant to trust social workers. In such cases, developing some degree of empathetic awareness of the cultural worldview in play is critical to achieving optimal outcomes. This view is echoed in the NASW *Code of Ethics* (2008), which enjoins social workers to develop their knowledge of clients' cultures and to provide culturally competent services that are sensitive to clients' cultural value systems (1.05b).

Interactions that are congruent with clients' value systems typically enhance client buy-in and engender positive outcomes. Knowledge of clients' worldviews helps practitioners to identify assets, respect client autonomy, and build therapeutic rapport. It helps social workers avoid interactions that impair the therapeutic alliance and facilitates the selection of culturally-sensitive interventions that are more likely to be adopted and faithfully implemented.

Spirituality frequently plays a fundamental role in shaping individuals' worldviews. As noted above, spirituality is expressed in particular religions, which tend to engender culturally distinct value systems (Van Hook, Hugen & Aguilar, 2001). These value systems can affect beliefs and practices in many areas of significance to social workers including, for example, perspectives about animals, burial practices, child birth, child care, communication styles, coping practices, death, diet, finances, grieving, healing, health, marital relations, medical care, military participation, recreation, schooling, and wellness.

The United States is among the most religiously diverse nations in the world. As is the case with many other countries, the past few decades has witnessed substantial growth in a variety of culturally distinct traditions in which religion and ethnicity are comingled. Such groups include Asian Muslims, Hispanic Catholics, Indian Hindus, Korean Presbyterians, Latino Pentecostals, Punjabi Sikhs, and Soviet Jews. These groups supplement existing religious subcultures in America, such as evangelical Christians, Latter Day Saints, traditional Catholics, and hundreds of Native tribal groups.

With each of these populations, their cultural values can differ from those affirmed in mainstream discourse. For instance, in many American Indians tribes, mental health cannot be understood apart from the spiritual. Assisting a Native individual wrestling with a mental illness—within the context of a Native worldview—may require incorporating tribally specific spiritual interventions into treatment. In other situations, routine practices may be contraindicated as they conflict with Native spiritual values.

Ignoring the existence of these spiritual values in practice settings impairs service provision (Gardner, 2011). In some cases, the failure to take these values into account can engender negative affect. Accordingly, it is necessary to inquire about clients' spiritual value systems. Learning how clients construct their spiritually animated worldviews assists social workers develop an empathetic understanding of rationales that inform their beliefs and practices. This knowledge allows practitioners to tailor service provision so that it engages, rather than conflicts, with clients' values. In turn, this type of culturally congruent practice leads to better outcomes.

POLICY REQUIREMENTS The final rationale for addressing spirituality is policy requirements. A number of agencies, professional organizations, and accrediting bodies stipulate that service provision should be tailored to incorporate client spirituality. In recognition of the importance of spirituality in practice, these entities explicitly address spirituality in their policy statements.

These policy recommendations serve to guide practice. The situation is analogous to the NASW ethical standards or the human rights of religious nondiscrimination and religious freedom reviewed above. In much the same way that professional ethical standards or the United Nation's Universal Declaration informs practice decisions, the following policies serve to direct conduct.

To assist practitioners interacting with clients, NASW issued a set of Standards for Cultural Competence in Social Work Practice (NASW Standards for Cultural Competence in Social Work Practice, 2001). These standards specifically mention the importance of spirituality and religion in the lives of clients.

The standards also state that the term culture includes ways in which people from various religious backgrounds experience the world around them. Thus, the delivery of culturally competent services incorporates attending to clients' spiritual value systems.

The CSWE Educational Policy and Accreditation Standards (2008) are designed to promote excellence in social work educational programs. These standards explicitly mention spirituality and/or religion three times. The explicit curriculum should include content designed to help future social workers engage religious diversity in practice (EP 2.1.4). Similarly, content regarding human behavior and the social environment should foster understanding of spiritual development (EP 2.1.7). In addition, programs should demonstrate their commitment to religious diversity in their larger educational environment (for example, demographic make-up of its faculty and selection of field education settings) (EP 3.1).

The Joint Commission, formerly known as the Joint Commission on Accreditation of Healthcare Organizations or JCAHO, is the largest health care accrediting body in the United States. It accredits most of the nation's hospitals and thousands of other health care organizations. It recommends that services be tailored to take into account clients' spiritual values. Similarly, at the local level, many agencies provide services that address spirituality as a matter of policy (Canda & Furman, 2010).

These various policies are not limited to organizations in the United States (Furness & Gilligan, 2010). For example, similar recommendations have been enumerated by various organizations in the United Kingdom as well as the World Health Organization (WHO). As an example of the former, the National Institute for Clinical Excellence (2004) recommends practitioners explore clients' spiritual needs and assets. The WHO Expert Committee on Cancer Pain Relief (1990) makes similar recommendations regarding palliative care. WHO grounds these recommendations in the internationally recognized right to religious freedom.

As this grounding implies, these policies are often implemented because various organizations recognize the importance of the rationales discussed above. Professional ethical standards that require non-discrimination when dealing with religion, the internationally recognized human right of religious freedom, the importance of respecting clients' spiritual self-determination, the salient role that spiritual assets can play in helping ameliorate problems, and the critical importance of tailoring services so they are congruent with clients' spiritual value systems are all widely affirmed. In turn, these rationales often form the basis for various policy statements, either explicitly or implicitly. As such, these five rationales are interlinked and mutually reinforcing. Together, they provide a comprehensive foundation for services that address spirituality.

Spiritual Assessment

To tailor service provision to incorporate client spirituality, a spiritual assessment is commonly recommended. Such an assessment involves gathering and synthesizing information about spirituality into a framework that provides the basis for subsequent practice decisions. A spiritual assessment is typically conducted as a part of a larger bio-psycho-social-spiritual evaluation. This type of holistic assessment provides practitioners with a more complete understanding of relevant factors in clients' lived realities.

The assessment focuses on understanding how spirituality informs clients' value systems. Social workers do not attempt to determine the veracity of clients' spiritual beliefs, an endeavor that lies outside the purview of their professional training and risks violating clients' spiritual autonomy. Rather, the aim is to understand how clients' spirituality shapes their worldviews with the goal of tailoring service provision accordingly. For instance, a strengths-oriented practitioner might attempt to understand how various spiritual practices function as assets with an eye toward leveraging those assets to help clients ameliorate problems.

Assessment is typically conceptualized as a two-stage process. Initially, a brief assessment is administered. The fact that this initial assessment entails a minimal time commitment means that it is possible to administer such an assessment to all clients. The purpose of the preliminary assessment is two-fold: (a) to determine the relevance of spirituality to service provision and (b) to ascertain whether a comprehensive assessment is needed.

As alluded to above, the use of a two-stage model helps to conserve practitioners' time for those individuals whose spirituality directly intersects service provision. In some cases, spirituality may be a marginal or non-existent dimension in clients' lives. Alternatively, spirituality may be personally important, but unrelated to service provision. In such instances, a brief assessment is typically sufficient.

A brief assessment also helps to legitimize the topic of spirituality in practice settings. Some clients assume that social workers are secular and/or hostile to spirituality. Such individuals are unlikely to broach the topic with practitioners unless first asked, and even then may exhibit considerable hesitancy in discussing spirituality. An assessment helps meta-communicate that the spiritual dimension of existence plays an important role along with the biological, psychological, and social dimensions.

If the brief assessment suggests the client's spirituality might intersect with service provision, then a comprehensive assessment is administered. A number of comprehensive assessment tools have appeared in the literature, some of which have undergone preliminary validation for use with specific populations, such as American Indians (Hodge & Limb, 2011). Perhaps the most popular approach to assessment is conducting a spiritual history, a process that is analogous to conducting a family history. Other conceptually distinct assessment approaches include spiritual lifemaps, spiritual genograms, spiritual eco-maps, and spiritual ecograms. Each approach is characterized by a certain set of advantages and limitations, allowing practitioners to select an assessment approach that best fits the unique needs of each individual client in a given clinical context.

A comprehensive assessment provides a vehicle to elicit clinically salient information that can be used to promote wellness. For example, medical social workers developing discharge plans might use the information obtained in an assessment to link patients with the spiritual supports needed to process the existential concerns that emerged during hospitalization. Similarly, school social workers might use the information to help a child who is bullied because of her spiritual values. A spiritual assessment also provides practitioners with the necessary knowledge to consider the use of spiritual interventions.

Spiritual Interventions

Spiritual interventions are clinical strategies that incorporate a spiritual dimension as a primary component of the intervention. Research suggests that many social workers use spiritual interventions. According to a number of studies, the majority of NASW affiliated practitioners utilize an array of spiritual interventions in their work with clients (Canda & Furman, 2010; Sheridan, 2009). Research also indicates that many practitioners in the UK and other nations also regularly employ spiritual interventions (Furman & Benson, 2006).

These same studies indicate that most social workers report receiving little, if any, training in spirituality during their educational training. This may be an artifact of the relatively recent emergence of spirituality as a legitimate topic in social work discourse. Nevertheless, concerns have been raised regarding the widespread use of spiritual interventions with minimal training.

GUIDELINES FOR USING SPIRITUAL INTERVENTIONS IN PRACTICE To help practitioners use spiritual interventions in an ethical and effective manner, four guidelines have appeared in the literature (Hodge, 2011). These guidelines, which are drawn from the evidence-based practice movement, can be summarized under the following rubrics: client preference, clinical expertise, cultural competency, and research evaluation. First, client preferences should be respected. Assuming an assessment reveals an interest in utilizing spirituality in clinical situations, the use of possible interventions is explored and informed consent obtained for any intervention selected. Informed consent is understood to be an ongoing process with practitioners monitoring clients throughout the implementation process to ensure that they remain fully supportive of the intervention.

A second factor to consider in the use of spiritual interventions is the practitioner's degree of clinical expertise. Spiritual interventions should typically be used only when sufficient training has been received to ensure that the intervention can be implemented in an ethical and professional manner. Some proficiency with the intervention under consideration is required. Practitioners ought to have some degree of training and experience using a given intervention.

A third consideration is cultural competency. Cultural competency is required to select and implement spiritual interventions within the context of clients' cultures. An intervention that is effective with a mainline Christian client may not be effective with a Hindu client. In order to implement an intervention effectively, practitioners require some knowledge of clients' spiritual value systems.

Finally, the research on spiritual interventions that are relevant to the presenting problem should be evaluated. Interventions should only be used if research suggests they will be effective with a given problem. It is widely recognized that epistemological assumptions influence understandings of what is considered to be good evidence. Nevertheless, some empirical rationale should exist if an intervention is to be considered in a clinical context. In other words, some empirical evidence ought to suggest that the intervention will be effective in addressing the client's presenting problem.

RESEARCH ON SPIRITUAL INTERVENTIONS A limited, but growing, body of research exists on spiritual interventions (Koenig et al., 2012). Using various types of experimental designs, a number of spiritual interventions have been evaluated. Included among these are 12-step programs, Buddhist-based mindfulness, forgiveness therapy, generic spiritual meditation, Hindu-based meditation, mantra-chanting, spiritual teaching, spiritual coping therapy, spiritually-focused therapy, and spiritually modified cognitive behavioral therapy (CBT). In aggregate, the use of these spiritual interventions has yielded generally positive outcomes.

Among the more effective interventions is spiritually modified CBT. In this therapeutic modality, standard CBT treatment protocols are modified with spiritual beliefs and practices drawn from clients' spiritual value systems. The cognitive restructuring strategies and the behavioral assignments are similar to those used in the traditional secular CBT pioneered by Ellis. However, once unproductive beliefs and behaviors are identified, they are replaced with salutary schema and actions that resonate with clients' spiritual values.

Although the evidenced-based practice movement remains controversial in some social work circles, it is notable that spiritually modified CBT meets the criteria for an efficacious treatment in at least one context. Specifically, it is an effective treatment for devout Christians coping with depression. Other outcomes that have been examined include anxiety disorder, bereavement, bipolar disorder, compulsive disorder, neurosis, perfectionism, schizophrenia, and stress. In addition to Christianity, this approach has been used with Buddhism, Taoism, Islam, and a generic form of spirituality. As implied above, outcome research using this modality has typically produced positive results.

Reflecting the broad cross-disciplinary acceptance of spirituality sparked by postmodernism, most of the research on spiritual interventions has been conducted outside the field of social work. Social workers have, however, contributed to the larger empirical knowledge base on spirituality. These contributions have frequently been facilitated by various organizations, networks, and journals.

Spiritually Animated Social Work Organizations

The social work profession is home to a number of spiritually animated organizations. These groups vary in size and reflect the diverse expressions of spirituality within the profession. Accordingly, their foci and purposes vary. Among the more prominent are the North American Association of Christians in Social Work (NACSW) and the Society for Spirituality and Social Work. Many smaller groups exist that also play vital roles including, for example, the Islamic Social Services Association (ISSA) and Integral Social Work network.

The oldest of these various organizations is NACSW, which was established in 1954 in the midst of the secularization era. The mission of this ecumenical organization is to equip its members to integrate Christian faith and professional social work practice. Toward this end, it sponsors annual conventions, provides CEUs, and publishes book as well as a quarterly academic journal—*Social Work & Christianity*.

The Society for Spirituality and Social Work was founded in 1990 by Ed Canda, at the cusp of the postmodern-influenced era that witnessed the accelerating reemergence of spirituality in the profession. The vision of the Society is to create connections and mutual support among social workers of many contrasting spiritual perspectives. It also sponsors an annual conference on spirituality in social work, typically in conjunction with the Canadian Society for Spirituality in Social Work, a sister organization that is oriented to professional social work in Canada.

The Islamic Social Services Association (ISSA)—established in 1999 by a group of Muslim social workers—split into two independent organizations in 2003: one in the U.S. and one in Canada. The founders' vision was to develop a network of Muslims in the human services to address the mental health, family issues, and other social welfare concerns that impact Muslims.

The Integral Social Work network is comprised of social workers interested in the application of Integral Theory to social work. Integral Theory was originally developed by Ken Wilber. Influenced by transpersonal psychology, it is a post-disciplinary meta-framework that incorporates the insights of diverse philosophical systems.

There are many other initiatives housed at various social work programs. For instance, the social work program at the Catholic University of America (CUA) is home to the Center for Spirituality and Social Work, which seeks to increase awareness of the role of both religious and non-religious expressions of spirituality in all aspects of life. CUA has also played an important role in the development of the quarterly academic periodical *The Journal of Religion & Spirituality in Social Work: Social Thought*, another disciplinary social work journal devoted to disseminating scholarship on spirituality.

As implied above, these organizations are not limited to the U.S. In addition to the Canadian groups mentioned above, organizations also exist in other parts of the world. For instance, in the UK, the Social Work Christian Fellowship (SWCF) was founded in 1964. In manner analogous to the other groups listed above, it provides professional and spiritual support to its members through a variety of national and local events around the U.K.

Social workers also participate in a myriad of spiritually animated groups hosted in other disciplines. These various groups, both inside and outside the profession, help support and nurture spirituality in social work. They also help equip social workers to tackle challenges and chart the future directions of the nascent spirituality movement.

Future Directions

The past few decades have witnessed considerable advancement in terms of the profession's acknowledgement and understanding of spirituality. Nevertheless, spirituality is still a relatively new area of academic interest in social work. In keeping with the recent appearance of spirituality in the professional conversation, this emerging movement faces a number of challenges as it seeks to develop and mature.

Many individuals have contributed to the emergence of spirituality as a valid topic in social work discourse. Among those who have played a major role in this process are the following seven individuals. As scholars whose efforts have helped create space for spirituality in social work discourse, they have been asked to share their perceptions on the critical steps required to advance spirituality in social work to the next stage in its professional development. Although articulated by individuals, these prescriptions reflect currents of thought affirmed by many social workers invested in spirituality.

In light of the ongoing problems regarding religious discrimination in the profession, Cnaan (2006) recommends research to assess the magnitude of the problem with the aim of ensuring that the basic human rights of spiritually motivated people are respected in social work. Ai (2006) highlights the need for rigorous, controlled outcome research on spiritual interventions with different religious groups. Drawing from transpersonal psychology, Derezotes (2006) suggests developing a third, spiritual methodology that bridges quantitative and qualitative approaches while simultaneously incorporating transrationale ways of knowing.

Russel (2006) emphasizes the need to integrate spirituality content comprehensively into social work education so that practitioners are prepared to work competently with clients. Furman and Benson (2006) stresses the need for large-scale quantitative and qualitative studies to understand the role of spirituality in direct practice and education, both in America and elsewhere. Graham (2006) proposes increased international collaborations between the Global North and Global South to enrich and diversify understandings of spirituality. Finally, to address the problems spawned by globalization, Canda (2005) calls for the continued growth in professional efforts to nurture appreciation for spiritual diversity in nations around the world.

REFERENCES

Ai, A. L. (2006). Faith matters, empirical research, and professional practice: Current needs and future steps. *Arête*, 30(1), 30–41.

Canda, E. R. (2005). The future of spirituality in social work: The farther reaches of human nurture. *Advances in Social Work*, 6(1), 97–108.

Canda, E. R., & Furman, L. D. (2010). *Spiritual diversity in social work practice: The heart of helping* (2nd ed.). New York, NY: Oxford University Press.

Cnaan, R. A. (2006). Faith in the closet: Reflections of a secular academic. *Arête*, 30(1), 19–29.

Cnaan, R. A., Wineburg, R. J., & Boddie, S. C. (1999). *The newer deal: Social work and religion in partnership*. New York, NY: Columbia University Press.

Crabtree, S. A., Husain, F., & Spalek, B. (2008). *Islam and social work: Debating values, transforming practice*. Bristol, England: Policy Press.

Crisp, B. R. (2010). *Spirituality and social work*. Surrey, England: Ashgate Publishing.

CSWE Educational Policy and Accreditation Standards. (2008). *Educational policy and accreditation standards*. Retrieved from http://www.cswe.org/File.aspx?id=64764

Derezotes, D. S. (2006). Individual consciousness and social responsibility: Spirituality in new-century social work. *Arête*, 30(1), 8–18.

Ellis, A. (1980). *The case against religion: A psychotherapist's view and the case against religiosity*. Austin, TX: American Atheist Press.

Freud, S. (1927/1964). *The future of an illusion, civilization and its discontents and other works* (J. Strachey, Trans.) (Vol. 21). London: Hogarth Press.

Furman, L. D., & Benson, P. W. (2006). Practice and educational considerations: Cross-national perspectives from the United States, the United Kingdom, and Norway. *Arête*, 30(1), 53–62.

Furness, S., & Gilligan, P. (2010). *Religion, belief and social work: Making a difference*. Bristol, UK: Policy Press.

Gardner, F. (2011). *Critical spirituality: A holistic approach to contemporary practice*. Surrey, England: Ashgate Publishing.

Gellner, E. (1992). *Postmodernism, reason and religion*. New York, NY: Routledge.

Graham, J. R. (2006). Spirituality and social work: A call for an international focus of research. *Arête*, 30(1), 63–77.

Grim, B. J., & Finke, R. (2010). *The price of freedom denied: Religious persecution and conflict in the twenty-first century*. New York, NY: Cambridge University Press.

Hanawalt, E. A., & Lindberg, C. (Eds.). (1994). *Through the eye of a needle: Judeo-Christian roots of social welfare.* Lanham, MD: Thomas Jefferson University Press.

Hodge, D. R. (2011). Using spiritual interventions in practice: Developing some guidelines from evidenced-based practice. *Social Work, 56*(2), 149–158.

Hodge, D. R., & Limb, G. E. (2011). Spiritual assessment and Native Americans: Establishing the social validity of a complementary set of assessment tools. *Social Work, 56*(3), 213–223.

Holloway, M., & Moss, B. (2010). *Spirituality and social work.* London, England: Palgrave Macmillan.

IFSW Ethics in Social Work, Statement of Ethical Principles. (2004). Retrieved from http://ifsw.org/policies/statement-of-ethical-principles/

Koenig, H. G., King, D., & Carson, V. B. (2012). *Handbook of religion and health* (2nd ed.). New York, NY: Oxford University Press.

Lyotard, J.-F. (1979/1984). *The postmodern condition: A report on knowledge* (G. Bennington & B. Massumi, Trans.). Minneapolis, MN: University of Minnesota Press.

Magnuson, N. (1977). *Salvation in the slums: Evangelical social work 1865–1920.* Grand Rapids, MI: Baker Book House.

Marty, M. E. (1980). Social service: Godly and godless. *Social Service Review, 54*(4), 463–481.

Miller, G. (2003). *Incorporating spirituality in counseling and psychotherapy.* Hoboken, NJ: John Wiley & Sons.

NASW Code of Ethics. (2008). Retrieved from http://www.socialworkers.org/pubs/code/code.asp

NASW Standards for Cultural Competence in Social Work Practice. (2001). Retrieved from http://www.socialworkers.org/practice/standards/NASWCulturalStandards.pdf

National Institute for Clinical Excellence. (2004). *Improving supportive and palliative care for adults with cancer.* Retrieved from http://www.nice.org.uk/nicemedia/live/10893/28816/28816.pdf

Newport, F. (2012). *God is alive and well: The future of religion in America.* New York, NY: Gallup Press

Pargament, K. I. (2007). *Spiritually integrated psychotherapy: Understanding and addressing the sacred.* New York, NY: Guilford Press.

Popple, P. R., & Leighninger, L. (2011). *Social work, social welfare, and American society* (8th ed.). Boston, MA: Allyn & Bacon.

Russel, R. (2006). Spirituality and social work: Current trends and future directions. *Arête, 30*(1), 42–52.

Sheridan, M. (2009). Ethical issues in the use of spiritually based interventions in social work practice: What we are doing and why. *Journal of Religion and Spirituality in Social Work, 28*(1/2), 99–126.

Smith, C. (Ed.). (1996). *Disruptive religion: The force of faith in social-movement activism.* New York, NY: Routledge.

Smith, C. (2003). *The secular revolution.* Berkeley, CA: University of California Press.

Smith, T. L. (1957). *Revivalism and social reform in mid-nineteenth-century America.* New York, NY: Abingdon Press.

Stark, R. (2003). *For the glory of God: How monotheism led to reformations, science, witch-hunts, and the end of slavery.* Princeton, NJ: Princeton University Press.

Taylor, R. J., Chatters, L. M., & Jackson, J. S. (2007). Religious and spiritual involvement among older African Americans, Caribbean Blacks, and non-Hispanic Whites: Findings from the National Survey of American Life. *Journal of Gerontology: Social Sciences, 62B*(4), S238–S250.

United Nations. (1948/1998). *Universal Declaration of Human Rights.* Retrieved from http://www.un.org/Overview/rights.html

Van Hook, M., Hugen, B., & Aguilar, M. A. (Eds.). (2001). *Spirituality within religious traditions in social work practice.* Pacific Grove, CA: Brooks/Cole.

World Health Organisation (WHO). (1990). *World Health Organisation expert committee: Cancer pain relief and palliative care.* Retrieved from http://whqlibdoc.who.int/trs/WHO_TRS_804.pdf

DAVID R. HODGE

STRENGTHS PERSPECTIVE

ABSTRACT: In social work practice, the strengths perspective has emerged as an alternative to the more common pathology-oriented approach to helping clients. Instead of focusing on clients' problems and deficits, the strengths perspective centers on clients' abilities, talents, and resources. The social worker practicing from this approach concentrates wholly on identifying and eliciting the client's strengths and assets in assisting them with their problems and goals (Saleebey, 2006). The focus here is on the historical development of the strengths perspective, practice techniques, current applications, and philosophical distinctiveness.

KEY WORDS: strengths perspective; strength-based case management; strengths-based practice; strengths

History

Although the profession of social work has a long history of recognizing client strengths, most social workers tend to focus on clients' problems and their dysfunctions (Weick, Rapp, Sullivan, & Kisthardt 1989). However, in 1982, the strengths perspective movement began to emerge from various faculty and staff members at the University of Kansas School of Social Welfare (Brun & Rapp 2001; Rapp, 1998; Saleebey, 1996), which encouraged social workers to shift from this problem-focused approach to helping. At that time, the school was awarded a small grant to provide case management services to people with psychiatric disabilities. Spearheading this project were faculty member Charles Rapp and doctoral student Ronna Chamberlain, who together decided to take a different approach to case management services by having case managers focus on their clients' strengths and clients' abilities to function successfully in the community (Brun & Rapp 2001; Rapp, 1998). Results from this project were successful, and this "strength-based case management" approach was implemented the following year in three other mental health centers in Kansas (Rapp, 1998). From the success of these projects, the strength-based approach started to develop, and other faculty members from KU School of Social Welfare began to apply it to other areas of social work practice.

By the late 1980s, KU faculty member Dennis Saleebey, Dean Ann Weick, and others at the school began developing and writing the conceptual understanding of the strengths perspective (Rapp, 1998; Weick et al., 1989). This effort culminated in the article "A Strengths Perspective for Social Work Practice," published in the journal *Social Work* (Weick et al., 1989) and the book *The Strengths Perspective in Social Work Practice* by Saleebey (1992). These writings aided in spreading the word about the strengths perspective and helped popularize the approach in the social work field. Interest in the strengths perspective continues to grow each year and its application continues to expand into the many different aspects of social work practice.

Definition

The strengths perspective is not so much a theory as it is a way of viewing clients that influences the social worker's approach to helping them. It is a set of principles and ideas that require social workers to help their clients identify and emphasize talents, skills, possibilities, and hopes. Cultural and personal narratives, along with family and community resources, are explored and drawn on to aid the clients (Saleebey, 1996).

The basic assumptions inherent in the strengths perspective address the clients' capabilities. One of the main assumptions is that all individuals possess talents and skills, some of which may be untapped, and that each therefore has the capacity to develop and improve. It is also assumed that growth is more likely to occur in the individual from focusing exclusively on clients' strengths rather than their deficits,. Finally, clients are viewed as equals and expected to help define the problem as well as its possible resolutions (Bell, 2003; Saleebey, 1992; Weick et al., 1989).

Saleebey (2006) recommends looking for clients' strengths and resources not only within individuals but also within their communities. The strengths perspective emphasizes knowledge gained from difficulties and struggles as well as from mentors and teachers. Realized strengths abound in all individuals when thinking about their various talents, virtues, personality traits, and spiritual beliefs. Strengths can be found in personal and cultural stories in addition to the various community resources that may be overlooked.

From these assumptions and ideas, Saleebey (2006) identifies six key principles of the strengths perspective which helped to further define this approach and serve as a guide. These principles include the following:

1. *Individual, family, and community strengths.* Social workers must view their clients as competent and possessing skills and strengths which may not be initially visible. In addition, clients may have family and community resources which need to be explored and utilized.

2. *Illnesses, abuses, and struggles can serve as opportunities.* Clients can not only overcome very difficult situations, but also learn new skills and develop positive protective factors. Individuals exposed to a variety of trauma are not always helpless victims or damaged beyond repair.

3. *Respect client aspirations and hold high expectations.* Too often professional "experts" hinder their clients' potential for growth by viewing clients' identified goals as unrealistic. Instead, social workers need to set high expectations for their clients so that the clients believe they can recover and that their hopes are tangible.

4. *Collaborate with clients.* Playing the role of expert or professional with all the answers does not allow social workers to appreciate their clients' strengths and resources. The strengths perspective emphasizes collaboration between the social worker and the client.

5. *Environmental resources.* Every community, regardless of how impoverished or disadvantaged, has something to offer in terms of knowledge, support, mentorship, and tangible resources. These resources go beyond the general social service agencies in the communities and can serve as a great resource for clients.

6. *Care for each other.* Strength perspective recognizes the importance of community and inclusion of all its members in society and working for social justice. This is built on the basic premise that caring for each other is a basic form of civic participation.

These key principles help guide social work practice from a strengths perspective. It should be noted, however, that these principles continue to evolve and be refined (Saleebey, 2006). What remains constant and central, though, is the strengths perspective's focus on clients' personal assets along with their environmental resources rather than on their pathology and limitations.

Change Philosophy and Techniques

The strengths perspective contends that focusing on clients' pathology and incompetencies hinders clients' progress toward growth. In contrast, underlying the change process in the strengths perspective is the belief that focusing entirely on clients' strengths will help bring about positive changes in the clients (Holmes & Saleebey 1993). This approach to practice provides a perspective from which to work with clients and has not developed specific techniques and skills to the same degree as in other practice models. However, Saleebey (2006) does identify some elements of strengths-based practice, namely, listening for and sharing client strengths, providing words and images that help identify client strengths, and collaboratively discovering client resources in their environment.

Besides Saleebey's (2006) elements of strengths-based practice, Rapp (1998) offers more concrete techniques to help social work case managers apply the strengths perspective framework to their practice. The strength-based case management model was developed in the early 1980s to work in community settings with people suffering from psychiatric disabilities (Rapp, 1998). It includes a set of practice methods based on the six strengths perspective principles described earlier. Rapp and Goscha (2006) identify five categories of practice methods which serve as a function of the strengths model for case management: (a) relationship building, (b) assessing client strengths, (c) planning client goals, (d) acquiring environmental resources, and (e) collaborating continuously with client.

Additionally, a review of the empirical studies on strengths-based case management by Staudt, Howard, and Drake (2001) identified and described how these studies defined strengths-based case management. These common themes included focusing on client strengths, providing services in community, focusing on client identified needs, helping clients acquire resources, letting clients determine goals and interventions.

Another tool to aid social workers practicing from a strengths perspective approach is to utilize a strengths assessment. Brun and Rapp (2001) recommend conducting a strengths assessment early on in the therapeutic work to help identify capabilities and resources the client can utilize. The focus of the assessment should be entirely on clients' abilities and assets, both personally as well as environmentally, which provides the foundation for a strengths-based practice. Information can be gathered on what clients want, what their current situation is like, and available resources and skills (Rapp & Goscha, 2006; Weick et al., 1989).

Current Applications

Over the years, researchers and practitioners have applied the strengths perspective approach to a wide variety of client populations and problems both domestically and internationally. The strengths-based practice model has been studied and applied to substance use (Siegel et al., 1995), community practice (Itzhaky & Bustin, 2002), social policy development (Chapin, 1995), elderly (Chapin & Cox, 2001; Perkins, & Tice 1999; Yip, 2005), domestic violence (Bell, 2003), families (Allison et al., 2003; Early & GlenMaye, 2000; Werrbach, 1996), and adolescents (Yip, 2006).

One of the earliest and most studied applications of the strengths perspective is with case managers working with adults having psychiatric disabilities. Rapp and Goscha (2006) summarize nine studies (Barry, Zeber, Blow, & Valenstein, 2003; Kisthardt, 1993; Macias, Farley, Jackson, & Kinney, 1997; Macias, Kinney, Farley, Jackson, & Vos, 1994; Modrcin, Rapp, & Poertner, 1988; Rapp & Chamberlain, 1985; Rapp & Wintersteen, 1989; Ryan, Sherman, & Judd, 1994; Stanard, 1999) that examined the effectiveness of the strengths-based case management model on people with psychiatric disabilities. Overall the review found support for the strengths-based case management model, but concerns about the lack of rigorous research designs, types of measures used, and small sample sizes warranted caution regarding the conclusiveness of the studies' results (Chamberlain & Rapp 1991; Rapp & Goscha 2006; Staudt et al., 2001).

Despite the popularity of the strengths perspective approach to social work practice, research on its effectiveness as a practice model has not been fully answered. For example, the review of nine strengths-based case management studies by Staudt et al. (2001) found similarities in how these studies operationalized and defined the techniques used in strengths-based case management practice, but noted that none of the studies provided examples of specific questions or protocols. The authors were critical of the lack of measurement of treatment fidelity in the studies they reviewed, noting that only three studies describe efforts to ensure adherence to treatment model. Furthermore the article questioned the uniqueness of the strengths-based case management practice model, citing similar features in other case management models. Subsequent books and articles (Rapp & Goscha, 2006; Saleebey, 2006; Yip, 2006) have been written to further elaborate and differentiate the practice model of strengths perspective as well as strengths-based case management. Additionally, efforts are under way to further operationalize and empirically test the effectiveness of the strengths-based case management approach through rigorous research designs, including the development of strengths-based case management fidelity measures (Green, McAllister, & Tarte, 2004; Rapp & Goscha, 2006).

Distinctiveness

The strengths perspective is clearly distinct from a medical model approach to helping which has significantly influenced social work practice, especially within the mental health field. This approach views clients from an illness and pathological standpoint. The social worker attempts to diagnose the clients' problem, develops a treatment plan, and evaluates the outcome (Shulman, 2006). This traditional stance of helping assumes that clients have problems that they are unable or unwilling to resolve and therefore, they need professional services. Many times, this view assumes that the existence of the problem and the need for the client to seek professional help indicate deficits or flaws in clients (Weick et al., 1989). In addition, the emphasis on the problems in the client creates a wave of pessimistic expectations about the client's capabilities and environment. Clients may then believe that because they have these problems, they are somehow deficient or abnormal. This ignores the idea that clients have tremendous assets and potential that may not be recognized (Saleebey, 2006).

Strengths perspective, in contrast to the medical model, provides a different way of viewing clients and the helping process in social work practice. It balances out this problem-focused emphasis in social work practice and provides an alternative framework for working with clients. Instead of focusing mainly on the problems of the clients, the strengths perspective is goal oriented and focuses primarily on the strengths of the clients, looking for talents, knowledge, capacities, and resources. Practicing from this perspective means the social worker is always exploring and utilizing clients' strengths and resources, both within the person and their environment, in helping them with their problems or goals (Saleebey, 2006; Sullivan, 1992).

Another major influence in social work practice, containing both similar and differing elements of the strengths perspective, is generalist social work practice. Generalist social work practice assesses clients' problems, strengths, and abilities to develop an intervention plan (Boyle, Hull, Mather, Smith, & Farley, 2006). The distinction between the strengths-based interventions and traditional generalist social work practice is the concerted emphasis on clients' strengths and resources rather than their problems and dysfunctions. This emphasis creates a different context for the social-worker–client relationship whereby the discussions and questions being asked have less to do with their inabilities and symptoms but instead on their resiliencies and resources (Saleebey, 1996; Weick et al., 1989).

Integration

The central idea of focusing on client strengths and assets emphasized in the strengths perspective has also been identified and discussed in other disciplines and practice models. For example, emerging from resiliency theory, resilience-based practice is another model in psychology and social work that explores protective factors, especially in at-risk adolescents (Saleebey, 2006). Resilience revolves around the idea of positive adaptive strategies clients use to overcome adverse situations or conditions (Greene, 2007). Similarly, empowerment-oriented practice also posits focusing on client strengths and environmental resources and shares many of the same commonalities as the strengths perspective (Chapin & Cox, 2001).

In psychology, the theory and practice of positive psychology has gained significant attention for its differing approach to working with clients. Snyder (2000) promoted hope as a core construct of positive psychology, acting as a motivator and key influence in client behavior. Similar to the strengths perspective, positive psychology centers on the ideas of optimism, resilience, hope, and motivation (Seligman & Csikszentmihalyi, 2000).

Other social work researchers and practitioners have also advocated incorporating the strengths perspective principles with their practice models as a way of expanding on the strengths-based approach. For example solution-focused brief therapy has been linked with the strengths perspective as a way to add specific practice techniques to build on clients' abilities and solutions to solve their problems (DeJong & Miller, 1995; Lee, Uken, & Sebold, 2004). Both are grounded in the social worker working collaboratively with the client to look for client's abilities and to focus on client's goals, rather than dwelling on the problems (Weick, Kreider, & Chamberlain, 2006). The difference lies in the specific questions and interviewing techniques solution-focused brief therapy uses that allows the conversation with the client to center on identifying solutions to the problems. Weick, Kreider, and Chamberlain (2006) explain:

> The strengths perspective tends to emphasize goal-setting as the strategy for moving toward a new future and identifying the strengths that will help lead there. Solution-focused therapy emphasizes solution-finding through a strategy of purposeful questions that are intended to develop a detailed picture of a future beyond the problem. (p. 123)

Other social workers have suggested the use of integrative relational approach to enhance the strengths perspective approach to practice because of its similarities in therapeutic communication with both the strengths perspective and solution-focused brief therapy (Ornstein & Ganzer, 2000).

REFERENCES

Allison, S., Stacey, K., Dadds, V., Roeger, L., Wood, A., & Martin, G. (2003). What the family brings: Gathering evidence for strengths-based work. *Journal of Family Therapy, 25*(3), 263–284.

Barry, K. L., Zeber, J. E., Blow, F. C., & Valenstein, M. (2003). Effect of strengths model versus assertive community treatment model on participant outcomes and utilization: Two year follow-up. *Psychiatric Rehabilitation Journal, 26*(3), 268–277.

Bell, H. (2003). Strengths and secondary trauma in family violence work. *Social Work, 48*(4), 513–522.

Boyle, S. W., Hull, G. H., Mather, J. H., Smith, L. L., & Farley, O. W. (2006). *Direct practice in social work.* Boston: Allyn and Bacon.

Brun, C., & Rapp, R. C. (2001). Strengths-based case management: Individuals' perspectives on strengths and the case manager relationship. *Social Work, 46*(3), 278–288.

Chamberlain, R., & Rapp, C. A. (1991). A decade of case management: A methodological review of outcome research. *Community Mental Health Journal, 27*(3), 171–188.

Chapin, R. (1995). Social policy development: The strengths perspective. *Social Work, 40*(4), 506–514.

Chapin, R., & Cox, E. O. (2001). Changing the paradigm: Strengths-based and empowerment-oriented social work with frail elders. *Journal of Gerontological Social Work, 36,* 165–179.

DeJong, P., & Miller, S. D. (1995). How to interview for client strengths. *Social Work, 40*(6), 729–736.

Early, T. J., & GlenMaye, L. F. (2000). Valuing families: Social work practice with families from a strengths perspective. *Social Work, 45*(2), 118–130.

Green, B. L., McAllister, C. L., & Tarte, J. M. (2004). The strengths-based practices inventory: A tool for measuring strengths-based service delivery in early childhood and family support programs. *Families in Society, 85*(3), 326–334.

Greene, R. R. (2007). *Social work practice: A risk and resilience perspective.* Belmont, CA: Thomson Brooks/Cole.

Holmes, G. E., & Saleebey, D. (1993). Empowerment, the medical model, and the politics of clienthood. *Journal of Progressive Human Services, 4,* 61–78.

Itzhaky, H., & Bustin, E. (2002). Strengths and pathological perspectives in community social work. *Journal of Community Practice, 10*(3), 61–73.

Kisthardt, W. (1993). The impact of the strengths model of case management from the consumer perspective. In M. Harris & H. Bergman (Eds.), *Case management: Theory and practice* (pp. 165–182). Washington, DC: American Psychiatric Association.

Lee, M. Y., Uken, A., & Sebold, J. (2004). Accountability for change: Solution-focused treatment with domestic violence offenders. *Families in Society, 85*(4), 463–476.

Macias, C., Farley, O. W., Jackson, R., & Kinney, R. (1997). Case management in the context of capitation financing: An evaluation of the strengths model. *Administration and Policy in Mental Health, 24*(6), 535–543.

Macias, C., Kinney, R., Farley, O. W., Jackson, R., & Vos, B. (1994). The role of case management within a community support system: Partnership with psychosocial rehabilitation. *Community Mental Health Journal, 30*(4), 323–339.

Modrcin, M., Rapp, C., & Poertner, J. (1988). The evaluation of case management services with the chronically mentally ill. *Evaluation and Program Planning, 11,* 307–314.

Ornstein, E. D., & Ganzer, C. (2000). Strengthening the strengths perspective: An integrative relational approach. *Psychoanalytic Social Work, 7*(3), 57–78.

Perkins, K., & Tice, C. (1999). Family treatment of older adults who misuse alcohol: A strengths perspective. *Journal of Gerontological Social Work, 31*(3/4), 169–185.

Rapp, C. A. (1998). *The strengths model: Case management with people suffering from severe and persistent mental illness.* New York: Oxford University Press.

Rapp, C. A., & Chamberlain, R. (1985). Case management services to the chronically mental ill. *Social Work, 30*(5), 417–422.

Rapp, C. A., & Goscha, R. J. (2006). *The strengths model: Case management with people with psychiatric disabilities* (2nd ed.). New York: Oxford University Press.

Rapp, C. A., & Wintersteen, R. (1989). The strengths model of case management: Results from twelve demonstrations. *Psychosocial Rehabilitation Journal, 13*(1), 23–32.

Ryan, C. S., Sherman, P. S., & Judd, C. M. (1994). Accounting for case management effects in the evaluation of mental health services. *Journal of Consulting and Clinical Psychology, 62*(5), 965–974.

Saleebey, D. (1992). *The strengths perspective in social work practice.* New York: Longman.

Saleebey, D. (1996). The strengths perspective in social work practice: Extensions and cautions. *Social Work, 41*(3), 296–305.

Saleebey, D. (2006). *The strengths perspective in social work practice* (4th ed.). Boston: Allyn and Bacon.

Seligman, M. P., & Csikszentmihalyi, M. (2000). Positive psychology. *American Psychologist, 55,* 5–14.

Shulman, L. (2006). *The skills of helping individuals, families, groups, and communities* (5th ed.). Belmont: Brooks/Cole.

Siegel, H. A., Fisher, J. H., Rapp, R. C., Kelliher, C. W., Wagner, J. H., O'Brien, W. F., et al. (1995). The strengths perspective of case management: A promising inpatient substance abuse treatment enhancement. *Journal of Psychoactive Drugs, 27,* 67–72.

Snyder, C. R. (2000). *Handbook of hope: Theory, measures, and applications.* San Diego: Academic Press.

Stanard, R. P. (1999). The effect of training in a strengths model of case management on outcomes in a community mental health center. *Community Mental Health Journal, 35*(2), 169–179.

Staudt, M., Howard, M. O., & Drake, B. (2001). The operationalization, implementation, and effectiveness of the strengths perspective: A review of empirical studies. *Journal of Social Service Research, 27*(3), 1–21.

Sullivan, W. P. (1992). Reclaiming the community: The strengths perspective and deinstitutionalization. *Social Work, 37*(3), 204–354.

Weick, A., Kreider, J., & Chamberlain, R. (2006). Solving problems from a strengths perspective. In D. Saleebey (Ed.), *The strengths perspective in social work practice* (4th ed., pp. 116–127). Boston: Allyn and Bacon.

Weick, A., Rapp, C., Sullivan, P., & Kisthardt, W. (1989). A strengths perspective for social work practice. *Social Work, 34*(4), 350–354.

Werrbach, G. B. (1996). Family-strengths-based intensive child case management. *Families in Society, 77*(4), 216–226.

Yip, K.-S. (2005). A strengths perspective in working with Alzheimer's disease. *The International Journal of Social Research and Practice, 4*(3), 434–441.

Yip, K.-S. (2006). A strengths perspective in working with an adolescent with self-cutting behaviors. *Child and Adolescent Social Work Journal, 23*(2), 134–146.

JOHNNY S. KIM

SURVIVORS OF SUICIDE, THOSE LEFT BEHIND WHEN SOMEONE DIES BY SUICIDE

ABSTRACT: Suicide is a more prevalent cause of death in many countries than automobile accidents, homicide, and breast cancer. Despite this, the experience of people left behind after a suicide is not well understood. This is a sociohistorical overview of suicide that places suicide death in a relevant cultural context, explores the bereavement experiences of those grieving a loss to suicide, and presents the debate about similarities and differences regarding suicide bereavement in relation to other forms of traumatic death. In addition, this examination looks at the role of social workers in working with people bereaved by suicide.

KEY WORDS: suicide; bereavement; survivors; postvention; grief; loss

Introduction

Each year over one million people worldwide die by suicide. Suicide, the intentional taking of one's own life, is the 11th leading cause of death in America. Approximately 38,000 people die by suicide each year in the United States, with a suicide occurring every 14.2 minutes, totaling over 100 deaths by suicide each day (McIntosh, 2012). Suicide in the early twenty-first century claims more American lives than breast cancer and automobile accidents and almost double the number of yearly homicides. Suicide is a leading cause of preventable death and occurs primarily in young people and during middle age, particularly for men. Similar trends exist in Australia (Australian Bureau of Statistics, 2013), the United Kingdom (Office for National Statistics, 2013), and Canada (Statistics Canada, 2012). When an individual dies by suicide, family members, friends, work colleagues, and other associates are left behind to grieve and try to understand why the person took his or her life. This overview provides a brief sociohistorical overview of suicide to place suicide death in a relevant cultural context, explores the bereavement experiences of those grieving a loss to suicide, presents the debate about similarities and differences regarding suicide bereavement in relation to other forms of traumatic death, and finally examines the role of social workers working in the field of suicide bereavement, whether in specialized fields or in other settings.

History

Suicide has existed throughout human history, yet how such a death is viewed by society has changed over time and is shaped by the cultural context in which the death occurs. In the past, reliable statistics of the number of suicide deaths were not kept. This remains the case in some (generally low- and middle-income) countries throughout the world. The historical literature that does report on suicide death examines the ways that society deals with suicide, rather than the number of people who die in this way. For example, in early societies, suicide death primarily occurred among the old, disabled, and humiliated. As society evolved, the reasons for suicide and the methods used have changed. In the early Middle Ages, suicide was generally seen as a cure for shame. Throughout history, suicide was seen as a criminal act, a type of murder, and a desperate, mortal sin in the opinion of some Christian churches. Suicide was punishable by the state through the reclaiming of personal possessions of the deceased and forbidding a church burial. During these times, the deceased's loved ones suffered punishment for the suicidal actions of their relative, and civil law had the power to enact severe sanctions against surviving family members (Minios, 1999).

During the industrialization of many countries, the growth of societies, and the emergence of large cities, the rate of suicide reached new heights, causing speculation that lonely people in cities became desperate and took their own lives. One early suicide theorist, Emile Durkheim, set out to try and explain suicide and why suicide occurs (Durkheim, 1857). Durkheim's widely known and enduring analysis locates the causes of suicide in the social realm, suggesting there are three causes. The first cause, known as "egotistic suicide," is said to occur when an individual lacks integration into society. The second, "altruistic suicide," is said to occur when an individual is highly integrated into society and is governed by social customs and habits, yet perceives his or her suicide to be "commanded" by a higher power, either religious or political. Third is "anomic suicide," when there is lack of regulation in society or when order is suddenly upset.

Durkheim's focus in his theory of suicide was on the manner in which interaction between an individual and society takes place. Since the 1990s, parts of his theory have been brought into question, in particular the ways in which Durkheim viewed the protective features of marriage (Lehmann, 1995). Although this questioning is likely caused by the dominant culture of the time, his theory provides a social lens in which to consider suicide and suicide-related behaviors. In direct contrast, more recent theories of suicide focus on the medicalization of suicide (among other conditions and behaviors) and are driven by the view that suicide is a symptom of a lack of reason, related to mental illness or mental disorder. This theory has led to the fundamental premise underlying suicide prevention activities in the early twenty-first century, placing the emphasis on the individual and particular risk factors he or she may exhibit and on intervention strategies to promote positive mental health, rather than broader societal influences.

Religious prohibitions against suicide are still common to try to deter individuals from ending their lives. In the early twenty-first century, many religious groups condemn the act of suicide but not the individual who died by suicide. This leads to a situation for the family in which normal grieving rituals can take place and offers an understanding that the death was the result of mental illness. This attitude can help family members feel that the death was not their fault and can help with community support following the death. Nevertheless, the powerful influence of history cannot be underestimated, with suicide death continuing to be stigmatized and family members' grieving affected. Importantly, most individuals working in the field supporting those bereaved by suicide, along with those bereaved, caution against use of the word "commit" when discussing someone who died by suicide because "commit" is related to the antiquated criminalization of suicide (Beaton, Forster, & Maple, 2013). Families bereaved by the suicide of a loved one react negatively when the word commit is used because they feel it is stigmatizing and more related to a crime or sin than to a hopeless person who saw no other solution to his or her problems.

Defining the Population

It has been estimated that there are six "survivors," that is, those bereaved, for every death by suicide (Shneidman, 1972). However, this understanding of the number of people affected by a suicide death is based on an estimate created by Dr. Edwin Shneidman in the 1970s, which was meant to be comparable to the number of extended family members who were eligible to receive compensation following an airline disaster. Researchers, support service personnel, and bereaved people all report this figure to be a significant underestimation. Although determining the actual population is challenging, some examples exist. In a recent phone survey in a southern U.S. state, 66% of people stated they knew someone who had attempted or died by suicide, 40% knew someone who had died, and 20% of people indicated they were a survivor in that one or more suicides had a profound effect upon them (Cerel, Maple, Van de Venne, & Aldrich, 2013). In the only nationally representative sample of self-identifying suicide-bereaved individuals published to date, Crosby and Sacks (2002) found exposure to suicide (in the 12 months prior to the interview) among 7% of surveyed households in the United States. Extrapolating this finding to the whole population of the United States results in 1 in 14 Americans being exposed to suicide in the survey year. Of the 7% of households reporting exposure to suicide, 1.1% reported it was a family member who died and 5.4% reported exposure to suicide of another person they knew. Again, extending this conclusion to the whole of U.S. population results in 3.3 million Americans experiencing the suicide death of a family member in that year. If approximately 30,000 people in America died by suicide that year, then at least 10 family members were affected for each death. Crosby and Sacks also reported on suicide risk among the population in their study exposed to suicide and concluded that exposed individuals were 1.6 times more likely to report suicidal ideation, 2.9 times more likely to have suicidal plans, and 3.7 times more likely to have made an attempt than those not exposed to suicide. Therefore, early estimates of six people affected appear to be underestimates in that when a suicide occurs, entire families, neighborhoods, schools, and communities are impacted, as well as individuals. Further, the effect that a suicide death has on an individual appears also to influence poor morbidity and mortality outcomes associated with the experience.

To allow a broader and deeper understanding of who is affected by suicide, a definition is required that is usefully broad, but at the same time provides people with the ability to self-identify their bereavement status. Several authors have offered definitions, including Andreissen (2009), who suggests that "a survivor is usually regarded as a person who has lost a significant other (or loved one) by suicide, and whose life is changed because of this loss" (p. 43). However, this definition excludes a broad definition of relationships between the person now deceased and the person bereaved. Jordan and McIntosh (2011a) offer the following: "Someone who experiences a high level of self-perceived psychological, physical, and/or social distress for a considerable length of time after exposure to the suicide of another person" (p. 7). This definition is problematic because it relies first on symptomatology and the lack of any way to operationalize "a high level" of distress and second on a "considerable length of time," not allowing the prediction of who will be a survivor among people who are exposed to suicide and experience immediate distress. A third useful definition is offered by Berman (2011), as follows: "survivors of suicide were defined as those believed to be *intimately and directly affected* by a suicide; that is, those who would self define as survivors after the suicide of another person" (p. 111, original italics). This definition is useful in that it relies on self-report for distress in the absence of knowing why some people are more distressed than others. It is also broad enough to capture those who may not be intimately related to the deceased, but are negatively affected nonetheless.

More research is needed to determine nomenclature that indicates a continuum through which

people can be identified as being "exposed to suicide" in the immediate aftermath of a suicide death; within those exposed, a proportion will be "affected by the suicide"; some of those affected will be "suicide bereaved, short term" and a smaller proportion will become "suicide bereaved, long term." This nomenclature has been described in detail by Cerel and colleagues (Cerel, McIntosh, Neimeyer, Maple, & Marshall, 2014).

In the proposed continuum of survivorship, Cerel et al. (2014) propose that those labeled as "exposed" would include those defined as suicide survivors by Jordan and McIntosh, but would also include those who "know of" or knew someone who died by suicide but did not experience (or would not likely experience) the severity of or longer term effects associated with this definition of survivors. Such reactions may represent typically more fleeting and shallow initial bereavement reactions, but likely indicates that a larger percentage of the population is exposed to suicide at some point in their lives.

Those identified as "affected" include people who are exposed to suicide who have a potential for the death to have a disruptive effect on their lives. These individuals might have some sort of reaction to the death, but not as much as someone thought to be suicide bereaved. People who are suicide bereaved are likely to experience posttraumatic stress disorder (PTSD), depression, or prolonged grief as a result of the death. Individuals who are suicide bereaved, long term, may experience suicidal ideation or behavior, may have the potential for posttraumatic growth as a result of the death, and, most importantly, identify the suicide as a defining experience in their lives. There is evidence to indicate that certain risk factors or mediators may exist that increase the likelihood of the bereaved individual experiencing the loss at different levels. These factors will most likely include kinship relationship and perceived emotional closeness to the deceased, previous experience with suicide, exposure to the trauma of the death, and demographics such as age and sex. Other variables that may play a role include perceived responsibility for the death and hostile social environments or stigma (real or perceived). Protective factors that are seen to play a role in the reaction of a suicide-bereaved individual include resources, support systems, and coping skills. These various groups may represent individuals of differing needs and reactions in their suicide bereavement and may help to lessen the inconsistencies of previous research findings and clinical experience. This will lead to better identification of those who would benefit from interventions and the kind of interventions most likely to assist them in their grief experience (Cerel et al., 2014).

Although this discussion presents ideas on a definition to better identify the ways in which people are affected by a suicide, it is necessary for the community of researchers, clinicians, and people who are themselves affected by suicide to agree on a definition of who is bereaved following a suicide death. This will allow research to determine the full impact of the death and identify people at highest risk and most in need of clinical intervention, thus informing evidence-based interventions that provide support services that are timely and appropriate to need. In the field of suicidology, the term for services offering support to those bereaved is "postvention".

Suicide Bereavement

Grief is the living response to loss. Grief usually follows the loss of certain primary relationships, but not when less intimate relationships are lost. Primary relationships may be defined as those that are close, face to face, emotionally important, or comprising a strong identification with the other person. The loss may be real or perceived, yet grief will still occur. Grief is a universally human phenomenon, yet it is experienced in a highly individualized and multidimensional manner. Grief encompasses sensory, behavioral, and cognitive systems showing emotional and often spiritual components. The type of death may influence the way in which the grief is experienced. Sudden, unexpected, or unnatural deaths may have elements of grief that differ from those experienced when a person dies in old age or after a long illness or when the death is anticipated. Culture and cultural norms also play a role in how grief is experienced. Some cultures have highly structured ways of demonstrating grief, sometimes with specific periods of time allocated for particular tasks. However, in many Western countries, the way in which grief is expressed is very personal.

Over time, many theorists have offered interpretations and explanations for the ways in which people grieve following a death. There are two theoretically derived frameworks for understanding grief, with many variations. The first framework is a stage-oriented model that has seen many evolutions and adaptations and continues to inform the social understanding of grief in both lay and professional circles. This framework was first noted by Freud (1917) in *Mourning and Melancholia*. Follow-up work by Bowlby (1980) extended the model to conceptualize death as a loss of attachment to the deceased. Bowlby argues that the bereaved person must adjust to this loss of attachment by detaching him- or herself from the deceased before being able to move forward from the bereaved state. Kubler-Ross (1969) suggests that this grief occurs in five stages. Although her research was based on the experiences of people anticipating their own death, rather than in response to the death of a loved one, these stages rapidly became the prominent and accepted model of grieving across the field of grief and bereavement. The stage framework, underpinned by a developmental process, is characterized by working through of a number of tasks associated with loss. Grief is assumed to be a linear process, with stages that will be moved through, in no particular order, before reaching the final goal of resolution. These stage models emphasize the breaking of bonds with the deceased, characterized by reaching a point of acceptance that he or she is gone.

Many, including Stroebe (2001), question some of the pivotal assumptions to stage-based models, indicating that there is little empirical evidence that working through grief is more effective for coming to terms with loss than not working through it. As a consequence of this critical analysis of the stage model, a newer framework in which the continuation of a bond with the deceased is acknowledged is now broadly recognized (Klass, Silverman, & Nickman, 1996). Although it does not completely discount aspects of the stages-and-phases framework, the continuing-bonds model acknowledges the presence of a continued connection with the deceased person once the physical bond is broken through death. Bauer and Bonanno (2001) propose that such continuing bonds enable the bereaved "to recognize the personal meaning of past goals and relationships and then to understand how those meanings can continue in the present" (p. 155).

The way in which grief is conceptualized is thought to be influenced by the manner in which the person died. Several factors are reported to be unique to bereavement through suicide because of the particular nature of the type of death (Jordan, 2001). In short, suicide death, along with accidental death, is viewed as a life cut short or a waste of life. Because suicide death is often sudden, there is little or no time to clear up any unfinished business with the deceased, which is particularly problematic when the prior relationship was ambivalent, antagonistic, or estranged (Ratnarajah, Maple, & Minichiello, 2014).

Several factors are often reported as being different with suicide deaths, with the seven most common elements including shock, guilt, blame, shame, stigma, lack of social support, and, for some, relief that the deceased person is no longer in pain or suffering

(Maple, Cerel, McKay, & Jordan, 2014). Each is briefly described below.

SHOCK. On finding out about the death, the bereaved individual has questions of where and how the suicide occurred. There may be high levels of shock experienced in response to learning of the suicide death. Following the initial shock upon learning of the death, there are questions about why the person chose to take his or her own life. Although much of the literature reports a need to come to an acceptable answer for the question of "why" a person ended his or her life, which is clearly an important part of the grieving process for survivors of suicide, research has thus far failed to examine why survivors need to explain the act or what purpose this serves internally. Shock has also been linked to the development of posttraumatic stress reactions and complicated grief reactions in those bereaved by suicide (Young et al., 2012).

Nevertheless, for most bereaved individuals the rationale used by the person now deceased remains a mystery. This holds true for situations where a note was not left behind, as well as for many where a presuicide message was recorded. Notes have been found in around 10% to 40% of suicide deaths but notes are often also found to be inadequate in explaining why a life was ended (Callanan & Davis, 2009; De Leo, Milner, & Sveticic, 2012; Gunn, Lester, Haines, & Williams, 2012; Leenaars, Girdhar, Dogra, Wenckstern, & Leenaars, 2010; Leenaars, Sayin, et al., 2010).

GUILT. First and foremost, guilt experienced by survivors of suicide is thought to be caused by a perceived inability to prevent the suicide from occurring. Suicide is generally viewed as preventable; thus, by natural extension, those who are close to the person now deceased feel they should have been able to intervene in some way to stop the actions. Guilt experienced following a death by suicide has been linked to poor health and well-being outcomes in the survivor (Li, Stroebe, Chan, & Chow, 2014).

BLAME. Many authors report survivors of suicide describing feelings of blame internally, within the family, or from the wider community (Jordan & McIntosh, 2011b). Horror may also be experienced upon realizing the pain the bereaved was experiencing before death that the survivor had not been aware of. There may be a tendency to blame the self, spouse, child, partner, or anyone who had been close to the deceased at the time of death. Blame also tends to increase stigma and decrease access to social support. In young people, this has been linked to self-imposed isolation from potential supports (Bartik, Maple, Edwards, & Keirnan, 2013).

SHAME. A survivor of suicide may also experience feelings of shame. Shame appears to be elevated among this group when compared with people bereaved through other deaths. Feelings of shame can lead to social isolation. Shame is often related to the cause of death as a stigmatized one, blame from others in the social network, and guilt about not being able to prevent the death.

STIGMA. Because of the complex dynamic of suicide deaths throughout history, stigma is often associated with suicide. People bereaved through suicide often report feelings of being stigmatized by the death of their loved one. Stigma is not always easy to detect. Some have questioned whether stigma is real and whether survivors of suicide must deal with it or whether they are self-stigmatizing. Either way, the feeling of being stigmatized has been related to the difficulties some suicide survivors have in talking about their experience (Maple, Edwards, Plummer, & Minichiello, 2010). Regardless of whether stigma is real or perceived, it can result in people who are suicide bereaved being social isolated at a time when most need access to social support networks (de Groot, de Keijser, & Neeleman, 2006).

Because suicide appears to be taboo, talking about it is often discouraged. Campbell (1997) suggests that "society's inability to deal with survivors in an honest and caring way remains a negative legacy of suicide" (p. 330). Public displays of grief are generally socially discouraged, and as such, survivors may feel awkward with previous social supports and find themselves drawn to support from people who have experienced similar losses.

SUPPORT FOR THOSE BEREAVED THROUGH SUICIDE. The value of social support has been measured in many areas of personal distress, including suicide survivors. In general, social support networks have been found to facilitate the grieving process and at the same time lower separation anxiety, feelings of rejections, and depression (Reed, 1998). Initially, support appears to be available for the bereaved (for example, immediately postdeath following the funeral); however, it often weakens over time. Further, although people within support networks may offer support, the bereaved may not know how to ask for the assistance they require. To further complicate the issues relating to social support for survivors of suicide, supporters may hold unrealistic or undesirable attitudes or misconceptions about the ways in which people react to suicide, potentially resulting in support attempts being inappropriate or inaccessible to the bereaved person.

RELIEF FOR SOME. Suicide death is typically thought of as unexpected and sudden. However, some families may feel relief, especially when the suicide death ended a troubled, painful history. This is not to suggest that the person will not be greatly missed, but rather that the family may experience reduced stress and be relieved that the individual is now free from distress. The notion that suicide may not be sudden and unexpected has received little attention. However, when it has been studied it has been shown to influence the way in which the resultant grief is experienced and is therefore an important consideration (Maple, Plummer, Edwards, & Minichiello, 2007) in the range of emotions experienced by those bereaved by suicide.

Within the family setting it is most common for survivors to feel anger and feelings of social stigmatization and to experience familial dysfunction both prior to and after the death. Following the death, prior events in the family may be reviewed individually or among family members as they search for explanations as to why the deceased family member ended his or her life (Ratnarajah et al., 2014). Cerel, Fristad, Weller, and Weller (2000) suggested three types of families in which the suicide of a parent had occurred: *functional* families, which are characterized by no evidence of preexisting family conflict or psychopathology, with the suicide often taking place in the context of chronic physical illness; *encapsulated* families, in which psychopathology and conflict were generally observed only in the deceased, not in other family members; and *chaotic* families, in which clear evidence of psychopathology in multiple family members or turmoil prior to suicide was present. Although research has not examined whether these three categories represent all families in which a suicide occurs, it is helpful to think about the variety of families who experience suicide.

In short, some aspects of the bereavement process appear to be unique to suicide. Suicide bereavement appears to cause an existential crisis in the bereaved as they struggle to find meaning in a world that feels meaningless while suffering feelings of blame, guilt,

and responsibility for the death. Given that more than 38,000 people die by suicide each year in the United States and using the often quoted, yet extremely conservative estimate of 6 people affected by each suicide death, at least 198,000 Americans are newly bereaved by suicide each year. In Australia, around 2,500 people die by suicide. Again, using this calculation of 6 people affected, these deaths result in at least 15,000 Australians newly bereaved. It is important to note that this is an annual addition to an already large population continuing to grieve prior deaths—because suicide bereavement affects individuals for a long time after the event and in profound ways.

PSYCHOLOGICAL OUTCOMES FOR SUICIDE-BEREAVED INDIVIDUALS. With the multitude of complex emotions suddenly confronting suicide-bereaved individuals, the trauma of the event may lead to additional psychopathology. Although there is limited evidence about how suicide bereavement differs from bereavement from other types of sudden traumatic deaths (Jordan, 2001; Jordan & McIntosh, 2011b), attention to the longer term morbidity associated with this experience is an important consideration.

Complicated or prolonged grief may be common for those bereaved by suicide, as for those survivors of other types of sudden and traumatic death. Prolonged grief disorder shares features of PTSD and depression and also involves intrusive yearning, longing for, or searching for the deceased (Prigerson et al., 2009). Symptoms of trauma that may be present include avoidance of reminders of the person who died, a feeling of purposelessness or futility, difficulty imagining life without the deceased, numbness, detachment, feelings of being stunned, dazed, or shocked, feeling like life is empty or meaningless, feeling like part of oneself has died, disbelief, excessive death-related bitterness or anger, and identification with symptoms or harmful behaviors resembling the behaviors experienced by the person who died before his or her death. Complicated grief has been shown to occur following the suicide of a family member and to increase the risk of suicidal ideation for those bereaved by a suicide; in addition, it appears to be related to the onset of depression, a prolonged course of depression, and PTSD. Complicated grief appears to be highest in those with the closest ties to the deceased, perhaps because suicide-related bereavement differs from other bereavements in regard to its nature, including the deceased's choice to end his or her life, the cultural and historical perceptions of suicide, and the involvement of officialdom based on legislative requirements to determine cause of death.

No overall difference in suicidal behavior and diagnosable depression in children bereaved from a suicide compared to children bereaved from other types of death has been found in the few studies focused on outcomes for children. However, compared to children bereaved from other types of death, children bereaved by suicide have been shown to experience increased levels of psychopathology, especially behavior problems, prior to the death, as well as increased behavioral and anxiety symptoms after the initial few months following the death (Ratnarajah & Schofield, 2008). This is an area worthy of future research attention.

DIFFERENCES IN SUICIDE BEREAVEMENT COMPARED WITH OTHER DEATHS.

In a comprehensive review of previously reported research, Jordan (2001) suggests three important differences evident in a person bereaved by suicide when assessing the research literature. These differences are that suicide survivors struggle to find meaning in the death, experience high levels of guilt at not being able to prevent the death, and experience higher levels of abandonment by the deceased. However, while recognizing that there are many similarities, Jordan maintains there are also important differences that must be acknowledged in the suicide bereaved. Thus, he concludes that the thematic content of the grief, the social processes the survivors must face, and the impact the death has on the family system are unique to this form of death.

The difference between suicide bereavement and bereavement following other deaths may appear less distinct based on the nature of the deaths to which suicide is often compared. The available literature compares suicide bereavement with other sudden and traumatic deaths such as death through homicide or motor-vehicle accident. Such comparisons may potentially dilute the difference and effects of sudden or traumatic bereavement from suicide by obscuring feelings of responsibility held by others toward the suicide victim, particularly in the case of young adults. These comparisons also obscure the inevitably confronting nature of suicide, that is, that the individual did not die by accident but purposely chose to take his or her own life. As Jordan (2001) proposes, it is important to understand whether significant differences exist because this will affect service delivery and planning. An approach focusing on understanding how grief affects individuals, rather than the manner in which the deceased died, to illuminate diversity in bereavement may be a critical step to designing effective policies and practices to support suicide survivors.

There is evidence that a person is more likely to die by suicide if a family member has died by suicide or has a history of psychiatric illness (Runeson & Asberg, 2003). Suicide survivors seem to be at risk for their own suicidal behavior, even where no familial relationship exists. In families, the mechanism of this transmission is both genetic/biological and cognitive/learned. Suicide rates have been shown to be twice as high in families where suicide death has occurred compared with families in which a suicide has not occurred (Roy & Segal, 2001; Statham et al., 1998). It also is possible that exposure to suicide in family members may sensitize people to the idea of suicide as a coping mechanism. This also can apply to others outside the immediate family who are at increased risk of suicide following exposure. This process, described by Joiner (Joiner, 2002; Van Orden et al., 2010), includes cognitive sensitization and opponent process theory. These processes sensitize people to suicide-related thoughts and behaviors, making these thoughts and behaviors more cognitively available as coping mechanisms. Further, as one becomes sensitized, emotion around the idea of suicide diminishes as it is repeated. The idea of suicide is primed, that is, more cognitively available, and perhaps less taboo for the family member, which then could be seen as a potential coping strategy when problems arise. The similarity of suicidal behavior over generations within a family or broader kinship group is evidence to support this model.

The interpersonal–psychological theory of suicidal behavior (Joiner, 2005) posits that for someone to end his or her life, he or she must experience a combination of perceived burdensomeness, thwarted belongingness, and acquired capacity for suicidal behavior. This acquired capacity may be especially primed by the experience of a loved one dying by suicide, which puts suicide survivors at special risk given their exposure. Although some will be affected in this way, others will not. Why some survivors are resilient whereas others are vulnerable is not yet understood.

Supporting Those Bereaved by Suicide

The needs of the bereaved are typically of concern to mental-health and counseling practitioners, including social workers in a variety of settings. Social workers must be aware of the issues outlined in this article because they will come across clients who are bereaved by suicides—whether or not these clients seek services for that loss. The total cost of unmet needs of those bereaved in terms of suffering, health problems, and economic losses is unknown and currently incalculable. The literature on effective interventions for those bereaved by suicide is sparse. Most survivors do not seek out mental-health treatment or formal or informal interventions. Yet given the high level of exposure to suicide, with some conservatively estimating that 1 in every 65 Americans will have been exposed (McIntosh, 2012) and research showing that over 40% of people know someone who has died by suicide (Cerel et al., 2013), a social worker in any field can assume that many clients will have been exposed to a suicide death at some time. This experience will have significantly affected the lives of some clients—even if it is not the presenting issue for service provision. Therefore, exploring a history of suicide bereavement should form part of any comprehensive social-work assessment. Although generalist service providers may come across people bereaved by suicide in their day-to-day work, services are emerging that directly respond to the needs of people bereaved by suicide. These services are known as postvention and refer to interventions that take place after a suicide for the surviving family, school, or community.

Postvention has been seen as a type of prevention in that survivors are at risk of future problems, including their own suicidal behavior. Historically, attempts to reach survivors for support following a suicide have been passive, often occurring weeks or months after the death. When postvention is passive, survivors themselves must find out about resources that might be available in their community. These resources include postings on agency websites, brochures or flyers at funeral homes, or newspaper advertisements for bereavement groups. Because most people bereaved immediately following a suicide do not know the term "survivor," it may be difficult for people to find appropriate sources of help.

Barriers to people getting help include stigma about suicide and not knowing about available resources or where to turn for help. A new type of postvention, called the active postvention model, was devised by Dr. Frank Campbell (2004) and has been disseminated across the United States and internationally. Active postvention allows services to occur as close to the time as death as possible, which can better help identify and assist survivors. There is an emerging evidence base that indicates that accessing support in close proximity to the time of the death appears to reduce the long-term morbidity and mortality associated with being bereaved by suicide. A similar model in several locations in Australia, offering support early following the suicide death, has been economically evaluated. Not only do these active postvention models offer timely support, but also the Australian StandBy Model appears to indicate that providing such a service is cost-effective. Unfortunately, these services are provided only in some localities and are not available to everyone who may benefit.

Traditional psychotherapy, both in individual and in family format, is preferred by some individuals and may be helpful. Where therapy is viewed most positively, it is often attributed to the therapist's knowledge and understanding of suicide bereavement as a unique form of grief and loss. If the therapist does not have this experience and knowledge base, therapy can be a negative experience. In some countries, including the United States, insurance coverage of mental-health care and the perceived stigma of being in therapy may prevent many survivors from accessing psychotherapy.

Peer-led or professional-led support groups, often called Survivor of Suicide groups, are the most common form of intervention received by people bereaved by suicide. Many view participation in support groups as an essential part of working through bereavement following suicide. Support groups are thought to be preferred because there is low or no cost and because they are convenient and less stigmatizing than formal mental-health treatments. Further, these groups are most often run by group leaders who are themselves bereaved by loss through suicide. In some instances, professional leadership occurs alongside lay leadership. There are over 400 support groups for survivors in America, with at least 1 group in each state. There are also online support groups available for people who prefer the anonymity and convenience of online support. A similar proportion of services are found in other countries, with more online support groups commencing. Online support groups are particularly useful for people who live in rural areas, who may be inhibited from attending support groups by distance and time. Support groups may be helpful because they allow members to feel a sense of identification with other group members who may have experienced similar situations. People in support groups can feel like they are benefitting both themselves and others from sharing their experiences and listening and providing advice to people newer to the process. Over time, people who have been in the group and who have been bereaved for a longer period of time can help newer members as they describe how they made it through especially difficult times or handled sensitive topics. This becomes a form of social support, which often extends to friendships outside the group. This social support may be helpful for survivors dealing with depression, loneliness, or life stress. Support groups can be located through the websites of the American Association of Suicidology (*http://www.suicidology.org*) and the American Foundation for Suicide Prevention (*http://www.afsp.org*). There is a limited research base to draw from to determine who is most helped by these support groups, which group practices are the most helpful, or how long survivors should continue to attend a group (Cerel, Padgett, Conwell, & Reed, 2009). Although reports that do provide information regarding participants' experiences are often positive, a lack of information from those who do not attend or only attend support groups for a short period and do not find them helpful makes it difficult to contextualize these reports.

Advocacy has been a source of support for some survivors, either on its own or in combination with individual or group therapy. Using their grief to advocate for local, regional, or national change, survivors have been at the forefront of the suicide prevention movement. In some instances, these efforts have resulted in a variety of policy and legislative successes. For example, during the 1990s in the United States, the introduction of congressional resolutions recognized suicide as a serious public-health challenge, which led to the passage of the Garrett Lee Smith Memorial Act in 2004. The Garrett Lee Smith Memorial Act, named after the son of Senator Smith of Oregon who died by suicide, was the first-ever authorization and appropriation for youth suicide prevention. The Garrett Lee Smith Act authorized $82 million over three years for youth suicide prevention programs, including grants to states, American Indian tribes, and colleges to support suicide prevention efforts. Services for survivors are part of these funds. Some survivors have reported that the act of creating political will and seeing change becomes a part of their healing experience. Other survivors use their grief to work in suicide prevention with the hope that other families will not have to experience the pain of losing a family member to suicide. There has been no research to date about the effect of survivors engaging in advocacy or prevention work.

Although the challenges for survivors are multifaceted and complex, some family members may experience what has been termed posttraumatic growth. Posttraumatic growth, a concept that has grown out of the positive psychology movement, has been described as psychological change that occurs as the result of a person's struggle with a stressful and traumatic event. This area requires further research to determine which survivors or what situations might be most associated with growth following a suicide. Social workers involved with supporting survivors must acknowledge the wide variation in experience and the needs of the individual client to support where they are in their bereavement and not assume that particular experiences, events, or situations will lead to expected outcomes.

The tendency to regard suicide survivors as a homogenous group overlooks the diversity of experiences and responses to suicide and the accompanying grief. In the early twenty-first century, it appears responses to those bereaved through suicide may be too limited. Recognizing the different needs of suicide-bereaved people is important in determining the appropriateness of the services delivered. Neimeyer (2000) suggests that for those experiencing an unproblematic reaction to the death of their loved one, conventional therapy is not indicated. Indeed, he suggests there are potential negative consequences from engaging an individual in therapy when it is not needed. In contrast, for individuals suffering an extreme grief reaction to a sudden and unexpected death, therapy can be useful.

It is likely that social workers, especially those in direct clinical practice, will be impacted by client suicide. Research indicates that 55% of social workers will experience at least one client suicide attempt and 31% will experience a client suicide completion during the course of their career (Ting, Sanders, Jacobson, & Power, 2006). Social workers who lose clients to suicide can experience reactions related to their professional identity as well as the personal experience of loss. A loss of a client to suicide can be related to feelings of professional incompetence and is an occasion in which it is appropriate to seek peer supervision or actual therapy (Clark, 2009). The American Association of Suicidology maintains a clinician/survivor task force that has a listserv on which clinicians can discuss their experiences as well as information about how to get help following a client suicide (*http://www.suicidology.org/c/document_library/get_file?folderId=236&name=DLFE-275.pdf*).

Conclusion

Those bereaved by suicide are the individuals left behind when a person dies by suicide. Suicide is no longer a criminalized act and many religious groups are moving toward helping those family members left behind by condemning the act of suicide, but not the individual who died. Up to a third of the population may feel the profound impact of a suicide in their social network within their lifetime. Postvention, the interventions that take place following a suicide, is becoming more active, including reaching out so survivors can get the help they need. Suicide survivors are at risk for their own suicidal behavior, depression, posttraumatic stress, and complicated grief. The most common form of treatment for suicide survivors is support groups. Advocacy and working for suicide prevention are other common sources of support.

Given the complex political and policy environments in which services are provided, along with funding and health-care provision costs, it is timely to provide a broad overview of the issues related to this complex grief and aftermath of a suicide death. Social workers are required to work in ethical and meaningful ways with those affected by suicide and self-harm and contribute to reducing stigma experienced by these individuals, families, and communities. With much of the social-work literature in the suicide domain focused on suicide prevention and intervention, it is timely to acknowledge both the full range of activities that must be addressed by the social-work profession and that suicide prevention and postvention are both issues central to social work.

REFERENCES

Andreissen, K. (2009). Can postvention be prevention? *Crisis, 30*(1), 43–47. doi:10.1027/0227-5910.30.1.43

Australian Bureau of Statistics. (2013). *3303.0 Causes of Death, Australia 2011*. Canberra: Australian Bureau of Statistics.

Bartik, W., Maple, M., Edwards, H., & Keirnan, M. (2013). Adolescent survivors of suicide: Australian young people's bereavement narratives. *Crisis, 34*(3), 211–217. doi:10.1027/0227-5910/a000185

Bauer, J., & Bonanno, G. (2001). Continuity amid discontinuity: Bridging one's past and present in stories of conjugal bereavement. *Narrative Inquiry, 11*(1), 123–158.

Beaton, S., Forster, P., & Maple, M. (2013). Suicide and language: Why we shouldn't use the "C" word. *InPsych: The Bulletin of the Australian Psychological Society, 35*(1), 30–31.

Berman, A. (2011). Estimating the population of survivors of suicide: Seeking an evidence base. *Suicide and Life-Threatening Behavior, 41*(1), 110–116.

Bowlby, J. (1980). *Attachment and loss, Vol. 3: Sadness and depression*. New York, NY: Basic Books.

Callanan, V. J., and Davis, M. S. (2009). A comparison of suicide note writers with suicides who did not leave notes. *Suicide & Life-Threatening Behavior, 39*(5), 558–568.

Campbell, F. (1997). Changing the legacy of suicide. *Suicide and Life-Threatening Behavior, 27*(4), 329–338.

Campbell, F. (2004). An active postvention program. *Crisis, 25*(1), 30–32.

Cerel, J., Fristad, M., Weller, E., & Weller, R. (2000). Suicide-bereaved children and adolescents: II. Parental and family functioning. *Journal of the American Academy of Child and Adolescent Psychiatry, 39*(4), 437–444.

Cerel, J., Maple, M., Van de Venne, J., & Aldrich, R. (2013). Exposure to suicide and identification as survivor: Results from a random-digit dial survey. *Crisis, 34*(6), 413–419.

Cerel, J., McIntosh, J., Neimeyer, R., Maple, M., & Marshall, D. (2014, 7 April). The continuum of survivorship: Definitional issues in the aftermath of suicide. *Suicide and Life-Threatening Behavior*. doi:10.1111/sltb.12093

Cerel, J., Padgett, J, Conwell, Y., & Reed, G. (2009). A call for research: The need to better understand the impact of support groups for suicide survivors. *Suicide and Life-Threatening Behavior, 39*(3), 269–281. PMID:19606919.

Clark, J. (2009). Clinical supervision after client suicide: Panacea or pretence? *Psychotherapy in Australia, 16*(1), 16–23.

Crosby, A., & Sacks, J. (2002). Exposure to suicide: Incidence and association with suicidal ideation and behavior: United States, 1994. *Suicide and Life-Threatening Behavior, 32*(3), 321–328.

de Groot, M., de Keijser, J., & Neeleman, J. (2006). Grief shortly after suicide and natural death: A comparative study among spouses and first-degree relatives. *Suicide and Life-Threatening Behavior, 36*(4), 418–431.

De Leo, D., Milner, A., and Sveticic, J. (2012). Mental disorders and communication of intent to die in Indigenous suicide cases, Queensland, Australia. *Suicide & Life-Threatening Behavior, 42*, 136–146.

Durkheim, E. (1857). *Suicide: A study in sociology*. London: Routledge & Kegan Paul.

Freud, S. (1917). Mourning and melancholia. In *The standard edition of the complete psychological works of Sigmund Freud, XIV* (pp. 237–258). London: Hogarth Press.

Gunn, J., Letser, D., Haines, J., & Williams, C. (2012). Thwarted belongingness and perceived burdensomeness in suicide notes. *Crisis, 33*(3), 178–181.

Joiner, T. E., Jr. (2002). The trajectory of suicidal behavior over time. *Suicide & Life-Threatening Behavior, 32*(1), 33–41.

Joiner, Jr., T. E., Conwell, Y., Fitzpatrick, K. K., Witte, T. K., Schmidt, N.B., Berlin, M.T., Fleck, M.P.A., Rudd, M.D. (2005). Four studies on how past and current suicidality relate even when "everything but the kitchen sink" is covaried. *Journal of Abnormal Psychology, 114*, 291–303.

Jordan, J. (2001). Is suicide bereavement different? A reassessment of the literature. *Suicide and Life-Threatening Behavior, 31*(1), 91–102.

Jordan, J., & McIntosh, J. (2011a). Suicide bereavement: Why study survivors of suicide loss? In J. Jordan & J. McIntosh (Eds.), *Grief after suicide: Understanding the* consequences and caring for the survivors (pp. 3–18). New York, NY: Routledge.

Jordan, J. R., & McIntosh, J. L. (2011b). *Grief after suicide: Understanding the consequences and caring for the survivors.* New York, NY: Brunner-Routledge.

Klass, D., Silverman, P., & Nickman, S. (Eds.). (1996). *Continuing bonds: New understandings of grief.* Washington, DC: Taylor & Francis.

Kubler-Ross, E. (1969). *On death and dying.* London: Tavistock.

Leenaars, A. A., Girdhar, S., Dogra, T. D., Wenckstern, S., & Leenaars, L. (2010a). Suicide notes from India and the United States: A thematic comparison. *Death Studies, 34*(5), 426–440.

Leenaars, A. A., Sayin, A., Candansayar, S., Leenaars, L., Akar, T., & Demirel, B. (2010b). Suicide in different cultures: A thematic comparison of suicide notes from Turkey and the United States. *Journal of Cross-Cultural Psychology, 41*(2), 253–263.

Lehmann, J. M. (1995) Durkheim's theories of deviance and suicide: A feminist reconsideration. *The American Journal of Sociology, 100*, 904–930.

Li, J., Stroebe, M., Chan, C., & Chow, A. (2014). Guilt in bereavement: A review and conceptual framework. *Death Studies, 38*(3), 165–171. doi:10.1080/07481187.2012.738770

Maple, M., Cerel, J., McKay, K., & Jordan, J. (2014). Uncovering and identifying the missing voices in suicide bereavement. *Suicidology Online, 5*(1), 1–12.

Maple, M., Edwards, H., Plummer, D., & Minichiello, V. (2010). Silenced voices: Hearing the stories of parents bereaved through the suicide death of a young adult child. *Health and Social Care in the Community, 18*(3), 241–248. doi:10.1111/j.1365-2524.2009.00886.x

Maple, M., Plummer, D., Edwards, H., & Minichiello, V. (2007). The effects of preparedness for suicide following the death of a young adult child. *Suicide and Life-Threatening Behavior, 37*(2), 127–134.

McIntosh, J. L. (2012, January 12). *U.S.A. suicide: 2009 official final data.* Retrieved from http://www.suicidology.org

Minios, G. (1999). *A history of suicide: Voluntary death in Western culture.* Baltimore, MD: John Hopkins University Press.

Neimeyer, R. (2000). Searching for the meaning of meaning: Grief therapy and the process of reconstruction. *Death Studies, 24*(6), 541–588.

Office for National Statistics. (2013). *Suicides in the United Kingdom, 2011: National records of Scotland, Northern Ireland Statistics and Research Agency and Office for National Statistics.* Retrieved from http://www.ons.gov.uk

Prigerson, H., Horowitz, M., Jacobs, S., Parkes, C., Aslan, M., Goodkin, K., et al. (2009). Prolonged grief disorder: Psychometric validation of criteria proposed for DSM-V and ICD-11. *PLoS Medicine, 6*(8), e1000121. doi:10.1371/journal.pmed.1000121

Ratnarajah, D., Maple, M., & Minichiello, V. (2014). Understanding family member suicide narratives by investigating family functioning history. *Omega: Journal of Death & Dying, 69*(1), 41–57.

Ratnarajah, D., & Schofield, M. (2008). Survivors' narratives of the impact of parental suicide. *Suicide and Life-Threatening Behavior, 38*(5), 618–630.

Reed, M. (1998). Predicting grief symptomatology among the suddenly bereaved. *Suicide and Life-Threatening Behavior, 28*(3), 285–300.

Roy, A., & Segal, N. L. (2001). Suicidal behavior in twins: A replication. *Journal of Affective Disorders, 66*(1), 71–74. doi:10.1016/S0165-0327(00)00275-5

Runeson, B., & Asberg, M. (2003). Family history of suicide among suicide victims. *American Journal of Psychiatry, 160*(8), 1525–1526.

Shneidman, E. (1972). Foreword. In A. Cain (Ed.), *Survivors of suicide.* Springfield, IL: Charles C. Thomas.

Statham, D. J., Heath, A. C., Madden, P. A., Bucholz, K. K., Bierut, L., Dinwiddie, S. H., et al. (1998). Suicidal behaviour: An epidemiological and genetic study. *Psychological Medicine, 28*(4), 839–855.

Statistics Canada. (2012). *Suicide rates: An overview.* Ottawa, Ontario: Author.

Stroebe, M. (2001). Bereavement research and theory: Retrospective and prospective. *American Behavioral Scientist, 44*(5), 854–865.

Ting, L., Sanders, S., Jacobson, J. M., & Power, J. R. (2006). Dealing with the aftermath: A qualitative analysis of mental health social workers' reactions after a client suicide. *Social Work, 51*(4), 329–341.

Van Orden, K. A., Witte, T. K., Cukrowicz, K. C., Braithwaite, S. R., Selby, E. A., & Joiner, T. E., Jr. (2010). The interpersonal theory of suicide. *Psychological Review, 117*(2), 575–600. doi:10.1037/a0018697

Young, I., Iglewicz, A., Glorioso, D., Lanouette, N., Seay, K., Ilapakurti, M., et al. (2012). Suicide bereavement and complicated grief. *Dialogues of Clinical Neuroscience, 14*(2), 177–186.

FURTHER READING

American Association of Suicidology: http://www.suicidology.org

Bolton, I., & Mitchell, C. (1983). *My son...my son...: A guide to healing after death, loss, or suicide.* Atlanta: Bolton Press.

Linn-Gust, M., & Cerel, J. (2011). *Seeking hope: Stories of the suicide bereaved.* Albuquerque, NM: Chellhead Works.

Suicide Prevention Resource Center. *After a suicide: A toolkit for schools:* http://www.sprc.org/sites/sprc.org/files/library/AfterSuicideToolkitforSchools.pdf. There are a number of programs in place for postvention, including a free toolkit for school personnel to utilize following a suicide in a school. This toolkit addresses crisis response in the immediate aftermath of the suicide and how to help students cope, including expressing their emotions and identifying strategies for managing them. It also discusses the issues of memorialization of the deceased student. The toolkit describes how it is important for schools to treat all deaths the same way in terms of memorialization because there is a balance between how to appropriately memorialize the student who has died and the risk of suicide contagion among at-risk surviving students. Despite this comprehensive resource, no existing research examines how postvention within a school impacts affected children.

JULIE CEREL AND MYFANWY MAPLE

SYSTEMATIC REVIEWS

ABSTRACT: Systematic reviews summarize a body of empirical evidence to address important questions for practice and social policy. Widely used to compile evidence about intervention effects in the helping professions, systematic reviews can also be used to assess rates, trends, associations, and variations on many topics. Credible reviews are based on the science of research synthesis, which provides the theoretical and empirical foundations that undergird efforts to minimize bias and error at each step in the review process to ensure that systematic reviews are comprehensive and their conclusions are accurate. Methods for the synthesis of quantitative studies are well developed. Meta-analysis, a set of statistical procedures, is often used in quantitative reviews, but meta-analysis is only one part of the systematic review process; other steps are needed to limit bias and error. Methods for systematic reviews of qualitative research are under development, as are strategies to combine quantitative and qualitative data in reviews.

KEY WORDS: evidence; empirical; literature review; meta-analysis; research

Systematic reviews take a scientific approach to the identification, critical appraisal, analysis, synthesis, and reporting of results of multiple studies on a single topic. The review process is treated like any other form of research: reviewers pose clear and answerable questions and take steps to obtain unbiased answers by finding relevant studies, reliably extracting information from those studies, and compiling and reporting results in a systematic and transparent manner. Following a long history of development in the helping professions and scientific disciplines, systematic reviews have flourished in the early 21st century with the advent of new scientific methods for research synthesis and the need to manage ever-increasing amounts of information on topics relevant for clinical practice and social policy.

History

Early attempts to organize results of previous research appeared in a few 18th- and 19th-century publications in medicine and psychology; more examples emerged in the early 20th century and by the 1930s the science of research synthesis was developing in agriculture, physics, psychology, education, medicine, and statistics (Chalmers, Hedges, & Cooper, 2002). The term "systematic review" appeared in the mid-1930s, but was not widely adopted until the 1990s, when it was used to draw a distinction between meta-analysis (the statistical synthesis of results from multiple studies) and "a process involving measures to control bias in research synthesis" (Chalmers et al., p. 16).

The publication in the 1970s of several large meta-analyses drew attention to the value of research synthesis in addressing important issues in the social sciences. Landmark publications included Smith and Glass's (1977) review of research on psychotherapy; Glass and Smith's (1978) review on effects of school class size on achievement; Rosenthal and Rubin's (1979) review on interpersonal expectancy effects; and Hunter, Schmidt, and Hunter's (1979) review of research on the validity of employment tests by race. These studies focused on the statistical synthesis of data and not on other steps in the review process. Formal statistical methods for meta-analysis followed (Hedges & Olkin, 1985).

In the 1980s, Cooper (1982) and others (for example, Light & Pillemer, 1984) developed scientific approaches to the entire review process. Cooper (1982, 1998) likened research synthesis to any other form of research, noting that reviews should follow all of the usual steps in the research process, including problem formulation, data collection, data evaluation, analysis and interpretation, and reporting. This raised issues about the scope and foci of reviews, procedures used to identify relevant studies, criteria for study inclusion and exclusion, reliability of attempts to extract data from studies, and so on.

The international Cochrane Collaboration was established in 1993 to produce systematic reviews of research on interventions in health care. The Cochrane Collaboration soon became a world leader in the development of methods for research synthesis. In addition to producing high-quality reviews on important topics in health care, Cochrane contributors organized and synthesized research on methodological issues to inform the conduct of future studies and systematic reviews. This led to the development of evidence-based standards for research and reviews (described below).

In the late 1990s, participants in the Cochrane Collaboration, prominent social-work scholars, and others recognized the need for systematic reviews on a wide range of topics in social work and social welfare, education, and criminology. As a result, the Campbell Collaboration was established in 1999 to produce systematic reviews in the fields of social care (Boruch, Petrosino, & Chalmers, 1999). In 2010, the Campbell Collaboration was expanded to include reviews on topics in international development and interventions in low- and middle-income countries. The Cochrane and Campbell groups continue to maintain close ties and set standards for best practice in systematic reviews.

In 2005, the Society for Research Synthesis Methodology was created to further the development and application of synthesis methods. This international, multidisciplinary group produces a journal (*Research Synthesis Methods*) that captures many new developments in the field. Other organizations involved in research synthesis include the U.K. Centre for Reviews and Dissemination, U.S. Agency for Healthcare Research and Quality, U.S. Centers for Disease Control, and the EPPI-Centre.

The science of research synthesis has flourished since the 1990s, with the publication of many influential texts and guidelines for the conduct, reporting, and critical appraisal of systematic reviews and meta-analysis (Bornstein, Hedges, Higgins, & Rothstein, 2009; Cooper, Hedges, & Valentine, 2009; Higgins & Green, 2011; Institute of Medicine (IOM), 2011; Moher, Liberati, Tetzlaff, Altman, & the PRISMA Group, 2009; Rothstein, Sutton, & Bornstein, 2005; Shea et al., 2007). Petticrew and Roberts (2006) and Littell and colleagues (Littell, Corcoran, & Pillai, 2008) described systematic reviews in the social sciences and social work.

To date, relatively few social-work scholars have conducted Cochrane or Campbell reviews (or systematic reviews that meet current international, interdisciplinary standards). Many schools of social work are beginning to teach systematic review methods (often at the doctoral level). This is a small, but rapidly growing area of social-work scholarship, influenced by interests in obtaining and using scientifically sound evidence summaries to inform social-work practice and social policy.

Uses

Systematic reviews can summarize empirical evidence on a wide range of topics relevant for policy and practice, including questions about the incidence or prevalence (rates) of various conditions, trends over time, correlates and predictors of outcomes (including risk and protective factors), the accuracy of diagnostic or prognostic tests, properties of measurement tools, the effectiveness or comparative effectiveness of interventions for various conditions, the durability of outcomes over time, moderators of treatment effects, and so forth. Systematic approaches have most often been used in reviews of research on effects of interventions in health care, mental health, education, social welfare, criminology, and environmental sciences, but many other topics are possible. Contrary to common misconceptions, systematic reviews are not limited to randomized controlled trials, questions about interventions, or "biomedical" models (Petticrew, 2001). For example, systematic reviews have been used to synthesize research on the following: (a) the proportion of children with secure attachments to their parents and/or nonparental caregivers, (b) associations between various attitudes and behaviors, and (c) factors associated with turnover and retention in human services (for references, see Littell et al., 2008).

By integrating results of multiple studies on the same topic, systematic reviews can provide readers with an overview of a large body of research, showing overall trends (for example, average rates or effects) and important variations across studies. This method allows us to better understand the consistency or inconsistency of important phenomena over time, subgroups, contexts, and cultures. In addition to summarizing what is known on a particular topic, systematic reviews and meta-analyses can address questions that have not yet been considered in any primary studies; that is, by capitalizing on natural variations among existing studies, reviewers can explore whether results vary systematically by characteristics of the studies, participants, interventions, settings, or timing. For example, Smedslund and colleagues (Smedslund et al., 2006) found that the welfare-to-work programs that have relatively better employment outcomes are those that provide assistance with job searches, use fewer sanctions, and have older participants.

Although most systematic reviews focus exclusively on quantitative research, there is increasing interest in the synthesis of qualitative studies, either alone or alongside systematic reviews of quantitative research. Barnett-Page and Thomas (2009) describe the numerous, overlapping approaches for qualitative synthesis. The choice of methods depends in part on the aims of the review (Hannes & Harden, 2011), but there is little empirical research and no consensus to suggest which of the many available methods is preferable for various purposes. Harden and colleagues (Harden, Brunton, Fletcher, & Oakley, 2009) provide an example of the use of multiple methods in research synthesis. They assessed interventions that address the social disadvantages associated with teenage pregnancy using (a) a systematic review and meta-analysis of quantitative studies to assess program effects along (b) a thematic synthesis of qualitative studies on the views of early parenthood among young people living in the United Kingdom.

Umbrella reviews compile results of several systematic reviews on the same topic, often to compare effects of different treatments for a particular condition (Ioannidis, 2009). Using available data, reviewers can create a network of comparisons among multiple treatment and control conditions. Network meta-analysis (also known as multiple-treatments or multiple-comparisons meta-analysis) uses both direct and indirect comparisons to rank the effectiveness of different interventions for the same condition (Ioannidis; Salanti, 2012).

Common Sources of Bias and Error in Research Reviews

Research reviews will be affected by problems in the conduct, reporting, and dissemination of prior research, as well as issues that arise in the review process itself. There is a growing body of methodological research on bias and error and how to minimize these problems in research reviews (Cooper et al., 2009; Higgins & Green, 2011; Littell et al., 2008). This body of evidence informs the practice of systematic reviews.

Biases can arise within primary studies in many ways. The threats-to-validity framework is a useful way to conceptualize different types and sources of bias (Shadish, Cook, & Campbell, 2002). The threats to validity that are most relevant for a specific study will depend on its purpose and methods. For example, selection bias is a common threat to the internal validity of studies aimed at assessing intervention effects (Larzelere, Kuhn, & Johnson, 2004). There are a variety of ways to control for or address selection bias in primary studies, but some methods are more reliable than others (Shadish, 2011). Reviewers should consider whether studies address relevant threats to internal, external, construct, and statistical conclusion validity when evaluating primary studies to be included in a review (but note that the lack of sufficient statistical power in the original studies can be overcome in some meta-analyses). Systematic reviewers deal with biases in primary studies in several ways: First, they set clear minimum standards for inclusion to weed out methodologically weak studies that cannot provide credible answers to the review questions. Second, they assess relevant risks of bias

(or other qualities) in each study included in the review and report results of this assessment. Finally, reviewers may conduct moderator analysis to assess the potential impact of specific study qualities on research results (Higgins & Green, 2011).

The results of any single study will be affected by the play of chance (random error). It is not possible to know how random error has affected the results of individual studies. Thus, single studies provide information that is of limited usefulness in making generalizations to other samples. However, when we pool results from multiple studies, we have much more information on the likely distribution of events or outcomes both within and across samples. Meta-analysis then allows reviewers to determine whether chance alone or other factors may account for differences across studies (Wilson, 2009).

Bias and error can also occur when reviewers search for studies, decide which studies to include and exclude, extract and code information from primary studies, analyze and synthesize the data, and report results. Fortunately, steps can be taken to minimize these problems.

To provide an accurate summary of prior research, a systematic review must include an unbiased sample of relevant studies. Such samples are not easily obtained because of well-documented biases in the reporting, publication, and dissemination of research results: approximately half of completed studies remain unpublished, but unpublished studies are not inherently inferior to published ones (Dwan et al., 2008). In fact, McLeod and Weisz (2004) found that unpublished dissertations tend to be methodologically superior to published studies, yet dissertations report significantly smaller effect sizes. In general, research results that are positive and statistically significant are more likely to be presented at conferences and published in journals than equally valid results that are not statistically significant or do not confirm research hypotheses (Scherer, Langenberg, & von-Elm, 2007; Song et al., 2009, 2010). Even when accepted for publication, studies with negative or null results take longer to appear in print (Hopewell, Clarke, Stewart, & Tierney, 2007), whereas studies with positive, significant results are cited and reprinted more often (Egger & Smith, 1998). Thus, it is easier to find studies with positive results and miss equally valid research with negative or null results.

According to Wilson (2009), "A biased collection of studies will lead to a biased review" (p. 437). Reviews based on published studies are likely to overestimate benefits of favored treatments and underestimate their potential harms (Hopewell, McDonald, Clarke,

& Egger, 2007). Indeed, the effects of many widely used treatments (including cognitive–behavioral treatments and other psychotherapies) have been overestimated in meta-analyses because of publication bias (Cuijpers, Smit, Bohlmeijer, Hollon, & Andersson, 2010). To counteract reporting, publication, and dissemination biases, systematic reviewers make special attempts to obtain unpublished and hard-to-find ("gray") literature. There are several strategies for doing this (discussed below).

Early reports suggested that publication and dissemination biases might be particularly problematic in English-language journals (Egger et al., 1997). However, a recent review found inconclusive evidence on this topic (Morrison et al., 2009).

Errors are common in the extraction of data from quantitative studies (Gøtzsche, Hrógjartsson, Maric, & Tendal, 2007). These errors can be reduced when two or more reviewers independently code information from primary studies, then compare notes, and resolve any differences with a third party if necessary (Buscemi, Hartling, Vandermeer, Tjosvold, & Klassen, 2005). (There is little or no evidence about the reliability of data extraction in qualitative syntheses.)

Narrative syntheses of results of quantitative studies and vote counting (tallying the number of studies that provide support for and against a hypothesis) can lead to inaccurate and misleading conclusions (Bushman & Wells, 2001; Carlton & Strawderman,1996; Cooper & Rosenthal, 1980). Narrative reviews are unduly affected by trivial properties of studies (Bushman & Wells), whereas vote counting fails to consider important variations in sample sizes and heterogeneity in assessing overall results.

Systematic Review Methods

Systematic reviews are conducted in phases that are parallel to the steps in primary research. These phases include problem formulation, the literature search, data evaluation, analysis and synthesis, interpretation, and reporting (Cooper et al., 2009).

Reviewers develop a detailed protocol, specifying the objectives and methods of the review. The protocol clarifies the scope and boundaries of the review with explicit inclusion and exclusion criteria, which describe the types of studies, populations or problems, interventions, comparisons, and outcomes that will and will not be included in the review. This limits reviewers' freedom to select studies on the basis of their results or on some other basis (Higgins & Green, 2011; Littell et al., 2008). The protocol also describes in detail the methods that will be used

to search for studies, screen titles and abstracts, determine study eligibility, reliably extract data, critically appraise studies, and analyze and synthesize results. To enhance transparency, protocols for systematic reviews should be publicly available before the review begins. If reviewers find that a change of plan is needed, changes can be explained in the final report. Protocols for systematic reviews can be found in the Cochrane Database of Systematic Reviews (http://www.cochrane.org), the Campbell Library (http://www.campbellcollaboration.org), and the International Prospective Register of Systematic Reviews (http://www.crd.york.ac.uk/PROSPERO).

Systematic reviewers work in teams and are often assisted by specialists or advisory panels. Review teams should include a librarian or information specialist (IOM, 2011). Substantive expertise is important, as is knowledge of primary research methodologies, systematic review methods, and meta-analysis. Some review teams or advisory boards include consumers or policy makers, along with substantive and methodological experts.

Team members develop and execute a strategy for finding potentially eligible studies for the review. Diverse sources and methods are required to obtain an unbiased sample of studies (Hammerstrøm, Wade, & Jørgensen, 2010). It is important to search multiple databases because each database only includes a subset of available studies. Crafting efficient (sensitive and specific) keyword search strings requires both knowledge of the substantive area and specialized knowledge of the content and structure of various databases. Keyword searches are carefully documented, so that that they can be reported accurately and updated later, as needed. In addition to keyword searches of multiple databases, hand searching of relevant journals is often needed to find eligible studies that are not properly indexed in electronic databases (Hopewell, Clarke, Lefebvre, & Scherer, 2007). Systematic reviewers make special attempts to locate relevant gray literature (unpublished and hard-to-find studies) to minimize the effects of reporting, publication, and dissemination biases on results of reviews (Chandler, Churchill, Higgins, Lasserson, & Tovey, 2012; Hopewell, Clarke, & Mallett, 2005; IOM, 2011; Rothstein, 2008; Rothstein et al., 2005; Wilson, 2009). Many reviewers contact experts (via email or listservs) with a call for unpublished studies that meet the review criteria.

Reviewers screen titles and abstracts, ruling out those that are obviously irrelevant. It is usually necessary to obtain the full text of documents to determine whether a study meets all of the review's eligibility criteria. Systematic reviewers assess the reliability of their inclusion and exclusion decisions. To do this, two or more reviewers make independent decisions about each study's eligibility for the review, then compare notes, assess interrater agreement (often using Cohen's κ), resolve differences (with a third reviewer if necessary), and document reasons for their decisions (Higgins & Green, 2011). Specific reasons for exclusion are given for every study that passes the initial screening phase, so that readers can find out why specific studies were excluded. The Preferred Reporting Items for Systematic Reviews and Meta-Analyses flowchart is used to document the flow of studies through the review process (Moher et al., 2009).

Reviewers extract key pieces of information from study documents onto structured paper or electronic coding forms. This process captures potentially important information about study design characteristics, data collection procedures, measures, treatment characteristics (if applicable), settings, participants, raw data, and statistical results. These data are then available for use in the analysis. Reviewers often seek additional information or clarification from studies' original investigators.

A critical appraisal of each study in the review is essential. Reviewers assess methodological characteristics of primary studies because study design and implementation issues affect the credibility and interpretation of results (Shadish, 2011; Shadish et al., 2002). There are many approaches to study quality assessment in systematic reviews (Jüni, Altman, & Egger, 2001; Jüni, Witschi, Bloch, & Egger, 1999). Some focus on overall design features, whereas others emphasize threats to validity or vulnerability to certain types of bias. The Cochrane risk-of-bias tool (Higgins & Green, 2011) can be used with nonrandomized studies with minor modifications (Shrier, 2011). There is a general consensus among methodologists and meta-analysts that study qualities should be assessed separately and should not be summed into overall study-quality scores (Jüni et al., 2001; Wells & Littell, 2009). The potential impact of specific study qualities on results may be examined with moderator analysis.

If possible, meta-analysis should be used to analyze and synthesize results across studies (Bornstein et al., 2009; Higgins & Green, 2011; Littell et al., 2008). Meta-analysis includes a wide range of techniques to describe overall averages, variations, and trends in a set of studies (Bornstein et al.). If a review contains heterogeneous results and a sufficient number of studies, moderator analysis can be used to explore possible explanations for observed varia-

tions in results across studies. Sensitivity analysis is used to assess decisions made in the review process, the potential effects of outliers, and problems of missing data.

There are a variety of methods to detect and correct for reporting and publication biases in systematic reviews and meta-analyses. Older methods, such as Failsafe N (or the file drawer number), are unreliable and have been replaced by newer analytic techniques (Rothstein, 2008; Rothstein et al., 2005).

Recent advances in network meta-analysis (also known as multiple-treatments or multiple-comparisons meta-analysis) allow reviewers to use both direct and indirect evidence to compare the relative effectiveness of multiple treatments for various conditions (Salanti, 2012). This approach is computationally complex, but it allows reviewers to rank the relative effectiveness of different treatments for the same condition. For example, Cipriani and colleagues (Cipriani et al., 2009) used this approach to assess the relative benefits and acceptability of 12 antidepressants in cases of major depression.

Standards and Guidelines

A number of organizations have produced guidelines and standards for reviews, but only some of these documents are based on the evidence from methodological research on ways to minimize bias and error in the review process. Evidence-based guidelines and standards for the conduct of systematic reviews of interventions are available from the Cochrane Collaboration (Chandler et al., 2012; Higgins & Green, 2011) and the IOM (2011). Evidence-based guidelines for reporting on systematic reviews and meta-analyses include the Preferred Reporting Items for Systematic Reviews and Meta-Analyses statement (Moher et al., 2009) and the Meta-analysis of Observational Studies in Epidemiology statement (Stroup et al., 2000). The Cochrane Collaboration has also produced guidelines for plain-language summaries of systematic reviews (*http://www.editorial-unit.cochrane.org/mecir*).

Guidelines for the Assessment of Multiple Systematic Reviews were developed by Shea and colleagues (Shea et al., 2007). The guidelines include 11 items that can be used to gauge the quality of a systematic review or meta-analysis (Littell & Shlonsky, 2011).

Advantages

Systematic reviews have many advantages over other review methods. They are more reliable and more accurate than traditional (haphazard) reviews, even when the latter are conducted by experts (Littell, 2008; Petticrew & Roberts, 2006). To the extent that explicit steps are taken to minimize bias and error, systematic reviews will produce more complete and accurate summaries of available evidence than narrative reviews of quantitative data, vote counting, or stand-alone meta-analyses (for example, meta-analyses that are limited to published studies). When properly executed, systematic reviews will produce the most comprehensive, transparent, and accurate research syntheses possible. Plain-language summaries of systematic reviews help policy makers and practitioners understand the best available evidence.

Limitations

Most systematic reviews are labor intensive and time-consuming; thus, they can be costly. The search for relevant studies (especially for unpublished and hard-to-find documents), duplicate extraction of data, and the careful execution and documentation of all systematic review procedures can be daunting. For this reason, systematic reviews are best conducted in teams that contain necessary expertise in information retrieval (library sciences), substantive knowledge of the topic, research methodology, systematic review methodology, and meta-analysis. Training in systematic review methods is available through the Cochrane and Campbell collaborations and others, often at low or no cost. If reviewers skip steps in the systematic review process, they are obligated to acknowledge the potential limitations that may follow in terms of increased risks of bias and error in the results and conclusions of their review (Moher et al., 2009).

Current Status

The use of systematic review methods is increasing, but their quality is uneven and there are concerns about continued use of nonsystematic (haphazard) review methods.

Moher and colleagues (Moher, Tetzlaff, Tricco, Sampson, & Altman, 2007) estimated that 2,500 systematic reviews were published in English and indexed in MEDLINE in 2004 alone. They noted important variations in the quality of reporting on these systematic reviews. Thus, this study was followed by improved guidelines for reporting on systematic reviews (the Preferred Reporting Items for Systematic Reviews and Meta-Analyses statement; Moher et al., 2009).

The Cochrane Collaboration has produced over 5,000 systematic reviews, primarily on the effectiveness of interventions for specific conditions. Given concerns about uneven quality of reviews, Cochrane authors recently published explicit methodological expectations for intervention reviews (Chandler et al., 2012). Cochrane authors are also developing a handbook to guide the conduct of systematic reviews on the accuracy of diagnostic tests.

The IOM released guidelines for systematic reviews in 2011, noting that many systematic reviews fall short of current guidance by failing to provide adequate documentation of search and screening methods, failing to acknowledge or address risks of reporting and publication biases, neglecting to appraise the quality of included studies, and failing to account for errors likely to occur in data extraction and meta-analysis. A systematic review "might lead to the wrong conclusions, and ultimately, the wrong clinical recommendations, if relevant data are missed, errors are uncorrected or unreliable research is used" (IOM, 2011, p. 82).

In social work, psychology, and related fields, the adoption of systematic review methods appears to be lagging behind that in the health fields. Meta-analyses of published studies continue to appear in journals, with insufficient attention to problems of publication bias. As systematic reviews have increased in popularity, the term systematic review has sometimes been misappropriated (that is, applied to reviews that are not truly systematic).

Just as researchers must be careful to limit bias and error in primary studies, reviewers must take explicit steps to ensure the integrity of their reviews. Fortunately, there is a growing body of evidence on the reliability and validity of quantitative methods of research synthesis, which has fueled the development of evidence-based standards for systematic reviews (for example, Chandler et al., 2012; IOM, 2011; Moher et al., 2009).

Implications for Social-Work Practice and Policy

Social work has long been interested in building an empirical evidence base to inform policy and practice. Single studies are insufficient for this purpose because they do not tell us whether results will be replicable in other samples or circumstances. Research reviews are necessary, but some reviews are more credible than others.

Research reviews should provide readers with comprehensive and unbiased summaries of a body of evidence; unfortunately, many published reviews fall far short of these goals (Gibbs, 2003; Petticrew & Roberts, 2006). Even when conducted by experts, haphazard reviews provide weak foundations for practice and policy because these reviews are subject to bias and error (Littell, 2008; Petticrew & Roberts).

Readers should expect systematic reviews to be comprehensive, transparent, and accurate. However, critical appraisal of review methods is necessary to assess the credibility of their conclusions (Littell & Shlonsky, 2011).

Good systematic reviews provide information that can be used by social workers, agency administrators, policy makers, and consumers to inform their decisions and priorities, aid in selecting among competing alternatives, identify areas for further development or research, and assist in decisions about the allocation of scarce resources (Shlonsky, Noonan, Littell, & Montgomery, 2011).

REFERENCES

Barnett-Page, E., & Thomas, J. (2009). *Methods for the synthesis of qualitative research: A critical review.* Southampton, U.K.: U.K. Economic and Social Research Council, National Centre for Research Methods.

Bornstein, M., Hedges, L. V., Higgins, J. P. T., & Rothstein, H. R. (2009). *Introduction to meta-analysis.* West Sussex, England: Wiley.

Boruch, R., Petrosino, A., & Chalmers, I. (1999). The Campbell Collaboration: A proposal for systematic, multinational, and continuous reviews of evidence. In P. Davis, A. Petrosino, & I. Chalmers (Eds.), *The effects of social and educational interventions: Developing an infrastructure for international collaboration to prepare, maintain and promote the accessibility of systematic reviews of relevant research* (pp. 1–22). London, U.K.: London University College London School of Public Policy.

Buscemi, N., Hartling, L., Vandermeer, B., Tjosvold, L., & Klassen, T. P. (2005). Single data extraction generated more errors than double data extraction in systematic reviews. *Journal of Clinical Epidemiology, 59,* 697–703.

Bushman, B. J., & Wells, G. L. (2001). Narrative impressions of literature: The availability bias and the corrective properties of meta-analytic approaches. *Personal and Social Psychology Bulletin, 27,* 1123–1130.

Carlton, P. L., & Strawderman, W. E. (1996). Evaluating cumulated research I: The inadequacy of traditional methods. *Biological Psychiatry, 39,* 65–72.

Chalmers, I., Hedges, L. V., & Cooper, H. (2002). A brief history of research synthesis. *Evaluation & the Health Professions, 25*(1), 12–37.

Chandler, J., Churchill, R., Higgins, J., Lasserson, T., & Tovey, D. (2012). *Methodological standards for the conduct of new Cochrane Intervention Reviews* (Version 2.2). Retrieved January 15, 2013, from http://www.editorial-unit.cochrane.org/sites/editorial-unit.cochrane.org/files/uploads/MECIR_conduct_standards%202.2%2017122012_0.pdf

Cipriani, A., Furukawa, T. A., Salanti, G., Geddes, J. R., Higgins, J. P. T., Churchill, R., et al. (2009). Comparative efficacy and acceptability of 12 new-generation antidepressants: A multiple-treatments meta-analysis. *The Lancet, 373,* 746–758.

Cooper, H. (1998). *Synthesizing research* (3rd ed.). Thousand Oaks, CA: Sage.

Cooper, H. M. (1982). Scientific guidelines for conducting integrative research reviews. *Review of Educational Research, 52*(2), 291–302.

Cooper, H. M., Hedges, L. V., & Valentine, J. C. (2009). *The handbook of research synthesis and meta-analysis* (2nd ed.). New York, NY: Russell Sage Foundation.

Cooper, H. M., & Rosenthal, R. (1980). Statistical versus traditional procedures for summarizing research findings. *Psychological Bulletin, 87*(3), 442–449.

Cuijpers, P., Smit, F., Bohlmeijer, E., Hollon, S. D., & Andersson, G. (2010). Efficacy of cognitive–behavioural therapy and other psychological treatments for adult depression: Meta-analytic study of publication bias. *The British Journal of Psychiatry, 196*(3), 173–178. doi:10.1192/bjp.bp.109.066001

Dwan, K., Altman, D. G., Arnaiz, J. A., Bloom, J., Chan, A.-W., Cronin, E., et al. (2008). Systematic review of the empirical evidence of study publication bias and outcome reporting bias. *PLoS ONE, 3*(8), e3081.

Egger, M., & Smith, G. D. (1998). Bias in location and selection of studies. *British Medical Journal, 316*(7124), 61–66.

Egger, M., Zellweger-Zahner, T., Schneider, M., Junker, C., Lengeler, C., & Antes, G. (1997). Language bias in randomised controlled trials published in English and German. *The Lancet, 350*(9074), 326–329.

Gibbs, L. E. (2003). *Evidence-based practice for the helping professions: A practical guide with integrated multimedia.* Pacific Grove, CA: Brooks/Cole–Thompson Learning.

Glass, G. V., & Smith, M. K. (1978). Meta-analysis of research on the relationship of class size and achievement. *Educational Evaluation and Policy Analysis, 1,* 2–16.

Gøtzsche, P. C., Hrógjartsson, A., Maric, K., & Tendal, B. (2007). Data extraction errors in meta-analyses that use standardized mean differences. *Journal of the American Medical Association, 298*(4), 430–437.

Hammerstrøm, K., Wade, A., & Jørgensen, A.-M. K. (2010). *Searching for studies: A guide to information retrieval for Campbell systematic reviews.* Retrieved January 15, 2013, from http://www.campbellcollaboration.org/resources/research/new_information_retrieval_guide.php

Hannes, K., & Harden, A. (2011). Multi-context versus context-specific qualitative evidence syntheses: Combining the best of both. *Research Synthesis Methods, 2,* 271–278.

Harden, A., Brunton, G., Fletcher, A., & Oakley, A. (2009). Teenage pregnancy and social disadvantage: Systematic review integrating controlled trials and qualitative studies. *British Medical Journal, 339,* b4254.

Hedges, L. V., & Olkin, I. (1985). *Statistical methods for meta-analysis.* Orlando, FL: Academic Press.

Higgins, J. P. T., & Green, S. (Eds.). (2011). *Cochrane Handbook for Systematic Reviews of Interventions* (Version

5.1.0). Retrieved January 15, 2013, from http://handbook.cochrane.org/

Hopewell, S., Clarke, M. J., Lefebvre, C., & Scherer, R. W. (2007). Handsearching versus electronic searching to identify reports of randomized trials. *Cochrane Database of Systematic Reviews, 2007*(2), MR000001.

Hopewell, S., Clarke, M., & Mallett, S. (2005). Grey literature and systematic reviews. In H. R. Rothstein, A. J. Sutton, & M. Bornstein (Eds.), *Publication bias in meta-analysis: Prevention, assessment and adjustments* (pp. 49–72). West Sussex, England: Wiley.

Hopewell, S., Clarke, M. J., Stewart, L., & Tierney, J. (2007). Time to publication for results of clinical trials. *Cochrane Database of Systematic Reviews, 2007*(2), MR000011.

Hopewell, S., McDonald, S., Clarke, M., & Egger, M. (2007). Grey literature in meta-analyses of randomized trials of health care interventions. *The Cochrane Database of Systematic Reviews, 2007*(2), MR000010.

Hunter, J. E., Schmidt, F. L., & Hunter, R. (1979). Differential validity of employment tests by race: A comprehensive review and analysis. *Psychological Bulletin, 86,* 721–735.

Institute of Medicine. (2011). *Finding what works in health care: Standards for systematic reviews.* Washington, DC: National Academy Press. Retrieved January 15, 2013, from http://www.iom.edu/srstandards

Ioannidis, J. P. A. (2009). Integration of evidence from multiple meta-analyses: A primer on umbrella reviews, treatment networks and multiple treatments meta-analyses. *Canadian Medical Association Journal, 181*(8), 488–493.

Jüni, P., Altman, D. G., & Egger, M. (2001). Assessing the quality of controlled clinical trials. *British Medical Journal, 323*(7303), 42–46.

Jüni, P., Witschi, A., Bloch, R., & Egger, M. (1999). The hazards of scoring the quality of clinical trials for meta-analysis. *Journal of the American Medical Association, 282,* 1054–1060.

Larzelere, R. E., Kuhn, B. R., & Johnson, B. (2004). The intervention selection bias: An under-recognized confound in intervention research. *Psychological Bulletin, 130,* 289–303.

Light, R. J., & Pillemer, D. B. (1984). *Summing up: The science of reviewing research.* Cambridge, MA: Harvard University Press.

Littell, J. H. (2008). Evidence-based or biased? The quality of published reviews of evidence-based practices. *Children and Youth Services Review, 30,* 1299–1317.

Littell, J. H., Corcoran, J., & Pillai, V. (2008). *Systematic reviews and meta-analysis.* New York, NY: Oxford University Press.

Littell, J., & Shlonsky, A. (2011). Making sense of meta-analysis: A critique of "Effectiveness of Long-Term Psychodynamic Psychotherapy." *Clinical Social Work Journal, 39,* 340–346.

McLeod, B. D., & Weisz, J. R. (2004). Using dissertations to examine potential bias in child and adolescent clinical

trials. *Journal of Consulting and Clinical Psychology, 72*(2), 235–251.

Moher, D., Liberati, A., Tetzlaff, J., Altman, D. G., & the PRISMA Group. (2009). Preferred reporting items for systematic reviews and meta-analyses: The PRISMA statement. *PLoS Med, 6*(7), e1000097. doi:10.1371/journal.pmed.1000097

Moher, D., Tetzlaff, J., Tricco, A. C., Sampson, M., & Altman, D. G. (2007). Epidemiology and reporting characteristics of systematic reviews. *PLoS Medicine, 4*(3), e78.

Morrison, A., Moulton, K., Clark, M., Polisena, J., Fiander, M., Mierzwinski-Urban, M., et al. (2009). *English-language restriction when conducting systematic review-based meta-analyses: Systematic review of published studies.* Ottawa, Ontario, Canada: Canadian Agency for Drugs and Technologies in Health.

Petticrew, M. (2001). Systematic reviews from astronomy to zoology: Myths and misconceptions. *British Medical Journal, 322,* 98–101.

Petticrew, M., & Roberts, H. (2006). *Systematic reviews in the social sciences: A practical guide.* Oxford, U.K.: Blackwell.

Rosenthal, R., & Rubin, D. B. (1979). Interpersonal expectancy effects: The first 345 studies. *Behavioral and Brain Sciences, 3,* 377–386.

Rothstein, H. R. (2008). Publication bias as a threat to the validity of meta-analytic results. *Journal of Experimental Criminology, 4,* 61–81.

Rothstein, H., Sutton, A. J., & Bornstein, M. (2005). *Publication bias in meta-analysis: Prevention, assessment, and adjustments.* Chichester, U.K.: Wiley.

Salanti, G. (2012). Indirect and mixed-treatment comparison, network, or multiple-treatments meta-analysis: Many names, many benefits, many concerns for the next generation evidence synthesis tool. *Research Synthesis Methods, 3,* 80–97.

Scherer, R. W., Langenberg, P., & von-Elm, E. (2007). Full publication of results initially presented in abstracts. *Cochrane Database of Systematic Reviews, 2007*(2), MR000005. doi:10.1002/14651858.MR000005.pub3

Shadish, W. R. (2011). Randomized controlled studies and alternative designs in outcome studies. *Research on Social Work Practice, 21,* 636–643.

Shadish, W. R., Cook, T. D., & Campbell, D. T. (2002). *Experimental and quasi-experimental designs for generalized causal inference.* Boston, MA: Houghton Mifflin.

Shea, B. J., Grimshaw, J. M., Wells, G. A., Boers, M., Andersson, N., Hamel, C., et al. (2007). Development of AMSTAR: A measurement tool to assess the methodological quality of systematic reviews. *BMC Medical Research Methodology, 7,* 10. Retrieved January 15, 2013, from http://www.biomedcentral.com/1471-2288/7/10

Shlonsky, A., Noonan, E., Littell, J., & Montgomery, P. (2011). The role of systematic reviews and the Campbell Collaboration in the realization of evidence-informed practice. *Clinical Social Work Journal, 39,* 362–368.

Shrier, I. (2011). Structural approach to bias in meta-analysis. *Research Synthesis Methods, 2,* 223–237.

Smedslund, G., Dalsbo, T. K., Hagen, K. B., Johme, T., Rud, M. G., & Steiro, A. (2006). Work programmes for welfare recipients. *Campbell Systematic Reviews, 2006, 9.* Retrieved from http://campbellcollaboration.org/lib/project/18/

Smith, M. L., & Glass, G. V. (1977). Meta-analysis of psychotherapy outcome studies. *American Psychologist, 32,* 752–760.

Song, F., Parekh, S., Hooper, L., Loke, Y. K., Ryder, J., Sutton, A. J., et al. (2010). Dissemination and publication of research findings: An updated review of related biases. *Health Technology Assessment, 14*(8), 1–220.

Song, F., Parekh-Bhurke, S., Hooper, L., Loke, Y., Ryder, J., Sutton, A., et al. (2009). Extent of publication bias in different categories of research cohorts: A meta-analysis of empirical studies. *BMC Medical Research Methodology, 9*(1), 79.

Stroup, D. F., Berlin, J. A., Morton, S. C., Olkin, I., Williamson, G. D., Rennie, D., et al. for the Meta-analysis of Observational Studies in Epidemiology (MOOSE) Group. (2000). Meta-analysis of observational studies in epidemiology: A proposal for reporting. *Journal of the American Medical Association, 283*(15), 2008–2012.

Wells, K., & Littell, J. H. (2009). Study quality assessment in systematic reviews of research on intervention effects. *Research on Social Work Practice, 19,* 52–62.

Wilson, D. B. (2009). Missing a critical piece of the pie: Simple document search strategies inadequate for systematic reviews. *Journal of Experimental Criminology, 5,* 429–440.

SUGGESTED LINKS

The Campbell Collaboration: http://www.campbellcollaboration.org

Research Synthesis Methods journal: http://onlinelibrary.wiley.com/journal/10.1002/%28ISSN%291759-2887

The Cochrane Collaboration: http://www.cochrane.org

Reporting Guidelines: http://www.equator-network.org/resource-centre/library-of-health-research-reporting/reporting-guidelines/systematic-reviews-and-meta-analysis/

JULIA H. LITTELL

T

TASK-CENTERED PRACTICE

ABSTRACT: Task-centered practice is a social work technology designed to help clients and practitioners collaborate on specific, measurable, and achievable goals. It is designed to be brief (typically 8–12 sessions), and can be used with individuals, couples, families, and groups in a wide variety of social work practice contexts. With nearly 40 years of practice and research arguing for its effectiveness, task-centered practice can rightfully claim to be one of social work's original "evidence-based practices," though the relative paucity of research on its effectiveness in this decade suggests that the approach itself may have become increasingly integrated into other brief social work technologies.

KEY WORDS: brief treatment; case work; contracts; goal setting; task-centered

Task-centered practice (TCP) is now well into its fourth decade as a social work practice model, and has matured as a social work generalist practice tool that can empower clients to solve a wide variety of problems. Originally formulated by Laura Epstein (1914–1996) and William Reid (1928–2003) at the University of Chicago's School of Social Service Administration (SSA), the approach has been adopted by schools of social work and social work practitioners internationally, and the key textbooks for TCP have been translated into numerous languages. Many popular recent social work brief treatment approaches, such as narrative therapy and solution-focused brief treatment, have incorporated facets of TCP, and many key ideas of TCP are being taught in American, European, and Asian schools of social work in generalist practice courses. However, despite the seeming prevalence of the approach in multiple international settings and its potential applicability to a wide variety of problems typically treated by social work practitioners, TCP struggles to gain the recognition and respect it deserves as a social work practice innovation.

Definitions and Descriptions

TCP involves a four-step process that trains social work practitioners to work closely with clients to establish distinct and achievable goals based on an agreed-upon presenting problem, usually called the target problem. Under TCP, a maximum of three target problems are identified by the client and the social worker collaborates with the client on devising tasks to work on those target problems. The social worker and client cocreate a contract that contains the target problem, tasks to be implemented by both client and practitioner to address the target problem, and overall goals of the treatment. At all times through the process, TCP emphasizes client preferences by asking clients what they most want to work on to address their problems. Client priorities and strengths are interwoven into the entire TCP process. Most TCP involves working briefly with clients, typically 8–12 sessions over the course of a six-month period (Reid & Epstein, 1972).

The phases of TCP are both straightforward and flexible enough to be applied in almost any social work practice context (Marsh & Doel, 2005). After the target problem has been successfully defined (Step 1) and goals have been established to help deal successfully with the target problem (Step 2), a contract is created between the practitioner and the client that includes a schedule to help facilitate the intended changes (also Step 2). After several sessions in which clients and practitioners share the outcomes of the specific tasks they agreed to carry out (Step 3), the sessions turn to focusing on how well the overall goals have accomplished and whether another task-centered goal-setting process is necessary or whether the social work intervention has been successful enough to consider termination (Step 4) (Reid & Epstein, 1972). TCP developers Epstein and Reid acknowledged that these steps, while meant to be sequential, can often overlap and require that practitioners be trained to maximize the potential benefit of each step in the process when helping a client.

Main Developers and Contributors

The TCP approach began with Epstein and Reid's work at SSA, with the major initial research and development of TCP taking place under their direction between 1970 and 1978. During that time, the SSA project had over 100 graduate students helping Reid, Epstein, and their research team test out TCP interventions in a variety of settings common to social work practice, for example, schools, child welfare agencies, and hospitals. Their initial findings demonstrated that TCP was a potentially effective and flexible modality to employ with a wide array of client populations and problems. Since that pioneering era of TCP, over 200 books, articles, and dissertations have been published describing the TCP approach and demonstrating its effects in a host of social work practice contexts. Reid and Epstein have continued to publish on TCP, and have been joined by Cynthia Bailey-Dempsey, Anne Fortune, Matthias Naleepa, Ronald Rooney, and Eleanor Tolson as major academic proponents of TCP (Fortune, McCallion, & Briar-Lawson, 2010).

Statistics and Demographics

TCP has become firmly ensconced in most generalist social work practice textbooks, and most students learn at least the rudiments of TCP in their introductory classes. Reid continued to write about TCP until his passing in 2003, and other TCP leaders continue to emphasize TCP's benefits in this new era of evidence-based practice. However, despite having TCP adherents in the academy, it is unclear what the perception is of TCP in the larger social work practitioner community. To some extent, TCP may be a victim of its own success in this respect. Many new social workers may just assume that the process of setting discrete measurable goals with clients on the basis of the clients' ideas about what they would like to change is simply good social work practice rather than being rooted in the principles of TCP.

Similarly, because advocates of TCP have always maintained that it is a social work technology that can be viewed as both a psychotherapeutic and a casework intervention, perhaps the other therapeutic techniques that many social workers favor today (solution-focused brief therapy, narrative therapy) are more prominent because they emphasize the application of clinical skills over casework methods, and thus appeal to the desire of some social workers to be therapists first, and social workers second. Interestingly, these other brief therapy methods borrow heavily from the core concepts of TCP (respecting client views of the problem, helping the client set goals that they want to work on), though proponents of these approaches seldom explicitly acknowledge their debt to TCP, preferring instead to emphasize constructivist therapeutic ideas and the importance of cognitive-behavioral therapy research largely conducted in psychology.

The comparison with cognitive-behavioral therapy is particularly interesting, as it is slightly older as a treatment technology than is TCP but has been given far more attention from both researchers and practitioners in social work and other mental health fields. This may be another example of social work not being able to celebrate and further refine one of its own contributions to the knowledge base.

Current Applications

Many social work practice settings are good fits for TCP. Hospital settings with the emphasis on brief treatment and discharge planning; schools, with the increasing emphasis on identifying specific behavioral and social/emotional goals for students to work on; private practice and community mental health settings wherein clients are encouraged to set concrete goals to fulfill the mandates of managed care and brief treatment; and gerontology settings wherein older clients and their families need help identifying target problems and marshalling their resources to address those problems in a step-by-step fashion are all good examples of settings wherein practitioners using TCP may be able to increase the effectiveness of their interventions with clients. Researchers have studied all these areas using TCP and have found that TCP bolsters client participations in treatment planning, increases prosocial behaviors, and empowers clients to accomplish the treatment goals they are most interested in achieving (Reid, 1997).

Current Evidence on TCP and Its Connection to Evidence-Based Practice (EBP)

Like all models of casework and clinical practice, TCP cannot claim to be universally effective for all clients and all problems. However, given the over 200 published works on it, TCP stands as one of the most studied "home-grown" social work technologies in the profession's history. Sadly, with the death of Reid, it seems that interest in further establishing the research base for TCP's effectiveness has slowed considerably. Since 2000, there have been fewer than 10 published works on TCP, and those works have been mostly in the form of books, book chapters, and conceptual pieces rather than experimental studies of TCP's effectiveness. Though the early pioneers of TCP research have written consistently of the need for further refinement and adaption of the model, few current researchers appear to be adding to the empirical research base of TCP. A recent book honoring the legacy of TCP described innovative applications of TCP in 10 countries in Europe and Asia, though no new experimental trials of TCP research were cited beyond the current literature available (Fortune, McCallion, & Briar-Lawson, 2010).

A book chapter on TCP by Reid published post-humously (2004) correctly identified TCP as an "exemplar" of evidence-based practice. Indeed, TCP can claim to be one of social work's earliest examples of an evidence-based practice that was tested rigorously (including randomized controlled trials) and found to have modest but nonetheless consistently powerful effects for clients when compared with control groups (Reid, 1997). In this respect, supporters of TCP can rightfully claim that there is empirical support for TCP, though they would also readily acknowledge that much more study needs to be done on what clients and problems may benefit most from TCP. However, proponents of even more transparent approaches, for example, the kind of evidence-informed practice that Gambrill, Gibbs, and other EBP proponents favor, may chafe at the implication in TCP that while social workers using TCP make every effort to include clients in formulating the target problem to work on, they still maintain their authority as the director of the TCP process rather than being equal co-collaborators (Gambrill, 2006).

Distinctiveness and Integrations of the TCP Model

Many of the central principles of TCP are now considered simply good social work practice; its influence has contributed to the theoretical move away by the profession from uniformly subscribing to a psychodynamic long-term treatment model embedded in the medical model to diagnose and treat clients. The client-centered qualities of TCP are congruent with social work's roots, in that TCP challenges social workers to start where the clients are and stay in that place until the clients feel their problem is solved. Experts in TCP freely acknowledge that TCP is less a stand-alone model than an approach that can be easily adapted into multiple social work practice frameworks and practice settings (Reid, 1992). This may ultimately be its major contribution to the field of social work practice: a sturdy yet flexible practice technology that contains enough rigor to be consistently effective but also enough space to be adapted creatively to an incredible number of social work practice contexts.

REFERENCES

Fortune, A. E., Mccallion, P., Briar-Lawson, K. (Eds.) (2010). *Social work practice for the twenty-first century*. New York: Columbia University Press.

Gambrill, E. (2006). Evidence-based practice and policy: Choices ahead. *Research on Social Work Practice, 16*, 338–357.

Marsh, P., & Doel, M. (2005). *The task-centred book*. London: Routledge Books.

Reid, W. J. (1992). *Task strategies: An empirical approach to clinical social work*. New York: Columbia University Press.

Reid, W. J. (1997). Research on task-centered practice. *Research in Social Work, 21*, 132–137.

Reid, W. J., & Epstein, L. (1972). *Task-centered casework*. New York: Columbia University Press.

FURTHER READING

Fortune, A. E. (1985). *Task-centered practice with families and groups*. New York: Springer.

Gibbons, J. S., Bow, I., Butler, J., & Powell, J. (1979). Clients' reactions to task-centered casework: A follow-up study. *British Journal of Social Work, 9*, 203–215.

Madden, L. L., Hicks-Coolick, A., & Kirk, A. B. (2002). An empowerment model for social welfare consumers. *Lippincott's Case Management, 7*, 129–136.

Reid, W. J. (2000). *The task planner: An intervention resource for human service professionals*. New York: Columbia University Press.

Rooney, R. H. (1992). *Strategies for work with involuntary clients*. New York: Columbia University Press.

"From the Task-Centered Approach to Evidence-Based and Integrative Practice" Symposium. http://ssacentennial.uchicago.edu/events/symposium-mccracken-rzepnicki.shtml

Institute for Research and Innovation in Social Sciences. http://content.iriss.org.uk/taskcentered/index.html

MICHAEL S. KELLY

TEAMS

ABSTRACT: Teams maximize the coordinated expertise of various professionals. Social work skills used with clients, especially contracting, monitoring team processes, managing conflict, creating a climate of openness, and developing and supporting group cohesion, need to be purposefully utilized in practice with teams. Social workers can improve team functioning by supporting families and clients as active team members and by addressing ethical issues, including confidentiality and the competence and ethics of team members. Although there is some outcome-based research on teams, more is needed. Emerging trends in this field include embedding the notion of teams in a wider web of collaborative activities, including those mandated by the Affordable Care Act, and giving attention to teams as a vital part of social work education.

KEY WORDS: collaboration; family; group; interdisciplinary; interprofessional; teamwork; community

Although interdisciplinary teams first emerged in health care in the 1940s as a response to increased specialization, they did not become commonplace until the 1960s and 1970s (Julia & Thompson, 1994). Teams developed in U.S. industry in the 1970s in response to Japanese success with quality circles, in contrast to hierarchical management structures in their manufacturing systems. In health and mental health care, teams emerged to combine specialized knowledge to meet the range of needs of an individual. More recently, accreditation bodies and governmental and private funding sources have mandated collaborative approaches to human services to reduce duplication and promote coordinated service provision; as a result, teams have become commonplace in a range of settings (Aldred-Crouch, Hickman, Kent, & Randall, 2010; Harr, Souza, & Fairchild, 2008; Jent, Merrick, Dandes, Lambert, Haney, & Cano, 2009; Payne, 2000; Proenca, 2000). In particular, primary care and community health initiatives have included collaboration as a critical element (Keefe, Geron & Enguidanos, 2009). Yet, as health care has shifted to a managed care structure with concomitant emphasis on cost containment, questions about the efficiency and effectiveness of team decision making are being raised. However, serious questioning of the use of interdisciplinary teams has been limited; despite the extensive personnel hours required, it remains at the center of service delivery in diverse settings. Therefore, social work practitioners need to understand principles and skills of interdisciplinary team practice to perform their functions effectively.

Teams Defined

The term *team* was originally derived from Old English and was first used to refer to "a group of animals harnessed together to draw some vehicle" (Dingwall, 1980, p. 135). Various labels have been used to describe teams of professionals, including multidisciplinary, interprofessional, transdisciplinary, and interdisciplinary. Distinctions among them are not well articulated in the literature; here, the term *interdisciplinary* is used primarily. It implies the following: a group of professionals from different disciplines; a common purpose; integration of various professional perspectives in decision making; interdependence, coordination, and interaction; active communication; role division based on expertise; a climate of collaboration (Abramson, 2002). A model for interdisciplinary teamwork among social workers and other professionals describes the following as components of this kind of collaboration: interdependence, newly created professional activities, flexibility, collective ownership of goals, and reflection on process (Bronstein, 2002, 2003).

Barriers to and Supports for Teamwork

Despite wide acceptance of teams as a mechanism of service delivery, much of the literature on teamwork addresses the obstacles encountered by teams. Bronstein (2002, 2003), however, defines these barriers in their inverse, as potential supports for teamwork; by understanding and addressing them, teamwork can be strengthened. The following are most often cited in the literature as potential barriers or supports: (a) structural characteristics (time and space for teamwork to occur; administrative support for teamwork; skilled team leadership, institutional value on diversity and equality); (b) professional roles (security in one's role; shared professional language and technologies; training for teamwork; dual affiliation with profession and team; role competition or blurring); (c) personal characteristics (interactional styles; mutual respect; liking one's team mates; issues of race, culture, and gender); and (d) prior history with teamwork (Abramson, 2002; Bronstein, 2002, 2003; Bronstein & Abramson, 2003; Chesluk and Holmboe, 2010; Drinka & Streim, 1994; Ivery, 2010; Gallagher, Malone & Ladner, 2009).

The impact of distinct professional socialization processes on team functioning is profound and rarely well understood. Professional socialization shapes values, language, preferred roles, methods of problem solving, and establishment of priorities. As one becomes a social worker or other professional, perspectives particular to that profession become so integrated with a role that awareness of these perspectives diminishes, and thus, they remain unexamined for their impact on collaboration (Abramson, 2002). Yet, distinctions in professional beliefs and approaches to treatment are often at the root of disagreements among team members, even if unrecognized as such (Abramson & Bronstein, 2004; Koenig, Chapin & Spano, 2010). In addition, professional education does not adequately teach students about the contributions made by other professions or about the skills needed for teamwork; instead, professional education usually emphasizes discipline-specific priorities (Forrest & Derrick, 2010; Interprofessional Education Collaborative Expert Panel (IECEP), 2011; Ramsammy, 2010). To compensate for the gaps in professional education, team members need to make systematic efforts to understand the socialization and distinct contributions of other professionals.

Skills in Teamwork

Although social work education, like other forms of professional training, rarely or only minimally teaches specific skills in teamwork, social work students do learn clinical and macro practice concepts and skills that can easily be adapted to work with teams. These include the following: careful listening; beginning where the client (that is, the team) is; respecting differences; maintaining a nonjudgmental stance; communicating empathically; reaching for feelings; assessing individuals, groups, and organizations, among others (Gallagher, Malone, & Ladner, 2009). In fact, Sargaent, Loney, and Murphy (2008) identified communication as a major contributor to effective collaboration while Couturier, Gagnon, Carrier, and Ethridge (2008) label the affective aspect of communication as the "relational" aspect of collaboration. Unfortunately, the relevance of these skills for teamwork is not frequently articulated in the classroom or practice arena. Social workers do not sufficiently recognize or acknowledge that these skills are transferable to their work with colleagues; nor do they always accept that strategic and thoughtful interventions are needed in their interactions with colleagues (Abramson & Bronstein, 2004).

Perhaps the most important social work skills for teamwork are those used in facilitating groups. Teams are unique among task groups in the direct connection between their performance and the impact of their decisions on clients. Once social workers accept the need to address process issues in teams, they can draw on their group work knowledge base to assist teams in addressing these issues (Abramson & Bronstein, 2004).

It is a natural extension to apply the contracting concepts that are used in group work to teamwork. Many of the difficulties faced by teams are based in unexamined assumptions and can be effectively addressed through a well-developed contracting discussion. Monitoring team processes is another critical team maintenance task for all team leaders and team members; yet, it is a responsibility often taken on reluctantly, if at all. Participants need to think simultaneously about treatment and team issues so that they are able to address team processes that obstruct the client-centered goals of the team. When working with client groups, social workers typically attend to interactions among clients while also addressing the topics being discussed; thus they can draw on similar skills in working with teams. In addition, their systems orientation can assist them in evaluating organizational factors that may impinge on team functioning.

Social workers can also play a key role in creating a team climate of openness, trust, and group cohesion. Cohesion has been identified as contributing to commitment to the team and to its effectiveness (Barrick, Stewart, Neubert, & Mount, 1998). Mutual support occurs when team members are "there" for one another as they deal with challenging patient or client or community circumstances and with the

disappointments and struggles that are part of their daily work lives (Gallagher, Malone, & Ladner, 2009). Such support provides the cushion that then allows team participants to assert their expectations of each other (Abramson & Bronstein, 2004).

Teams that successfully manage conflict find their cohesion as a group greatly enhanced as well by their capacity to deal with differing points of view. The development of consensus in decision-making and growth in team functioning often depend on the ability of group members to confront conflict within the group directly. The inability to deal with conflict within the team is perhaps the most critical obstacle to effective collaboration. A number of sources address strategies that can contribute to conflict resolution in teams (Abramson, 2002; Toseland & Rivas, 2012).

Integrating Clients and Families into Teams

Effective teamwork is synonymous with an approach that views clients and families as critical team members (Winek, Dome, Gardner, Sackett, Zimmerman, & Davis, 2010). For meaningful participation to take place, team professionals, clients, and families need to engage jointly in the process of goal definition, attainment, and evaluation. Social workers can assure that clients and families are supported to find their own voices in team meetings (Biggs, Simpson, & Gaus, 2010).

The notion of families as collaborative team members has gone beyond the professional literature and has a presence in the popular literature. As this occurs, it is likely that clients and families will demand increasing substantive involvement in decisions about their own and their loved ones' care. A December 16, 2006, *New York Times* article by Clemetson states that 21 states have adopted team approaches wherein family members involved with the foster care system help in "decisions about where endangered children should live ... even families under scrutiny from state agencies can help make positive decisions for their children" (pp. A1, A13). Research studies, primarily in child welfare, are starting to evaluate the impact on teams of participation by clients and families (for example, Crea, Usher, & Wildfire, 2009). Results indicate benefits from their involvement through an array of structures including wraparound services and family group conferencing, and indicate a positive trend related to improvement of child management skills by foster parents, greater sense of efficacy and improved perceptions of well-being by those involved, as well as changes in child behavior (Ogles et al., 2006; Pennell & Anderson, 2005).

It is important, however, to recognize the challenges of fully involving clients and families as team members, especially in light of their time-limited involvement with the team and their perceived power deficit. A literature review of the conceptual basis for interprofessional collaboration found no definitions of collaboration that either adequately reflect the patient or family's perspective or successfully conceptualize their role on the team (D'Amour, Ferrade-Videla, San Martin Rodriguez, & Beaulieu, 2005). In fact, Gallagher, Malone, & Ladner (2009) note that, despite federal mandates and professional standards regarding the inclusion of families in team decision making, a review of the literature indicates that families are not yet successfully integrated into the process.

Ethical Issues in Teamwork
The integration of client and family into the team is a key arena where ethical issues can arise in teamwork. Unfortunately, most professionals, including social workers, have been highly influenced by the medical model that emphasizes professional expertise and implicitly and often explicitly minimizes the role of clients and family in the decisions made about them (Opie, 2000; Freidson, 1984). How often does a team even share its assessment of the client's situation with the client and family, no less involve them as active participants in deciding what should be assessed or what options should be considered for addressing the problems identified?

Issues of confidentiality are embedded in the very nature of teamwork; do most clients understand that they are discussed in team meetings or that some professionals attend who are not directly involved in their care? How comfortable would clients and families be with team discussions if they were more aware of their existence? Information should be provided routinely to clients to explain the team approach, to communicate clearly how confidentiality is maintained, and to identify the contributions of interprofessional discussion to helping them meet their goals.

The ways that team members conduct themselves on the team can also raise ethical questions. Alliances among subgroups of team members or hierarchical or status issues can distort or dominate team decision-making as can personal relationships between or among team members. Unethical or incompetent behavior by a team member may be apparent to others on the team but remain unaddressed because of lack of clear accountability channels or discomfort in raising the concern. The codes of ethics of other professional groups (American Medical Association: *http://www.ama-assn.org*; American Psychiatry Association: *http://www.psych.org/*; American Nurses Association: *http://www.nursingworld.org/MainMenuCategories/*

EthicsStandards/CodeofEthicsforNurses; American Psychological Association, *http://www.apa.org/ethics*) are similar to the National Association of Social Workers' Code of Ethics in warning of conflicts of interest and in spelling out professional responsibilities to perform competently and to report colleagues who are unethical or incompetent.

Research on Team Effectiveness
Remarkably little empirical examination of the operating assumptions regarding teamwork has been undertaken. Interest in studying teamwork seems somewhat higher in United Kingdom, Australia, and New Zealand than in the United States, judging by the disproportionate number of studies originating in those countries. When research has been conducted, team processes have more often been evaluated than the impact of teamwork on client outcomes. Process evaluations focus on the interaction in a team (communication patterns, cohesion, norms, roles, leadership, level of investment), while outcome evaluation addresses the extent to which the team is effectively fulfilling its client care function (Toseland & Rivas, 2012). There are some studies that examine process for its impact on outcome. One such study evaluated the impact on patient outcomes by training health-care teams in continuous quality improvement methods (Irvine Doran et al., 2002). This study found that only 9 of 25 teams were successful in improving outcomes; the markers of these successful teams included success at problem-solving, more functional group interactions, and physician participation. Another study (Oliver, Bronstein, & Kurzejeski, 2005) found quality of hospice care related to effective management of conflict and referrals to social workers by other professionals.

Enough research on team functioning and outcomes has been published to allow for several review articles. Faulkner and Amodeo (1999) reviewed studies of teamwork effectiveness and found very few that met their design criteria. They identified substantial inconsistencies in definitions of the team across various studies, which made comparisons of findings difficult and found none that looked directly at the relationship between these conditions and client outcomes. Schmitt (2001) reviewed studies over the previous 15 years and identified the methodological challenges of making the connection between teamwork and client outcomes. She notes the difficulties in integrating process variables with outcome variables, in developing conceptual clarity and valid measurement tools, in applying field experimental or control group multisite designs and in sifting out the impact of confounding factors. Both she and Lemieux-Charles and McGuire (2006), who reviewed the literature on health team effectiveness, note the research complexities posed by the multidimensionality of teamwork. Lemieux-Charles and McGuire did find evidence of positive teamwork on clinical outcomes and patient quality of life and satisfaction; its impact on cost factors was more mixed, although the longitudinal studies of geriatric evaluation teams in the Veterans' Administration health care system have demonstrated significant reductions in costs of care (Englehardt, Toseland, Gao, & Banks, 2006).

Conversely, Cummings (2009) did not find that use of a similar mental health geriatric interdisciplinary team (MHGIT) reduced hospitalizations, and thus cost, for mentally ill elders; however, she did find that depression was decreased and quality of life improved for clients of a MHGIT. Watson's (2010) study with a different population examined the impact of crisis intervention teams in a police department, and found that such teams increased linkages to mental health services and improved safety in calls involving persons with mental illness. It is essential that more empirical studies be conducted on the impact of teamwork on client outcomes; if not, this labor-intensive mechanism of service delivery may not have the future it deserves. However, even teams without research capacities can use a team assessment tool (see Bronstein, 2002, Dattner Consulting, 2007, Gallagher, Malone & Ladner, 2009, or Mellin, Bronstein, Anderson-Butcher, Amorose, Ball, & Green, 2010, for examples) as part of a formal team evaluation process. It is possible to correlate team functioning with client outcomes through use of a brief checklist to evaluate various aspects of care in order to identify patterns in client outcomes that relate to team functioning.

Emerging Trends in Teamwork

Emerging and critical trends in teamwork include an increase in research, greater emphasis on teamwork in professional education, including interdisciplinary education efforts, a more expansive definition of collaboration, and greater inclusion of clients and family in teams, and an emphasis on interdisciplinary teams in the Affordable Care Act.

The Affordable Care Act (ACA) (also referred to as health care reform or Obamacare) stresses the role and importance of the interdisciplinary team in health care delivery. Teamwork is noted as a key element in the ACA's discussion of cost containment, care coordination, patient centered medical homes and accountable care organizations. For example, the ACA

specifically authorizes "a federal grant program to support Community Health Teams to help coordinate care and provide access to a range of services, including preventive care." It goes on to state, "teams must comprise an interdisciplinary, inter-professional group of health care providers... representing a significant opportunity for inter-sectoral collaboration" (Boufford, Finkelstein, & Garcia, 2012). Including patients and families as team members is also cited as a requirement of the Affordable Care Act. There are other indicators as well that the social work role on teams may expand. For example, the relationship between social work and medicine has been evolving to a more collaborative model (Abramson & Mizrahi, 2003), and several studies have found the role of social workers to be highly valued by many of their physician colleagues (Mizrahi & Rizzo, 2008; Abramson & Mizrahi, 2003).

To further support the successful functioning of interdisciplinary teams, additional research on their work needs to be conducted and explicitly tied to client outcomes. The differences and similarities of teamwork in an array of settings need to be explored to develop generic models for practice as well as knowledge about how to shape teams to create the best fit with the needs of particular client populations and settings. Although there is much clinical wisdom and many case studies that guide this work, we need to increase efforts to develop evidence-based models to define and guide best practices. Instruments exist in social work and related fields to assess teamwork, but they rely largely on self-reporting. Although research on teamwork has matured and expanded to include contextual factors, specific areas cited in the literature as influences on teamwork should be empirically examined for their impact on team processes and outcomes, specifically, differential professional socialization, structural and organizational dimensions, contracting processes, the balance between task and process emphasis in teams, conflict management strategies and personal characteristics (Abramson & Bronstein, 2004; Bronstein & Abramson, 2009).

In addition to further research efforts, social work educators can make more explicit linkages for students between their generic social work knowledge and skills and their work on interdisciplinary teams (Howe et al., 2001). Outside the classroom, field instructors can also foster this linkage in their supervision of students in internship. For example, field instructors can require that students do process recordings of team meetings. If this aspect of their practice is elevated in importance to that given direct work with clients, and if students are evaluated on their performance in collaborative arenas, they will be eager to learn teamwork and collaborative skills. Field and classroom instructors should also articulate and consistently reinforce the connections between the group work skills students are using in their clinical work, and the skills needed as team members. While increasing numbers of social work educators are paying attention to interdisciplinary collaboration as part of the social work curriculum, there is not agreement about where and how to best teach these skills (Bronstein, Mizrahi, Korazim-Korosoy, & McPhee, 2010).

Last, it is critical to keep in mind that interdisciplinary teamwork is only one "type" of collaboration; it is not exercised in a void and is best achieved when interlocking with a number of other "types" of collaboration. These other forms of collaboration require many of the same skills necessary for inter-disciplinary teamwork (Payne, 2000). Lawson (2008) categorizes these collaborative types as intraorganizational, interorganizational, or inter-agency and community-based, among others. The more we value and develop skills in each of these kinds of collaboration, the more we also develop our abilities in the others, and become more effective members and facilitators of interdisciplinary teams—a central component of quality social work practice and service delivery in the 21st century.

REFERENCES

Abramson, J. S. (2002). Interdisciplinary team practice. In G. Greene & A. Roberts (Eds.), *Social work desk reference* (pp. 44–50). New York, NY: Oxford University Press.

Abramson, J. S., & Bronstein, L. R. (2004). Group process dynamics and skills in interdisciplinary teamwork. In C. Garvin, M. Galinsky, & L. Gutierrez (Eds.), *Handbook of social work with groups.* New York, NY: Guilford.

Abramson J. S., & Mizrahi, T. (2003). Collaboration between social workers & physicians: Application of a typology. *Social Work in Health Care, 37*(2), 71–100.

Aldred-Crouch, M., Hickman, S., Kent, B. & Randall, E. (2010). The health-mental health connection: Integrated behavioral health collaborative care. *NASW Health Section Connection, 1,* 3–5.

Barrick, M., Stewart, G., Neubert, M., & Mount, M. (1998). Relating member ability anpersonality to work-team processes and team effectiveness. *Journal of Applied Psychology, 83*(3), 377–391.

Biggs, M., Simpson, C., & Gaus, M. (2010). Using a team approach to address bullying of students with Asperger's Syndrome in activity-based settings. *Children & Schools, 32*(3), 135–142.

Boufford, J.I., Finkelstein, R., & Garcia, A. (2012). *Federal health care reform in New York State: A population health perspective.* New York, NY: NYS Health Foundation & New York Academy of Medicine.

Bronstein, L. R. (2002). Index of interdisciplinary collaboration. *Social Work Research, 26*(2), 113–126.

Bronstein, L. R. (2003). A model for interdisciplinary collaboration. *Social Work, 48*(3), 297–306.

Bronstein, L. R. & Abramson, J. S. (2009). Interdisciplinary teamwork. In A. Gitterman & R. Salmon (Eds.), *Encyclopedia of Social Work with Groups.* New York, NY: Routledge.

Bronstein, L. R. & Abramson, J. S. (2003). Understanding socialization of teachers and social workers: Groundwork for collaboration in the schools. *Families in Society, 84*(3), 1–8.

Bronstein, L.R., Mizrahi, T., Korazim-Korosoy, Y., & McPhee, D. (2010). Interdisciplinary collaboration in social work education in the U.S., Israel, and Canada: Deans' and directors' perspectives. *International Social Work, 53*(4), 457–473.

Chesluk, B. & Holmboe, E.S. (2010). How teams work—or don't—in primary care: A field study on internal medicine practices. *Health Affairs, 29*(5), 874–879.

Clemetson, L. (2006, December 16). Giving troubled families a say in what's best for the children. *New York Times,* pp. A1, A13.

Couturier, Y., Gagnon, D., Carrier, S., & Ethridge, F. (2008). The interdisciplinary condition of work in relational professions of the health and social care field: A theoretical standpoint. *Journal of Interprofessional Care, 22*(4), 341–351.

Crea, T., Usher, C., & Wildfire, J. (2009). Implementation fidelity of team decision-making. *Children and Youth Services Review, 31,* 119–124.

Cummings, S. M. (2008): Treating older persons with severe mental illness in the community: Impact of an interdisciplinary geriatric mental health team. *Journal of Gerontological Social Work, 52*(1), 17–31.

D'Amour, D., Ferrade-Videla, M., San Martin Rodriguez, L., & Beaulieu, M. D. (2005). The conceptual basis for interprofessional collaboration: Core concepts and theoretical frameworks. *Journal of Interprofessional Care, 19* (Suppl. 1), 116–131.

Dattner Consulting. Sample Leader. *Feedback Report* (2007). Retrieved from http://www.dattnerconsulting.com/leader.pdf

Dingwall, R. (1980). Problems of teamwork in primary care. In S. Lonsdale, A. Webb, & T. L. Briggs (Eds.), *Teamwork in the personal and social services and health care* (pp. 111–137). London, UK: Personal Social Services Council.

Englehardt, J. B., Toseland, R. W., Gao, J., & Banks, S. (2006). Long term effects of outpatient geriatric evaluation and management on health care utilization and survival. *Research on Social Work Practice, 16*(1), 20–27.

Faulkner, S. R., & Amodeo, M. (1999). Interdisciplinary teams in health care and human services settings: Are they effective? *Health and Social Work, 24*(3), 210–219.

Forrest, C. & Derrick, C. (2010). Interdisciplinary education in end-of-life care: Creating new opportunities for social work, nursing, and clinical pastoral education students. *Journal of Social Work in End of Life & Palliative Care, 6,* 91–116.

Freidson, E. (1984). The changing nature of professional control. *Annual Review of Sociology, 10*, 1–20.

Gallagher, P.A., Malone, D. M. & Ladner, J.R. (2009). Social-psychological support personnel: Attitudes and perceptions of teamwork supporting children with disabilities. *Journal of Social Work in Disability & Rehabilitation*, 8,1–20.

Harr, C., Souza, L. & Fairchild, S. (2008). International models of hospital interdisciplinary teams for the identification, assessment and treatment of child abuse. *Social Work in Health Care, 46*(4), 1–16.

Howe, J. L., Schwartz, H. L., Hyer, K., Mellor, J., Lindemann, D. A., & Luptak, M. (2001). Educational approaches for preparing social work students for interdisciplinary teamwork on geriatric health care teams. *Social Work in Health Care, 32*(4), 19–42.

Interprofessional Education Collaborative Expert Panel (2011). *Core competencies for interprofessional collaborative practice: Report of an expert panel*. Washington, DC: Interprofessional Education Collaborative.

Irvine Doran, D. M., Baker, G. R., Murray, M., Bohnen, J., Zahn, C., Sidani, S., & Carryer, J. Achieving (2002). Clinical improvement: An interdisciplinary intervention. *Health Care Management Review, 27*(4), 42–56.

Ivery, J. (2010). Partnerships in transition: Managing organizational and collaborative change. *Journal of Human Behavior in the Social Environment, 20*, 20–37.

Keefe, B., Geron, S. M. & Enguidanos, S. (2009). Integrating social workers into primary care: Physician and nurse perceptions of roles, benefits, and challenges. *Social Work in Health Care, 48*(6), 579–96.

Koenig, T. L., Chapin, R. & Spano, R. (2010). Using multidisciplinary teams to address ethical dilemmas with older adults who hoard. *Journal of Gerontological Social Work, 53*(2), 137–147.

Lawson, H. A. (2008). Collaborative practice. In T. Mizrahi & L. Davis (Eds.), *Encyclopedia of social work* (20th ed.). New York, NY: Oxford University Press & The National Association of Social Workers.

Lemieux-Charles, L., & McGuire, W. (2006). What do we know about health care team effectiveness: A review of the literature. *Medical Care Research and Review, 63*(3), 263–300.

Jent, J., Merrick, M., Dandes, S., Lambert, W., Haney, M, & Cano, N. (2009). Multidisciplinary assessment of child maltreatment: A multi-site pilot descriptive analysis of the Florida Child Protection Team model. *Children and Youth Services Review 31*, 896–902

Julia, M. C., & Thompson, A. (1994). Group process and interprofessional teamwork. In R. M. Casto, M. C. Julia, L. Platt, G. Harbaugh, A. Thompson, T. Jost, et al. (Eds.), *Interprofessional care and collaborative practice* (pp. 35–41). Pacific Grove, CA: Brooks/Cole.

Mellin, E., Bronstein, L.R., Anderson-Butcher, D., Amrose, A., Green, J., & Ball, A. (2010). Measuring interprofessional team collaboration in expanded school mental health: Model refinement and scale development. *Journal of Interprofessional Care, 24*(5), 514–523.

Mizrahi, T. & Rizzo, V. M. (2008). Perspectives on the roles and values of social work practice in neighborhood health centers and implications for the reimbursement of services. *Social Work and Public Health, 23*, 99–125.

Ogles, B. M., Carlston, D., Hatfield, D., Melendez, G., Dowell, K., & Fields, S. A. (2006). The role of fidelity and feedback in the wraparound approach. *Journal of Child and Family Studies, 15*(1), 115–129.

Oliver, D., Bronstein, L. R., & Kurzejeski, L. (2005). Examining variables related to successful collaboration on the hospice team. *Health and Social Work, 30*(4), 279–286.

Opie, A. (2000). *Thinking teams/thinking clients: Knowledge-based teamwork*. New York, NY: Columbia University Press.

Payne, M. (2000). *Teamwork in multiprofessional care*. Chicago, IL: Lyceum Books.

Pennell, J., & Anderson, G. (Eds.). (2005). *Widening the circle: The practice and evaluation of family group conferencing with children, youths and their families*. Washington, DC: NASW Press.

Proenca, E. J. (2000). Community orientation in hospitals: An institutional and resource dependence perspective. *Health Services Research, 35*(5), 210–218.

Ramsammy, L. (2010). Interprofessional education and collaborative practice. *Journal of Interprofessional Care, 24*(2), 131–138.

Sargaent, J., Loney, E., & Murphy, G. (2008). Effective interprofessional teams: "Contact is not enough" to build a team. *Journal of Continuing Education in the Health Professions, 28*(4), 228–234.

Schmitt, M. H. (2001). Collaboration improves the quality of care: Methodological challenges and evidence from US health care research. *Journal of Interprofessional Care, 15*(1), 47–66.

Toseland, R., & Rivas, R. (2012). *An introduction to group work practice* (7th ed.). Boston, MA: Pearson Education.

Watson, A. (2010). Research in the real world: Studying Chicago police department's crisis intervention team program. *Research on Social Work Practice 20*, 536.

Winek, J. L., Dome, L. J., Gardner, J. R., Sackett, C. R., Zimmerman, M. J. & Davis, M. K. (2010). Support Network Intervention Team: A Key Component of a Comprehensive Approach to Family-Based Substance Abuse Treatment. *Journal of Groups in Addiction & Recovery, 5*, 45–69.

FURTHER READING

Abramson, J. S., & Rosenthal, B. B. (1995). Interdisciplinary and interorganizational collaboration. In T. Mizrahi & L. Davis (Eds.), Encyclopedia of Social Work (19th ed.), pp. 1479–1489. Washington, DC: NASW.

American Medical Association Code of Ethics: http://www.ama-assn.org/ama/pub/physician-resources/medical-ethics/code-medical-ethics.page

American Nurses Association: http://www.nursingworld.org/MainMenuCategories/EthicsStandards/CodeofEthicsforNurses

American Psychiatry Association Code of Ethics: http://www.apa.org/ethics/code/index.aspx

Bronstein, L. R., McCallion, P., & Kramer, E. (2006). Developing an aging prepared community: Collaboration among counties, consumers, professionals and organizations. *Journal of Gerontological Social Work*, 48(1/2), 193–202.

Bronstein, L. R., & Wright, K. (2006). The impact of prison hospice: Collaboration among social workers and other professionals in a criminal justice setting that promotes care for the dying. *Journal of Social Work in End-of-Life and Palliative Care*, 2(4), 85–102.

Cashman, S. B., Reidy, P., Cody, K., & Lemay, C. A. (2004). Developing and measuring progress toward collaborative, integrated, interdisciplinary health care teams. *Journal of Interprofessional Care*, 18(2), 183–196.

Curran, V. R., Deacon, D. R., & Fleet, L. (2005). Academic administrators' attitudes towards interprofessional education in Canadian Schools of health professional education. *Journal of Interprofessional Care, Suppl. 1*, 76–86.

Drinka, T. J. K., & Clark, P. G. (2000). *Health care and teamwork: Interdisciplinary practice and teaching*. Westport, CT: Auburn House.

Dattner Consulting, LLC: http://www.dattnerconsulting.com

Fleming, J. L., & Monda-Amaya, L. (2001). Process variables critical for team effectiveness. Remedial and Special Education, 22(3), 158–172.

Garland, C., Frank, A., Buck, D., & Seklemian, P. (1995). *Skills inventory for teams*. Lightfoot, VA: Child Development Resources Training Center.

Human Resources: http://humanresources.about.com/od/involvementteams/a/team_culture.htm

Kivimaki, M., Kuk, G., Elovainio, M., & Thomson, L. (1997). The team climate inventory (TCI)—Four or five factors? Testing the structure of TCI in samples of low and high complexity jobs. *Journal of Occupational and Organizational Psychology*, 70, 375–390.

Knox, K. S., & Roberts, A. R. (2005). Crisis intervention and crisis team models in schools. *Children and Schools*, 27(2), 93–100.

Mailick, M. D., & Ashley, A. A. (1981). Politics of interprofessional collaboration: Challenge to advocacy. *Social Casework: The Journal of Contemporary Social Work*, 62(3), 131–136.

Mizrahi, T., & Abramson, J. S. (1985). Sources of strain between physicians and social workers: Implications for social workers in health care settings. *Social Work in Health Care*, 10(3), 33–51.

NASA Headquarters Library: http://www.hq.nasa.gov/office/hqlibrary/ppm/ppm5.htm

Questia: http://www.questia.com/library/health-care-teams.jsp

Reese, D. J., & Sontag, M. A. (2001). Successful interprofessional collaboration on the hospice team. *Health and Social Work*, 26(3), 167–175.

Sands, R., Staffor, J., & McClelland, M. (1990). I beg to differ: Conflict in the interdisciplinary team. *Social Work in Health Care*, 14(3), 55–72.

Seaburn, D. B., Lorenz, A. D., Gunn, W. B., Gawinski, B. A., & Mauksch, L. B. (1996). *Models of collaboration*. New York: Basic Books.

Specht, H. (1985). The interpersonal interactions of professionals. *Social Work*, 30(3), 225–230.

Suter, E., Arndt, J., Arthur, N., Parboosingh, J., Taylor, E., & Deutschander, S. (2009). Role understanding and effective communication as core competencies for collaborative practice. *Journal of Interprofessional Care*, 23(1), 41–51.

Vinokur-Kaplan, D. (1995). Treatment teams that work (and those that don't): An application of Hackman's group effectiveness model to interdisciplinary teams in psychiatric hospitals. *Journal of Applied Behavioral Science*, 31(3), 303–327.

Watson, W., Johnson, L., & Merritt, D. (1998). Team orientation, self-orientation and diversity in task groups. *Group and Organization Management*, 23, 161–188.

Waugaman, W. (1994). Professionalization and socialization in inter-professional collaboration. In R. M. Casto, M. C. Julia, L. Platt, G. Harbaugh, A. Thompson, T. Jost, et al. (Eds.), *Interprofessional care and collaborative practice* (pp. 23–31). Pacific Grove, CA: Brooks/Cole.

Xyrichis, A., & Lowton, K. (2008). What fosters or prevents interprofessional teamworking in primary and community care? A literature review. *International Journal of Nursing Studies*, 45(1), 140–153.

Julie Abramson and Laura Bronstein

TECHNOLOGY: TECHNOLOGY IN MACRO PRACTICE

Abstract: Information technology has had a profound effect on social work practice with larger systems. These tools improve traditional practice and allow new forms of practice. This review looks at the use of technology in macro social work practice. It examines the role of technology in social administration, community practice, and social policy practice; discusses current practice and tools; and discusses the challenges faced in the use of technology in macro practice.

Key Words: information technology; macro social work; social administration; community practice; social policy practice

Administrative Practice

Technology has had a substantial impact on the way that agencies are managed, reflecting the growth of e-commerce and e-government. Most organizations have a series of databases that support their work, which have developed into Management Information

Systems (MIS) efforts (Schoech, 1999). These systems are intended to support management decision-making by providing timely, decision-relevant information. At first relatively simple arrangements that collected, processed, and reported programmatic and financial data, they were often difficult for managers to use in guiding their organizations because the information provided was often not always what was needed for critical decisions. They have evolved into decision support systems that support management decision-making as well as data warehousing and Knowledge Management Systems that can support organizational learning (Schoech, Fitch, MacFadden, & Schkade, 2002). These developments have tailored technology to the decision-making environment and created ways to better use and preserve the information that the organization depends upon. Often these efforts attempt to provide relevant information across organizational boundaries. Advanced statistical techniques, such as data mining, allow extraction of important information from large datasets created in the knowledge management process. More and more organizations are moving to cloud computing as a means to support diverse operations, and the integration with emerging health care information systems will lead to additional modifications.

There are also efforts to bring together information from across organizations where individual units have data systems that cannot communicate with one another. This makes it difficult to provide strategic information to higher levels of management, and workers in complementary departments cannot have access to needed information. In response to this problem, organizations have developed Enterprise Resource Planning Systems that combine many of the local systems into an organizational strategy. Internal communication is often facilitated through e-mail, wireless, and Intranet-based systems. Customer Relationship Management Systems are also important components of human services organizations. These systems combine databases with other technology to manage the organizations' relationships with its clients.

Technology also supports marketing, fund-raising, and financial management (Cortés & Rafter, 2007). Organizational websites have become increasingly important tools in promoting the agency in the community and many agencies have developed Content Management Systems to organize the information they provide. Some use technology to segment their market and develop messages that appeal to those segments. Marketing can also include e-mail newsletters, streaming video, and other appeals. The Web 2.0 or social media revolution has moved many agency marketing efforts toward Facebook and other social networking sites, videos, and other tools (Wymer & Grau, 2011).

Technology is also providing a way to raise funds, solicit volunteers, and recruit employees. E-fundraising has become an important source of funding for many agencies (Grobman & Grant, 2006; Wymer & Grau, 2011). Some of the approaches include secure donation systems, shop-for-a-cause approaches, and online charity auctions. Some organizations use e-mail to raise money. In addition to online systems, technology can be used to support more traditional fundraising by facilitating prospect research.

Spreadsheets and other forms of financial management software facilitate the management of money within an agency. The growth of mobile applications has accelerated in the past decade and continues to develop. Smartphones, laptop computers, tablet computers, and other mobile devices can do most of the things that other computers can do and bring the advantage of easy mobility.

Larger agencies have information technology staff and may even have a department. Smaller organizations often rely on consultants or application service providers, which are organizations that provide all or part of the organization's technology on an outsourced basis (Cortés & Rafter, 2007).

Finally, technology has facilitated the development of virtual organizations, which develop a network to perform the organization's work. Nearly every task is outsourced to another entity and work is coordinated through the network (Cooper & Muench, 2000).

Community Practice

Community organization or development has also been influenced by new technology (Hick & McNutt, 2002). This not only makes current practice more effective but also allows community practitioners to extend their work into new areas, such as virtual communities.

Traditional social planning and community organizing or development have benefited from the growth of community data libraries, organizations that aggregate data on the community's situation, and the development of Geographic Information Systems (GIS). Geographic Information Systems provide the capacity to map data and a wealth of analytical facility with spatial statistics, which can facilitate decision-making (Hiller, 2007; Queralt & Witte, 1998).

Community computer networks and community technology centers were early, important ways to reduce access disparities and also create stronger communities. Technology has been a critical part of "Smart Communities" efforts and programs to promote local civic participation.

Finally, there are the beginnings of work in virtual communities. There is accumulating evidence that one can build community in cyberspace. For example, virtual volunteering has grown in importance and represents an exciting new way for people to become involved. Virtual volunteers participate over the Internet doing things that traditional volunteers do.

Social Policy Practice and Advocacy

The technological revolution in advocacy and political practice has matured into an accepted practice with a wide variety of available tactics and techniques (Hick & McNutt, 2002). While the use of technology for political advocacy emerged in the late 1980s, the last 10 or so years have seen it evolved into an important part of social movement efforts, political campaigning, and issue advocacy. Technology can assist advocates in gathering information, informing the public, organizing constituents, and applying pressure to decision-makers. E-mail, websites, and discussion lists form the initial foundation of practice.

Newer techniques reflect the social media or Web 2.0 emphasis on social networking, pooling of collective intelligence, and user-generated content. These include wikis, blogs, social networking sites, microblogging, online games, social bookmarking systems, and video or image sharing sites (Germany, 2006). Starting with the 2004 Howard Dean democratic primary campaign, the 2008 and 2010 election campaigns demonstrated a significant move forward of the role of technology, particularly social media, in political action. This was paralleled by similar developments in issue advocacy campaigns (McNutt & Menon, 2008) One of the more significant developments in this area was the emergence of virtual advocacy organizations, such as Move On. These organizations, unlike many traditional social movement organizations, exist as virtual organizations almost totally in cyberspace. There is also evidence that technology-assisted leaderless organizations are emerging in the social movement arena (Earl & Kimport, 2011).

The question of effectiveness is difficult for any type of advocacy practice (McNutt, 2006), but recent findings suggest that decision makers are influenced by this technology (Congressional Management Foundation, 2005; Larsen & Rainie, 2002).

Summary

Information technology is an important factor in society and has had an impact on people and professions throughout the world. In social work, technology has allowed fundamental improvements in social work practice to occur.

There are certain risks and issues to any new development. Living in a connected world has consequences such as privacy violations, cybercrime and cyber terrorism, surveillance, and accidental release of confidential information. The digital divide means that a part of the population will not have access to the benefits of technology. While much of what technology can provide is beneficial, there is always a potential downside.

Since the 1980s, technology has become a greater part of people's lives. They work online and engage in commerce online; many become educated via technology and, especially in the wake of the social media revolution, many devote a significant portion of time to virtual activities and relationships. Any profession that deals with people will have to engage this part of the social environment or become irrelevant. Technology will become a more pervasive part of macro social work as time moves forward. It will become less a separate entity and more the way that practice is conducted. The other side is that if social workers lack the training to take advantage of technology, they may be replaced by professions that do.

Technology continues to develop at an impressive rate. Hardware is likely to become more capable and more mobile. Software will become more intelligent, easier to use, and more collaborative.

Technology has created new opportunities, capabilities, and challenges for macro social workers. It is a central force for improving the quality of macro social work practice and making life better for the people we serve.

REFERENCES

Bergan, D. E. (2009). Does grassroots lobbying work? A field experiment measuring the effects of an e-mail lobbying campaign on legislative behavior. *American Politics Research*, 37(2), 327–352.

Congressional Management Foundation. (2005). *Communicating with Congress: How Capitol Hill is coping with the surge in citizen advocacy*. Washington, DC: Author.

Cooper, W. W., & Muench, M. L. (2000). Virtual organizations: Practice and the literature. *Journal of the Organizational Computing and Electronic Computing*, 10(3), 189–208.

Cortés, M., & Rafter, K (Eds.). (2007). *Nonprofits and technology: emerging research for usable knowledge*. Chicago, IL: Lyceum Books.

Earl, J., & Kimport, K. (2011). *Digitally enabled social change: Activism in the Internet age*. Cambridge, MA: MIT Press.

Germany, J. B. (Ed.). (2006). *Person-to-person-to-person: Harnessing the political power of online social networks and user-generated content*. Washington, DC: Institute for

Politics, Democracy and the Internet, George Washington University.

Hick, S., & McNutt, J. G. (Eds.). (2002). *Advocacy, activism, and the Internet: Community organization and social policy.* Chicago, IL: Lyceum Books.

Hiller, A. (2007). Why social work needs mapping. *Journal of Social Work Education, 43*(2), 205–221.

Larsen, E., & Rainie, L. (2002). *Digital town hall: How local officials use the Internet and the civic benefits they cite from dealing with constituents online.* Washington, DC: Pew Internet and American Life Project.

McNutt, J. G. (2006). Building evidence-based advocacy in cyberspace: A social work imperative for the new millennium. *Journal of Evidence-Based Social Work, 3*(2/3), 91–102.

McNutt, J. G. (2011). Is social work advocacy worth the cost? Issues and barriers for an economic analysis of social work political practice. *Research on Social Work Practice, 21*(4), 397–403.

McNutt, J. G., & Menon, G. M. (2008). Cyberactivism and Progressive Human Services. *Families and Society, 89*(1), 33–38.

Queralt, M., & Witte, A. D. (1998). A map for you? Geographic information systems in the social services. *Social Work, 43*(5), 455–469.

Schoech, D. (1999). *Human services technology: Understanding, designing, and implementing computer and Internet applications in the social services.* New York: Haworth Press.

Schoech, D., Fitch, D., MacFadden, R., & Schkade, L. L. (2002). From data to intelligence: Introducing the intelligent organization. *Administration in Social Work, 26*(1), 1–21.

Wymer, W. W., & Grau, S. L. (2011). *Connected causes: Online marketing strategies for nonprofit organizations.* Chicago, IL: Lyceum Books.

Further Reading

Benkler, Y. (2006). *The wealth of networks: How social production transforms markets and freedom.* New Haven, CT: Yale University Press.

Grobman, G. M., & Grant, G. B. (2006). *Fundraising online: Using the Internet to raise serious money for your nonprofit organization.* Harrisburg, PA: White Hat Communications.

Kanter, B., & Fine, A. H. (2010). *The network nonprofit: Connecting with social media to drive change.* San Francisco: Jossey-Bass.

Rainie, L., & Wellman, B. (2012). *Networked: The new social operating system.* Cambridge, MA: MIT Press.

Smith, A., Schlozman, K. L., Verba, S., & Brady, H. (2009). *The Internet and civic engagement.* Washington, DC: Pew Internet and American Life Projects. Available at http://www.pewinternet.org/Reports/2009/15--The-Internet-and-Civic-Engagement.aspx

Suggested Links

Websites

Berkman Center for Internet and Society: http://cyber.law.harvard.edu/home/

NetSquared: http://www.netsquared.org
New Social Worker: http://blog.socialworker.com/
Pew Internet and American Life Project: http://www.pewinternet.org
TechSoup: http://www.techsoup.org/

Videos

Clay Shirky: How the Internet will (one day) transform government. (2012): http://www.ted.com/talks/clay_shirky_how_the_internet_will_one_day_transform_government.html

Jennifer Pahlka: Coding a better government. (2012): http://www.ted.com/talks/jennifer_pahlka_coding_a_better_government.html

John G. McNutt

TRANSDISCIPLINARY AND TRANSLATIONAL RESEARCH

Abstract: This overview examines the nature of transdisciplinary and translational priorities in the context of changing forms of research and assessments of the relationship of research to societal impact. It first describes shifts away from single disciplinary to more integrative disciplinary approaches to science and discusses emerging forms of integrative research, distinguishing and illustrating multidisciplinary, interdisciplinary, and transdisciplinary approaches. It then turns to describing the social forces behind the acceleration of science into service, illustrating what are referred to as *translational gaps* and efforts to bridge them. Within social work, methods attentive to adaptation for diverse settings, organizational dissemination and implementation, and community partnership models have become prominent. The article concludes with attention to the development of an educational pipeline that prepares professionals as well as researchers for capable, confident participation into this environment of transdisciplinary and translational approaches.

Key Words: research; translational; transdisciplinary; interprofessional; evaluation; implementation; collaboration

> Shifts in the ways that science is being undertaken and marshalled toward social change argue for a new kind of professional competence... stimulat(ing) reflectiveness regarding social work's preparedness to support and indeed amplify a robust culture of high impact science.... (Nurius & Kemp, 2012, p. 548)

Science is no longer monopolized by any one discipline. Nor can many pressing social and environmental problems be solved by a single discipline, field of study, profession, or sector. Increasingly, science is collaborative, based in partnerships—across disciplines and with community stakeholders—focused on more effectively tackling challenging real-world problems. It increasing involves discipline-spanning approaches to a wide range of societal, population, and community problems. Emerging efforts focus on building sustainable bridges across disciplines (in order to develop more complete solutions), across phases of research (where findings too often do not progress from discovery to delivery—for instance, from basic research to applied research to implementation in usual settings), and between academic researchers and a wide range of community stakeholders (Nurius & Kemp, 2013). This growing emphasis on transdisciplinary and translational research is evident across scientific levels: from federal research funders such as the National Institutes of Health and National Science Foundation and on through major foundations, nonprofit organizations, and local public sectors seeking to bridge the "know-do" gap (Lynch, 2006) and enhance collective impact (Kania & Kramer, 2011; Social Research Unit, 2011).

This changing "scientific marketplace" has significant implications for social work and its potential for impacting the problems and issues that are its central concerns. In a 2011 Invited Presidential Address to the Society of Social Work and Research, King Davis urged the profession to assertively strengthen its contributions to and its ability to make good use of 21st-century transformations in the forms, exchanges, and applications of research. Similar imperatives are reflected in calls to (re)shape social work science (Soydan, 2012), develop the transdisciplinary tools necessary for progress on intransigent social and health problems (Gehlert et al., 2010), strengthen social work's ability to translate research to more efficiently meet practice needs (Palinkas & Soydan, 2012), and strategically focus social work science and service toward solving pressing "grand" challenges (Uehara et al., 2013).

In many respects the profession is already oriented toward these emerging research and practice imperatives. It has long emphasized ecological frameworks that acknowledge multiple levels of influence, the importance of history and context, and the complex, interlocking systems shaping research and practice. From its earliest professional beginnings, it has consistently linked science and service (Almgren, Kemp, &

Eisinger, 2000; Kirk & Reid, 2002). Inherently interdisciplinary, the profession also draws on a range of research modalities. *Encyclopedia of Social Work* articles, for example, encompass quantitative and qualitative research, action- and community-based participatory research, agency-based research, survey research, practice and intervention research, and research ethics. Nonetheless, Davis (2011) and others highlight gaps in social work's readiness to fully engage in the transdisciplinary and translational environment of the changing scientific marketplace, and those observations about the profession are not relegated only to those working most directly as researchers. In 21st-century contexts, skill sets conducive to being credible, effective communicators of the discipline's vision of values-anchored science are important for social workers across professional roles and fields of practice—from practitioners to administrators to researchers—particularly when they may be the only social worker at the table (Kemp & Nurius, 2013).

Paralleling and intersecting these research developments, interprofessional education and collaborative, team-based practice are likewise emerging as central to effective, responsive social and health care (see, for example, Frenk, Chen, Bhutta, Cohen, Crisp, Evans, et al., 2010; King et al., 2009). Across the social and health care professions, increasing emphasis is placed on skillful interprofessional teamwork, particularly where problems and needs are complex and interlocking (in elder care, for example, or where chronic health conditions such as diabetes and heart disease intersect with poverty-related stressors). Teams that include community and lay providers are also becoming more important as a means of enhancing outreach, support, and access to care for marginalized and underserved groups (Ruddy & Rhee, 2005).

The practical relevance of transdisciplinary and translational research and practice comes into focus within the specific realities of social work practice. The interlocking challenges confronting child-welfare-involved families (and thus the child welfare system), for example, range from the impacts of trauma and early adversity on children's development to the weathering effects of chronic structural deprivation. In turn, the scope and complexity of families' needs is mirrored in the challenges entailed in implementing effective interventions in the equally complex organizations charged with serving them. Just this one service system stands as a vivid example that no single discipline is adequate to the task of capturing the complex etiologies underlying child-welfare-system involvement or designing the range of policy and practice interventions entailed in serving children and families with multiple needs. Similarly, this service is emblematic of the value of high-quality translational research responsive to both the difficult demands facing public child welfare practitioners and the needs and perspectives of the system's diverse and typically highly marginalized client families. In child welfare, therefore, as is in fields such as health care and aging, the need for innovative, broad-based research and practice collaborations is increasingly emphasized (DiLorenzo, White, Morales, Paul, & Shaw, 2013).

This article provides an overview of the transdisciplinary and translational priorities that are becoming central to research and to the relationship of research to societal impact. It describes how the field is shifting away from single discipline to more integrative disciplinary approaches to science. It defines key terms related to transdisciplinary science, distinguishing among multidisciplinary, interdisciplinary, and transdisciplinary research and providing an illustration of the latter. It then discusses translational research, describing the social forces urging accelerated translation of science into service, and illustrating what are referred to as translational gaps and efforts to bridge them. In summary, it assesses the changing nature of social work within this climate, as well as the changing nature of an educational pipeline that prepares professional as well as research-prepared social workers for transdisciplinary and translational science and practice (Fong, 2012).

Evolving Research Models: From Silos to Bridges

Since the late 19th century, modern universities have been organized around singular disciplines, an organizational structure that helped solidify and deepen disciplinary identities, content knowledge, and methodological tools. Departments of sociology, psychology, and public health, for example, are typically associated with particular aspects of social and health phenomena. Examined against the need for greater progress in addressing the world's most complex and intractable problems, however—whether poverty, health disparities, war, famine, or global climate change—the limits of this unidisciplinary, silo-like approach to education and research are increasingly apparent. Narrowly specialized and segmented expertise "can place serious limits on our research horizons by restricting the types of questions we can ask, the methods and concepts we use, the answers we believe and our criteria for truth and validity" (Lyall & Fletcher, 2013, p. 2).

Analyses and interventions that fail to integrate factors representing multiple domains (often drawn from differing disciplines—that is, transdisciplinarity) or to foresee implementation challenges down the line (that is, translational insights) risk unforeseen negative impacts. Economic science, for example, is critical to evaluating the outcomes of social policies such as welfare reform. Yet research that focuses on how recipients respond to the incentives built into welfare programs without also attending to the causes and consequences of poverty can miss critically important factors affecting outcomes such as child well-being. As Henly (2013) has demonstrated, damaging gaps can occur when economically oriented welfare reform researchers and researchers attentive to family and child development and outcomes fail to integrate their models, questions, or evidence. Similarly, there is growing recognition that success in reducing or preventing health disparities—an area in which the United States has made little progress despite decades of effort—is dependent on the ability to address multiple, complex, and interlocking influences, from cells to societies (Gehlert, 2012).

Defining Levels of Disciplinary Integration in Research

Common terms for disciplinary collaborations—*multidisciplinary, interdisciplinary, transdisciplinary* and *cross-disciplinary*—are often used interchangeably. Definitions are, however, sharpening in response to efforts to distill what forms of training and teamwork are best suited for different types of goals. The following definitions build from those suggested by Gehlert et al. (2010), Nash (2008), Rosenfield (1992), and Stokols (2006). The umbrella term *cross-disciplinary* is here used to include all types.

LEVEL 1: MULTIDISCIPLINARY In a *multidisciplinary* collaboration, participants from different fields bring their respective disciplinary expertise to an effort yet stay predominantly within their disciplinary spheres, working separately or sequentially but with limited interaction. A group might produce an edited book, for example, which illustrates multiple perspectives on a common problem (for example, child maltreatment, juvenile delinquency, poverty). As a whole the book provides complementary perspectives on a central issue, but the authors and chapters are not structured to "speak" to one another. Fields may also be multidisciplinary in that multiple disciplines contribute or participate. Frequently, however, participants formulate and address distinct research questions, often coming to separate conclusions that are disseminated through their own disciplinary journals or conferences. Metaphorically, if one thinks of a unidisciplinary perspective as a single piece of fruit, one might think of a multidisciplinary approach as represented by a fruit platter. Multiple components, collectively, provide an array of flavors, but they reside alongside one another within their respective skins (inspired by Hall, 2013).

The limitations of multidisciplinarity are increasingly recognized. As Lynch (2006) trenchantly observed, "simply bolting other disciplines onto our research like some multidisciplinary Mechano set, which had a genetics piece, a psychology piece, a social piece and a biology piece, did not really deliver what we were after" (p. 1120). At the same time, attempts to integrate and make sense of separate bodies of work beyond what any single discipline can achieve are hampered by differences in theories, approaches to problems, questions, research metrics and analyses, and interpretive frameworks. Unless these differences are addressed, they tend to limit investigation of or insights into interactions between various domains or levels of factors. Social work doctoral programs, for example, frequently encourage students to take courses from other departments. However comparatively fewer social work programs offer courses, assignments, or experiences that provide opportunities for cross-discipline groups of students to learn about and begin to integrate one another's disciplines—that is, to undertake interdisciplinarity.

Level 2: Interdisciplinary

In *interdisciplinary* collaborations, participants work together not only to bring multiple forms of expertise to bear on an issue but to also engage across disciplines and influence one another. To extend the fruit metaphor, interdisciplinary collaborations turn fruit platters into fruit salads. In such collaborations, researchers intentionally exchange knowledge from one discipline to another, typically learning enough to have working familiarity with one another's conceptual frameworks, language, and methodological tools. The functional relationships and products are much more "mixed together." This may result in the creation of new disciplines such as bioengineering, health economics, or environmental science. Members of interdisciplinary teams or disciplines generally come with the expectation that they will draw on their disciplinary strengths *and* be prepared to link with other disciplinary frameworks and methods toward a common goal. Learning to communicate effectively within and across disciplinary differences is strongly emphasized. In the practice arena, emerging models of interprofessional education and practice likewise emphasize the importance of interdependence among varied professionals aimed at strengthening service systems, improving care, and increasing access for underserved groups (World Health Organization, 2010).

Level 3: Transdisciplinary

Transdisciplinary collaborations and training "transcend" participating disciplines with the goal of generating bodies of knowledge and methodological approaches that more fully capture complexity. By synthesizing theoretical and methodological tools from different disciplines, these collaborations aim to more effectively address a defined problem area. Transdisciplinarity overlaps interdisciplinarity but aims for deeper levels of integration, typically requiring time, commitment of effort, patience, and a strong common vision. Taking the fruit metaphor one step further, transdisciplinarity turns the fruit salad into a fruit smoothie. Transdisciplinary collaborators create a common language, formulate shared questions, develop a holistic conceptual framework, and plan research and dissemination projects that carefully build upon one another.

In social work, transdisciplinary models are perhaps most evident in health-related research, where funding has supported centers that are focused on population health and disparities with an eye to much more fully integrating social determinants with health science models. These centers have fostered multilevel research that combines population, social and behavioral, clinical, and biological theory and methods with a focus on disparities in health services (Warnecke et al., 2008). Similar transdisciplinary models are also emerging in areas such as prevention of high-risk behaviors (Fishbein & Ridenour, 2013). Beyond social work, transdisciplinarity is a hallmark of sustainability science (Lang, Wiek, Bergmann, Stauffacher, Martens, Moll et al., 2012), a field that increasingly is engaging social work attention (Schmitz, Matyók, Sloan, & James, 2012).

Illustrating Transdisciplinarity

These newer forms of research collaboration can be illustrated using the example of the Center for Interdisciplinary Health Disparities Research (CIHDR) at the University of Chicago, funded by the National Institutes for Health as part of an initiative to address health disparities through transdisciplinary research. Years of conventional research effort had resulted in limited progress in reducing disparate health outcomes, in part due to the multiple forces involved and the complex interactions among these multiple drivers. Recognizing the limitations of earlier approaches, this NIH initiative fostered the development of teams from multiple disciplines, working across multiple projects to (1) more fully capture and interconnect biological, behavioral, and social contributors to health disparities; and (2) guide policy and practice directives responsive to these more encompassing models.

Research that focused on reducing breast cancer mortality among African American women illustrates this approach. A central question united the CIHDR investigators and their community partners: why, despite the fact that white women are more likely to have breast cancer, are African American women more likely to die from it? Building on knowledge that breast cancer development is predicated on specific genetic interactions, the CIHDR team developed four mutually informative, interdependent research projects. Two projects included genetics analysis, such as how aspects of the environment such as stressors and maternal behavior affected genetic expression and tumor growth. Figuratively speaking, such biological phenomena are often referred to as "downstream," in contrast to the "upstream" influence of physical, social, and political

environments. Additional projects were situated to capture the aspects of upstream environments likely to have figural roles in breast cancer development (for example, housing and community characteristics, social connections, services access). This purposefully multilevel approach allowed the teams to build in measures through which outcomes at a cellular level could be progressively linked to mezzo- and macro-level factors. For more detail on the projects, how the teams worked, and the use of this kind of research to support new interventions and training models, see Gehlert et al. (2010) (also Gehlert, 2012; Gehlert & Browne, 2013).

Figure 1 presents a simplified pictorial representation, by level of analysis, of the four projects undertaken by the transdisciplinary CIHDR team. Each tier includes complexity in its own right, in addition to the complex nature of interactions among the levels (for more detail see Warnecke et al., 2008).

Projects 1 and 4 used animal models (rat studies) to explore connections between the psychosocial environment and mammary tumor development. This approach allowed the team to realistically undertake a life-span approach to mammary tumor development (within a 2- to 4-year window), as well as experimental manipulation of social conditions (for instance,

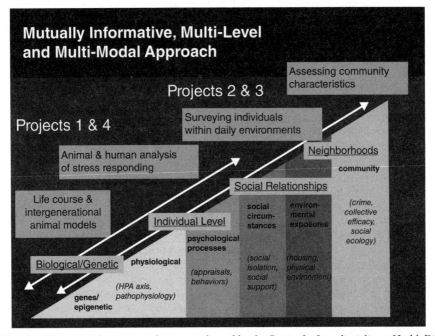

Figure 1.   Illustrating transdisciplinary research team work used by the Center for Interdisciplinary Health Disparities Research. Adapted from: Gehlert, S., Murray, A., Sohmer, D., McClintock, M., Conzen, S., & Olopade, O. (2010). The importance of transdisciplinary collaborations for understanding and resolving health disparities. *Social Work in Public Health*, 25(3–4), 408–422.

different types of stressors, social isolation), while being able to control for other factors and thus separate out causal mechanisms. These studies trace the ways in which environmental factors influence psychological and physiological mechanisms that, in turn, affect genetic activity related to cancer development. Paralleling the animal model studies, Projects 2 and 3 followed a sample of African American women with newly developed breast cancer living in 15 different urban neighborhoods. These projects captured social and psychological functioning as well as neighborhood and community data, using multiple methods including community ethnography (Salant & Gehlert, 2008). All four projects used theoretical and measurement approaches that helped the team to interrelate these data, incrementally building greater clarity about mechanisms that "crossed levels" and thus served to transfer stress and risk from environments into embodied biology.

This kind of ecological system thinking has long been central to social work. In order to specify with precision the cross-level series of causal mechanisms that lead to inequalities, however, the urgent trend is toward more comprehensive teamwork. By staying in constant communication, the CIHDR team has evolved toward more cross-project work and toward intervention development, testing, and advocacy for policy and system change. Emergent models such as that represented by CIHDR are thus more quickly and effectively "moving" science into practical application and demonstrable population benefit.

Understanding Translational Science
Like most professions and applied sciences, social work has long struggled with chasms separating research from practice and service provision. Research and practice activities are often undertaken in different settings, by different sets of individuals, with overlapping yet distinctly different priorities and training, and limited opportunities for systematic, sustained communication and collaboration. Social work routinely pursues partnered research within agencies, communities, and systems, yet knowledge producers and knowledge implementers face a host of barriers to bridging their work and maintaining a dialogue that sustains mutual relevance and comprehensibility (Proctor 2007). These challenges are particularly acute when it comes to building and sustaining collaborative relationships with community stakeholders.

Funders, legislators, and other stakeholders have expressed growing concern about these gaps, noting that investments in research are often not matched by the benefits to constituents. Social and health service providers, advocates, and the public are likewise keenly aware of problems with the fit, relevance, and timeliness of the evidence that reaches them, and of impediments to its implementation (Green, Ottoson, Garcia, & Hiatt, 2009). Practitioners and community stakeholders are removed from research activities to which they could be contributing valuable field-relevant knowledge. Furthermore, only a modest percentage of scientific knowledge "gets through" to application in the field. Reports have identified a 15- to 20-year gap between knowledge generated from research and the application of that knowledge in social and health care settings (Green, 2008; Hogan, 2003). This means that practitioners in usual care settings lag many years behind in getting access to the science that should be informing their practice (Brekke, Ell, & Palinkas, 2007).

How to Think about Translational Gaps
The goal of translational science is to better understand the nature of these impediments, to develop solutions that accelerate the movement of research to applied societal benefit, and to build partnerships between research and practice constituents to facilitate and sustain this acceleration (Woolf, 2008). Stimulated by health researchers aiming to hasten health-enhancing and life-saving advances, much of the early work on translational science was framed in clinical and biomedical terminology (Zerhouni, 2003). However, translational science is rapidly migrating into fields such as mental health and child welfare, demonstrating the broad applicability of these frameworks (Brekke, Ell, & Palinkas, 2007; *Child Maltreatment*, 2012).

The National Institutes of Health "road map," aimed at transforming U.S. health care through translational science commitments, identifies three T's or translational gaps (Dougherty & Conway, 2008). Translation 1 (T1) represents the gap between basic science and clinical research. In biomedical fields, this often involves translating laboratory "bench" research into human models or conceptualization of clinical interventions with patients, or both. Translation 2 (T2) represents the gap between clinical research (which often involves efficacy testing under highly controlled designs like randomized clinical trials) and clinical effectiveness in usual care settings, including the development of practice guidelines and tools for patients, practitioners, and policy makers. Translation 3 (T3) activities focus on moving interventions into larger systems—addressing, for example, the "how" of managing health care delivery such that evidence-informed interventions are provided with fidelity and reliability and indeed improve health outcomes. Focusing on the gaps, or "roadblocks," between sets of activities in the many phases of research, from basic science to sustainable application, should allow better understanding of the factors that contribute to these separations, stronger "road maps" that help to minimize blockages, and faster practical benefit.

Figure 2 provides a more nuanced illustration of the range of gaps in the research continuum—each of which needs to be bridged to accelerate the journey from basic research to demonstrable population or societal benefit. Some overlap is evident between the levels portrayed in Figure 1 and the phases of research and its application and infusion into practice portrayed in Figure 3. Individuals and groups working within basic research—whether that be biomedical, developmental, or economic—are often from different disciplines, with quite different skill sets than those working on effectiveness testing (for example, assessing the outcomes when interventions developed in controlled studies are applied in typical practice settings) or those focusing on system change (for example, reorienting training, supervision, and field supports in child welfare; see Marcenko, Hook, Romich, & Lee, 2012). Translational research encourages individuals working at different points in the continuum to be more explicitly cognizant of the whole, including developing skills in engaging with researchers in other phases of research and with stakeholders.

The translational continuum is bidirectional. Not uncommonly, findings at later points in the continuum bring to the surface realizations that require going "back to the drawing board" of earlier work (Fraser, Richman, Galinsky, & Day, 2009). The process of moving new interventions from controlled testing into usual practice settings frequently identifies differences among client populations that require rethinking and possibly modifying the intervention to achieve satisfactory levels of effectiveness. Cultural adaptation of evidence-based interventions is thus emerging as a critical dimension of translational research and practice (Cabassa & Baumann, 2013).

Stakeholder engagement is likewise increasingly seen as central to meaningful and sustainable research-practice translation (Callard, Rose, & Wykes, 2012). Reversing the conventional assumption that knowledge flows unidirectionally from research to practice, bidirectional relationships between practitioners, stakeholders, and researchers are seen as vital to strengthening the development, use, and dissemination of tested, culturally responsive interventions. Newer generations of evidence-based practices, for example, focus less on adherence to manualized interventions and more on ensuring that interventions balance efficacy with responsiveness to local issues and needs. In this context, practitioners and end users are increasingly engaged as active partners: providing vital information about where and how interventions should be tailored to meet diverse needs, shaping the research process by generating questions and practice innovations, and participating as members of research teams (Salisbury Forum Group, 2011; McKay et al., 2010).

Investments in cultural responsiveness and stakeholder involvement require not only intervention designs responsive to diverse populations and "messy" usual care settings but research methods that better accommodate community and provider priorities (Glasgow, Magid, Beck, Ritzwoller, & Estabrooks, 2005; Landsverk, Brown, Reutz, Palinkas, & Horwitz, 2011). Central to these developments has been growing use of community-based participatory research (CBPR) methods. CBPR principles guide researchers toward forms of communication, co-construction, and collaboration that are critical to community acceptance and sustainable implementation and to ensuring effectiveness within diverse populations and complex contexts (Minkler & Wallerstein, 2010; Wallerstein & Duran, 2010). Palinkas & Soydan (2012) provide guidance for CBPR application within translation and

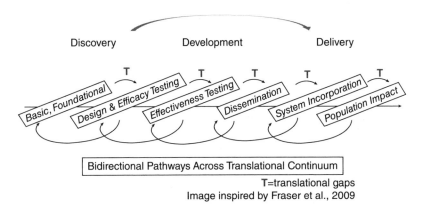

Figure 2. Illustrating phases of research and translational (T) gaps to bridge toward optimizing the benefit of science to societal benefit

implementation frameworks, as well as illustrations of recent social work projects.

Key developments in translational science thus include acknowledgment of the inherently iterative, engaged nature of applied research in realms such as social and health care (Green, 2008; Proctor, 2004), wider use of participatory models, more practical research designs, and an emphasis on models that are sustainable in complex real-world systems (Glasgow & Emmons, 2007; Spoth et al., 2013). Complementing and extending these efforts, implementation research addresses translational gaps related to the movement from intervention research (both controlled efficacy testing and more usual care setting effectiveness testing) to dissemination, organizational or system incorporation, and the capacity to evaluate large-scale impact (e.g., Proctor et al., 2009). In implementation research the translational gaps or challenges relate to processes of taking evidence regarding promising interventions through a complex array of contextual layers. In the social work context, these include factors such as agency or organizational contexts and processes, community characteristics, economic considerations, policy mandates or premises, systems thinking, uncertainties regarding broad-based efficacy and acceptability, and questions as to comparative effectiveness. The need for new kinds of teamwork that span these myriad gaps is a rapidly growing priority. Implementation research is thus an expanding arena of research trans-

lation within social work, with book-length guidance increasingly available (for example, Brownson, Colditz, & Proctor, 2012; Palinkas & Soydan, 2012).

By juxtaposing Figures 1 and 2, one can see that transdisciplinary and translational research have intertwined aims and strategies. Efforts to foster both more comprehensive, multilevel perspectives on social welfare and public health problems and more expedient, field-relevant pathways from research to practice require new kinds of partnerships and new ways of thinking about the relationships between research and impact. The surge of interest in collective impact represented in Hanleybrown, Kania, and Kramer (2012) and Kania and Kramer (2011), for example, emphasizes large-scale social change built upon broad cross-sector coordination—around issues such as education reform, obesity prevention, fair labor market models, and many other tenacious social problems familiar to social work. Such collaborations frequently entail radically new ways of partnering and using data and information. These, in turn, have implications for social work's capacity to function effectively in these cutting-edge efforts—whether in research, administrative, policy, or practice roles.

One additional illustration may be helpful in conveying the idea of translation gaps. The CIHDR health disparities research described above includes designing, funding, launching, and evaluating innovative interventions. Figure 3 highlights the connections between

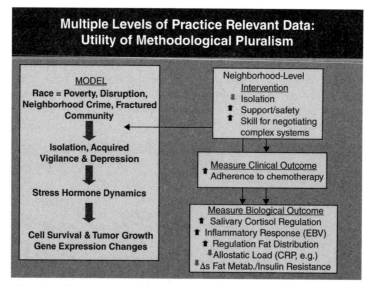

Figure 3. Illustrating the value of understanding data across multiple complex levels in translating transdisciplinary findings into effective interventions; the Center for Interdisciplinary Health Disparities Research.
Adapted from: Gehlert, S., Murray, A., Sohmer, D., McClintock, M., Conzen, S., & Olopade, O. (2010). The importance of transdisciplinary collaborations for understanding and resolving health disparities. *Social Work in Public Health*, 25(3–4), 408–422.

structural and environmental conditions and biopsychosocial factors in accounting for racial differences in breast cancer outcomes. Although the model used here as an example focuses on breast cancer, it has much broader applicability. It shows, for instance, that interventions aimed at decreasing health disparities should address neighborhood-level factors (for example, reducing isolation, fostering system supports, enabling system navigation) as upstream targets of what are often treated as a highly individual level health issues (for example, getting mammograms, medical treatment adherence).

Conceptually, the connective threads from structural and environmental forces to health outcomes are provided by models of life course stress embodiment (Furumoto-Dawson, Gehlert, Sohmer, Olopade, & Sacks, 2007; Nurius & Hoy-Ellis, 2013). These theoretical frameworks direct attention to biological changes and trajectories alongside and indeed interwoven with behavioral, social, and environmental factors. In fact, intervention effects, even those directed at more macro or meso levels, may reveal initial effects at the biological level, as sensitive indicators of change that precede changes at cognitive-learning, behavioral, social network, psychological, family, or community levels. Future practitioners working in arenas related to poverty, health inequalities, child and family well-being, school- or work-related issues, and a host of other social welfare concerns are thus likely to find that their training needs to include the ability to think across and understand data at multiple levels of complex ecologies. Research on stress embodiment—the mechanisms through which toxic and pernicious stress "gets under the skin," "poisons the brain," and subsequently affects a broad range of developmental, health, and functioning outcomes—is one example of powerful findings highly relevant to social workers working with vulnerable populations spanning many specific domains of practice and policy (see Lende, 2012; Shonkoff et al., 2012).

Building Transdisciplinary and Translational Capacity

The social work profession is "well placed to produce the socially engaged, accountable... research knowledge best suited to contemporary markets" (Sharland, 2012, p. 101). Its social justice mission, collaborative interdisciplinary character, long history of community-based engagement, and deep investment in the science and practice of people in context align closely with emerging emphases and imperatives. Consequently, major social work organizations have been focusing strategically on increasing social work's perceived relevance as a key player in contemporary impact-oriented research and practice efforts. The Grand Challenges initiative sponsored by the American Academy of Social Work and Social Welfare (Uehara et al., 2013), for example, calls for social work to play more central, transformative, and collaborative roles in addressing the most pressing issues of this time, and notes the centrality to these efforts of "innovative, collaborative, interdisciplinary work" (p. 167).

The transdisciplinary and translational priorities embedded in these efforts are relevant to social workers across many roles and settings. Collaboration and teamwork are as much features of contemporary health and human services practice as they are of contemporary research. Effective research to practice translation similarly relies on practitioners sensitized to the complexities of developing and implementing interventions in diverse contexts. The need for transdisciplinary and translational capacity and confidence thus applies equally, if differentially, to social work practitioners as well as researchers. Recognizing this, attention to the topics addressed in this entry is growing at all levels of social work education, from undergraduate and graduate to doctoral and postdoctoral (Bellamy et al, 2013; Fong, 2013). These and related efforts to amplify social work's transdisciplinary and translational capacities are key to the profession's readiness to collectively engage with others toward ambitious and sustainable solutions.

REFERENCES

Almgren, G., Kemp, S. P., & Eisinger, A. (2000). The legacy of Hull House and the Children's Bureau in the American mortality transition. *Social Service Review, 74*(1), 1–27.

Bellamy, J. L., Mullen, E. J., Satterfield, J. M., Newhouse, R. P., Ferguson, M., Brownson, R. C., & Spring, B. (2013). Implementing evidence-based practice education in social work: A transdisciplinary approach. *Research on Social Work Practice, 23*, 426-436.

Brekke, J. S., Ell, K., & Palinkas, L. A. (2007). Translational science at the National Institute of Mental Health: Can social work take its rightful place? *Research on Social Work Practice, 17*(1), 123–133.

Brownson, R., Colditz, G., & Proctor, E. (Eds.). (2012). *Dissemination and implementation research in health: Translating science to practice.* New York: Oxford University Press.

Cabassa, L. J., & Baumann, A. (2013, August 19). A two-way street: Bridging implementation science and cultural adaptations of mental health treatments. *Implementation Science, 8,* 90. doi:10.1186/1748-5908-8-90. Retrieved May 7, 2014, from http://www.implementationscience.com/content/8/1/90

Callard, F., Rose, D., & Wykes, T. (2012). Close to the bench as well as at the bedside: Involving service users in all phases of translational research. *Health Expectations, 15*(4), 389–400.

Child Maltreatment. (2012). Special journal issue: Disseminating child maltreatment interventions: Research on implementing evidence-based programs, *17*(1).

Davis, K. (2011). The youngest science: Social work research as product and process in a competitive scientific market. Invited Presidential Address, Society for Social Work & Research.

DiLorenzo, P., White, C. R, Morales, A., Paul, A., & Shaw, S. (2013). Innovative cross-system and community approaches for the prevention of child maltreatment. *Child Welfare, 92*(2), 161–178.

Dougherty, D., & Conway, P. H. (2008). The "3T's" road map to transform U.S. health care: The "how" of high-quality care. *JAMA: Journal of the American Medical Association, 299*(19), 2319–2321.

Fishbein, D. H., & Ridenour, T. A. (2013). Advancing transdisciplinary translation for prevention of high-risk behaviors: Introduction to the special issue. *Prevention Science, 14*(3), 201–205.

Fong, R. (2013). Framing doctoral education for a science of social work: Positioning students for the scientific career, promoting scholars for the academy, propagating scientists of the profession, and preparing stewards of the discipline. *Research on Social Work Practice.* Published online before print December 16, 2013. doi:10.1177/1049731513515055

Fong, R. (2012). Framing education for a science of social work: Missions, curriculum, and doctoral training. *Research on Social Work Practice, 22*(5), 529–536.

Fraser, M. W, Richman, J. M., Galinsky, M. J, & Day, S. H. (2009). *Intervention research: Developing social programs.* New York: Oxford University Press.

Frenk, J., Chen, L., Bhutta, Z. A., Cohen, J., Crisp, N., Evans, T., et al. (2010). Health professionals for a new century: Transforming education to strengthen health systems in an interdependent world. *Lancet, 376*(9756), 1923–1958.

Furumoto-Dawson, A., Gehlert, S., Sohmer, D., Olopade, O., & Sacks, T. (2007). Early-life conditions and mechanisms of population health vulnerabilities. *Health Affairs, 26*(5), 1238–1248.

Gehlert, S. (2012). Shaping education and training to advance transdisciplinary health research. *Transdisciplinary Journal of Engineering and Science, 3*, 1–10.

Gehlert, S., & Browne, T. (2013). Transdisciplinary training and education. In D. Haire-Joshu & T. D. McBride (Eds.), *Transdisciplinary public health: Research, education, and practice* (pp. 31–51). San Francisco, CA: Jossey-Bass

Gehlert, S., Murray, A., Sohmer, D., McClintock, M., Conzen, S., & Olopade, O. (2010). The importance of transdisciplinary collaborations for understanding and resolving health disparities. *Social Work in Public Health, 25*(3–4), 408–422.

Glasgow, R. E., & Emmons, K. M. (2007). How can we increase translation of research into practice? Types of evidence needed. *Annual Review of Public Health, 28*, 413–433.

Glasgow, R. E., Magid, D. J., Beck, A., Ritzwoller, D., & Estabrooks, P. A. (2005). Practical clinical trials for translating research to practice: Design and measurement recommendations. *Medical Care, 43*(6), 551–557.

Green, L. W. (2008). Making research relevant: If it is an evidence-based practice, where's the practice-based evidence? *Family Practice, 25*(suppl. 1), i20–i24.

Green, L. W., Ottoson, J., Garcia, C., & Robert, H. (2009). Diffusion theory and knowledge dissemination, utilization, and integration in public health. *Annual Review of Public Health, 30*, 151.

Hall, K. L. (2013). *Transdisciplinary research: Conceptual and practical issues.* Paper presented at the Transdisciplinary Translation for Prevention of High Risk Behaviors Conference. Retrieved May 7, 2014, from http://www.ttpr.org/images/2013_Presentation/_Keynote_Hall_2013.pdf

Hanleybrown, F., Kania, J., & Kramer, M. (2012). Channeling change: Making collective impact work. *Stanford Social Innovation Review.* Retrieved May 7, 2014, from http://www.ssireview.org/blog/entry/channeling_change_making_collective_impact_work

Henly, J. R. (2013). Scientific exemplars in social work: Poverty and child well-being. Paper presented at the Islandwood Science in Social Work Roundtable, Bainbridge, Washington.

Hogan, M. F. (2003). New Freedom Commission report: The president's New Freedom Commission: Recommendations to transform mental health care in America. *Psychiatric Services, 54*(11), 1467–1474

Kania, J., & Kramer, M. (2011). Collective impact. *Stanford Social Innovation Review, 1*(9), 36–41.

Kemp, S. P. & Nurius, P. S. (in press). Preparing emerging scholars for transdisciplinary research: A developmental approach to doctoral education. *Journal of Teaching in Social Work.*

Kemp, S. P., & Nurius, P. S. (2013). Practical reason within and across disciplinary borders: A response to Longhofer and Floersch. *Research on Social Work Practice.* Published online before print November 5, 2013, as doi:10.1177/1049731513509898

King, G., Tucker, M., Duwyn, B., Desserud, S., & Shillington, M. (2009). The application of a transdisciplinary model for early intervention services. *Infants and Young Children, 22*(3), 211–223.

Kirk, S. A., & Reid, W. J. (2002). *Science and social work: A critical appraisal.* New York: Columbia University Press.

Landsverk, J., Brown, C. H., Reutz, J. R., Palinkas, L., & Horwitz, S. M. (2011). Design elements in implementation research: A structured review of child welfare and child mental health studies. *Administration and Policy in Mental Health and Mental Health Services Research, 38*(1), 54–63.

Lang, D. J., Wiek, A., Bergmann, M., Stauffacher, M., Martens, P., Moll, P., et al. (2012). Transdisciplinary research in sustainability science: Practice, principles, and challenges. *Sustainability Science, 7* (Suppl. 1), 25–43.

Lende, D. H. (2012). Poverty poisons the brain. *Annals of Anthropological Practice, 36*(1), 183–201.

Lyall, C., & Fletcher, I. (2013). Experiments in interdisciplinary capacity-building: The successes and challenges of large-scale interdisciplinary investments. *Science and Public Policy, 40*(1), 1–7.

Lynch, J. (2006). It's not easy being interdisciplinary. *International Journal of Epidemiology, 35*(5), 1119–1122.

McKay, M. M., Gopalan, G., Franco, L. M., Kalogerogiannis, K., Umpierre, M., Olshtain-Mann, O., et al. (2010). It takes a village to deliver and test child- and family-focused services. *Research on Social Work Practice, 20*(5), 476–482.

Marcenko, M. O., Hook, J., Romich, J. L, & Lee, J. S. (2012). Multiple jeopardy: Poor, economically disconnected, and child welfare involved. *Child Maltreatment, 17*(3), 195–206.

Minkler, M., & Wallerstein, N. (Eds.). (2010). *Community-based participatory research for health: From process to outcomes.* San Francisco, CA: Jossey-Bass.

Nash, J. M. (2008). Transdisciplinary training: Key components and prerequisites for success. *American Journal of Preventive Medicine, 35*(2), S133–S140.

Nurius, P. S., & Hoy-Ellis, C. P. (2013). Stress effects and health. In C. Franklin (Ed.), *Encyclopedia of Social Work Online.* National Association of Social Workers Press and Oxford University Press.

Nurius, P. S. & Kemp, S. P. (2012). Social work, science, social impact: Crafting an integrative conversation. *Research on Social Work Practice, 22*(5), 548–552.

Nurius, P. S. & Kemp, S. P. (2013). Transdisciplinarity and translation: Preparing social work doctoral students for high impact research. *Research on Social Work Practice.* First published online before print November 19, 2013, as doi:10.1177/1049731513512375

Palinkas, L. A., & Soydan, H. (2012). *Translation and implementation of evidence-based practice.* New York: Oxford University Press.

Proctor, E. K. (2004). Leverage points for the implementation of evidence-based practice. *Brief Treatment and Crisis Intervention, 4*(3), 227.

Proctor, E. K. (2007). Implementing evidence-based practice in social work education: Principles, strategies, and partnerships. *Research on Social Work Practice, 17*(5), 583–591.

Proctor, E. K., Landsverk, J., Aarons, G., Chambers, D., Glisson, C., & Mittman, B. (2009). Implementation research in mental health services: An emerging science with conceptual, methodological, and training challenges. *Administration and Policy in Mental Health and Mental Health Services Research, 36*(1), 24–34.

Rosenfield, P. L. (1992). The potential of transdisciplinary research for sustaining and extending linkages between the health and social sciences. *Social Science & Medicine, 35*(11), 1343–1357.

Ruddy, G., & Rhee, K. S. (2005). Transdisciplinary teams in primary care for the underserved: A literature review. *Journal of Health Care for the Poor and Underserved, 16*(2), 248–256.

Salant, T., & Gehlert, S. (2008). Collective memory, candidacy, and victimization: Community epidemiologies of breast cancer risk. *Sociology of Health & Illness, 30*(4), 599–615.

Salisbury Forum Group. (2011). The Salisbury statement. *Social Work and Society, 9*(1), 4–9.

Schmitz, C. L., Matyók, T., Sloan, L. M., & James, C. (2012). The relationship between social work and environmental sustainability: Implications for interdisciplinary practice. *International Journal of Social Welfare, 21*(3), 278–286.

Sharland, E. (2012). All together now? Building disciplinary and inter-disciplinary research capacity in social work and social care. *British Journal of Social Work, 42*(2), 208–226.

Shonkoff, J. P., Garner, A. S., Siegel, B. S., Dobbins, M. I., Earls, M. F., McGuinn, L., et al. (2012). The lifelong effects of early childhood adversity and toxic stress. *Pediatrics, 129*(1), e232–e246.

Social Research Unit. (2011). *Achieving lasting impact at scale: Part 1.* A convening hosted by the Bill and Melinda Gates Foundation, Seattle, WA, November 1–2, 2011. Synthesis and summary by the Social Research Unit at Dartington, UK.

Soydan, H. (Ed.) (2012). Shaping a science of social work. *Research on Social Work Practice, Special Issue, 22*(5).

Spoth, R., Rohrbach, L. A., Greenberg, M., Leaf, P., Brown, C. H., Fagan, A., et al. (2013). Addressing core challenges for the next generation of Type 2 translation research and systems: The translation science to population impact (TSci Impact) framework. *Prevention Science, 14*(4), 1–33.

Stokols, D. (2006). Toward a science of transdisciplinary research. *American Journal of Community Psychology, 38*, 63–77.

Uehara, E., Flynn, M., Fong, R., Brekke, J., Barth, R. P., Coulton, C., & Walters, K. (2013). Grand challenges for social work. *Journal of the Society for Social Work and Research, 4*(3), 165-170.

Wallerstein, N., & Duran, B. (2010). Community-based participatory research contributions to intervention research: The intersection of science and practice to improve health equity. *American Journal of Public Health, 100*(S1), S40–S46.

Warnecke, R. B., Oh, A., Breen, N., Gehlert, S., Paskett, E., Tucker, K. L., et al. (2008). Approaching health disparities from a population perspective: The National Institutes of Health Centers for Population Health and Health Disparities. *American Journal of Public Health, 98*(9), 1608–1615.

Woolf, S. H. (2008). The meaning of translational research and why it matters. *JAMA: Journal of the American Medical Association, 299*(2), 211–213.

World Health Organization. (2010). *Health Workforce: Framework for action on interprofessional education and collaborative practice.* Retrieved May 7, 2014, from http://www.who.int/hrh/resources/framework_action/en/

Zerhouni, E. (2003, October 3). The NIH roadmap. *Science*, pp. 63–72.

FURTHER READING

Brekke, J. S. (2012). Shaping a science of social work. *Research on Social Work Practice*, 22(5), 455–464.

Frodeman, R., Klein, J. Y., & Mitcham, C. (Eds.) (2010). *Oxford handbook of interdisciplinarity*. Oxford: Oxford University Press.

Haire-Joshu, D., & McBride, T. D. (Eds.) (2013). *Transdisciplinary public health: Research, education, and practice*. San Francisco, CA: Jossey Bass.

Mor Barak, M. & Brekke, J. S. (2014). Social work science and identity formation for doctoral scholars within intellectual communities. *Research on Social Work Practice*, 24(5), 616–624.

O'Rourke, M., Crowley, S., Eigenbrode, S. D., & Wulfhorst, J. D. (Eds.). (2014). *Enhancing communication and collaboration in interdisciplinary research*. Los Angeles: Sage.

Powell, B. J., McMillen, J. C., Proctor, E. K., Carpenter, C. R., Griffey, R. T., Bunger, A. C., et al. (2012). A compilation of strategies for implementing clinical innovations in health and mental health. *Medical Care Research and Review*, 69(2), 123–157.

PAULA S. NURIUS AND SUSAN P. KEMP

TRAUMA-INFORMED CARE

ABSTRACT: The concepts of trauma and trauma-informed care have evolved greatly since the late twentieth century. Following the Vietnam War, professional understanding of post-traumatic stress disorder (PTSD) increased. The greater understanding of trauma and its effects on war veterans has extended to informing our comprehension of trauma in the civilian world and with children and families who have experienced abuse, neglect, and other traumatic events. This elevated insight has led to the development of evidence-based models of trauma treatment along with changes in organizational policies and practices designed to facilitate resilience and recovery. This article highlights the concept of trauma-informed care by providing an overview of trauma and its effects, then providing a comprehensive description of our understanding of trauma-informed care across child- and family-serving systems.

KEY WORDS: post-traumatic stress disorder; psychological safety; resilience; trauma; trauma-informed care; trauma-informed systems; well-being

Trauma-Informed Care

The concepts of *trauma-informed care* have evolved over the past 30 years from a variety of streams of thought and innovation. They are now being applied in a wide range of settings, from mental health and substance-abuse treatment providers to child welfare systems and even schools and criminal justice institutions. In the simplest terms, the concept of trauma-informed care is straightforward. If professionals were to pause and consider the role trauma and lingering traumatic stress plays in the lives of the specific client population served by an individual, professional, organization, or an entire system, how would they behave differently? What steps would they take to avoid, or at least minimize, adding new stress or inadvertently reminding their clients of their past traumas? How can they better help their traumatized clients heal? In effect, by looking at how the entire system is organized and services are delivered through a "trauma lens," what should be done differently? The answer can be used to guide practice, policy, procedures, and even how the physical caregiving environment is structured.

Foundations of Trauma-Informed Care

Long before anyone used the term "trauma-informed," caring professionals and committed volunteers were instinctively acting in a trauma-informed manner. Much of this was influenced by the emergence of the feminist movement and the increasingly influential voice of survivors of interpersonal trauma, as seen in the rape crisis centers and the domestic violence movements of the 1970s (Burgess & Holmstrom, 1974) and the dramatic growth of child-advocacy centers and multidisciplinary teams in child abuse in the 1980s. These natural incubators for trauma-informed innovation and practice were "married" in the 1990s with the growing body of science and trauma-specific empirical research into how human beings respond in the aftermath of traumatic events, and how professionals and concerned activists could help them move toward recovery. That stream of research began with interest in combat-related post-traumatic stress after the Vietnam War. By the mid-1980s, the focus had expanded and was adopted by the wider mental health community as a relevant construct for understanding the cascade of symptoms often noted after rapes, shootings, and other major traumatic life events. In 1985, the International Society for Traumatic Stress was founded in the United States and served as a focal point for professionals searching for answers to support highly traumatized populations. By 1989, the United States Department of Veterans Affairs had created the National Center for Post-Traumatic Stress Disorder (*www.ptsd.va.gov*). In the 1990s, the

Substance Abuse and Mental Health Administration (SAMHSA), within the U.S. Department of Health and Human Services, recognized the role of trauma in a significant number of women's issues and gender-specific treatments. Over the next 20 years, a huge expansion of knowledge about trauma and traumatic stress occurred. This included not only better diagnostic criteria but also the development of empirically tested treatments for PTSD and other related trauma symptoms.

What Is Trauma?

Defining trauma is not without its controversies. Those who approach it from a clinical perspective tend to view trauma as a combination of a terrible event or series of events that involve real or perceived threats of death or serious injury, or threat to the physical integrity of the person or others, *and* from which that person experiences overwhelming fear, hopelessness, helplessness, or horror. This type of overwhelming stress, especially when it occurs over and over, as is common in many individuals served by the social work community, can create significant long-term impacts, including changes in the physiology of the brains of developing children. Some survivors of trauma, however, favor a definition that places greater emphasis on the subjective experience and the level of stress an individual perceives, independent of an event or series of events that threaten the individual with death, serious injury, or loss of their physical integrity such as a highly emotional argument with a family member (Substance Abuse and Mental Health Services Administration, 2012).

Prevalence of Trauma

Most individuals seeking public behavioral health services and other public services, such as homeless and domestic violence services, have histories of physical and sexual abuse, and witnessing or experiencing domestic violence, and they often live in neighborhoods where community violence is ever present. These individuals often present with co-occurring disorders such as chronic health conditions, substance abuse, eating disorders, and HIV/AIDS. In fact, 50% to 70% of women in psychiatric hospitals, 40% to 60% of women receiving outpatient mental health services, and 55% to 90% of women with substance abuse disorders report being physically or sexually abused, or both, in their lives (Substance Abuse and Mental Health Services Administration, 2007). While trauma occurs throughout the lifespan, for many seeking the services of social workers and other helping

professionals, the trauma began in childhood. Studies have reported high rates of trauma among children in the United States since the 1950s (Landis, 1956). For example, in one study, the authors found that 25% of their sample of 9- to 16-year-olds had recently experienced a potentially traumatic event (Costello, Erkanli, Fairbank, & Angold, 2002). Child abuse and neglect is an all-too-common form of trauma. In 2011, there were approximately 3.4 million reports of abuse or neglect that covered 6.2 million children (U.S. Department of Health and Human Services [DHHS], 2011). Another study found that approximately 15.5 million children were estimated to live in homes where they were exposed to at least one incidence of domestic violence in the previous year (McDonald, Jouriles, Ramisetty-Mikler, et al., 2006.). Anda and Felitti (2003) found that 21% of a 17,000-person sample drawn from adults enrolled in a San Diego Health Maintenance Organization reported being sexually abused; 26% were physically abused; and 13% lived in a home with domestic violence as a child. These and other studies reveal that a substantial number of children have experienced abuse or exposure to other traumatic events prior to their eighteenth birthday.

Not only are these forms of trauma common, they are among the most emotionally devastating and have been linked to a host of negative outcomes in childhood, from emotional and behavioral problems to impaired school performance (Conradi & Wilson, 2010; Ethier, Lemelin, & Lacharite, 2004). Without effective intervention, there is compelling evidence of long-term adverse consequences of untreated trauma lasting into adulthood that include substance abuse, suicidality, serious mental illness, and long-term physical health factors associated with early death (Felitti, Anda, Nordenberg, Williamson, et al., 1998; Anda, Dong, Brown, et al., 2009).

Whether children or adults, those who have experienced a traumatic event are likely to come into contact with multiple systems. Child welfare services alone come into contact with over 6 million children a year (US DHHS, 2011), and there are as many as 223,000 children placed in the protective custody of state or local governments at any one time (US DHHS, 2012). Youth involved in the juvenile justice system also present with high rates of trauma. In one study of a juvenile justice population, 92.5% of participants had experienced one or more traumatic events in their lifetime, and 11.2% of the sample met criteria for PTSD in the past year (Abram, Teplin, Charles, et al., 2004). By virtue of the events that brought the children into contact with these systems, and the additional traumas the system may impose (removal from the home, changes in placement, instability of relationships, use of seclusion and restraint, risk of re-abuse, inconsistent caregivers and caseworkers, separation of siblings, and so forth), virtually all have suffered major trauma.

Unique Response to Highly Stressful Events

Trauma, however, does not affect everyone in the same way. Some people experience a terrible event but suffer no long-term adverse emotional effects, while the same event have a devastating impact on the individual standing next to them. Traumatic response is highly individualized and shaped by a wide range of factors, from genetics, to previous life experiences, to support systems available in the aftermath of the event. How helping professionals respond also influences the long-term impact of traumatic events for the better, when delivered in a trauma-informed environment, or for the worse, if delivered in a trauma-insensitive manner, as has been the case for much of history.

The Emergence of Trauma-Informed Care

In 1994, the Substance Abuse and Mental Health Services Administration (SAMHSA) convened the Dare to Vision conference, which explored the high prevalence of physical and sexual abuse among women served by the public mental health system. This event provided a forum for survivors to discuss their trauma histories and how trauma impacted their physical and mental health. It highlighted the re-victimization many experienced in residential or inpatient settings through the use of such practices as seclusion and restraint. By the late 1990s and early 2000s, a variety of professionals began to articulate the importance of the organizational context in the delivery of services to individuals who have experienced significant traumatic life events (Bloom, 1997; Harris & Fallot, 2001; Covington, 2002; Rivard, Bloom, & Abramovitz, 2003; Ko, Ford, Kassam-Adams N., et al., 2008; Bloom, 2010). The concepts at the core of "trauma-informed care" began to take greater shape and spread with the launch in 1998 of the Women, Co-Occurring Disorders and Violence Study, sponsored by SAMHSA (see www.wcdvs.com for more information), which integrated service system strategies for women with co-occurring mental health and substance abuse disorders who have also been victims of trauma. This study, carried out in 27 sites over five years in two phases (fourteen Phase One women sites, nine Phase Two women sites, and four Phase Two children's sites), provided recommendations for "trauma-integrated services counseling." This important study laid out a framework of principles for this population, complete with guidance for providers to be cognizant of their own practices and policies that might put women in danger physically and psychologically, add new traumatic experiences, or unnecessarily trigger memories of past traumatic events. The study highlighted the importance of "all service interventions [being] gender-specific, culturally competent, trauma-informed and trauma-specific, comprehensive, integrated, and [with] consumer/survivor/recovering women involved" (U.S. Department of Health and Human Services, Substance Abuse and Mental Health Services Administration, 2007, p. 1). This study and others brought attention to the need for trauma-informed care in the adult world.

In 2001, the U.S. Congress and SAMHSA established the Donald J. Cohen National Child Traumatic Stress Initiative, and, through it, the National Child Traumatic Stress Network (NCTSN, www.nctsn.org). This national network, under the leadership of the National Center for Child Traumatic Stress at Duke University and the University of California–Los Angeles (UCLA), initially focused on the mission of raising "the standard of care and improve access to services for traumatized children, their families and communities throughout the United States." Toward that end, the NCTSN concentrated on the identification and spread of empirically supported trauma-specific mental health interventions such as TraumaFocused Cognitive Behavioral Therapy (Deblinger, Lippmann, & Steer, 1996; Cohen, Deblinger, Mannarino, & Steer, 2004; Cohen, Mannarino, & Staron, 2006) Deblinger, Mannarino, Cohen, & Steer (2006); Cohen, Mannarino & Iyengar (2011), and Child-Parent Psychotherapy (Lieberman, Weston, & Pawl, 1991; Cicchetti, Toth, & Rogosch, 1999; Toth, Maughan, Manly, Spagnola, & Cicchetti, 2002; Lieberman, Ghosh Ippen, & Van Horn, 2006). By 2003, however, the NCTSN increasingly recognized that system issues could support or undermine effective trauma-specific treatments and began to explore the organization and system context in which trauma-specific interventions were being delivered, with the establishment of the Systems Integration Committee (Taylor & Siegfried, 2005). In short order, that effort was replaced by system-specific initiatives within the NCTSN designed to facilitate the NCTSN mission within the context of specific systems, including child welfare, juvenile justice, schools, and health care (Ko, Ford, Kassam-Adams, et al., 2008). In these efforts, the lessons learned in the Women with Co-Occurring Disorders Study and early adopters of trauma-informed care in the adult trauma world, along with the practical experience implementing trauma-specific interventions in child-serving environments, were integrated to create a trauma-informed perspective to serving traumatized children and their families.

As the term "trauma-informed care" took root in both adult- and child-serving worlds, distinctions began to be drawn between related, but discrete, perspectives. These ranged from "trauma-informed care" to "trauma-informed practice," "trauma-informed organizations," "trauma-specific treatments," "trauma-informed systems," and "trauma-informed approaches"; all linked by the concept of "trauma-informed."

What Does It Mean to Be Trauma-Informed?

Many organizations and authors have offered definitions or a list of elements about what constitutes trauma-informed care or the related concepts of trauma-informed practice, organizations, and systems. In 2005, SAMHSA established the National Center for Trauma- Informed Care (NCTIC). The NCTIC suggested that every part of an organization seeking to be trauma-informed—its organizational structure, its management systems, and its service delivery—be

> assessed and potentially modified to include a basic understanding of how trauma affects the life of an individual seeking services. Trauma-informed organizations, programs, and services are based on an understanding of the vulnerabilities or triggers of trauma survivors that traditional service delivery approaches may exacerbate, so that these services and programs can be more supportive and avoid re-traumatization. (National Center for Trauma-Informed Care, 2012)

Fallot and Harris (2009) suggest that trauma-informed care is built on five core values: (1) safety, (2) trustworthiness, (3) choice, (4) collaboration, and (5) empowerment. Here *safety* means both physical and emotional safety, while *trustworthiness* relates to the clarity of expectations, providing consistent service delivery across the organization, and maintaining boundaries. Fallot and Harris's view of trauma-informed care emphasizes the active role of the person receiving the services or support. The concept of *choice* is important because it gives the consumer control over the services they receive. *Control* is significant because, as a victim of trauma, client control was taken from the during the traumatic event, whether through a rape, physical assault, or even a natural disaster. *Collaboration* emphasizes the need for client involvement and sharing of power, while *empowerment* relates to the development and enhancement of consumer skills.

In a working paper, US Department of Health and Human Servicese (USHHS/SAMHSA, 2012) suggests that a trauma-informed approach is guided by 10 principles:

1. Safety: throughout the organization, staff and the people they serve feel physically and psychologically safe; the physical setting is safe and interpersonal interactions promote a sense of safety.
2. Trustworthiness and transparency: organizational operations and decisions are conducted with transparency and the goal of building and maintaining trust among staff, clients, and family members of people being served by the organization.
3. Collaboration and mutuality: there is true partnering and leveling of power differences between staff and clients and among organizational staff from direct care staff to administrators; there is recognition that healing happens in relationships and in the meaningful sharing of power and decision-making.
4. Empowerment: throughout the organization and among the clients served, individuals' strengths are recognized, built on, and validated and new skills developed as necessary.
5. Voice and choice: the organization aims to strengthen the staff's, clients', and family members' experience of choice and recognize that every person's experience is unique and requires an individualized approach.
6. Peer support and mutual self-help: are integral to the organizational and service delivery approach and are understood as a key vehicle for building trust, establishing safety, and empowerment.
7. Resilience and strengths based: a belief in resilience and in the ability of individuals, organizations, and communities to heal and promote recovery from trauma; builds on what clients, staff and communities have to offer rather than responding to their perceived deficits.
8. Inclusiveness and shared purpose: the organization recognizes that everyone has a role to play in a trauma-informed approach; one does not have to be a therapist to be therapeutic.
9. Cultural, historical, and gender issues: the organization addresses cultural, historical, and gender issues; the organization actively moves past cultural stereotypes and biases (e.g. based on race, ethnicity, sexual orientation, age, geography, etc.), offers gender responsive services, leverages the healing value of traditional cultural connections, and recognizes and addresses historical trauma.

10. Change process: is conscious, intentional, and ongoing; the organization strives to become a learning community, constantly responding to new knowledge and developments (What are the key principles of a trauma-informed approach? section)

Meanwhile, the National Child Traumatic Stress Network (NCTSN, 2012, What is a trauma-informed child- and family-service system? section, para. 1) defines the trauma-informed child-and family-serving system as one in which

> all parties involved recognize and respond to the impact of traumatic stress on those who have contact with the system including children, caregivers, and service providers. Programs and agencies within such a system infuse and sustain trauma awareness, knowledge, and skills into their organizational cultures, practices, and policies. They act in collaboration with all those who are involved with the child, using the best available science, to facilitate and support the recovery and resiliency of the child and family.

The NCTSN goes on to suggest that a service system with a trauma-informed perspective is one in which programs, agencies, and service providers (NCTSN, 2012):

1. routinely screen for trauma exposure and related symptoms;
2. use culturally appropriate evidence-based assessment and treatment for traumatic stress and associated mental health symptoms;
3. make resources available to children, families, and providers on trauma exposure, its impact, and treatment;
4. engage in efforts to strengthen the resilience and protective factors of children and families impacted by and vulnerable to trauma;
5. address parent and caregiver trauma and its impact on the family system;
6. emphasize continuity of care and collaboration across child-service systems; and
7. maintain an environment of care for staff that addresses, minimizes, and treats secondary traumatic stress, and that increases staff resilience.

Some organizations, like the National Center for Children in Poverty (NCCP), have outlined a trauma-informed approach into a policy framework (Cooper, Masi, Dababnah, Aratani, & Knitzer, 2007). The NCCP advocates that:

1. All federal, tribal, state, and local policies should reflect a trauma-informed perspective. A trauma-informed response encompasses a fundamental understanding of trauma and how it shapes an individual who has experienced it.
   a. Policies should support delivery systems that identify and implement strategies to prevent trauma, increase capacity for early identification and intervention, and provide comprehensive treatment.
   b. Policies should support and require that strategies are designed to prevent and eliminate treatment practices that cause trauma or re-traumatization.
   c. Policies should reinforce the core components of best practices in trauma-informed care: prevention; developmentally appropriate, effective strategies; cultural and linguistic competence; and family and youth engagement.
2. Policy and practice should be reflective of trauma-informed principles and be developmentally appropriate, based on a public health framework, and engage children, youth, and their families in healing.
   a. Policies should focus on prevention of trauma and developing strategies to identify and intervene early for children, youth, and their families exposed to trauma or at risk of exposure to trauma.
   b. Policies should focus on enhancing child, youth, and family engagement strategies to support informed trauma care delivery.
   c. Policies should support strategies that encompass family-based approaches to trauma intervention.
3. Trauma-informed and related policies must include responsive financing, cross-system collaboration and training, accountability, and infrastructure development.
   a. Policies should ensure that funding is supportive of trauma-informed care and based upon sound fiscal strategies.
   b. Policies should make funding contingent upon eliminating harmful practices that cause trauma and re-traumatization across child-serving settings.
   c. Policies should support comprehensive workforce investment strategies. (Cooper et al, 2007, pp. 1–2)

Emerging Themes

While the actual words vary considerably across definitions and perspectives on trauma-informed care, and the related topics of trauma-informed practice, trauma-informed approach, trauma-informed organizations and systems, some common themes emerge as the essential elements of trauma-informed care (Child Welfare Committee, National Child Traumatic Stress Network, & The California Social Work Education Center, 2012; Chadwick Trauma Informed Systems Project, 2013).

MAXIMIZE PHYSICAL AND PSYCHOLOGICAL SAFETY

At its most fundamental level, recovery from trauma requires a sense of safety, and trauma-informed providers must recognize safety is both physical and psychological. Removing a child from an abusive home, for example, and placing him or her in a physically safe foster home where the child will not be maltreated may achieve physical safety but does not guarantee the child will feel safe. In fact, the very process of securing physical safety may intensify the child's fears and insecurity and feelings of being out of control, helpless, and inherently unsafe. Without a sense of safety, not only will the client not progress, but the anxiety and stress it creates will add new trauma, amplify old trauma, and impact their behavior, often emerging as unhealthy maladaptive behaviors replayed long after the physical threat is gone.

The term *psychological safety* means a "sense of safety, or the ability to feel safe, within one's self and safe from external harm" (Chadwick Trauma-Informed Systems Project, 2013, p. 13) This type of safety occurs on an emotional level and is not defined by objective observable reality. It has direct implications for physical safety and is critical for optimal functioning as well as physical and emotional growth. A lack of psychological safety can impact an individual's and family's interactions with all others, including those trying to help them, and can lead to a variety of maladaptive strategies for coping with the anxiety associated with feeling unsafe. These survival strategies may include high-risk and counterproductive behaviors, such as substance abuse, aggression and violence, high-risk-taking activities, and self-mutilation. The child (and his or her siblings) may continue to feel psychologically unsafe long after the physical threat has been removed or he or she has been relocated to a physically safe environment. In reality, the client may feel psychologically unsafe for a number of reasons. These may include factors the system can control, such as the placement environment and how professionals help the client regulate their emotions. Even after the client gains some degree of security, a *trigger*, such as a person, place, or event, may unexpectedly remind him or her of the trauma and draw his or her attention back to intense and disturbing memories that overwhelm his or her ability to cope, again creating a sense of fear and anxiety. At other times, a seemingly innocuous event or sensory stimulus like an odor, sound, touch, taste, or particular scene may act as a trigger and be a subconscious reminder of the trauma. In either of these situations, a physiological response is sparked due to the body's biochemical system reacting as if the trauma were reoccurring. A trauma-informed provider understands that these pressures may help explain a client's or family member's behavior and can use this knowledge to help her or him better manage triggers and to feel safe.

As a result, trauma-informed care means considering not only how safe the service delivery environment actually is, but also how safe it is *perceived* to be by the clients being served; how trauma reminders and trauma triggers are managed; how the physical environment is structured to make the client feel safe; how culturally, developmentally, and linguistically congruent the service delivery system is with the client population served, and what can be done to maximize the sense of safety and security for both clients and service providers.

PARTNER WITH CLIENTS

Consumers being served, and often their family members, who have been involved in the service system have a unique perspective. This experience can help the client and family guide their own services, and provide valuable feedback on how the system can better address trauma among those served, as well as others impacted by the experience. As articulated in the foundational work on trauma-informed systems by Fallot and Harris and advanced strongly by SAMHSA and the NCTIC, consumers should be given choices and an active voice in decision-making on both an individual and systemic level (*choice* and *collaboration*). This can help them reclaim the power (*empowerment*) that was taken away from them during the trauma, enhance their resilience, and provide important information to providers and the system. A sense of control and empowerment also helps build a sense of psychological safety as described above, and facilitates the client's engagement and active participation in service delivery.

IDENTIFY TRAUMA-RELATED NEEDS OF CLIENTS

The first step in helping those that have been impacted by abuse, neglect, violence, and other trauma is understanding *how* trauma impacts them and their families on an individual level. Social workers and other helping professionals should use that knowledge to help educate the clients and their family, when appropriate, about the impact of trauma and how it influences their life and short- and long-term recovery. While much has been written on the subject, the NCTSN has done an excellent job of summarizing this in *Core Concepts of Understanding Traumatic Stress Responses in Childhood*. While written from a child trauma point of view, many of these concepts apply to adult trauma victims as well.

The 12 core concepts: Concepts for understanding traumatic stress responses in children and families. Core Curriculum on Childhood Trauma.[1]

1. **Traumatic experiences are inherently complex.** Every traumatic event—even events that are relatively circumscribed—is made up of different traumatic moments. These moments may include varying degrees of objective life threat, physical violation, and witnessing of injury or death. Trauma-exposed children experience subjective reactions to these different moments that include changes in feelings, thoughts, and physiological responses; and concerns for the safety of others. Children may consider a range of possible protective actions during different moments, not all of which they can or do act on. Children's thoughts and actions (or inaction) during various moments may lead to feelings of conflict at the time, and to feelings of confusion, guilt, regret, and/or anger afterward. The nature of children's moment-to-moment reactions is strongly influenced by their prior experience and developmental level. Events (both beneficial and adverse) that occur in the aftermath of the traumatic event introduce additional layers of complexity. The degree of complexity often increases in cases of multiple or recurrent trauma exposure, and in situations where a primary caregiver is a perpetrator of the trauma.

2. **Trauma occurs within a broad context that includes children's personal characteristics, life experiences, and current circumstances.** Childhood trauma occurs within the broad ecology of a child's life that is composed of both child-intrinsic and child-extrinsic factors. Child-*intrinsic* factors include temperament, prior exposure to trauma, and prior history of psychopathology. Child-*extrinsic* factors include the surrounding physical, familial, community, and cultural environments. Both child-

intrinsic and child-extrinsic factors influence children's experience and appraisal of traumatic events; expectations regarding danger, protection, and safety; and course of post-trauma adjustment. For example, both child-intrinsic factors such as prior history of loss; and child-extrinsic factors such as poverty may act as vulnerability factors by exacerbating the adverse effects of trauma on children's adjustment.

3. **Traumatic events often generate secondary adversities, life changes, and distressing reminders in children's daily lives.** Traumatic events often generate secondary adversities such as family separations, financial hardship, relocations to a new residence and school, social stigma, ongoing treatment for injuries and/or physical rehabilitation, and legal proceedings. The cascade of changes produced by trauma and loss can tax the coping resources of the child, family, and broader community. These adversities and life changes can be sources of distress in their own right and can create challenges to adjustment and recovery. Children's exposure to trauma reminders and loss reminders can serve as additional sources of distress. Secondary adversities, trauma reminders, and loss reminders may produce significant fluctuations in trauma survivors' post-trauma emotional and behavioral functioning.

4. **Children can exhibit a wide range of reactions to trauma and loss.** Trauma-exposed children can exhibit a wide range of post-trauma reactions that vary in their nature, onset, intensity, frequency, and duration. The pattern and course of children's post-trauma reactions are influenced by the type of traumatic experience and its consequences, child-intrinsic factors including prior trauma or loss, and the post-trauma physical and social environments. Post-traumatic stress and grief reactions can develop over time into psychiatric disorders, including post-traumatic stress disorder (PTSD), separation anxiety, and depression. Post-traumatic stress and grief reactions can also disrupt major domains of child development, including attachment relationships, peer relationships, and emotional regulation, and can reduce children's level of functioning at home, at school, and in the community. Children's post-trauma distress reactions can also exacerbate preexisting mental health problems including depression and anxiety. Awareness of the broad range of children's potential reactions to trauma and loss is essential to competent assessment, accurate diagnosis, and effective intervention.

5. **Danger and safety are core concerns in the lives of traumatized children.** Traumatic experiences can undermine children's sense of protection and safety, and can magnify their con-

---

1 NCTSN Core Curriculum on Childhood Trauma Task Force (2012). *The 12 core concepts: Concepts for understanding traumatic stress responses in children and families. Core Curriculum on Childhood Trauma*. Los Angeles, CA, and Durham, NC: UCLA–Duke University National Center for Child Traumatic Stress.

cerns about dangers to themselves and others. Ensuring children's physical safety is critically important to restoring the sense of a protective shield. However, even placing children in physically safe circumstances may not be sufficient to alleviate their fears or restore their disrupted sense of safety and security. Exposure to trauma can make it more difficult for children to distinguish between safe and unsafe situations, and may lead to significant changes in their own protective and risk-taking behavior. Children who continue to live in dangerous family and/or community circumstances may have greater difficulty recovering from a traumatic experience.

6. **Traumatic experiences affect the family and broader caregiving systems.**

Children are embedded within broader caregiving systems, including their families, schools, and communities. Traumatic experiences, losses, and ongoing danger can significantly impact these caregiving systems, leading to serious disruptions in caregiver–child interactions and attachment relationships. Caregivers' own distress and concerns may impair their ability to support traumatized children. In turn, children's reduced sense of protection and security may interfere with their ability to respond positively to their parents; and other caregivers' efforts to provide support. Traumatic events—and their impact on children, parents, and other caregivers—also affect the overall functioning of schools and other community institutions. The ability of caregiving systems to provide the types of support that children and their families need is an important contributor to children's and families' post-trauma adjustment. Assessing and enhancing the level of functioning of caregivers and caregiving systems are essential to effective intervention with traumatized youths, families, and communities.

7. **Protective and promotive factors can reduce the adverse impact of trauma.**

Protective factors buffer the adverse effects of trauma and its stressful aftermath, whereas *promotive* factors generally enhance children's positive adjustment regardless of whether risk factors are present. Promotive and protective factors may include *child-intrinsic* factors such as high self-esteem, self-efficacy, and possessing a repertoire of adaptive coping skills. Promotive and protective factors may also include *child-extrinsic* factors such as positive attachment with a primary caregiver, possessing a strong social support network, the presence of reliable adult mentors, and a supportive school and community environment. The presence and strength of promotive and protective factors—both before and after traumatic events—can enhance children's ability to resist, or to quickly recover (by resiliently "bouncing back") from the harmful effects of trauma, loss, and other adversities.

8. **Trauma and post-trauma adversities can strongly influence development.**

Trauma and post-trauma adversities can profoundly influence children's acquisition of developmental competencies and their capacity to reach important developmental milestones in such domains as cognitive functioning, emotional regulation, and interpersonal relationships. Trauma exposure and its aftermath can lead to developmental disruptions in the form of regressive behavior, reluctance or inability to participate in developmentally appropriate activities, and developmental accelerations such as leaving home at an early age and engagement in precocious sexual behavior. In turn, age, gender, and developmental period are linked to risk for exposure to specific types of trauma (e.g., sexual abuse, motor vehicle accidents, and peer suicide).

9. **Developmental neurobiology underlies children's reactions to traumatic experiences.**

Children's capacities to appraise and respond to danger are linked to an evolving neurobiology that consists of brain structures, neurophysiological pathways, and neuroendocrine systems. This "danger apparatus" underlies appraisals of dangerous situations, emotional and physical reactions, and protective actions. Traumatic experiences evoke strong biological responses that can persist and that can alter the normal course of neurobiological maturation. The neurobiological impact of traumatic experiences depends in part on the developmental stage in which they occur. Exposure to multiple traumatic experiences carries a greater risk for significant neurobiological disturbances, including impairments in memory, emotional regulation, and behavioral regulation. Conversely, ongoing neurobiological maturation and neural plasticity also create continuing opportunities for recovery and adaptive developmental progression.

10. **Culture is closely interwoven with traumatic experiences, response, and recovery.**

Culture can profoundly affect the meaning that a child or family attributes to specific types of traumatic events such as sexual abuse, physical abuse, and suicide. Culture may also powerfully influence the ways in which children and their families respond to traumatic events, including the ways in which they experience and express distress, disclose personal information to others, exchange support, and seek help. A cultural group's experiences with historical or multigenerational trauma can also affect their responses to trauma and loss, their world view, and their expectations regarding the self, others, and social institutions.

Culture also strongly influences the rituals and other ways through which children and families grieve over and mourn their losses.

11. **Challenges to the social contract, including legal and ethical issues, affect trauma response and recovery.**

Traumatic experiences often constitute a major violation of the expectations of the child, family, community, and society regarding the primary social roles and responsibilities of influential figures in the child's life. These life figures may include family members, teachers, peers, adult mentors, and agents of social institutions such as judges, police officers, and child welfare workers. Children and their caregivers frequently content with issues involving justice, obtaining legal redress, and seeking protection against further harm. They are often acutely aware of whether justice is properly served and the social contract is upheld. The ways in which social institutions respond to breaches of the social contract may vary widely and often take months or years to carry out. The perceived success or failure of these institutional responses may exert a profound influence on the course of children's post-trauma adjustment, and on their evolving beliefs, and attitudes and values regarding family, work, and civic life.

12. **Working with trauma-exposed children can evoke distress in providers that makes it more difficult for them to provide good care.**

Mental healthcare providers must deal with many personal and professional challenges as they confront details of children's traumatic experiences and life adversities, witness children's and caregivers' distress, and attempt to strengthen children's and families' belief in the social contract. Engaging in clinical work may also evoke strong memories of personal trauma- and loss-related experiences. Proper self-care is an important part of providing quality care and of sustaining personal and professional resources and capacities over time.

A key to trauma-informed care is recognizing many, but not all, clients have trauma-related needs and would benefit from a trauma-specific intervention. To identify who would benefit from a trauma-specific intervention and to guide future interactions with those with a trauma history in a way that does not exacerbate past traumas or unnecessarily trigger trauma memories, a broad trauma-screening system is indicated. Where possible, a trauma-informed approach suggests the use of a reliable and valid screening tool for identifying the client's trauma history and traumatic stress responses, and to make direct referrals for assessment and treatment when indicated (Conradi, Wherry, & Kisiel, 2011).

Enhance Client Well-Being and Resilience

Some individuals who have experienced maltreatment and subsequent trauma are more resilient than others; most often, these individuals have both internal and external resources, such as strong relationships; success in school, work, or other activities; and a temperament that helps them manage stress more readily. It is important for the social worker or other helping professional to recognize and build on the client's existing strengths, while linking them to trauma-informed services when needed. Trauma-informed care seeks to support positive relationships in the client's life and minimize disruptions of what is familiar, and to make sure that positive figures, including parents, children, teachers, neighbors, siblings, and other relatives, remain involved in client's lives.

For many clients, recovery requires the support of specially trained mental health professionals who are schooled in evidence-based treatment models that are tailored to meet the needs of the clients. Any decision to treat a client with a history of significant trauma should be based on a thorough assessment that yields a clear picture of their unique strengths and needs. For children, this type of multidimensional assessment algorithm is exemplified by the Trauma Assessment Pathway (Chadwick Center for Children and Families, 2009; Taylor, Gilbert, Mann, & Ryan, 2005; Igelman, Taylor, & Gilbert, 2007) developed at the Chadwick Center for Children and Families at Rady Children's Hospital in San Diego (*www.chadwickcenter.org*) with support from SAMHSA. The assessment should be designed to match the client to the evidence-based or evidence-informed treatment model best suited for their unique needs. It is important to remember that trauma often co-occurs with other major behavioral health disorders. In some cases, trauma serves as a precursor for another disorder like substance abuse. In other cases, another disorder, such as some forms of serious mental illness, may precede the trauma events or develop independently of the trauma history, and the assessment must explore those connections.

Recovery from trauma often requires the right evidence-based or evidence-informed mental health treatment, delivered by a skilled therapist, that helps the client reduce the overwhelming emotions related to the trauma, manage the behavioral and emotional symptoms of traumatic stress, address any traumatic grief issues the traumas produced, cope with trauma triggers, and make new meaning of his or her trauma history. The treatment also may need to address a second co-occurring disorder first, or a treatment model should be selected that addresses the co-occurring disorder in a trauma context, such as how Seeking Safety addresses substance abuse (Najavits, Weissbecker, & Clark, 2007; Najavits, 2009).

There are numerous evidence-based treatment models now available that have been empirically tested with highly traumatized children and adults and fit well in a trauma-informed environment. Seeking out the empirical evidence on each possible model can be overwhelming for those actively involved in service delivery. Fortunately, there are multiple Internet-based clearinghouses that contain trauma-specific interventions in which the research reviews have already been conducted (see *www.nrepp.samhsa.gov*; *www.cebc4cw.org*; *www.colorado.edu/cspv*; and *www.samhsa.gov/nctic*).

ENHANCE FAMILY WELL-BEING AND RESILIENCE

When it comes to child trauma victims and many adults, especially transition-age youths, families are a critical part of their recovery and enhance their natural resilience. However, families may find it difficult to be protective if they have been affected by trauma themselves, and they may need help and support in order to draw on their natural strengths.

- Asking parents and other caregivers about their history of trauma provides critical information to social workers or other helping professionals about their behavior and needs, as well as helping inform service planning for all family members. It is common for the parents of traumatized children and young adults to share a significant trauma history. Sometimes that history is based in childhood experiences such as physical or sexual abuse, or it may be contemporary, such as ongoing intimate-partner violence.
- Providing effective trauma-informed education and professionally delivered trauma-informed services to parents enhances their protective capacities, thereby increasing their children's resilience and feelings of safety, permanency, and well-being. Additionally, educating other caregivers, foster parents, members of the child's safety network and the parent's support system enhances their protective capacities, thereby reducing the risk that the child will be inadvertently exposed to trauma triggers or have their behaviors, which may be trauma-related, misidentified as "bad" and subject the child to inappropriate and trauma-insensitive discipline or punishment.
- Those working with these families must recognize that caregivers may also experience secondary traumatic stress related to their children's trauma, and provide them with appropriate training and supports.

ENHANCE THE WELL-BEING AND RESILIENCE OF THOSE WORKING IN THE SYSTEM

While the origins of trauma-informed care are clearly centered on the clients served, it is apparent that the professionals working with highly traumatized populations are also profoundly affected by the experience. Those experiences can influence their judgments on the job, invade their private lives, and shape their worldview at home as well as at work. Those working in a trauma-informed environment must be aware of this sometimes-insidious side effect of serving this population. Trauma-informed organizations must consider their staff's physical *and* psychological safety. Actively working to increase staff resilience to secondary traumatic stress (STS) involves seeking ways to reduce the risk of STS among all personnel—from the receptionists, to transcriptionists, to the frontline professionals and their supervisors; identifying the early signs of STS among personnel; minimizing the impact of STS; and promoting effective interventions for secondary traumatic stress. Helping staff manage professional and personal stress and addressing the impact of secondary traumatic stress on both individuals and on the system as a whole is beneficial for all levels, from client to community.

PARTNER WITH AGENCIES AND SYSTEMS THAT INTERACT WITH CLIENTS

Because trauma can impact many aspects of an individual's life, it is important that those aspiring to provide trauma-informed care partner with others in parallel service systems in identifying and addressing trauma. Working with allied professionals who know the clients and family can help in developing an appropriate service plan and prevent potentially competing priorities.

Failure to work together can not only undermine all the efforts to provide trauma-informed care, but actually can inadvertently add new traumas. Well-meaning agencies or professionals pursuing their own mission and goals independently can work at cross-purposes and trigger traumatic reactions, causing more harm. In fact, this was the genesis of the child-advocacy center movement (see www.*nationalcac.org* and *www.nationalchildrensalliance.org*) which began when the grandmother of an abused child in Huntsville, Alabama, protested to the district attorney how uncoordinated agencies in child protection, law enforcement, health care, and prosecution were not only operating independently, but were making things worse for her grandchild. The result was a national movement starting in the 1980s to create a multidisciplinary investigative team response to child-abuse allegations. This model was designed so that all aspects of the forensic investigation process were reconfigured to be child-centered, with tasks focused on providing all services in a single location, reducing unnecessary duplication of interviews, and having representatives from all involved agencies co-located. All this was done to enhance the possibility the system did not re-traumatize the child through lack of coordination and communication among the professionals.

A truly trauma-informed system is one in which all the disparate elements understand trauma, and, as articulated by the NCTSN, "infuse and sustain trauma awareness, knowledge, and skills into their organizational cultures, practices, and policie" (NCTSN, 2012, What is a trauma-informed child- and family-service system? section, para. 1). To achieve this lofty goal, those aspiring to deliver true trauma-informed care need to establish strong partnerships with others serving the same clients and families. Service providers should develop common protocols and frameworks where possible for documenting trauma history, exchanging information, coordinating assessments, and planning and delivering services.

Moving to Trauma-Informed Care

Several organizations have developed formal self-assessment tools to help organizations and systems assess the degree to which they have become trauma-informed or are ready to move in that direction. Among the stronger assessments are Community Connections' *Creating Cultures of Trauma-Informed Care: a Self-Assessment and Planning Protocol* (Fallot & Harris, 2009); the Chadwick Center's *Community Trauma-Informed Assessment Protocol* (Hendricks, Conradi, & Wilson, 2011) and *Trauma System Readiness Tool* (Hendricks, Conradi, & Wilson, 2011); the National Center on Family Homelessness's *Trauma-Informed Organizational Toolkit* (Guarino et al., 2009); and Western Michigan University's *Trauma-Informed System Change Instrument* (Richardson, Coryn, Henry, Black-Pond, & Unrau, 2010). The NCTSN has developed training resources to support transformation efforts at the system level, with *Caring for Children Who Have Experienced Trauma: A Resource Parent Curriculum,* and *Child Welfare Trauma Training Tookit* (Child Welfare Committee, National Child Traumatic Stress Network, & The California Social Work Education Center, 2013). Early studies show these type resources show promise in practice change efforts (Kramer, Sigel, Conners-Burrow, Savary, & Tempel, 2013).

Conclusion

Trauma-informed care is not so much a new model of service delivery as it is an approach to service delivery. It weaves trauma knowledge and sensitivity into existing actions and models in a way that avoids or minimizes negative side-effects of intervention and increases the likelihood of meaningful engagement and effective implementation of other models. Effective trauma-informed care does rely on the capacity to deliver evidence-based and evidence-informed trauma-specific interventions when needed, but it goes further in viewing the whole service-delivery experience through a trauma lens. Trauma-informed care engages the customers and clients as partners, empowering them to help guide their intervention and seeking out the unique path to safety and resilience that will give the clients the capacity to face and overcome trauma triggers and new adversities in the future.

REFERENCES

Abram, K. M., Teplin, L. A., Charles, D. R., et al. (2004). Posttraumatic stress disorder and psychiatric comorbidity among detained youths. *Archives of General Psychiatry, 61*, 403–410.

Anda, R. F., Dong, M., Brown, D. W., et al. (2009). The relationship of adverse childhood experiences to a history of premature death of family members. *BMC Public Health, 1*, 106–115.

Anda, R. A., & Felitti, V. J. (2003). Origins and essence of the study. *ACE Reporter, 1*(1), 1–3.

Bloom, S. (1997). *Creating sanctuary: Toward the evolution of sane societies.* London: Taylor & Francis.

Bloom, S. (2010). Organizational stress as a barrier to trauma-informed service delivery. In M. Becker & B. Levin, *A public health perspective of women's mental health* (pp. 295–311). New York: Springer.

Burgess, A. W., & Holmstrom, L. L. (1974). Rape trauma syndrome. *American Journal of Psychiatry, 131*, 981–986.

Chadwick Center for Children and Families. (2009). *Assessment-based treatment for traumatized children: A trauma assessment pathway* (TAP). San Diego, CA: Author.

Chadwick Trauma-Informed Systems Project. (2013). *Creating trauma-informed child welfare systems: A guide for administrators* (2nd ed.). San Diego, CA: Chadwick Center for Children and Families.

Child Welfare Committee, National Child Traumatic Stress Network, & The California Social Work Education Center. (2012). *Child welfare trauma training toolkit: Comprehensive guide* (3rd ed.). Los Angeles, CA, and Durham, NC: National Center for Child Traumatic Stress.

Child Welfare Committee, National Child Traumatic Stress Network, & The California Social Work Education Center. (2013). *Child welfare trauma training toolkit* (2nd ed.). Los Angeles, CA, and Durham, NC: National Center for Child Traumatic Stress.

Cicchetti, D., Toth, S. L., & Rogosch, F. A. (1999). The efficacy of toddler-parent psychotherapy to increase attachment security in offspring of depressed mothers. *Attachment & Human Development, 1*(1), 34–66.

Cohen, J. A., Deblinger, E., Mannarino, A. P., & Steer, R. (2004). A multisite, randomized controlled trial for children with sexual abuse-related PTSD symptoms. *Journal of the American Academy of Child & Adolescent Psychiatry, 43,* 393–402.

Cohen, J. A., Mannarino, A. P., & Iyengar, S. (2011). Community treatment of posttraumatic stress disorder for children exposed to intimate partner violence. *Archives of Pediatrics & Adolescent Medicine, 165*(1), 16–21.

Cohen, J. A., Mannarino, A. P., & Knudsen, K. (2004) Treating childhood traumatic grief: A pilot study. *Journal of the American Academy of Child & Adolescent Psychiatry, 43,* 1225–1233.

Cohen, J. A., Mannarino, A. P., & Staron, V. (2006). A pilot study of modified cognitive behavioral therapy for childhood traumatic grief (CBT-CTG). *Journal of the American Academy of Child & Adolescent Psychiatry, 45*(12), 1465–1473.

Conradi, L., Wherry, J., & Kisiel, C. (2011). Linking child welfare and mental health using trauma-informed screening and assessment practices. *Child Welfare, 90*(6), 129–148.

Conradi, L., & Wilson, C. (2010). Managing traumatized children: A trauma systems perspective. *Current Opinion in Pediatrics, 22,* 621–625.

Cooper, J. L., Masi, R., Dababnah, S., Aratani, Y., & Knitzer, J. (2007). *Unclaimed children revisited working paper no. 2:, Strengthening policies to support children, youth, and families who experience trauma.* New York: National Center for Children in Poverty.

Costello, E. J., Erkanli, A., Fairbank, J. A., & Angold, A. (2002). The prevalence of potentially traumatic events in childhood and adolescence. *Journal of Traumatic Stress, 15,* 99–112.

Covington, S. S. (2002). Helping women recover: Creating gender-responsive treatment. In S. Straussner and S. Brown (Eds.), *Handbook of women's addictions treatment* (pp. 52–72). San Francisco: Jossey-Bass.

Deblinger, E., Lippmann, J., & Steer, R. (1996). Sexually abused children suffering posttraumatic stress symptoms: Initial treatment outcome findings. *Child Maltreatment, 1*(4), 310–321.

Deblinger, E., Mannarino, A. P., Cohen, J. A., & Steer, R. A. (2006). A multisite, randomized controlled trial for children with sexual abuse-related PTSD symptoms: Examining predictors of treatment response. *Journal of the American Academy of Child and Adolescent Psychiatry, 45,* 1474–1484.

Ethier, L. S., Lemelin, J., & Lacharite, C. A. (2004). A longitudinal study of the effects of chronic maltreatment on children's behavioral and emotional problems. *Child Abuse and Neglect, 28,* 1265–1278.

Fallot, R. D., & Harris, M. (2009). *Creating cultures of trauma-informed care (CCTIC): A self-assessment and planning protocol.* Washington, DC: Community Connections.

Felitti, V. J., Anda, R. F., Nordenberg, D., Williamson, D. F., et al. (1998). Relationship of childhood abuse and household dysfunction to many of the leading causes of death in adults: The Adverse Childhood Experiences (ACE) study. *American Journal of Preventive Medicine, 14,* 245–258.

Guarino, K., Soares, P., Konnath, K., Clervil, R., & Bassuk, E. (2009). *Trauma-informed organizational toolkit.* Rockville MD: Center for Mental Health Services, SAMHSA.

Harris, M., & Fallot, R. (2001). *Using trauma theory to design service systems.* San Francisco: Jossey-Bass.

Hendricks, A., Conradi, L., & Wilson, C. (2011). Creating trauma-informed child welfare systems using a community assessment process. *Child Welfare, 90*(6), 187–206.

Igelman, R., Taylor, N., Gilbert, A., et al. (2007). Creating more trauma-informed services for children using assessment-focused tools. *Child Welfare, 86,* 15–33.

Ko, S. J., Ford, J. D., Kassam-Adams, N., et al. (2008). Creating trauma-informed systems: Child welfare, education, first responders, health care, juvenile justice. *Professional Psychology: Research & Practice, 39,* 396–404.

Kramer, T., Sigel, B., Conners-Burrow, N., Savary, P., & Tempel, A. (2013). A statewide introduction of trauma-informed care in child welfare. *Children & Youth Services Review, 35,* 19–24.

Landis, J. T. (1956). Experiences of 500 children with adult sexual deviation. *Psychiatric Quarterly Supplement, 30*(1), 91–109.

Lieberman, A. F., Ghosh Ippen, C., & Van Horn, P. (2006). Child-parent psychotherapy: Six- month follow-up of a randomized controlled trial. *Journal of the American Academy of Child & Adolescent Psychiatry, 45*(8), 913–918.

Lieberman, A. F., Weston, D. R., & Pawl, J. H. (1991). Preventive interaction and outcome with anxiously attached dyads. *Child Development, 62,* 199–209.

McDonald, R., Jouriles, E., Ramisetty-Mikler, S., et al. (2006). Estimating the number of American children living in partner violent families. *Journal of Family Psychology, 30,* 137–142.

Najavits, L. M. (2009). Seeking Safety: An implementation guide. In A. Rubin & D. W. Springer (Eds.), Substance Abuse Treatment for Youth and Adults: *The clinician's guide to evidence-based practice* (311-348). Hoboken, NJ: John Wiley.

Najavits, L. M., Weissbecker I., & Clark, C. (2007). The impact of violence and abuse on women's physical health: Can trauma-informed treatment make a difference? *Journal of Community Psychology, 35,* 909–923.

National Center for Trauma-Informed Care. (2012). Retrieved November 18, 2012, from www.mentalhealth.samhsa.gov/nctic/trauma.asp

National Child Traumatic Stress Network. (2012). *Creating trauma-informed child- and family-serving systems: A definition.* Retrieved January 15, 2013, from http://www.nctsn.org/resources/topics/creating-trauma-informed-systems

NCTSN Core Curriculum on Childhood Trauma Task Force. (2012). *The 12 core concepts: Concepts for understanding traumatic stress responses in children and families. Core Curriculum on Childhood Trauma.* Los Angeles, CA, and Durham, NC: UCLA-Duke University National Center for Child Traumatic Stress.

Richardson, C., Henry, B.-P., & Unrau, Y. (2010). Trauma-informed system change instrument. Western Michigan University, unpublished manuscript.

Rivard, J. C., Bloom, S. L., Abramovitz, R., et al. (2003). Assessing the implementation and effects of a trauma-focused intervention for youths in residential treatment. *Psychiatric Quarterly*; *74*, 137–154.

Taylor, N., Gilbert, A., Mann, G., & Ryan, B. E. (2005). Unpublished manuscript. San Diego: Chadwick Center for Children & Families, Rady Children's Hospital.

Taylor, N., & Siegfried, C. (2005). *Helping children in child welfare system heal from trauma: A systems integration approach*. Los Angeles, CA & Durham, NC: National Center for Child Traumatic Stress (NCTSN).

Toth, S. L., Maughan, A., Manly, J. T., Spagnola, M., & Cicchetti, D. (2002). The relative efficacy of two interventions in altering maltreated preschool children's representational models: Implications for attachment theory. *Development & Psychopathology*, *14*, 877–908.

U.S. Department of Health and Human Services, Administration on Children, Youth and Families. (n.d.). *General findings from the federal child and family services review*. Washington DC: Government Printing Office; Retrieved May 3, 2010, from http://www.acf.hhs.gov/sites/default/files/cb/summary_of_the_results_of_the_2001_2004_cfsr.pdf

U.S. Department of Health and Human Services; Administration for Children and Families; Administration on Children, Youth and Families; Children's Bureau (2011). Child maltreatment. Retrieved March 2, 2016, from http://www.acf.hhs.gov/sites/default/files/cb/cm11.pdf

U.S. Department of Health and Human Services, Substance Abuse and Mental Health Services Administration (2007). *Lessons learned from the Women, Co-Occurring Disorders, and Violence Study: Exploring how to best serve women survivors of violence and trauma who have substance abuse and mental health disorders*. Rockville, Maryland: Author.

U.S. Department of Health and Human Services. Substance Abuse and Mental Health Services Administration (2012). *Trauma definition, part two: A trauma-informed approach*. Retrieved December 2, 2012, from http://www.samhsa.gov/traumajustice/traumadefinition/approach.aspx

FURTHER READING

California Evidence-Based Clearinghouse for Child Welfare (CEBC): http://www.cebc4cw.org

Center for the Study and Prevention of Violence: http://www.colorado.edu/cspv/.

Chadwick Center for Children and Families at Rady Children's Hospital in San Diego: http://www.chadwickcenter.org.

National Center for Post-Traumatic Stress Disorder: http://www.ptsd.va.gov

National Center for Trauma-Informed Care: http://www.samhsa.gov/nctic/.

National Child Traumatic Stress Network: http://www.nctsn.org

National Children's Advocacy Center: http://www.nationalcac.org.

National Children's Alliance: http://www.nationalchildrensalliance.org.

National Registry of Evidence-based Programs and Practices: http://www.nrepp.samhsa.gov/.

CHARLES WILSON, DONNA M. PENCE, AND LISA CONRADI

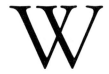

WOMEN: PRACTICE INTERVENTIONS

ABSTRACT: Gender hierarchy is the most pervasive source of inequality in the world. In view of the commitment of social work to the goal of justice, redressing the consequences of inequality among the most disenfranchised should be at the core of professional intervention. Rather than discussing the merits of specific types of practice intervention adopted by social workers, I focus on strategies and knowledge-gathering techniques relevant to empowering women, with an emphasis on five social work methods.

KEY WORDS: gender hierarchy; women inequality; class, race, and gender oppression; social justice professional goal; psychological and social empowerment strategies

The Professional Commitment to Social Justice for Women

Issues of women's social and economic oppression are at the core of the professional goal of social justice (for example, Gil, 1998; Jordan, 1990; Piven & Cloward, 1997; Wakefield, 1988). The codes and standards of the National Association of Social Workers lay out the goal:

- Promote the general welfare of society, from local to global levels, and the development of people, their communities, and environments. Social workers should advocate for living conditions conducive to the fulfillment of basic human needs and should promote social, economic, political, and cultural values and institutions that are compatible with the realization of social justice.
- Facilitate informed participation by the public in shaping social policies and institutions.
- Engage in social and political actions that seek to ensure that all people have equal access to resources, employment, services, and opportunities they require to meet their basic human needs and to develop fully. Social workers should be aware of the impact of the political arena on practice and should advocate for changes in policy and legislation to improve social conditions in order to meet basic human needs and promote social justice (2003, pp. 394–395).

Wakefield's (1988) argument that professional goals are much more crucial to the legitimacy of a profession than are methods of intervention is crucial in this context. The effectiveness of strategies of intervention evolves over time with knowledge expansion and in response to social change. The social justice goal, on the other hand, defines permanently the profession of social work guiding all its activities and definitively practice with women.

Societal Issues Impacting Practice with Women

Nussbaum (1999) argues that forces of social and economic inequalities impinging on women form the major social justice issue in any society. A culture that has justified, over centuries, the assignment of roles on the basis of sexual characteristics remains resistant to societal change because of the nature of the gendered culture (Fausto-Sterling, 2000). The interaction of class, race, and gender exacerbates the level of disadvantage (Arrighi, 2001; McAdoo, 2002). Despite real progress of women in economic autonomy, educational access, and legal statutes, the fact remains that the Equal Rights Amendment, which would have granted full social citizenship to women, failed to pass into law. Equity legislation resulting from the pressure of women's groups deals with discrete issues on a case-by-case basis.

The weakness of this one-step-at-a-time approach to helping women improve their status in a gendered society shows up in the prolonged fight for equal pay for equal work since the 1970s. The female–male wage gaps hover at 80%, with progress at less than 5% since the mid-1990s (Leonhardt, 2006). What is more, new freedoms in the economic and family spheres are ambiguous. The double burden of women in the work force is a direct result of the care responsibilities assigned to them. The United States is the only developed country in the West without public childcare (Figueira-McDonough, 2007).

A few facts portray the magnitude of the economic gaps and economic and social stressors that face women. About 2 million poor women live 50% below the poverty level, and among homeless single parents with children the overwhelming majority are women, many of whom are running away from abusive homes

(Jones-DeWeever, Peterson, & Song, 2002; National Law Center of Homeless and Poverty, 2002); 60% of women on welfare have experienced physical violence (Davis, 1999); women prisoners have been sexually abused by their guards in state prisons (Geer, 2000; Human Rights Watch, 1996); 1 in every 3 girls below the age of 18, 34% before the age of 12, have been sexually abused (KidSafe Project, 2001).

Choosing Appropriate Practices for Women

Since society may be biased against women's rights, social workers need to review models of intervention with a skeptical mind. Theories developed mainly by men, for example, interpret the world from their point of view. Training in critical thinking is indispensable for social workers, since most institutions with power over women (poor and non-Whites) often uphold biased assumptions.

Critical thought involves a two-track process: (a) inquiry into the authorship of the theories and their historical and cultural contexts, focusing on the dangers of partial and context-dependent knowledge, and (b) careful analysis of the internal logical coherence of the theories and the empirical evidence for alternative theories (Calhoun, 1995; Talaska, 1990). Applied to gender theories, the skeptical procedure has two foci: (a) the extent to which theories were developed by men, on the basis of limited experience and research, nonetheless claiming universal application, and (b) the exploration of alternative theories geared to women's experiences, together with examination of the evidence behind them and the alternatives they offer for practice. Each type of intervention has its own conceptual requirement for contributing to social justice.

Different Methods of Social Work Practice and Applied Empowering Knowledge

INDIVIDUAL PRACTICE: MUTUALITY, RESPECT, AND COLLABORATION The relationship between the social worker and the client is the core of individual practice that can inform and transform the meaning of experiences. For women, especially marginalized women, personal experience is the lived version of socioeconomic reality. Difficulties undergone by marginalized women should not be dissected in terms of what is wrong, deficient, or missing according to the dominant culture but as signs of survival in the face of oppression and as potentially healthy protest against patriarchal norms. The canon of knowledge from which the therapist derives her understanding of behavior must be reshaped to include subjugated knowledge from the margins.

Feminist psychotherapies may heighten awareness of women's repression and the reactions to it, speeding the evolution of coping mechanisms. Cognitive and behavior therapies may develop habits and behaviors—assertiveness, pursuit of success—that make women better able to compete and hold their own in a man's world. Therapies inspired by essentialist theories may contribute to the valuation of women's culture and solidarity. Such approaches can strengthen women, but they do not necessarily deprivatize what has been silenced and kept secret in the lives of women.

Basic to the therapeutic relationship is recognition of the distance between a professional, usually from a higher socioeconomic background and invested with institutional authority, and the client. This gap puts the social worker at a disadvantage inasmuch as a full comprehension of the meaning attached to the client's issues is a precondition for authentic communication and development of the therapeutic relationship.

Principles of qualitative research, often applied in anthropology, offer valuable guidelines to bridge this distance. They are characterized by acceptance of the lack of knowledge about cultures outside one's experience, a nonjudgmental inquiry about patterns of behavior, and dependence on insiders to explain the meanings of observed patterns and desired outcomes. The strength of this approach is the maximization of knowledge when prior knowledge is low (Runkel & McGrath, 1972).

Transferred to socioclinical intervention, the strategy encompasses respect for the client, interpretation of her problem and its meaning as understood from her perspective, and its desired resolution. The following procedures, derived in part from critical and structural theories in social work, have the potential to increase trust and honest collaboration in the therapeutic relationship (Gambrill, 2006, pp. 385–394; Jackson & Servaes, 1999; Mullaly, 2007; Wood, 2006):

- Maintain interaction as a process of mutual learning, avoiding the professional–client hierarchy.
- Accept the experiential knowledge of clients and their analysis of the problem.
- Validate the client's resilience and the range of possibilities the client sees as appropriate to respond to her needs.
- Discuss contextual causes of the problem, highlighting social structural constraints.
- Share client files with them and open the files to corrections and explanations.

For oppressed clients, such as refugees, African Americans, immigrants, and lesbians living in poverty and exposed to violence, these principles foster a validation of their worth that is a precondition to psychological empowerment.

Group Work: Communication, Relationship, and Mutual Support

Group work gained prominence after World War II and for a couple of decades was an important action method of intervention (Toseland, 1995). Eventually, however, it was transformed into group therapy (Middleman & Goldman, 1987). Feminist theory renewed interest in this method and introduced innovations in group work. Comparative group studies, popular in social work research, have contributed to greater specification in interventions. When focusing on gender group composition, they have allowed researchers to estimate the effects of the same intervention on mixed groups, male only, and female only groups (Bride, 2001; Zelvin, 1999).

However, the greatest contribution to the theory and practice of group work with women came from research done at the Stone Center at Wellesley and Harvard (Gilligan, 1996; Miller & Silver, 1991). This decades-long program of research revealed the centrality of relational context and communication on the development of women. Social workers added new questions about the impact of gender identity and location to group intervention (Gutiérrez et al., 1998; Maxine & Nisivoccia, 2005). Group work is a method that can address issues of powerlessness through consciousness-raising and self-identification; it can concentrate on repressed socialization and experiences of oppression.

Insights derived form these studies underscore the major advantages of this type of intervention:

- Women respond better in relational settings that support communication.
- Group membership can give a sense of protection and empowerment to powerless individuals (Gitterman & Shulman, 2005).

The professional literature is rich in examples suggesting different strategies that assess the consequences of the gender composition of groups, often crucial to the success of interventions. Although all the elements of group practice have to be adjusted to the relational imperative in women's development, the process of member selection is very important to this adjustment.

Many groups are formed out of a common trauma or by the referral of practitioners knowledgeable about clients' needs. In such cases the group worker can follow a clearer pattern of intervention, as exemplified in the work of Schiller and Zimmer (2005) with sexual abuse survivors.

Working with natural groups requires both a longer period of acceptance of the leader and agreement on goals of immediate interest to the group. Lee's work (2005) with homeless young women illustrates this process.

To evaluate the impact of recent changes on disenfranchised women, the use of focus groups is a useful type of practice. The selection of members is more open, and group duration is shorter, than is typically the case with types of groups. An example of this is an assessment of the consequences of the implementation of Temporary Assistance for Needy Families (TANF) in an extremely antiwelfare state (Luna, 2005; Luna & Figueira-McDonough, 2002). Women from poor neighborhoods with high rates of welfare recipients were invited to attend these groups and express their reaction to the welfare reform. The advantage of focus groups over techniques such as surveys is that they encourage interaction that stimulates the expression of feelings, reactions, and desired outcomes. They represent an important strategy for reaching out into new areas of women's oppression.

Community Practice: Women's Grassroots Strength

The method of community organization takes in a variety of strategies. As with all social work practice, an assessment of the client's strengths is essential prior to intervention. In the case of communities this means gauging the resources that can be mobilized collectively for dealing with local problems. Relevant community resources include local grassroots and formal organizations and the links they may have with influential external allies (Figueira-McDonough, 2001). Such stocktaking is particularly important when working in low-income communities that may have hidden strengths.

As with other social work macro methods, there has been a male bias in reporting on community achievements. The bias derives less from intentional dismissal of women's contributions than from the tendency of formal leadership, planning processes, organizational deals, and political agreements—functions habitually carried out by men—to get the limelight (Smith, 1990). The consensus has been that women's activity goes on primarily at the grassroots level (Weil, Gable, & Williams, 1998); a team of women studying and analyzing community projects brought to the forefront the breadth of women's grassroots activism.

Historical research on protests unearthed by Abramovitz (1996) has challenged the stereotype of the passive nature of poor women. Abramovitz found that women were at the forefront of protests, both as leaders and followers, concerning food prices, crime, dilapidated housing, and cuts in social benefits. Nancy Naples has devoted much of her work to examining the activism of poor women during and after the War on Poverty (Naples, 1991, 1998). These "grassroots warriors" fought for federal grants that supported community activities, and they planned and staffed the programs supported by these grants. As the War on Poverty was dismantled, groups of women kept donating their time and searched for alternative funds to keep the services going. Naples found that this communitarian activism was often transmitted to their daughters.

Stoutland (1997) discovered a similar pattern in a study of the Community Development Corporation in Boston. Women were at the center of collective action. They were overwhelmingly the tenants' organization activists, a fact confirmed by other Community Development Corporations (Heskin, 1991, Leavitt & Saeger, 1990). Seitz's analysis (1995) of the local strike of the United Mine Workers in southwest Virginia uncovered the pivotal role of miners' wives in a part of the country known for its patriarchal culture. As the strike heated up, the women shifted from cooking meals and doing sewing for extra income to less traditional activities: they picketed the houses of mine owners and managers, boycotted businesses opposed to the strike, barred police access to the strikers, and dampened internal violence among the despairing miners. Finally, when the miners' demands were not met, the women took over the mine headquarters, and the conflict was settled at last.

Feldman (2004) also reported women's active resistance in Chicago's public housing controversies, and Finn (2002) has explored the resilience of women's groups in community building in a dangerous and unstable setting. The literature is in accord that women's activism is triggered by concern over the welfare of family and children. Women are the foot soldiers of community activism, and their indispensable contributions often go unnoticed. Greater attention is paid to grant-making, deals with business, government and religious organizations—all activities frequently dominated by men (Schorr, 1997).

Social workers cannot neglect the grassroots dimension of community practice. Some preliminary strategies suggest themselves:

- Analyze demographic data about the stability of the resident population (often associated with community attachment) and of local plants, indicating the geographical proximity of housing units (a predictor of interaction). Both indicators, stability and proximity, are pertinent to the formation of grassroots ties.

- Interview community leaders to find out about informal organizations that address women-related issues.
- Identify localities where women congregate (stores, churches, parks, welfare offices, and so forth) and gather information about their pressing concerns (Naples, 2003).

Organizational Practice: Commitment to Social Work Values and Women's Rights

Howe (1980) criticized the liberal professional organizational practice model that pervaded the training of social workers. She argued that while social workers operated mainly in organizational settings, in such contexts the assumptions of traditional, free-standing liberal professions were not met. Hence, an organizational professional model should be adopted. Despite the popularity of private practice and the increase of organizational courses in many schools of social work, Howe's observations remain valid.

Organizational theory and research have expanded considerably, and students are offered a huge variety of models of analysis. In a review of this development, Netting and Rokwell (1998) note that the variety of the structural models has metamorphosed from their origins in the first half of the 20th century. Weber's ideal model was a response to the industrial expansion and the optimization of efficient production. The rational factory required a centralized hierarchy of decisions, implemented by strict rules for mass workers. Preexisting organizations such as the military and the church inspired this design, and the male imprint was undisputable. Recent innovations in organizational theory, influenced by open system, power dynamics, and organizational culture approaches, have been more responsive to the variety of goals of contemporary organizations, and more inclusive of women.

The relevance of organizational practice for women social workers stems directly from two facts. Women social workers in service organizations make up the majority of the rank and file staff, and many of these organizations, especially in the public sector, serve mostly poor women.

The role and power of women in nonprofit organizations are well documented (Oddental & O'Neil, 1994). Recent research on women has turned up important clues about leveraging women's organizational leadership and participatory management styles in order to enhance both communication and creative outcomes (Barrett & Davidson, 2006; Buzzanell, 2006). This holds promise for greater gender equality in organizational life. Kravetz's account (2004) of the evolution of feminist service organizations is an inspiring example. In addition, proposals for sharing organizational tasks with informal groups, as well as for capitalizing on the complementary strengths of primary and secondary groups, have been advanced as breakthroughs for human service organizations (Mulroy & Shay, 1997; Specht & Courtney, 1994).

Because they exemplify tremendous obstacles to progress in this type of practice with women, public service organizations are worth considering in detail. These organizations are likely to be structured by hierarchical decision-making and strict rules of implementation. Upholding professional values and working effectively with disempowered women clients will almost certainly necessitate major changes.

Jordan (1998) suggests that social workers have more power in the implementation of policies than they realize. Public services are in charge of implementing goals that are general and standardized; yet the specific circumstances they are supposed to address are complex and often idiosyncratic. The on-site skills of social workers can help render publicly endorsed goals workable.

From this perspective, social workers have both power and responsibility for policy outcomes (Jordan & Jordan, 2000; Mullaly, 2007). With power comes a degree of discretion. For example, a social worker in a youth program may or may not send a teenager back to an institution when a child violates curfew, as mandated by current statutes. The professional may decide that the spirit of the law does not apply in light of the particular circumstances that led to the breaking of the curfew. The social worker must of course justify such decisions on a case-by-case basis. In some public service organizations no discretion may be allowed. Routine enforcement of rigid rules of intervention will clash with social work values and the rights of clients. Under these conditions, the social worker has three options: submit, quit, or assert her professional role.

The first two responses may be the easiest and the most frequent. Submissive social workers or untrained case workers replacing them are known to contribute to the alienation of clients. In both cases, poor women in programs are shortchanged (Gray, 2005; Thretheway, 1997; Whitley & Dressel, 2002). Although difficult, the third option can have a positive impact on social services, as well as for the social work rank-and-file and service recipients. Asserting professional roles may involve:

- organizing professional groups within the agency to resist unprofessional regulation. Group resistance is stronger than individual resistance and is more disruptive for the organization.
- establishing links with other organizations or groups that face similar obstacles to their commitment to clients' rights.
- proving that the regulations in place subvert or contradict the public service goal.

Promoting solidarity among the social work rank-and-file with the support of professional associations is a vital step toward the first strategy. Gray (2005) argues that the National Association of Social Workers should recommend practice standards for social workers in public services. Infractions of these standards could legitimize resistance to poorly designed regulations. Consulting with other human service professions with experience in labor resistance strategies is also valuable. Interorganizational know-how and experience about the interdependence of services could facilitate the identification of potential external allies.

Opportunities for public service reform increase when the institutions are found to be deficient in fulfilling their mandate (Jordan & Jordan, 2000). So, while the third strategy could probably be the most effective, it is also hard to pull off. It requires an in-depth analysis of the policy under which the service was established in order to clarify its goals. It also requires a thorough examination of service outcomes. This could include analysis of administrative data, a survey of recipients regarding expectations and outcomes, and the use of case vignettes (McMillen et al., 2005).

Policy Practice: Top-Down and Bottom-Up Influence

Two sets of deficiencies prevail in the sources of injustice that social workers have been increasingly concerned about since the mid-nineties: economic inequality and poverty and the policies that reinforce them (Hopps & Morris, 2000; Reisch & Gambrill, 1998; Van Wormer, 2004). Intertwined with these are the negative ideologies popularized by powerful groups about the poor (Gramsci, 1971; Lakoff, 2002) and their political marginality. This combination of factors underpins the enactment of policies with heavy burdens and few benefits for the poor (Schneider & Ingram, 1993).

The goal of policy practice in social work is to prevent or alter policies that have damaging consequences for powerless groups and to promote those that benefit them. In a gender hierarchical society, attention to policy impacts on poor women is central to this practice (Arrighi, 2001). Examining the effects of the 1996 Welfare Reform Act covering poor parents, 87% of whom are poor single mothers, serves as a template for other policies that affect negatively women in poverty.

Legislative practice, a type of top-down influence, has improved greatly since the last two decades of the past century, and carefully designed strategies have been developed recently for social workers (for example, Jansson, 2003). They include careful study of the legislation under review, research on the positions of decision-makers regarding past human service issues and legislation, reaching out for influential allies, matching lobbyists' skills to legislators' characteristics, the ability to cooperate with groups with partial overlapping interests, and so on. The National Association of Social Workers and its state chapters help in this process, especially through their political action committees.

Schneider (2002) has argued convincingly that social work legislative policy should focus on state legislatures. Schneider's position is particularly relevant in the case of the 1996 Welfare Reform Act that transferred many responsibilities to the states. It is significant for the topic at hand that nearly 90% of the recipients of this program are women (Jones De Weever et al., 2003).

Studies comparing the welfare of recipients before and after the reform with regard to levels of poverty, employment stability, and quality of childcare show marginal improvement after the reform or even deterioration (Jones-DeWeever, Peterson, & Song, 2002; Weil & Finegold, 2001). However, some states showed creativity and strategic coherence by evaluating the outcome of their interventions (Nox, 2002). This evidence corroborates Greenberg's conclusion (2001) that the lack of systematic evaluation of programs and sharing of successful interventions is the greatest weakness of the new welfare regime. Improvement in these areas is a must for improving the well-being of recipients.

Judicial intervention, another type of top-down influence, has been successful in protecting the rights of clients. For example, in some states, settlements opened up access to services for non-English speakers. Injunctions lifted the requirement, set by private contractors, of drug testing for prospective workers. The discontinuation of Medicaid coverage for individuals caring for children receiving government assistance was stopped. Finally, legislative decisions to lower the income cap for certain benefits were declared unconstitutional (Welfare Information Network, 2004).

Records of the hearings on the Temporary Assistance for Needy Families Act confirm that the negative image of women in poverty is widespread. Legislators routinely defined poor single mothers as deviants, attributing their problems to laziness and sexual intemperance. These views, in turn, justified punitive features of the policy (for example, Segal & Kitty, 2003). The added burdens and decreased benefits decreed by TANF can be attributed in part to this sort of stereotyping.

This suggests the importance, for top-down policy practice, of evaluating outcomes for TANF programs. It also highlights the need to correct misinformed and discriminatory views about single mothers in poverty. For social workers in policy practice committed to improve TANF at the sate level, three strategies may be relevant.

1. Involvement in program outcome evaluations and identification of strategies for empowering women and enhancing their welfare. This entails a search of findings that relate concrete types of interventions to the goals of work stability and income above poverty. Examples of such evidence in Minneapolis, Wisconsin, and Michigan are promising (Solomon, 2006; Welfare Information Network, 2001), as is the implementation of a TANF-like policy in Britain (Nelson & Whales, 2006).

2. Review of evidence about policy implementations that infringe on human and civil rights granted by state constitutions. Information along these lines can contribute to effective judicial practice (Figueira-McDonough, 2006, pp. 369–372).

3. Collection and distribution of statistics can counter the distorted image of single mothers in poverty. Media coverage that conveys the lived experience of these mothers is crucial. Prime examples are articles with pictures likely to attract readers, such as those used by the *New York Times* in reporting on "the neediest cases." Theatrical adaptations—for example, of Ehrenreich's *Nickel and Dimed* (2001) or of Nia Orm's *Please Take a Number* (2007)—also reach the public. They help ordinary citizens to participate in the experiences of women in poverty and foster understanding of the problems they face.

Social movements represent a type of bottom-up policy influence. The civil rights movement, the women's movement, and their impact on extending rights to marginalized populations are classic examples. The ingredients of success are clearly established: (a) widely known incidents recognized as cases of social injustice, (b) close interaction among the population suffering the injustice, (c) the emergence of leaders respected by the group, and (d) proposals to address the source of injustice (Gamson, 1995).

The women's movement pressed for the creation of volunteer services to deal with the neglected needs of women: rape crisis centers, women's health clinics, women's substance abuse and domestic abuse programs. Today such programs are institutionalized and they have affected policies across many states for the better (Kravetz, 2004). Another successful example is Mothers Against Drunk Driving (MADD). With chapters all over the country, Mothers Against Drunk Driving has become a major force in legislation on drunk driving and regulations on the sale of alcohol.

Social workers have a long history of participating in movements for social justice. Their involvement has been individual or through groups committed to the goals of the movement (Reisch & Andrews, 2001). To what extent can the practice skills of social workers contribute to movements that influence policies affecting women in poverty? Fine-tuning the two interventions just outlined may be a viable direction.

Organizational practice that focuses on improving the delivery of services in social service programs can go beyond the mismatch between policy goals and program implementation to question the justice of the policy itself. Diane Pearce (who coined the phrase *feminization of poverty*) has devised a creative strategy for improving TANF. Unlike others, she does not attack the work requirement of the program. She focuses instead on the goal, proclaimed by the policy, of achieving self-sufficiency for welfare recipients. She has developed an operational definition of the economic requirements for self-sufficiency (food, health, housing, transportation, and so forth). Since the cost of these basic resources varies significantly across states, she contends that the requirements for self-sufficiency have to be calculated locally. Groups committed to the improvement of TANF have adopted her strategy in many states (Pearce, 2002).

Similarly, community practice can contribute to social movements that matter to the well-being of women. Informal grassroots associations among women have proven their power in addressing issues that matter to them. Connecting these groups across communities around a shared concern is a catalytic strategy for women's movements. Analysts of the demise of the War on Poverty claim that the rapid dismantling of programs could have been prevented if affected communities had joined in concerted resistance (Halpern, 1995).

A contemporary example is the creation and development of a Montana-based grassroots advocacy and educational organization that emerged to respond to inequities in the state implementation of TANF (Finn, Castellanos, McOmber, & Kahan, 2000). Founded by two managers of the Job Opportunities and Basic Skills (JOBS) and with a board made up of single mothers living on below-poverty incomes, membership grew

steadily, and so did the development of programs. The account of the learning process in dealing with the legislature affecting TANF recipients is impressive. The women often testified in favor of legislation on a number of bills that could affect favorably low-income mothers.

The Continuum of Empowerment Interventions for Women

The empowerment of women, especially of socioeconomically marginalized women, is an expected outcome of social work interventions, founded on the professional principle of social justice. The ultimate goal, Gil (1998) argues, is to eliminate the structure of oppression. Linkages among the macrointerventions toward this end goal can be discerned in the foregoing proposals. But interventions targeted to individual empowerment often lack explicit links to social empowerment.

Dietz (2000) notes that women's traumas are often internalizations of external structures of domination. Lee's account (2005) of her practice with women in extreme poverty demonstrates how group success has to be accompanied by contextual changes in programs and policies. Thus, individual interventions should include features designed to promote the connection between psychological and social empowerment. In their intervention with individuals, social workers may encourage and facilitate contacts with groups facing similar problems. Easing the transition toward self-support groups would also become a step in the direction of social empowerment in the group work process. In both instances, information about and access to local activist groups engaged in changing structures at the root of individual problems would advance the connection between psychological and social empowerment.

REFERENCES

Abramovitz, M. (1996). *Under attack, fighting back: Women and welfare in the United States.* New York: Monthly Review Press.

Arrighi, B. (2001). *Understanding inequality: The intersection of race/ethnicity, class, and gender.* Lanham, MD: Rowman & Littlefield.

Barrett, M., & Davidson, M. J. (2006). *Gender and communication at work.* Burlington, VT: Ashgate.

Bride, B. E. (2001). Single gender treatment of substance abuse: Effects on treatment retention and completion. *Social Work Research, 25*(4), 223–232.

Buzzanell, P. M. (2006). *Rethinking organizational and managerial communication from feminist perspectives.* Thousand Oaks, CA: Sage.

Calhoun, C. (1995). *Critical social theory.* Oxford: Blackwell.

Davis, E. (1999). The economics of abuse: How violence perpetuates women's poverty. In R. A. Brandwein (Ed.), *Battered women, children, and the welfare reform: The ties that bind* (pp. 17–30). Thousand Oaks, CA: Sage.

Dietz, C. A. (2000). Responding to oppression and abuse: A feminist challenge to clinical social work. *Affilia, 15*(3), 369–389.

Ehrenreich, B. (2001). *Nickel and dime: On (not) getting by in America.* New York: Holt.

Fausto-Sterling, A. (2000). *Sexing the body: Gender politics and construction of sexuality.* New York: Basic Books.

Feldman, R. M. (2004). *The dignity of resistance: Women residents' activism in Chicago public housing.* New York: Cambridge University Press.

Figueira-McDonough, J. (2001). *Community analysis and praxis: Towards a grounded civil society.* New York: Taylor & Francis.

Figueira-McDonough, J. (2006). *The welfare state and social work: Pursuing social justice.* Thousand Oaks, CA: Sage.

Figueira-McDonough, J. (2007). Childcare and the potential of breaking intergenerational poverty. In B. A. Arrighi & D. J. Maume (Eds.), *Child poverty in America today* (Vol. 1, pp. 171–187). Westport, CT: Praeger.

Finn, J., Castellanos R., McOmber, T., & Kahan K. (2000). Working for equality and economic liberation: Advocacy and education for welfare reform. *Affilia, 15*(2), 294–310.

Finn, J. L. (2002). Raíces: Gender-conscious community building in Santiago, Chile. *Affilia, 25*(4), 448–470.

Gambrill, E. (2006). *Social work practice: A critical thinker's guide.* New York: Oxford University Press.

Gamson, W. A. (1995). Constructing social protest. In H. Johnson & B. Kladermans (Eds.), *Social movements and culture* (pp. 85–106). Minneapolis: University of Minneapolis Press.

Geer, M. A. (2000, Spring). Human rights and wrongs in our backyard: Incorporating international human rights protections under domestic civil rights law—A case study of women in the United States prisons. *Harvard Human Rights Journal, 13,* 71–140.

Gil, D. (1998). *Confronting injustice and oppression: Concepts and strategies for social workers.* New York: Columbia University Press.

Gilligan, C. (1996). The centrality of relationships in human development: A puzzle, some evidence and a theory. In G. G. Noam & K. W. Fisher (Eds.), *Development and vulnerability in close relationships* (pp. 237–261). Mahwey, NJ: Erlbaum.

Gitterman, A., & Shulman L. (2005). The life model, oppression, vulnerability and resilience, mutual aid and the mediating function. In A. Gitterman & L. Shulman (Eds.), *Mutual aid groups, vulnerable and resilient populations and the life cycle* (pp. 139–165). New York: Columbia University Press.

Gramsci, A. (1971). *Selections from the prison notebooks of Antonio Gramsci In* (Q. Hoare & G. N. Smith, Trans.). (Eds.) New York: International Press.

Gray, K. A. (2005). Pride, prejudice, and a dose of shame: The meaning of public assistance. *Affilia, 20*(3), 329–345.

Greenberg, M. (2001). Welfare reform and devolution: Looking forward and backward. *Brookings Review, 19*(3), 20–24.

Gutiérrez, L., Reed B. G., Ortega R., & Lewis E., (1998). Teaching about groups in a gendered world. In J. Figueira-McDonough, F. E. Netting, & A. Nichols-Casebolt (Eds.), *The role of gender in practice knowledge: Claiming half the human experience* (pp. 169–200). New York: Garland.

Halpern, R. (1995). *Rebuilding the inner city.* New York: Columbia University Press.

Heskin, A. D. (1991). *The struggle for community.* Boulder, CO: Westview.

Hopps, J. G., & Morris R. (2000). *Social work at the millennium.* New York: Free Press.

Howe, E. (1980). Public professions and the private model of professionalism. *Social Work, 25*(2), 179–191.

Human Rights Watch. (1996). *All too familiar, sexual abuse of women prisoners in U.S. state prisons.* New York: Author, Women Rights Project.

Jackson, T. L., & Servaes J. (1999). *Theoretical approaches to participatory communication.* Cresskill, NJ: Hampton.

Jansson, B. S. (2003). *Becoming an effective policy advocate: From policy practice to social justice.* Pacific Grove, CA: Brooks/Cole.

Jones-DeWeever, A., Peterson J., & Song X. (2002). Before and after welfare reform: The work and well-being of low-income single parent families. Report series on low income families and children. Washington, DC: Institute for Women' Policy Research. http://www.iwpr.org

Jordan, B. (1990). *Social work in an unjust society.* London: Harvester Wheatsheaf.

Jordan, B. (1998). *The new politics of welfare: Social justice in a global context.* Thousand Oaks, CA: Sage.

Jordan, B., & Jordan C. (2000). *Social work and the third way: Tough love as social policy.* Thousand Oaks, CA: Sage

KidSafe Project. (1997–2001). Child sexual abuse statistics. Washington, DC: National Institute of Justice. http:// republican.ses.ca.gov/web/36/projectkidsafe/stats.asp

Kravetz, D. (2004). *Tales from the trenches: Politics and the practice in feminist service organizations.* Lanham, MD: University Press of America.

Lakoff, G. (2002). *Moral politics: How liberals and conservatives think.* Chicago: University of Chicago Press.

Leavitt, J., & Saeger S. (1990). *From abandonment to hope: Community households in Harlem.* New York: Columbia University Press.

Lee, J. (2005). No place to go: Women and children. In A. Gitterman & L. Shulman (Eds.), *Mutual aid groups, vulnerable and resilient populations and the life cycle* (pp. 373–399). New York: Columbia University Press.

Leonhardt, D. (2006, December 24). Scant progress on closing gap in women's pay. *New York Times,* pp. 1, 18.

Luna, Y. (2005). *Social constructions, social control, and resistance: An analysis of welfare reform as a hegemonic process.* Unpublished doctoral dissertation, Arizona State University, Tempe.

Luna, Y., & Figueira-McDonough, J. (2002). Charity, ideology, and exclusion: Continuities and resistance in U.S. welfare reform. In J. Figueira-McDonough & R. C. Sarri (Eds.), *Women at the margins: Neglect, punishment, and resistance* (pp. 321–345). New York: Haworth.

Maxine, L., & Nisivoccia D. (2005). When the world no longer feels safe. In A. Gitterman & L. Shulman (Eds.), *Mutual aid groups, vulnerable and resilient populations and the life cycle* (pp. 139–165). New York: Columbia University Press.

McAdoo, H. P. (2002). The storm is passing over: Marginalized African American women. In J. Figueira-McDonough & R. C. Sarri (Eds.), *Women at the margins: Neglect, punishment, and resistance* (pp. 87–99). New York: Haworth.

McMillen, J. C., Proctor E. K., Megivern D., Striley C. W., Cabassa L. J., Munson M. R., et al. (2005). Quality care in the social services: Research agenda and methods. *Social Work Research, 19*(3), 181–191.

Middleman, R., & Goldberg G. (1987). Social practice with groups. In A. Middleman (Ed.), *Encyclopedia of social work* (18th ed., pp. 714–729). Silver Springs, MD: NASW Press.

Miller, J. B., & Silver I. P. (1991). A relational reframing of therapy. Work in progress, No. 52. Wellesley, MA: Stone Center Working Paper Series.

Mullaly, R. (2007). *New structural social work.* New York: Oxford University Press.

Mulroy, E. A., & Shay S. (1997). Nonprofit organizations and innovation. A model of neighborhood-based collaboration to prevent child maltreatment. *Social Work, 42,* 515–524.

Naples, N. (1991). Just what needed to be done: Political practice of women community workers in low-income neighborhoods. *Gender and Society, 5*(9), 478–496.

Naples, N. (1998). *Grassroots warriors: Activist mothers, community work and the war on poverty.* New York: Routledge.

Naples, N. (2003). *Feminism and method: Ethnography, discourse analysis, and activist research.* New York: Routledge.

National Association of Social Workers. (2003). Social workers ethical responsibilities to the broader society. In *Social work speaks: Policy statements* (pp. 381–395). Washington, DC: NASW Press.

National Law Center of Homeless and Poverty. (2002). Homeless poverty in America. http://www.nlchp.org/FA-HPLA

Nelson, E., & Whales J. (2006, December). With U.S. methods, Britain posts gains in fighting poverty. *The Wall Street Journal, 22,* pp. 1, 10.

Netting, F. E., & Rokwell M. K. (1998). Integrating gender into human service organization, administration and planning curricula. In J. Figueira-McDonough, F. E. Netting, & A. Nicchols-Casebolt (Eds.), *The role of gender in practice knowledge: Claiming half the human experience* (pp. 287–321). New York: Garland.

Nox, V. (2002, Summer). Money also matters. *American Prospect,* A26–A31.

Nussbaum, M. C. (1999). *Sex and social justice.* New York: Oxford University Press.

Oddental, T., & O'Neil, M. (1994). *Women and power in the nonprofit sector.* San Francisco, CA: Jossey Bass.

Orm, N. (2007). Please take a number. http://www.niaorms.com

Pearce, D. M. (2002). Welfare reform now that we know it: Enforcing women's poverty and preventing self sufficiencyc. In J. Figueira-McDonough & R. C. Sarri (Eds.), *Women at the margins: Neglect, punishment, and resistance.* New York: Haworth.

Piven, F. F., & Cloward R. A. (1997). *The breaking of the American social compact.* New York: Free Press.

Reisch, M., & Gambrill E. (1998). *Social work in the 21st century.* Thousand Oaks, CA: Pine Forge.

Reisch, M., & Andrews J. (2001). *The road not taken: A history of radical social work in the United States.* New York: Brunner-Routledge.

Runkel, P. J., & McGrath, J. E. (1972). *Research on human behavior.* New York: Holt, Rinehart and Winston.

Schiller, L. Y., & Zimmer B. (2005). Sharing secrets. The power of women's groups for sexual abuse survivors. In A. Gitterman & L. Shulman (Eds.), *Mutual aid groups, vulnerable and resilient populations and the life cycle* (pp. 290–319). New York: Columbia University Press.

Schneider, A., & Ingram H. (1993). Social construction of target populations: Implications for politics and policy. *American Political Science Review, 87*(2), 334–346.

Schneider, R. (2002). Influencing "state" policy: Social arena for the 21st century. *Social Policy Journal, 1*(1), 113–116.

Schorr, L. B. (1997). *Common purpose: Strengthening families and neighborhoods to rebuild America.* New York: Doubleday.

Segal, E., & Kitty K. M. (2003). Political promises for welfare reform. *Journal of Poverty, 7*(1/2), 51–67.

Seitz, V. R. (1995). *Women, development and communities for empowerment in Appalachia.* Albany: State University of New York Press.

Smith, D. F. (1990). *The conceptual practice of power: A feminist sociology of knowledge.* Boston, MA: Northeastern University Press.

Solomon, D. (2006, December 15). The interim solution: For welfare clients, temporary jobs can be a roadblock. *The Wall Street Journal,* pp. 1, 16.

Specht, H., & Courtney M. (1994). *Unfaithful angels: How social work abandoned its mission.* New York: Free Press.

Stoutland, S. E. (1997). *Neither urban jungle nor urban village: Women, families and urban development.* New York: Garland.

Talaska, R. (1990). *Critical reasoning in contemporary culture.* Albany: State University of New York Press.

Thretheway, A. (1997). Resistance, identity, and empowerment: A postmodern feminist analysis of human service organization. *Communication Monographs, 64,* 281–301.

Toseland, R. (1995). *An introduction to group work.* Boston, MA: Allyn & Bacon.

Van Wormer, K. (2004). *Confronting oppression, restoring justice: From policy analysis to social action.* Alexandria, VA: Council on Social Work Education.

Wakefield, J. C. (1988). Psychotherapy, distributive justice and social work: Distributive justice as a conceptual framework for social work (Part I). *Social Service Review, 62,* 187–210.

Weil, A., & Finegold K. (2001). *Welfare reform: The next act.* Washington, DC: The Urban Institute Press.

Weil, M., Gable D. N., & Williams E. S. (1998). Women, communities and development. In J. Figueira-McDonough, F. E. Netting, & A. Nichols-Casebolt (Eds.), *The role of gender in practice knowledge: Claiming half the human experience* (pp. 242–286). New York: Garland.

Welfare Information Network. (2004). The effect of litigation on the design and administration of welfare policies and programs. *Resources for Welfare Decision Making, 8, 3.* http://financeprogectinfo.org

Welfare Information Network. (2001). Earnings supplements and income disregards can ease transition from welfare to work. *Resources for Welfare Decision Making, 5*(12). http://financeproject.org

Whitley, D. M., & Dressel P. M. (2002). The controllers and the controlled. In J. Figueira-McDonough & R. C. Sarri (Eds.), *Women at the margins: Neglect, punishment, and resistance* (pp. 103–123). New York: Haworth.

Wood, G. (2006). *The structural approach to direct practice: A social constructionist approach.* New York: Columbia University Press.

Zelvin, E. (1999). Applying relational theory to the treatment of women's addictions. *Affilia, 14*(1), 1–23.

JOSEFINA FIGUEIRA-MCDONOUGH

Topical Outline of Entries

Directory of Contributors

JULIE ABRAMSON
University at Albany, State University of New York;
Emeritus
   Task-Centered Practice

RUDOLPH ALEXANDER JR.
The Ohio State University
   Criminal Justice: Overview

PAULA ALLEN-MEARES
University of Illinois at Chicago
   School Social Work

JEANE W. ANASTAS
New York University
   Ethics in Research

REBECCA S. ASHERY
Retired; consultant
   Primary Health Care

DARLYNE BAILEY
Bryn Mawr College
   Leadership, Foundations of

LAURA R. BRONSTEIN
Binghamton University, State University of New York
   Task-Centered Practice

BONNIE E. CARLSON
Arizona State University
   Intimate Partner Violence

JULIE CEREL
University of Kentucky
   Survivors of Suicide, Those Left Behind When
      Someone Dies by Suicide

LISA CONRADI
Chadwick Center for Children and Families, Rady
Children's Hospital, San Diego
   Trauma-Informed Care

LOIS F. COWLES
Idaho State University, Emerita, and St. Thomas Clinic
   Health Care: Practice Interventions

TERRY L. CROSS
National Indian Child Welfare Association
   Cultural Competence

DIANE DE ANDA
UCLA, Emerita
   Adolescents: A Historical Overview of
      Developmental Theories

PETER DE JONG
Calvin College
   Interviewing

ALAN DETTLAFF
University of Illinois at Chicago
   Disproportionality and Disparities

JAMES W. DRISKO
Smith College
   Common Factors in Psychotherapy

NABILA EL-BASSEL
Columbia University
   Practice Interventions and Research

JOSEFINA FIGUEIRA-MCDONOUGH
Arizona State University, Emerita
   Women: Practice Interventions

JANET L. FINN
University of Montana
   Social Justice

ROWENA FONG
University of Texas at Austin
   Disproportionality and Disparities

CYNTHIA FRANKLIN
University of Texas at Austin
   Family Therapy

SUSAN FRAUENHOLTZ
University of Kansas
   Child and Adolescent Mental-Health Disorders

DOROTHY N. GAMBLE
University of North Carolina, Chapel Hill
   Community: Practice Interventions

CAREL B. GERMAIN
University of Connecticut
   Ecological Framework

ALEX GITTERMAN
University of Houston
   Ecological Framework

EDA G. GOLDSTEIN
New York University, Emerita
   Psychosocial Framework

JESSE J. HARRIS, COL. USA RET.
University of Maryland
   Military Social Work

LYNNE M. HEALY
University of Connecticut
   International Social Work: Overview

JOHN M. HERRICK
Michigan State University, Emeritus
   Social Policy: Overview

JOSEPH HIMLE
University of Michigan
   Cognitive Behavioral Therapy

DAVID R. HODGE
Arizona State University
   Spirituality in Social Work

NANCY R. HOOYMAN
University of Washington
   Aging: Overview

LAURA M. HOPSON
University of Alabama
   Family Therapy

HEATHER HORTON
University at Albany, State University of New York
   Group Work

MATTHEW O. HOWARD
University of North Carolina, Chapel Hill
   Evidence-Based Practice

RICHARD ISRALOWITZ
Ben-Gurion University, Beer Sheva, Israel
   Alcohol and Drug Problems:
      An Overview

MAXINE JACOBSON
PRAXIS - Building Knowledge for Action
   Social Justice

JEFFREY M. JENSON
University of Denver
   Evidence-Based Practice

MICHAEL S. KELLY
Loyola University Chicago
   Task-Centered Practice

SUSAN KEMP
University of Washington
   Transdisciplinary and Translational Research

JOHNNY S. KIM
University of Denver
   Strengths Perspective

MARY ELLEN KONDRAT
University of Kansas
   Person-in-Environment

HAL A. LAWSON
University at Albany, State University of New York
   Collaborative Practice

EUN-KYOUNG OTHELIA LEE
University of North Carolina, Charlotte
   Multiculturalism

KAREN KYEUNGHAE LEE
University of Kansas
   Major Depressive Disorder and Bipolar Mood
      Disorders

MO YEE LEE
Ohio State University
   Solution-Focused Brief Therapy

LORI LESTER
Independent Scholar, Ft. Walton Beach, FL
   Advocacy

JULIA H. LITTELL
Bryn Mawr College
   Systematic Reviews

SADYE L. M. LOGAN
University of South Carolina
   Family: Overview

MARGARET LOMBE
Boston College
   Rights-Based Framework and Social Work

JENNIFER L. MAGNABOSCO
*U.S. Department of Veterans Affairs; California
Mental Health Services Authority*
   Outcome Measures in Human Services

GERALD P. MALLON
Hunter College, City University of New York
   Lesbian, Gay, BiSexual and Transgender
     (LGBT) Families and Parenting

MYFANWY MAPLE
University of New England
   Survivors of Suicide, Those Left Behind When
     Someone Dies by Suicide

JOHN G. MCNUTT
University of Delaware
   Social Work Practice: History and Evolution
   Technology: Technology in Macro Practice

RUTH MCROY
Boston College
   Disproportionality and Disparities
   Multiculturalism

AMY MENDENHALL
University of Kansas
   Child and Adolescent Mental-Health
     Disorders

DORLEE MICHAELI
Center for Financial Social Work
   Financial Social Work

DAVID P. MOXLEY
University of Oklahoma
   Action Research

JORDANA MUROFF
Boston University
   Cognitive Behavioral Therapy

FLORENCE ELLEN NETTING
Virginia Commonwealth University, Emerita
   Macro Social Work Practice

DORINDA N. NOBLE
Texas State University–San Marcos
   Children: Overview

PAULA S. NURIUS
University of Washington
   Transdisciplinary and Translational
     Research

JULIA OCHIENG
Virginia Commonwealth University
   Advocacy

THOMAS PACKARD
San Diego State University
   Organizational Change in Human Service
     Organizations

DEBORAH K. PADGETT
New York University
   Qualitative Research

KYLE L. PEHRSON, COL. USA RET.
Brigham Young University
   Military Social Work

DONNA M. PENCE
San Diego State University
   Trauma-Informed Care

MARK R. RANK
Washington University in St. Louis
   Poverty

FREDERIC G. REAMER
Rhode Island College
   Ethics and Values
   The NASW Code of Ethics
   Social Work Malpractice, Liability, and
     Risk Management

VIRGINIA RONDERO HERNANDEZ
Fresno State University
   Generalist and Advanced Generalist
     Practice

FARIYAL ROSS-SHERIFF
Howard University
   Human Trafficking: Overview

GINA MIRANDA SAMUELS
University of Chicago
   Multiethnic and Multiracialism

ROSEMARY C. SARRI
University of Michigan, Emerita
   Juvenile Justice: Overview

ROBERT L. SCHNEIDER
Virginia Commonwealth University, Emeritus
   Advocacy

UMA A. SEGAL
University of Missouri–St. Louis
   Immigration Policy

TRACY M. SOSKA
University of Pittsburgh
 Housing

HALUK SOYDAN
University of Southern California
 Intervention Research

GAIL STEKETEE
Boston University
 Cognitive Behavioral Therapy

SHULAMITH LALA ASHENBERG STRAUSSNER
New York University
 Alcohol and Drug Problems: An Overview

PAUL H. STUART
Florida International University
 Social Work Profession: History

RONALD W. TOSELAND
University at Albany, State University of New York
 Group Work

KATRINA M. UHLY
Northeastern University
 Leadership, Foundations of

DOROTHY VAN SOEST
University of Washington
 Oppression

ERIC F. WAGNER
Florida International University
 Motivational Interviewing

ADDIE WEAVER
University of Michigan
 Cognitive Behavioral Therapy

MARIE WEIL
University of North Carolina,
Chapel Hill
 Community: Practice Interventions

SUSAN J. WELLS
University of British Columbia
 Child Abuse and Neglect

JESSICA SCHAFFNER WILEN
Bryn Mawr College
 Leadership, Foundations of

CHARLES WILSON
Chadwick Center for Children and Families, Rady
Children's Hospital, San Diego
 Trauma-Informed Care

REETA WOLFSOHN
Center for Financial Social Work
 Financial Social Work

Index

Page numbers in *italics* refer to figures and tables. Page ranges in **bold** indicate main entries.